Maternity Nursing

Deitra Leonard LOWDERMILK
RNC, PhD, FAAN

Clinical Professor Emerita, School of
  Nursing
University of North Carolina at Chapel Hill
Chapel Hill, North Carolina

Shannon E. PERRY
RN, CNS, PhD, FAAN

Professor Emerita, School of
  Nursing
San Francisco State University
San Francisco, California

Associate Editors

Kathryn Rhodes Alden, RN, MSN, IBCLC

Clinical Assistant Professor, School of
  Nursing
University of North Carolina at Chapel
  Hill
Chapel Hill, North Carolina
Lactation Consultant, Rex Healthcare
Raleigh, North Carolina

Kitty Cashion, RN, BC, MSN

Clinical Nurse Specialist
University of Tennessee
  Health Science Center
Department of Obstetrics &
  Gynecology
Division of Maternal-Fetal
  Medicine
Memphis, Tennessee

Robin Webb Corbett, RN,C, PhD

Associate Professor, School of Nursing
East Carolina University
Greenville, North Carolina

7th

seventh edition

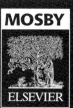

MOSBY

ELSEVIER

MOSBY
ELSEVIER

11830 Westline Industrial Drive
St. Louis, Missouri 63146

MATERNITY NURSING, SEVENTH EDITION   ISBN-13: 978-0-323-03366-4
Copyright © 2006, 2003, 1999, 1995, 1991, 1987, 1983 by Mosby, Inc.   ISBN-10: 0-323-03366-0

Notice

Knowledge and best practice in this field are constantly changing. As new research and experience broaden our knowledge, changes in practice, treatment, and drug therapy may become necessary or appropriate. Readers are advised to check the most current information provided (i) on procedures featured or (ii) by the manufacturer of each product to be administered, to verify the recommended dose or formula, the method and duration of administration, and contraindications. It is the responsibility of the practitioner, relying on his or her own experience and knowledge of the patient, to make diagnoses, to determine dosages and the best treatment for each individual patient, and to take all appropriate safety precautions. To the fullest extent of the law, neither the Publisher nor the Authors assume any liability for any injury and/or damage to persons or property arising from or related to any use of the material contained in this book.

ISBN-13: 978-0-323-03366-4
ISBN-10: 0-323-03366-0

Acquisitions Editor: Catherine Jackson
Senior Developmental Editor: Laurie K. Gower
Publishing Services Manager: Jeff Patterson
Senior Project Manager: Anne Konopka
Senior Designer: Amy Buxton

Printed in Canada

Last digit is the print number: 9 8 7 6 5 4 3 2 1

Working together to grow
libraries in developing countries

www.elsevier.com | www.bookaid.org | www.sabre.org

ELSEVIER   BOOK AID International   Sabre Foundation

for Instructors

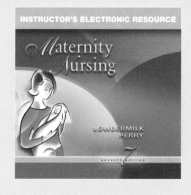

INSTRUCTOR'S ELECTRONIC RESOURCE

0-323-04340-2

Available in CD and online formats, this helpful instructor's package provides all of the tools needed to quickly and consistently develop lectures and student assignments and evaluate student comprehension. The Instructor's Manual includes chapter outlines and teaching strategies, activities for students, case studies, curriculum guides for courses of various lengths, and open-book quizzes. The ExamView Test Bank contains questions in NCLEX® format, including new alternate format questions, and an answer key with page references to the text, rationales, and NCLEX® coding. Also included are a full-color Image Collection and PowerPoint Lecture Slides for building presentations and developing lectures.

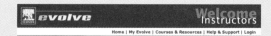

EVOLVE COURSE MANAGEMENT SYSTEM

http://evolve.elsevier.com/Lowdermilk/Maternity/

Evolve is an interactive teaching and learning environment that works in coordination with Maternity Nursing, 7th edition, providing Internet-based course content that reinforces and expands on the concepts that instructors deliver in class. In addition to the resources available to students, instructors are able to access all of the components of the Instructor's Electronic Resource, including the computerized test bank and PowerPoint slides. Instructors can also use Evolve to: publish class syllabi, outline, and lecture notes; set up "virtual office hours" and email communication; share important dates and information through the online class Calendar; and encourage student participation through Chat Rooms and Discussion Boards. Instructors are encouraged to contact their sales representative for more information about integrating Evolve into their curriculum.

Contents

About the Authors

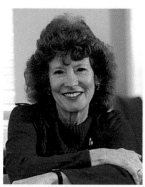

Deitra Lowdermilk is Clinical Professor Emerita, School of Nursing, University of North Carolina at Chapel Hill (UNC CH). She received her BSN from East Carolina University and her MEd (and Minor in Obstetric Nursing) and PhD in Education from UNC CH. She is certified in In-Patient Obstetrics by the National Certification Corporation (NCC). She is a Fellow in the American Academy of Nursing. In addition to being a nurse educator for over 34 years, Dr. Lowdermilk has clinical experience as a public health nurse, a staff nurse in labor and delivery, postpartum, and newborn units, and has worked in gynecologic surgery and cancer care units. Dr. Lowdermilk continues to teach undergraduate maternal-newborn theory and clinical experiences for the 24- and 14-month BSN program options at UNC CH.

Dr. Lowdermilk has been recognized for her expertise in nursing education. She has repeatedly been selected as Classroom and Clinical Teacher of the Year by graduating seniors. She was a recipient of the Educator of the Year Award from both the District IV Association of Women's Health, Obstetric, and Neonatal Nurses (AWHONN) and the North Carolina Nurses Association. She also received the 2005 AWHONN Excellence in Education Award.

She is active in AWHONN, having served as a Chair of the North Carolina Section of AWHONN and has served as chair and member of various committees in AWHONN at the national, district, state, and local levels. She has served as guest editor for the *Journal of Obstetric, Gynecologic, and Neonatal Nursing (JOGNN)* and served on editorial boards for other publications. She has been a board member and officer for other nursing organizations in North Carolina.

Dr. Lowdermilk's most significant contribution to nursing has been to promote excellence in nursing practice and education in women's health through integration of knowledge into practice. She has published extensively in nursing texts, served as associate editor for two texts, including Maternal Child Nursing Care, third edition, and is co-author of Maternity and Women's Health Care, eighth edition. She has published articles in refereed journals and made presentations nationally and internationally. She has published computer-assisted instruction programs, one of which received a Media Award for Excellence in Nursing Journalism from Sigma Theta Tau International. She has made invited presentations at national and international meetings, as well as presented continuing education programs. She has also served as a consultant to nursing schools in the United States, Australia, Thailand, and Taiwan. In 2005 she received the first Distinguished Alumni Award from East Carolina University School of Nursing for her exemplary contributions to the nursing profession in the area of maternal-child care and the community.

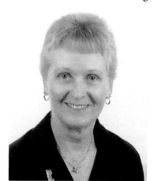

Shannon Perry is Professor Emerita, School of Nursing, San Francisco State University. She received her diploma in nursing from St. Joseph Hospital School of Nursing, Bloomington, Illinois; a Baccalaureate in Nursing from Marquette University, Milwaukee, Wisconsin; an MSN in Maternal-Child Nursing from the University of Colorado Medical Center, Denver, Colorado; and a PhD in Educational Psychology with a specialization in child development from Arizona State University, Tempe, Arizona. She completed a 2-year postdoctoral fellowship in perinatal nursing at the University of California, San Francisco, as a Robert Wood Johnson Clinical Nurse Scholar.

Dr. Perry has had clinical experience as a staff nurse, head nurse, and supervisor in surgical nursing, obstetrics, pediatrics, gynecology, and neonatal nursing. She has taught nursing in schools of nursing in several states. She is a Fellow in the American Academy of Nursing, has been an officer or board member in a number of professional organizations, recently completed a 2-year term on the National League for Nursing Board of Governors, and is nursing consultant to the International Education Research Foundation. She is interested in international nursing, has traveled extensively learning about nursing and health care in various countries, and has taught international nursing courses in which she traveled with nursing students to the United Kingdom, Italy, Thailand, Ghana, and China.

Her current research interests include the history of nursing and evidence-based practice. She has published widely on perinatal topics and on the nurse as an expert witness. Dr. Perry is also co-author on two other successful Elsevier titles: *Maternity & Women's Health Care,* eighth edition, and *Maternal Child Nursing Care,* third edition.

About the Associate Editors

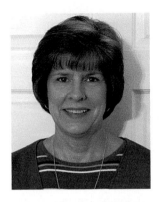

Kathryn Rhodes Alden is Clinical Assistant Professor, University of North Carolina at Chapel Hill School of Nursing. She received her BSN from the University of North Carolina at Charlotte and her MSN from the University of North Carolina at Chapel Hill. She has completed the course work for a doctorate in adult education from North Carolina State University and is currently working on the dissertation.

Ms. Alden has had clinical experience as a staff nurse in pediatrics and neonatal intensive care. She has worked in administrative and quality improvement roles in nursing. She has taught in the baccalaureate nursing program at the University of North Carolina at Charlotte. For the past 17 years, Ms. Alden has served on faculty at the University of North Carolina at Chapel Hill School of Nursing, where she teaches maternal-newborn nursing to undergraduate students and serves as academic counselor for the nursing school. She has been recognized and awarded for her clinical teaching expertise.

Ms. Alden is an international board certified lactation consultant and works part-time as a lactation consultant for Rex Healthcare in Raleigh, North Carolina. She has provided continuing education programs on breastfeeding throughout the state of North Carolina.

She has authored numerous chapters in maternity texts for Elsevier on endocrine and metabolic disorders of pregnancy as well as newborn nutrition, assessment, and nursing care.

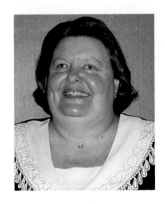

Kitty Cashion is Clinical Nurse Specialist, Maternal-Fetal Medicine Division, University of Tennessee Health Science Center, Memphis, College of Medicine, Department of Obstetrics and Gynecology. She received her BSN from the University of Tennessee College of Nursing in Memphis and her MSN in Parent-Child Nursing from Vanderbilt University School of Nursing in Nashville, Tennessee. Ms. Cashion is certified as a High Risk Perinatal Nurse through the American Nurses Credentialing Center (ANCC).

Ms. Cashion's job responsibilities at the University of Tennessee include providing education regarding low and high risk obstetrics to staff nurses in West Tennessee community hospitals. In addition, she works part-time as a staff nurse in Labor and Delivery at The Regional Medical Center at Memphis (The MED), and teaches Labor and Delivery clinical for students at Northwest Mississippi Community College in Senatobia, Mississippi, and Union University in Germantown, Tennessee.

Ms. Cashion has been an active AWHONN member, holding office at both the local and state levels. She has also served as an officer and board member of the Tennessee Perinatal Association and as an active volunteer for the Tennessee Chapter, March of Dimes Birth Defects Foundation.

Ms. Cashion has contributed to several obstetric nursing textbooks. She recently co-authored a series of Virtual Clinical Excursions workbooks to accompany four obstetric nursing textbooks published by Elsevier.

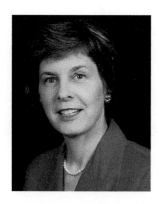

Robin Webb Corbett is Associate Professor of Nursing, East Carolina University, Greenville, North Carolina. She received her BSN from Atlantic Christian College, Wilson, North Carolina; an MSN in Parent-Child Nursing from East Carolina University, Greenville, North Carolina; and a PhD in Nursing Research with a focus in clinical research from the University of South Carolina, Columbia, South Carolina.

Dr. Corbett has extensive clinical experience as a nurse in obstetrics, pediatrics, critical care, and community health and home health nursing. She is a member of Sigma Theta Tau International, has been an officer or board member in a number of professional organizations, and is currently chair of the Edgecombe County Board of Health. She is interested in the practice of pica and has researched this topic extensively in varied populations.

Her current research interests include nutritional decision making and behaviors and nutritional interventions in rural, socioeconomically disadvantaged populations. Dr. Corbett's other contributions include chapters in *Maternal, Fetal, and Neonatal Physiology: A Clinical Perspective,* second edition and *Pharmacology: A Nursing Process Approach,* fifth edition.

Contributors & Reviewers

CONTRIBUTORS

Kelly Ann Crum, RN, MSN
Instructional Specialist, RN Faculty
University of Phoenix Online
Phoenix, Arizona

Pat Mahaffee Gingrich, RN-C, MSN, WHNP
Clinical Assistant Professor, School of Nursing
University of North Carolina at Chapel Hill
Chapel Hill, North Carolina

Barbra W. Manning, RN, MSN
OB/Peds Coordinator, Division of Nursing
Northwest Mississippi Community College
Senatobia, Mississippi

Donna Bossick Rowe, RN, BSN
Nurse Clinician I, James A. Taylor Student Health Service
Adjunct Instructor, School of Nursing
University of North Carolina at Chapel Hill
Chapel Hill, North Carolina

REVIEWERS

Cindy Borgers, RNC, MSN, NNP
Assistant Professor, Division of Nursing
Baptist College of Health Sciences
Memphis, Tennessee

Carolyn F. Covington, PhD, MSN, RN
Assistant Professor, Division of Nursing
Howard University
Washington, District of Columbia

Jo Garner, RN, BSN
Clinical Nurse II
UNC Hospitals
Chapel Hill, North Carolina

Brenda Hanson-Smith, DNS, RNC, OGNP, CLC
Professor of Nursing
California State University
Sacramento, California

Helen Jones, PhD, MN
Chair, Health Science Education Department
Raritan Valley Community College
Somerville, New Jersey

Elizabeth T. Jordan, DNSc, RNC
Course Coordinator, School of Nursing
Johns Hopkins University
Baltimore, Maryland

Jeanne Linhart, BS, MSN, FNP
Associate Professor of Nursing
Rockland Community College
Suffern, New York

Edward L. Lowdermilk, BS, RPh
Pharmacist/Consultant
Piedmont Health Services
Carrboro, North Carolina

Toni Manogin, RN, BSN, MSN
Assistant Professor, School of Nursing
Southern University
Baton Rouge, Louisiana

Lisa Scheresky-O'Neil, RN, MSN
Assistant Professor, Department of Nursing
Montana State University–Northern
Havre, Montana

Preface

This seventh edition of *Maternity Nursing* focuses on the care of women during their reproductive years. Childbearing issues and concerns, including neonatal care, are the primary focus, but the promotion of wellness and the management of common women's health problems are also addressed.

The specialty of maternity and women's health nursing offers both challenges and opportunities. Nurses are challenged to assimilate knowledge and develop the technical and critical thinking skills needed to apply that knowledge to practice. Each woman presents a new challenge because her individual needs must be identified and met. However, the opportunities are sufficiently extraordinary to make this one of the most fulfilling specialties of nursing practice.

The goal of nursing education is to prepare today's student to meet the challenges of tomorrow. This preparation must extend beyond the mastery of facts and skills. Nurses must be able to combine competence with caring and critical thinking. They must address both the physiologic and the psychosocial needs of patients. They must look beyond the condition and see the woman as an individual with distinctive needs but also in the context of her family, her culture, and her community. Above all, nurses must strive to improve nursing practice on the basis of evidence.

In a time of shrinking financial and personnel resources for health care, nurses can use evidence-based practice to produce measurable outcomes that can validate their unique role in the health care delivery system.

Maternity Nursing was developed to provide students with guidance for acquiring the knowledge and skills they need to become competent, critically thinking, caring nurses. This edition has been revised and refined in response to comments and suggestions from educators, clinicians, and students. It includes the most accurate, current, and clinically relevant information available. Many exciting changes are noted throughout the book. However, we have retained the underlying philosophy that has been the strength of the previous editions: Pregnancy and childbirth and developmental changes in a woman's life are natural processes. We have also retained a strong integrated focus on the family and evidence-based practice.

Approach

Professional nursing practice continues to evolve and adapt to society's changing health priorities. The rapidly changing health care delivery system offers new opportunities for nurses to alter the practice of maternity and women's health nursing and to improve the way care is given. Consumers of maternity and women's health care vary in age, ethnicity, culture, language, social status, marital status, and sexual preference. They seek care from obstetricians, gynecologists, family practice physicians, nurse-midwives, nurse practitioners, and other health care providers in a variety of health care settings, including the home. Increasingly, many are self-treating, using a variety of alternative and complementary therapies.

Nursing education must reflect these changes. Clinical education must be planned to offer students a variety of maternity and women's health care experiences in settings that include hospitals and birth centers, homes, clinics and private physicians' offices, shelters for the homeless or women in need of protection, and other community-based settings. The changing needs of nursing students also must be addressed. Today's nursing students are challenged to learn more than ever before and often in less time than their predecessors. Students are diverse. They may be high school graduates, college students, or older adults with families. They may be men or women. They may have college degrees in other fields and be interested in switching to a nursing career through a traditional or accelerated nursing curriculum, or they may pursue education online. They may represent various cultures; English may not be their primary language.

This seventh edition of *Maternity Nursing* is designed to meet the changing needs of women during their childbearing years and students in all types of nursing programs. This edition presents tighter, focused content in a clearly written and easily readable manner while retaining the comprehensiveness of previous editions.

To ensure a logical and consistent presentation of material, *Care Management* has been used again as an organizing framework for discussion in the nursing care chapters. This approach incorporates the nursing process and collaborative care approach to demonstrate how nurses work with other health care providers to give the most comprehensive care to women and newborns. Assessment, nursing diagnoses, expected outcomes, nursing and collaborative interventions, and evaluation of care are highlighted throughout the chapters for emphasis. Nursing plans of care and care paths reinforce the problem-solving approach to patient care. In chapters that focus on complications of childbearing and reproductive conditions, medical care is often the priority for patient care. Therefore in these discussions the specific condition is discussed first, followed by discussion of medical and nursing management, including home care.

Health care today emphasizes *wellness*. This focus is an integral part of our philosophy. Likewise, the developmental changes that a woman experiences throughout her life are considered natural and normal. In women's health care the goal is promotion of wellness for the woman through knowledge of her body and its normal functions throughout her reproductive years. Health care also helps her develop an awareness of conditions that require professional intervention. The unit on women's health care emphasizes the wellness aspect of care. This unit has been placed before the units on pregnancy because many of the aspects of assessment and care can be applied to later chapters. Pregnancy and childbirth are also part of a natural developmental process. We believe that students need to thoroughly understand and recognize the normal processes before they can identify complications and comprehend their implications for care. Therefore we present the entire normal childbearing cycle before discussing potential complications.

Teaching for self-care is an essential component of nursing care for women and newborns. In recognition of integrative health care models that provide both traditional and nontraditional health care and in seeking to provide options for women that encourage them to take more responsibility for their health, we have integrated and highlighted new content on alternative and complementary therapies; an icon is placed in the margin to call attention to these therapies. The chapter on women's health promotion and screening emphasizes teaching for self-care to promote wellness and encourage preventive care. The chapter entitled Transition to Parenthood focuses on teaching for new mothers and infants at home. Special boxed features highlight teaching guidelines and patient self-care throughout the text. Information in these boxes can be used in inpatient and home care settings. To implement *preventive care*, perinatal and women's health nurses must be able to recognize signs and symptoms of emergent problems. Throughout the discussion of assessment and care, we alert the nurse to signs of potential problems and provide boxed information highlighting warning signs and emergency situations. Today's perinatal and women's health nurses will encounter women from diverse backgrounds. The family chapter includes a discussion of cultural implications and focuses on specific customs related to childbearing and women's health. This chapter also stresses the importance of assessing both the nurse's and the patient's cultural beliefs. *Cultural considerations* are integrated throughout the text to emphasize the wide range of ethnic diversity and its effects on maternity and women's health. Boxes throughout the text highlight cultural aspects of care. More English-Spanish Guidelines/Guías boxes have been added to provide students with common terms, statements, and questions to be used to make assessments and provide teaching. The chapter on care in the community and home prepares the student to provide maternity and women's health care in a variety of settings. *Community aspects of care* are also integrated throughout nursing care chapters to emphasize that care can take place wherever the woman and her family may be.

To truly meet the specific needs of each woman, the nurse must include family members and significant others in the plan of care. *Family dynamics* are rarely more prominent than in pregnancy and childbirth. The nurse is often the family's primary advocate. A separate chapter on the family, as well as integrated family considerations throughout the chapters on pregnancy, labor and birth, postpartum, and newborn care, demonstrates the importance of the entire family. Issues concerning grandparents, siblings, and different family constellations are addressed.

Evidence-based practice is an integral part of nursing education and practice. Evidence-based practice is incorporated by including evidence-based practice boxes in each chapter and placing an icon next to content for which there is research evidence of its effectiveness. Students and practicing nurses will be challenged to think critically and improve nursing practice by questioning traditional nursing practices that have no scientific basis. Maternity and women's health nurses confront ethical and legal challenges daily and increasingly will face situations involving genetics issues. Nurses must develop a reflective stance that assesses the new reproductive and women's health technologies and policies in light of their potential to influence human well-being. Information on legal tips and ethical considerations is integrated throughout the text to emphasize these issues as they relate to maternal and women's health nursing. Content on genetics and the nurse's role has been updated.

Features

This seventh edition features a contemporary design and spacious presentation. Students will find that the logical, easy-to-follow headings and attractive *full-color* design highlight important content and increase visual appeal. Hundreds of color photographs, many of them new, and drawings throughout the text illustrate important concepts and techniques to further enhance comprehension.

Each chapter includes a list of ***Key Terms and Definitions*** that alerts students to new vocabulary; these terms are then boldfaced within the chapter. ***Learning Objectives*** focus students' attention on the important content to be mastered. ***Electronic Resources*** that can be found on the companion website and/or the interactive companion CD are listed at the beginning of each chapter to provide the student with additional information. Each chapter ends with ***Community Activity, Key Points,*** which summarize important content, and ***Answer Guidelines to Critical Thinking Exercises***. A ***Resources*** list includes websites and/or contact information for organizations and educational resources available for the topics discussed. ***References*** have been updated significantly, with most citations being less than 5 years old and all chapters including citations within 1 year of publication. The following are more of the outstanding features:

- *Care Management* is the organizing framework used consistently to discuss nursing care. The five steps of the nursing process are incorporated into this framework.
- *Plans of Care* are included to help students apply the nursing process in the clinical setting. The Plans of Care use only NANDA-approved nursing diagnoses, describe expected outcomes for patient care, provide rationales for interventions, and include evaluation of care.
- *Care Paths* and *Procedure* boxes for care are included to provide students with examples of various approaches to the implementation of care.
- English-Spanish *Guidelines/Guías* boxes provide common phrases in English and Spanish for patient assessments and teaching.
- *Patient Instructions for Self-Care* boxes emphasize guidelines for the patient to practice self-care and provide information to help students transfer learning from the hospital to the home setting.
- *Emergency* boxes alert students to the signs and symptoms of various emergency situations and provide interventions for immediate implementation
- *Nurse Alerts* highlight critical information for the student.
- *Evidence-Based Practice* is incorporated throughout in **NEW** boxes that integrate findings from studies on selected clinical practices and changing practice. In addition, research findings summarized in the *Cochrane Pregnancy and Childbirth Database* that confirm effective practices or identify practices that have unknown, ineffective, or harmful effects are integrated throughout the text and identified by this icon in the margin.
- *Signs of Potential Complications* are included in chapters that cover uncomplicated pregnancy and childbirth, because although childbearing is a normal process, complications may occur.
- *Alternative and Complementary Therapies* are discussed for many women's health and pregnancy-related problems and are identified in the text by a **NEW** icon in the margin.
- *Cultural Considerations* boxes describe beliefs and practices about pregnancy, childbirth, parenting, and women's health concerns and the importance of understanding cultural variations when providing care.
- *Legal Tips* and *Ethical Considerations* are integrated throughout to provide students with relevant information to deal with these important areas in the context of maternity and women's health nursing.
- *Medication Guide* boxes include key information about medications used in maternity and women's health care, including their indications, adverse effects, and nursing considerations.
- *Critical Thinking Exercises* are integrated into the chapters to guide the students in applying their knowledge and in increasing their ability to think critically about maternity and women's health care issues. Answers to these exercises are provided at the end of the chapter.

- *Community Activity* exercises are new to each chapter and focus on maternal and newborn activities that can be pursued in local community settings.
- *Historic Milestones in Maternity Care* is NEW in Chapter 1.
- *Teaching Guidelines* emphasize the information needed by the nurse to teach the patient about self-care and health promotion.

Organization

This seventh edition of *Maternity Nursing* is composed of seven units organized to enhance understanding and learning and to facilitate easy retrieval of information.

Unit I, *Introduction to Maternity Nursing,* begins with an overview of contemporary maternity and women's health nursing practice. It then addresses the family as a unit of care, incorporating cultural aspects of care. The unit concludes with a chapter on community and home care that provides an understanding of these practice settings in relation to maternity and women's health nursing.

Unit II, *Reproductive Years,* is a reorganized unit on women's health. Three chapters discuss health promotion, physical assessment of women, and common reproductive concerns.

Unit III, *Pregnancy,* describes nursing care of the woman and her family from conception through preparation for childbirth. Genetics content has been expanded. A chapter on maternal and fetal nutrition emphasizes the important aspects of care, highlights cultural variations on diet, and stresses the importance of early recognition and management of nutritional problems.

Unit IV, *Childbirth,* focuses on collaborative care among physicians, nurse-midwives, nurses, and women and their families during the processes of labor and birth. Separate chapters deal with the nurse's role in management of discomfort during labor and childbirth and fetal monitoring. These chapters familiarize students with current childbirth practices and focus on interventions to support and educate the woman and her family.

Unit V, *Postpartum Period,* deals with a time of significant change for the entire family. The mother requires both physical and emotional support as she adjusts to her new role. Chapters on assessment and care during the fourth trimester focus on these needs. The chapter on transition to parenthood discusses family dynamics in response to the birth of a child and describes ways nurses can facilitate parent-infant adjustment, including anticipatory guidance for the first few days at home and home follow-up care.

Unit VI, *The Newborn,* addresses physiologic adaptations of the newborn and assessment and care of the newborn. Information on the nutritional needs of the newborn and nursing care associated with breastfeeding and formula feeding are highlighted in a separate chapter.

Unit VII, *Complications of Childbearing,* discusses the conditions that place the woman, fetus, infant, and family at risk. This unit includes a chapter on high risk assessment of pregnancy complications, two chapters on pregnancy at risk (preexisting and gestational conditions), a chapter on labor and birth complications, a chapter on postpartum complications, and two chapters on newborn complications. Care management focuses on achieving the best possible outcomes and supporting the woman and family when expectations are not met. Loss and grief issues of the family experiencing a fetal or neonatal loss are discussed in a separate chapter.

The text concludes with a detailed, cross-referenced Index and Glossary.

Teaching and Learning Package

Several ancillaries to this text have been developed to assist instructors and students in the teaching and learning process.

The *Instructor's Resource Manual* and *Test Bank* are keyed chapter by chapter to the text to help coordinate course objectives to chapter content. Each chapter includes an outline of content with course guidelines, suggested learning activities, and a summary of key concepts. The test bank portion includes approximately 800 updated questions that parallel the NCLEX format. The answer key provides page references and coding of questions according to the NCLEX test plan category of cognitive level.

A *Curriculum Guide* that includes a proposed class schedule and reading assignments for courses of varying lengths is provided. This gives educators suggestions for using the text in the most essential manner or in a more comprehensive way. *Open-Book Quizzes* are also provided.

An *Electronic Image Collection* is another valuable tool for instructors that provides easy access to electronic images from the main textbook. Each image can easily be imported to a slide, transparency, or PowerPoint presentation to enhance lecture materials. *PowerPoint Lecture Slides* for building presentations and developing lectures are also included.

A separate *Student Study Guide* includes Chapter Review Activities and Critical Thinking Exercises to reinforce learning and evaluate comprehension. The *Study Guide* can be used for homework assignments or for remedial practice. The exercises in the guide were developed to assist students in synthesizing knowledge of maternity and women's health care and to foster critical thinking.

A new *Clinical Companion* provides students with an accessible, quick reference to the information needed in the clinical setting.

The *Companion CD* packaged with the text provides the student with case studies; critical thinking questions with categories and rationales; video segments, including births and assessments; a care plan constructor; illustrated skills, and an English-Spanish audio glossary.

The *Evolve* website includes case studies, review questions, and WebLinks.

Acknowledgments

The seventh edition of *Maternity Nursing* would not have been possible without the contributions of many people. First we want to thank the many nurse educators, clinicians, and nursing students who made comments and suggestions about the manuscript that led to this collaborative effort. We wish to welcome Kathy Alden, Kitty Cashion, and Robin Webb Corbett in their roles as Associate Editors for this seventh edition. Special thanks goes to the contributors of the sixth edition. Their expertise and knowledge of current clinical practice and research added to the relevance and accuracy of the materials presented and provided a strong base for the revision. We especially thank Patricia Gingrich for contributing to the Evidence-Based Practice boxes, Jo Garner for assisting with Spanish translations, and Ed Lowdermilk for assisting with the Medication Guides.

We are also appreciative of the critiques given by the reviewers, especially in their attention to validating the accuracy of the content and their challenge to present content differently and include new ideas. These combined efforts have resulted in a revision that incorporates the most recent research and current information about the practice of maternity and women's health care. We offer thanks for shared expertise and photographs to the staff and patients of the University of North Carolina at Chapel Hill Women's Hospital; Leonard Nihan (Sea-Band International); Polly Perez (Cutting Edge Press); and Barbara Harper (Global Maternal/Child Health Association, Inc.).

We would also like to thank the following photographers: Kim Molloy, Knoxville, IA; Jonas N. McCoy, Raleigh, NC; Michael S. Clement, MD, Mesa, AZ; Leslie Canerday, Phoenix, AZ; Ed Lowdermilk, Chapel Hill, NC; Amy and Ken Turner, Cary, NC; Ellen Lewis, Irvine, CA; Judy Meyr, St. Louis, MO; Judy Bamber, San Jose, CA; Tammie McGee, Millbrae, CA; Sharon Johnson, Petaluma, CA; Wendy Wetzel, Flagstaff, AZ; Patricia Hess, San Francisco, CA; Brian Sallee, Las Vegas, NV; Sara Kossuth, Los Angeles, CA; Julie Perry Nelson, Gilbert, AZ; Tricia Olson, North Ogden, UT; Rosemary Toohill, LeRoy, IL; Bob and Jill McConnell, Bloomington, IL; Mary Gastelum, Heyworth, IL; Joan R. Vogel, Boca Raton, FL; Chris Rozales, San Francisco, CA; Christine Brockett, Boulder, CO; Susan McGuire, Lexington, IL; Eugene Doerr, Leitchfield, KY; Mahesh Kotwal, MD, Phoenix, AZ; Rebekah Vogel, Fort Collins, CO; H. Gil Rushton, MD, Washington, DC; Edward S. Tank, MD, Portland, OR; David A. Clarke, Philadelphia, PA; and Dale Ikuta, San Jose, CA.

We would like to especially thank Marjorie Pyle, RNC, Lifecircle, Costa Mesa, CA for her many photographic contributions to our texts since the third edition. We wish her enjoyment in her retirement.

Special words of gratitude are extended to Catherine Jackson, Acquisitions Editor; Laurie Gower, Senior Developmental Editor; Jeff Patterson, Publishing Services Manager; Anne Konopka, Senior Project Manager; and Amy Buxton, Senior Designer, for their encouragement, inspiration, and assistance in the preparation and production of this text. These talented and hardworking people helped change our manuscript into a beautiful book by editing the manuscript, designing an attractive format for our special features, and overseeing the production of the book from start to finish. We continue to be especially thankful to Laurie Gower, who always had time to answer our questions, kept track of innumerable details, found just the right photo or resource, obtained that elusive permission, and always reassured us that we were doing a great job and were going to finish on time. We also thank Michael Ledbetter, Publisher, and Sally Schrefer, Executive Vice-President, for their support and encouragement throughout the project.

Deitra Leonard Lowdermilk
Shannon E. Perry

Special Features

Learning Objectives
begin each chapter to focus attention on the important content to be mastered.

CHAPTER 3

Community and Home Care

SHANNON E. PERRY

LEARNING OBJECTIVES

- Compare community-based health care and community health (population- or aggregate-focused) care.
- Identify key components of the community assessment process.
- List indicators of community health status and their relevance to perinatal health.
- Describe data sources and methods for obtaining information about community health status.
- Identify predisposing factors and characteristics of vulnerable populations.
- List the potential advantages and disadvantages of home visits.

- Explore telephonic nursing care options in perinatal nursing.
- Describe how home care fits into the maternity continuum of care.
- Identify and define common perinatal conditions amenable to home care.
- Discuss safety and infection control principles as they apply to the care of patients in their homes.
- Describe the nurse's role in perinatal home care.

KEY TERMS AND DEFINITIONS

continuum of care Range of clinical services provided for an individual or group that reflects care given during a single hospitalization or care for multiple conditions over a lifetime
home health care Care that is provided within the home
key informants Individuals in positions of leadership who can provide information about a situation
levels of prevention Consists of three levels; primary prevention is promoting general health and well-being; secondary prevention involves early detection of health problems so that treatment can begin before significant disability occurs; tertiary prevention is the treatment and rehabilitation of persons who have developed disease

telephonic nursing Services such as "warm lines," nurse advice lines, and telephonic nursing assessments
vulnerable populations Groups who are at higher risk of developing physical, mental, or social health problems or who are more likely to have worse outcomes from these health problems than the population as a whole
walking survey Using one's senses while traveling through a community to obtain information about sociocultural characteristics and the environment, housing, transportation, and local community agencies

ELECTRONIC RESOURCES

Additional information related to the content in Chapter 3 can be found on

the companion website at **evolve**
http://evolve.elsevier.com/Lowdermilk/Maternity/
• NCLEX Review Questions
• WebLinks

or on the interactive companion CD
• NCLEX Review Questions
• Critical Thinking Exercise—Community Resources for Families
• Plan of Care—Community and Home Care

Electronic Resources
related to chapter content are included at the beginning of each chapter and highlighted throughout the text.

EVIDENCE-BASED PRACTICE
Decreasing the Discomfort and Pain of Mammography

BACKGROUND
- Mammography, the radiographic screening test for breast cancer, has been shown by randomized, controlled trials to decrease mortality rates. Each breast is pressed between two plates horizontally, then vertically, and a low-level x-ray is taken of each view. Mammography can find breast lumps that are too small to be palpable, thus enabling life-saving surgery to remove the cancer before it metastasizes. In spite of all these advantages, studies show that some women never return after their first mammogram. From 32% to 53% of women reported discomfort or pain with the procedure. It is important to make mammograms acceptable to the women who need them as a screening tool. Causes of pain may include the level of compression of the breast, a woman's expectations of the procedure, her level of confidence in the procedure and the technician, breast density, and timing of the mammogram during the woman's menstrual cycle. It is important to measure the pain accurately, with a standardized scale that has demonstrable reliability and validity (meaning, a tool that measures exactly what it claims to measure and nothing else).

OBJECTIVES
- The reviewers were seeking evidence of interventions that might relieve the discomfort and pain of mammography. Interventions might include technique and manner of staff and facility, the woman's preparation for the procedure (including analgesia and alternative therapy), the procedure itself, and her participation in the procedure. Outcomes would be pain and discomfort, and some way to standardize these measures. Quality of mammogram is also an important outcome, because false-positive results and recalls decrease the woman's confidence in the process.

METHODS
Search Strategy
- The search was extensive and used Cochrane, EBM Reviews, AMED, CANCERLIT, CINAHL, Current Contents, EMBASE, HealthSTAR, PREMEDLINE, MEDLINE, PsycINFO, dissertation and theses databases, and five journals, as well as relevant organizations and specialists. Search keywords were *pain*, *mammogram*, and *screen*, and the search was limited to humans and females. Three randomized, controlled trials were included in the review, dated 1993 to 1998, representing 574 women.

Statistical Analyses
- Meta-analysis was not possible because of the heterogeneity of the trials. Discomfort scales were not standardized, ranging from "comfortable–not comfortable" to a six-point visual analog scale from comfortable to very uncomfortable.

FINDINGS
- Trial findings are presented separately.
- Study 1 compared the comfort level of technician compression of one breast with patient-controlled compression of the other breast, with each woman to serve

as her own control for comparison. Women reported significantly less pain in self-controlled compression than when the technician compressed the other breast, regardless of which went first. The qualities of the mammogram images were equal when the technician went first, but were of significantly poorer quality when the patient controlled the first compression. This suggests that there was some modeling during the first compression, so that the women knew approximately how much compression was desirable.
- Study 2 was a master's thesis and compared the discomfort level in women who were given acetaminophen before the procedure with the control group with no pretreatment. There were no differences in discomfort levels between groups.
- Study 3 measured the discomfort levels of a standard mammogram compression on one breast with a standard compression that was loosened for one second on the other breast. No significant differences were found. More than half (57%) noted no difference, 23% felt the firmer compression to be the more uncomfortable side, and 20% felt the loosened compression to be the more uncomfortable side.

LIMITATIONS
- The small number of trials, and their small numbers of subjects, limits the power of the findings. Pain and discomfort could lend themselves well to standardized scales, which could then be metaanalyzed across trials, increasing their generalizability. Even though pain is discussed, the measures are all of discomfort, and they are not standardized. The quality of mammogram interpretation across trials was also not addressed.

CONCLUSIONS
- There are not enough data to draw conclusions about how to reduce the discomfort of mammograms. Increasing the woman's control of the procedure seemed to decrease her discomfort, but mild analgesics did not.

IMPLICATIONS FOR PRACTICE
- Some women may find the experience less unpleasant if they are given the option to control their own mammograms. The role of perception of control in alleviating pain is well documented in patient-controlled analgesia. Preparing a woman for a mammogram should include an honest description of the procedure and the sensations.

IMPLICATIONS FOR FURTHER RESEARCH
- More replication and further research into creative intervention to alleviate mammogram discomfort is needed. Measures of women's attitudes and confidence in the procedure still need research. This seems an ideal area in which to explore alternative interventions, such as hypnosis, guided imagery, aromatherapy, massage, temperature, acupressure, music, and distraction. Research may show that pretreatment with other analgesics, such as nonsteroidal antiinflammatory drugs (NSAIDs), holds more promise than pretreatment with acetaminophen.

Reference: Miller D et al: Interventions for relieving the pain and discomfort of screening mammography (Cochrane Review). In *The Cochrane Library*.

Evidence-Based Practice
boxes highlight both research and critical thought processes that support and guide the outcomes of nursing care.

PATIENT INSTRUCTIONS FOR SELF-CARE
Breast Self-Examination

1 The best time to do breast self-examination is about a week after your period, when breasts are not tender or swollen. If you do not have regular periods or sometimes skip a month, do it on the same day every month. If you are breastfeeding or no longer menstruating, choose a date and examine your breasts at the same time each month.
2 Lie down and put a pillow under your right shoulder. Place your right arm behind your head (Fig. 1).

Fig. 1

3 Use the finger pads of your three middle fingers on your left hand to feel for lumps or thickening. Your finger pads are the top third of each finger.
4 Press firmly enough to know how your breast feels. If you're not sure how hard to press, ask your health care

provider or try to copy the way your health care provider uses the finger pads during a breast examination. Learn what your breast feels like most of the time. A firm ridge in the lower curve of each breast is normal.
5 Move around the breast in a set way. You can choose either circles (Fig. 2, A), vertical lines (Fig. 2, B), or wedges (Fig. 2, C). Do it the same way every time. It will help you to make sure that you've gone over the entire breast area and to remember how your breast feels.
6 Gently compress the nipple between your thumb and forefinger and look for discharge.
7 Now examine your left breast using the finger pads of your right hand.
8 If you find any changes, see your health care provider right away.
9 You may want to check your breasts while standing in front of a mirror right after you do your breast self-examination each month. See if there are any changes in the way your breasts look: dimpling of the skin, changes in the nipple, or redness or swelling.
10 You may also want to do an extra breast self-examination while you're in the shower (Fig. 3). Your soapy hands will glide over the wet skin, making it easy to check how your breasts feel.
11 It is important to check the area between the breast and the underarm and the underarm itself. Also examine the area above the breast to the collarbone and the shoulder.

Fig. 2

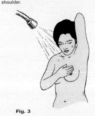

Fig. 3

---

pregnancy does not occur, menstruation follows. Menstruation is the periodic uterine bleeding that begins approximately 14 days after ovulation. The average length of a menstrual cycle is 28 days, but variations are common. The first day of bleeding is designated as day 1 of the menstrual cycle, or menses (Fig. 4-7). The average duration of menstrual flow is 5 days (range of 3 to 6 days), and the average blood loss is 50 ml (range of 20 to 80 ml), but these vary greatly.

The woman's age, physical and emotional status, and environment also influence the regularity of her menstrual cycles.

Hypothalamic-pituitary cycle. Toward the end of the normal menstrual cycle, blood levels of estrogen and progesterone fall. Low blood levels of these ovarian hormones stimulate the hypothalamus to secrete gonadotropin-releasing hormone (GnRH). In turn, GnRH stimulates anterior pituitary secretion of follicle-stimulating hormone

Patient Instructions for Self-Care
boxes promote patient wellness and encourage preventive care.

English-Spanish Guidelines boxes assist students in translating key words and phrases to better serve Spanish-speaking patients.

GUIDELINES/GUÍAS

Prenatal Interview

- Have you had a pregnancy test?
- *¿Ha tenido una prueba del embarazo?*
- When was your last menstrual period?
- *¿Cuándo fue su última menstruación (regla)?*
- Have you been pregnant before?
- *¿Ha quedado embarazada antes?*
- How many times?
- *¿Cuántas veces?*
- How many children do you have?
- *¿Cuántos hijos tiene usted?*
- Have you ever had a miscarriage (spontaneous abortion)?
- *¿Ha perdido un bebé alguna vez? (¿Ha tenido un aborto espontáneo?)*
- Have you ever had a therapeutic abortion?
- *¿Ha tenido un aborto provocado?*
- Have you ever had a stillborn?
- *¿Ha tenido un niño que nació sin vida?*
- Have you ever had a cesarean?
- *¿Ha tenido una operación cesárea?*
- Have you had any problems with past pregnancies?
- *¿Ha tenido problemas durante sus embarazos anteriores?*
- Do you take drugs? Prescription medicine?
- *¿Usa drogas? ¿Medicina recetada?*
- If so, which type of medicine do you use and for what?
- *Qué clases de medicina toma? ¿Para qué las toma?*
- Do you drink alcohol? Do you smoke?
- *¿Toma bebidas alcohólicas? ¿Fuma?*

during the initial interview, the nurse's reference to cues, such as a MedicAlert bracelet, prompts the woman to explain allergies, chronic diseases, or medications being taken (e.g., cortisone, insulin, or anticonvulsants).

The nature of previous surgical procedures also should be described. If a woman has undergone uterine surgery or extensive repair of the pelvic floor, a cesarean birth may be necessary; appendectomy rules out appendicitis as a cause of right lower quadrant pain in pregnancy; and spinal surgery may contraindicate the use of spinal or epidural anesthesia. Any injury involving the pelvis is noted.

Often women who have chronic or handicapping conditions forget to mention them during the initial assessment because they have become so adapted to them. Special shoes or a limp may indicate the existence of a pelvic structural defect, which is an important consideration in pregnant women. The nurse who observes these special characteristics and inquires about them sensitively can obtain individualized data that will provide the basis for a comprehensive nursing care plan. Observations are vital components of the interview process because they prompt the nurse and woman to focus on the specific needs of the woman and her family.

Nutritional history. The woman's nutritional history is an important component of the prenatal history because her nutritional status has a direct effect on the growth and development of the fetus. A dietary assessment can reveal special diet practices, food allergies, eating behaviors, the practice of pica (Corbett, Ryan, & Weinrich, 2003), and other factors related to her nutritional status. Pregnant women are usually motivated to learn about good nutrition and respond well to nutritional advice generated by this assessment.

History of drug and herbal preparations use. A woman's past and present use of legal (over-the-counter [OTC] and prescription medications; herbal preparations; caffeine; alcohol; nicotine) and illegal (marijuana, cocaine, heroin) drugs must be assessed because many substances cross the placenta and may therefore harm the developing fetus. Periodic urine toxicology screening tests are often recommended during the pregnancies of women who have a history of illegal drug use. Results of such tests have been used for criminal prosecution, which results in a breach in patient-provider relationship and in ethical responsibilities to the patient (Foley, 2002; Harris & Paltrow, 2003). Nurses may have ethical concerns if pregnant women are not informed of the possibility of random urine testing for presence of drugs. The other side of this concern is the unborn child and whether the mother has a duty not to harm him or her.

LEGAL TIP **Informed Consent for Drug Therapy**

Hospitals must obtain informed consent from a pregnant woman before she can be tested for drug use (Kehringer, 2003).

Family history. The family history provides information about the woman's immediate family, including parents, siblings, and children. These data help identify familial or genetic disorders or conditions that could affect the present health status of the woman or her fetus.

Social, experiential, and occupational history. Situational factors such as the family's ethnic and cultural background and socioeconomic status are assessed while the history is obtained. The following information may be obtained in several encounters. The woman's perception of this pregnancy is explored by asking her such questions as the following: Is this pregnancy planned or not, wanted or not? Is the woman pleased, displeased, accepting, or nonaccepting? What problems related to finances, career, or living accommodations may arise as a result of the pregnancy? The family support system is determined by asking her such questions as the following: What primary support is available to her? Are changes needed to promote adequate support? What are the existing relationships among the mother, father or partner, siblings, and in-laws? What preparations are being made for her care and that of dependent family members during labor and for the care of the infant after birth? Is financial, educational, or other support needed from the community? What are the woman's ideas about

Text continued on p. 246.

Legal Tips provide students with relevant information regarding legal aspects in the context of maternity and women's health nursing.

Medication Guides provide students with key information about medications and their effects on the woman and her newborn.

Critical Thinking Exercises depict real-life situations that challenge students to choose the best interventions and make good clinical judgments.

warming process is monitored to progress slowly over a period of 2 to 4 hours.

Therapeutic interventions

It is the nurse's responsibility to perform certain interventions immediately after birth to provide for the safety of the newborn.

Eye prophylaxis. The instillation of a prophylactic agent in the eyes of all neonates is mandatory in the United States as a precaution against ophthalmia neonatorum (Fig. 19-4). This is an inflammation of the eyes resulting from gonorrheal or chlamydial infection contracted by the newborn during passage through the mother's birth canal. The agent used for prophylaxis varies according to hospital protocols, but the usual agent is erythromycin, tetracycline, or silver nitrate. In some institutions, eye prophylaxis is delayed until an hour or so after birth so that eye contact and parent-infant attachment and bonding are facilitated. The Centers for Disease Control and Prevention specifies that it should be given as soon as possible after birth; if instillation is delayed, there should be a monitoring process in place to ensure that all newborns are treated (Workowski & Levine, 2002) (Medication Guide). In the United States, if parents object to eye prophylaxis, they may be asked to sign an informed refusal form, and their refusal will be noted in the infant's record.

Topical antibiotics such as tetracycline and erythromycin, silver nitrate, and a 2.5% povidone-iodine solution (currently unavailable in commercial form in the United State) have not proved to be effective in the treatment of chlamydial conjunctivitis.

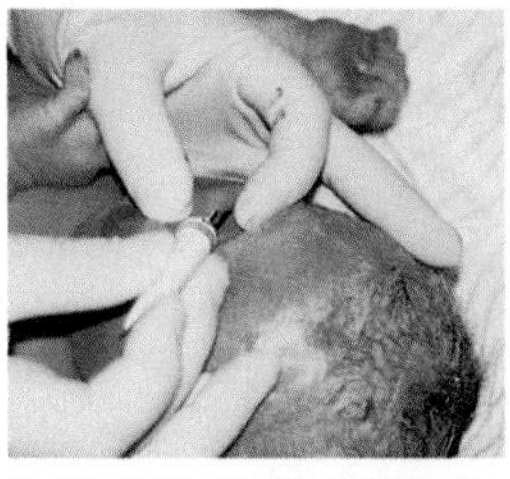

Fig. 19-4 Instillation of medication into eye of newborn. Thumb and forefinger are used to open the eye; medication is placed in the lower conjunctiva from the inner to the outer canthus. (Courtesy Marjorie Pyle, RNC, Lifecircle, Costa Mesa, CA.)

Medication Guide

Eye Prophylaxis: Erythromycin Ophthalmic Ointment, 0.5%, and Tetracycline Ophthalmic Ointment, 1%

ACTION

- These antibiotic ointments are both bacteriostatic and bactericidal. They provide prophylaxis against *Neisseria gonorrhoeae* and *Chlamydia trachomatis.*

INDICATION

- These medications are applied to prevent ophthalmia neonatorum in newborns of mothers who are infected with gonorrhea, conjunctivitis and chlamydia.

NEONATAL DOSAGE

- Apply a 1- to 2-cm ribbon of ointment to the lower conjunctival sac of each eye; also may be used in drop form.

ADVERSE REACTIONS

- May cause chemical conjunctivitis that lasts 24 to 48 hours; vision may be blurred temporarily.

NURSING CONSIDERATIONS

- Administer within 1 to 2 hr of birth. Wear gloves. Cleanse eyes if necessary before administration. Open eyes by putting a thumb and finger at the corner of each lid and gently pressing on the periorbital ridges. Squeeze the tube and spread the ointment from the inner canthus of the eye to the outer canthus. Do not touch the tube to the eye. After 1 min, excess ointment may be wiped off. Observe eyes for irritation. Explain treatment to parents.
- Eye prophylaxis for ophthalmia neonatorum is required by law in all states of the United States.

A 14-day course of oral erythromycin or an oral sulfonamide may be given for chlamydial conjunctivitis (AAP & ACOG, 2002) (see Medication Guide).

Vitamin K administration. For the first few days after birth the newborn is at risk for prolonged clotting and bleeding because of vitamin K deficiency. Vitamin K is poorly transferred across the placenta or through breast milk, and the infant's intestines are not yet colonized by microflora that synthesize vitamin K. Administering vitamin K intramuscularly is routine in the newborn period. A single parenteral dose of 0.5 to 1 mg of vitamin K is given soon after birth to prevent hemorrhagic disorders (Kliegman, 2002; Miller & Newman, 2005). By day 8, normal newborns are able to produce their own vitamin K (Medication Guide).

NURSE ALERT *Vitamin K is never administered by the intravenous route for prevention of hemorrhagic disease of the newborn except in some cases of a preterm infant who has no muscle mass. In such cases, the medication should be diluted and given over 10 to 15 minutes, with the infant being closely monitored with a cardiorespiratory monitor. Rapid bolus administration of vitamin K may cause cardiac arrest.*

National groups supporting home birth are the Home Oriented Maternity Experience (HOME) and the National Association of Parents for Safe Alternatives in Childbirth (NAPSAC). These groups work to foster more humane childbearing practices at all levels, integrating the alternatives for childbirth to meet the needs of the total population.

With a home birth the family is in control of the experience, and the birth may be more physiologically natural in familiar surroundings. The mother may be more relaxed than she would be in the hospital environment. The family can assist in and be a part of the birth, and the mother-father and partner-infant (and sibling-infant) contact is immediate and sustained. Home birth may be less expensive than a hospital confinement. Serious infection may be less likely (assuming strict aseptic principles are followed) because it is usual for people to be relatively immune to the bacteria in their own homes.

Although some physicians and nurses support home births that use good medical and emergency backup systems, many regard this practice as exposing the mother and the fetus to unnecessary danger. Therefore home births are not widely accepted by the North American medical community. This makes it difficult for a family to find a qualified health care provider willing to give prenatal care and to attend the birth. Backup emergency care by a physician in a hospital may be difficult to arrange in advance. If an emergency birth is necessary, no effective way exists to do this rapidly in the home setting.

Factors increasing the safety of birth at home. Most health care providers agree that if home birth is the woman's choice, certain criteria promote a safe home birth experience. The woman must be comfortable with her decision to have her baby at home. She should be in good health. Home birth is not indicated for women with a high risk pregnancy. A drive to the hospital (if needed) should take no more than 10 to 15 minutes. The woman should be attended by a well-trained physician or midwife with adequate medical supplies and resuscitation equipment, including oxygen.

Critical Thinking Exercise

Deciding about a Home Birth

Millie, 28 years old and gravida 1, para 0, is interested in having a home birth. She is currently 14 weeks pregnant, and her pregnancy is progressing normally. According to an ultrasound examination she has one fetus, which is of appropriate size for gestational age with no detectable anomalies. She asks a nurse in the obstetric clinic how to find a midwife who will attend a home birth.

1 Evidence—Is there sufficient evidence to draw conclusions about the safety of a home birth for Millie?
2 Assumptions—Describe the underlying assumptions for each of the following issues:
   a. Assessments that are necessary to identify whether it is feasible and safe for Millie to have a home birth
   b. Supports necessary for a home birth
   c. How to identify providers who are willing to attend a home birth
   d. Ethics of the nurse assisting Millie to find a midwife who will attend a home birth
3 What implications and priorities for nursing care can be drawn at this time?
4 Does the evidence objectively support your conclusion?
5 Are there alternative perspectives to your conclusion?

COMMUNITY ACTIVITY

Select an immigrant or other minority group in your community and identify childbirth-related beliefs and practices that are unique to that group. Are there stores in the area that sell items that meet the needs of that group? Does the community center have activities or classes that are directed toward that group? Are there childbirth education programs available that provide essential information while incorporating cultural patterns? As a nurse, what could you contribute to the community that would help meet the needs of that group?

Key Points

- The prenatal period is a preparatory one both physically, in terms of fetal growth and parental adaptations, and psychologically, in terms of anticipation of parenthood.
- Parent-child, sibling-child, and grandparent-child relationships are affected by pregnancy.
- Discomforts and changes of pregnancy can cause anxiety to the woman and her family and require sensitive attention and a plan for teaching self-care measures.
- Education about healthy ways of using the body (e.g., exercise, body mechanics) is essential given maternal anatomic and physiologic responses to pregnancy.
- Important components of the initial prenatal visit include detailed and carefully recorded findings from the interview, a comprehensive physical examination, and selected laboratory tests.
- Even in normal pregnancy the nurse must remain alert to hazards such as supine hypotension,

Continued

Full-color photographs and **illustrations** help clarify information.

Nurse Alerts point out critical information students should not overlook when treating patients.

Community Activity boxes focus on maternal and newborn activities that can be pursued in local community settings.

Contents

UNIT **TWO**
Reproductive Years

 Assessment and Health Promotion, 63

 Common Reproductive Concerns, 100

 Contraception, Abortion, and Infertility, 134

UNIT THREE
Pregnancy

 7   Genetics, Conception, and Fetal Development, 175

 8   Anatomy and Physiology of Pregnancy, 208

 9   Nursing Care during Pregnancy, 231

 10   Maternal and Fetal Nutrition, 288

UNIT FOUR
Childbirth

11   Labor and Birth Processes, 316

UNIT FIVE
Postpartum Period

UNIT **SEVEN**
Complications of Childbearing

21 **Assessment for Risk Factors, 648**

22 **Pregnancy at Risk: Preexisting Conditions, 673**

23 **Pregnancy at Risk: Gestational Conditions, 715**

Companion CD Contents

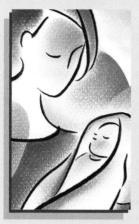

Contemporary Maternity Nursing

SHANNON E. PERRY

LEARNING OBJECTIVES

- *Describe the scope of maternity nursing.*
- *Evaluate contemporary issues and trends in maternity nursing.*
- *Describe sociopolitical issues affecting the care of women and infants.*
- *Compare selected biostatistical data among races and countries.*

- *Examine social concerns in maternity nursing.*
- *Explain quality management and standards of practice in the delivery of nursing care.*
- *Debate ethical issues in perinatal nursing.*
- *Examine the Healthy People 2010 goals related to maternal and infant care.*

KEY TERMS AND DEFINITIONS

best practice A program or service that has been recognized for excellence

clinical benchmarking Standards based on results achieved by others

Cochrane Pregnancy and Childbirth Database Database of up-to-date systematic reviews and dissemination of reviews of randomized controlled trials of health care

evidence-based practice Practice based on knowledge that has been gained through research and clinical trials

failure to rescue Concept that the quality and quantity of nursing care can be measured by comparing the number of surgical patients who develop common complications who survive versus those who do not survive

integrative health care Complementary and alternative therapies in combination with conventional Western modalities of treatment

low-birth-weight (LBW) infants Babies born weighing less than 2500 g

outcomes-oriented care Measures effectiveness of care against benchmarks or standards

preterm infants Infants born before 38 weeks of gestation

standard of care Level of practice that a reasonable, prudent nurse would provide

telemedicine Use of communication technologies and electronic information to provide or support health care when participants are separated by distance

ELECTRONIC RESOURCES

Additional information related to the content in Chapter 1 can be found on

the companion website at **evolve**
http://evolve.elsevier.com/Lowdermilk/Maternity/
- NCLEX Review Questions
- WebLinks

or on the interactive companion CD
- NCLEX Review Questions

*M*aternity nursing focuses on the care of childbearing women and their families through all stages of pregnancy and childbirth, as well as the first 4 weeks after birth. Throughout the prenatal period, nurses, nurse practitioners, and nurse-midwives provide care for women in clinics and physicians' offices and teach classes to help families prepare for childbirth. Nurses care for childbearing families during labor and birth in hospitals, in birthing centers, and in the home. Nurses with special training may provide intensive care for high risk neonates in special care units and for high risk mothers in antepartum units, in critical care obstetric units, or in the home. Maternity nurses teach about pregnancy; the process of labor, birth, and recovery; and parenting skills; and provide continuity of care throughout the childbearing cycle. The Vision for Women and Their Health of the International Confederation of Midwives provides an excellent model for nurses who care for women and children (Box 1-1).

Tremendous advances in the care of mothers and their infants have taken place during the past 150 years (Box 1-2). However, in the United States serious problems exist related to the health and health care of mothers and infants. Lack of access to prepregnancy and pregnancy-related care for all women and lack of reproductive health services for adolescents are major concerns. Sexually transmitted infections, including acquired immunodeficiency syndrome (AIDS), continue to adversely affect reproduction. One fifth of all people in the United States, 58 million people, lack health insurance for a year or more sometime during their life (Marwick, 2002).

Racial and ethnic diversity are increasing within North America. It is estimated that by the year 2050, 50% of the U.S. population will be European-American, 15% will be African-American, 24% will be Hispanic, and 8% will be Asian-American (U.S. Census Bureau, 2004). Health care providers will be challenged to provide culturally sensitive health care.

Although the United States has made great strides in public health, significant disparities exist in health outcomes among people of various racial and ethnic groups. In addition, people may have lifestyles, health needs, and health care preferences related to their ethnic or cultural backgrounds. They may have dietary preferences and health practices that are not understood by caregivers. To meet the health care needs of a culturally diverse society, the nursing workforce must reflect the diversity of its patient population.

This chapter presents a general overview of issues and trends related to the health and health care of women and infants during the maternity cycle.

CONTEMPORARY ISSUES AND TRENDS

Structure of Health Care Delivery

The changing health care delivery system offers opportunities for nurses to alter nursing practice and improve the way care is delivered through managed care, integrated delivery systems (IDSs), and redefined roles. Nurses have been critically important in developing strategies to improve the well-being of women and their infants and have led the efforts to implement clinical practice guidelines and to practice using an evidence-based approach. Through professional associations, nurses can have a voice in setting standards and in influencing health policy by actively participating in the education of the public and of state and federal legislators.

Changes in the health care market are influencing the way health care providers can care for their patients. Health spending varies considerably among nations (Table 1-1). In the United States during 2001 health spending accounted for 13.9% of the gross domestic product (GDP); in Canada 9.7% of the GDP was spent on health care (Reinhardt, Hussey, & Anderson, 2004). A national nursing shortage exists, and nurses are working longer hours. The longer hours jeopardize patient safety (Rogers, Hwang, Scott, Aiken, & Dinges, 2004). A minimum nurse-patient ratio has been legislated.

The role of the nurse is evolving from primary caregiver to the leader of an interdisciplinary care team. Documentation of patient outcomes has become essential (see later discussion). Advanced practice roles will increase as nurses assume more responsibility for patient care.

BOX 1-1

The Vision for Women and Their Health

The International Confederation of Midwives envisions a world where

Women are respected and treated as persons in their own right in all societies.

Women stand as equal partners with men in the world order.

Women are recognized as crucial to the health of any nation.

Women and their families are part of a health care system with high-quality care and easy access when needed.

Women have the right to choose from among safe options for care throughout their lives, including high-quality, state-of-the-art care from competent providers who truly care about the woman and her health.

Women are educated and empowered to delight in a strong sense of self, to trust their bodies, to plan their pregnancies, and to make wise choices in their health care.

Women experience a reasonable standard of living, including a clean and safe environment, healthy food, and a reasonable place to live.

Women need have no fear for their lives or the lives of their babies when they are pregnant.

Women believe that birth is normal and prefer to avoid unnecessary intervention.

From The International Confederation of Midwives: Internet document available at www.internationalmidwives.org/vision.htm (accessed June 15, 2002).

BOX 1-2

Historic Milestones in the Care of Mothers and Infants

1847—James Young Simpson in Edinburgh, Scotland, used ether for an internal podalic version and birth; the first reported use of obstetric anesthesia

1861—Ignaz Semmelwies wrote *The Cause, Concept, and Prophylaxis of Childbed Fever*

1906—First program for prenatal nursing care established

1908—Childbirth classes started by the American Red Cross

1909—First White House Conference on Children convened

1911—First milk bank in the United States established in Boston

1912—U.S. Children's Bureau established

1916—Margaret Sanger established first U.S. birth control clinic in Brooklyn, New York

1923—First U.S. hospital center for premature infant care established at Sarah Morris Hospital in Chicago

1933—*Natural Childbirth* published by Grantly Dick-Read

1941—Penicillin used as a treatment for infection

1953—Virginia Apgar, an anesthesiologist, published Apgar scoring system of neonatal assessment

1955—Jonas Salk's injected polio vaccine was found to be safe and effective

1956—Oxygen determined to cause retrolental fibroplasia (RLF) (now known as *retinopathy of prematurity* [ROP])

1958—Edward Hon reported on the recording of the fetal electrocardiogram (ECG) from the maternal abdomen (first commercial electronic fetal monitor produced in the late 1960s)

1958—Ian Donald, a Glasgow physician, was the first to report clinical use of ultrasound to examine the fetus

1959—*Thank You, Dr. Lamaze* published by Marjorie Karmel

1959—Cytologic studies demonstrated that Down syndrome is associated with a particular form of nondisjunction now known as *trisomy 21*

1960—American Society for Psychoprophylaxis in Obstetrics (ASPO/Lamaze) formed

1960—International Childbirth Education Association formed

1960—Birth control pill introduced in the United States

1962—Thalidomide found to cause birth defects

1962—Albert Sabin's oral polio vaccine replaced the Salk vaccine

1963—Title V of the Social Security Act amended to include comprehensive maternity and infant care for women who were low income and high risk

1965—Supreme Court ruled that married people have the right to use birth control

1967—$Rh_o(D)$ immune globulin produced

1967—Reva Rubin published article on Maternal Role Attainment

1968—Rubella vaccine became available

1969—Nurses Association of the American College of Obstetricians and Gynecologists (NAACOG) founded; renamed Association of Women's Health, Obstetric and Neonatal Nurses (AWHONN) and incorporated as a 501(c)3 organization in 1993

1972—Special Supplemental Nutrition Program for Women, Infants, and Children (WIC) started

1973—Abortion legalized

1974—First standards for obstetric, gynecologic, and neonatal nursing published by NAACOG

1975—The Pregnant Patient's Bill of Rights published by the International Childbirth Education Association

1978—Louise Brown, first test-tube baby, born

1989—Gene for cystic fibrosis identified

1991—Society for Advancement of Women's Health Research founded

1992—Office of Research on Women's Health authorized by U.S. Congress

1993—Human embryos cloned at George Washington University

1993—Family and Medical Leave Act enacted

1998—Newborns' and Mothers' Health Act put into effect

2000—Working draft of sequence and analysis of human genome completed

TABLE 1-1

International Comparison of Percentage of Gross Domestic Product Spent on Health Care in 2001

COUNTRY	PERCENTAGE
United States	13.9
Switzerland	11.1
Germany	10.7
Canada	9.7
France	9.5
Australia	9.2
New Zealand	8.1
Japan	8.0
United Kingdom	7.6

Source: Reinhardt, U., Hussey, P., & Anderson, G. (2004). U.S. Health care spending in an international context. *Health Affairs, 23*(3), 10-25.

Integrative Health Care

Integrative health care encompasses complementary and alternative therapies in combination with conventional Western modalities of treatment. Many popular alternative healing modalities offer human-centered care based on philosophies that recognize the value of the patient's input and honor the individual's beliefs, values, and desires (Fig. 1-1). The focus of these modalities is on the whole person, not just on a disease complex (Box 1-3). Patients often find that alternative modalities are more consistent with their own belief systems and also allow for more patient autonomy in health care decisions. Complementary and alternative therapies are identified throughout the text with an icon ✎.

Increasing numbers of U.S. adults are seeking alternative and complementary health care, which exceeds visits paid

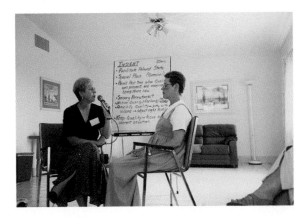

Fig. 1-1   Nurse and patient during guided imagery session. (Courtesy Nurses Certificate Program in Interactive Imagery, Foster City, CA.)

to U.S. primary care physicians. Use of complementary and alternative therapies is increasing rapidly in Canada (Verhoef & Findlay, 2003). Approximately 40% of the general population uses complementary and alternative therapies (Barrett, 2003), and most of these users do not tell their physicians. Annual expenditures related to alternative therapies are estimated at $27 billion, over half of which consists of out-of-pocket expenses not covered by medical insurance (Eisenberg et al., 1998). Throughout the world the use of traditional medicine presents unique challenges in terms of policy, efficacy, accessibility, and utilization (World Health Organization, 2002).

In 1992 the National Institutes of Health (NIH) developed the Office of Alternative Medicine (OAM). Mandated by Congress, the OAM was designed to support research and evaluation of various alternative and complementary modalities and to provide information to health care consumers about such modalities. In 1998 Congress instituted the National Center for Complementary and Alternative Medicine (NCCAM), which incorporates the work of the OAM in its mission and function.

BOX 1-3

Five Types or Classifications of Complementary or Alternative Therapies

> **Alternative medical systems** (e.g., homeopathic and naturopathic medicine; traditional Chinese medicine)
> **Mind-body interventions** (e.g., patient support groups, cognitive-behavioral therapy; meditation, prayer, art, music, dance)
> **Biologically based therapies** (e.g., herbs, foods, vitamins)
> **Manipulative and body-based methods** (e.g., chiropractic or osteopathic manipulation, massage)
> **Energy therapies** (e.g., qi gong, reiki, therapeutic touch, use of electromagnetic fields)

Source: Hawks, J., & Moyad, M. (2003). CAM: Definition and classification overview. *Urology Nursing, 23*(3), 221-223.

Childbirth Practices

Prenatal care may promote better pregnancy outcomes by providing early risk assessment and promoting healthy behaviors such as improved nutrition and smoking cessation. In 2003 84.1% of all women received care in the first trimester and 3.5% had late or no prenatal care. There is disparity in use of prenatal care in the first trimester by race and ethnicity: non-Hispanic whites (89%), non-Hispanic blacks (76%), and Hispanic (77.4%) (Martin, Kochanek, Strobino, Guyer, & MacDorman, 2005).

Women can choose physicians or nurse-midwives as primary care providers. In 2002, physicians attended 91% and nurse-midwives attended 8% of all births (Martin et al., 2003). Hospital births accounted for 99% of births. Of the out-of-hospital births, 65% were in the home, 27% in freestanding birth centers, and 2% in clinics or doctors' offices (Martin et al., 2003). Cesarean births increased to 27.6% of live births in the United States in 2003, the highest rate ever in the United States, whereas the rate of vaginal births after cesarean (VBACs) declined to 10.6% (Martin et al., 2005). Women who choose nurse-midwives as their primary providers actively participate in childbirth decisions and receive fewer interventions such as epidural analgesia for labor (Jackson et al., 2003) (Table 1-2).

Changes are occurring in the conduct of the second stage of labor (from 10 cm dilation to birth of the baby); positions are varied, with more emphasis on upright posture. The arbitrary limit of 2 hours for the second stage is less rigid, as delayed pushing (waiting until the forces of labor propel the fetus down in the birth canal instead of encouraging pushing as soon as the cervix is 10 cm dilated) is instituted. Delayed pushing conserves the energy of the mother, results in fewer instrumental deliveries, and is less costly. The rates of episiotomy are declining, resulting in fewer severe perineal lacerations. Midwives perform fewer episiotomies than do physicians.

The method of analgesia varies, depending on the condition and choice of the mother and the preferences of the providers. Mothers typically are awake and aware during labor and birth. Contrasting philosophies exist regarding analgesia during labor. Some women prefer to experience the sensations of birth with little or no analgesia; others opt for

---

TABLE 1-2

Percent of Women Undergoing Various Obstetric Procedures

PROCEDURE	PERCENT
Electronic fetal monitoring	85.2
Ultrasound	68.0
Induction of labor	20.6
Stimulation of labor	17.3
Tocolysis	2.1
Amniocentesis	2.0

Data from Martin, J., et al. (2003). Births: Final data for 2002. *National Vital Statistics Reports, 52*(10), 1-114.

epidural analgesia to provide comfort and control over their behavior during the experience.

With family-centered care, fathers, partners, grandparents, siblings, and friends may be present for labor and birth. Fathers or partners may be present for cesarean births. Father participation may include cutting the umbilical cord (Fig. 1-2). Doulas—trained and experienced female labor attendants—provide a continuous, one-on-one, caring presence throughout the labor and birth. Newborn infants remain with the mother and are encouraged to breastfeed immediately after birth. Parents participate in the care of their infants in nurseries and neonatal intensive care units. Kangaroo care, parent holding an infant skin-to-skin, is supported for preterm infants.

Childbirth education and parenting classes encourage the participation of a support person, teach breathing and relaxation techniques, and give general information about birth, infant development, and parenting. Other classes or parent support groups may be organized for the weeks and months after birth.

In some cases a woman labors, gives birth, and recovers in the same room (labor-delivery-recovery); she may stay in the same room for the entire birth experience (labor-delivery-recovery-postpartum). Instead of having one nurse care for the baby and another nurse care for the mother, some hospitals have one nurse care for both the mother and baby (couplet or mother-baby care). In some hospitals, central nurseries have been eliminated, and babies "room-in" with their mothers. Many hospitals use lactation consultants to assist mothers with breastfeeding.

Discharge of a mother and baby within 24 hours of birth has created a growing need for follow-up or home care. In some settings, discharge may occur as early as 6 hours after birth. Legislation has been enacted to ensure that mothers and babies are permitted to stay in the hospital at least 48 hours after vaginal birth and 96 hours after cesarean birth. Focused and efficient teaching is necessary to enable the parents and infant to make a safe transition from hospital to home. Nurses may use follow-up telephone calls or home visits to assist families needing information and reassurance.

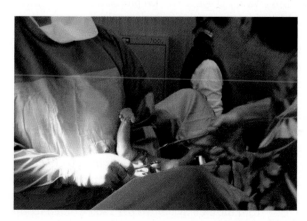

Fig. 1-2 Father cutting cord of his newborn daughter. (Courtesy Tricia Olson, North Ogden, UT.)

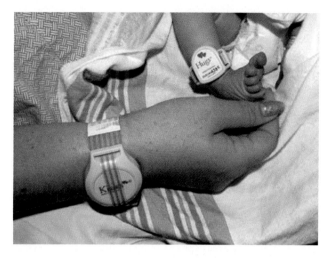

Fig. 1-3 Infant security system. (Courtesy Shannon Perry, Phoenix, AZ.)

Neonatal security in the hospital setting is of concern. Cases of "baby-napping" and of sending parents home with the wrong baby have been reported. Security systems are common in nurseries and mother-baby units (Fig. 1-3), and nurses are required to wear photo identification or some other security badge.

Certified Nurse-Midwives

Certified nurse-midwives (CNMs) are registered nurses with education in the two disciplines of nursing and midwifery. Certified midwives (direct-entry midwives) are educated only in the discipline of midwifery. In the United States, certification of midwives is through the American College of Nurse-Midwives, the professional association for midwives in the United States. The Royal College of Midwives is the professional association for midwives in the United Kingdom. In Canada, the Association of Ontario Midwives is the professional association, and the College of Midwives of Ontario is the regulatory body for midwives in Ontario; the other provinces of Canada have similar regulatory bodies. Many national associations belong to the International Confederation of Midwives, which is composed of 83 member associations from 70 countries in the Americas and Europe, Africa, and the Asia-Pacific region.

Views of Women

Women must be viewed holistically and in the context in which they live. Their physical, mental, and social factors must be considered because these interdependent components influence health and illness. Even the language health care professionals use to describe women and their problems needs to be examined (Freda, 1995). For example, practitioners describe women who have an "incompetent cervix," who "fail to progress," or who have an "arrest" of labor. They may describe a fetus as having intrauterine growth "retardation." They also "allow" women a "trial" of labor. Freda suggests that practitioners use phrases such as "women who have recurrent premature dilation of the cervix" or "fetuses whose intrauterine growth has been restricted." There is a movement to refer to spontaneous pregnancy loss as a "miscarriage" instead of the more politically charged "abortion," especially when talking to patients (Freda, 1999).

Breastfeeding in the Workplace

Women are a significant proportion of the workforce. Companies are recognizing that it is good business to retain good employees and are making provisions for women returning to work after childbirth. Lactation rooms that provide space and privacy for pumping are available at many work sites and on college campuses (Fig. 1-4). In some instances, breastfeeding women bring their babies to work. Since 1999, by law, women may breastfeed in federal buildings and on federal property. Some states have enacted legislation to ensure that mothers can breastfeed their babies in public places. These efforts may help mothers breastfeed longer and meet the recommendation of the American Academy of Pediatrics that breastfeeding continue for at least 1 year.

Family Leave

The Family and Medical Leave Act of 1993 provides for up to 12 weeks of unpaid leave to eligible employees for birth, adoption, or foster placement; for care of a child, spouse, or parent who is seriously ill; or for the employee's own illness. This is of great benefit to women because they are usually the primary caretakers of family members.

Violence

Violence is a major factor affecting pregnant women. This includes battering (which may increase during pregnancy), rape or other sexual assaults, and attacks with various weapons. Approximately 8% of pregnant women are battered. Violence is associated with complications of pregnancy such as bleeding, miscarriage, and preterm labor and birth.

HIV and AIDS in Pregnancy and the Newborn

Cases of perinatally acquired human immunodeficiency virus (HIV) infection and AIDS peaked in 1992; since then the rate of AIDS among infants has continued to decline. Treatment with zidovudine of mothers who tested positive for HIV before giving birth has resulted in a dramatic decrease in the number of infants infected with the virus; highly active antiretroviral therapy (HAART) and elective cesarean birth reduce the rate of mother-to-child transmission of HIV (European Collaborative Study, 2005). Universal HIV testing and access to quality prenatal care will contribute to reducing the transmission of HIV and prolonging survival. For women in labor who have had no prenatal care, rapid HIV testing is available (European Collaborative Study, 2005).

International Concerns

Female genital mutilation, infibulation, and *circumcision* are terms used to describe procedures in which part or all of the female external genitalia are removed for cultural reasons (Ahmed & Abushama, 2005; Momoh, 2004). Worldwide, many women undergo such procedures. With the growing number of immigrants from African and other countries in which female genital mutilation is practiced, nurses will increasingly encounter women who have undergone the procedure. Ethical dilemmas arise when the woman requests that after birth the perineum be repaired as it was after infibulation and the health care provider believes that such repair is unethical. The International Council of Nurses and other health professionals have spoken out against the procedures as harmful to women's health.

Healthy People 2010 Goals

Healthy People 2010 is the nation's agenda for improving health. It has two overarching goals: to increase the quality and years of healthy life and to eliminate health disparities. Within *Healthy People 2010* are 467 objectives to improve health, which are organized into 28 specific focus areas including one related to maternal, infant, and child health (Box 1-4). Current information about the goals of *Healthy People 2010* is available on the Internet at www.health.gov/healthypeople.

Trends in Fertility and Birthrate

Fertility trends and birthrates reflect women's needs for health care. Box 1-5 defines biostatistical terminology useful in analyzing maternity health care. In 2003 the fertility rate—the number of births per 1000 women from 15 to 44 years of age—was 66.1 (Martin et al., 2005). This is a slight increase from the 64.8 live births per 1000 women reported in 2002. The highest birthrates (number of births per 1000 women) were for women between ages 25 and 29 (115.7 per

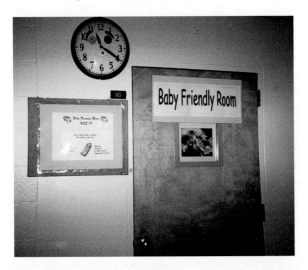

Fig. 1-4 Room on a university campus dedicated to parents and infants. The room contains comfortable furniture, a breast pump, a refrigerator, a baby changing table, and a television and VCR for instructional purposes. The room is available to students, faculty, and staff. (Courtesy Shannon Perry, Phoenix, AZ.)

1000), but the birthrate for women 40 to 44 years old (8.7 per 1000) continues to increase (Martin et al., 2003). One third (34.6%) of all births in the United States in 2003 were to unmarried women, with much variation in proportion among racial groups (African-American 68.5%, Hispanic 45%, non-Hispanic white 23.5%) (Martin et al., 2005). Births to unmarried women are often related to less favorable outcomes, such as low birth weight or preterm birth, because there are typically a large number of teenagers in the unmarried group.

The rates of pregnancy and abortion among adolescents have declined (Martin et al., 2005) but are still higher in the United States than in any other industrialized country.

BOX 1-5

Maternal-Infant Biostatistical Terminology

Abortus: An embryo or fetus that is removed or expelled from the uterus at 20 weeks of gestation or less, weighs 500 g or less, or measures 25 cm or less
Birthrate: Number of live births in 1 year per 1000 population
Fertility rate: Number of births per 1000 women between the ages of 15 and 44 years (inclusive), calculated on a yearly basis
Infant mortality rate: Number of deaths of infants under 1 year of age per 1000 live births
Maternal mortality rate: Number of maternal deaths from births and complications of pregnancy, childbirth, and puerperium (the first 42 days after termination of the pregnancy) per 100,000 live births
Neonatal mortality rate: Number of deaths of infants under 28 days of age per 1000 live births
Perinatal mortality rate: Number of stillbirths and the number of neonatal deaths per 1000 live births
Stillbirth: An infant who, at birth, demonstrates no signs of life, such as breathing, heart beat, or voluntary muscle movements

Incidence of Low Birth Weight

Babies born weighing less than 2500 g are classified as low-birth-weight (LBW) infants, and their risks for morbidity and mortality increase. In 2002 the incidence of LBW was 7.8%, and the incidence of very low birth weight (VLBW; less than 1500 g) was 1.4% (Martin et al., 2005). There is racial disparity in the incidence of LBW. African-American babies are twice as likely as Caucasian babies to be LBW and to die within the first year of life. By race, the incidence of LBW in 2002 for African-American births was 13.3%; for Hispanic births, 6.5%; and for Caucasian births, 6.8%. Cigarette smoking is associated with LBW, prematurity, and intrauterine growth restriction. In 2003, 11% of pregnant women smoked, a proportion that has declined from 19.5% since 1989 (Martin et al., 2005).

The proportion of preterm infants (i.e., those born before 38 weeks of gestation) in 2002 was 17.8% for non-Hispanic black births, 11.9% for Hispanic births, and 11.3% for non-Hispanic white births (Martin et al., 2005). Multiple births accounted for 3.3% of births in 2002, with most of the increase associated with increased use of fertility drugs and older age at childbearing (Martin et al., 2005).

Infant Mortality in the United States

A common indicator of the adequacy of prenatal care and the health of a nation as a whole is the infant mortality rate, the number of deaths of infants younger than 1 year of age per 1000 live births. The infant mortality rate in the U.S. for 2002 was 7.0, the first increase in this rate in over 40 years (Martin et al., 2005). The infant mortality rate continues to be higher for non-Hispanic black babies (13.9 per 1000) than for non-Hispanic whites (5.8 per 1000) and Hispanic (5.6 per 1000) babies (Martin et al., 2005). Limited maternal education, young maternal age, unmarried status, poverty, and lack of prenatal care appear to be associated with higher infant mortality rates. Poor nutrition, smoking and alcohol use, and maternal conditions such as poor health or hypertension are also important contributors to infant mortality. A shift from the current emphasis on high-technology medical interventions to a focus on improving access to preventive care for low-income families is necessary to reduce the disparity. Research on racial disparities must increase.

International Trends in Infant Mortality

The infant mortality rate of Canada (5.2 per 1000 in 2001) ranks nineteenth and that of the United States ranks twenty-seventh when compared with other industrialized nations (Martin et al., 2005). One reason for this is the high rate of LBW infants in the United States compared with other countries.

Maternal Mortality Trends

Worldwide, approximately 1600 women die each day of problems related to pregnancy or childbirth; many of these deaths are preventable. In the United States in 2002, the annual maternal mortality rate (number of maternal deaths per 100,000 live births) was 8.9 (Kochanek, Murphy, Anderson, & Scott, 2004). The United States is tied for seventeenth among developed countries. Reduction of maternal mortality rates is a key goal of the Millennium Development Goals (2004).

There are significant racial differences in the rates: African-American women have a maternal mortality rate four times higher than that of Caucasian women. The maternal mortality rate was 30 per 100,000 for African-American women, in contrast with 8.1 per 100,000 for Caucasian women (Chang et al., 2003). The predominant causes of these deaths are embolism, hemorrhage, gestational hypertension, and infection (Chang et al., 2003). The *Healthy People 2010* goal of 3.3 maternal deaths per 100,000 poses a significant challenge. To achieve this goal, early diagnosis and appropriate intervention must occur. Worldwide strategies to reduce maternal mortality rates include improving access to skilled attendants at birth, providing postabortion care, improving family planning services, and providing adolescents with better reproductive health services (Millennium Development Goals, 2004).

Involving Consumers and Promoting Self-Care

Self-care is appealing to both patients and the health care system because of its potential to reduce health care costs. Maternity care is especially suited to self-care because childbearing is essentially health focused, women are usually well when they enter the system, and visits to health care providers can present the opportunity for health and illness interventions. Measures to improve health and reduce risks associated with poor pregnancy outcomes and illness can be addressed. Topics such as nutrition education, stress management, smoking cessation, alcohol and drug treatment, improvement of social supports, and parenting education are appropriate for such encounters.

Efforts to Reduce Health Disparities

Significant disparities in morbidity and mortality rates are experienced by African-Americans, Native Americans, Hispanics, Alaska Natives, and Asian and Pacific Islanders. Shorter life expectancy, higher infant and maternal mortality rates, more birth defects, and more sexually transmitted infections are found among these groups. The cause-specific mortality ratio was three to four times higher for black women when compared with white women for each cause of death (Chang et al., 2003). The disparities are thought to result from a complex interaction among biologic factors, environment, and health behaviors. Disparities in education and income are associated with differences in occurrence of morbidity and mortality. NIH has a commitment to improve the health of minorities and provides funding for research and training of minority researchers. The National

Institute of Nursing Research has included the goal of reducing disparities in its strategic plan and supports research for that purpose. The nation must make a concerted effort to eliminate health disparities.

Health Literacy

Almost half of all American adults have difficulty in understanding and using health information (Nielsen-Bohlman, Panzer, & Kindig, 2004). Health literacy is "the degree to which individuals have the capacity to obtain, process, and understand basic health information and services needed to make appropriate health decisions" (Ratzan & Parker, 2000). Literacy encompasses a set of skills including reading, writing, mathematics, and speech and speech comprehension. Health literacy involves a spectrum of abilities, ranging from reading an appointment slip to interpreting medication instructions. These skills must be assessed routinely to recognize a problem and accommodate patients with limited literacy skills. An excellent resource is *Teaching Patients with Low Literacy Skills* (2nd ed.) (Doak, Doak, & Root, 1996).

Individuals and groups for whom English is a second language often lack the skills necessary to seek medical care and function adequately in the health care setting. Lack of English fluency is a barrier, and communication difficulties continue to affect access to care, particularly in such areas as making appointments, applying for services, and obtaining transportation. As a result of the increasingly multicultural

 Critical Thinking Exercise

Health Literacy

Yu Mei speaks English as her second language; she speaks Cantonese at home. She has been diagnosed with a urinary tract infection. While giving Yu Mei instructions about perineal hygiene and medication administration, the nurse notes that Yu Mei listens intently to her instructions, nods affirmatively, and looks at the patient information handout.

1 Evidence—Is there sufficient evidence to draw conclusions about Yu Mei's comprehension of the oral and written instructions?
2 Assumptions—What assumptions can be made about patient understanding of the information and instructions?
  a. Mode of patient education
  b. Reading and comprehension
  c. Processing of information
  d. Nonverbal language
  e. Clarity and use of words
  f. Use of interpreters
3 What implications and priorities for nursing care can be drawn at this time?
4 Does the evidence objectively support your conclusion?
5 Are there alternative perspectives to your conclusion?

U.S. population, there is a more urgent need to address health literacy as a component of culturally and linguistically competent care. Health care providers contribute to health literacy by using simple common words, avoiding jargon, and assessing whether the patient is understanding the discussion. Speaking slowly and clearly and focusing on what is important will increase understanding (Roberts, 2004).

High-Technology Care

Advances in scientific knowledge and the large number of high risk pregnancies have contributed to a health care system that emphasizes high-technology care. Maternity care has been extended to preconception counseling, more and better scientific techniques to monitor the mother and fetus, more definitive tests for hypoxia and acidosis, and neonatal intensive care units. Point-of-care testing is available. Personal data assistants are used to enhance comprehensive care (Lewis & Sommers, 2003); the electronic medical record is being used. Virtually all women are monitored electronically during labor despite the lack of evidence of efficacy of such monitoring.

Telemedicine is an umbrella term for the use of communication technologies and electronic information to provide or support health care when the participants are separated by distance. Telemedicine permits specialists, including nurses, to provide health care and consultation when distance separates them from those needing care. For example, Baby CareLink (Gray et al., 2000) is an Internet-based program that incorporates teleconferencing and the World Wide Web to enhance interactions among health care providers, families, and community providers. It includes distance learning, virtual home visits, and remote monitoring of the infant after discharge. This technology has the potential to save billions of dollars annually spent on health care.

Strides are being made in identifying genetic codes, and genetic engineering is taking place. In general, high-technology care has flourished while "health" care has been relatively neglected. These technologic advances have also contributed to higher health care costs. Nurses must use caution and prospective planning and assess the effect of the emerging technology.

Community-Based Care

A shift in settings, from acute care institutions to the home, has been occurring. Even childbearing women at high risk are cared for in the home. Technology previously available only in the hospital is now found in the home. This has affected the organizational structure of care, the skills required to provide such care, and the cost to consumers.

Home health care also has a community focus. Nurses are involved in caring for women and infants in homeless shelters, in caring for adolescents in school-based clinics, and in promoting health at community sites, churches, and shopping malls. Nursing education curricula are increasingly community based.

Increase in High Risk Pregnancies

The number of high risk pregnancies has increased, which means that a greater number of women are at risk for poor pregnancy outcomes. Escalating drug use (ranging from 11% to 27% of pregnant women, depending on geographic location) has contributed to higher incidences of prematurity, LBW, congenital defects, learning disabilities, and withdrawal symptoms in infants. Alcohol use in pregnancy has been associated with miscarriages, mental retardation, LBW, and fetal alcohol syndrome.

The two most frequently reported maternal medical risk factors are hypertension associated with pregnancy and diabetes. The birthrate of higher-order multiples (triplet, quadruplet, and greater) rose 2% from 2000 to 2001 (Martin et al., 2005). Multiple births now account for 3.2% of all births (Martin et al., 2005). The cesarean birthrate increased to 27.6% of all births in 2003, with primary cesareans rising to 19.1% and VBACs dropping to 10.6% (Martin et al., 2005). This cesarean rate is significantly higher than the *Healthy People 2010* goal of 15%. Births of babies born vaginally assisted with forceps or with vacuum extraction decreased to 5.9% (Arias, MacDorman, Strobino, & Guyer, 2003).

High Cost of Health Care

Health care is one of the fastest-growing sectors of the U.S. economy. The United States spends proportionally more on health care than any of the other 190 countries that make up the World Health Organization (Reinhardt, Hussey, & Anderson, 2004). A shift in demographics, an increased emphasis on high-cost technology, and the liability costs of a litigious society contribute to the high cost of care. Most researchers agree that the cost of caring for the increased number of LBW infants in neonatal intensive care units contributes significantly to the overall health care costs.

Midwifery care has helped contain some health care costs. However, not all insurance carriers reimburse nurse practitioners and clinical nurse specialists as direct care providers. Nor do they reimburse for all services provided by nurse-midwives, a situation that continues to be a problem. Nurses must become involved in the politics of cost containment because they, as knowledgeable experts, can provide solutions to many of the health care problems at a relatively low cost.

Early postpartum discharge programs also are used to reduce costs. The American Academy of Pediatrics has published minimal criteria for early discharge of a newborn (American Academy of Pediatrics Committee on Fetus and Newborn, 2004) (see Box 16-2.)

Limited Access to Care

Barriers to access must be removed so pregnancy outcomes can be improved. The most significant barrier to access is the inability to pay. Lack of transportation and dependent child care are other barriers. In addition to a lack of insurance and high costs, a lack of providers for low-income women exists. Many physicians either refuse to take Medicaid patients or take only a few such patients. This presents a serious problem because a significant proportion of births are to mothers who receive Medicaid.

TRENDS IN NURSING PRACTICE

The increasing complexity of care for maternity and women's health patients has contributed to specialization of nurses working with these patients. This specialized knowledge is gained through experience, advanced degrees, and certification programs. Nurses in advanced practice (e.g., nurse practitioners and nurse-midwives) may provide primary care throughout a woman's life, including during the pregnancy cycle. In some settings, the clinical nurse specialist and nurse practitioner roles are blended, and nurses deliver high-quality, comprehensive, and cost-effective care in a variety of settings. Lactation consultants provide services in the postpartum unit or on an outpatient basis, including home visits.

Nursing Interventions Classification

When the National Institute of Medicine proposed that all patient records be computerized by the year 2000, a need for a common language to describe the contributions of nurses to patient care became evident. Nurses from the University of Iowa developed a comprehensive standardized language that describes interventions that are performed by generalist or specialist nurses. This language is included in the Nursing Interventions Classification (NIC) (Dochterman & Bulachek, 2004). Interventions commonly used by maternal-child nurses include those in Box 1-6.

Evidence-Based Practice

Evidence-based practice—providing care based on evidence gained through research and clinical trials—is being increasingly emphasized. Although not all practice can be evidence based, practitioners must use the best available information on which to base their interventions. The Association of Women's Health, Obstetric and Neonatal Nurses (AWHONN) *Standards and Guidelines for Professional Nursing Practice in the Care of Women and Newborns* (1998) and the *Standards for Professional Perinatal Nursing Practice and Certification in Canada* (2002) include an evidence-based approach to practice. Discussion of nursing care and evidence-based nursing boxes throughout this text provide examples of evidence-based practice in perinatal nursing.

AWHONN has conducted six research-based practice projects (Box 1-7). These projects were conducted in several states, and staff nurses were involved in their implementation and in data collection. The AWHONN practice guidelines incorporate evidence-based practices for second-stage labor management, continence for women, breastfeeding

---

BOX 1-6

Childbearing Care Interventions

LEVEL 1 DOMAIN: FAMILY
- Care that supports the family

LEVEL 2 CLASS: CHILDBEARING CARE
- Interventions to assist in the preparation for childbirth and management of the psychologic and physiologic changes before, during, and immediately after childbirth

LEVEL 3: INTERVENTIONS
- Amnioinfusion
- Birthing
- Bleeding reduction: antepartum uterus
- Bleeding reduction: postpartum uterus
- Breastfeeding assistance
- Cesarean section care
- Childbirth preparation
- Circumcision care
- Electronic fetal monitoring: antepartum
- Electronic fetal monitoring: intrapartum
- Environmental management: attachment process
- Family integrity promotion: childbearing family
- Family planning: contraception
- Family planning: infertility
- Family planning: unplanned pregnancy
- Fertility preservation

- Genetic counseling
- Grief work facilitation: perinatal death
- High risk pregnancy care
- Intrapartal care
- Intrapartal care: high risk delivery
- Kangaroo care
- Labor induction
- Labor suppression
- Lactation suppression
- Newborn care
- Newborn monitoring
- Nonnutritive sucking
- Phototherapy: neonate
- Postpartal care
- Preconception counseling
- Pregnancy termination care
- Prenatal care
- Reproductive technology management
- Resuscitation: fetus
- Resuscitation: neonate
- Risk identification: childbearing family
- Surveillance: late pregnancy
- Tube care: umbilical line
- Ultrasonography: limited obstetric

From Dochterman, J., & Bulachek, G. (2004). *Nursing interventions classification (NIC)* (4th ed.). St. Louis: Mosby.

BOX 1-7

Association of Women's Health, Obstetric and Neonatal Nurses Research-Based Practice Programs

> Transition of the Preterm Infant to an Open Crib
> Management of Women in Second-Stage Labor
> Continence for Women
> Neonatal Skin Care
> Cyclic Pelvic Pain and Discomfort Management
> Setting Universal Cessation Counseling, Education, and Screening Standards: Nursing Care for Pregnant Women Who Smoke (SUCCESS)

---

support, midlife well-being, perianesthesia care, neonatal skin care, and cardiac health. By using such guidelines and published reports, nurses can develop protocols and procedures based on published research and incorporate an evidence base into their practice. AWHONN research priorities include the aforementioned topics, as well as family violence, fetal surveillance, genetics, infertility, and early parenting (Box 1-8). The incorporation of research findings into practice is essential in developing a science-based practice.

Introduction to Evidence-Based Practice Reviews

Evidence-based practice review groups systematically examine all relevant research studies on a certain topic and efficiently communicate their findings to the professionals who make clinical decisions and write protocols for clinical practice. Many studies are too small to be generalizable to the general population. With the studies combined, several smaller studies together achieve more "power," or predictive value. The review by Brown, Small, Faber, Krastev, and Davis (2002), for example, combined eight smaller trials with a total of 3600 women (Evidence-Based Practice box).

A review group may choose to review only randomized trials, because these are the most generalizable to the larger population. In addition, they may choose only controlled trials (one group gets the intervention and one group, the control, does not), which makes a stronger case that any difference between the groups is actually a result of the intervention rather than to some other influence. In the study in the Evidence-Based Practice box, the studies ranged from 1962 to 2000 and were from North America, Sweden, the United Kingdom, and Australia. The standard length of stay after normal birth ranged from 2 to 5 days, and early discharge ranged from 6 hours to 4 days, so considerable overlap prevented some calculations from all the studies together. In this case the reviewers combined studies with similar definitions.

Conclusions are the review committee's best recommendations for clinical practice, based on the best available evidence. Reviewers may find that some of our long-standing assumptions about clinical care are not beneficial, or may even be harmful for mother or baby. In the Brown and colleagues (2002) review, the trend was toward improvement in most outcome measures with early discharge, but there were no statistically significant differences. Therefore the conclusion is that early discharge appears to do no harm, but adverse outcomes cannot be ruled out because of limitations in the studies.

BOX 1-8

Association of Women's Health, Obstetric and Neonatal Nurses Research Priorities for Women's and Neonatal Health

STRATEGIES TO PROMOTE HEALTHY BEHAVIORS IN WOMEN ACROSS THE LIFESPAN
- Prevention of unintended pregnancy
- Cardiovascular health, including smoking cessation
- Weight management and nutrition
- Menstrual and menopausal adjustment and symptom management
- Cancer screening and risk reduction
- Chronic illness self-care (e.g., diabetes)
- Social risks (poverty, addiction, sexual risks, violence)
- Promotion of women's mental health and stress management

REDUCING HEALTH DISPARITIES
- Delivering culturally competent care
- Enhancing access to and use of health care
- Reducing disparities in rates of low birth weight
- Improving breastfeeding rates among low-income and minority women

- Reducing genetically determined risk through appropriate screening

MODELS OF NURSING CARE DELIVERY
- Strategies to increase diversity of the nursing workforce
- Effect of workforce diversity on patient outcomes
- Comparative studies of quality, patient outcomes, and cost across the following:
  - Providers (physicians, nurses, advanced practice nurses)
  - Delivery settings (medical centers, birth centers, primary care, home care)
  - Practice decisions and decision making (levels and types of clinical decision making and interventions)
  - Staff development and support models
  - Models of care delivery in prenatal and antepartum care

Approved by AWHONN Research Committee, July, 2001.

EVIDENCE-BASED PRACTICE
Early Postnatal Discharge of Healthy Mothers and Babies

BACKGROUND

- Since the 1970s the trend has been toward shorter postpartum length of stay. Current average stays in the United States are typically 12 to 24 hours for uncomplicated vaginal births and 48 to 72 hours for uncomplicated cesarean births. Many have debated the consequences to mothers and babies of this change in practice. Risks include delay in detecting maternal and infant morbidity, readmission of mothers and babies, breastfeeding problems, decreased maternal satisfaction in care, and decreased confidence in infant care. Advantages included family-centered bonding, better sleep for the mother in her own home, decreased exposure to nosocomial infections for mother and baby, increased maternal satisfaction in care, and decreased cost.

OBJECTIVES

- Specific research questions include identifying whether early postnatal discharge leads to any of the following:
  1 Increased maternal or infant readmissions or physical problems
  2 Increased maternal fatigue, depression, or anxiety
  3 Breastfeeding problems
  4 Change in maternal satisfaction levels with health care
  5 Increased paternal anxiety
  6 Increased costs, including any prenatal teaching and support after discharge

METHODS
Search Strategy

- The search strategy included searching in the Cochrane, Medline, CINAHL, and EMBASE databases. Search keywords were *postnatal care, postpartum, puerpera, childbirth, length of stay, discharge, hospitalization,* and *readmission.*
- The reviewers selected eight randomized, controlled studies, involving a total of 3600 women and their babies. The studies were published from 1962 to 2000 and involved Australia, Canada, the United States, the United Kingdom, and Sweden. All studies had some cointervention to accompany early discharge, such as antenatal education and postdischarge midwife or nurse visits or calls.

Statistical Analysis

- Reviewers independently analyzed the studies and then met to resolve disagreements. "Early" and "standard" time frames overlapped, so the reviewers agreed to accept the "standard" of the setting of each study. Statistical analysis enabled comparison of outcomes, such as readmissions or breastfeeding problems, of early versus standard discharge patients (using the standards of that particular study).

FINDINGS

- The reviewers found no significant differences between early versus standard discharge groups in numbers of readmissions of infants or mothers. One study found significantly increased depression scores (indicating more depression) in the standard discharge group at 1 month. There was no significant difference in maternal fatigue. Both groups were the most exhausted the day after discharge.
- Early discharge mothers were more confident at 1 week, but there was no difference between the groups by 1 month.
- Trends were mixed for breastfeeding, which may reflect the cultural differences of the time frame (1950s to present) and countries. The reviewers identified no significant differences.
- There was a trend toward higher maternal satisfaction with care in the early discharge group that was not statistically significant.
- Fathers spent significantly more time with the baby who was discharged early. No data about paternal anxiety were found.
- One study showed that early discharge cost was considerably less than standard care, even with the costs of multiple home visits and acute care visits factored in.

LIMITATIONS

- Many studies had low recruitment rates (only 24% to 44%) and high exclusion rates after randomization and withdrawals for reasons such as not following the assigned protocol. Some women changed their minds about their length of stay or developed problems and stayed longer. Cointerventions included some combination of prenatal education and from one to seven postnatal visits by midwives or nurses. Available postnatal primary and specialist medical support varied. Definitions of "standard" versus "early" discharge overlapped. The three studies that measured depression scores did not use validated depression screening tools. The studies were too heterogeneous to assess breastfeeding success or maternal satisfaction with care. Few studies reported costs.

CONCLUSIONS

- The review committee finds no evidence of adverse outcomes from early discharge. However, methodologic limitations may obscure adverse outcomes.

IMPLICATIONS FOR PRACTICE

- Health care providers can include in their prenatal education the information that all women feel the most exhausted on the first day after discharge. Maternal confidence seems to increase with time after discharge. Early discharge may allow more time for paternal bonding before the father must return to work.

IMPLICATIONS FOR FURTHER RESEARCH

- The authors call for large, well-designed trials, using standardized approaches, factoring in the likely attrition rates. Much remains to be clarified in further research regarding the importance of postdischarge nursing and midwifery care.

Reference: Brown, S. et al. (2002). Early postnatal discharge from hospital for healthy mothers and term infants (Cochrane Review). In *The Cochrane Library,* Issue 2, 2005. Chichester, UK: John Wiley & Sons.

Cochrane Pregnancy and Childbirth Database

The Cochrane Pregnancy and Childbirth Database was first planned in 1976 with a small grant from the World Health Organization to Dr. Iain Chalmers and colleagues at Oxford. In 1993, the Cochrane Collaboration was formed, and the Oxford Database of Perinatal Trials became known as the Cochrane Pregnancy and Childbirth Database. The Cochrane Collaboration oversees up-to-date, systematic reviews of randomized controlled trials of health care and disseminates these reviews. The premise of the project is that these types of studies provide the most reliable evidence about the effects of care.

The evidence from these studies should encourage practitioners to implement useful measures and to abandon those that are useless or harmful. Studies are ranked in six categories:

1. Beneficial forms of care
2. Forms of care that are likely to be beneficial
3. Forms of care with a trade-off between beneficial and adverse effects
4. Forms of care with unknown effectiveness
5. Forms of care that are unlikely to be beneficial
6. Forms of care that are likely to be ineffective or harmful

Practices that have been reviewed by the Collaboration are identified with a symbol ❋ throughout this text.

Outcomes-Oriented Practice

Outcomes of care (that is, the effectiveness of interventions and quality of care) are receiving increased emphasis. Outcomes-oriented care measures effectiveness of care against benchmarks or standards. It is a measure of the value of nursing using quality indicators and answers the question, "Did the patient benefit or not benefit from the care provided?" (Moorhead, Johnson, & Maas, 2004). The Outcome Assessment Information Set (OASIS) is an example of an outcome system important for nursing. Its use is required by the Centers for Medicare and Medicaid Services, formerly the Health Care Financing Administration (HCFA), in all home health organizations that are Medicare accredited. The Nursing Outcomes Classification (NOC) is an effort to identify outcomes and related measures that can be used for evaluation of care of individuals, families, and communities across the care continuum (Moorhead, Johnson, & Maas, 2004). An example of outcomes classification is provided in Table 1-3.

Best Practices as Goal of Care

A program or service that has been recognized for excellence is considered to be a best practice. A best practice must provide a better or a new way to achieve goals and be sound from operational, clinical, and financial perspectives. To determine best practices, information is collected from similar institutions. Staff members then identify solutions that have been successful in addressing specific needs and select one that incorporates the best resolutions of the problem that fit the agency's unique population and mission characteristics. The agency continually compares its performance against the best in the industry and the best of a specific function.

Clinical Benchmarking

Clinical benchmarking is a process used to compare one's own performance against the performance of the best in an area of service. Benchmarking supports and promotes continual quality improvement and helps the organization remain competitive in the health care market.

Collaborative benchmarking involves sharing strategies and outcomes and leads to the development of new best practices (Clinical Benchmarking, 2005). Areas of practice routinely monitored in perinatal nursing include hospital length of stay, maternal mortality rate, infant mortality rate, cesarean birth rate, epidural rate, and episiotomy rate.

A Global Perspective

Advances in medicine and nursing have resulted in increased knowledge and understanding in the care of mothers and infants and reduced perinatal morbidity and mortality rates. However, these advances have affected predominantly the industrialized nations. For example, the majority of the 3.2 million children living with HIV or AIDS acquired the infection through perinatal transmission and live in sub-Saharan Africa. This illustrates the inequities that exist between industrialized and resource-poor parts of the world (Cohan, 2003).

As the world becomes smaller because of travel and communication technologies, nurses and other health care providers are gaining a global perspective and participating in activities to improve the health and health care of people worldwide (Katz & Hirsch, 2003). Nurses participate in medical outreach, providing obstetric, surgical, ophthalmologic, orthopedic, or other services; attend international meetings; conduct research; and provide international consultation. International student and faculty exchanges occur (Perry & Mander, 2005) (Fig. 1-5). More articles about health and health care in various countries are appearing in nursing journals. Several schools of nursing in the United States are World Health Organization Collaborating Centers.

Millennium Development Goals

The member states of the United Nations adopted the Millennium Declaration in September 2000. The Millennium Development Goals are a guide to implementing the Millennium Declaration. The goals are to (1) eradicate extreme poverty and hunger, (2) achieve universal primary education, (3) promote gender equality and empower women, (4) reduce child mortality, (5) improve maternal health, (6) combat HIV and AIDS, malaria, and other diseases, (7) ensure environmental sustainability, and (8) develop a global partnership for development. The target date for achievement of the goals is 2015. The goals help to define a yardstick with which

TABLE 1-3

Nursing Outcomes Classification

TAXONOMY

Level 1: Domain IV—Health Knowledge and Behavior
Outcomes that describe attitudes, comprehension, and actions with respect to health and illness

Level 2: Q—Health Behavior
Outcomes that describe an individual's actions to promote, maintain, or restore health

Level 3: 1607—Prenatal Health Behavior

Care Recipient: | Data Source:

Scale(s)—*Never demonstrated* to *Consistently demonstrated*

Definition: Personal actions to promote a healthy pregnancy and a healthy newborn

Outcome Target Rating: | Maintain at _____ | Increase to _____

Prenatal Health Behavior Overall Rating	Never demonstrated 1	Rarely demonstrated 2	Sometimes demonstrated 3	Often demonstrated 4	Consistently demonstrated 5	
Indicators:						
160701 Maintains healthy preconceptual state	1	2	3	4	5	NA
160702 Uses proper body mechanics	1	2	3	4	5	NA
160703 Keeps appointments for prenatal care	1	2	3	4	5	NA
160704 Maintains healthy weight gain pattern	1	2	3	4	5	NA
160705 Receives proper dental care	1	2	3	4	5	NA
160706 Uses seat belt appropriately	1	2	3	4	5	NA
160707 Attends childbirth education classes	1	2	3	4	5	NA
160709 Participates in regular exercise	1	2	3	4	5	NA
160710 Maintains adequate nutrient intake for pregnancy	1	2	3	4	5	NA
160711 Practices safe sex	1	2	3	4	5	NA
160721 Uses medications as prescribed	1	2	3	4	5	NA
160712 Consults health care professional concerning use of nonprescription drugs	1	2	3	4	5	NA
160713 Avoids environmental hazards	1	2	3	4	5	NA
160714 Avoids exposure to infectious diseases	1	2	3	4	5	NA
160715 Avoids recreational drugs	1	2	3	4	5	NA
160716 Abstains from alcohol	1	2	3	4	5	NA
160717 Abstains from tobacco use	1	2	3	4	5	NA
160718 Avoids teratogenic agents	1	2	3	4	5	NA
160719 Avoids abusive situations	1	2	3	4	5	NA

Outcome Content References: Bell, R., & O'Neill, M. (1994). Exercise and pregnancy: A review. *Birth, 21*(2), 85-95; Crowell, D. (1995). Weight change in the postpartum period: A review of the literature. *Journal of Nurse-Midwifery, 40*(5), 418-423; Freda, M. et al. (1993). What pregnant women want to know: A comparison of client and provider perceptions. *Journal of Obstetric, Gynecologic, and Neonatal Nursing, 22*(3), 237; Kearney, M. et al. (1995). Salvaging self: A grounded theory of pregnancy on crack cocaine. *Nursing Research, 44*(4), 208-213; McFarlane, J. et al. (1996). Abuse during pregnancy: Associations with maternal health and infant birth weight. *Nursing Research, 45*(1), 37-42; Olds, S. et al. (1996). *Maternal-newborn nursing: A family-centered approach* (5th ed.). Menlo Park, CA: Addison-Wesley; Shapiro, H. (1993). Prenatal education in the work place. *AWHONN's Clinical Issues in Perinatal and Women's Health Nursing 4*(1), 113-121; Summers, L. (1993). Preconception care: An opportunity to maximize health in pregnancy. *Journal of Nurse-Midwifery, 38*(4), 188-198.
Source: Moorhead, S., Johnson, M., & Maas, M. (2004). *Nursing outcomes classification (NOC)* (3rd ed.). St Louis: Mosby.

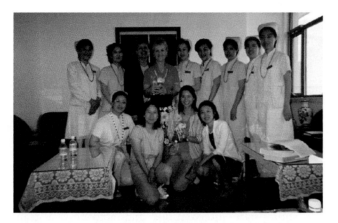

Fig. 1-5 U.S. nursing students and faculty posing with head nurses in a pediatric hospital in China as part of an international perspectives in nursing course. (Courtesy Shannon Perry, Phoenix, AZ.)

to measure results. With the rich resources of many developed countries, poorer countries can be provided with additional resources and assistance (Millennium Development Goals, 2004).

STANDARDS OF PRACTICE AND LEGAL ISSUES IN DELIVERY OF CARE

Nursing standards of practice in perinatal nursing have been described by several organizations, including the American Nurses Association (ANA), which publishes standards for maternal-child health nursing; AWHONN, which publishes standards of practice and education for perinatal nurses and women's health (Box 1-9); the American College of Nurse Midwives (ACNM), which publishes standards of practice for midwives; and the National Association of Neonatal Nurses (NANN), which publishes standards of practice for neonatal nurses. These standards reflect current knowledge, represent levels of practice agreed on by leaders in the specialty, and can be used for clinical benchmarking.

In addition to these more formalized standards, agencies have their own policy and procedure books that outline standards to be followed in that setting. In legal terms, the **standard of care** is that level of practice that a reasonably prudent nurse would provide. In determining legal negligence, the care given is compared with the standard of care. If the

---

BOX 1-9

Standards of Care for Women and Newborns

STANDARDS THAT DEFINE THE NURSE'S RESPONSIBILITY TO THE PATIENT
Assessment
- Collection of health data of the woman or newborn

Diagnosis
- Analysis of data to determine nursing diagnosis

Outcome Identification
- Identification of expected outcomes that are individualized

Planning
- Development of a plan of care

Implementation
- Performance of interventions for the plan of care

Evaluation
- Evaluation of the effectiveness of interventions in relation to expected outcomes

STANDARDS OF PROFESSIONAL PERFORMANCE THAT DELINEATE ROLES AND BEHAVIORS FOR WHICH THE PROFESSIONAL NURSE IS ACCOUNTABLE
Quality of Care
- Systemic evaluation of nursing practice

Performance Appraisal
- Self-evaluation in relation to professional practice standards and other regulations

Education
- Participation in ongoing educational activities to maintain knowledge for practice

Collegiality
- Contribution to the development of peers, students, and others

Ethics
- Use of Code for Nurses to guide practice

Collaboration
- Involvement of patient, significant others, and other health care providers in the provision of patient care

Research
- Use of research findings in practice

Resource Utilization
- Consideration of factors related to safety, effectiveness, and costs in planning and delivering patient care

Practice Environment
- Contribution to the environment of care delivery

Accountability
- Legal and professional responsibility for practice

Source: Association of Women's Health, Obstetric and Neonatal Nurses (AWHONN). (1998). *Standards and guidelines for professional nursing practice in the care of women and newborns* (5th ed.). Washington, DC: AWHONN.

standard was not met and harm resulted, negligence occurred. The number of legal suits in the perinatal area has typically been high. As a consequence, malpractice insurance costs are high for physicians, nurse-midwives, and nurses who work in labor and delivery.

LEGAL TIP Standard of Care

When you are uncertain about how to perform a procedure, consult the agency procedure book and follow the guidelines printed therein. These guidelines are the standard of care for that agency.

Risk Management

Risk management is an evolving process that identifies risks, establishes preventive practices, develops reporting mechanisms, and delineates procedures for managing lawsuits. Nurses should be familiar with concepts of risk management and their implications for nursing practice. These concepts can be viewed as systems of checks and balances that ensure high-quality patient care from preconception until after birth. Effective risk management minimizes the risk of injury to patients and the number of lawsuits against nurses. Each facility or site develops site-specific risk management procedures based on accepted standards and guidelines. The procedures and guidelines must be reviewed periodically.

To decrease risk of errors in the administration of medications, the Joint Commission on Accreditation of Healthcare Organizations (JCAHO) has developed a list of abbreviations, acronyms, and symbols *not* to use (Table 1-4). In addition, each agency must develop its own list.

Sentinel Events

JCAHO describes a sentinel event as "an unexpected occurrence involving death or serious physical or psychological injury, or the risk thereof. Serious injury specifically includes loss of limb or function." These events are called "sentinel" because they signal a need for an immediate investigation and response (JCAHO, 2002).

Failure to Rescue

Failure to rescue is used to "evaluate the quality and quantity of nursing care by comparing the number of surgical patients who develop common complications who survive versus those who do not" (Simpson, 2005). As mothers and babies are generally healthy, complications leading to death in obstetrics are comparatively rare. Simpson (2005) proposes evaluating the perinatal team's ability to decrease risk of adverse outcomes by measuring processes involved in common complications and emergencies in obstetrics. Key components of failure to rescue are (1) careful surveillance and identification of complications, and (2) acting quickly to initiate appropriate interventions and activating a team response. For the perinatal nurse, this involves timely identification of complications, appropriate interventions, and efforts of the team to minimize patient harm. Maternal complications that are appropriate for process measurement are placental abruption, postpartum hemorrhage, uterine rupture, eclampsia, and amniotic fluid embolism (Simpson, 2005). Fetal complications include nonreassuring fetal heart rate pattern, prolapsed umbilical cord, shoulder dystocia, and uterine hyperstimulation (Simpson, 2005). Perinatal nurses can use these complications to develop a list of expectations for monitoring, timely identification, interventions, and roles of team members. The list can be used to evaluate the perinatal team's response.

ETHICAL ISSUES IN PERINATAL NURSING

Ethical concerns and debates have multiplied with the increased use of technology and with scientific advances. For example, with reproductive technology, pregnancy is now possible in women who thought they would never bear children, including some who are menopausal or postmenopausal. Should scarce resources be devoted to achieving pregnancies in older women? Is giving birth to a child at an older age worth the risks involved? Should older

---

TABLE 1-4

JCAHO "Do Not Use" List

ABBREVIATION	POTENTIAL PROBLEM	PREFERRED TERM
U (for unit)	Mistaken as zero, four, or cc.	Write "unit."
IU (for international unit)	Mistaken as IV (intravenous) or 10 (ten).	Write "international unit."
Q.D., Q.O.D. (Latin abbreviations for once daily and every other day)	Mistaken for each other. The period after the Q can be mistaken for an "I." The "O" can be mistaken for "I."	Write "daily" and "every other day."
Trailing zero (X.0 mg); lack of leading zero (.X mg)	Decimal point is missed.	Never write a zero by itself after a decimal point (X mg), and always use a zero before a decimal point (0.X mg).
MS MSO$_4$ MgSO$_4$	Confused for one another. Can mean morphine sulfate or magnesium sulfate.	Write "morphine sulfate" or "magnesium sulfate."

Source: "Do not use" list required in 2004. *LTC Update,* Issue 3, 2003.

parents be encouraged to conceive a baby when they may not live to see the child reach adulthood? Should a woman who is HIV positive have access to assisted reproduction services? Should third-party payers assume the costs of reproductive technology? With induced ovulation and in vitro fertilization, multiple pregnancies occur, and multifetal pregnancy reduction (selectively terminating one or more fetuses) may be considered. Innovations such as intrauterine fetal surgery, fetoscopy, therapeutic insemination, genetic engineering, stem cell research, surrogate childbearing, surgery for infertility, "test tube" babies, fetal research, and treatment of VLBW babies have resulted in questions about informed consent and allocation of resources. The introduction of long-acting contraceptives has created moral choices and policy dilemmas for health care providers and legislators; that is, should some women (substance abusers, women with low incomes, or women who are HIV positive) be required to take the contraceptives? With the potential for great good that can come from fetal tissue transplantation, what research is ethical? What are the rights of the embryo? Should cloning of humans be permitted? Discussion and debate about these issues will continue for many years. Nurses and patients, as well as scientists, physicians, attorneys, lawmakers, ethicists, and clergy, must be involved in the discussions.

RESEARCH IN PERINATAL NURSING

Research plays a vital role in the establishment of a maternity nursing science. Nurses should promote research funding and conduct research on maternity and women's health, especially concerning the effectiveness of nursing strategies for these patients. Research can validate that nursing care makes a difference. For example, although prenatal care is clearly associated with healthier infants, no one knows exactly which nursing interventions produce this outcome. Many possible areas of research exist in maternity and women's health care. The clinician can identify problems in the health and health care of women and infants. Through research, nurses can make a difference for these patients.

Ethical Guidelines for Nursing Research

Nurses must protect the rights of human subjects (that is, patients) in all of their research. For example, nurses may collect data on or care for patients who are participating in clinical trials. The nurse ensures that the participants are fully informed and aware of their rights as subjects. Research with perinatal patients may create ethical dilemmas for the nurse. For example, participating in research may cause additional stress to a woman concerned about outcomes of genetic testing or one who is waiting for an invasive procedure. Obtaining amniotic fluid samples or performing cordocentesis poses risks to the fetus. The nurse may be involved in determining whether the benefits of research outweigh the risks to the mother and the fetus. Following the ANA ethical guidelines in the conduct, dissemination, and implementation of nursing research helps nurses ensure that research is conducted ethically.

COMMUNITY ACTIVITY

Examine a daily newspaper for 7 days. Identify articles reporting topics related to maternity or reproductive health.
- How many articles did you identify? What are the topics? Are they local or national issues?
- Is the reporter a health reporter? A local or national columnist? Male or female?
- What is the "slant" of the articles? Are the reports favorable to women and reproductive health? Does the viewpoint of the articles limit reproductive freedom or infringe on women's rights?
- What conclusions can you draw related to the treatment of women's issues and reproductive health in your community?

Key Points

- Maternity nursing focuses on women and their infants and families during the childbearing cycle.
- Nurses caring for women can play an active role in shaping health care systems to be responsive to the needs of contemporary women.
- Childbirth practices have changed to become more family focused and to allow alternatives in care.
- Canada ranks nineteenth and the United States ranks twenty-seventh among industrialized nations in infant mortality.
- Integrative medicine combines modern technology with ancient healing practices and encompasses the whole of body, mind, and spirit.

- Evidence-based practice, outcomes orientation, best practices, and clinical benchmarking are emphasized in current practice.
- Risk management and learning from sentinel events can improve quality of care.
- *Healthy People 2010* provides goals for maternal and infant health.
- Research plays a vital role in improving the health of women and infants.
- Ethical concerns have multiplied with increasing use of technology and scientific advances.

Answer Guidelines to Critical Thinking Exercise

Health Literacy

1 No. The nurse should assess Yu Mei's understanding of the instructions—for example, by asking Yu Mei to tell the nurse how she will practice perineal hygiene and take her medications.

2 a. Patients must be able to read and understand written information if the nurse is relying on that mode of patient education.
   b. Looking at the written instructions does not indicate that Yu Mei can read or understand English or can comprehend the information that is in the material.
   c. Patients of different cultures may process information differently.
   d. Patients' nonverbal language may vary based on their culture.
   e. Patients are more likely to understand information if it is given clearly and slowly, while using simple and common words.
   f. Interpreters (unless professional) may not translate completely and accurately.

3 Yu Mei must receive information about perineal hygiene and taking her prescribed medications. She must have information about contraindications and side effects of the medication. She needs to know when to call her health care provider.

4 Yes. Standards of practice guide patient education and administration of medication.

5 Nodding may mean that Yu Mei is listening, not that she understands the nurse's instructions. Respect for authority dictates that she not question the nurse. Sensitivity to diversity and culture is necessary in a setting where patients are from a variety of cultures and speak other languages. Interpreters who are not family members should be available; patients have the right to an interpreter. Nurses in this type of setting should increase their language capabilities and work with other staff members to prepare patient education materials in a variety of languages to meet the needs of the patients they see.

Resources

Alternative Health News Online
www.altmedicine.com

Alternative Medicine Foundation
www.amfoundation.org

Alternative Medicine: Health Care Information Resources
http://hsl.mcmaster.ca/tomflem/altmed.html

American College of Nurse Midwives
www.acnm.org

American Massage Therapy Association
www.amtamassage.org

Ask NOAH: Complementary and Alternative Medicine
www.noah-health.org

Association of Nurse Advocates for Childbirth Solutions
www.anacs.org

Benchnet, the Benchmarking Exchange
Benchmarking and Best practices Network
www.benchnet.com

Birthing from Within
www.birthpower.com

CAM on PubMed
www.nlm.nih.gov/nccam/camonpubmed.html

Childbirth.org
www.childbirth.org

Clinical Benchmarking
P.O. Box 65
Glen Ellyn, IL 60138
800-808-3076
630-690-7596 (fax)
http://clinmarking.com

Doulas of North America
P. O. Box 626
Jasper, IN 47547
888-788-DONA (3662)
812-634-1494 (fax)
www.dona.org

Emerging Infectious Diseases
Centers for Disease Control and Prevention
www.cdc.gov/ncidod/eid/index.htm

Global Health Council
www.globalhealth.org

HerbMed
www.herbmed.org

Homebirth Information
www.changesurfer.com/Hlth/homebirth.html

International Council of Nurses
3, Place jean Marteau
1201-Geneva
Switzerland
41-22-908-01-00
41-22-908-01-01 (fax)
www.icn.ch

Internet Health Library
www.internethealthlibrary.com

MEDLINEplus: Alternative Medicine
www.nlm.nih.gov/medlineplus

Midwives Alliance of North America
P.O. Box 6310
Charlottesville, VA 22906
www.mana.org

National Association of Childbearing Centers
www.birthcenters.org

National Center for Complementary and Alternative Medicine
National Institutes of Health
P.O. Box 7923
Gaithersburg, MD 20898-7923
888-644-6226
866-464-3616 (fax)
http://nccam.nih.gov/

National Institutes of Health
Office of Dietary Supplements
http://dietary-supplements.info.nih.gov/

Ounce of Prevention Fund
122 S. Michigan Ave., Suite 2050
Chicago, IL 60603-6107
312-922-3863
http://www.ounceofprevention.org

Patient Safety Network (PSNET)
http://psnet.ahrq.gov

Promising Practices Network
(Highlights programs and practices that research indicates are
    effective in improving outcomes for children, youth, and
    families)
www.promisingpractices.net

Touch Research Institutes (University of Miami, School of
    Medicine)
www.miami.edu/touch-research/

UNICEF
www.unicef.org

Waterbirth International
http://waterbirth.org/spa/index.php

WholeHealthMD
46040 Center Oak Plaza, Suite 130
Sterling, VA 20166
www.wholehealthmd.com

World Health Organization
Avenue Appia 20
1211 Geneva 27
Switzerland
www.who.org

References

Ahmed, B., & Abushama, M. (2005). Female genital mutilation and childbirth. *Saudi Medical Journal, 26*(3), 376-378.

American Academy of Pediatrics Committee on Fetus and Newborn (2004). Policy Statement. Hospital stay for healthy term newborns. *Pediatrics, 113*(5), 1434-1436.

Arias, E., MacDorman, M., Strobino, D., & Guyer, B. (2003). Annual summary of vital statistics–2002. *Pediatrics, 112*(6 Pt 1), 1215-1230.

Association of Women's Health, Obstetric and Neonatal Nurses (AWHONN). (1998). *Standards and guidelines for professional nursing practice in the care of women and newborns* (5th ed.). Washington, DC: AWHONN.

Association of Women's Health, Obstetric, and Neonatal Nurses (AWHONN). (2002). *Standards for professional perinatal nursing practice and certification in Canada.* Washington, DC: AWHONN.

Barrett, B. (2003). Alternative, complementary, and conventional medicine: Is integration upon us? *Journal of Alternative and Complementary Medicine, 9*(3), 417-427.

Brown, S., Small, R., Faber, B., Krastev, A., & Davis, P. (2002). Early postnatal discharge from hospital for healthy mothers and term infants (Cochrane Review). In *The Cochrane Library,* Issue 2, 2005. Chichester, UK: John Wiley & Sons.

Chang, J., Elam-Evans, L., Berg, C., Herndon, J., Flowers, L., Seed, K., Syverson, C. (2003). Pregnancy-related mortality surveillance–United States, 1991-1999. *Morbidity and Mortality Weekly Report Surveillance Summaries, 52*(SS02), 1-8.

Clinical Benchmarking. (2005). *Clinical benchmarking.* Internet document available at http://clinmarking.com (accessed April 9, 2005).

Cohan, D. (2003). Perinatal HIV: Special considerations. *Topics in HIV Medicine, 11*(6), 200-213.

"Do not use" list required in 2004. *LTC Update,* Issue 3. Internet document available at www.jcaho.org/accredited+organizations/long+term+care/ltc+update/2003 issue3/npsg_04.htm (accessed April 4, 2004).

Doak, C., Doak, L., & Root, J. (1996). *Teaching patients with low literacy skills* (2nd ed.). Philadelphia: Lippincott Williams & Wilkins.

Dochterman, J., & Bulachek, G. (2004). *Nursing interventions classification (NIC)* (4th ed.). St. Louis: Mosby.

Eisenberg, D., Davis, R., Ettner, S., Appel, S., Wilkey, S., Van Rompay, M., Kessler, R. (1998). Trends in alternative medicine use in the United States, 1990-1997: Results of a follow-up national survey. *Journal of the American Medical Association, 280*(18), 1569-1575.

European Collaborative Study. (2005). Mother-to-child transmission of HIV infection in the era of highly active antiretroviral therapy. *Clinical Infectious Diseases, 40*(3), 458-465.

Freda, M. (1995). Arrest, trial, and failure. *Journal of Obstetric, Gynecologic, and Neonatal Nursing, 24*(5), 393-394.

Freda, M. (1999). MCN editorial: The power of words. *MCN American Journal of Maternal Child Nursing, 24*(1), 63.

Gray, J., Safran, C., Davis, R., Pompilio-Weitzner, G., Stewart, J., Zaccagnini, L., Pursley, D. (2000). Baby CareLink: Using the Internet and telemedicine to improve care for high-risk infants. *Pediatrics, 106*(6), 1318-1324.

Hawks, J., & Moyad, M. (2003). CAM: Definition and classification overview. *Urology Nursing, 23*(3), 221-223.

Jackson, D., Lang, J., Swartz, W., Ganiats, T., Fullerton, J., Ecker, J., Nguyen, U. (2003). Outcomes, safety and resource utilization in a collaborative care birth center program compared with traditional physician-based perinatal care. *American Journal of Public Health, 93*(6), 999-1006.

Joint Commission on Accreditation of Healthcare Organizations (JCAHO). (2002). *Sentinel event policy and procedures. Revised: July 2002.* Internet document available at www.jcaho.org (accessed April 9, 2005).

Katz, J., & Hirsch, A. (2003). When global health is local health. *American Journal of Nursing, 103*(1), 75-79.

Kochanek, K., Murphy, S., Anderson, R., & Scott, C. (2004). Deaths: Final data for 2002, *National Vital Statistics Reports, 53*(5), 1-115.

Lewis, J., & Sommers, C. (2003). Personal data assistants: Using new technology to enhance nursing practice. *MCN American Journal of Maternal Child Nursing, 28*(2), 66-73.

Martin, J. et al. (2003). Births: Final data for 2002. *National Vital Statistics Reports, 52*(10), 1-114.

Martin, J., Kochanek, K., Strobino, D., Guyer, B., & MacDorman, M. (2005). Annual summary of vital statistics–2003. *Pediatrics, 115*(3), 619-634.

Marwick, C. (2002). A total of 58 million Americans lack health insurance. *British Medical Journal, 325*(7366), 678.

Millennium Development Goals. (September, 2004). Internet document available at www.developmentgoals.org (accessed April 9, 2005).

Momoh, C. (2004). Female genital mutilation. *Current Opinion in Obstetrics and Gynecology, 16*(6), 477-480.

Moorhead, S., Johnson, M., & Maas, M. (2004). *Nursing outcomes classification (NOC)* (3rd ed.). St. Louis: Mosby.

National Center for Complementary and Alternative Medicine (NCCAM). (2002). Internet document available at http://nccam.nih.gov (accessed November 25, 2004).

Nielsen-Bohlman, L., Panzer, A., & Kindig, D. (Eds.). (2004). *Health literacy: A prescription to end confusion* (pp. 31-58). Washington, DC: Institute of Medicine.

Perry, S., & Mander, R. (2005). A global frame of reference: Learning from everyone, everywhere. *Nursing Education Perspectives, 26*(3), 148-151.

Ratzan, S., & Parker, R. (2000). Introduction. In C. Selden et al. (Eds.), *National Library of Medicine current bibliographies in medicine: Health literacy* (Vol. NLM), Pub. No. CBM 2000-1. Bethesda, MD: National Institutes of Health, U.S. Department of Health and Human Services.

Reinhardt, U., Hussey, P., & Anderson, G. (2004). U.S. health care spending in an international context. *Health Affairs, 23*(3), 10-25.

Roberts, K. (2004). Simplify, simplify: Tackling health literacy by addressing reading literacy. *American Journal of Nursing, 104*(3), 118-119.

Rogers, A., Hwang, W., Scott, L., Aiken, L., & Dinges, D. (2004). The working hours of hospital staff nurses and patient safety. *Health Affairs (Millwood), 23*(4), 202-232.

Simpson, K. (2005). Failure to rescue in obstetrics. *MCN American Journal of Maternal Child Nursing, 30*(1), 76.

U.S. Census Bureau. (2004). *U.S. interim projections by age, sex, race, and Hispanic origin.* Internet document available at www.census.gov/ipc/www/usinterimproj/(accessed April 13, 2004).

United States Department of Health and Human Services (USDHHS). (2000). *Healthy People 2010* (Conference ed.) (Vols. 1 and 2). Washington, DC: U.S. Government Printing Office.

Verhoef, M., & Findlay, B. (2003). Maturation of complementary and alternative healthcare in Canada. *Healthcare Papers, 3*(5), 56-61.

World Health Organization. (May 2, 2002). *Traditional medicine: Growing needs and potential: WHO Policy Perspectives on Medicine.* Geneva: WHO. Internet document available at www.who.int/medicines/organization/trm/orgtrmmain.shtml (accessed November 25, 2004).

CHAPTER 2

The Family and Culture

SHANNON E. PERRY

LEARNING OBJECTIVES

- *Describe the main characteristics of contemporary family forms.*
- *Identify key factors influencing family health.*
- *Explain family functions that contribute to the well-being of family members and society.*
- *Explain family dynamics and how family dynamics contribute to accomplishing family functions.*

- *Compare theoretic approaches for working with childbearing families.*
- *Relate the impact of culture on childbearing families.*
- *Discuss cultural competence in relation to one's own nursing practice.*

KEY TERMS AND DEFINITIONS

acculturation Changes that occur within one group or among several groups when people from different cultures come in contact with one another

assimilation Process that occurs when a cultural group loses its identity and becomes part of the dominant culture

binuclear family Family after divorce, in which the child is a member of both the maternal and paternal nuclear households

cultural competence Awareness, acceptance, and knowledge of cultural differences and adaptation of services to acknowledge and support the culture of the patient

cultural context Setting in which one considers the individual's and the family's beliefs and practices (culture)

cultural knowledge Includes beliefs and values about each facet of life and is passed from one generation to the next

cultural relativism Refers to learning about and applying the standards of another person's culture to activities within that culture

ethnocentrism Belief in the rightness of one's culture's way of doing things

extended family Family that includes nuclear family and other people related by blood

family dynamics Interaction and communication among family members

family functions Affective, socialization, reproductive, economic, and health care functions that contribute to the well-being of the family

genogram Pictorial representation of family relationships and health history

homosexual (lesbian or gay) family Consists of same-sex adults and children from previous heterosexual unions, conceived through therapeutic insemination, or adopted

nuclear family Family that consists of parents and their dependent children

reconstituted family Also called blended, combined, or remarried family; includes stepparents and stepchildren

single-parent family Family in which child lives with one parent because of divorce, separation, or desertion, birth to a single parent; or adoption

subculture Group existing within a larger cultural system that retains its own characteristics

ELECTRONIC RESOURCES

Additional information related to the content in Chapter 2 can be found on

the companion website at *evolve*
http://evolve.elsevier.com/Lowdermilk/Maternity/
- NCLEX Review Questions
- WebLinks

or on the interactive companion CD
- NCLEX Review Questions
- Critical Thinking Exercise—Cultural Health and the Family
- Plan of Care—Incorporating the Infant into the Family
- Plan of Care—The Family Newly Immigrated from a Non—English-Speaking Country

THE FAMILY IN CULTURAL AND COMMUNITY CONTEXT

The family is one of society's most important institutions. It represents a primary social group that influences and is influenced by other people and institutions. The family assumes major responsibility for the introduction and socialization of children. It transmits its fundamental cultural background to its members. The family and its cultural context play an important role in defining the work of maternity nurses. Family structure and function, care-seeking behavior, and relationships with providers are all influenced by culturally related health beliefs and values. Ultimately all of these factors have the power to affect maternal and child health outcomes. It is therefore important to recognize these influences, discuss current trends in families, and explore nursing implications.

DEFINING FAMILY

The family has traditionally been viewed as the primary unit of socialization, the basic structural unit within a community. Family preserves and transmits culture. Family plays a pivotal role in health care, representing the primary target of health care delivery for maternal and newborn nurses. Most models of health behavior view family as a "system" within the larger social framework of a community. These definitions and understandings affect our approaches to health and health care of individuals within the family unit.

The family assumes major responsibility for the introduction and socialization of children. It transmits its fundamental cultural background to its members. Despite modern stresses and strains, the family, through its structure and function, forms a social network that acts as a potent support system for its members. The current emphasis in working with families is on wellness and empowerment for families to achieve control over their lives (Evidence-Based Practice box). More challenging issues such as poverty, teenage pregnancy, drug addiction, incest, abuse, and violence require increasing attention.

Family Organization and Structure

Census data indicate significant alterations in the definition and social configuration of families over the past several decades. The Urban Institute recognizes four categories of families: the two-parent family, the single-parent family, blended families, and no-parent families (Staveteig & Wigton, 2000). A broader view of the contemporary family is as "a group of two or more persons related by blood, marriage, adoption, or emotional commitment who have a permanent relationship and who work together to meet life goals and needs" (Brooks, 2002).

When members are gained or lost through events (e.g., marriage, divorce, birth, death, abandonment, or incarceration), the family composition is altered and roles must be redefined or redistributed. Children may belong to several different family groups during their lives.

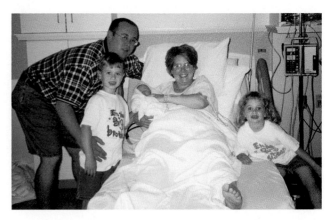

Fig. 2-1 Nuclear family. (Courtesy Jill and Robert McConnell, Bloomington, IL.)

Nuclear family

The nuclear family has long represented the traditional American family in which male and female partners and their children live as an independent unit, sharing roles, responsibilities, and economic resources (Fig. 2-1). In contemporary society, this idealized family structure actually represents only a relatively small number of families. Two-parent families (biologic or adoptive parents) account for approximately 64% of American families, representing 72% of Caucasian, 60% of Latino, and 29% of African-American families (Staveteig & Wigton, 2000). The binuclear family is an alternate form of the traditional nuclear family arrangement that results from divorce. Children of remarried parents then become members of both the maternal and paternal nuclear households. In joint custody the court assigns divorcing parents equal rights to and responsibilities for the minor child or children.

Extended family

Many nuclear families have other relatives living in the same household. These extended family members, called *kin*, are grandparents, aunts or uncles, or other people related by blood (Fig. 2-2). For some groups, such as African-American and Latin-American women, the family kin

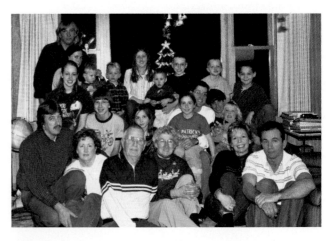

Fig. 2-2 Extended family. (Courtesy Rosemary Toohill, Le Roy, IL.)

BACKGROUND

- Cervical cancer is the third most common cancer worldwide, with 400,000 cases and 200,000 deaths every year. Most, if not all, cervical cancers are caused by human papillomavirus (HPV). Risk factors for cervical cancer include smoking, early sexual activity, multiple lifetime sexual partners, sexually transmitted infection, and impaired immunologic status. Primary prevention of cervical cancer involves avoiding the risk factors. Secondary prevention includes achieving regular cervical screening. The Papanicolaou (Pap) test can increase survival rates, depending on the skill of the clinician collecting the endocervical and ectocervical cells from the transformation zone and the skill of the cytologist evaluating the smear. Typing for HPV can also screen for the aggressive types, of which types 16 and 18 cause 80% of all cervical cancers. Cervical screening is generally recommended every 1 to 3 years for women age 20 to 65 years. Compliance ranges from 84% in England, which has a well-established national screening program, to about 5% in developing countries, where 80% of all cervical cancer cases occur. In most countries, being older, less well educated, of lower socioeconomic status, and from a rural environment is associated with the poorest screening rate. Barriers to screening include feelings of embarrassment and vulnerability; cost; lack of perceived benefit; fear of cancer; and, in the case of HPV typing, connotation of sexual promiscuity.
- Critics of cervical screening point out the false-negative results (averaging 20% to 60% of all Pap tests) and the possible harm they may cause: anxiety, false alarm, unnecessary colposcopy or biopsy, overtesting, and overtreatment. Some lower-grade cervical lesions resolve spontaneously. Treatment can injure cervical structure and function. Women need to be informed of these risks before testing.

OBJECTIVES

- The reviewers' goal was to examine the interventions that promote both compliance with cervical screening recommendations and informed consent. The following types of interventions were sought: invitations, reminders, educational materials, positive or negative message framing, counseling, risk factor assessment, procedures to ease the screening procedure, and economic incentives. Primary outcomes included receiving a cervical screen and obtaining informed consent about the details of the procedure and its risks and benefits. Reviewers hoped for intermediate outcomes of appointments booked, intentions to attend screening, knowledge of screening, and satisfaction with screening, as well as costs.

METHODS
Search Strategy

- Reviewers searched Cochrane, MEDLINE, BIDS, CANCERLIT, DHSS data, Dissertation Abstracts, HealthStat, ASSIA, Pascal, SIGLE, CINAHL, Sociofile, PsycINFO, SHARE, NHS CRD DARE, and National Research Register, as well as bibliographies, specialists, and the *Journal of American Screening*. Keywords included *vaginal smears, Pap tests, Papanicolaou, cytology, pap smear*, with *attitude, accept, encourage, improve, promote, uptake, and utilization*. The

reviewers found 35 controlled studies, representing over 57,000 women from the United States, Australia, the United Kingdom, Canada, Italy, and Belgium. Of these trials, 27 were randomized and eight were quasi-randomized.

Statistical Analysis

- Similar data were pooled. Reviewers calculated relative risks for dichotomous (categoric) data, and weighted mean differences for continuous data. Results outside the 95% confidence interval were accepted as significantly different.

FINDINGS

- Women were significantly more likely to use cervical screening when they received an invitation, especially when the letter was from the woman's general practitioner health care provider and when they were provided with a fixed appointment in the letter. There was a trend toward greater participation when the letter revealed the gender of the clinician who would be taking the smear, and when using a health promotion nurse, but none of these reached the level of statistical significance. Response to telephone calls was equivocal. There was a greater response from women who received educational materials than controls. There was limited evidence of a beneficial effect of having a lay community member involved in promoting the screening.

LIMITATIONS

- None of the studies were in developing countries. Invitations may not work in an area of frequent migration, illiteracy, or transportation from remote areas. Many address lists were outdated, and therefore many subjects were lost to follow-up. None of the trials examined informed consent related to risks and benefits. The assumption throughout the trials was that screening was always beneficial. The reviewers noted methodologic problems with the trial sizes, randomization, blinding of assessors, concealment of treatment allocation, and numbers lost to follow-up, as well as the way the statistical analysis of some of the data was handled.

CONCLUSIONS

- Invitations and educational material appear to be effective at increasing participation in cervical screening in developed countries. Modifications of these methods may increase use of cervical screening in developing countries. Revealing the gender of the clinician and making a fixed appointment seem to be promising.

IMPLICATIONS FOR PRACTICE

- To increase rates of cervical screening, health care providers can institute a program of written invitations with fixed appointments. The letter should include the gender of the health care provider. Educational materials should be distributed widely.

IMPLICATIONS FOR FURTHER RESEARCH

- Trials that account for the methodologic problems of randomization, concealment, blinding the assessor, and follow-up would strengthen the data pool. Research is still needed on informed consent. Much more information is needed about promotional interventions in developing countries, which stand to benefit greatly from cervical screening.

Reference: Forbes, C., Jepson, R., & Martin-Hirsch, P. (2001). Interventions targeted at women to encourage the uptake of cervical screening (Cochrane Review). In *The Cochrane Library*, Issue 2, 2004. Chichester, UK: John Wiley & Sons.

network is an important resource in terms of preventive health behavior. Through its kinship network, the extended family provides role models and support to all its members. In the extended family, childrearing is often a shared responsibility. The extended family is becoming more common as the U.S. population ages. The need to care for elderly parents within the same household often creates a "sandwich generation" in which parents of the nuclear family provide care for their children as well as for elderly grandparents or other relatives.

Single-parent family

Single-parent families are composed of an unmarried biologic or adoptive parent who may or may not be living with other adults. The single-parent family may result from the loss of spouse by death, divorce, separation, or desertion; from either an unplanned or a planned pregnancy; or from the adoption of a child by an unmarried woman or man. This family structure is becoming more prevalent, with current estimates at one fifth of Caucasian families, one third of Hispanic families, and more than half of African-American families in the United States. Although the number of single-parent households has decreased for most groups, the number of single-parent families among African-American households has remained fairly steady at approximately 55% (Staveteig & Wigton, 2000).

Current research takes opposing perspectives on the merits and challenges of single-parent households. In many cases the single-parent family tends to be vulnerable economically and socially, creating an unstable and deprived environment for the growth potential of children. Research demonstrates the impact of single-parenthood not only in economic instability but also in relation to health status, school achievement, and high risk behaviors for affected children. Single mothers are more likely to live in poverty and have poor perinatal outcomes.

In recent years, single parenting has become a common and acceptable choice in society. Individuals for whom the single-parent family is a chosen lifestyle often enjoy a free and open system for the development of parents and children. In these families decision making and communication are seen as joint commitments between parent and child. The parent-child relationship is considered a major source of life fulfillment. The most frequently identified strength in these families is emotional closeness.

Binuclear family

A binuclear family is a family after divorce, in which the child is a member of both maternal and paternal nuclear households. In these families the degree of cooperation between parents varies. In joint custody the court assigns divorcing parents equal rights to and responsibilities for the minor child or children. These alternate family forms are efforts on the part of those concerned to view divorce as a process or reorganization and redefinition of a family rather than as a family dissolution.

Reconstituted family

Reconstituted or blended families, those formed as the result of divorce and remarriage, consist of unrelated family members (stepparents, stepchildren, and stepsiblings) who join together to create a new household. These family groups frequently involve a biologic or adoptive parent whose spouse has not adopted the child.

Homosexual (lesbian and gay) family

Other family configurations that are less well documented include families in which the parents are cohabiting and an increasing number of homosexual (lesbian and gay) families, who may live together with or without children (Federal Interagency Forum on Children and Family Statistics, 2004). Children in homosexual (lesbian and gay) families may be the offspring of previous heterosexual unions, conceived by one member of a lesbian couple through therapeutic insemination, or adopted. These trends reflect the increased opportunities for alternate forms of parenthood within our society, owing both to more liberal social mores and to technologic and medical advances that offer the possibility of parenthood to single men and women. Despite increasing recognition of the biologic and psychologic needs of homosexual families, social acceptance and attitudes of health care providers often present significant barriers to quality health care.

Family Functions

Although family functions have evolved and adapted over time in response to social and economic changes (Friedman, Bowden, & Jones, 2002), the family progresses through its life cycle (Table 2-1) and continues to carry out certain functions for the well-being of family members and the wider society.

Family functions are described as affective, socialization, reproductive, economic, and health care functions (Friedman, Bowden, & Jones, 2002). The affective function is one of the most vital and focuses on meeting family members' needs for affection and understanding. The socialization function refers to the learning experiences provided within the family to teach children their culture and how to function and assume adult social roles and is a lifelong process. The reproductive function ensures family continuity over the generations and the survival of society (Fig. 2-3). Economic functions involve the family's provision and allocation of sufficient resources. Health care functions are met by the provision of such physical necessities as food, clothing, shelter, and health care.

Some functions are emphasized more in one phase of a family's life cycle; others are continuous for the family's survival and progress. Many functions previously performed almost exclusively by one gender (e.g., child care and financial support) are today shared between genders. Although goals for socialization and childrearing practices differ from culture to culture, in most societies the family appears to have three major objectives in relation to children: caregiving, nurturing, and training.

Stages of the Family Life Cycle

STAGE OF FAMILY LIFE CYCLE	EMOTIONAL PROCESS OF TRANSITION: KEY PRINCIPLES	SECOND-ORDER CHANGES IN FAMILY STATUS REQUIRED TO PROCEED DEVELOPMENTALLY
Leaving home: single young adults	Accepting emotional and financial responsibility for self	Differentiation of self in relation to family of origin Development of intimate peer relationships Establishment of self through work and financial independence
Joining of families through marriage: new couple	Commitment to new system	Formation of marital system Realignment of relationships with extended families and friends to include spouse
Families with young children	Accepting new members into system	Adjusting marital system to make space for child(ren) Joining in childrearing, financial, and household tasks Realignment of relationships with extended family to include parenting and grandparenting roles
Families with adolescents	Increasing flexibility of family boundaries to include children's independence and grandparents' frailties	Shifting of parent-child relationships to permit adolescent to move in and out of system Refocus on midlife marital and career issues Beginning shift toward joint caring for older generation
Launching children and moving on	Accepting multitude of exits from and entries into the family system	Renegotiation of marital system as a dyad Development of adult-to-adult relationships between grown children and their parents Realignment of relationships to include in-laws and grandchildren Dealing with disabilities and death of parents (grandparents)
Families in later life	Accepting shifting of generational roles	Maintaining own and/or couple's functioning and interests in face of physiologic decline; exploration of new familial and social role options Support for a more central role of middle generation Making room in the system for wisdom and experience of elderly members; supporting older generation without overfunctioning for them Dealing with loss of spouse, siblings, and other peers and preparation for own death; life review and integration

From Carter, B., & McGoldrick, M. (1999). *The expanded family life cycle: Individual, family, and social perspectives* (3rd ed.). Boston: Allyn & Bacon.

Family Dynamics

Families work cooperatively to accomplish family functions. Through family dynamics (interactions and communication), family members assume appropriate social roles. Social roles in the family are learned in pairs (e.g., mother-father, parent-child, and brother-sister). Role pairing enables social interactions to take place in an orderly, predictable manner; the roles are said to be complementary. Some families maintain a traditional pairing of roles, whereas other families change behavior patterns to suit a change in family lifestyle. Rather than mother-father and brother-sister, the roles may be mother-daughter or mother-son. Negotiation brings these pair roles into a new alignment. Negotiation is essential to maintain family equilibrium.

Ideally, the family uses its resources to provide a safe, intimate environment for the biopsychosocial development of the family members. The family provides for the nurturing of the newborn and the gradual socialization of the growing child. Children form their earliest and closest relationships with their parents or parenting persons; these affiliations continue throughout a lifetime. For better or worse, parent-child relationships influence self-worth and the ability to form later relationships. The family also influences the child's perceptions of the outside world. The family provides the growing child with an identity that possesses both a past and a sense of the future. Cultural values and rituals are passed from one generation to the next through the family (Friedman, Bowden, & Jones, 2002).

Through everyday interactions the family develops and uses its own patterns of verbal and nonverbal communication. These patterns give insight into the emotional exchange within a family and act as reliable indicators of interpersonal

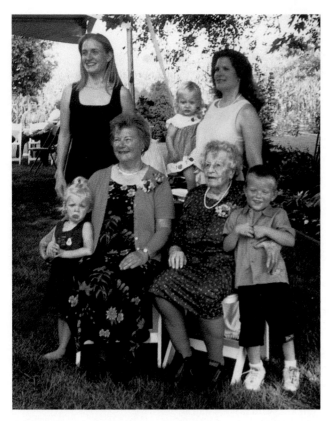

Fig. 2-3 Five generations of a family. (Courtesy Mary Gastelum, Heyworth, IL.)

functioning. Family members not only react to the communication or actions of other family members, but also interpret and define them.

Over time the family develops protocols for problem solving, particularly regarding important decisions such as having a baby, buying a house, or sending children to college. The criteria used in making decisions are based on family values and attitudes about the appropriateness of the behavior and the moral, social, political, and economic events of society. The power to make critical decisions is given to a family member through tradition or negotiation. This power is not always stated. Power reflects the family's concepts of male or female dominance and cultural practices, social customs, and community norms. As a result, family members attain certain statuses or hierarchies. They play out these statuses by assuming various roles. Most families have a member who "takes charge" or "is supportive" or "can't be expected to do anything."

The Family in Society

The social context for the family can be viewed in relation to social and demographic trends that define the population as a whole. Current U.S. census data indicate that the racial and ethnic diversity of the population has grown dramatically in the last three decades. This increased diversity—first manifested among children, and soon to be evident in the older population—is projected to increase in the future.

Each family sets up boundaries between itself and society. People are conscious of the difference between "family members" and "outsiders," or people without kinship status. Some families isolate themselves from the outside community; others have a wide community network to help in times of stress. Although boundaries exist for every family, family members set up channels through which they interact with society. These channels also ensure that the family receives its share of social resources.

THEORETIC APPROACHES TO UNDERSTANDING FAMILIES

A family theory can be used to describe families and how the family unit responds to events both within and outside the family. Each family theory makes certain assumptions about the family and has inherent strengths and limitations. Most nurses use a combination of theories in their work with families. A brief discussion of a theory commonly used with families, systems theory, and the implications of this theory for maternal-child nursing is presented. A brief synopsis of several other theories useful in working with families is included in Table 2-2.

Family Systems Theory

Among the caring disciplines, a systems approach to understanding the family is almost universally applied. Many systems concepts are central to the delivery of holistic nursing care. These include recognition that changes occurring in one member affect the entire family, and an appreciation that nurses who work with families also enter into a systemic relationship with them. This is especially true for nurses who provide perinatal nursing care through community- or home-based agencies. Understanding how family members influence and interact with one another can help the nurse develop empathy with and respect for different ways of functioning.

When applied to families, the systems theory allows nurses to "view the family as a unit and thus focus on observing the interaction among family members rather than studying family members individually" (Wright & Leahey, 2000). Within a systems framework, the individual takes on several roles as a unique and important person in his or her own system and as part of one or more subsystems within the larger family. For example, an individual may belong to one of several subsystems, such as a child subsystem or a parental subsystem. When considering more than one generation of a family, a married woman may belong to a parental subsystem in her own home and to a subsystem of children when considered in relationship to her own parents.

Wright and Leahey (2000) outlined the key characteristics of family systems theory:

- A family system is part of a larger suprasystem and is composed of many subsystems.

TABLE 2-2

Theories and Models Relevant to Family Nursing Practice

THEORY	SYNOPSIS OF THEORY
Family Life Cycle (Developmental) Theory (Carter & McGoldrick, 1999)	Families move through stages. The family life cycle is the context in which to examine the identity and development of the individual. Relationships among family members go through transitions. Although families have roles and functions, a family's main value is in relationships that are irreplaceable. The family involves different structures and cultures organized in various ways. Developmental stresses may disrupt the life cycle process.
Family Stress Theory (Boss, 2002)	Concerned with ways families react to stressful events. Family stress can be studied within the internal and external contexts in which the family is living. The internal context involves elements that a family can change or control, such as family structure, psychologic defenses, and philosophic values and beliefs. The external context consists of the time and place in which a particular family finds itself and over which the family has no control, such as the culture of the larger society, the time in history, the economic state of society, maturity of the individuals involved, success of the family in coping with stressors, and genetic inheritance.
McGill Model of Nursing (Allen, 1997)	Strength-based focus in clinical practice with families rather than a deficit approach. Identification of family strengths and resources; provision of feedback about strengths; assistance given to family to develop and elicit strengths and use resources.
Health Belief Model (Becker, 1974; Janz & Becker, 1984)	The goal of the model is to reduce cultural and environmental barriers that interfere with access to health care. Key elements of the Health Belief Model include the following: perceived susceptibility, perceived severity, perceived benefits, perceived barriers, cues to action, and confidence.
Human Developmental Ecology (Bronfenbrenner, 1979; Bronfenbrenner, 1989)	Behavior is a function of interaction of traits and abilities with the environment. Major concepts include ecosystem, niches (social roles), adaptive range, and ontogenetic development. Individuals are "embedded in a microsystem (role and relations), a mesosystem (interrelations between two or more settings), an exosystem (external settings that do not include the person), and a macrosystem (culture)" (Klein & White, 1996). Change over time is incorporated in the chronosystem.

- The family as a whole is greater than the sum of its individual members.
- A change in one family member affects all family members.
- The family is able to create a balance between change and stability.
- Family members' behaviors are best understood from a view of circular rather than linear causality—that is, an individual's behavior affects and is affected by the behavior of others.

The family systems theory encourages nurses to view individual family members as part of a larger family system influenced by and influencing others. Application of these concepts can guide assessment and interventions for the family. For example, the childbearing family interacts as a system with many elements in the environmental suprasystem, including the health care community. The extent to which this suprasystem influences the family in matters such as prenatal care, childbirth education, and infant care depends on the family's boundary permeability. A relatively closed family may want instructions only from others within the family, whereas a relatively open family may be more receptive to instructions from health care providers.

Using Theories to Guide Practice

People interact effectively with each other in many ways. The nurse must understand that countless factors influence ways in which family members relate among themselves and with the health care community. Some of these factors include the natural history of the family, culture, roles, values, beliefs, and traditional customs. Because so many variables affect ways of relating, the nurse must be aware that most family members will interact and communicate with each other in ways that are very different from those of the nurse's own family of origin. Most families will hold at least some beliefs about health that are very different from those of the nurse. In some instances their beliefs will conflict with principles of health care management predominant in the Western health care system. Therefore, to be effective in working with families, the nurse must possess a degree of personal openness and acceptance and be willing to work with families in a way that is respectful and adapts to their ways of learning and communicating.

Because family relationships are always complex, viewing the interaction of the whole family helps nurses to understand more fully the functioning of individual family members. A family that has recently immigrated to this country may want to receive health information only from others within the family or the immediate cultural community, whereas a family that has more experience in dealing with the American health care system may be more receptive to nurses who are culturally different. When interacting with family members, the nurse becomes part of a system with them. The behaviors and interaction style of the nurse affect not just the individual who is identified as the "patient" but also contribute to family members' responses to each other. Finally, the quality of the nurse-family system strongly influences how the family will interact with the greater health care community in the future.

Knowing about the phases of the life cycle can assist nurses in providing anticipatory guidance for families. For example, helping childbearing families prepare for the birth of a newborn may minimize the development of crises (Plan of Care–Incorporating the Infant into the Family). By using developmental theory, a nurse can anticipate that a family who has a child with a serious anomaly might experience a crisis or state of disequilibrium because the birth of an ill child is not a normative event. Because such a family may revert to a state of dependence, the nurse will realize that their need for extra support and nurturing from the nurse is a natural response to stress.

Because today's families experience a great deal of pressure, they must develop effective stress-management strategies. Maternity nurses working in community settings may care for families in a full range of situations including healthy but highly stressed families and families coping with the extraordinary stress of ill infants or mothers who have recently had major surgical procedures such as cesarean births. Nurses can assist families in changing their stress levels by helping families control internal and external context factors. The

---

PLAN OF CARE   *Incorporating the Infant into the Family*

NURSING DIAGNOSIS Readiness for enhanced family coping related to adaptation of family to new infant

Expected outcome *Family members will verbalize that individual and family goals are met during a smooth transition of new family member into the home.*

Nursing Interventions/*Rationales*

- Assess type and amount of support available to family on a daily basis during the postpartum period *to facilitate adaptation of the family to situation of a new member.*
- Encourage family to use past successful coping mechanisms *to enhance ability to cope with new situation and promote self-esteem.*
- Encourage mother to use family and other support or services to carry out daily household tasks *to permit her to focus on herself and infant.*
- Suggest that woman take time to rest when infant sleeps *to conserve energy for healing and limit responsibility to herself and infant.*
- Assess family structure and relationships, including culture, *to evaluate if longer period of adjustment may be expected.*
- Teach family about sensory needs and capabilities of infant *to motivate family to meet infant's needs and set realistic expectations for infant's capabilities.*
- Refer to parent support group or community agencies, as needed, *to facilitate and validate ongoing positive adjustment of family to new family member.*

NURSING DIAGNOSIS Ineffective role performance related to developmental challenge of addition of new family member

Expected outcome *Each family member will verbalize realistic expectations regarding his or her role in the family and formulate a plan to incorporate role into overall family goals.*

Nursing Interventions/*Rationales*

- Assess family structure, roles, and each member's perception of his or her role in the family *to evaluate the impact of the new member on the structure and roles of the family as perceived by the members.*
- Evaluate individual's perception of goals and new roles during this transition *to promote early intervention and correct any misinterpretation.*
- Encourage discussion of family members' thoughts and feelings regarding this transition *to promote open communication and trust.*
- Provide positive reinforcement for family members' actions that promote a positive environment for the infant *to increase self-esteem and provide encouragement.*
- Refer to community support groups *to provide group reinforcement and further assistance.*
- Give information about sibling and grandparent classes and support groups as available *to promote empowerment and self-esteem for significant others in the family.*

CD: Plan of Care—Incorporating the Infant into the Family

nurse can intervene through educational strategies to correct misconceptions and reduce stress. Explaining normal infant growth and development (maturation) may reduce the stress of parenting.

In planning the care of a family or an individual family member, the nurse may find it useful to view the family at a developmental phase in the life cycle, facing stressful life events, and operating as a system. A family assessment tool such as the one outlined by Friedman (1998) (Fig. 2-4) can be used as a guide for assessing aspects of the family discussed in this chapter. A family genogram (family tree format depicting relationships of family members over at least three generations) (Fig. 2-5) provides valuable information about a family and can be placed in the nursing care plan for easy access by care providers.

By using the Health Belief Model as a guide to assessment, nurses can better address concerns specific to an individual from a different cultural group, motivating the individual to take action on his or her own behalf. Understanding a woman's concerns from her own point of view can help the nurse to provide interventions that will place women at ease in the health care setting. For example, the nurse can modify or adjust care in assessing uterine involution as part of postpartum care for a woman who holds traditional Mexican beliefs and fears of having cold enter her uterus during a normal examination. The culturally competent nurse can close the door to the room, pull curtains to minimize air flow around the woman, position the woman so that the perineum is facing away from the door or air vents, and keep the perineum draped so that the examination takes place with a minimum of exposure.

Within the larger society, individuals and families have a variety of stressors that affect their ability to function and to engage consistently in behaviors that will promote health and wellness. These individuals and families fall into high risk or vulnerable populations. Their stresses relate to many aspects of life: ethnic and cultural minority status, immigration status, poverty, challenges with English language fluency and literacy, malnutrition, and limited access to housing.

Some families have multiple stressors, placing them at especially high risk for poor health outcomes. It should be noted, however, that not only low-income or minority groups are at high risk for morbidity and mortality. Some stressors affect families in all strata of society. Those who are well educated and in a higher socioeconomic class can also have life stressors that make them highly vulnerable to health problems. These antecedents to vulnerability include mental illness; substance use; domestic violence; and reduced access to medical care because of unemployment, loss of medical insurance, or inadequate insurance coverage. Nurses cannot make the assumption that a family is immune to vulnerability because its members live in an exclusive neighborhood, are well educated, and are fully employed. The concepts of high risk and vulnerability potentially apply to everyone.

CULTURAL FACTORS RELATED TO FAMILY HEALTH ■

Cultural Context of the Family

Culture has many definitions. Thomas (2001) defined culture as "a unified set of values, ideas, beliefs, and standards of behavior shared by a group of people; it is the way a person accepts, orders, interprets, and understands experiences throughout the life course." Culture includes values, beliefs and practices that are acquired over a lifetime through interactions with others from that culture. Culture gives meaning to what people do in their everyday lives. The political, social, and economic context of people's lives also is part of the cultural experience and helps shape a person's interpretation of every life experience.

Culture is influenced by religion, environment, and historic events, and plays a powerful role in the individual's behavior and patterns of human interaction. Culture is not static; it is an ongoing process that influences people throughout their entire life, from birth to death. Culture is an essential element of what defines us as people.

Cultural knowledge includes beliefs and values about each facet of life and is passed from one generation to the next. Cultural beliefs and traditions relate to food, language, religion, art, health and healing practices, kinship relationships, and all other aspects of community, family, and individual life. Culture also has been shown to have a direct effect on health behaviors. Values, attitudes, and beliefs that are culturally acquired may influence perceptions of illness, as well as health care–seeking behavior and response to treatment (National Academy Press, 2002). The impact of these influences must be assessed by health professionals in providing health care and developing effective intervention strategies (Cultural Considerations).

Many subcultures may be found within each culture. Subculture refers to a group existing within a larger cultural system that retains its own characteristics. A subculture may be an ethnic group or a group organized in other ways. In the United States, there are many ethnic subcultures (e.g., African-Americans, Asian-Americans, Hispanics), as well as subcultures within these groups. In addition, the Caucasian population in America has diverse and multiple subcultures (e.g., Italian, Russian, German). Because every identified cultural group has subcultures, and because it is impossible to study every subculture in depth, greater differences may exist among and between groups than is generally acknowledged.

Each subculture holds rich and complex traditions, including health practices that have proved effective over time. These traditions vary from group to group. In a multicultural society, many groups can influence traditions and practices. As cultural groups come in contact with one another, acculturation and assimilation may occur.

Acculturation refers to changes that occur within one group or among several groups when people from different

The Friedman Family Assessment Model (Short Form)

Identifying Data

1. Family name
2. Address and phone
3. Family composition
4. Type of family form
5. Cultural (ethnic) background
6. Religious identification
7. Social class status
8. Family's recreational or leisure-time activities

Developmental Stage and History of Family

9. Family's present developmental stage
10. Extent of family developmental tasks fulfillment
11. Nuclear family history
12. History of family of origin of both parents

Environmental Data

13. Characteristics of home
14. Characteristics of neighborhood and larger community
15. Family's geographic mobility
16. Family's associations and transactions with community
17. Family's social support system or network

Family Structure

18. Communication patterns
    Extent of functional and dysfunctional communication
    (types of recurring patterns)
    Extent of emotional (affective) messages and how expressed
    Characteristics of communication within family subsystems
    Extent of congruent and incongruent messages
    Types of dysfunctional communication processes seen in family
    Areas of open and closed communication
    Familial and contextual variables affecting communication
19. Power structure
    Power outcomes
    Decision-making process
    Power bases
    Variables affecting family power
    Overall family system and subsystem power
    (Family power continuum placement)
20. Role structure
    Formal role structure
    Informal role structure
    Analysis of role models (optional)
    Variables affecting role structure
21. Family values
    Compare the family to American or family's reference group values and/or identify important family values and their importance (priority) in family.
    Congruence between the family's values and the family's reference group or wider community

Congruence between the family's values and family member's values
Variables influencing family values
Values consciously or unconsciously held
Presence of value conflicts in family
Effect of the above values and value conflicts on health status of family

Family Functions

22. Affective function
    Family's need–response patterns
    Mutual nurturance, closeness, and identification
    Separateness and connectedness
23. Socialization function
    Family child-rearing practices
    Adaptability of child-rearing practices for family form and family's situation
    Who is (are) socializing agent(s) for child(ren)?
    Value of children in family
    Cultural beliefs that influence family's child-rearing patterns
    Social class influence on child-rearing patterns
    Estimation about whether family is at risk for child-rearing problems and if so, indication of high risk factors
    Adequacy of home environment for children's need to play
24. Health care function
    Family's health beliefs, values, and behavior
    Family's definitions of health–illness and their level of knowledge
    Family's perceived health status and illness susceptibility
    Family's dietary practices
    Adequacy of family diet (recommended 3-day food history record)
    Function of mealtimes and attitudes toward food and mealtimes
    Shopping (and its planning) practices
    Person(s) responsible for planning, shopping, and preparation of meals
    Sleep and rest habits
    Physical activity and recreation practices (not covered earlier)
    Family's drug habits
    Family's role in self-care practices
    Medically based preventive measures (physicals, eye and hearing tests, and immunizations)
    Dental health practices
    Family health history (both general and specific diseases— environmentally and genetically related)
    Health care services received
    Feelings and perceptions regarding health services
    Emergency health services
    Source of payments for health and other services
    Logistics of receiving care

Family Stress and Coping

25. Short- and long-term familial stressors and strengths
26. Extent of family's ability to respond, based on objective appraisal of stress-producing situations
27. Coping strategies utilized (present/past)
    Differences in family members' ways of coping
    Family's inner coping strategies
    Family's external coping strategies
28. Dysfunctional adaptive strategies utilized (present/past; extent of usage)

Family Composition Form

Name (last, first)	Gender	Relationship	Date/place of birth	Occupation	Education
1. (Father)					
2. (Mother)					
3. (Oldest child)					
4.					
5.					
6.					
7.					
8.					

Fig. 2-4 The Friedman Family Assessment Model (Short Form). (From Friedman, M. [1998]. *Family nursing theory and assessment* [4th ed.]. New York: Appleton & Lange.)

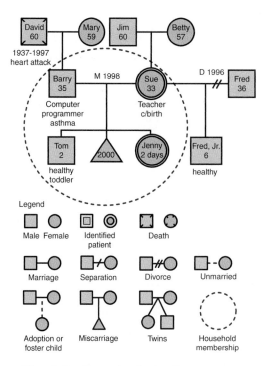

Legend

☐ Male ○ Female | ☐ ◉ Identified patient | ◪ ◔ Death

Marriage | Separation | Divorce | Unmarried

Adoption or foster child | Miscarriage | Twins | Household membership

Fig. 2-5 Example of a family genogram.

cultures come in contact with one another. People may retain some of their own culture while adopting some of the cultural practices of the dominant society. This familiarization among cultural groups results in some overt behavioral similarity, especially in mannerisms, styles, and practices. Dress, language patterns, food choices, and health practices

Cultural Considerations

Questions to Elicit Cultural Expectations about Childbearing

1 What do you and your family think you should do to remain healthy during pregnancy?
¿Qué piensan usted y su familia que usted debe hacer para mantenerse sana durante el embarazo?

2 What are the things you can do or cannot do to improve your health and the health of your baby?
¿Cuáles son las cosas que usted puede hacer o dejar de hacer para mejorar su salud y la salud de su bebé?

3 Who do you want with you during your labor?
¿Quién le acompañará durante el trabajo de parto?

4 What actions are important for you and your family to do after the baby's birth?
¿Qué deben hacer usted y su familia después del nacimiento del bebé?

5 What do you and your family expect from the nurse(s) caring for you?
¿Qué tipo de cuidados esperan usted y su familia de los enfermeros que le atienden?

6 How will family members participate in your pregnancy, childbirth, and parenting?
¿Cómo participarán los miembros de su familia en el embarazo, el nacimiento, y el cuidado del niño?

especially show differences among cultural groups. In the United States, acculturation is generally thought to take three generations. An adult grandchild of an immigrant is usually fully Americanized. An example of acculturation is the adoption of ethnic food practices in the United States.

During times of family transitions such as childbearing, or during crisis or illness, a woman may rely on old cultural patterns even after she has become acculturated in many ways. This is consistent with family developmental theory that states that during times of stress, people revert to practices and behaviors that are most comfortable and familiar.

Assimilation, on the other hand, occurs when a cultural group loses its identity and becomes part of the dominant culture. According to Friedman, Bowden, and Jones (2002), "assimilation denotes the more complete and one-way process of one culture being absorbed into the other." Assimilation is the process by which groups "melt" into the mainstream, thus accounting for the notion of a "melting pot," a phenomenon that has been said to occur in the United States. This is illustrated by individuals who identify themselves as being of "Irish" or "German" descent, without having any remaining cultural practices or values linked specifically to that culture, such as food preparation techniques, style of dress, or proficiency in the language associated with their reported cultural heritage. Spector (2004) asserts that in the United States the melting pot, with its dream of a common culture, is a myth. Instead, a mosaic phenomenon exists in which we must both accept and appreciate the differences among people.

The family process within its cultural context is a central concern in nursing, especially when the nurse is providing care to the childbearing family. A critical life experience, such as childbearing, is often bound by traditional beliefs and practices. A culture's beliefs and practices regarding childbearing are embedded in its economic, religious, kinship, and political structures. All cultures have behavioral norms and expectations for each stage of the perinatal cycle. These norms and expectations relate to each culture's view of how people stay healthy and prevent illness. Patients have the right to expect that their physiologic and psychologic health care needs will be met and that their cultural beliefs will be respected. Cultural sensitivity, compassion, and a critical awareness of family dynamics and social stressors that will affect health-related decision making are critical components in developing an effective plan of care (Plan of Care—The Family Newly Immigrated from a Non-English-Speaking Country).

Understanding the concepts of ethnocentrism and cultural relativism may be helpful to nurses caring for families in a multicultural society.

Ethnocentrism is a belief in the rightness of one's culture's way of doing things. Essentially, ethnocentrism supports the notion that "my group is the best." Although the United States is a culturally diverse nation, the prevailing practice of health care is based on beliefs and practices held by members of the dominant culture, primarily Caucasians

PLAN OF CARE *The Family Newly Immigrated from a Non–English-Speaking Country*

NURSING DIAGNOSIS Impaired verbal communication related to inability to speak or understand English

Expected Outcome *Family and health care providers will communicate using bilingual health care providers or interpreters.*

Nursing Interventions/*Rationales*

- Determine language of patient *to provide a basis for facilitating communication.*
- Enlist assistance of bilingual health care provider or interpreter *to complete assessment and health teaching.*
- Prepare health education materials in languages of patients commonly seen in the agency *to facilitate patient education.*
- Use gestures and other nonverbal techniques such as pictures and diagrams *to enhance understanding.*
- Listen actively *to indicate concern for family and reduce anxiety.*

NURSING DIAGNOSIS Risk for loneliness related to separation from family and country of origin

Expected Outcome *Family members will form new relationships within the community and reduce their loneliness.*

Nursing Interventions/*Rationales*

- Provide emotional support *to assist family in developing coping skills.*
- Introduce family to a support group of people from a similar culture *to enhance developing relationships and provide comfort.*
- Promote family involvement in new parent groups or neighborhood activities *to enhance participation in activities that enhance parenting skills, support the development of relationships, and help reduce loneliness.*
- Refer to clergy of choice for spiritual support *to enhance coping skills.*

of European descent. This practice is based on the biomedical model that focuses on curing disease states. From this biomedical perspective, pregnancy and childbirth are viewed as processes with inherent risks that are most appropriately managed by using scientific knowledge and advanced technology. This medical perspective stands in direct contrast with the belief systems of many cultures. For many women, birth is a completely normal process that can be managed with a minimum of involvement from health practitioners. When encountering behavior in women unfamiliar with the biomedical model, the nurse may become frustrated and impatient. The nurse may label the woman's behavior inappropriate and believe that it conflicts with "good" health practices. If the Western health care system provides the nurse's only standard for judgment, the behavior of the nurse is called *ethnocentric.*

Cultural relativism is the opposite of ethnocentrism. It refers to learning about and applying the standards of another person's culture to activities within that culture. To be culturally relativistic, the nurse recognizes that people from different cultural backgrounds comprehend the same objects and situations differently. In other words, culture determines a person's viewpoint.

Cultural relativism does not require nurses to accept the beliefs and values of another culture. Instead, nurses recognize that the behavior of others may be based on a system of logic different from their own. Cultural relativism affirms the uniqueness and value of every culture.

Childbearing Beliefs and Practices

Nurses working with childbearing families care for families from many different cultures and ethnic groups. To provide culturally competent care, the nurse must assess the beliefs

and practices of patients. A nurse should consider all aspects of culture, including communication, space, time orientation, and family roles, when working with childbearing families.

Communication

Communication often creates the most challenging obstacle for nurses working with patients from diverse cultural groups. This is because communication is not merely the exchange of words. Instead it involves (1) understanding the individual's language, including subtle variations in meaning and distinctive dialects; (2) appreciation of individual differences in interpersonal style; and (3) accurate interpretation of the volume of speech, as well as the meanings of touch and gestures. For example, members of some cultural groups tend to speak more loudly, with great emotion, and with vigorous and animated gestures when they are excited; this is true whether their excitement is related to positive or negative events or emotions. It is important, therefore, for the nurse to avoid rushing to judgment regarding a patient's intent when the patient is speaking, especially in a language not understood by the nurse. In such situations it is critical that the nurse avoid instantaneous responses that may well be based on an incorrect interpretation of the patient's gestures and meaning. Instead, the nurse should withhold an interpretation of what has been communicated until it is possible to clarify the patient's intent. The nurse needs to enlist the assistance of a person who can help and verify with the patient the true intent and meaning of the communication.

Use of interpreters

Inconsistencies between the language of patients and the language of providers present a significant barrier to effective health care. Because of the diversity of cultures and languages within the U.S. and Canadian populations, health care agencies are increasingly seeking the services of interpreters (of oral communication from one language to another) or translators (of written words from one language to another) to bridge these gaps and fulfill their obligation for culturally and linguistically appropriate health care (Box 2-1).

Finding the best possible interpreter in the circumstance also is critically important. A number of personal attributes and qualifications contribute to an interpreter's potential to be effective. Ideally, interpreters should have the same native language and be of the same religion or have the same country of origin as the patient. Interpreters should have specific health-related language skills and experience and help bridge the language and cultural barriers between the patient and the health care provider. The person interpreting also should be mature enough to be trusted with private information.

However, because the nature of nursing care is not always predictable and because nursing care that is provided in a home or community setting does not always allow expert, experienced, or mature adult interpreters, ideal interpretive services sometimes are impossible to find when they are needed. In crisis or emergency situations, or when family members are having extreme stress or emotional upset, it may be necessary to use relatives, neighbors, or children as interpreters. If this situation occurs, the nurse must ensure that the patient is in agreement and comfortable with using the available interpreter to assist.

When using an interpreter, the nurse respects the family by creating an atmosphere of respect and privacy. Questions should be addressed to the woman and not to the interpreter. Even though an interpreter will of necessity be exposed to sensitive and privileged information about the family, the nurse should take care to ensure that confidentiality

---

BOX 2-1

Working with an Interpreter

STEP 1: BEFORE THE INTERVIEW

A Outline your statements and questions. List the key pieces of information you want or need to know.

B Learn something about the culture so that you can converse informally with the interpreter.

STEP 2: MEETING WITH THE INTERPRETER

A Introduce yourself to the interpreter and converse informally. This is the time to find out how well he or she speaks English. No matter how proficient or what age the interpreter is, be respectful. Some ways to show respect are to ask a cultural question to acknowledge that you can learn from the interpreter, or you could learn one word or phrase from the interpreter.

B Emphasize that you do want the patient to ask questions because some cultures consider this inappropriate behavior.

C Make sure the interpreter is comfortable with the technical terms you need to use. If not, take some time to explain them.

STEP 3: DURING THE INTERVIEW

A Ask your questions and explain your statements (see Step 1).

B Make sure that the interpreter understands which parts of the interview are most important. You usually have limited time with the interpreter, and you want to have adequate time at the end for patient questions.

C Try to get a "feel" for how much is "getting through." No matter what the language is, if in relating information to the patient the interpreter uses far fewer or far more words than you do, "something else" is going on.

D Stop every now and then and ask the interpreter, "How is it going?" You may not get a totally accurate answer, but you will have emphasized to the interpreter your strong

desire to focus on the task at hand. If there are language problems: (1) speak *slowly;* (2) use gestures (e.g., fingers to count or point to body parts); and (3) use pictures.

E Ask the interpreter to elicit questions. This may be difficult, but it is worth the effort.

F Identify cultural issues that may conflict with your requests or instructions.

G Use the interpreter to help problem solve or at least give insight into possibilities for solutions.

STEP 4: AFTER THE INTERVIEW

A Speak to the interpreter and try to get an idea of what went well and what could be improved. This will help you to be more effective with this or another interpreter.

B Make notes on what you learned for your future reference or to help a colleague.

Remember

Your interview is a *collaboration* between you and the interpreter. *Listen* as well as speak.

Notes

1 The interpreter may be a child, grandchild, or sibling of the patient. Be sensitive to the fact that the child is playing an adult role.

2 Be sensitive to cultural and situational differences (e.g., an interview with someone from urban Germany will likely be different from an interview with someone from a transitional refugee camp).

3 Younger females telling older males what to do may be a problem for both a female nurse and a female interpreter. This is not the time to pioneer new gender relations. Be aware that in some cultures it is difficult for a woman to talk about some topics with a husband or a father present.

Courtesy Elizabeth Whalley, PhD, San Francisco State University, San Francisco, CA.

is maintained. A quiet location free from interruptions is the ideal place for interpretive services to take place. In addition, culturally and linguistically appropriate educational materials that are easy to read, with appropriate text and graphics, should be available to assist the woman and her family in understanding health care information. When using interpretive services, the nurse demonstrates respect for the woman and helps her maintain a sense of dignity by taking care to do all of the following:

- Respect the woman's wishes
- Involve her in the decision about who will be the most appropriate person to interpret under the circumstances
- Provide as much privacy as possible
- Use culturally appropriate learning aides

Personal space

Cultural traditions define the appropriate personal space for various social interactions. Although the need for personal space varies from person to person and with the situation, the actual physical dimensions of comfort zones differ from culture to culture. Actions such as touching, placing the woman in proximity to others, taking away personal possessions, and making decisions for the woman can decrease personal security and heighten anxiety. Conversely, if nurses respect the need for distance, they allow the woman to maintain control over personal space and support personal autonomy, thereby increasing her sense of security. For example, many Asian groups have reserved attitudes about physical contact, and touching a woman may at times create anxiety when health care is delivered. To provide care, nurses must touch patients. However, they frequently do so without any awareness of the emotional distress they may be causing their patients.

Time orientation

Time orientation also is a fundamental way in which culture affects health behaviors. People in cultural groups may be relatively more oriented to past, present, or future. Those who focus on the past strive to maintain tradition or the status quo and have little motivation for formulating future goals. In contrast, individuals who focus primarily on the present neither plan for the future nor consider the experiences of the past. These individuals do not necessarily adhere to strict schedules and are often described as "living for the moment" or "marching to the beat of their own drummer." Individuals oriented to the future maintain a focus on achieving long-term goals.

The time orientation of the childbearing family may affect nursing care. For example, talking to a family about bringing the infant to the clinic for follow-up examinations (events in the future) may be difficult for the family that is focused on the present concerns of day-to-day survival. Because a family with a future-oriented sense of time plans far in advance, thinking about the long-term consequences of present actions, they may be more likely to return as scheduled for follow-up visits. Despite the differences in time orientation, each family may be equally concerned for the well-being of its newborn.

Family roles

Family roles involve the expectations and behaviors associated with a member's position in the family (e.g., mother, father, grandparent). Social class and cultural norms also affect these roles, with distinct expectations for men and women clearly determined by social norms. For example, culture may influence whether a man actively participates in pregnancy and childbirth, yet maternity care practitioners working in the Western health care system expect fathers to be involved. This can create a significant conflict between the nurse and the role expectations of very traditional Mexican or Arab families, who usually view the birthing experience as a female affair. The way that health care practitioners manage such a family's care molds its experience and perception of the Western health care system.

In maternity nursing the nurse supports and nurtures the beliefs that promote physical or emotional adaptation to childbearing. However, if certain beliefs might be harmful, the nurse should carefully explore them with the woman and use them in the reeducation and modification process. Strategies for care delivery and providing appropriate care are presented in Box 2-2.

Table 2-3 provides examples of some cultural beliefs and practices surrounding childbearing. The cultural beliefs and customs in this table are categorized based on distinct cultural traditions and are not practiced by all members of the cultural group in every part of the country. Women

---

BOX 2-2

Strategies for Care Delivery and Providing Appropriate Care

STRATEGIES FOR CARE DELIVERY
- Break down the language barriers
- Explain your rationale and reasons for suggestions
- Integrate folk and Western treatments
- Enlist the family caretaker and others
- Get consent from the right person
- Provide language-appropriate materials

PROVIDING APPROPRIATE CARE
- Ask about traditional beliefs, such as the role of hot and cold
- Be sensitive regarding interpreters and language barriers
- Ask about important dietary practices, particularly related to events such as childbirth
- Ask about group practices and beliefs
- Ask about a woman's fears, and those of her family, regarding an unfamiliar care setting

From Mattson, S. (2000). Providing culturally competent care: Strategies and approaches for perinatal clients. *AWHONN Lifelines, 4*(5), 37-39.

from these cultural and ethnic groups may adhere to some, all, or none of the practices listed.

In using Table 2-3 as a guide, the nurse should use caution to avoid making stereotypic assumptions about any person based on sociocultural-spiritual affiliations. Nurses should exercise sensitivity in working with every family, being careful to assess the ways in which they apply their own mixture of cultural traditions.

DEVELOPING CULTURAL COMPETENCE

Cultural competence has many names and definitions, all of which have subtle shades of difference, but which are essentially the same: multiculturalism, cultural sensitivity, and intercultural effectiveness. The culturally competent person thinks, feels, and acts in ways that acknowledge, respect and build upon ethnic, [socio]cultural, and linguistic diversity. Culturally competent professionals act to meet the needs of the patient and are respectful of ways and traditions that may be very different from their own. In today's society it is of critical importance that nurses develop more than technical skill. Nurses at every level of preparation, and throughout their professional lives, must engage in a continual process of developing and refining attitudes and behaviors that will promote culturally competent care.

In addition to issues of preserving and promoting human dignity, the development of cultural competence is of equal importance in terms of health outcomes. Nurses who relate effectively with patients are able to motivate them in the direction of health-promoting behaviors. Cultural competence then becomes an issue of cost-effectiveness as well.

Pathways to the Development of Cultural Competence

Cultural competence proceeds along a continuum. Programs that promote values important to the cultural identity of the community build on the values of mutual support, cohesiveness, and self-sufficiency and therefore result in better health outcomes for community members. The use of community advocates most effectively reaches underserved populations through a network of existing social relationships. This can be especially true in isolated communities such as those that exist in remote or rural areas. Using local health workers builds on preexisting trust relationships. Moreover, local health workers are in a position to reinforce health teaching and best practices in health maintenance even when nurses or other heath professionals are absent.

TABLE 2-3

Traditional* Cultural Beliefs and Practices: Childbearing and Parenting

PREGNANCY	CHILDBIRTH	PARENTING
HISPANIC		
(Based primarily on knowledge of Mexican-Americans; members of the Hispanic community have their origins in Spain, Cuba, Central and South America, Mexico, Puerto Rico, and other Spanish-speaking countries.)		
Pregnancy	*Labor*	*Newborn*
Pregnancy desired soon after marriage	Use of "partera" or lay midwife preferred in some places; may prefer presence of mother rather than husband	Breastfeeding begun after third day; colostrum may be considered "filthy" or "spoiled"
Late prenatal care	After birth of baby, mother's legs brought together to prevent air from entering uterus	Olive oil or castor oil given to stimulate passage of meconium
Expectant mother influenced strongly by mother or mother-in-law	Loud behavior in labor	Male infant not circumcised
Cool air in motion considered dangerous during pregnancy		Female infant's ears pierced
Unsatisfied food cravings thought to cause a birthmark	*Postpartum*	Belly band used to prevent umbilical hernia
Some pica observed in the eating of ashes or dirt (not common)	Diet may be restricted after birth; for first 2 days only boiled milk and toasted tortillas permitted (special foods to restore warmth to body)	Religious medal worn by mother during pregnancy; placed around infant's neck
Milk avoided because it causes large babies and difficult births	Bed rest for 3 days after birth	Infant protected from "evil eye"
Many predictions about sex of baby	Keep warm	Various remedies used to treat "mal ojo" (evil eye) and fallen fontanel (depressed fontanel)
May be unacceptable and frightening to have pelvic examination by male health care provider	Delay bathing	
Use of herbs to treat common complaints of pregnancy	Mother's head and feet protected from cold air; bathing permitted after 14 days	
Drinking chamomile tea thought to ensure effective labor	Mother often cared for by her own mother	
	Forty-day restriction on sexual intercourse	

*Variations in some beliefs and practices exist within subcultures of each group.

Continued

TABLE 2-3

Traditional* Cultural Beliefs and Practices: Childbearing and Parenting—cont'd

PREGNANCY	CHILDBIRTH	PARENTING

AFRICAN-AMERICAN

(Members of the African-American community, many of whom are descendants of slaves, have different origins. Today a number of black Americans have emigrated from Africa, the West Indian Islands, the Dominican Republic, Haiti, and Jamaica.)

Pregnancy	Labor	Newborn
Acceptance of pregnancy depends on economic status	Use of "Granny midwife" in certain parts of United States	Feeding very important: "Good" baby thought to eat well
Pregnancy thought to be state of "wellness," which is often the reason for delay in seeking prenatal care, especially by lower-income African-Americans	Varied emotional responses: some cry out, some display stoic behavior to avoid calling attention to selves	Early introduction of solid foods
"Old wives' tales" include beliefs that having a picture taken during pregnancy will cause stillbirth and reaching up will cause cord to strangle baby	Woman may arrive at hospital in far-advanced labor	May breastfeed or bottle-feed; breastfeeding may be considered embarrassing
Craving for certain foods, including chicken, greens, clay, starch, and dirt	Emotional support often provided by other women, especially the woman's own mother	Parents fearful of spoiling baby
Pregnancy may be viewed by African-American men as a sign of their virility	**Postpartum**	Commonly call baby by nicknames
Self-treatment for various discomforts of pregnancy, including constipation, nausea, vomiting, headache, and heartburn	Vaginal bleeding seen as sign of sickness; tub baths and shampooing of hair prohibited	May use excessive clothing to keep baby warm
	Sassafras tea thought to have healing power	Belly band used to prevent umbilical hernia
	Eating liver thought to cause heavier vaginal bleeding because of its high "blood" content	Abundant use of oil on baby's scalp and skin
		Strong feeling of family, community, and religion

ASIAN-AMERICANS

(Typically refers to groups from China, Korea, the Philippines, Japan, Southeast Asia [particularly Thailand], Indochina, and Vietnam.)

Pregnancy	Labor	Newborn
Pregnancy considered time when mother "has happiness in her body"	Mother attended by other women, especially her own mother	Concept of family important and valued
Pregnancy seen as natural process	Father does not actively participate	Father is head of household; wife plays a subordinate role
Strong preference for female health care provider	Labor in silence	Birth of boy preferred
Belief in theory of hot and cold	Cesarean birth not desired	May delay naming child
May omit soy sauce in diet to prevent dark-skinned baby	**Postpartum**	Some groups (e.g., Vietnamese) believe colostrum is dirty; therefore they may delay breastfeeding until milk comes in
Prefer soup made with ginseng root as general strength tonic	Must protect self from yin (cold forces) for 30 days	
Milk usually excluded from diet because it causes stomach distress	Ambulation limited	
Inactivity or sleeping late may cause difficult delivery	Shower and bathing prohibited	
	Warm room	
	Diet:	
	Warm fluids	
	Some women are vegetarians	
	Korean mother served seaweed soup with rice	
	Chinese diet high in hot foods	
	Chinese mother avoids fruits and vegetables	

TABLE 2-3

Traditional* Cultural Beliefs and Practices: Childbearing and Parenting—cont'd

PREGNANCY	CHILDBIRTH	PARENTING
EUROPEAN-AMERICAN		
(Members of the European-American [Caucasian] community have their origins in countries such as Ireland, Great Britain, Germany, Italy, and France.)		
Pregnancy	*Labor*	*Newborn*
Pregnancy viewed as a condition that requires medical attention to ensure health	Birth is a public concern	Increased popularity of breastfeeding
	Technology dominated	Breastfeeding begins as soon as possible after childbirth
Emphasis on early prenatal care	Birthing process in institutional setting valued	
Variety of childbirth education programs available, and participation encouraged	Involvement of father expected	*Parenting*
	Physician seen as head of team	Motherhood and transition to parenting seen as stressful time
Technology driven		Nuclear family valued, although single parenting and other forms of parenting more acceptable than in the past
Emphasis on nutritional science	*Postpartum*	
Involvement of the father valued	Emphasis or focus on early bonding	
Written source of information valued	Medical interventions for dealing with discomfort	
	Early ambulation and activity emphasized	Women often deal with multiple roles
	Self-care valued	Early return to prenatal activities
NATIVE AMERICAN		
(Many different tribes exist within the Native American culture; viewpoints vary according to tribal customs and beliefs.)		
Pregnancy	*Labor*	*Newborn*
Pregnancy considered as a normal, natural process	Prefers female attendant, although husband, mother, or father may assist with birth	Infant not fed colostrum
		Use of herbs to increase flow of milk
Late prenatal care	Birth may be attended by whole family	Use of cradle boards for infant
Avoid heavy lifting	Herbs may be used to promote uterine activity	Babies not handled often
Herb teas encouraged	Birth may occur in squatting position	
	Postpartum	
	Herb teas to stop bleeding	

Data from Amaro, H. (1994). Women in the Mexican-American community: Religion, culture, and reproductive attitudes and experiences. *Journal of Comparative Psychology, 16*(1), 6-19; Bar-yam, N. (1994). Learning about culture: A guide for birth practitioners. *International Journal of Childbirth Education, 9*(2), 8-10; Galanti, G. (1997). *Caring for patients from different cultures: Case studies from American hospitals.* (2nd ed.). Philadelphia: University of Pennsylvania Press; D'Avanzo, C., & Geissler, E. (2003). *Pocket guide to cultural assessment* (3rd ed.). St. Louis: Mosby; Mattson, S. (1995). Culturally sensitive prenatal care for Southeastern Asians. *Journal of Obstetric, Gynecologic, and Neonatal Nursing, 24*(4), 335-341; Spector, R. (2004). *Cultural diversity in health and illness.* (6th ed.). Upper Saddle River, NJ: Prentice Hall Health; and Williams, R. (1989). Issues in women's health care. In B. Johnson (Ed.), *Psychiatric mental health nursing: Adaptation and growth.* Philadelphia: JB Lippincott.
NOTE: Most of these cultural beliefs and customs reflect the traditional culture and are not universally practiced. These lists are not intended to stereotype patients but rather to serve as guidelines while discussing meaningful cultural beliefs with a patient and her family. Examples of other cultural beliefs and practices are found throughout this text.
*Variations in some beliefs and practices exist within subcultures of each group.

Integrating Cultural Competence with the Nursing Care Plan

In many cultures, family members make most of the decisions for the patient, and therefore the central relationship between the nurse and patient is mediated directly by the family. The nurse must recognize the cultural importance of family in supporting the patient, guiding decision making, and preserving cultural integrity in the health care interaction.

All nursing care is delivered in multiple cultural contexts. These contexts include the cultures of the patient, of the nurse, and of the health care system, as well as the larger culture of the society in which health care is delivered. If any of these cultural groups is excluded from the nurse's assessment and consideration, nursing care may fail to achieve its goals and may be culturally insensitive.

Implications for Nursing

To provide culturally competent care, nurses must develop awareness of various cultures and sensitivity to differences; gain knowledge of values, beliefs, and lifeways of other groups; develop skills in cultural assessment as a basis for intervention; and engage in direct cultural encounters or immersion in cultural experiences. These approaches build

Critical Thinking Exercise

Family Roles and Functions

Marta is a 23-year-old married woman. She is having a protracted labor with fetal distress, and the obstetrician has recommended a cesarean birth. The obstetrician talked with Marta and her husband, Cesar, and coming out of her room, asked the nurse to get the operative permit signed. When the nurse approached Marta for her signature, Cesar said, "Here, I will sign it." Marta explained that "Cesar makes all the decisions in our family." The nurse responded that, "Oh, no. Marta has to sign it. Just sign right here." Was the nurse's response appropriate?

1 Evidence—Is there sufficient evidence to draw conclusions about the appropriateness of the nurse's response?
2 Assumptions—What assumptions can be made about the appropriateness of the response in relation to:
  a. Legal requirements for informed consent
  b. Who is the decision maker in the family
  c. The patient's preferences
  d. Culture of the patient and family
  e. Values of the patient
3 What implications and priorities for nursing care can be drawn at this time?
4 Does the evidence objectively support your conclusion?
5 Are there alternative perspectives to your conclusion?

a basis for effective care strategies, enabling the nurse to promote self-care and effective lifestyle changes (Pender, Murdaugh, & Parsons, 2002). Cross-cultural experiences also present an opportunity for the health care professional to expand cultural sensitivity, awareness, and skills. Increasingly, schools of nursing are providing cross-cultural and international experiences for their students (Perry & Mander, 2005).

All cultures maintain behavioral norms and expectations for each stage of the perinatal cycle. These norms and expectations evolve from a culture's view of how people stay healthy and prevent illness. A culture's economic, religious, kinship, and political structures pervade its beliefs and practices regarding childbearing. To practice with cultural competence, nurses must understand the ways in which people of different cultures perceive life events and the health care system. Patients have a right to expect that their physiologic and psychologic health care needs will be met and that their cultural and spiritual beliefs will be respected.

CARE MANAGEMENT

Assessment and Nursing Diagnoses

When nurses develop plans of care for patients and families who are culturally different from themselves or from the dominant culture of the community, they should be certain to include an assessment that addresses psychosocial issues related to that diversity.

No plan of care is complete without attention to nursing diagnoses that address cultural diversity issues.

- *Impaired verbal communication related to*
  —inability to speak or understand English
- *Risk for loneliness related to*
  —separation from family and country of origin
- *Social isolation related to*
  —separation from family and friends because of immigration status
- *Chronic sorrow related to*
  —refugee status, separation from family, and death of family members

Expected Outcomes of Care

Examples of expected outcomes for perinatal patients include that the woman and/or family will do the following:
- Verbalize understanding of treatments
- Report decreased anxiety about procedures she will perform (e.g., insulin injection)
- Perform procedures accurately (e.g., blood glucose monitoring), as evidenced by return demonstration
- Use support systems to cope effectively with problems (e.g., pregnancy complications, newborn complications or treatments)
- Verbalize decreased role strain

Plan of Care and Interventions

The nursing plan of care is developed in collaboration with the patient, based on the health care needs of the individual.

Evaluation

Evaluation is based on the expected outcomes of care. The plan is revised as necessary.

COMMUNITY ACTIVITY

In a prenatal clinic, interview families from at least two different cultural backgrounds.
- What do they believe will keep them healthy in pregnancy?
- What are the roles of men and women in childbirth? Who should be present at birth?
- What is the role of technology in the childbirth process?
- Are there restrictions on activity and diet in the postpartum period?
- What is the preferred method of infant feeding? How soon after birth should breastfeeding begin?
- Are there special foods that should be eaten during pregnancy or after childbirth?
- What will keep the infant healthy after birth?
- Did the responses to these questions differ significantly between the two families? Did the responses differ from what you have learned as the "correct way" to keep healthy? How can you use this information?

CD: Critical Thinking Exercise—Cultural Health and the Family

Key Points

- Contemporary American society recognizes and accepts a variety of family forms.
- The family is a social network that acts as an important support system for its members.
- Ideally, the family provides a safe, intimate environment for the biopsychosocial development of its children and adult members.
- Family theories provide nurses with useful guidelines for understanding family function.
- Family socioeconomics, response to stress, and culture are key factors influencing family health.

- The reproductive beliefs and practices of a culture are embedded in its economic, religious, kinship, and political structures.
- To provide quality care to women in their childbearing years and beyond, nurses should be aware of the cultural beliefs and practices important to individual families.
- Nurses must develop cultural competence and integrate it into the nursing plan of care.

Answer Guidelines to Critical Thinking Exercise

Family Roles and Functions

1 Yes. The nurse's response is not appropriate. Legally in the United States the patient must sign the consent for her surgery (unless she is unconscious or incapacitated). However, in some cultures and some families, the decision maker may be another person such as the husband or parent. The obstetrician should explain the situation to Marta and Cesar, obtain Cesar's consent, and then have Marta sign the consent form.

2 a. Legal requirements for obtaining informed consent must be met.
  b. The patient may not always be the decision maker.
  c. The wishes of the patient must be ascertained.
  d. To provide culturally competent care, the family's culture, roles, and responsibilities must be respected.
  e. Patients may have values that do not fit with the Western biomedical model of care.

3 To protect the mother and the fetus, the fetus must be delivered. This requires informed consent for the procedure. The priority for the nurse is to ensure that Marta and Cesar have a clear understanding of the need for the procedure and that a written consent is obtained. (A physician is responsible for obtaining informed consent; a nurse can obtain a signature on a consent form.)

4 Yes, the evidence supports this conclusion.

5 The values of patients and their families may differ from those of health care providers. Ultimately, the patient has the right to consent to or refuse treatment even if health care providers believe that the decision is wrong or may result in harm. In some situations, health care providers have sought a court order for a cesarean in the belief that it is their responsibility to save the life of the fetus. This drastic step should be avoided if at all possible.

Resources

Child and Family Policy Center
218 6th Ave., Suite 1021
Des Moines, IA 50309-4013
515-280-9027
515-244-8997 (fax)
www.cfpciowa.org

Federal Interagency Forum on Children and Family Statistics
www.childstats.gov

The Harriet and Robert Heilbrunn Department of Population and
  Family Health
http://cpmcnet.columbia.edu/dept/sph/popfam/

Health Literacy Toolbox
www.nationalhealthcouncil.org/pubs/hlt_spring_2004.pdf

Indian Health Services
www.ihs.gov

Institute for the Support of Latino Families and Communities
www.uiowa.edu/~nrcfcp/latino

Institute for Urban Family Health
16 East 16th St.
New York, NY 10003
212-633-0800
212-691-4610 (fax)
www.institute2000.org/

Kaiser Family Foundation
www.kff.org/

Maternal and Child Health Bureau
http://mchb.hrsa.gov/

Maternal and Neonatal Health Resources
www.jhuccp.org

National Alliance for Hispanic Health
1501 Sixteenth St., NW
Washington, DC 20036
202-387-5000
www.hispanichealth.org

National Center for the Study of Adult Learning and Literacy
www.hsph.harvard.edu/healthliteracy/

The National Multicultural Institute
www.nmci.org

National Resource Center on Family Centered Practice (NRC/FCP)
www.uiowa.edu/~nrcfcp

Women's Health in the United States: Health Coverage and Access to Care
www.kff.org/about/womenshealth.cfm

Urban Institute
National Survey of America's Families
http://newfederalism.urban.org/nsaf/

References

Allen, M. (1997). Comparative theories of the expanded role in nursing and implications for nursing practice: A working paper. *Nursing Papers, 9*(2), 38-45.

Amaro, H. (1994). Women in the Mexican-American community: Religion, culture, and reproductive attitudes and experiences. *Journal of Comparative Psychology, 16*(1), 6-19.

Bar-yam, N. (1994). Learning about culture: A guide for birth practitioners. *International Journal of Childbirth Education, 9*(2), 8-10.

Becker, M. (1974). The Health Belief Model and sick role behavior. *Health Education Monographs, 2,* 409-419.

Boss, P. (2002). *Family stress management* (2nd ed.). Thousand Oaks, CA: Sage.

Bronfenbrenner, U. (1979). *The ecology of human development: Experiments by nature and design.* Cambridge, MA: Harvard University Press.

Bronfenbrenner, U. (1989). Ecological systems theory. In R. Vasta (Ed.), *Annals of child development* (Vol 6, pp. 187-249), Greenwich, CT: JAI.

Brooks, E. (2002). Family assessment and cultural diversity. In S. Clemen-Stone, S. McGuire, & D. Eigsti (Eds.), *Comprehensive community health nursing: Family, aggregate, and community practice* (6th ed.). St. Louis: Mosby.

Carter, B., & McGoldrick, M. (1999). *The expanded family life cycle: Individual, family, and social perspectives* (3rd ed.). Boston: Allyn & Bacon.

D'Avanzo, C., & Geissler, E. (2003). *Pocket guide to cultural assessment* (3rd ed.). St. Louis: Mosby.

Federal Interagency Forum on Children and Family Statistics. (2004). *Population and family characteristics.* Internet document available at www.childstats.gov (accessed November 28, 2004).

Forbes, C., Jepson R., & Martin-Hirsch, P. (2001). Interventions targeted at women to encourage the uptake of cerevical screening (Cochrane Review). In *The Cochrane Library,* Issue 2, 2004. Chichester, UK: John Wiley & Sons.

Friedman, M. (1998). *Family nursing theory and assessment* (4th ed.). New York: Appleton & Lange.

Friedman, M., Bowden, V., & Jones, E. (2002). *Family nursing: Research, theory, and practice* (5th ed.). Upper Saddle River, NJ: Prentice Hall.

Galanti, G. (1997). *Caring for patients from different cultures: Case studies from American hospitals* (2nd ed.). Philadelphia: University of Pennsylvania Press.

Janz, N., & Becker, M. (1984). The Health Belief Model: A decade later. *Health Education Quarterly, 11*(1), 1-47.

Klein, D., & White, J. (1996). *Family theories: An introduction.* Newbury Park, CA: Sage.

Mattson, S. (1995). Culturally sensitive prenatal care for Southeastern Asians. *Journal of Obstetric, Gynecologic, and Neonatal Nursing, 24*(4), 335-341.

Mattson, S. (2000). Providing culturally competent care: Strategies and approaches for perinatal clients. *AWHONN Lifelines, 4*(5), 37-39.

National Academy Press. (2002). *From generation to generation: The health and well-being of children in immigrant families.* Internet document available at http://search.nap.edu/html/generation/summary.html (accessed November 28, 2004).

Pender, N., Murdaugh, C., & Parsons, M. (2002). *Health promotion in nursing practice.* Upper Saddle River, NJ: Prentice Hall Health.

Perry, S., & Mander, R. (2005). A global frame of reference: Learning from everyone, everywhere. *Nursing Education Perspectives, 26*(3), 148-151.

Spector, R. (2004). *Cultural diversity in health and illness* (6th ed.). Upper Saddle River, NJ: Prentice Hall Health.

Staveteig, S., & Wigton, A. (2000). *Key findings by race and ethnicity: Findings from the National Survey of America's Families.* Washington, DC: Urban Institute. Internet document available at www.urban.org (accessed November 28, 2004).

Thomas, N. (2001). The importance of culture throughout all of life and beyond. *Holistic Nursing Practice, 15*(2), 40-46.

Williams, R. (1989). Issues in women's health care. In B. Johnson (Ed.), *Psychiatric mental health nursing: Adaptation and growth.* Philadelphia: JB Lippincott.

Wright, L., & Leahey, M. (2000). *Nurses and families: A guide to family assessment and intervention* (3rd ed.). Philadelphia: FA Davis.

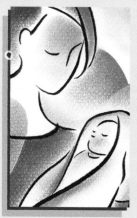

CHAPTER 3

Community and Home Care

SHANNON E. PERRY

LEARNING OBJECTIVES

- Compare community-based health care and community health (population- or aggregate-focused) care.
- Identify key components of the community assessment process.
- List indicators of community health status and their relevance to perinatal health.
- Describe data sources and methods for obtaining information about community health status.
- Identify predisposing factors and characteristics of vulnerable populations.
- List the potential advantages and disadvantages of home visits.

- Explore telephonic nursing care options in perinatal nursing.
- Describe how home care fits into the maternity continuum of care.
- Identify and define common perinatal conditions amenable to home care.
- Discuss safety and infection control principles as they apply to the care of patients in their homes.
- Describe the nurse's role in perinatal home care.

KEY TERMS AND DEFINITIONS

continuum of care Range of clinical services provided for an individual or group that reflects care given during a single hospitalization or care for multiple conditions over a lifetime

home health care Care that is provided within the home

key informants Individuals in positions of leadership who can provide information about a situation

levels of prevention Consists of three levels; primary prevention is promoting general health and well-being; secondary prevention involves early detection of health problems so that treatment can begin before significant disability occurs; tertiary prevention is the treatment and rehabilitation of persons who have developed disease

telephonic nursing Services such as "warm lines," nurse advice lines, and telephonic nursing assessments

vulnerable populations Groups who are at higher risk of developing physical, mental, or social health problems or who are more likely to have worse outcomes from these health problems than the population as a whole

walking survey Using one's senses while traveling through a community to obtain information about sociocultural characteristics and the environment, housing, transportation, and local community agencies

ELECTRONIC RESOURCES

Additional information related to the content in Chapter 3 can be found on

the companion website at **evolve**
http://evolve.elsevier.com/Lowdermilk/Maternity/
- NCLEX Review Questions
- WebLinks

or on the interactive companion CD
- NCLEX Review Questions
- Critical Thinking Exercise—Community Resources for Families
- Plan of Care—Community and Home Care

*H*ealth care in the United States has evolved rapidly in recent years, with notable shifts in both the nature of health priorities and the ways that health care is delivered to populations, families, and individuals. Greater emphasis is placed on the prevention of disease and disability, rather than the curative focus of past decades.

Most health care for women occurs outside the acute care setting. The movement to reduce health care costs has shortened hospitalization time and led to an increase of home- and community-based options for the provision of care. The increased emphasis on brief hospital stays reduces the financial burden for individuals, agencies, and insurance carriers. Hospital stays after childbirth may be abbreviated. By minimizing inpatient length of stay, much of acute care nursing has been transferred to home-based nursing services in local communities.

The U.S. national health objectives in *Healthy People 2010* focus attention on the unequal distribution of disease and disability and the need to reach out to vulnerable populations not being adequately served by the current health system (U.S. Department of Health and Human Services [USDHHS], 2000a). Hospital-based nurses are increasingly involved in follow-up of patients and families after discharge.

Trends in maternal and infant health in the United States reveal that progress has been made in relation to reduced infant and fetal deaths, use of prenatal care, and rates of cesarean births (see Chapter 1), but notable gaps remain in many other target areas. Some critical measures, such as low birth weight (LBW) and very low birth weight (VLBW), have increased, with significant disparities in infant mortality rates between Caucasians and other racial and ethnic groups in the United States. Despite favorable trends in early prenatal care and cesarean births, maternal mortality has not decreased significantly since 1982, with disproportionate rates among African-American and Hispanic women (Martin, Kochanek, Strobino, Guyer, & MacDorman, 2005; Minino et al., 2002). That many of these outcomes are preventable through access to prenatal care and use of preventive health practices clearly demonstrates the need for comprehensive, community-based care for mothers, infants, and families.

Changing demands on the community-based nurse evolve out of these societal, economic, and health-related trends. Acuity of illness of home care patients may be far greater than in the past, requiring the community nurse to become more adept in maternal assessment, direct care, and teaching. Assessment of the neonate requires knowledge of parameters for measuring the health of a newborn within the first days of life. Skill in assisting with breastfeeding is essential. Knowledge of an ever-widening array of diverse family traditions, beliefs, and expectations related to childbearing becomes even more critical for the nurse to facilitate effectively the transition required when a family moves through the stages of incorporating a new family member.

Community and family cannot be considered separately. Furthermore, as population demographics change, nurses are assuming greater roles in assessing community health status and providing health promotion and disease prevention interventions across the perinatal health continuum. Chapter 2 contains an overview of family and cultural theory and assessment. This chapter discusses the integration of community and home care within the context of family-focused nursing in relation to *Healthy People 2010* and perinatal health outcomes. Methods of community assessment and the special perinatal health needs of vulnerable aggregates in the population are discussed.

HEALTH AND WELLNESS IN THE COMMUNITY

In the context of community-based health care, both the aggregate (group of people who have shared characteristics) and the population become the focus of intervention. Health professionals are required not only to determine health priorities but also to develop successful plans of care to be delivered in the health clinic, the community health center, or the patient's home.

Public Health Services

Public health services are essential to provide for the needs of the community, especially for those who do not have the resources to access needed health care. Communities must do assessments to determine the needs of the populations they serve. Basic and essential services are listed in Box 3-1. Individual communities may identify other needs.

BOX 3-1

Essential Public Health Services

1. Monitor health status to identify community health problems.
2. Diagnose and investigate health problems and health hazards in the community.
3. Enforce laws and regulations that protect health and ensure safety.
4. Inform, educate, and empower people about health issues.
5. Mobilize community partnerships to identify and solve health problems.
6. (a) Link people to needed personal health services and
   (b) Assure the provision of health care when otherwise unavailable.
7. Evaluate effectiveness, accessibility, and quality of personal and population-based health services.
8. Assure a competent public health and person health care workforce.
9. Develop policies and plans that support individual and community health efforts.
10. Research for new insights and innovative solutions to health problems.

Source: Essential Public Health Services Work Group of the Public Health Functions Steering Committee. Internet document available at www.phf.org/essential.htm (accessed April 12, 2005).

Community Health Status Indicators

The data collected about communities can be compared with state or national standards to assess the well-being of the population as a whole and answer questions such as the following: Do most women begin prenatal care in the first trimester? What are the fetal and infant mortality rates?

Box 3-2 displays a set of community health status indicators developed by a committee of experts from many community health-related organizations. Infant mortality, because it is affected by the preconceptional health and prenatal and intrapartal care of the mother, as well as living conditions for the infant after birth, is a statistic widely used to compare the health status of different populations. Three of the five indicators of risk (i.e., incidence of low birth,

---

BOX 3-2

Consensus Set of Indicators* for Assessing Community Health Status

INDICATORS OF HEALTH STATUS OUTCOME

1. Race- or ethnicity-specific infant mortality, as measured by the rate (per 1000 live births) of deaths among infants younger than 1 year of age

Death rates (per 100,000 population)† for

2. Motor vehicle crashes
3. Work-related injury
4. Suicide
5. Lung cancer
6. Breast cancer
7. Cardiovascular disease
8. Homicide
9. All causes

Reported incidence (per 100,000 population) of

10. Acquired immunodeficiency syndrome
11. Measles
12. Tuberculosis
13. Primary and secondary syphilis

INDICATORS OF RISK FACTORS

14. Incidence of LBW, as measured by percentage of total number of live-born infants weighing less than 2500 g at birth
15. Births to adolescents (females age 10 to 17 years) as a percentage of total live births
16. Prenatal care, as measured by percentage of mothers delivering live infants who did not receive prenatal care during first trimester
17. Childhood poverty, as measured by the proportion of children younger than 15 years of age living in families at or below the poverty level
18. Proportion of persons living in counties exceeding U.S. Environmental Protection Agency standards for air quality during previous year

From US Department of Health and Human Services. (1991). Consensus set of indicators for assessing community health status, *Morbidity and Mortality Weekly Report, 40*(27), 449.
LBW, Low birthweight.
*Position or number of the indicator does not imply priority.
†Age-adjusted to the 1940 standard population.

---

adolescent pregnancy, and early prenatal care) refer to maternal-infant health. Poverty and a high percentage of young children in a community are strongly associated with significant community health needs.

VULNERABLE POPULATIONS ■

Several broad categories of high risk or vulnerable populations, i.e., those more likely to develop health problems or who are more likely to have worse outcomes from these health problems than the population as a whole, are of special interest to perinatal nurses working in the community. These include the categories discussed in the following sections.

Women

One of the primary factors compromising women's health is lack of access to acceptable-quality health care, which may take many forms: lack of health insurance, living in a medically underserved area, or an inability to obtain needed services, particularly basic services such as prenatal care. For example, some rural areas have few obstetricians, pediatricians, and nurse-midwives; women may have to travel hundreds of miles for this kind of care. Women often have lower incomes and less education and are therefore considered at high risk. Infant mortality is nearly two times higher for mothers without a high school education (USDHHS, 2000b).

Within the larger group of vulnerable women, a number of subgroups present challenges to the community-based perinatal nurse.

Adolescent girls

Youths and adults younger than 24 years of age are the least medically served of all age groups in the United States. Lifestyle choices related to substance use, sexually transmitted infections, and human immunodeficiency virus (HIV) represent high risk behaviors with both immediate and long-term health consequences. Many engage in "survival sex," exchanging sexual favors for food, clothing, and shelter, making them vulnerable to sexually transmitted infections and unintended pregnancies. Young women, particularly African-Americans and Hispanics, are less likely to have access to routine care and often fail to seek care because of inability to pay, lack of transportation, or confidentiality issues.

Minority women

In the United States, disparities continue to exist in health and health care. Higher infant and maternal mortality rates are evident in African-American and Hispanic women and among some Native American and Alaskan Native communities. Women with underlying health conditions are at especially high risk for poor obstetric outcomes for both themselves and their infants. They have high rates of preterm labor and gestational hypertension and often have intrauterine growth restriction resulting in the birth of infants who are small for gestational age. These are the patients for whom the community-based perinatal nurse will be providing care, and their needs are complex, demanding expertise and high levels of skill.

Women and poverty

In 2002, 13.5 million women were living with incomes below the federal poverty level, with a 19.5% poverty rate reported for women aged 18 to 24 years (Health Resources and Services Administration [HRSA], 2004). Because these are also the years of greatest childbearing, many women and their infants have unmet needs. A significant proportion of women are underinsured or uninsured.

Homeless women

An estimated 2.5 to 3.5 million people are homeless nationally, with 6.5% of adults reporting homelessness each year. This includes increasing numbers of women, children, and adolescents who are disenfranchised from their homes, families, and services for various reasons, resulting in a 17% increase in the demand for family assistance (Bureau of Primary Health Care, 2001). Depending on the cause of homelessness and the availability of services, a person may be homeless for weeks or months, intermittently, or on a prolonged basis.

The most significant causes of homelessness in the United States relate to mental illness (approximately 50%) and substance use (nearly 75% among homeless men). Violent relationships and a history of abuse are significant contributing factors to homelessness for women.

Although the homeless population is generally higher in urban areas, a growing number of the homeless are found in rural agricultural, mining, and fishing regions, where they seek temporary employment. Often these families remain hidden within the community. Sometimes the family stays in a local hotel (paying on a daily basis while they work), lives out of a car, resides in an unoccupied building, or camps in a national park. Couples with children form the largest group among rural homeless. Lack of visibility and community resources in rural areas frequently results in longer periods of poverty and homelessness for these families (Bushy, 2000).

Health issues among the homeless are numerous, resulting primarily from a lack of preventive care and a lack of resources in general. Because very few are able to access primary care, most of the homeless are forced to use the emergency room for routine health problems. Mental health and substance abuse services for the homeless are extremely limited in many communities, in particular in medically underserved rural regions of the United States (Bureau of Primary Health Care, 2001).

For women the emotional and psychologic trauma of the homeless experience is often exacerbated by physical or sexual assault; 36% of homeless women report being a victim of a crime while living on the streets. Approximately 24% of women become pregnant while they are homeless. Although many women are eligible for Medicaid and public health services, few receive prenatal care.

Incarcerated women

In 2002 there were 165,800 women incarcerated in the United States. Non-Hispanic black women aged 30 to 34 years experience the highest rate of incarceration (HRSA, 2004). Mental illness and HIV infection are significant health problems among female inmates, with 23.6% of female inmates mentally ill and more than 5% infected with HIV.

Migrant women

An estimated 3 to 5 million people, 21% of whom are women, are classified as migrant farm workers in the United States (Economic Research Service, 2003). Migrant laborers establish temporary residence in various areas on a seasonal basis to obtain employment. Although many acquire temporary housing for at least 6 months, others move continuously throughout the year. Diverse ethnic groups are represented among migrants: African-Americans, European-Americans, Hispanics, Haitians, and Southeast Asians.

Migrant laborers and their families face many problems, including financial instability, child labor, poor housing, lack of education, language and cultural barriers, and limited access to health and social services (McGuire, 2002). Poor dental health, diabetes, hypertension, malnutrition, tuberculosis, and parasitic infections are common health issues among migrant populations. The average life expectancy for migrant laborers is 49 years (as compared with 79 years for the population as a whole). Substance abuse and domestic violence are significant problems.

Numerous reproductive health issues exist for migrant women, including less consistent use of contraception and increased rates of sexually transmitted infections. Migrants are less likely to receive early prenatal care and have a greater incidence of inadequate weight gain during pregnancy than do other poor women. The infant mortality rate among migrant workers is estimated to be 25 times higher than the national average (Murray, Zentner, & Samiezade-Yazd, 2001).

Federally funded migrant health centers have been established in many regions of the United States, but they are unable to meet the demands of the 3 to 5 million migrants. Many seek care at local hospitals and clinics in the areas in which they work, but access is limited by lack of time and financial constraints. Even if services are free, the loss of wages incurred in leaving the field is a deterrent to preventive care. Lack of trust or fear of being reported to the Immigration and Naturalization Services prevents many undocumented workers from seeking care.

Rural versus Urban Community Settings

Rural refers to a town or community area that has a population of less than 2500 or to a county with fewer than 50,000 people. Approximately 21% of the population live in rural areas (HRSA, 2004). A number of common characteristics define rural groups: they lack anonymity, are isolated, and tend to be content to live independently (Bushy, 2000; Murray, Zentner, & Samiezade-Yazd, 2001). They are more

Critical Thinking Exercise

Health Needs of a Migrant Worker

The home care agency receives a referral for a home visit to a 16-year-old Vietnamese-speaking mother, Linh, who is a migrant worker. She has a 2-week-old infant and is expected to return to the fields to work. Before visiting Linh, the nurse establishes as priorities to promote breast-feeding, encourage use of birth control, and involve the father of the baby in child care.

1 Evidence—Is there sufficient evidence to draw conclusions about the appropriateness of the nurse's plan of care?

2 Assumptions—What assumptions can be made about the needs of this mother and baby in regard to the following issues?
   a. The priorities for care
   b. Conditions for effective breastfeeding
   c. Feasibility of maintaining breastfeeding while working in the field
   d. Cultural relevancy of involving the father

3 What implications and priorities for nursing care can be drawn at this time?

4 Does the evidence objectively support your conclusion?

5 Are there alternative perspectives to your conclusion?

likely to be diagnosed with hypertension and cancer (HRSA, 2004). Geographic and socioeconomic factors present barriers to accessing prenatal care and other health care associated with transportation and provider inaccessibility.

Refugees and Immigrants

Refugees are defined as those who are displaced suddenly or forced to leave their country of origin because of persecution, civil unrest, or war. Families are thus forced from their own homes to seek residence and employment elsewhere (Murray, Zentner, & Samiezade-Yazd, 2001). Often these groups are extremely impoverished and face extreme physical and emotional stress when they arrive in the United States. Some refugees have a history of arrival in a new country by precarious means, such as crossing wide oceans in fragile boats. Many survivors of such journeys have memories of relatives and friends who died at sea. Many have been raped by modern pirates who prey on those who are desperate for a better life. The traumatic stress of having witnessed the murders of their families as a result of war haunts many refugees. Many have profound grief over the loss of loved ones, their homelands, and all they owned. Both refugees and immigrants are saddened by the knowledge that it will be difficult or impossible to go "home" to the people, traditions, and customs that were familiar and comforting.

Along with their profound resilience and determination, refugees and immigrants have brought rich diversity to the United States in several important dimensions, including cultural heritage and customs, economic productivity, and enhanced national vitality. At the same time, multiple challenges accompany the dramatic influx of individuals and families from other countries.

In general, refugees are more likely to live in poverty than are immigrants (Murray, Zentner, & Samiezade-Yazd, 2001). Over time, measures of health and well-being actually decline for the immigrant population as they become part of American society (National Academy Press [NAP], 2002). Many of the conditions or illnesses that they acquire contribute to the persistence of disparities in maternal and neonatal health outcomes for both immigrants and refugees.

Implications for Nursing

Working in the community or in the home with the full spectrum of family organizational styles, vulnerable populations, and cultural groups presents challenges for the nurse. Whether it involves perinatal care focused on women and their newborns, or women's health care directed toward treatment and prevention of other health conditions such as communicable diseases and sexually transmitted infections, nursing must be accomplished with a high degree of professionalism. Cultural sensitivity, compassion, and a critical awareness of family dynamics and social stressors that will affect health-related decision making are critical components in developing an effective plan of care.

Although the long-term consequences of contemporary immigration for U.S. society are unclear, the successful incorporation of immigrant families depends on the resources, benefits, and policies that ensure their healthy development and successful social adjustment. Culturally competent health care and involvement of the immigrant community in health care programs are recommended strategies for improving the access to and effectiveness of health care for this population (NAP, 2002).

The use of camp volunteers, known as "romatoras," has been effective in assisting families living in migrant worker camps to obtain prenatal, postpartum, and infant care (see Resources at the end of the chapter). Working in partnership with health professionals such as nurses, lay camp aides have been used effectively for outreach and health education; however, more strategies are needed to link traditional practices with the formal health care system. Guidance and information about other health resources are available to health care providers through the National Migrant Resource Program and the Migrant Clinicians Network.

Nurses working with homeless women and families are challenged to treat them with dignity and respect to establish a therapeutic relationship. Case management is recommended to coordinate the services and disciplines that may be involved in meeting the complex needs of these families. Whenever possible, health services must be provided when the woman seeks treatment, as this may be the only opportunity to provide health information and intervention. Building on existing coping strategies and strengths, the health care provider helps the woman and her family to reconnect with a social support system. Nurses also have an important role in advocating for funding to support homeless health services and to improve access to preventive care for all homeless populations.

Women who are incarcerated are exposed to stress and violence and have limited access to health care, especially for treatment for mental disorders. Nurses who work in prisons and jails must be creative in their approaches to providing health care for this vulnerable group of women.

Nurses have established and maintained a variety of clinics where the homeless, migrants, immigrants, and those living in poverty have access to care. Outreach must continue, as women who are eligible for services often do not access the services for a variety of reasons.

ASSESSING THE COMMUNITIES IN WHICH FAMILIES LIVE

Mothers assume much of the health-related decision making for their families, with up to 83% of them having sole or shared responsibility for financial decisions affecting family health. A significant link exists between the maternal roles of health care provider and decision maker and family health behavior. The health and well-being of women and children will be in jeopardy as long as the communities in which they live are ill prepared to provide the quantity and quality of services they need.

Important measures of community health include access to care, level of provider services available, and other social and economic factors. For women and infants, access to a consistent source of care is critical. Those with a regular source of care are more likely to use preventive services and receive timely treatment for illness and injury, but 13.9% of women are uninsured (9% of non-Hispanic white, 17.9% of Black, 18.0% of Asian/Pacific Islander, and 29.5% of Hispanic female) (HRSA, 2004). More Medicaid-covered women as compared with privately insured women lack access to a usual source of care or rely primarily on emergency services. Consequently, many of these women have unmet health or dental needs. In 2002, 12% of women reported not having seen a dentist for 5 years or having never seen one (HRSA, 2004).

Methods of Community Assessment

Community, in its broadest definition, refers to a geographically defined area; its residents; their cultural, religious, and ethnic characteristics; and the activities or functions through which the needs of the residents are met. The health of individuals or groups is inextricably linked to the health status of each community.

With the community as the focus of perinatal health care, the nurse must become familiar with the neighborhoods and resources that influence patients. Community assessment is a complex although well-defined process through which the unique characteristics of the populations and their special needs are identified to plan and evaluate health services for the community as a whole. The desired outcome of this process is identification of direct service, as well as advocacy needs of the targeted aggregate or group and improved health for the community as a whole (Kuehnert, 2002).

Data Collection and Sources of Community Health Data

A community assessment framework or model provides criteria for conducting a community assessment, identifies types and methods of data collection, and organizes the data of a community assessment (Ervin, 2002) (Fig. 3-1).

Data collection is often the most time-consuming phase of the community assessment process, but it provides an important definition and description of the community (Ervin, 2002). A broad range of health information is available for nurses in conducting a community assessment. The most critical indicators of perinatal health in a community are related to access to health care; maternal mortality; infant mortality; low birth weight; first trimester prenatal care; and rates for mammography, Papanicolaou tests, and other similar screening tests. Nurses may use these indicators as a reflection of access, quality, and continuity of health care in a community.

The U.S. government census provides data on population size, age ranges, sex, racial and ethnic distribution, socioeconomic status, educational level, employment, and housing characteristics. Summary data are available for most large metropolitan areas, arranged by zip code and census tract, which usually corresponds to a neighborhood (approximately 3000 to 6000 people). Looking at individual census tracts within a community helps to identify subpopulations or aggregates whose needs may differ from those of the larger community. For example, women at high risk for inadequate prenatal care according to age, race, and ethnic or cultural group may be readily identified, and outreach activities may be appropriately targeted.

City, county, and state health departments provide annual reports of births and deaths. Maternal and infant death rates are particularly important, as they reflect health outcomes that may be preventable (McDevitt & Wilbur, 2002). Local health departments also compile extensive statistics about the birth complications, causes of death, and leading causes of morbidity and mortality for each age group. The National Health Survey, which describes national health trends, is published annually by the National Center for Health Statistics.

Other sources of useful information are hospitals and voluntary health agencies. The March of Dimes Birth Defects Foundation, for example, has supported perinatal needs assessments in many communities across the United States. Other community health resources include health care providers or administrators, government officials, religious leaders, and representatives of voluntary health agencies. Community or county health councils exist in many areas, with oversight of specific health initiatives or programs for that region. These key informants often provide a unique perspective that may be inaccessible through other sources.

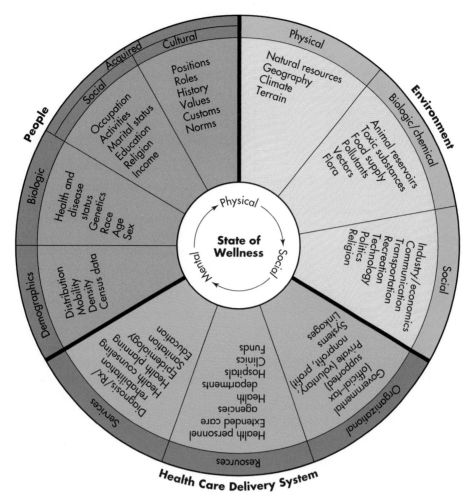

Fig. 3-1 Community health assessment wheel. (Clemen-Stone, S. [2002]. Community assessment and diagnosis. In S. Clemen-Stone, S. McGuire, & D. Eigsti, [Eds.]. *Comprehensive community health nursing: Family, aggregate, and community practice* [6th ed.]. St. Louis: Mosby.)

The perinatal health nurse also may explore community health program reports, records of preventive health screenings, and other informal data. Established programs often provide good indicators of the health promotion and disease prevention characteristics of the population.

Professional publications are a rich and readily accessible source of information for all nurses. In addition to nursing and public health journals, behavioral and social science literature offers diverse perspectives on community health status for specific populations and subgroups. The Internet has increased the availability and accessibility of national, state, and local health data as well. Use of Web-based resources for health information requires some caution, however, as the reliability and the validity of the data are difficult to verify. Some guidelines for evaluation of Internet health resources can be found at the Health on the Net Web site at www.hon.org. Additional health websites are identified at the end of the chapter.

Data collection methods may be either qualitative or quantitative, including visual surveys that can be completed by walking through a community, participant observation, interviews, focus groups, and analysis of existing data. Potential patients and health care consumers may be asked to participate in focus groups or community forums to present their views on needed community services and programs. Formal surveys, conducted by mail, by telephone, or by face-to-face interviews, can be a valuable source of information not available from national databases or other secondary sources. Several drawbacks exist with this method: surveys are generally expensive to develop and time consuming to administer. In addition to the cost of such surveys, poor response rates often preclude a sufficiently representative response on which to base nursing interventions.

A **walking survey** is generally conducted by a walk-through observation of the community (Box 3-3), taking note of specific characteristics of the population, economic and social environment, transportation, health care services, and other resources. This method allows the nurse to collect subjective data and may facilitate other aspects of the assessment (Ervin, 2002). Fig. 3-2 is an example of an

BOX 3-3

Community Walk-Through

- *Physical environment*—Older neighborhood or newer addition? Sidewalks, streets, and buildings in good or poor repair? Billboards and signs? What are the billboards and signs advertising? Are lawns kept up? Is there trash in the streets? Parks or playgrounds? Parking lots? Empty lots?
- *People in the area*—Old, young, homeless, children, predominant ethnicity, language?
- *Services available*—Restaurants: chain, local, ethnic? Grocery stores: neighborhood or chain? Department stores, gas stations, real estate or insurance offices, travel agencies, pawn shops, liquor stores, discount or thrift stores, newspaper stands?
- *Social and religious*—Clubs, bars, fraternal organizations (e.g., Elks, American Legion), museums, churches, synagogues, mosques?
- *Health services*—Drug stores, doctors' offices, clinics, dentists, mental health services, veterinarians, urgent care facilities, hospital, shelters?
- *Transportation*—Cars, bus, taxi, light rail, sidewalks, bicycle paths, access for disabled persons?
- *Education*—Schools, before and after school programs, child care, libraries, bookstores? What is the reputation of the schools?
- *Government*—What is the governance structure? Is there a mayor? City council? Are meetings open to the public?
- *Safety*—How safe is the community? What is the crime rate? What types of crimes are committed? Are police visible? Is there a fire station?
- *Evaluation of the community based on your observations*—What is your impression of the community? Is the environment pleasing? Are services and transportation adequate? How difficult is it for residents to obtain needed services—i.e., how far do they have to travel? Would you want to live in this community? Why or why not?

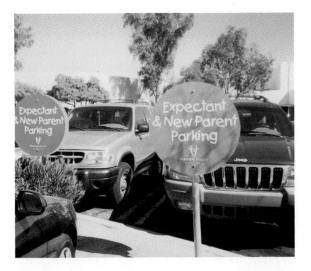

Fig. 3-2 Community accommodation for expectant and new parents. (Courtesy Shannon Perry, Phoenix, AZ.)

accommodation for expectant and new mothers that might be noticed during such a survey.

Participant observation is another useful assessment method in which the nurse actively participates in the community to understand the community more fully and to validate observations.

Finally, as part of the assessment process, nurses working in multiethnic and multicultural groups need an in-depth assessment of culturally driven behaviors. Needs assessment for these groups should focus on epidemiologic data and population needs and interests.

Analysis and synthesis of data obtained during the assessment process helps to generate a comprehensive picture of the community's health status, needs, and problem areas, as well as its strengths and resources for addressing these concerns. The goal of this process is to assign priorities to community health needs and to develop a plan of action for correcting them. A comparison of community health data with state and national statistics may be useful in identification of appropriate target populations, as well as interventions to improve health outcomes.

Successful community-based health initiatives involve understanding of community relationships and resources, as well as participation of community leaders (Lauderdale, 2001). Failure to recognize and involve individuals, families, and communities in the process often results in failed or short-lived health interventions (Bruhn, 2001).

Comprehensive community assessment and the use of timely, high-quality data sources can help prevent poor birth outcomes and promote maternal health by identifying aggregates at risk and giving direction to preventive interventions. Often the outcomes of local and state assessments are used to determine policy and resource allocation, which directly or indirectly affect health for the most needy and vulnerable populations. Decisions related to funding of community health promotion initiatives also are linked to these data sources.

LEVELS OF PREVENTIVE CARE

Population-based care involves prevention activities focused on target needs identified in the community assessment process. These levels of prevention provide a framework for nursing interventions. Primary prevention involves health promotion and disease prevention activities to decrease the occurrence of illness and enhance general health and quality of life. Sometimes referred to as "true prevention," primary prevention precedes disease or dysfunction and encourages individuals to achieve the optimal level of health possible. This includes the use of specific health protections such as recommended immunizations, infant car seats, and school health education to prevent tobacco use.

Early detection of health problems is the focus of secondary prevention. Persons who are asymptomatic or who have nonspecific disease symptoms are targeted to receive curative treatment and reduce disease prevalence. At this level, various methods of health screening and testing facilitate early treatment of the pathologic process. The goal is to shorten disease duration and severity, thus enabling an individual to return to normal function as quickly as possible (Murray, Zentner, & Samiezade-Yazd, 2001).

Tertiary prevention follows the occurrence of a defect or disability that is permanent and irreversible. Persons who have developed disease are provided with treatment and rehabilitation to prevent complications and further deterioration and to maintain their optimal level of function.

Primordial prevention is a form of early intervention designed to prevent the development of risk factors. It is the promotion of healthy behaviors to preclude susceptibility to disease.

Because most women are healthy during pregnancy, maternal-newborn nursing emphasizes primary and secondary prevention activities regardless of where care is provided. Tertiary prevention is frequently the focus for the ill patient at home or in the hospital. Nurses can emphasize primordial prevention through anticipatory guidance and other forms of health teaching. Good nutrition and exercise are important components of primordial prevention.

COMMUNITY HEALTH PROMOTION

The emphasis on community-based health promotion has grown in recent years, with recognition that many health issues require the collaborative efforts of a diverse community network to achieve public health goals. Pender, Murdaugh, and Parsons (2002) noted the benefits of community-based, coordinated health promotion programs with the potential for widespread change in community health status. These efforts are particularly relevant in relation to maternal-newborn health, which encompasses multiple public health issues: lack of health insurance, teen pregnancy, substance abuse, and the consequences of inadequate prenatal care.

Health promotion efforts for childbearing families are primarily focused on early intervention through prenatal care and prevention of complications during the perinatal period. Often this early exposure to health information sets the stage for a successful birth and positive outcomes for mother and baby. Involving expectant mothers and fathers in identification of their learning needs is an essential first step to securing their participation in the health promotion process.

A wide variety of strategies have been used to disseminate heath information to women in the community. Prenatal classes are a well-established mechanism for increasing awareness of healthy behaviors during pregnancy and preparing parents for the care of themselves and their newborn during the postpartum period. Mass media efforts such as those presented by the March of Dimes "Baby Your Baby" advertisements are clear, consumer-friendly messages designed to reach a large target audience. Other venues include public health education in newspapers and magazines and health department programs such as the Special Supplemental Nutrition

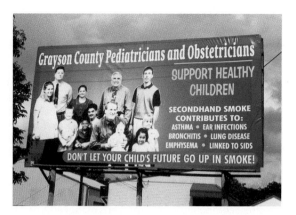

Fig. 3-3 Billboard illustrating the hazards of smoking. (Courtesy Joan R. Vogel, Boca Raton, FL.)

Program for Women, Infants, and Children (WIC), which offers a variety of health education and written information to mothers. The Association of Women's Health, Obstetric and Neonatal Nurses' (AWHONN's) 2004 education guide, *Every Woman: The Essential Guide for Healthy Living,* is an evidence-based practice guide distributed to women by their nurses.

Many communities have organized coalitions to address specific health promotion agendas related to sharing information, educating community members, or advocating for health policies around maternal and child health issues. An example of this is Healthy Start, a community-based initiative to reduce infant mortality and improve the health and well-being of women, children, and families. Smoking presents major health risks for women, fetuses, and infants. There are major smoking cessation efforts directed toward pregnant women (Fig. 3-3). Adolescent health is another broad target area for community health promotion efforts, including both health education and policy initiatives. Issues related to adolescent sexuality, teen pregnancy, and substance abuse are particularly problematic, requiring aggressive prevention programs and community outreach.

Community-based health promotion for childbearing families is often a challenge, because those who are most in need are less able to access such services. For example, low-income, uneducated, or homeless women, who frequently delay seeking prenatal care, also are disenfranchised in relation to other health promotion activities. Failure to address these social and environmental barriers and inability to engage the target audience often limits the benefits and sustainability of health promotion initiatives (Bruhn, 2001). Efforts should therefore be focused on increasing awareness of health promotion activities, as well as ensuring access for all community groups.

PERINATAL CONTINUUM OF CARE

Within the community, perinatal care is provided on a continuum. A continuum of care is defined as a range of clinical services provided for an individual or group that reflects

CD: Critical Thinking Exercise—Community Resources for Families

EVIDENCE-BASED PRACTICE
Parenting Groups for Teenage Parents

BACKGROUND

- In the developed world, teen pregnancy is highest in the United States (55 per 1000 women age 15 to 19 years), followed by New Zealand (33 per 1000) and Canada (25 per 1000). The United Kingdom (23 per 1000) has the highest rate in Europe. Where deprivation and poverty are high, so is teen pregnancy. There is evidence that teen mothers have lower aspirations for themselves and come from family backgrounds of low educational expectations. Early parenthood brings the needs of the still-developing teen in direct competition with the needs of the fetus and baby and usually truncates the mother's opportunities. Younger parents may lack realistic expectations of child development and parenting and disciplinary skills. They may experience stress, depression, low self-esteem, and socioeconomic deprivation. Infants of teen mothers may have developmental delays, behavioral problems, intellectual deficits, and lower educational achievement. Child abuse may be present for all these reasons, rather than young parental age alone. The prevention of teen pregnancy remains the primary intervention to prevent these vulnerabilities. After birth, however, early interventions such as parenting programs show promise as a way to compensate for a lack of life exposure and perspective in the immature and inexperienced parent.

OBJECTIVES

- The reviewers' goal was to assess the impact of parenting skills education on the health and well-being of teen parents and their babies. The ideal interventions would be individually or group formatted, offered during pregnancy or after birth to teen parents, and structured to improve parenting attitudes, skills, or knowledge. Outcomes sought were maternal anxiety, stress, depression, self-esteem, sense of parenting competence, and parenting and child development knowledge, and infant cognitive, social, and mental development.

METHODS
Search Strategy

- The authors searched Cochrane, MEDLINE, EMBASE, CINAHL, Psyclit, Sociofile, Social Science Citation Index, ASSIA, National Research Registry, ERIC, and reference lists. Search keywords included *parent, program, train, education, promotion, health, adolescent, mother, teen, father, pregnancy,* and combinations of these words.
- Four randomized, controlled trials were selected, for a subject pool of 247 teen mothers who volunteered for a parenting program. The studies were published between 1977 and 1999 and were all from the United States. The trials used a variety of settings, including a school, a health setting, a residential maternity home, community health clinics, and family support centers.

Statistical Analysis

- The reviewer calculated a treatment effect for each available and reliable outcome. This enabled assessment of how strongly the intervention was associated with the outcomes.

FINDINGS

- When compared with the controls, the parenting intervention group showed a significant increase in maternal sensitivity, identity as a mother, parenting knowledge, maternal-child interaction, mealtime attitudes and communication, and cognitive growth fostering capacities. There were trends toward improvement in maternal self-confidence and motivation, but not to the level of statistical significance. Infants whose mothers were receiving the parenting intervention had nonsignificant trends toward responsiveness to parent, clearer interaction, and language scores, up to 2 years of age.

LIMITATIONS

- The small number of studies, and the fact that they were all from the same country, limits generalizability of the results. Some of the data were collected with tools that had no reported reliability or validity. The treatment effects may have seemed stronger than they actually were, because of the statistical handling of cluster randomization (groups in a school who were divided into groups by classroom), dropouts, and subjects lost to follow-up. Dropout rates were marked in one study (33%) but remarkably low in the other three studies, considering that dropout rates are usually increased with teenagers, low socioeconomic status, and ethnic minorities.
- There were no data on fathers. All the subjects were volunteers, and so may have self-selected for motivation, the maturity to identify their own deficits, self-esteem, or some other confounding influence. A strength of the review was the variety of settings in which pregnant teens were seen.

CONCLUSIONS

- Interventions facilitating parenting skills for vulnerable teen parents foster improved outcomes for both the mother and (probably) the child.

IMPLICATIONS FOR PRACTICE

- Interventions to foster parenting skills should be provided for teen parents. Health care providers need to give some thought to which setting might maximize the effects of which interventions. Some coordination among various providers is required. Teen fathers, often absent because of lack of commitment, mistrust in the services, illiteracy, and personality, need interventions tailored to their special needs as teens and parents.

IMPLICATIONS FOR FURTHER RESEARCH

- More trials are needed, with attention to large numbers, minimizing dropouts, and statistical rigor for confounding effects. Some methods to recruit and randomize non-volunteers would improve the generalizability of the results. Of particular interest are the influences of peers in the group. The skill of the facilitator is critical to the process and tone of the group, but none of the studies discussed this variable. Data on the long-term outcomes of the children are needed.

Reference: Coren, E., & Barlow, J. (2001). Individual and group-based parenting programmes for improving psychosocial outcomes for teenage parents and their children (Cochrane Review). In *The Cochrane Library,* Issue 2, 2004. Chichester, UK: John Wiley & Sons.

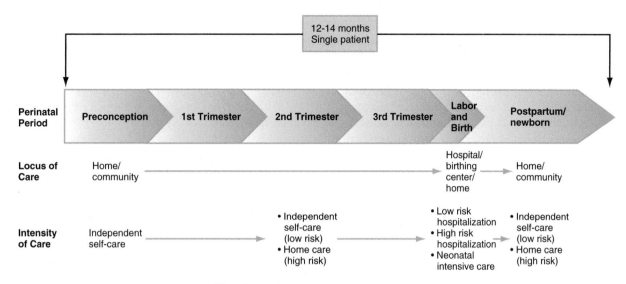

Fig. 3-4 Perinatal continuum of care.

care given during a single hospitalization or care for multiple conditions over a lifetime. Home care is one delivery component available along the perinatal continuum of care (Fig. 3-4). This continuum begins with family planning and continues with preconception care, prenatal care, intrapartum care, postpartum care, newborn care, interconception care, and infant care until the infant is 1 year old. Independent self-care, ambulatory care, home care, low risk hospitalization, or specialized intensive care may be appropriate at different points along this continuum.

Clinical integration of services can improve services. The goals of clinical integration are improved coordination of care and care outcomes; better communication among health care providers; increased patient, payer, and provider satisfaction; and reduced cost. With clinical integration, the focus changes from illness to health, from the individual to the population, and from care provided in one setting to care across the continuum. The following factors make home care an important area in perinatal services:

- Interest in family birthing alternatives
- Shortened hospital stays
- New technologies that allow sophisticated assessments and treatments to be performed in the home
- Reimbursement by third-party payers

Modern home care nursing has its foundation in public health nursing, which provided comprehensive care to sick and well patients in their own homes. Specialized maternity home care nursing services began in the 1980s, when public health maternity nursing services were limited and services had not kept pace with the changing practices of high risk obstetrics and emerging technology. Lengthy antepartal hospitalizations for such conditions as preterm labor and gestational hypertension created nursing care challenges for staff members of inpatient units. Many women expressed their concern for the negative effect of antepartal hospitalizations on the family. Although clinical indications showed that a

new nursing care approach was needed, home health care did not become a viable alternative until third-party payers (i.e., public or private organizations or employer groups that pay for health care) pushed for cost containment in maternity services.

COMMUNICATION TO BRIDGE THE CONTINUUM

As maternity care continues to consist of frequent and brief contacts with health care providers throughout the prenatal and postpartum periods, services that link maternity patients throughout the perinatal continuum of care have assumed increasing importance. These services include critical pathways, telephonic nursing assessments, discharge planning, specialized education programs, parent support groups, home visiting programs, nurse advice lines, and perinatal home care. Some hospitals provide cross-training for hospital-based nurses to make postpartum home visits or to staff outpatient centers for postpartum follow-up.

Telephonic Nursing Care

Telephonic nursing care through services such as warm lines, nurse advice lines, and telephonic nursing assessments is a valuable means of managing health care problems and bridging the gaps among acute, outpatient, and home care services. Some providers are using the Internet to communicate with patients who have an Internet service provider (ISP). Nursing care that occurs by telephone is interactive and responsive to immediate health care questions about particular health care needs. Warm lines are telephone lines that are offered as a community service to provide new parents with support, encouragement, and basic parenting education. Nurse advice lines, or toll-free nurse consultation services, often are supported by third-party payers or nurse case managers employed by health maintenance organizations (HMOs) or managed care organizations (MCOs) and are designed to provide answers to medical questions. These nurses are prepared to guide callers through urgent health care situations, suggest treatment options, and provide health education. Telephonic nursing assessments, or nurse consultation, assessment, and health education that take place during a telephone conversation, can be added to the plan of care in conjunction with skilled nursing visits or may be a separate nursing contact for the woman. Telephonic nursing assessments are commonly used after a postpartum home care visit to reassess a woman's knowledge about the signs and symptoms of adequate hydration in breastfeeding or after initiating home phototherapy to assess the caregiver's knowledge regarding problems with equipment.

GUIDELINES FOR NURSING PRACTICE

Although the home care industry continues to grow rapidly, perinatal home care nursing practice is still emerging. AWHONN (1998) defined *home care* as

> the provision of technical, psychologic, and other therapeutic support in the patient's home rather than in an institution. The scope of nursing care delivered in the home is necessarily limited to practices deemed safe and appropriate to be carried out in an environment that is physically separated from a health care institution and its resources. . . . Nursing practice at home is consistent with federal and state regulations . . . that direct home care practice. The nurse demonstrates practice competence through formalized orientation and ongoing clinical education and performance evaluation in the respective home care agency. Standards for practice from key specialty organizations such as AWHONN, the American College of Obstetricians and Gynecologists (ACOG), the American Academy of Pediatrics (AAP), and the Intravenous Nursing Society (INS) provide the basis for clinical protocols and pathways and organizational programs in home care practice. The Joint Commission on Accreditation of Health Care Organizations (JCAHO) provides criteria for home care operations based on Centers for Medicare and Medicaid Services regulations.

AWHONN (1994) developed standards of practice and identified essential knowledge and skills to provide safe perinatal home care. Health care agencies and individuals can use these to assess the nurse's skills and learning needs.

A wide range of professional health care services and health products can be delivered or used in the home with technology and telecommunication. For example, telehealth and telemedicine make it possible for patients in the home to be interviewed and assessed by a specialist located hundreds of miles away. Some view home health care as an extension of in-hospital care. Essentially, the primary difference between health care in a hospital and home care is the absence of the continuous presence of professional health care providers in a patient's home. Generally, but not always, home health care entails intermittent care by a professional who visits the patient's home for a particular reason and/or provides care on site for fewer than 4 hours at a time. The home health care agency maintains on-call professional staff to assist home care patients who have questions about their care and in emergencies, such as equipment failure.

HOME CARE PERINATAL SERVICES

Home care perinatal services may be provided by hospital-based programs, independent proprietary (for-profit) agencies or nonprofit home care agencies, and official or tax-supported agencies. Innovative programs may be supported by research grants for a period of years, but ultimately they must be sponsored by an agency with long-term funding. Home visits have both advantages and disadvantages. The pregnant woman is able to maintain bed rest if indicated, and vulnerable neonates are not exposed to the weather or external sources of infection. The nurse can observe and interact with family members in their most natural and secure environment. Adequacy of resources and safety factors can be assessed. Teaching can be tailored to the actual home conditions, and other family members can be included. A home visit is less expensive than a day's hospitalization, but a 60- to 90-minute visit requires 2.5 to 3 hours of nursing time, including travel and documentation. Travel time may be even greater when a patient resides in a rural area because of distance, travel, and weather-related factors. It is more cost-effective for the health care provider to see patients in an office, where professional time is not spent in travel. Availability of nurses with expertise in maternity care may be limited, and concerns about the nurse's physical safety in some communities may limit visits.

Visits for outreach and health promotion are an integral part of community (or public) health nursing. In countries with national health systems, a nurse or midwife may see all women during pregnancy and after birth. In the United States, visits of this sort have been provided mainly to low-income families without health insurance and Medicaid recipients who use the clinics provided by local health departments. Until recently, private insurers did not reimburse for health promotion visits. MCOs now recognize that anticipatory guidance can be cost-effective, but home visitation programs for the most part still target specific high risk populations, such as adolescents and women at risk for preterm labor.

Home care agencies are subject to regulation by governmental and professional organizations. They provide interdisciplinary services including social work, nutrition, and occupational and physical therapy. Increasingly their case loads are made up of patients who require high-technology care, such as infusions or home monitoring. Although the home health nurse develops the care plan, all care must be ordered by a physician. Additionally, interventions must meet the insurer's criteria for reimbursement, and services are limited to registered patients. Preconception care and low risk antepartum care can usually be provided more efficiently in offices and are not currently reimbursable. High risk antepartum care is often provided by home care agencies. For example, women with hyperemesis gravidarum who require parenteral nutrition may be treated at home. Conditions requiring bed rest, such as preterm labor and hypertension, are other common indications for home care. Other conditions may include cardiac disease, substance abuse, and diabetes in pregnancy.

Some insurers reimburse for at least one postpartum visit to families after early discharge or in the presence of high risk factors. Home phototherapy is used for treatment of neonatal hyperbilirubinemia and to avoid separation of mother and infant. Many other neonates who require long-term high-technology care also are managed with home care. The American Academy of Pediatrics Council on Child and Adolescent Health (1998) recommends home visits as an effective early intervention strategy to improve child health in families at risk.

Patient Selection and Referral

The office- or hospital-based nurse is often the key person in making effective referrals to home care. When a referral to home care is considered, the following factors are evaluated:

- Health status of mother and fetus or infant: Is the condition serious enough to warrant home care? Is it stable enough for intermittent observation to be sufficient?
- Availability of professionals to provide the needed services within the patient's community
- Family resources, including psychosocial, social, and economic resources: Will the family be able to provide care between nursing visits? Are relationships supportive? Is third-party reimbursement available, or can it be negotiated with the insurer? Could a voluntary or tax-supported community agency provide needed care without payment?
- Cost-effectiveness: Is it more reasonable for the patient to receive these services at home or to go to a local outpatient facility to receive them?

Community referrals should not be limited to women with physiologic complications of pregnancy that require medical treatment. Patients at risk (e.g., young adolescents, families with a history of abuse, members of vulnerable population groups, developmentally disabled individuals) may need follow-up care at home. In consultation with the social worker, the hospital-based nurse should become familiar with agencies in the community that accept such referrals. When the patient lives in a rural area, hospital-based nurses should familiarize themselves with available formal and informal resources in that community, as these may be different from those in a more populated setting (Bushy, 2000).

Standardized referral forms simplify the referral process and ensure that all needed information will be forwarded to the home health agency. The nursing assessment should include the woman's physical and psychologic status, her level of knowledge about self-care activities, her willingness to learn, the availability of caregivers and social support in the home, and her level of comfort with home care. If the referral is for a mother and infant home care visit, the nursing assessment should include data about the newborn.

High-technology home care requires additional information to be collected from the medical record and consultation with the referring physician and other members of the health care team before a home care referral is made. Additional data include the medical diagnosis, medical prognosis, prescribed therapies, medication history, drug-dosing information, potential ancillary supplies, type of infusion access device, and the available systems of social support for the patient and family. The nursing assessment and therapies data provide baseline information for the home care nurse and other types of health care providers involved in the care plan.

Whenever a referral is called in to a home health care agency, a member of the nursing or admission staff determines the agency's ability to accept the patient for service. The use of telecommunication such as fax machines, cellular phones, and the Internet to transmit information has eliminated delays in initiating home care services, even in more remote rural areas.

Preparing for the Home Visit

The home care nurse reviews the available clinical data, demographic information, and completed plan of care form and consults with the home care pharmacist or other health care team members who have previously contacted the woman to determine the goals of the visit. At this point the nurse uses the medical diagnosis and place on the perinatal continuum as a starting point to organize the woman's care. The nurse reviews agency policies and procedures, professional literature about diagnosis, and community resources as part of the previsit preparation work (Box 3-4).

Before going on a home visit, the nurse contacts the woman to make necessary arrangements and obtain detailed instructions on the location of the home. Contact by telephone has several goals besides establishing a convenient time to visit and exact directions; it also sets the stage for the first home care visit.

The nurse identifies himself or herself by name, title, and agency. He or she then explains who referred the woman to the agency for home care and the purpose of the home care visits. The nurse briefly explains what will occur during the visit and approximately how long the visit will last. The woman should be asked to restrain any pets during the visit. Last, the nurse asks about health supplies that may be needed for the woman's care.

Before the first visit the home care nurse collects the woman's clinical record, patient education materials, medical supplies, and equipment necessary for the visit. Medications and specialized equipment should be ordered before the visit and delivered at the time of the scheduled visit.

BOX 3-4

Protocol for Perinatal Home Visits

PREVISIT INTERVENTIONS

1 Contact family to arrange details for home visit.
   a. Identify self, credentials, and agency role.
   b. Review purpose of home visit follow-up.
   c. Schedule convenient time for visit.
   d. Confirm address and route to family home.
2 Review and clarify appropriate data.
   a. Review all available assessment data for mother and fetus or infant (e.g., referral forms, hospital discharge summaries, family-identified learning needs).
   b. Review records of any previous nursing contacts.
   c. Contact other professional caregivers as necessary to clarify data (e.g., obstetrician, nurse-midwife, pediatrician, referring nurse).
3 Identify community resources and teaching materials appropriate to meet needs already identified.
4 Plan the visit, and prepare bag with equipment, supplies, and materials necessary for assessments of mother and fetus or infant, actual care anticipated, and teaching.

IN-HOME INTERVENTIONS: ESTABLISHING A RELATIONSHIP

1 Reintroduce self and establish purpose of visit for mother, infant, and family; offer family opportunity to clarify their expectations of contact.
2 Spend brief time socially interacting with family to become acquainted and establish trusting relationship.

IN-HOME INTERVENTIONS: WORKING WITH FAMILY

1 Conduct systematic assessment of mother and fetus or newborn to determine physiologic adjustment and any existing complications.
2 Throughout visit, collect data to assess the emotional adjustment of individual family members to pregnancy or birth and lifestyle changes. Note evidence of family-newborn bonding and sibling rivalry; note relationships among mother, father, children, and grandparents.
3 Determine adequacy of support system.
   a. To what extent does someone help with cooking, cleaning, and other home management tasks?
   b. To what extent is help being provided in caring for the newborn and any other children?
   c. Are support persons encouraging the new mother to care for herself and get adequate rest?
   d. Who is providing helpful information? Emotional support?
4 Throughout the visit, observe home environment for adequacy of resources:
   a. Space: privacy, safe play of children, sleeping
   b. Overall cleanliness and state of repair
   c. Number of steps pregnant woman/new mother must climb

   d. Adequacy of cooking arrangements
   e. Adequacy of refrigeration and other food storage areas
   f. Adequacy of bathing, toilet, and laundry facilities
   g. Arrangements in home for newborn: sleeping, bathing, formula preparation (if needed), layette items, and diapers
5 Throughout the visit, observe home environment for overall state of repair and existence of safety hazards:
   a. Storage of medications, household cleaners, and other substances hazardous to children
   b. Presence of peeling paint on furniture, walls, or pipes
   c. Factors that contribute to falls, such as dim lighting, broken steps, scatter rugs
   d. Presence of vermin
   e. Use of crib or playpen that fails to meet safety guidelines
   f. Existence of emergency plan in case of fire; fire alarm or extinguisher
6 Provide care to mother, newborn, or both as prescribed by their respective primary care provider or in accord with agency protocol.
7 Provide teaching on basis of previously identified needs.
8 Refer family to appropriate community agencies or resources, such as warm lines and support groups.
9 Ascertain that woman knows potential problems to watch for and whom to call if they occur.
10 Ensure that used disposable items have been handled appropriately and that reusable items are cleaned and repacked appropriately in the nurse's bag.

IN-HOME INTERVENTIONS: ENDING THE VISIT

1 Summarize the activities and main points of the visit.
2 Clarify future expectations, including schedule of next visit.
3 Review teaching plan and provide major points in writing.
4 Provide information about reaching the nurse or agency if needed before the next scheduled visit.

POSTVISIT INTERVENTIONS

1 Document the visit thoroughly, using the necessary agency forms to serve as a legal record of the visit and to allow third-party reimbursement, as possible.
2 Initiate the plan of care on which the next encounter with the woman and family will be based.
3 Communicate appropriately (by telephone, letter, progress notes, or referral form) with primary care provider, other health professionals, or referral agencies on behalf of woman and family.

CARE MANAGEMENT ■

First Home Care Visit

Making the first home care visit can be stressful for the nurse and the woman. The home care nurse is faced with an unknown environment controlled by the woman and her family. The woman and her family also experience feelings about the unknown, such as anxiety about the way the nurse will treat them or what the nurse will do during the visit. The challenge for the home care nurse is to establish a nurse-patient relationship and provide the prescribed home care services within the time provided for the initial home visit. One of the most important roles of the home care nurse is modeling health-related behaviors for the patient and others who are in the home during the visit.

Introductions generally begin the visit; the nurse identifies himself or herself and the home care agency. The woman introduces herself and the other family members who are present. Sometimes the woman may feel uncertain of her role or be uncomfortable in taking the lead in introductions, so other people in the home may not be introduced to the nurse. In these situations the nurse can politely ask about other people in the home and their relationship to the woman.

During the first visit to the home, the home care nurse completes extensive documentation with the patient (Fig. 3-5). Before performing any services, the nurse must obtain written agreement and consent for the home health care services. This consent-for-care serves two major purposes: agreement for care and authorization to release medical information. Many third-party payers require written documentation of the services provided; therefore the agency obtains authorization from the woman to give information to her physician and any individual or company involved in payment for the services. Agencies that bill third-party payers for the rendered services will include agreement language for assignment of benefits and financial remuneration. By agreeing to assign insurance benefits to the agency, the woman allows her insurance company to pay the home health care agency directly.

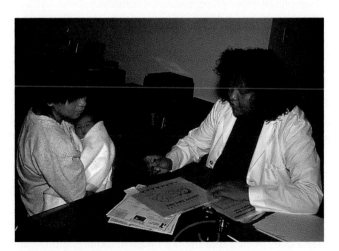

Fig. 3-5 Home care nurse visiting with woman and her infant. (Courtesy Michael S. Clement, MD, Mesa, AZ.)

All patients have the right to participate actively in their plan of care. These patient rights and responsibilities should begin the discussion about the nurse and patient roles during this initial visit.

Assessment and Nursing Diagnoses

The primary goals of the assessment phase are to develop a trusting relationship and collect data by various methods to obtain a comprehensive patient profile. It may not be feasible or appropriate to collect in-depth information about all areas of assessment during the first visit. In many instances, however, the nurse may be limited to one visit and must obtain information pertinent to the current situation in that hour.

The establishment of a trusting relationship begins with the previsit telephone call. An interview style that reflects sensitivity; a nonjudgmental, accepting attitude; and respect for the woman's rights facilitates the development of that trusting relationship. A skillful interviewer avoids barriers to communication such as false reassurance, advice giving, excessive talking, and the showing of approval or disapproval. This nurse-patient relationship continues to develop over the course of home visits.

The nurse is a guest in the woman's home and should show respect for her and her belongings. Some adaptation of the home visit schedule may be made if numerous distractions interrupt a visit, such as caring for the needs of small children. The nurse may ask to have the volume of the television reduced or suggest moving to another room where it is more quiet and private.

The major areas of the assessment are demographics, medical history, general health history, medication history, sociocultural assessment, home and community environment, and physical assessment. Some of this information can be obtained from patient records sent to the home care agency at the time of referral or from the previsit interview. These data will be used to develop the nursing care plan and complete the plan of care, which is required for many licensed home health care agencies. Two areas requiring further discussion are the social assessment and the home environment assessment.

Social assessment includes information regarding the number of people in the family, the roles of each household member, which family members or individuals have taken on the roles of caregivers, and the woman's social support network (Box 3-5). Identifying the roles of each member is helpful for developing the plan of care.

Physical assessment of the home environment is an essential element of the home care assessment. The major areas of the home environment assessment include physical features of the home, access to the home, sanitary conditions, the presence of utilities (e.g., indoor plumbing, telephone, electricity), safety features, and access to transportation and emergency support. Although some of this information can be collected during an interview, physically

BOX 3-5

Psychosocial Assessment

LANGUAGE
- Identify the primary language spoken in the home.
- Assess whether there are any language barriers to receiving support.

COMMUNITY RESOURCES AND ACCESS TO CARE
- Identify primary and secondary means of transportation.
- Identify community agencies the family currently uses for health care and support.
- Assess cultural and psychosocial barriers to receiving care.

SOCIAL SUPPORT
- Determine the people living with the pregnant woman.
- Identify who assists with household chores.
- Identify who assists with child care and parenting activities.
- Identify to whom the pregnant woman turns when problems occur or during a crisis.

INTERPERSONAL RELATIONSHIP
- Identify the way decisions are made in the family.
- Identify the family's perception of the need for home care.
- Identify roles of adults in caring for family members.

CAREGIVER
- Identify the primary caregiver for home care treatments.
- Identify other caregivers and their roles.
- Assess the caregiver's knowledge of treatments and care process.
- Identify potential strain from the caregiver role.
- Identify the level of satisfaction with the caregiver role.

STRESS AND COPING
- Identify what the woman perceives as lifestyle changes and their impact on her and her family.
- Identify the changes she and her family have made to adjust to her health condition and home health care treatments.

inspecting many areas of the home essential to care is a critical part of developing an accurate nursing plan of care. Before any physical inspection, the home care nurse should ask the woman or the caregiver for permission and assistance in identifying areas in the home that will be involved in the caregiving activities. During the physical inspection, careful consideration should be taken to avoid moving personal belongings that are not affected by the care.

Each plan of care has a different emphasis in the home environment. For example, women receiving infusion therapy for hyperemesis gravidarum need a safe place to store medications and infusion supplies that is out of reach of small children living in the home. The home care nurse should incorporate the agency policies and procedures for the storage and handling of infusion supplies into her walk-through inspection. During the walk-through, the home care nurse looks at the potential storage areas that are dry, that are clean, and where the temperature can be maintained. The home care nurse should include an inspection of work areas, such as countertops, tabletops, sinks, and trash areas, that the woman or caregiver may use for mixing medications, changing infusion tubing, handling supplies, or disposing of used equipment and supplies.

The homes of patients using electronic home health care equipment, such as phototherapy equipment or infusion pumps, require physical inspection of electrical outlets, electrical cords, and extension cords that will be used. Homes with faulty electrical wiring may place the patient at risk for being involved in an electrical fire. Faulty wiring may require inspection and repair by a professional electrician before electronic devices are used. Findings from the assessment are incorporated into the plan of care.

Nursing diagnoses are derived from the data collected at the first home visit. Nursing diagnoses for perinatal home health care patients include the following:

- *Deficient knowledge related to*
  —therapeutic regimen management (e.g., nausea and vomiting, preterm labor, gestational diabetes)
  —newborn care and feeding
- *Compromised family coping related to*
  —lack of child care while mother is on bed rest
  —care of newborn receiving oxygen therapy
- *Impaired home maintenance, deficient diversional activity related to*
  —prolonged bed rest at home or in the hospital
- *Impaired parenting related to*
  —maternal immaturity and lack of family support

Expected Outcomes of Care

Examples of expected outcomes for perinatal patients include that the woman and/or her family will do the following:
- Verbalize understanding of treatments
- Use support systems to cope effectively with problems (e.g., pregnancy complications, newborn complications or treatments)
- Perform procedures accurately (e.g., blood glucose monitoring) as evidenced by return demonstration
- Verbalize decreased role strain

Plan of Care and Interventions

The nursing plan of care is developed in collaboration with the patient, based on the health care needs of the individual. Home care nurses working in home health care agencies regulated by the Centers for Medicare and Medicaid Services use a plan of care that includes patient demographics, the health care provider's orders, home care goals, and the level of functioning. This document is initiated at the time of referral to the home care agency and must be updated every 60 days or as specified by state regulations.

The frequency of the skilled nursing visit may vary with the individual plan of care and reimbursement criteria established by the third-party payers (Plan of Care).

Nurse safety and infection control are two important aspects specific to home care.

Safety issues for the home care nurse

The nurse should be fully aware of the home environment and neighborhood in which the home care is being provided. Unlike hospitals, in which the environment is more predictable and controlled, the patient's neighborhood and home have the potential for uncertainty. Home care nurses should take necessary safety precautions and avoid dangerous areas.

Agencies that serve patients in high crime areas may conduct a violence potential assessment by telephone before the visit and enlist the patient's cooperation in minimizing risk. Others have hired full-time security personnel to accompany nurses on their visits. Personal strategies recommended for nurses visiting families with a history of violence or substance abuse include (1) self-awareness; (2) environmental assessment; (3) using listening and observation skills with patients to be aware of behavioral changes indicating aggression or lack of impulse control; (4) planning for dealing with aggressive behavior (e.g., allowing personal space and taking a nonaggressive stance); (5) making visits in pairs; and (6) having access to a cellular phone at all times.

Personal safety. The home care nurse must be aware of personal safety behaviors before going on a home visit. Dress should be casual but professional in appearance, with a name identification tag. Limited jewelry should be worn. Valuable personal items, such as an expensive purse or coat, should not be worn on a visit. Carrying an extra set of car keys in the nursing home care bag saves time and frustration if the nurse becomes locked out of the automobile. Automobile keys spread between the fingers with sharp ends outward can be used as a weapon if necessary. The same commonsense behaviors and precautions that guide a person's behavior when alone in any setting should be followed by home care nurses.

The agency should have a copy of the nurse's home care itinerary, including contact telephone numbers if a patient

---

✍ PLAN OF CARE | *Community and Home Care*

NURSING DIAGNOSIS **Readiness for enhanced family coping related to family growth and development in new community**
Expected Outcome *Family will identify at least three community groups that can serve as appropriate resources for an expectant family with small children.*

Nursing Interventions/*Rationales*

- Assess family structure and availability of significant others, friends, or family members to assist family with new baby and siblings *to provide database for further interventions.*
- Encourage family to enlist assistance of individuals who are available to help family at birth of new baby *to provide physical and emotional support.*
- Using therapeutic communication, assist the family to assess coping strategies used in the past for new situations *to provide clarification and promote empowerment of family in new situations.*
- Suggest strategies to find resources available in the community *to assist family during pregnancy, with new baby, and with small siblings.*
- Give information regarding community workshops, classes, or support groups *to promote networking, community bonding, and support.*

NURSING DIAGNOSIS **Ineffective community management of therapeutic regimen**
Expected Outcome *The community will develop programs to meet the needs of new members of the community.*

Nursing Interventions/*Rationales*

- Conduct a needs assessment of the community *to identify priority needs for new members of the community.*
- Initiate health education programs based on topics identified in the needs assessment *to meet the needs of members of the community.*
- Prepare patient education materials in a variety of languages *to enhance understanding of community members.*
- Identify risks in the community (e.g., environmental hazards, drug sales) *to provide a target for community improvement.*
- With community leaders, develop a plan to cope with and reduce environmental hazard *to improve public health and safety.*
- Develop a monitoring or surveillance system *to ensure that progress will continue and new problems will be identified.*

NURSING DIAGNOSIS **Ineffective community coping**
Expected Outcome *Health status of the community will improve.*

Nursing Interventions/*Rationales*

- Initiate health screening programs for community members *to identify effects of environmental hazards in the community.*
- Work with politicians and policy makers to develop the community *to provide a safe environment with means of economic survival for community members.*
- Initiate programs such as Block Watch, Safe Houses, and Neighborhood Watch *to enhance the safety of the environment.*
- Work with community leaders to develop or clean up playgrounds *to provide a safe place for children to play.*
- With community leaders, develop community grass roots initiatives *to enable community members to take ownership in the community.*
- Identify sites of lead exposure *to decrease the potential for lead poisoning in children.*
- Participate in immunization or vaccination clinics *to reduce the risk in the community of infectious diseases.*

CD: Plan of Care—Community and Home Care

does not have a telephone and information on the nurse's car (make, model, color, and license plate number). Many home care nurses carry agency-provided pagers or cellular telephones that allow the agency to contact the nurse throughout the day to give information about patient updates, changes in orders or services, schedule changes, and new patients who require an initial visit. The telephone also is useful to notify patients when the nurse is delayed.

The automobile used for the home care visits, whether a personal or an agency-owned vehicle, should have regular preventive maintenance checks, an adequate fuel level, and road safety items stored in the trunk. Items to carry in the vehicle include change for telephone calls and tolls, maps, emergency telephone numbers, a flashlight, a first aid kit, flares, a blanket, and equipment for inclement weather conditions. When a visit is made to a patient in a more remote rural setting, other travel considerations may be needed, as well as additional supplies or medication to be taken to the patient (Bushy, 2003).

Home care nurses should park and lock their cars in a safe place that is visible from the street and the patient's home and away from hidden alleys. While driving to the patient's home, the nurse should assess the neighborhood for safety, especially if the neighborhood is unfamiliar. All valuable items should be stored out of sight before the nurse leaves the office. While walking to the patient's home, nurses should not walk near groups of strangers hanging out in doorways or alleys, enter into vacant buildings, or enter a yard that has an unrestrained dog. The home or building should not be entered if the nurse has any safety concerns. Responsibility for safety of home care staff is the responsibility of the agency (McPhaul, 2004). All home care agencies should have policies to follow in such situations.

Unsafe situations in the patient's home. Once inside the woman's home, the nurse may encounter unsafe situations such as the presence of weapons, abusive behavior, or health hazards. Each potentially hazardous situation must be dealt with according to agency policies and procedures. If abuse or neglect is reasonably suspected, the home care nurse should follow home care agency and state and federal regulations for reporting and documenting the situation. Nurses should maintain their own safety first and act accordingly throughout the visit.

Infection control

The nurse carries the necessary supplies and equipment to provide nursing care to the woman. Home care bags should contain infection control supplies, such as personal protection equipment; disposable nonsterile, sterile, and utility gloves; disinfectants; disposable cardiopulmonary resuscitation (CPR) masks; gowns; shoe covers; caps; leakproof and puncture-resistant specimen containers; sharps container; dry hand disinfectants; and leakproof barriers. Proper infection control techniques should be used in stocking, storing, handling, and transporting this bag. When a procedure

is to be performed, the nurse should set up a clean area for necessary supplies. A "dirty" area is designated with a trash bag for the collection of soiled equipment and supplies. Hands are washed before all supplies and equipment for the visit are removed from the bag and placed in a clean area.

The importance of infection control does not diminish because nursing care is provided in the patient's home rather than in a hospital. Patients are not likely to become infected because of their home environment, but the nurse may be exposed to an infectious disease.

Standard Precautions should be used whenever a treatment is performed because it is difficult to determine which patients have a communicable disease (see Box 6-5).

Handwashing remains the single most important infection-control procedure, and the caregiver is in a position to educate about the importance of this practice in preventing disease. Hands should be washed thoroughly for 15 to 20 seconds before and after each patient contact. Wearing gloves does not eliminate the necessity for handwashing. If running water or clean facilities are unavailable, the hands can be cleaned with a self-drying antiseptic solution.

Using gloves reduces the incidence of exposure to bloodborne pathogens. Gloves should be selected according to the nursing activity to be performed. Nonsterile latex or vinyl gloves should be worn for each procedure that has the potential for contact with bodily substances (e.g., performing venipunctures, heel sticks on the newborn, perineal care). Sterile gloves should be worn for clinical procedures requiring sterile technique, such as insertion of peripherally inserted central lines and certain dressing changes. General purpose utility gloves should be used for housekeeping activities, such as cleaning equipment or spills. Nonsterile and sterile gloves should be discarded after each use in a leak-resistant waste receptacle. Utility gloves may be disinfected and reused.

Disposable personal protection equipment should be removed after each use and discarded in a plastic trash container. Safety glasses or goggles can be cleaned with soap and water after each use.

Whenever specimens are collected, Standard Precautions should be used. Any specimen of bodily fluids should be placed in a leakproof bag and secured in a puncture-proof container. The outside of the container is washed off, if it was soiled, before the container is transported. Specimens should be labeled with the woman's or infant's name and additional identifying information according to the home health care agency or laboratory policies. If specimens are being transported, they should be placed in a container on a flat surface in the vehicle. An insulated container may be used to keep specimens cool in transit. The nurse should be aware of the time-sensitive nature of laboratory procedures for certain types of specimens.

Sharps containers are puncture-proof and leakproof containers labeled with a biohazard sign on the outside and should be used to collect needles and sharp objects (Fig. 3-6). Patients are instructed to fill containers between two thirds

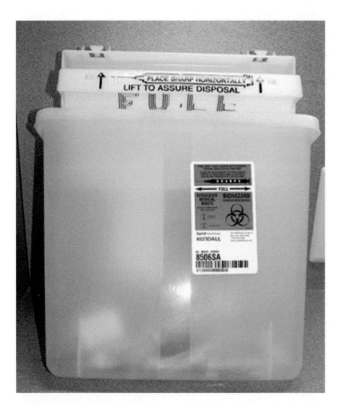

Fig. 3-6 Sharps container. (Courtesy Shannon Perry, Phoenix, AZ.)

and three fourths full to prevent spillage of their contents. As part of the patient teaching process, information about storage and handling is covered by the home care nurse. When the container reaches its maximal capacity, it should be returned to the home health care agency and replaced. Medical waste, such as urine and secretions, can be discarded through the sewer or septic system.

Contaminated dressings and disposable supplies should be placed in a leakproof plastic bag and securely fastened for disposal at the patient's home. The patient should be instructed regarding the proper disposal of medical waste in the home. Agency policies and procedures and local waste management ordinances should be consulted before the patient is instructed.

Nursing Considerations

In home care the woman or family members are responsible for administration of medications in the absence of the nurse. A careful medication history should be obtained to see if the woman is taking her medications correctly and understands the desired action and potential side effects. Sometimes when orders are changed, women continue to take both the old and new prescriptions, which can lead to dangerous overdoses or medication interactions. The nurse ensures that there is an adequate supply and a safe place for proper storage of medications to prevent deterioration or accidental ingestion by children or pets. The nurse

inquires about any other medications that the woman might be taking concurrently. Over-the-counter drugs or herbal supplements may not be considered medications by the women and not mentioned unless such information is specifically asked for. Even more important is ensuring that the patient and her caregivers fully understand the information that they are exposed to by health care providers.

High-technology home care involves many diagnostic and therapeutic procedures. A focused physical assessment is always part of the visit. Nurses involved in perinatal home care must be skilled in prenatal, postpartal, and newborn assessment. Many women require additional diagnostic tests. The nurse may need to collect blood or other specimens. Portable fetal monitoring equipment or even ultrasound can be used in the home for fetal assessment. Home infusion for women with hyperemesis gravidarum often replaces hospitalization. Women with preterm labor may receive parenteral tocolytic therapy. Phototherapy or apnea monitors can be provided in the home for newborns. The power supply and wiring must be reliable. Family members may need to be taught to monitor equipment between nurse visits and to prevent accidental damage.

Medical emergencies may occur during or between the nurse's visits to the home. Prior planning and education can reduce the risk of problems. All parents of newborns should know infant CPR. There should be immediate telephone access to call for emergency medical assistance. Women and their families should be taught to recognize danger signs related to their condition. For example, women at risk for preterm labor should learn to palpate the uterus and recognize contractions in the absence of pain; women with diabetes must learn the signs of hypoglycemia and what to do if it occurs; women with preeclampsia must know the danger signs that indicate worsening of their condition and to notify the health care provider immediately. In a more remote rural community that does not have an obstetrician in the region, the nurse may need to assist the patient's family to arrange for "boarding" somewhere that is closer to a medical specialist.

Patient and family education in home care includes information about the specific high risk condition(s) involved, implications for pregnancy outcome, and measures for self-monitoring. Verbal explanations should be supplemented with clearly written instructions. General information to promote well-being, such as about nutrition and common discomforts of pregnancy, also should be included. The need for preparation for childbirth can be addressed by using books or videos that are supplemented by individual teaching at home. Coping with bed rest or other limitation of activity is a problem for many women with high risk pregnancies. The nurse may share strategies that others have used, help with time management, and provide information about support services. Teaching about infant care or the special needs of the preterm infant may be appropriate during the prenatal period.

Clear documentation of assessments, problems identified, treatments and interventions performed, and the patient's responses is essential. Third-party payers base reimbursement on the nurse's written record of providing skilled nursing care and assessments that support the woman's continuing need for those services. The nurse must promptly inform the health care provider by telephone or facsimile of any significant changes. When new orders are transmitted by telephone, a written copy must be sent for the physician's signature.

The home care nurse continually reassesses the patient's condition and response to the interventions during every home visit and revises the nursing diagnoses and plan of care. Nursing documentation should reflect an objective description of the nursing assessment data collected at each visit. Statements such as "no change" or "same as last visit" do not accurately reflect the monitoring of the patient condition that occurred during the skilled nursing visit. Once the home care outcomes are achieved and the patient is discharged from the home care agency, documentation should include information about the patient's status at the time of discharge, progress toward attaining health care goals, and plans for follow-up care.

The role of the clinical record in home care has been affected by social, economic, and legal health care changes. Appropriate care should be taken to complete the necessary home health care records accurately and in a timely manner. Documentation guidelines include writing or dictating notes or using a laptop computer at the patient's home or shortly after the visit.

Evaluation

Evaluation is based on the expected outcomes of care. The plan is revised as necessary.

> ## COMMUNITY ACTIVITY
>
> Identify at least two cultural groups in your community. Read your local newspaper and identify articles describing health needs of vulnerable populations within these two groups in your community. Consult the yellow pages of the telephone book. Are there agencies in your area that specifically deal with meeting those needs? If you encountered a patient with one of the needs, to whom would you refer her?

Key Points

- A community is defined as a locality-based entity composed of systems of societal institutions, informal groups, and aggregates that are interdependent and whose function is to meet a wide variety of collective needs.
- Of necessity, most changes aimed at improving community health involve partnerships among community residents and health workers.
- Methods of collecting data useful to the nurse working in the community include walking surveys, analysis of existing data, informant interviews, and participant observation.
- Vulnerable populations are groups who are at higher risk for developing physical, mental, or social health problems.
- Perinatal home care is a unique nursing practice that incorporates knowledge from community health nursing, acute care nursing, family therapy, health promotion, and patient education.

- Social and economic factors affect the scope of perinatal nursing practice.
- Perinatal home care can be provided for women and infants throughout the perinatal period, beginning before conception and ending in the postpartum period.
- Perinatal home care nurses should incorporate personal safety and infection control practices in the nursing plan of care.
- Telephonic nurse advice lines, telephonic nursing assessments, and warm lines are low-cost health care services that facilitate continuous patient education, support, and health care decision making, even though health care is delivered in multiple sites.
- Communication protocols among members of the home health care team are critical to diminish fragmentation and duplication of health care services.

Answer Guidelines to Critical Thinking Exercise

Health Needs of a Migrant Worker

1 No, there is not sufficient evidence. The nurse needs to establish baseline data and understanding of the mother within her culture and perform an assessment before mutual goal setting.
2 a. The goals must be realistic, not just idealistic.
   b. Both mother and infant need adequate nutrition and rest.

   c. Maintaining breastfeeding while working long hours in the field is difficult if not impossible.
   d. Including other family members in the care of the infant will assist the mother. Including the father may be neither culturally appropriate nor possible given his work hours.

3 Priority for care is to ensure that the infant and mother obtain adequate nutrition. If the mother cannot breastfeed, a safe source of nutrition must be provided. Refrigeration must be available, as well as a source of safe water. WIC may be a source of formula for the infant and food for the mother. In this setting, powdered formula may be the safest form of milk because each feeding can be prepared at the time of feeding.

4 Yes. Standards of care dictate that the mother and infant need adequate nutrition, as well as sleep and rest.

5 There are no data to indicate whether or not the father of the baby is involved or that his involvement is culturally appropriate. Because the mother is Vietnamese speaking, a nurse who speaks Vietnamese or an interpreter must be involved. There also may be need for a bed and clothing and other supplies for the infant. Sources of family support should be ascertained. Whether there are other community agencies or groups that can provide assistance should be ascertained.

Resources

Bushy A. (2002). *Resource manual: Rural minorities, their health issues and resources.* Kansas City, MO: National Rural Health Association.

Centers for Medicare and Medicaid Services
7500 Security Blvd
Baltimore, MD 21244-1850
www.cms.hhs.gov

Community Health Status Indicators
Public Health Foundation
1300 L. St., NW, Suite 800
Washington, DC 20005
www.phf.org

National Association of County and City Health Officials
1100 17th St., NW, Second Floor
Washington, DC 20036
202-783-5550
202-783-1583 (fax)
www.naccho.org

The Children's Partnership
2000 P St., NW, Suite 330
Washington, DC 20036
202-429-0033
202-429-0974 (fax)
www.childrenspartnership.org

The Provider's Guide to Quality and Care
Management Sciences for Health
784 Memorial Dr.
Cambridge, MA 02139
617-250-9500
617-250-9090 (fax)
http://www.msh.org

U.S. Department of Health and Human Services
Centers for Disease Control and Prevention
1600 Clifton Rd.
Atlanta, GA 30333
404-639-3311
www.cdc.gov

U.S. Department of Health and Human Services
Health Resources and Services Administration (HRSA)
Parklawn Building
5600 Fishers Ln
Rockville, MD 20857
www.hrsa.gov/

U.S. Department of Health and Human Services
Office on Women's Health. (2001). *Women's health issues: An overview*
Internet document available at www.womenshealth.gov (accessed November 28, 2004).

References

American Academy of Pediatrics Council on Child and Adolescent Health. (1998). The role of home-visitation programs in improving health outcomes for children and families. *Pediatrics, 101*(3 Pt 1), 486-489.

Anderson, E., & McFarlane, J. (2004). *Community as partner: Theory and practice in nursing* (4th ed.). Philadelphia: Lippincott Williams & Wilkins.

Association of Women's Health, Obstetric and Neonatal Nurses (AWHONN). (1994). *Didactic content and clinical skills verification for professional nurse providers of perinatal home care.* Washington, DC: AWHONN.

Association of Women's Health, Obstetric and Neonatal Nurses (AWHONN). (1998). *Standards and guidelines for professional nursing practice in the care of women and newborns* (5th ed.). Washington, DC: AWHONN.

Association of Women's Health, Obstetric and Neonatal Nurses (AWHONN). (2004). *Every woman: The essential guide for healthy living* (5th ed.). Washington, DC: AWHONN.

Bruhn, J. (2001). Ethical issues in intervention outcomes. *Family & Community Health, 23*(4), 24-35.

Bureau of Primary Health Care. (2001). *Homeless population statistics.* Washington, DC: Bureau of Primary Health Care. Internet document available at www.hrsa.bphc.gov (accessed November 29, 2004).

Bushy, A. (2000). *Orientation to nursing in the rural community.* Thousand Oaks, CA: Sage.

Bushy, A. (2003). Strategies to facilitate communication with clients of another culture. *Lippincott's Case Management, 8*(5), 214-223.

Clemen-Stone, S. (2002). Community assessment and diagnosis. In S. Clemen-Stone, S. McGuire, & D. Eigsti (Eds.), *Comprehensive community health nursing: Family, aggregate, and community practice* (6th ed.). St. Louis: Mosby.

Coren, E., & Barlow, J. (2001). Individual and group-based parenting programmes for improving psychosocial outcomes for teenage parents and their children (Cochrane Review). In *The Cochrane Library,* Issue 2, 2004. Chichester, UK: John Wiley & Sons.

Economic Research Service. (2003). *Farm labor: Demographic characteristics of hired farmworkers.* U.S. Department of Agriculture. Internet document available at www.ers.usda.gov/Briefing/Farmlabor/ Demographics (accessed April 10, 2005).

Ervin, N. (2002). *Advanced community health nursing practice: Population-focused care.* Upper Saddle River, NJ: Prentice Hall Health.

Essential Public Health Services Work Group of the Public Health Functions Steering Committee. Internet document available at www.phf.org/essential.htm (accessed April 12, 2005).

Health Resources and Services Administration. (2004). *Women's Health USA 2004.* Vienna, VA: U.S. Department of Health and Human Services.

Kuehnert, P. (2002). Overview of program planning. In N. Ervin (Ed.), *Advanced community health nursing practice.* Upper Saddle River, NJ: Prentice Hall Health.

Lauderdale, M. (2001). Issues in securing the community's sanction before making an intervention. *Family & Community Health, 23*(4), 1-8.

Martin, J., Kochanek, K., Strobino, D., Guyer, B., & MacDorman, M. (2005). Annual summary of vital statistics–2003. *Pediatrics, 115*(3), 619-634.

McDevitt, J., & Wilbur, J. (2002). Locating sources of data. In N. Ervin (Ed.), *Advanced community health nursing practice: Population-focused care.* Upper Saddle River, NJ: Prentice Hall Health.

McGuire, S. (2002). Occupational health nursing. In S. Clemen-Stone, S. McGuire, & D. Eigsti (Eds.), *Comprehensive community health nursing: Family, aggregate, & community practice* [6th ed.]. St. Louis: Mosby.

McPhaul, K. (2004). Home care security. *American Journal of Nursing, 104*(9), 96.

Minino, A., et al. (2002). Deaths: Final data for 2000. *National Vital Statistics Report, 50*(15), 1-119.

Murray, R., Zentner, J., & Samiezade-Yazd, C. (2001). Sociocultural influences on the person and family. In R. Murray & J. Zentner (Eds.), *Health promotion strategies through the lifespan* (7th ed.). Upper Saddle River, NJ: Prentice Hall Health.

National Academy Press. (2002). *From generation to generation: The health and well-being of children in immigrant families.* Internet document available at http://search.nap.edu/html/generation/summary.html (accessed November 29, 2004).

Pender, N., Murdaugh, C., & Parsons, M. (2002). *Health promotion in nursing practice,* Upper Saddle River, NJ: Prentice Hall Health.

U.S. Department of Health and Human Services. (1991). Consensus set of indicators for assessing community health status. *Morbidity and Mortality Weekly Report, 40*(27), 449.

U.S. Department of Health and Human Services (USDHHS). (2000a). *Healthy people 2010: Understanding and improving health.* Washington, DC: U.S. Department of Health and Human Services, U.S. Government Printing Office.

U.S. Department of Health and Human Services (USDHHS). (2000b). Chapter 16: Maternal, infant, and child health. In *Healthy People 2010.* Internet document available at www.health.gov/healthypeople/Document/HTML/Volume2/16MICH.htm (accessed November 28, 2004).

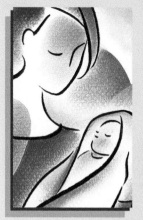

CHAPTER 4

Assessment and Health Promotion

DEITRA LEONARD LOWDERMILK

LEARNING OBJECTIVES

- Identify the structures and functions of the female reproductive system.
- Compare the hypothalamic-pituitary, ovarian, and endometrial cycles of menstruation.
- Identify the four phases of the sexual response cycle.
- Identify reasons why women enter the health care delivery system.
- Discuss financial, cultural, and gender barriers to seeking health care.
- Explain conditions and characteristics that increase health risks.

- Outline the components of taking a woman's history and performing a physical examination.
- Discuss how assessment and physical examination can be adapted for women with special needs.
- Identify the correct procedure for assisting with and collecting specimens for Papanicolaou testing.
- Review health promotion and prevention suggestions for the common health risks.

KEY TERMS AND DEFINITIONS

breast self-examination (BSE) Systematic examination of the breasts by the woman

climacteric The period of a woman's life when she is passing from a reproductive to a nonreproductive state, with regression of ovarian function; the cycle of endocrine, physical, and psychosocial changes that occurs during the termination of the reproductive years; also called *climacterium*

cycle of violence Violence against a woman (usually) occurs in a pattern consisting of three phases: period of increasing tension, the abusive episode, and a period of contrition and kindness

Kegel exercises Pelvic muscle exercises to strengthen the pubococcygeal muscles

menarche Onset, or beginning, of menstrual function

menopause From the Greek words *mensis* (month) and *pausis* (cessation), the actual permanent cessation of menstrual cycles; so diagnosed after 1 year without menses

menstrual cycle A complex interplay of events that occur simultaneously in the endometrium, the hypothalamus and pituitary glands, and the ovaries that results in ovarian and uterine preparation for pregnancy

menstruation Periodic vaginal discharge of bloody fluid from the nonpregnant uterus that occurs from the age of puberty to menopause

ovulation Periodic ripening and discharge of the ovum from the ovary, usually 14 days before the onset of menstrual flow

Papanicolaou (Pap) test (or smear) Microscopic examination using scrapings from the cervix, endocervix, or other mucous membranes that will reveal, with a high degree of accuracy, the presence of premalignant or malignant cells

perimenopause Period of transition of changing ovarian activity before menopause and through the first few years of amenorrhea

preconception care Care designed for health maintenance and health promotion for the general and reproductive health of all women of childbearing potential

prostaglandins (PGs) Substances present in many body tissues; have roles in many reproductive tract functions; used to induce abortions and for cervical ripening for labor induction

sexual response cycle The phases of physical changes that occur in response to sexual stimulation and sexual tension release

squamocolumnar junction Site in the endocervical canal where columnar epithelium and squamous epithelium meet; also called *transformation zone*

vulvar self-examination (VSE) Systematic examination of the vulva by the woman

Many women initially enter the health care system because of some reproductive system–related situation, such as pregnancy; irregular menses; desire for contraception; or episodic illness, such as vaginal infection. Once women are in the system, however, it is incumbent on health care providers to recognize the need for health promotion and preventive health maintenance and to provide these services as part of lifelong care for women. This chapter reviews female anatomy and physiology, including the menstrual cycle. Physical assessment and screening for disease prevention for women in their reproductive years is presented. Barriers to seeking health care and an overview of conditions and circumstances that increase health risks in the childbearing years are discussed. Anticipatory guidance suggestions for health promotion and prevention are also included.

FEMALE REPRODUCTIVE SYSTEM

External Structures

The external genital organs, or vulva, include all structures visible externally from the pubis to the perineum: the mons pubis, labia majora, labia minora, clitoris, vestibular

glands, vaginal vestibule, vaginal orifice, and urethral opening (Fig. 4-1) The mons pubis is a fatty pad that lies over the anterior surface of the symphysis pubis. In the postpubertal female, the mons is covered with coarse curly hair. The labia majora are two rounded folds of fatty tissue covered with skin that extend downward and backward from the mons pubis. The labia are highly vascular structures that develop hair on the outer surfaces after puberty. They protect the inner vulvar structures. The labia minora are two flat, reddish folds of tissue visible when the labia majora are separated. Anteriorly, the labia minora fuse to form the prepuce (hoodlike covering of the clitoris) and the frenulum (fold of tissue under the clitoris). The labia minora join to form a thin flat tissue called the *fourchette* underneath the vaginal opening at midline. The clitoris is located underneath the prepuce. It is a small structure composed of erectile tissue with numerous sensory nerve endings.

The vaginal vestibule is an almond-shaped area enclosed by the labia minora that contains openings to the urethra, Skene glands, vagina, and Bartholin glands. The urethra is not a reproductive organ but is considered here because of its location. It usually is found approximately 2.5 cm below the clitoris. The Skene glands are located on each side of the urethra and produce mucus, which aids in lubrication of

CD: Anatomy Review—External Female Genitalia

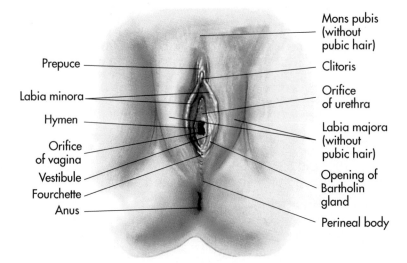

Fig. 4-1 External female genitalia.

the vagina. The vaginal opening is in the lower portion of the vestibule and varies in shape and size. The hymen, a connective tissue membrane, surrounds the vaginal opening. Bartholin glands (see Fig. 4-1) lie under the constrictor muscles of the vagina and are located posteriorly on the sides of the vaginal opening, although the ductal openings are usually not visible. During sexual arousal the glands secrete a clear mucus to lubricate the vaginal introitus.

The area between the fourchette and the anus is the *perineum*, a skin-covered muscular area that covers the pelvic structures. The perineum forms the base of the perineal body, a wedged-shaped mass that serves as an anchor for the muscles, fascia, and ligaments of the pelvis. The pelvic organs are supported by muscles and ligaments that form a sling.

Internal Structures

The internal structures include the vagina, uterus, uterine tubes, and ovaries. The vagina is a fibromuscular, collapsible tubular structure that extends from the vulva to the uterus and lies between the bladder and rectum. During the reproductive years the mucosal lining is arranged in transverse folds called *rugae*. These rugae allow the vagina to expand during childbirth. Estrogen deprivation that occurs after childbirth, during lactation, and at menopause causes dryness and thinness of the vaginal walls and smoothing of the rugae. Vaginal secretions are acidic (pH 4 to 5), so the vagina's susceptibility to infections is reduced. The vagina serves as a passageway for menstrual flow, as a female organ of copulation, and as a part of the birth canal for vaginal childbirth. The uterine cervix projects into a blind vault at the upper end of the vagina. Anterior, posterior, and lateral pockets called *fornices* surround the cervix. The internal pelvic organs can be palpated through the thin walls of these fornices.

The uterus is a muscular organ shaped like an upside-down pear that sits midline in the pelvic cavity between the bladder and rectum above the vagina. Four pairs of ligaments support the uterus: the cardinal, uterosacral, round, and broad. Single anterior and posterior ligaments also support the uterus. The cul-de-sac of Douglas is a deep pouch, or recess, posterior to the cervix and formed by the posterior ligament.

The uterus is divided into two major parts: an upper triangular portion called the *corpus* and a lower cylindric portion called the *cervix* (Fig. 4-2). The fundus is the dome-shaped top of the uterus and is the site where the uterine tubes enter the uterus. The isthmus (lower uterine segment) is a short, constricted portion that separates the corpus from the cervix.

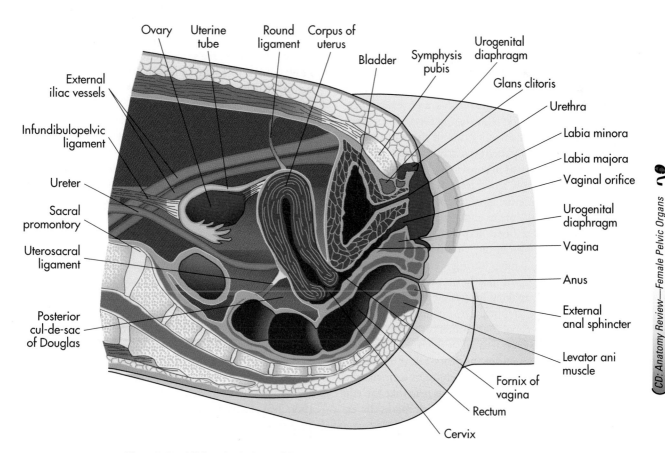

Fig. 4-2 Midsagittal view of female pelvic organs, with woman lying supine.

CD: Anatomy Review—Female Pelvic Organs

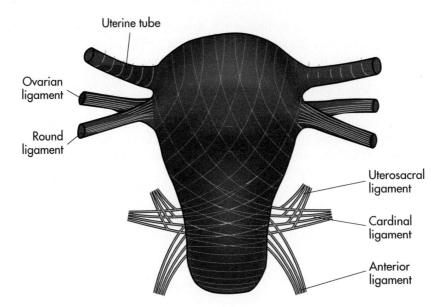

Fig. 4-3   Schematic arrangement of directions of muscle fibers. Note that uterine muscle fibers are continuous with supportive ligaments of uterus.

The uterus serves for reception, implantation, retention, and nutrition of the fertilized ovum and later the fetus during pregnancy and expulsion of the fetus during childbirth. It also is responsible for cyclic menstruation.

The uterine wall consists of three layers: the endometrium, the myometrium, and part of the peritoneum. The endometrium is a highly vascular lining made up of three layers, the outer two of which are shed during menstruation. The myometrium is made up of layers of smooth muscles that extend in three different directions (longitudinal, transverse, and oblique) (Fig. 4-3). Longitudinal fibers of the outer myometrial layer are found mostly in the fundus, and this arrangement assists in expelling the fetus during the birth process. The middle layer contains fibers from all three directions, which form a figure-eight pattern encircling large blood vessels. This arrangement assists in constricting blood vessels after childbirth and controls blood loss. Most of the circular fibers of the inner myometrial layer are around the site where the uterine tubes enter the uterus and around the internal cervical os (opening). These fibers help keep the cervix closed during pregnancy and prevent menstrual blood from flowing back into the uterine tubes during menstruation.

The cervix is made up of mostly fibrous connective tissues and elastic tissue, making it possible for the cervix to stretch during vaginal childbirth. The opening between the uterine cavity and the canal that connects the uterine cavity to the vagina (endocervical canal) is the internal os. The narrowed opening between the endocervix and the vagina is the external os, a small circular opening in women who have never been pregnant. The cervix feels firm (like the end of a nose) with a dimple in the center, which marks the external os.

The outer cervix is covered with a layer of squamous epithelium. The mucosa of the cervical canal is covered with columnar epithelium and contains numerous glands that secrete mucus in response to ovarian hormones. The squamocolumnar junction, where the two types of cells meet, is usually located just inside the cervical os. This junction is also called the *transformation zone* and is the most common site for neoplastic changes; cells from this site are scraped for the Papanicolaou (Pap) test (see p. 90).

The uterine tubes (fallopian tubes) attach to the uterine fundus. The tubes are supported by the broad ligaments and range from 8 to 14 cm in length. The uterine tubes provide a passage between the ovaries and the uterus for the passage of the ovum.

The ovaries are almond-shaped organs located on each side of the uterus below and behind the uterine tubes. During the reproductive years, they are approximately 3 cm long, 2 cm wide, and 1 cm thick; they diminish in size after menopause. The two functions of the ovaries are ovulation and production of estrogen, progesterone, and androgen.

Bony Pelvis

The bony pelvis serves three primary purposes: protection of the pelvic structures, accommodation of the growing fetus during pregnancy, and anchorage of the pelvic support structures. Two innominate (hip) bones (consisting of ilium, ischium, and pubis), the sacrum, and the coccyx make up the four bones of the pelvis (Fig. 4-4). Cartilage and ligaments form the symphysis pubis, sacrococcygeal, and two sacroiliac joints that separate the pelvic bones. The pelvis is divided into two parts: the false pelvis and the true pelvis (Fig. 4-5). The false pelvis is the upper portion above the pelvic brim or inlet. The true pelvis is the lower curved bony canal, which includes the inlet, the cavity, and the outlet through which the fetus passes during vaginal birth.

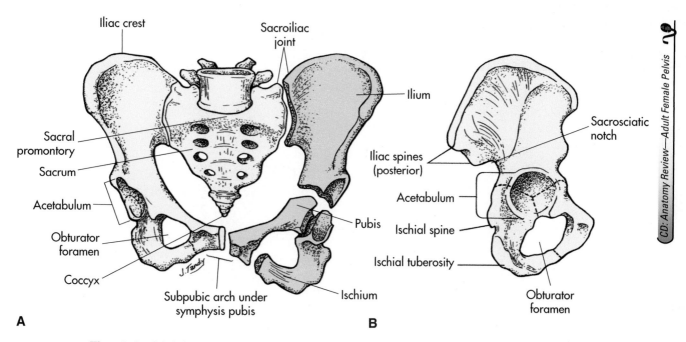

Fig. 4-4 Adult female pelvis. **A,** Anterior view. **B,** External view of innominate bone (fused).

Variations that occur in the size and shape of the pelvis are usually a result of age, race, and injury. Pelvic ossification is complete by approximately 20 years of age.

Breasts

The breasts are paired mammary glands located between the second and sixth ribs (Fig. 4-6). Approximately two thirds of the breast overlies the pectoralis major muscle, between the sternum and midaxillary line, with an extension to the axilla referred to as the *tail of Spence.* The lowest third of the

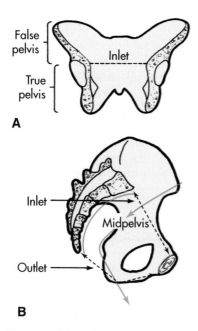

Fig. 4-5 Female pelvis. **A,** Cavity of false pelvis is shallow. **B,** Cavity of true pelvis is an irregularly curved canal *(arrows).*

breast overlies the serratus anterior muscle. The breasts are attached to the muscles by connective tissue called fascia.

The breasts of healthy mature women are approximately equal in size and shape but are often not absolutely symmetric. The size and shape vary depending on the woman's age, heredity, and nutrition. However, the contour should be smooth with no retractions, dimpling, or masses. Estrogen stimulates growth of the breast by inducing fat deposition in the breasts, development of stromal tissue (i.e., increase in its amount and elasticity), and growth of the extensive ductile system. Estrogen also increases the vascularity of breast tissue. The increase in progesterone at puberty causes maturation of mammary gland tissue, specifically the lobules and acinar structures. During adolescence, fat deposition and growth of fibrous tissue contribute to the increase in the gland's size.

Each mammary gland is made of 15 to 20 lobes, which are divided into lobules. Lobules are clusters of acini. An acinus is a saclike terminal part of a compound gland emptying through a narrow lumen or duct. The acini are lined with epithelial cells that secrete colostrum and milk. Just below the epithelium is the myoepithelium (*myo,* or muscle), which contracts to expel milk from the acini.

The ducts from the clusters of acini that form the lobules merge to form larger ducts draining the lobes. Ducts from the lobes converge in a single nipple (mammary papilla) surrounded by an areola. Just as the ducts converge, they dilate to form common lactiferous sinuses, which are also called ampullae. The lactiferous sinuses serve as milk reservoirs. Many tiny lactiferous ducts drain the ampullae and exit in the nipple.

The glandular structures and ducts are surrounded by protective fatty tissue and are separated and supported by

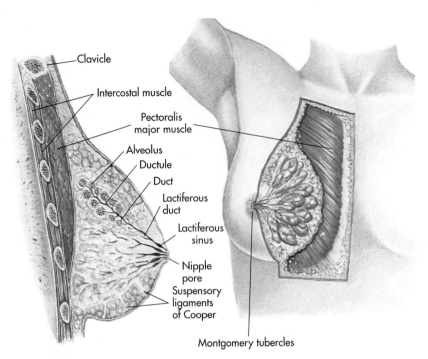

Fig. 4-6 Anatomy of the breast, showing position and major structures. (From Seidel, H., Ball, J., Dains, J., & Benedict, G. [2003]. *Mosby's guide to physical examination* [5th ed.]. St. Louis: Mosby.)

fibrous suspensory Cooper's ligaments. Cooper's ligaments provide support to the mammary glands while permitting their mobility on the chest wall (see Fig. 4-6). The round nipple is usually slightly elevated above the breast. On each breast the nipple projects slightly upward and laterally. It contains 15 to 20 openings from lactiferous ducts. The nipple is surrounded by fibromuscular tissue and covered by wrinkled skin (the areola). Except during pregnancy and lactation, there is usually no discharge from the nipple.

The nipple and surrounding areola are usually more deeply pigmented than the skin of the breast. The rough appearance of the areola is caused by sebaceous glands, Montgomery tubercles (see Fig. 4-6), directly beneath the skin. These glands secrete a fatty substance thought to lubricate the nipple.

The vascular supply to the mammary gland is abundant. The skin covering the breasts contains an extensive superficial lymphatic network that serves the entire chest wall and is continuous with the superficial lymphatics of the neck and abdomen. In the deeper portions of the breasts, the lymphatics form a rich network as well. The primary deep lymphatic pathway drains laterally toward the axillae.

The breasts change in size and nodularity in response to cyclic ovarian changes throughout reproductive life. Increasing levels of both estrogen and progesterone in the 3 to 4 days before menstruation increase vascularity of the breasts, induce growth of the ducts and acini, and promote water retention. As a result, breast swelling, tenderness, and discomfort are common symptoms just before the onset of menstruation. After menstruation, cellular proliferation begins to regress, acini begin to decrease in size, and retained water is lost. In time, after repeated hormonal stimulation, small persistent areas of nodulations may develop just before and during menstruation, when the breast is most active. The physiologic alterations in breast size and activity reach their minimum level approximately 5 to 7 days after menstruation stops. Therefore breast self-examination (BSE) is best carried out during this phase of the menstrual cycle (see Patient Instructions for Self-Care box).

Menstruation
Menarche and puberty

Puberty is a broad term that denotes the entire transitional stage between childhood and sexual maturity. Although young girls secrete small, rather constant amounts of estrogen, a marked increase occurs between 8 and 11 years of age. The term menarche denotes first menstruation. In North America this occurs in most girls at about 13 years of age.

Although pregnancy can occur in exceptional cases of true precocious puberty, most pregnancies in young girls occur after the normally timed menarche. All girls would benefit from knowing pregnancy can occur at any time after the onset of menses.

Menstrual cycle

Initially, menstrual periods are irregular, unpredictable, painless, and anovulatory. After the ovary produces adequate cyclic estrogen to make a mature ovum, periods tend to be regular and ovulatory. The menstrual cycle is a complex interplay of events that occur simultaneously in the endometrium, hypothalamus and pituitary glands, and ovaries. The menstrual cycle prepares the uterus for pregnancy. When

PATIENT INSTRUCTIONS FOR SELF-CARE
Breast Self-Examination

1 The best time to do breast self-examination is about a week after your period, when breasts are not tender or swollen. If you do not have regular periods or sometimes skip a month, do it on the same day every month. If you are breastfeeding or no longer menstruating, choose a date and examine your breasts at the same time each month.

2 Lie down and put a pillow under your right shoulder. Place your right arm behind your head (Fig. 1).

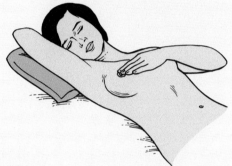

Fig. 1

3 Use the finger pads of your three middle fingers on your left hand to feel for lumps or thickening. Your finger pads are the top third of each finger.

4 Press firmly enough to know how your breast feels. If you're not sure how hard to press, ask your health care provider or try to copy the way your health care provider uses the finger pads during a breast examination. Learn what your breast feels like most of the time. A firm ridge in the lower curve of each breast is normal.

5 Move around the breast in a set way. You can choose either circles (Fig. 2, *A*), vertical lines (Fig. 2, *B*), or wedges (Fig. 2, *C*). Do it the same way every time. It will help you to make sure that you've gone over the entire breast area and to remember how your breast feels.

6 Gently compress the nipple between your thumb and forefinger and look for discharge.

7 Now examine your left breast using the finger pads of your right hand.

8 If you find any changes, see your health care provider right away.

9 You may want to check your breasts while standing in front of a mirror right after you do your breast self-examination each month. See if there are any changes in the way your breasts look: dimpling of the skin, changes in the nipple, or redness or swelling.

10 You may also want to do an extra breast self-examination while you're in the shower (Fig. 3). Your soapy hands will glide over the wet skin, making it easy to check how your breasts feel.

11 It is important to check the area between the breast and the underarm and the underarm itself. Also examine the area above the breast to the collarbone and to the shoulder.

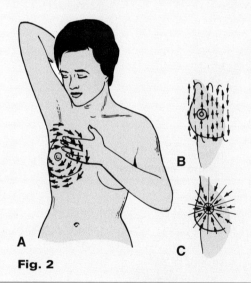

A   **B**   **C**   **Fig. 2**

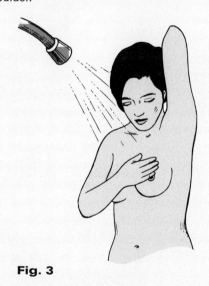

Fig. 3

pregnancy does not occur, menstruation follows. **Menstruation** is the periodic uterine bleeding that begins approximately 14 days after ovulation. The average length of a menstrual cycle is 28 days, but variations are common. The first day of bleeding is designated as day 1 of the menstrual cycle, or menses (Fig. 4-7). The average duration of menstrual flow is 5 days (range of 3 to 6 days), and the average blood loss is 50 ml (range of 20 to 80 ml), but these vary greatly.

The woman's age, physical and emotional status, and environment also influence the regularity of her menstrual cycles.

Hypothalamic-pituitary cycle.   Toward the end of the normal menstrual cycle, blood levels of estrogen and progesterone fall. Low blood levels of these ovarian hormones stimulate the hypothalamus to secrete gonadotropin-releasing hormone (GnRH). In turn, GnRH stimulates anterior pituitary secretion of follicle-stimulating hormone

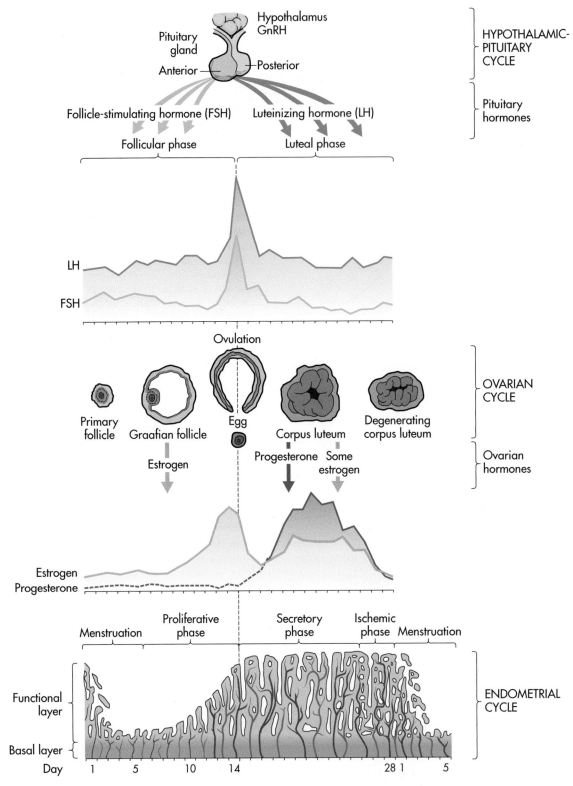

Fig. 4-7 Menstrual cycle: hypothalamic-pituitary, ovarian, and endometrial.

(FSH). FSH stimulates development of ovarian graafian follicles and their production of estrogen. Estrogen levels begin to fall, and hypothalamic GnRH triggers the anterior pituitary release of luteinizing hormone (LH). A marked surge of LH and a smaller peak of estrogen (day 12; see Fig. 4-7)

precede the expulsion of the ovum (ovulation) from the graafian follicle by approximately 24 to 36 hours. LH peaks at approximately the thirteenth or fourteenth day of a 28-day cycle. If fertilization and implantation of the ovum do not occur by this time, the corpus luteum regresses. Levels of progesterone and estrogen decline, menstruation occurs, and the hypothalamus is once again stimulated to secrete GnRH. This process is termed the *hypothalamic-pituitary cycle.*

Ovarian cycle. The primitive graafian follicles contain immature oocytes (primordial ova). Before ovulation, from 1 to 30 follicles begin to mature in each ovary under the influence of FSH and estrogen. The preovulatory surge of LH affects a selected follicle. The oocyte matures, ovulation occurs, and the empty follicle begins its transformation into the corpus luteum. This follicular phase (preovulatory phase) (see Fig. 4-7) of the ovarian cycle varies in length from woman to woman and accounts for almost all variations in ovarian cycle length. On rare occasions (approximately 1 in 100 menstrual cycles), more than one follicle is selected and more than one oocyte matures and undergoes ovulation.

After ovulation, estrogen levels drop. For 90% of women, only a small amount of withdrawal bleeding occurs, so it goes unnoticed. In 10% of women there is sufficient bleeding for it to be visible, resulting in what is known as *midcycle bleeding.*

The luteal phase begins immediately after ovulation and ends with the start of menstruation. This postovulatory phase of the ovarian cycle usually requires 14 days (range of 13 to 15 days). The corpus luteum reaches its peak of functional activity 8 days after ovulation, secreting both estrogen and progesterone. Coincident with this time of peak luteal functioning, the fertilized ovum is implanted in the endometrium. If no implantation occurs, the corpus luteum regresses, steroid levels drop, and menstruation occurs.

Endometrial cycle. The four phases of the endometrial cycle are (1) the menstrual phase, (2) the proliferative phase, (3) the secretory phase, and (4) the ischemic phase (see Fig. 4-7). During the menstrual phase, shedding of the functional two thirds of the endometrium (the compact and spongy layers) is initiated by periodic vasoconstriction in the upper layers of the endometrium. The basal layer is always retained, and regeneration begins near the end of the cycle from cells derived from the remaining glandular remnants or stromal cells in the basalis.

The proliferative phase is a period of rapid growth lasting from about the fifth day to the time of ovulation. The endometrial surface is completely restored in approximately 4 days, or slightly before bleeding ceases. From this point on, an eightfold to tenfold thickening occurs, with a leveling off of growth at ovulation. The proliferative phase depends on estrogen stimulation derived from ovarian follicles.

The secretory phase extends from the day of ovulation to approximately 3 days before the next menstrual period. After ovulation, larger amounts of progesterone are produced. The fully matured secretory endometrium reaches the thickness of heavy, soft velvet. It becomes luxuriant with blood and glandular secretions, a suitable protective and nutritive bed for a fertilized ovum.

Implantation of the fertilized ovum generally occurs about 7 to 10 days after ovulation. If fertilization and implantation do not occur, the corpus luteum, which secretes estrogen and progesterone, regresses. With the rapid fall in progesterone and estrogen levels, the spiral arteries go into spasm. During the ischemic phase, the blood supply to the functional endometrium is blocked and necrosis develops. The functional layer separates from the basal layer, and menstrual bleeding begins, marking day 1 of the next cycle (see Fig. 4-7).

Other cyclic changes. When the hypothalamic-pituitary-ovarian axis functions properly, other tissues undergo predictable responses. Before ovulation the woman's basal body temperature (BBT) is often below 37° C; after ovulation, with rising progesterone levels, her BBT rises. Changes in the cervix and cervical mucus follow a generally predictable pattern. Preovulatory and postovulatory mucus is viscous (thick), so sperm penetration is discouraged. At the time of ovulation, cervical mucus is thin and clear. It looks, feels, and stretches like egg white. This stretchable quality is termed *spinnbarkeit.* Some women experience localized lower abdominal pain, termed *mittelschmerz,* that coincides with ovulation.

Climacteric. The climacteric is a transitional phase during which ovarian function and hormone production decline. This phase spans the years from the onset of premenopausal ovarian decline to the postmenopausal time when symptoms stop. Menopause refers to the last menstrual period. Unlike menarche, however, menopause can be dated only with certainty 1 year after menstruation ceases. The average age at natural menopause is 51.4 years, with an age range of 35 to 60 years. Menopause is preceded by a period known as the perimenopause, during which ovarian function declines. Ova slowly diminish, and menstrual cycles are anovulatory, resulting in irregular bleeding; the ovary stops producing estrogen, and eventually menses no longer occurs. This period lasts about 4 years (Stenchever, Droegemueller, Herbst, & Mishell, 2001).

Prostaglandins

Prostaglandins (PGs) are oxygenated fatty acids classified as hormones. The different kinds of PGs are distinguished by letters (PGE, PGF), numbers (PGE_2), and letters of the Greek alphabet ($PGF_{2\alpha}$). PGs are produced in most organs of the body, but most notably by the endometrium. Menstrual blood is a potent prostaglandin source. Prostaglandins affect smooth muscle contractility and modulation of hormonal activity. Indirect evidence supports PGs' effects on ovulation, fertility, changes in the cervix and cervical mucus that affect receptivity to sperm, tubal and uterine motility, sloughing of endometrium (menstruation), onset of abortion (spontaneous and induced), and onset of labor (term and preterm).

Sexual Response

The hypothalamus and anterior pituitary gland in females regulate the production of FSH and LH. The target tissue for these hormones is the ovary, which produces ova and secretes estrogen and progesterone. A feedback mechanism involving hormone secretion from the ovaries, hypothalamus, and anterior pituitary aids in the control of the production of sex cells and steroid sex hormone secretion.

Although the first outward appearance of maturing sexual development occurs at an earlier age in females, both females and males achieve physical maturity at approximately 17 years of age. However, individual development varies greatly. Anatomic and reproductive differences notwithstanding, women and men are more alike than different in their physiologic response to sexual excitement and orgasm. For example, the glans clitoris and the glans penis are embryonic homologues. Not only is there little difference between female and male sexual response, but the physical response is essentially the same whether stimulated by coitus, fantasy, or masturbation. Physiologically, according to Masters (1992), sexual response can be analyzed in terms of two processes: vasocongestion and myotonia.

Sexual stimulation results in vasocongestion (congestion of blood vessels, usually venous) that causes vaginal lubrication and engorgement and distention of the genitals. This venous congestion occurs to a lesser degree in the breasts and other parts of the body. Arousal is characterized by myotonia (increased muscular tension), resulting in voluntary and involuntary rhythmic contractions. Examples of sexually stimulated myotonia are pelvic thrusting, facial grimacing, and spasms of the hands and feet (carpopedal spasms).

The sexual response cycle is divided into four phases: excitement phase, plateau phase, orgasmic phase, and resolution phase. The four phases occur progressively with no sharp dividing line between any two phases. Specific body changes take place in sequence. The time, intensity, and duration for cyclic completion also vary for individuals and situations. Table 4-1 compares male and female body changes during each of the four phases of the sexual response cycle.

TABLE 4-1

Four Phases of Sexual Response

REACTIONS COMMON TO BOTH SEXES	REACTIONS IN FEMALES	REACTIONS IN MALES
EXCITEMENT PHASE		
Heart rate and blood pressure increase. Nipples become erect. Myotonia begins.	Clitoris increases in diameter and swells. External genitals become congested and darken. Vaginal lubrication occurs; upper two thirds of vagina lengthen and extend. Cervix and uterus pull upward. Breast size increases.	Erection of the penis begins; penis increases in length and diameter. Scrotal skin becomes congested and thickens. Testes begin to increase in size and elevate toward the body.
PLATEAU PHASE		
Heart rate and blood pressure continue to increase. Respirations increase. Myotonia becomes pronounced; grimacing occurs.	Clitoral head retracts under the clitoral hood. Lowest third of vagina becomes engorged. Skin color changes occur—red flush may be observed across breasts, abdomen, or other surfaces.	Head of penis may enlarge slightly. Scrotum continues to grow tense and thicken. Testes continue to elevate and enlarge. Preorgasmic emission of two or three drops of fluid appears on the head of the penis.
ORGASMIC PHASE		
Heart rate, blood pressure, and respirations increase to maximum levels. Involuntary muscle spasms occur. External rectal sphincter contracts.	Strong rhythmic contractions are felt in the clitoris, vagina, and uterus. Sensations of warmth spread through the pelvic area.	Testes elevate to maximum level. Point of "inevitability" occurs just before ejaculation and an awareness of fluid in the urethra. Rhythmic contractions occur in the penis. Ejaculation of semen occurs.
RESOLUTION PHASE		
Heart rate, blood pressure, and respirations return to normal. Nipple erection subsides. Myotonia subsides.	Engorgement in external genitalia and vagina resolves. Uterus descends to normal position. Cervix dips into seminal pool. Breast size decreases. Skin flush disappears.	Fifty percent of erection is lost immediately with ejaculation; penis gradually returns to normal size. Testes and scrotum return to normal size. Refractory period (time needed for erection to occur again) varies according to age and general physical condition.

REASONS FOR ENTERING THE HEALTH CARE SYSTEM

Women's health assessment and screening focus on a systems evaluation beginning with a careful history and physical examination. During the assessment and evaluation, the responsibility for self-care, health promotion, and enhancement of wellness are emphasized. Nursing care includes assessment, planning, education, counseling, and referral as needed, as well as commendations for good self-care that the woman has practiced. This enables women to make informed decisions about their own health care.

Preconception Counseling

Preconception health promotion provides women and their partners with information that is needed to make decisions about their reproductive future. Preconception counseling guides couples on how to prevent unintended pregnancies, stresses risk management, and identifies healthy behaviors that promote the well-being of the woman and her potential fetus (Moos, 2003).

The initiation of activities that promote healthy mothers and babies must occur before the period of critical fetal organ development, which is between 17 and 56 days after fertilization. By the end of the eighth week after conception and certainly by the end of the first trimester, any major structural anomalies in the fetus are already present. Because many women do not realize that they are pregnant and do not seek prenatal care until well into the first trimester, the rapidly growing fetus may be exposed to many types of intrauterine environmental hazards during this most vulnerable developmental phase. Therefore preconception health care should occur well in advance of an actual pregnancy (Hobbins, 2003).

Critical Thinking Exercise

Preconception Counseling

Margo is a 37-year-old woman who has never been pregnant and is now considering whether or not to attempt to conceive. She has come to the clinic for a Pap test. She asks the nurse what she needs to consider to be in a healthy state before conceiving. What advice or counseling would you give Margo?

1 Evidence—Is there sufficient evidence to draw conclusions about what intervention is needed?
2 Assumptions—Describe underlying assumptions about the following issues:
   a. Risk factor assessment for disease prevention
   b. Health promotion for pregnancy
   c. Critical periods of fetal organ development
   d. Pregnancy after age 35
3 What implications and priorities for nursing care can be drawn at this time?
4 Does the evidence objectively support your conclusion?
5 Are there alternative perspectives to your conclusion?

Preconception care is important for women who have had a problem with a previous pregnancy (e.g., miscarriage, preterm birth). Although causes are not always identifiable, in many cases problems can be identified and treated and may not recur in subsequent pregnancies. Preconception care is also important to minimize fetal malformations. There are many examples illustrating effects of maternal age or illnesses; conditions that produce anomalies in the fetus (teratogenic agents), such as drugs, viruses, chemicals, or genetically inherited diseases; and conditions that might be harmful to the woman should a pregnancy occur. In many instances, counseling can allow for behavior modification before damage is done or a woman can make an informed decision about her willingness to accept potential hazards (Postlethwaite, 2003).

A suggested model for preconception care of women of reproductive age targets all women from menarche to menopause. Providing optimal health care for women whether or not they desire to conceive can result in a high level of preconception wellness (Moos, 2003). Suggested components of preconception care, such as health promotion, risk assessment, and interventions, are outlined in Box 4-1.

Pregnancy

A woman's entry into health care is often associated with pregnancy, either for diagnosis or for actual care. Suspicion of pregnancy occurs most commonly when a woman is late with her menses. It is highly desirable for a woman to enter prenatal care within the first 12 weeks of pregnancy. This allows for early pregnancy counseling, especially for the woman who has had no preconception care. Extensive discussion of pregnancy is found in Unit Three.

Well-Woman Care

Current trends in the health care of women have expanded beyond a reproductive focus. A holistic approach to women's health care includes a woman's health needs throughout her lifetime. This view is one that goes beyond simply her reproductive needs. Women's health assessment and screening focus on a multisystem evaluation emphasizing the maintenance and enhancement of wellness (Moos, 2003).

Fertility Control and Infertility

More than half of the pregnancies in the United States each year are unintended even with birth control use (Kowal, 2004). Education is the key to encouraging women to make family planning choices based on preference and actual risk-to-benefit ratios. Women who enter the health care system seeking contraceptive counseling can be assisted to use a chosen method correctly (see Chapter 6 for further discussion).

Women also enter the health care system because of their desire to achieve a pregnancy. Approximately 15% of couples in the United States have some degree of infertility. Infertility can cause emotional pain for many couples, and the inability to produce an offspring sometimes results in feelings of failure and inordinate stress on the relationship. Steps toward prevention of infertility should be undertaken as part

---

BOX 4-1

Components of Preconception Care

HEALTH PROMOTION: GENERAL TEACHING

- Nutrition
  - Healthy diet, including folic acid
  - Optimal weight
- Exercise and rest
- Avoidance of substance abuse (tobacco, alcohol, "recreational" drugs)
- Use of safer sex practices
- Attending to family and social needs

RISK FACTOR ASSESSMENT

- Medical history
  - Immune status (e.g., rubella, hepatitis B)
  - Family history (e.g., genetic disorders)
  - Illnesses (e.g., infections)
  - Current use of medication (prescription, nonprescription)
- Reproductive history
  - Contraceptive
  - Obstetric
- Psychosocial history
  Spouse or partner and family situation, including intimate partner violence

- Availability of family or other support systems
- Readiness for pregnancy (e.g., age, life goals, stress)
- Financial resources
- Environmental (home, workplace) conditions
  - Safety hazards
  - Toxic chemicals
  - Radiation

INTERVENTIONS

- Anticipatory guidance or teaching
- Treatment of medical conditions and results
  - Medications
  - Cessation or reduction in substance use and abuse
  - Immunizations (e.g., rubella, tuberculosis, hepatitis)
- Nutrition, diet, and weight management
- Exercise
- Referral for genetic counseling
- Referral to and use of:
  - Family planning services
  - Family and social needs management

---

of ongoing routine health care, and such information is especially appropriate in preconception counseling. For additional information about infertility, see Chapter 6.

Menstrual Problems

Irregularities or problems with the menstrual period are among the most common concerns of women and often cause them to seek help within the health care system. Common menstrual disorders include amenorrhea, dysmenorrhea, premenstrual syndrome, endometriosis, and menorrhagia or metrorrhagia. These problems are discussed in Chapter 5.

Perimenopause

Although fertility is greatly reduced during the perimenopausal period, women are urged to maintain some method of birth control because pregnancies still can occur. Most women seeking health care at this time do so because of irregular bleeding that may accompany the perimenopause. Others are concerned about vasomotor symptoms (hot flashes and flushes). All women need to have factual information, the dispelling of myths, a thorough examination, and periodic health screenings.

BARRIERS TO SEEKING HEALTH CARE

Financial Issues

The United States spends almost 15% of its gross domestic product on health, far more than any other industrialized nation in the world, yet major problems still exist.

Employment-based financing of health insurance has resulted in a system in which one's health insurance is linked to a job, and the system is working well for fewer and fewer people, especially women. Fourteen percent of young women have no health insurance, and 5 million more have coverage so inadequate that it does not even include maternity care (National Women's Law Center, 2000).

In the United States disparity among races and socioeconomic classes affects many facets of life, including health. With limited money and awareness, there is a lack of access to care, delay in seeking care, few prevention activities, and little accurate information about health and the health care system. Women use health services more often than do men but are more likely than men to have difficulty in financing the services; they are twice as often underinsured (i.e., have limited coverage with high-cost co-payments or deductibles). Women make up the majority of Medicaid recipients; however, only 42% of poor women are eligible. Medicaid includes special benefits for pregnant women, but they are limited to treatment of pregnancy-related conditions and terminate 60 days after birth. Current questions abound regarding possible changes in the Medicaid coverage related to care for mother and child during the maternity cycle. More and more states are requiring their Medicaid recipients to enroll in managed care programs; whether this improves access and outcomes is yet to be determined.

Insurance coverage varies significantly by age, marital status, race, and ethnicity. Caucasians of all ages are more likely than African-Americans and other racial or ethnic groups to have private insurance. Single, separated, or divorced individuals are less likely to have insurance. Often, unmarried teenagers, who are usually covered by their parents' medical insurance, do not have maternity coverage because policies have inclusion statements that cover only the employee or spouse.

Midwifery care has helped contain some health care costs, but reimbursement issues still exist in some areas. Nursing data must be identified and placed in a database to be included in public policy decisions; nursing variables such as patient education and supportive care must become part of the national data-gathering system. Nurses should deal with the politics involved in cost-containment health care policies, because they, as knowledgeable experts, can provide solutions to many of the health care problems at a relatively low cost.

Cultural Issues

Although they are most significant, financial considerations are not the only barriers to obtaining quality health care. As our nation becomes more racially, ethnically, and culturally diverse, the health of minority groups becomes a major issue. Providers must consider culturally based differences that could affect the treatment of diverse groups of women, and the women themselves must discuss with their health care providers the practices and beliefs that could influence their management responses or willingness to comply (Mattson, 2000). For example, women in some cultures value privacy to such an extent that they are reluctant to disrobe and as a result avoid physical examination unless absolutely necessary. Other women rely on their husbands to make major decisions, including those affecting the woman's health. Religious beliefs may dictate a plan of care, as with birth control measures or blood transfusions. Some cultural groups prefer folk medicine, homeopathy, or prayer to traditional Western medicine, and yet others attempt combinations of some or all practices.

Gender Issues

Gender influences provider-patient communication and may influence access to health care in general. The most obvious gender consideration is that between men and women. Researchers have reported significant male-female differences in receipt of major diagnostic and therapeutic interventions, especially with cardiac and kidney problems. Women tend to use primary care services more often (and, some believe, more effectively) than men. The sex of the provider plays a role, because studies have shown that female patients have tests such as the Pap test and mammogram more consistently if they are seen by female providers.

Sexual orientation may produce another barrier. Lesbian women have primary erotic attractions and relations with other women. Some lesbians may not disclose their orientation to health care providers because they may be at risk for hostility, inadequate health care, or breach of confidentiality. To offset stereotypes, it is necessary for providers to develop an approach that does not assume that all patients are heterosexual (Bonvicini & Perlin, 2003). Primary care of lesbians is not different from that for any other group of women, and lesbian patients have the same basic physical and psychologic needs as any woman.

HEALTH RISKS IN THE CHILDBEARING YEARS

Maintaining optimal health is a goal for all women. Essential components of health maintenance are identification of unrecognized problems and potential risks and the education/promotion needed to reduce them. This is especially important for women in their childbearing years because conditions that increase a woman's health risks are not only of concern to her well-being but also are potentially associated with negative outcomes for both mother and baby in the event of a pregnancy. Prenatal care is the prime example of prevention that is practiced after conception. However, prevention and health maintenance are needed before pregnancy because many of the mother's risks can be identified and eliminated or at least modified. An overview of conditions and circumstances that increase health risks in the childbearing years follows.

Age
Adolescence

All teens undergo progressive growth of sexual characteristics and also undertake developmental tasks of adolescence, such as establishing identity, developing sexual preference, emancipating from family, and establishing career goals. Some of these situations can produce great stress for the adolescent, and the health care provider should treat her very carefully. Female teenagers who enter the health care system usually do so for screening (Pap tests start three years after sexual activity begins or by age 21) or because of a problem such as episodic illness or accidents. Gynecologic problems are often associated with menses (either bleeding irregularities or dysmenorrhea), vaginitis or leukorrhea, sexually transmitted infections (STIs), contraception, or pregnancy. The adolescent is also at risk for major depressive disorder (Hauenstein, 2003).

Teenage pregnancy.   Pregnancy in the teenager who is 16 years of age or younger often introduces additional stress into an already stressful developmental period. The emotional level of such teens is commonly characterized by impulsiveness and self-centered behavior, and they often place primary importance on the beliefs and actions of their peers. In attempts to establish a personal and independent identity, many teens do not realize the consequences of their behavior, and planning for the future is not part of their thinking processes.

Teenagers usually lack the financial resources to support a pregnancy and may not have the maturity to avoid teratogens or to have prenatal care and instruction or follow-up care. Children of teen mothers may be at risk for abuse or neglect because of the teen's inadequate knowledge of growth, development, and parenting.

Young and middle adulthood

Because women ages 20 to 40 have need for contraception, pelvic and breast screening, and pregnancy care, they may prefer to use their gynecologic or obstetric provider also as their primary care provider. During these years, the woman may be "juggling" family, home, and career responsibilities with resulting increases in stress-related conditions. Health maintenance includes not only pelvic and breast screening but also promotion of a healthy lifestyle, that is, good nutrition, regular exercise, no smoking, moderate or no alcohol consumption, sufficient rest, stress reduction, and referral for medical conditions and other specific problems. Common conditions in well-woman care include vaginitis, urinary tract infections, menstrual variations, obesity, sexual and relationship issues, and pregnancy.

Parenthood after age 35 years. The woman older than 35 is at risk for age-related conditions that can affect pregnancy. For example, a woman with type 2 diabetes may not have had expression of her diabetes at age 22 but may have full-blown disease at age 38. Other chronic or debilitating diseases or conditions increase in severity with time, and these, in turn, may predispose to increased risks during pregnancy. Of significance to women in this age group is the risk for having a baby with certain genetic anomalies (e.g., Down syndrome), and the opportunity for genetic counseling should be available to all (Viau, Padula, & Eddy, 2002) (see Chapter 7).

Late reproductive age

Women of later reproductive age are often experiencing change and reordering personal priorities. Generally, the goals of education, career, marriage, and family have been achieved, and now the woman has increased time and opportunity for new interests and activities. Conversely, divorce rates are high at this age, and children leaving home may produce an "empty nest syndrome," resulting in levels of depression. Chronic diseases also become more apparent. Most problems for the well woman are associated with perimenopause (e.g., bleeding irregularities, vasomotor symptoms). Health maintenance screening continues to be of importance because some conditions such as breast disease or ovarian cancer occur more often during this stage.

Social and Cultural Factors

Differences exist among people from different socioeconomic levels and ethnic groups with respect to risk for illness and distribution of disease and death. Some diseases are more common among people of selected ethnicity, for example, sickle cell anemia in African-Americans, Tay-Sachs disease in Ashkenazi Jews, adult lactase deficiency in Chinese, beta thalassemia in Mediterranean peoples, and cystic fibrosis in northern Europeans. Cultural and religious influences also increase health risks because the woman and her family may have life and societal values and a view of health and illness that dictate practices different from those expected in the Judeo-Christian Western model. These may include food taboos or frequencies, methods of hygiene, effects of climate, care-seeking behaviors, willingness to undergo screening and diagnostic procedures, and value conflicts.

Socioeconomic contrasts result in major health differences as exemplified in birth outcomes. The rates of perinatal and maternal deaths, preterm births, and low-birth-weight babies are considerably higher in disadvantaged populations (Martin, Kochanek, Strobino, Guyer, & MacDorman, 2005). Social consequences for poor women as single parents are great because many mothers with few skills are caught in the bind of having insufficient income to afford child care. These families generate fewer and fewer resources and increase their risks for health problems. Multiple roles for women in general produce overload, conflict, and stress, resulting in higher risks for psychosocial health care.

Substance Use and Abuse

The inappropriate use of illicit and prescription drugs continues to increase and is found in all ages, races, ethnic groups, and socioeconomic strata. Addiction to substances is seen as a biopsychosocial disease with several factors leading to risk. These include biogenetic predisposition, lack of resilience to stressful life experiences, and poor social support. Women are less likely than men to abuse drugs, but the rate in women is increasing significantly. Substance-abusing pregnant women create severe problems for themselves and their offspring, including interference with optimal growth and development and addiction. In many instances the use of substances is identified through screening programs in prenatal clinics and obstetric units.

Smoking

Cigarette smoking is a major preventable cause of death and illness. Smoking is linked to cardiovascular heart disease, various types of cancers (especially lung and cervical), chronic lung disease, and negative pregnancy outcomes. Tobacco contains nicotine, which is an addictive substance that creates a physical and a psychologic dependence. Among adolescents and young adults, more women than men smoke (American Cancer Society [ACS], 2005). Cigarette smoking impairs fertility in both women and men, may reduce the age for menopause, and increases the risk for osteoporosis after menopause. Passive, or secondhand, smoke contains similar hazards and presents additional problems for the smoker, as well as harm for the nonsmoker. Smoking during pregnancy is known to cause a decrease in placental perfusion and is a cause of low birth weight (Behrman & Shiono, 2002).

Alcohol

About 1% to 2% of women of childbearing age have alcohol-related problems. Alcohol abuse during pregnancy has been associated with fetal growth restriction, altered facies, and developmental problems, specifically mental retardation (Eustace, Kang, & Coombs, 2003). Women who are problem drinkers are often depressed, have more motor vehicle injuries, and have a higher incidence of attempted suicide than women in the general population. Also, they are at particular risk for alcohol-related liver damage.

Caffeine

Caffeine is a stimulant that is found in society's most popular drinks: coffee, tea, and soft drinks. It is a stimulant that can affect mood and interrupt body functions by producing anxiety and sleep interruptions. Heart arrhythmias may be made worse by caffeine, and there can be interactions with certain medications such as lithium. Birth defects have not been related to caffeine consumption; however, high intake has been related to a slight decrease in birth weight and may also increase the risk of miscarriage (Cnattingius, 2000).

Prescription drugs

Psychotherapeutic drugs. Stimulants, sleeping pills, tranquilizers, and pain relievers are used by a small percent of American women. Such drugs can bring relief from undesirable conditions such as insomnia, anxiety, and pain, but because the drugs have mind-altering capacity, misuse can produce psychologic and physical dependency in the same manner as illicit drugs. Risk-to-benefit ratios should be considered when such drugs are used for more than very short periods of time. All of these categories of drugs have some effect on the fetus when taken during pregnancy, and their use should be monitored very carefully.

Depression is the most common mental health problem in women. Everyone has a case of the "blues" periodically, but true depression impairs the ability to live a normal life and involves symptoms of pervasive sadness, isolation, fatigue, changes in eating and sleeping patterns, and general negativity. Severely depressed people are at risk for suicide. Drugs used to treat depression include tricyclic antidepressants (see Chapter 25).

Illicit drugs

Cocaine. Cocaine is a powerful central nervous system stimulant that is addictive because of the tremendous sense of pleasure or good feeling that it creates. It can be snorted, smoked, or injected. Cocaine affects all of the major body systems. Among other complications, it produces cardiovascular stress that can lead to heart attack or stroke, liver disease, central nervous system stimulation that can cause seizures, and even perforation of the nasal septum. Users are often poorly nourished and commonly have STIs. If the user is pregnant, there is an increased incidence of miscarriage, preterm labor, small-for-dates babies, abruption of placenta, and stillbirth. Anomalies have also been reported (Briggs, Freeman, & Yaffe, 2002; Niebyl, 2002).

Heroin. Heroin is an opiate that is usually injected but can be smoked or snorted. It produces euphoria, relaxation, relief from pain, and "nodding out" (apathy, detachment from reality, impaired judgment, and drowsiness). Signs and symptoms are constricted pupils, nausea, constipation, slurred speech, and respiratory depression (Stuart and Laraia, 2001). Users are at increased risk for acquiring human immunodeficiency virus (HIV) and hepatitis B, C, and D viruses, primarily because of sharing needles that contain contaminated blood. Perinatal effects include interference with fetal growth, premature rupture of membranes, preterm labor, and prematurity.

Marijuana. Marijuana is a substance derived from the cannabis plant. It is usually rolled into cigarettes and smoked, but it may also be mixed into food and eaten. It produces an intoxicating and sensory-distorting "high." Marijuana smoke has the same characteristics as tobacco smoke: both readily cross the placenta and have the effect of increasing carbon monoxide levels in the mother's blood, which reduces the oxygen supply to the fetus. Fetal abnormalities are possible (Stuart & Laraia, 2001).

Other illicit drugs. A number of other street drugs pose risk to users. Variations of stimulants, such as "speed," methamphetamine ("meth"), and "ice," produce signs and symptoms similar to cocaine. Sedatives such as "downers," "yellow jackets," or "red devils" are used to "come down" from a high. Hallucinogens alter perception and body function. Phencyclidine hydrochloride (PCP; angel dust) and lysergic acid diethylamide (LSD) produce vivid changes in sensation, often with agitation, euphoria, paranoia, and a tendency toward antisocial behavior. Their use may lead to flashbacks, chronic psychosis, and violent behavior (Stuart & Laraia, 2001).

Nutrition

Good nutrition is essential for optimal health. A well-balanced diet helps prevent illness and also is used to treat certain health problems. Conversely, poor eating habits, eating disorders, and obesity are linked to disease and debility.

Nutritional deficiencies

Overt disease caused by lack of certain nutrients is rarely seen in the United States; however, insufficient amounts or imbalances of nutrients do pose problems for individuals and families. Overweight or underweight status, malabsorption, listlessness, fatigue, frequent colds and other minor infections, constipation, dull hair and thin nails, and dental caries are examples of problems that can be related to nutrition and indicate the need for further nutritional assessment. Poor nutrition, especially related to obesity and high fat and cholesterol intake, may lead to more serious conditions and is said to contribute to four of the 10 leading causes of death in the United States: diseases of the heart, malignant neoplasms, cerebrovascular diseases, and diabetes (Hoyert, Kung, & Smith, 2005).

Obesity

During the past 20 years there has been a dramatic increase in obesity in the United States. It is estimated that 25% of women older than 20 years are obese (body mass index [BMI], 30 or higher), and 51% of women older than 20 years are overweight (BMI, 25 to 25.9) (Kealy, 2003; National Center for Chronic Disease Prevention and Health Promotion, 2000). In the United States the prevalence of obesity is highest among non-Hispanic black women, followed by Hispanic women and non-Hispanic white women (Flegal, Carroll, Ogden, & Johnson, 2002). The BMI is defined as a measure of an adult's weight in relation to his or her height, specifically the adult's weight in kilograms divided by the square of his or her height in meters (see Chapter 10).

Overweight and obesity are known risk factors for diabetes, heart disease, stroke, hypertension, gallbladder disease, osteoarthritis, sleep apnea, and some types of cancer (uterine, breast, colorectal, kidney, and gallbladder) (ACS, 2005). In addition, obesity is associated with high cholesterol, menstrual irregularities, hirsutism (excessive body and facial hair), stress incontinence, depression, complications of pregnancy, increased surgical risk, and shortened life span (U.S. Department of Health and Human Services & U.S. Department of Agriculture, 2005). Pregnant women who are morbidly obese are at increased risk for hypertension, diabetes, gallbladder disease, postterm pregnancy, and musculoskeletal problems (Cesario, 2003).

Other considerations

Other dietary extremes also can produce risk. For example, insufficient amounts of calcium can lead to osteoporosis, too much sodium can aggravate hypertension, and megadoses of vitamins can cause adverse effects in several body systems. Fad weight-loss programs and "yo-yo dieting" (repeated weight gain and weight loss) result in nutritional imbalances and, in some instances, medical problems. Such diets and programs are not appropriate for weight maintenance. Adolescent pregnancy produces special nutritional requirements because the metabolic needs of pregnancy are superimposed on the teen's own needs for growth and maturation at a time when eating habits are less than ideal.

Anorexia nervosa

Some women have a distorted view of their bodies and, no matter what their weight, perceive themselves to be much too heavy. As a result, they undertake strict and severe diets and rigorous extreme exercise. This chronic and rarest of eating disorders is known as *anorexia nervosa.* A coexisting depression usually accompanies anorexia. Women can carry this condition to the point of starvation, with resulting endocrine and metabolic abnormalities. If nutritional status is not corrected, significant complications of arrhythmias, cardiomyopathy, and congestive heart failure occur and, in the extreme, can lead to death. The condition commonly begins during adolescence in young women who have some degree of personality disorder. They gradually lose weight over several months, have amenorrhea, and are abnormally concerned with body image. The condition requires both psychiatric and medical interventions.

Bulimia nervosa

Bulimia refers to secret, uncontrolled binge eating alternating with methods to prevent weight gain: self-induced vomiting, taking laxatives or diuretics, strict diets, fasting, and rigorous exercise. Bulimia usually begins in early adulthood (ages 18 to 25) and is found primarily in females. Complications can include dehydration and electrolyte imbalance, gastrointestinal (GI) abnormalities, dental problems, and cardiac arrhythmias.

Physical Fitness and Exercise

Exercise contributes to good health by lowering risks for a variety of conditions that are influenced by obesity and a sedentary lifestyle. It is effective in the prevention of cardiovascular disease and in the management of chronic conditions such as hypertension, arthritis, diabetes, respiratory disorders, and osteoporosis. Exercise also contributes to stress reduction and weight maintenance. Women report that engaging in regular exercise improves their body image and self-esteem and acts as a mood enhancer. Aerobic exercise produces cardiovascular involvement because increasing amounts of oxygen are delivered to working muscles. Anaerobic exercise, such as weight training, improves individual muscle mass without stress on the cardiovascular system. Because women are concerned about both cardiovascular and bone health, weight-bearing aerobic exercises such as walking, running, racket sports, and dancing are preferred. Excessive or strenuous exercise can lead to hormonal imbalances, resulting in amenorrhea and its consequences. Physical injury is also a potential risk.

Stress

The modern woman faces increasing levels of stress and as a result is prone to a variety of stress-induced complaints and illnesses. Stress often occurs because of multiple roles in which coping with job and financial responsibilities conflict with parenting and home. To add to this burden, women are socialized to be caretakers, which is emotionally draining in itself. Also, they find themselves in positions of minimal power that do not allow them to have control over their everyday environments. Some stress is normal and, in fact, contributes to positive outcomes. Many women thrive in busy surroundings. However, excessive or high levels of ongoing stress trigger physical reactions in the body, such as rapid heart rate, elevated blood pressure, slowed digestion, release of additional neurotransmitters and hormones, muscle tenseness, and weakened immune system. Consequently, constant stress can contribute to clinical illnesses such as flare-ups of arthritis or asthma, frequent colds or infections, GI upsets, cardiovascular problems, and infertility. Psychologic signs such as anxiety, irritability, eating disorders, depression, insomnia, and substance abuse also have been associated with stress.

Sexual Practices

Potential risks related to sexual activity are undesired pregnancy and STIs. The risks are particularly high for adolescents and young adults, who engage in sexual intercourse at earlier and earlier ages (Hutchinson, Sosa, & Thompson, 2001). Adolescents report many reasons for wanting to be sexually active, among which are peer pressure, desire to love and be loved, experimentation, enhancement of self-esteem, and enjoyment. However, many teens do not have the decision-making or values-clarification skills needed to take this important step at a young age and also lack a good knowledge base regarding contraception and STIs. They also do not believe that becoming pregnant or getting an STI will happen to them.

Although some STIs can be cured with antibiotics, many can cause significant problems. Possible sequelae include infertility, ectopic pregnancy, neonatal morbidity and mortality, genital cancers, acquired immunodeficiency syndrome, and even death (Centers for Disease Control and Prevention [CDC], 2002) (see Chapter 23). No method of contraception offers complete protection.

Medical Conditions

Most women of reproductive age are relatively healthy. However, certain medical conditions that occur during pregnancy can have deleterious effects on both mother and fetus. Of particular concern are risks from all forms of diabetes, urinary tract disorders, thyroid disease, hypertensive disorders of pregnancy, cardiac disease, and seizure disorders. Effects on the fetus vary and include intrauterine growth restriction, macrosomia, anemia, prematurity, immaturity, and stillbirth. Effects on the mother can also be severe. See Chapter 22 for information on specific conditions.

Gynecologic Conditions Affecting Pregnancy

Gynecologic conditions may contribute negatively to pregnancy by causing infertility, miscarriage, preterm labor, and fetal and neonatal problems. Most of these conditions are discussed in Chapter 5 and include pelvic inflammatory disease, endometriosis, STIs and other vaginal infections, uterine fibroids, and uterine deformities such as bicornuate uterus. Gynecologic cancers also affect women's health. Risk factors depend on the type of cancer.

Cervical cancer

Human papillomavirus (HPV) infection is the most common cause of cervical cancer. At least 15 types of HPV are associated with an increase in cervical cancer; types HPV 16 and HPV 18 are related to over 60% of cervical cancers (ACS, 2005). Other risks for cervical cancer include early age of first sexual intercourse, cigarette smoking, HIV infection, possible other STIs (e.g., chlamydia), and multiple sexual partners. In the United States, African-American women have the highest rate of invasive cancer of the cervix. Abnormal spotting or vaginal bleeding is the primary symptom (ACS, 2005).

Endometrial cancer

The most common malignancy of the reproductive system is endometrial cancer. Estrogen-related exposures such as nulliparity, unopposed estrogen therapy, infertility, early menarche, and late menopause are the most significant risk factors. Other risk factors include obesity, hypertension, diabetes, and family history of breast or ovarian cancer. Use of birth control pills and pregnancy appear to provide some protection against endometrial cancer. It occurs most frequently in Caucasian women and after menopause. Abnormal uterine bleeding is the cardinal sign (ACS, 2005).

Ovarian cancer

Ovarian cancer is the most malignant of all gynecologic cancers, accounting for the most deaths from these cancers. Risk factors include family history of ovarian or breast cancer and having no children or having them late in life. Abdominal enlargement accompanied by persistent vague digestive symptoms is the most common sign (ACS, 2005).

Other gynecologic cancers

Cancer of the vulva, vagina, and uterine tubes accounts for less than 6% of all female reproductive cancers. Cancers of the vulva and vagina have been linked to HPV and herpes simplex virus, but the cause of uterine tube cancer is unknown. These cancers occur most often in postmenopausal women. Lesions are often the first sign of vulvar cancer. Women with vaginal or uterine tube cancer may be asymptomatic or have vaginal bleeding (DiSaia & Creasman, 2002).

Other Cancers
Lung cancer

Lung cancer is the leading cause of cancer deaths in women. Cigarette smoking is the most important risk factor. Other risks include exposure to certain industrial substances, organic chemicals (e.g., radon, asbestos), and radiation. Symptoms include a persistent cough, blood-tinged sputum, chest pain, and recurring pneumonia or bronchitis (ACS, 2005). Survival rates are low because most cancers are not detected while they are still localized.

Breast cancer

Cancer of the breast is the second leading cause of cancer deaths in women. Mortality rates since 1991 have declined, probably as a result of earlier detection and improved treatment (ACS, 2005). Risk factors include family history, inherited genetic mutations (BRCA1 and BRCA2), early menarche, late menopause, nulliparity or having children later in life, and possibly postmenopausal use of estrogen. The incidence is highest in Caucasian and lowest among Native-American women. The earliest sign is having an abnormality that shows up on a mammogram before it can be detected by the woman or a clinician (ACS, 2005). (See further discussion in Chapter 5.)

Colon cancer

Colon cancer is the third most common cancer in women. Risk factors include a personal or family history of colorectal cancer or polyps; inflammatory bowel disease; and a high-fat, low-fiber diet. The incidence is highest in African-American women. Signs include rectal bleeding, blood in the stool, and a change in bowel habits (ACS, 2005).

EVIDENCE-BASED PRACTICE
Decreasing the Discomfort and Pain of Mammography

BACKGROUND

- Mammography, the radiographic screening test for breast cancer, has been shown by randomized, controlled trials to decrease mortality rates. Each breast is pressed between two plates horizontally, then vertically, and a low-level x-ray is taken of each view. Mammography can find breast lumps that are too small to be palpable, thus enabling life-saving surgery to remove the cancer before it metastasizes. In spite of all these advantages, studies show that some women never return after their first mammogram. From 32% to 53% of women reported discomfort or pain with the procedure. It is important to make mammograms acceptable to the women who need them as a screening tool. Causes of pain may include the level of compression of the breast, a woman's expectations of the procedure, her level of confidence in the procedure and the technician, breast density, and timing of the mammogram during the woman's menstrual cycle. It is important to measure the pain accurately, with a standardized scale that has demonstrable reliability and validity (meaning, a tool that measures exactly what it claims to measure and nothing else).

OBJECTIVES

- The reviewers were seeking evidence of interventions that might relieve the discomfort and pain of mammography. Interventions might include technique and manner of staff and facility, the woman's preparation for the procedure (including analgesia and alternative therapy), the procedure itself, and her participation in the procedure. Outcomes would be pain and discomfort, and some way to standardize these measures. Quality of mammogram is also an important outcome, because false-positive results and recalls decrease the woman's confidence in the process.

METHODS
Search Strategy

- The search was extensive and used Cochrane, EBM Reviews, AMED, CANCERLIT, CINAHL, Current Contents, EMBASE, HealthSTAR, PREMEDLINE, MEDLINE, PsycINFO, dissertation and theses databases, and five journals, as well as relevant organizations and specialists. Search keywords were *pain, mammogram,* and *screen,* and the search was limited to humans and females. Three randomized, controlled trials were included in the review, dated 1993 to 1998, representing 574 women.

Statistical Analyses

- Meta-analysis was not possible because of the heterogeneity of the trials. Discomfort scales were not standardized, ranging from "comfortable–not comfortable" to a six-point visual analog scale from comfortable to very uncomfortable.

FINDINGS

- Trial findings are presented separately.
- Study 1 compared the comfort level of technician compression of one breast with patient-controlled compression of the other. This design enabled the woman to serve as her own control for comparison. Women reported significantly less pain in self-controlled compression than when the technician compressed the other breast, regardless of which went first. The qualities of the mammogram images were equal when the technician went first, but were of significantly poorer quality when the patient controlled the first compression. This suggests that there was some modeling during the first compression, so that the women knew approximately how much compression was desirable.
- Study 2 was a master's thesis and compared the discomfort level in women who were given acetaminophen before the procedure with the control group with no pretreatment. There were no differences in discomfort levels between groups.
- Study 3 measured the discomfort levels of a standard mammogram compression on one breast with a standard compression that was loosened for one second on the other breast. No significant differences were found. More than half (57%) noted no difference, 23% felt the firmer compression to be the more uncomfortable side, and 20% felt the loosened compression to be the more uncomfortable side.

LIMITATIONS

- The small number of trials, and their small numbers of subjects, limits the power of the findings. Pain and discomfort could lend themselves well to standardized scales, which could then be metaanalyzed across trials, increasing their generalizability. Even though pain is discussed, the measures are all of discomfort, and they are not standardized. The quality of mammogram interpretation across trials was also not addressed.

CONCLUSIONS

- There are not enough data to draw conclusions about how to reduce the discomfort of mammograms. Increasing the woman's control of the procedure seemed to decrease her discomfort, but mild analgesics did not.

IMPLICATIONS FOR PRACTICE

- Some women may find the experience less unpleasant if they are given the option to control their own mammograms. The role of perception of control in alleviating pain is well documented in patient-controlled analgesia. Preparing a woman for a mammogram should include an honest description of the procedure and the sensations.

IMPLICATIONS FOR FURTHER RESEARCH

- More replication and further research into creative intervention to alleviate mammogram discomfort is needed. Measures of women's attitudes and confidence in the procedure still need research. This seems an ideal area in which to explore alternative interventions, such as hypnosis, guided imagery, aromatherapy, massage, temperature, acupressure, music, and distraction. Research may show that pretreatment with other analgesics, such as nonsteroidal antiinflammatory drugs (NSAIDs), holds more promise than pretreatment with acetaminophen.

Reference: Miller, D., Martin, I., & Herbison, P. (2003). Interventions for relieving the pain and discomfort of screening mammography (Cochrane Review). In *The Cochrane Library,* Issue 2, 2004. Chichester, UK: John Wiley & Sons.

Environmental and Workplace Hazards

Environmental hazards in the home, workplace, and community can contribute to poor health at all ages. Environmental hazards can affect fertility, fetal development, live birth, and the child's future mental and physical development. Everyone is at risk from air pollutants, such as tobacco smoke, carbon monoxide, smog, suspended particles (dust, ash, and asbestos), and cleaning solvents; noise pollution; pesticides; chemical additives; and poor preparation of food. Workers also face safety and health risks caused by ergonomically poor workstations and stress. It is important that risk assessments continue to be in effect to identify and understand environmental public health problems.

Violence against Women

Violence against women is a major health care problem in the United States, affecting over 4 million women each year and resulting in millions of dollars in annual medical costs (Tjaden & Thoennes, 2000). It is the second leading cause of injuries to women ages 15 to 44 in the United States (National Women's Health Information Center [NWHIC], 2003). Women of all races and of all ethnic, educational, religious, and socioeconomic backgrounds are affected. The magnitude of the problem may be far greater than the statistics indicate, because violent crimes against women are underreported as a result of fear, lack of understanding, and stigma surrounding violent situations.

Maternity and women's health nurses, by the very nature of their practice, are in a unique position to conduct case finding, provide sensitive care to women experiencing abusive situations, engage in prevention activities, and influence health care and public policy toward decreasing the violence.

Intimate partner violence

Intimate partner violence (IPV), wife battering, spouse abuse, and *domestic violence* or *family violence* are all terms applied to a pattern of assaultive and coercive behaviors that includes physical, sexual, and psychologic attacks, as well as economic coercion usually inflicted by a male partner in a marriage or other heterosexual, significant, intimate relationship. IPV is the preferred term.

Relationship violence rarely consists of a single episode, but rather is a pattern that may start with intimidation or threats and progress to more aggressive physical and sexual acts, resulting in injury to the woman. Common elements of battering are economic deprivation, sexual abuse, intimidation, isolation, and stalking and terrorizing victims and their children. Pregnancy is often a time when violence begins or escalates (NWHIC, 2003) (see Chapter 9).

Characteristics of women in battering relationships. Every segment of society is represented among abused women; race, religion, social background, age, and educational level are not significant factors in differentiating women at risk. Battered women may believe they are to blame for the situation because they are "not good enough wives." Many women have low self-esteem and may have histories of domestic violence in their families of origin. Social isolation seems to be another characteristic of battered women, which may result from stigma, fear, or restrictions placed on them by their partners.

Cycle of violence: the dynamics of battering. According to the cycle of violence concept, battering is neither random nor constant; rather, it occurs in repeated cycles (Fig. 4-8). A three-phase cyclic pattern to the battering behavior has been described as a period of increasing tension leading to the battery, which is then followed by a

CD: Critical Thinking Exercise—Women's Health and Safety

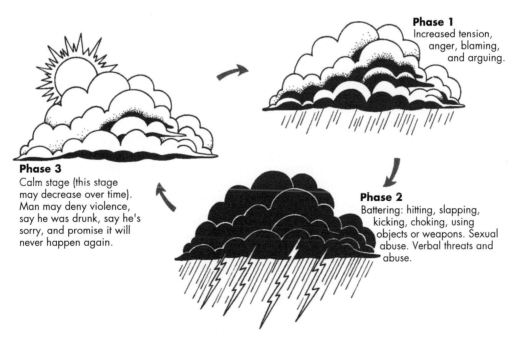

Phase 1
Increased tension, anger, blaming, and arguing.

Phase 2
Battering: hitting, slapping, kicking, choking, using objects or weapons. Sexual abuse. Verbal threats and abuse.

Phase 3
Calm stage (this stage may decrease over time). Man may deny violence, say he was drunk, say he's sorry, and promise it will never happen again.

Fig. 4-8 Cycle of violence. (From Helton, A. [1987]. *A protocol of care for the battered woman.* White Plains, NY: March of Dimes Birth Defects Foundation.)

period of calm and remorse in which the male partner displays kind, loving behavior and pleas for forgiveness. This "honeymoon" phase lasts until stress or other factors cause conflict and tension to mount again toward another episode of battering. Over time, the tension and battering phases last longer and the calm phase becomes shorter until there is no honeymoon phase (Walker, 1984).

Sexual abuse and rape

Many female sexual abuse and assault victims experience posttraumatic stress disorder (PTSD) (NWHIC, 2003). Up to 27% of women have experienced childhood sexual abuse (Molnar, Buka, & Kessler, 2001). Common psychopathologic consequences are dissociative identity disorder, borderline personality disorder, and generalized anxiety disorder. Although pregnant or postpartum patients with these diagnoses may come to the attention of maternity nurses, women who experience symptoms of PTSD, sexual dysfunction, depression, anxiety, or substance abuse problems are more likely to be seen in gynecologic practice.

Rape is an act of violence rather than a sexual act. Rape is a legal and not a medical entity and in its strictest sense is the penile penetration of the female sex organ or labia without her consent. *Sexual assault,* a term used interchangeably with *rape,* is also an act of force and has a much broader definition to include unwanted or uncomfortable touches, kisses, hugs, petting, intercourse, or other sexual acts. States may also use different legal definitions of rape.

Hymenal penetration or ejaculation does not have to occur to qualify as rape. The key feature to establish rape is the absence of consent: threat or coercion implies the lack of consent. The victim who is mentally retarded, who is unconscious or otherwise physically unable to move, who has taken drugs or who has been drugged without her knowledge, or who is a minor (statutory rape) is not capable of giving consent. The court must prove absence of consent; thus the term *alleged rape* or *alleged sexual assault* is used in medical records.

Medical considerations for the rape victim include treatment of physical injuries, prophylactic treatment for STIs, and prophylaxis for pregnancy (emergency contraception) (see Chapter 6). Emergency departments and ambulatory care facilities usually follow protocols for examination, collection of evidence and photographing injuries, treatment, and providing information on community resources for victims of violence.

HEALTH ASSESSMENT

Interview

At a woman's first visit, she is often expected to fill out a form with biographic and historical data before meeting with the examiner. The nurse is usually responsible for ensuring that the woman's name, age, marital status, race, ethnicity, address, phone numbers, occupation, and date of visit are

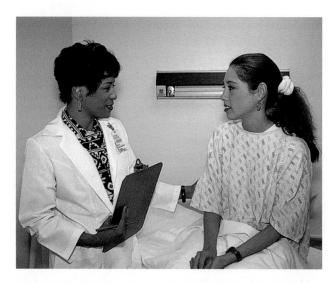

Fig. 4-9 Nurse interviews woman as part of annual physical examination. (From Potter, P., and Perry, A. [1997]. *Fundamentals of nursing: concepts, process, and practice* [4th ed.]. St. Louis: Mosby.)

recorded. The interview should be conducted in a private, comfortable, and relaxed setting and in an unhurried manner (Fig. 4-9). The woman is addressed by her title and name (e.g., Mrs. Chang), and the nurse introduces herself or himself using name and title. It is important to phrase questions in a sensitive and nonjudgmental manner. The woman's culture should be considered in case modifications in the examinations should be needed (Mattson, 2003). For example, a female examiner may be preferred or it may be inappropriate for the woman to disrobe completely for an examination. The nurse is cognizant of a woman's vulnerability and assures her of strict confidentiality. Many women are uninformed, misguided by myths, or afraid they will appear ignorant by asking questions about sexual or reproductive functioning. The woman is assured that no question is irrelevant. The history begins with an open-ended question such as, "What brings you in to the office/clinic/hospital today? Anything else? Tell me about it."

Communication may be hindered by different beliefs even when the nurse and patient speak the same language. Examples of communication variations are listed in the Cultural Considerations box.

Women with Special Needs

Women with emotional or physical disorders have special needs. Women who are visually, aurally, emotionally, or physically disabled should be respected and involved in the assessment and physical examination to the full extent of their abilities. The assessment and physical examination can be adapted to each woman's individual needs.

Communication with a woman who is hearing impaired can be accomplished without difficulty. Most of these women read lips, write, or both; therefore an interviewer who speaks and enunciates each word slowly and in full view may be easily understood. If a woman is not comfortable

EVOLVE/CD: Case Study—Health Assessment

Cultural Considerations

Communication Variations

- *Conversational style and pacing:* Silence may show respect or acknowledgment that the listener has heard. In cultures in which a direct "no" is considered rude, silence may mean no. Repetition or loudness may mean emphasis or anger.
- *Personal space:* Cultural conceptions of personal space differ, based on one's culture. Someone may be perceived as distant for backing off when approached or aggressive for standing too close.
- *Eye contact:* Eye contact varies among cultures from intense to fleeting. In an effort to refrain from invading personal space, avoiding direct eye contact may be a sign of respect.
- *Touch:* The norms about how people should touch each other vary among cultures. In some cultures, physical contact with the same sex (embracing, walking hand in hand) is more appropriate than that with an unrelated person of the opposite sex.
- *Time orientation:* In some cultures, involvement with people is more valued than being "on time." In other cultures, life is scheduled and paced according to clock time, which is valued over personal time

Reference: Mattson, S. (2000). Striving for cultural competence: Providing care for the changing face of the U.S. *AWHONN Lifelines, 4*(3), 48-52.

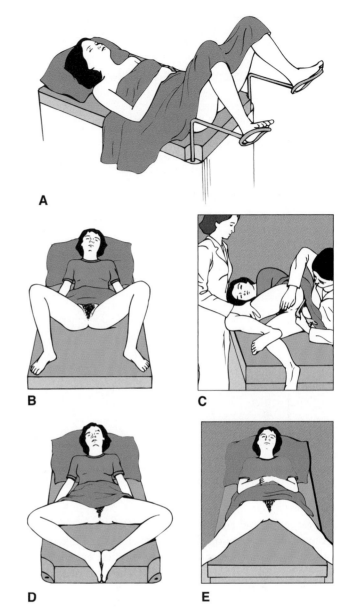

Fig. 4-10 Lithotomy and variable positions for women who have a disability. **A,** Lithotomy position. **B,** M-shaped position. **C,** Side-lying position. **D,** Diamond-shaped position. **E,** V-shaped position.

with lip reading, she may use an interpreter. The visually impaired woman needs to be oriented to the examination room and may have her guide dog with her. As with all patients, the visually impaired woman needs a full explanation of what the examination entails before proceeding. For example, before touching the woman, the nurse explains, "Now I am going to place a cuff on your right arm to take your blood pressure." Ask the woman if she would like to touch each of the items that will be used in the examination to reduce her anxiety.

Many physically disabled women cannot comfortably lie in the lithotomy position for the pelvic examination. Specially designed examination tables are available in some clinics. When this equipment is not available, several alternative positions may be used, including a lateral (side-lying) position, a V-shaped position, a diamond-shaped position, and an M-shaped position (Fig. 4-10). Ask the woman what has worked best for her previously. If she has not had a pelvic or a comfortable examination in the past, show her a picture of various positions and ask her which one she prefers. The nurse's support and reassurance can help the woman to relax, which will make the examination go more smoothly.

Abused women

Nurses should screen all women entering the health care system for potential abuse. It is important to keep in mind the possibility that violence against this woman may have occurred. Help for the woman may depend on the sensitivity with which the nurse screens for abuse, the discovery of abuse, and subsequent intervention. The nurse must be familiar with the laws governing abuse in the state in which she or he practices.

Pocket cards listing emergency numbers (abuse counseling, legal protection, and emergency shelter) may be available by calling the local police department or women's shelter or going to an emergency department or 24-hour clinic. It is helpful to have these on hand in the setting where screening is done. An abuse assessment screen can be used as part of the interview or written history (Fig. 4-11). If a male partner is present, he should be asked to leave the room, because the woman may not disclose experiences of abuse in his presence or he may try to answer questions for her to protect himself.

ABUSE ASSESSMENT SCREEN

1. Have you ever been emotionally or physically abused by your partner or someone important to you?

YES ☐   NO ☐

2. Within the last year, have you been hit, slapped, kicked, or otherwise physically hurt by someone?

YES ☐   NO ☐

If YES, by whom _____

Number of times _____

Mark the area of injury on body map.

3. Within the last year, has anyone forced you to have sexual activities?

YES ☐   NO ☐

If YES, by whom _____

Number of times _____

4. Are you afraid of your partner or anyone you listed above?

YES ☐   NO ☐

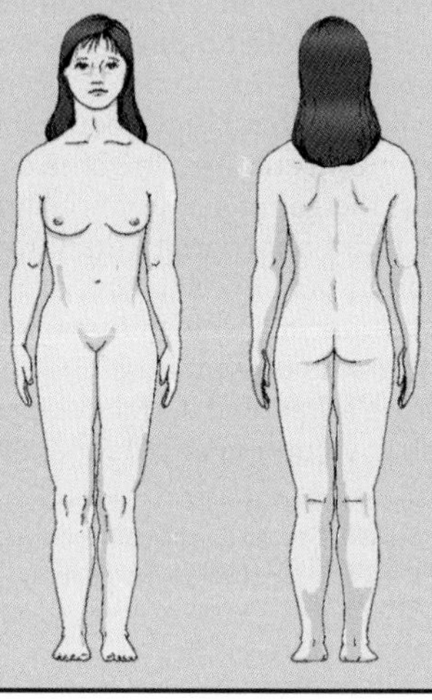

Fig. 4-11 Abuse assessment screen. (Modified from the Nursing Research Consortium on Violence and Abuse.)

Fear, guilt, and embarrassment may keep many women from giving information about family violence. Clues in the history and evidence of injuries on physical examination should give a high index of suspicion. The areas most commonly injured in women are the head, neck, chest, abdomen, breasts, and upper extremities. Burns and bruises in patterns resembling hands, belts, cords, or other weapons and multiple traumatic injuries may be seen.

Adolescents

As a young woman matures, she should be asked the same questions that are included in any history. Particular attention should be paid to hints about risky behaviors, eating disorders, and depression. Do not assume that a teenager is not sexually active. After rapport has been established, it is best to talk to a teen with the parent (or partner or friend) out of the room. Questions should be asked with sensitivity and in a gentle and nonjudgmental manner (Seidel, Ball, Dains, & Benedict, 2003).

History

A medical history usually includes the following:
1. *Identifying data.* Name, age, race, living household preference, occupation, religion, culture, and ethnicity are obtained.

2. *Chief complaint(s).* A verbatim response to the question, "What problem or symptom brought you here today?"

3. *History of present illness.* A chronologic narrative that includes onset of the problem, the setting in which it developed, its manifestations, and any treatments received are noted. The woman's state of health before the onset of the present problem is determined. If the problem is long-standing, the reason for seeking attention at this time is elicited. The principal symptoms should be described with regard to the following:
   - Location
   - Quality
   - Quantity or severity
   - Timing (onset, duration, frequency)
   - Setting
   - Factors that aggravate or relieve
   - Associated manifestations

4. *Past medical history.* Determine general state of health and strength:
   - Infectious diseases: measles, mumps, rubella, whooping cough, chicken pox, rheumatic fever, scarlet fever, diphtheria, polio, tuberculosis (TB), hepatitis
   - Chronic disease and system disorders: arthritis, cancer, diabetes, heart, lung, kidney, seizures, stroke, or ulcers

- Adult injuries, accidents, illnesses, disabilities, hospitalizations, or blood transfusions

5. *Present health status.*
   - Allergies: medications, previous transfusion reactions, or environmental allergies
   - Immunizations: diphtheria, pertussis, tetanus, polio; measles, mumps, rubella (MMR); hepatitis B, varicella, influenza, and pneumococcal vaccine; last TB skin test
   - Screening tests: Pap test (smear), mammogram, stool for occult blood, sigmoidoscopy or colonoscopy, chest x-ray study, hematocrit, hemoglobin, rubella titer, urinalysis and cholesterol test; blood type and Rh; last eye examination; last dental examination
   - Environmental and chemical hazards: home, school, work, and leisure setting; exposure to extreme heat or cold, noise, industrial toxins such as asbestos or lead, pesticides, diethylstilbestrol (DES), radiation, cat feces, or cigarette smoke
   - Use of safety measures: seat belts, bicycle helmets, designated driver
   - Exercise and leisure activities: regular
   - Sleep patterns: length and quality
   - Sexuality: Is she sexually active? With men, women, or both? Safer sex practices?
   - Diet, including beverages: 24-hour dietary recall
   - Medications: name, dose, frequency, duration, reason for taking, and compliance with prescription medications; home remedies, over-the-counter drugs, vitamin and mineral supplements used over a 24-hour period; herbal therapies
   - Nicotine, alcohol, illicit or recreational drugs: type, amount, frequency, duration, and reactions
   - Caffeine: coffee, tea, cola, or chocolate intake

6. *Past surgical history.* Type, date, reason, outcome, and any complications should be noted.

7. *Family history.* Information about age and health of family members may be presented in narrative or genogram: age, health status, or death of parents, siblings, spouse, children. Check for history of diabetes, heart disease, hypertension, stroke, respiratory disorders, renal disorders, thyroid disorders, cancer, bleeding disorders, hepatitis, allergies, asthma, arthritis, TB, epilepsy, mental illness, HIV, and other conditions.

8. *Social history.* Note birthplace, education, employment, marital status, living accommodations, children, persons at home, and hobbies. Does she enjoy what she is doing?
   - Screen for abuse: Has she ever been hit, kicked, slapped, or forced to have sex against her wishes? Has she been verbally or emotionally abused? Does she have a history of childhood sexual abuse? If yes, has she received counseling or does she need referral?

9. *Review of systems.* It is probable that all questions in each system will not be included every time a history

is taken. Some questions regarding each system should be included in every history. The essential areas to be explored are listed in the following head-to-toe sequence. If a woman gives a positive response to a question about an essential area, more detailed questions should be asked.

- General: weight change, fatigue, weakness, fever, chills, or night sweats
- Skin: skin, hair and nail changes, itching, bruising, bleeding, rashes, sores, lumps, or moles
- Lymph nodes: enlargement, inflammation, pain, suppuration (pus), or drainage
- Head, eyes, ears, nose, and throat (HEENT): head—trauma, vertigo (dizziness), convulsive disorder, syncope (fainting), headache location, frequency, pain type, nausea or vomiting, or visual symptoms; eyes—glasses, contact lenses, blurriness, tearing, itching, photophobia, diplopia, inflammation, trauma, cataracts, glaucoma, or acute visual loss; ears—hearing loss, tinnitus (ringing), vertigo, discharge, pain, fullness, recurrent infections, or mastoiditis; nose and sinuses—trauma, rhinitis, nasal discharge, epistaxis, obstruction, sneezing, itching, allergy, or smelling impairment; mouth, throat, and neck—hoarseness, voice changes, soreness, ulcers, bleeding gums, goiter, swelling, or enlarged nodes
- Breasts: masses, pain, lumps, dimpling, nipple discharge, fibrocystic changes or implants; BSE practice
- Respiratory: shortness of breath, wheezing, cough, sputum, hemoptysis, pneumonia, pleurisy, asthma, bronchitis, emphysema, or TB; date and result of last chest x-ray film
- Cardiac: hypertension, rheumatic fever, murmurs, angina, palpitations, dyspnea, tachycardia, orthopnea, edema, chest pain, cough, cyanosis, cold extremities, ascites, intermittent claudication (calf pain), phlebitis, or skin color changes
- GI: appetite, nausea, vomiting, indigestion, dysphagia, abdominal pain, ulcers, hematochezia (bleeding with stools), melena (black, tarry stools), bowel habit changes, diarrhea, constipation, bowel movement frequency, food intolerance, hemorrhoids, jaundice, or hepatitis; sigmoidoscopy, colonoscopy, barium enema, or ultrasound
- Genitourinary (GU): frequency, hesitancy, urgency, polyuria, dysuria, hematuria, nocturia, incontinence, stones, infection, or urethral discharge; dysmenorrhea, intermenstrual bleeding, dyspareunia, discharge, sores, itching, STIs, gravidity (G), parity (P), problems in pregnancy, contraception, menopause, hot flashes, or sweats (may be included here or as part of endocrine assessment)
- Vascular: leg edema, claudication, varicose veins, thromboses, or emboli
- Endocrine: heat or cold intolerance, dry skin, excessive sweating, polyuria, polydipsia, polyphagia,

thyroid problems, diabetes, or secondary sex characteristic changes; age at menarche, length and flow of menses, last menstrual period (LMP), age at menopause, libido, or sexual concerns

- Hematologic: anemia, easy bruising, bleeding, petechiae, purpura, or transfusions
- Musculoskeletal: muscle weakness, pain, joint stiffness, scoliosis, lordosis, kyphosis, range-of-motion instability, redness, swelling, arthritis, or gout
- Neurologic: loss of sensation, numbness, tingling, tremors, weakness, vertigo, paralysis, fainting, twitching, blackouts, seizures, convulsions, loss of consciousness or memory
- Psychiatric: moodiness, depression, anxiety, obsessions, delusions, illusions, or hallucinations

Physical Examination

Objective data are recorded by system or location. A general statement of overall health status is a good way to start. Findings are described in detail.

- General appearance: age, race, sex, state of health, stature, development, dress, hygiene, affect, alertness, orientation, cooperativeness, and communication skills
- Vital signs: temperature, pulse, respiration, blood pressure
- Height and weight
- Skin: color; integrity; texture; hydration; temperature; edema; excessive perspiration; unusual odor; presence and description of lesions; hair texture and distribution; nail configuration; color, texture, condition of nails or presence of nail clubbing
- Head: size, shape, trauma, masses, scars, rashes or scaling; facial symmetry; presence of edema or puffiness
- Eyes: pupil size, shape, reactivity; conjunctival injection; scleral icterus; fundal papilledema; hemorrhage; lids; extraocular movements; visual fields and acuity
- Ears: shape and symmetry, tenderness, discharge, external canal, and tympanic membranes; hearing: Weber should be midline (loudness of sound equal in both ears) and Rinne negative (no conductive or sensorineural hearing loss); should be able to hear whisper at 3 feet
- Nose: symmetry, tenderness, discharge, mucosa, turbinate inflammation, frontal and maxillary sinus tenderness; discrimination of odors
- Mouth, throat: hygiene, condition of teeth, dentures, appearance of lips, tongue buccal and oral mucosa, erythema, edema, exudate, tonsillar enlargement, palate, uvula, gag reflex, or ulcers
- Neck: mobility, masses, range of motion, trachea deviation, thyroid size, carotid bruits
- Lymphatic: cervical, intraclavicular, axillary, trochlear, or inguinal adenopathy; size, shape, tenderness, and consistency

- Breasts: skin changes, dimpling, symmetry, scars, tenderness, discharge or masses; characteristics of nipples and areolae
- Heart: rate, rhythm, murmurs, rubs, gallops, clicks, heaves, or precordial movements
- Peripheral vascular: jugular vein distention, bruits, edema, swelling, vein distention, Homans sign, or tenderness of extremities
- Lungs: chest symmetry with respirations, wheezes, crackles, rhonchi, vocal fremitus, whispered pectoriloquy, percussion, and diaphragmatic excursion; breath sounds equal and clear bilaterally
- Abdomen: shape, scars, bowel sounds, consistency, tenderness, rebound, masses, guarding, organomegaly, liver span, percussion (tympany, shifting, dullness), costovertebral angle tenderness
- Extremities: edema, ulceration, tenderness, varicosities, erythema, tremor, or deformity
- GU: external genitalia, perineum, vaginal mucosa, cervix, inflammation, tenderness, discharge, bleeding, ulcers, nodules, masses, internal vaginal support, bimanual and rectovaginal examination; palpation of cervix, uterus, and adnexa
- Rectal: sphincter tone, masses, hemorrhoids, rectal wall contour, tenderness, and stool for occult blood
- Musculoskeletal: posture, symmetry of muscle mass, muscle atrophy, weakness, appearance of joints, tenderness or crepitus, joint range of motion, instability, redness, swelling, or spine deviation
- Neurologic: mental status, orientation, memory, mood, speech clarity and comprehension, cranial nerves II through XII, sensation, strength, deep tendon and superficial reflexes, gait, balance, and coordination with rapid alternating motions

Pelvic Examination

Many women are intimidated by the gynecologic portion of the physical examination. The nurse in this instance can take an advocacy approach that supports a partnership relationship between the woman and the care provider (see Guidelines/Guías box). It is especially important to prepare the adolescent for her first speculum examination because she will develop perceptions that will remain with her for future examinations. What the examination entails should be discussed with the teen while she is dressed. Models or illustrations can be used to show exactly what will happen. All of the necessary equipment should be assembled so that there are no interruptions. Pediatric specula that are 1 to 1.5 cm wide can be inserted with minimal discomfort. If the teen is sexually active, a small adult speculum may be used.

The woman is assisted into the lithotomy position (see Fig. 4-10, *A*) for the pelvic examination. When she is in the lithotomy position, the woman's hips and knees are flexed with the buttocks at the edge of the table, and her feet are supported by heel or knee stirrups.

GUIDELINES/GUÍAS
Physical Examination

- Take off all your clothes, please.
- *Quítese toda la ropa, por favor.*

- Put on the gown, please.
- *Póngase la bata, por favor.*

- I am going to examine you.
- *Le voy a examinar.*

- You will feel less discomfort if you relax.
- *Se sentirá más cómoda si se relaja el cuerpo.*

- Lie down, please.
- *Acuéstese, por favor.*

- Put your feet in the stirrups.
- *Póngase los pies en los estribos.*

- Open your legs, please.
- *Sepárese las piernas, por favor.*

- I am going to take a sample from the lining of the cervix (Pap test).
- *Le voy a tomar una muestra del cuello uterino (el examen de Papanicolao).*

- We will test this sample for cancer.
- *Haremos un análisis de esta muestra para determinar si hay cáncer.*

- It won't hurt.
- *No le va a doler.*

- Everything looks fine.
- *Todo está bien.*

- You may get dressed.
- *Puede vestirse.*

Some women prefer to keep their shoes or socks on, especially if the stirrups are not padded. Many women express feelings of vulnerability and strangeness when in the lithotomy position. During the procedure the nurse assists the woman with relaxation techniques.

One method of helping the woman relax is to have her place her hands on her chest at about the level of the diaphragm, breathe deeply and slowly (in through her nose and out through her O-shaped mouth), concentrate on the rhythm of breathing, and relax all body muscles with each exhalation (Barkauskas, Baumann, & Darling-Fisher, 2002). This breathing technique is particularly helpful for the adolescent or the woman whose introitus may be especially tight or for whom the experience may be new or may provoke tension. Some women relax when they are encouraged to become involved with the examination with a mirror placed so that they can view the area being examined. This type of participation helps with health teaching as well. Distraction is another technique that can be used effectively (e.g., placement of interesting pictures on the ceiling over the head of the table).

Many women find it distressing to attempt to converse in the lithotomy position. Most women appreciate an explanation of the procedure as it unfolds, as well as coaching for the type of sensations they may expect. Generally, however, women prefer not to have to respond to questions until they are again upright and at eye level with the examiner. Questioning during the procedure, especially if they cannot see their questioner's eyes, may make women tense.

External inspection

The examiner sits at the foot of the table for the inspection of the external genitals and for the speculum examination. To facilitate open communication and to help the woman relax, the woman's head is raised on a pillow and the drape is arranged so that eye-to-eye contact can be maintained. In good lighting, external genitals are inspected for sexual maturity, clitoris, labia, and perineum. After childbirth or other trauma there may be healed scars.

External palpation

The examiner proceeds with the examination using palpation and inspection. The examiner wears gloves for this portion of the assessment. Before touching the woman, the examiner explains what is going to be done and what the woman should expect to feel (e.g., pressure). The examiner may touch the woman in a less sensitive area such as the inner thigh to alert her that the genital examination is beginning. This gesture may put the woman more at ease. The labia are spread apart to expose the structures in the vestibule: urinary meatus, Skene glands, vaginal orifice, and Bartholin glands (Fig. 4-12). To assess the Skene glands, the examiner inserts one finger into the vagina and "milks" the area of the urethra. Any exudate from the urethra or the Skene glands is cultured. Masses and erythema of either structure are assessed further. Ordinarily the openings to the Skene glands are not visible; prominent openings may be seen if the glands are infected (e.g., with gonorrhea). During the examination the examiner keeps in mind the data from the review of systems, such as history of burning on urination.

The vaginal orifice is examined. Hymenal tags are normal findings. With one finger still in the vagina, the examiner

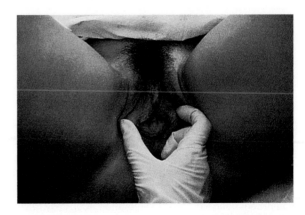

Fig. 4-12 External examination. Separation of the labia. (From Edge, V., & Miller, M. [1994]. *Women's health care.* St. Louis: Mosby.)

repositions the index finger near the posterior part of the orifice. With the thumb outside the posterior part of the labia majora, the examiner compresses the area of Bartholin glands located at the 8 o'clock and 4 o'clock positions and looks for swelling, discharge, and pain.

The support of the anterior and posterior vaginal wall is assessed. The examiner spreads the labia with the index and middle finger and asks the woman to strain down. Any bulge from the anterior wall (urethrocele or cystocele) or posterior wall (rectocele) is noted and compared with the history, such as difficulty to start the stream of urine or constipation.

The perineum (area between the vagina and anus) is assessed for scars from old lacerations or episiotomies, thinning, fistulas, masses, lesions, and inflammation. The anus is assessed for hemorrhoids, hemorrhoidal tags, and integrity of the anal sphincter. The anal area is also assessed for lesions, masses, abscesses, and tumors. If there is a history of STI, the examiner may want to obtain a culture specimen from the anal canal at this time. Throughout the genital examination, the examiner notes the odor. Odor may indicate infection or poor hygiene.

Vulvar self-examination. The pelvic examination provides a good opportunity for the practitioner to emphasize the need for regular **vulvar self-examination (VSE)** and to teach this procedure. Because there has been a dramatic increase in cancerous and precancerous conditions of the vulva in recent years, a VSE should be performed as an integral part of preventive health care by all women who are sexually active or 18 years of age or older, monthly between menses or more frequently if there are symptoms or a history of serious vulvar disease. Most lesions, including malignancy, condyloma acuminatum (wartlike growth), and Bartholin cysts, can be seen or palpated and are easily treated if diagnosed early.

The examination can be performed by the practitioner and woman together, using a mirror. A simple diagram of the anatomy of the vulva can be given to the woman, with instructions to perform the examination herself that evening to reinforce what she has learned. She does the examination in a sitting position with adequate lighting, holding a mirror in one hand and using the other hand to expose the tissues surrounding the vaginal introitus. She then systematically examines the mons pubis, clitoris, urethra, labia majora, perineum, and perianal area and palpates the vulva, noting any changes in appearance of abnormalities, such as ulcers, lumps, warts, and changes in pigmentation.

Internal examination

A vaginal speculum consists of two blades and a handle and comes in a variety of types and styles. A vaginal speculum is used to view the vaginal vault and cervix (Procedure box—Assisting with Pelvic Examination). The closed speculum is gently placed into the vagina and inserted to the back of the vaginal vault. The blades are opened to reveal the cervix and are locked into the open position. The cervix is inspected for position and appearance of the os: color, lesions, bleeding, and discharge (Fig. 4-13). Cervical findings

---

Procedure

Assisting with Pelvic Examination

- Wash hands. Assemble equipment (see Fig.).
- Ask woman to empty her bladder before the examination (obtain clean-catch urine specimen as needed).
- Assist with relaxation techniques. Have the woman place her hands on her chest at about the level of the diaphragm,

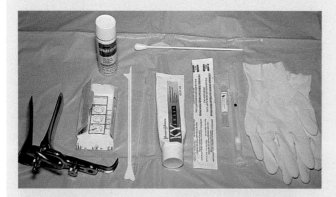

Equipment used for pelvic examination. (Courtesy Michael S. Clement, MD, Mesa, AZ.)

breathe deeply and slowly (in through her nose and out through an O-shaped mouth), concentrate on the rhythm of breathing, and relax all body muscles with each exhalation (Barkauskas, Baumann, & Darling-Fisher 2002).
- Encourage the woman to become involved with the examination if she shows interest. For example, a mirror can be placed so that she can see the area being examined.
- Assess for and treat signs of problems such as supine hypotension.
- Warm the speculum in warm water if a prewarmed one is not available.
- Instruct the woman to bear down when the speculum is being inserted.
- Apply gloves and assist the examiner with collection of specimens for cytologic examination, such as a Pap test. After handling specimens, remove gloves and wash hands.
- Lubricate the examiner's fingers with water or water-soluble lubricant before bimanual examination.
- Assist the woman at completion of the examination to a sitting position and then a standing position.
- Provide tissues to wipe lubricant from perineum.
- Provide privacy for the woman while she is dressing.

that are not within normal limits include ulcerations, masses, inflammation, and excessive protrusion into the vaginal vault. Anomalies, such as a cockscomb (a protrusion over the cervix that looks like a rooster's comb), a hooded or collared cervix (seen in DES daughters), or polyps are noted.

Collection of specimens.   The collection of specimens for cytologic examination is an important part of the gynecologic examination. Infection can be diagnosed through examination of specimens collected during the pelvic examination. Possible infections include *Candida albicans, Trichomonas vaginalis,* bacterial vaginosis, β-hemolytic streptococci, *Neisseria gonorrhoeae, Chlamydia trachomatis,* and

herpes simplex virus (see Chapter 5). Once the diagnoses have been made, treatment can be instituted. Carcinogenic conditions, potential or actual, can be determined by examination of cells from the cervix (e.g., Pap test, HPV DNA test) collected during the pelvic examination (see Procedure box–Papanicolaou [Pap] Test).

Vaginal examination

After the specimens are obtained, the vagina is viewed when the speculum is rotated. The speculum blades are unlocked and partially closed. As the speculum is withdrawn, it is rotated and the vaginal walls are inspected for color, lesions, rugae, fistulas, and bulging.

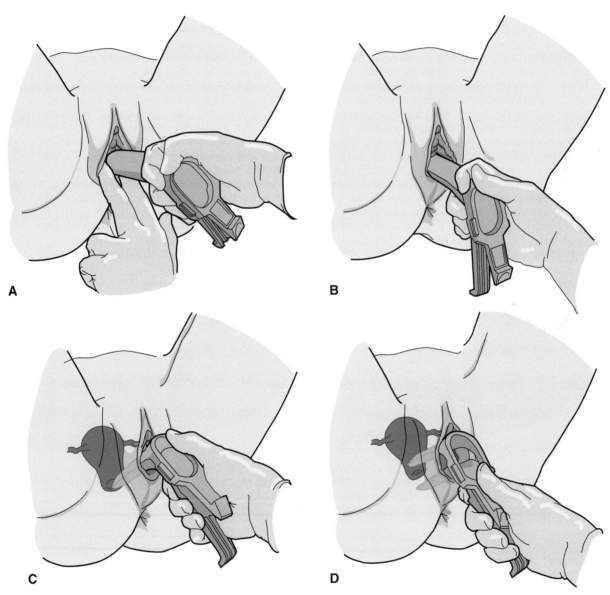

Fig. 4-13   Insertion of speculum for vaginal examination. **A,** Opening of the introitus. **B,** Oblique insertion of the speculum. **C,** Final insertion of the speculum. **D,** Opening of the speculum blades. (From Barkauskas, V., Baumann, L., & Darling-Fisher, C. [2002]. *Health and physical assessment* [3rd ed.]. St. Louis: Mosby.)

Procedure

Papanicolaou (Pap) Test

- In preparation, make sure the woman has not douched, used vaginal medications, or had sexual intercourse for 24 to 48 hours before the procedure (Gingrich, 2004). Reschedule the test if the woman is menstruating. Midcycle is the best time for the test.
- Explain to the woman the purpose of the test and what sensations she will feel as the specimen is obtained (e.g., pressure but not pain).
- The woman is assisted into a lithotomy position. A speculum is inserted into the vagina.
- The cytologic specimen is obtained before any digital examination of the vagina is made or endocervical bacteriologic specimens are taken. A cotton swab may be used to remove excess cervical discharge before the specimen is collected.
- The specimen is obtained by using an endocervical sampling device (Cytobrush, Cervex-Brush, papette, or broom) (see Fig.). If the two-sample method of obtaining cells is used, the cytobrush is inserted into the canal and rotated 90 to 180 degrees, followed by a gentle smear of the entire transformation zone by using a spatula. Broom devices are inserted and rotated 360 degrees five times. They obtain endocervical and ectocervical samples at the same time. If the patient has had a hysterectomy, the vaginal cuff is sampled. Areas that appear abnormal on visualization will require colposcopy and biopsy. If using a one-slide technique, the spatula sample is smeared first. This is followed by applying the cytobrush sample (rolling the brush in the opposite direction from which it was obtained), which is less subject to drying artifact; then the slide is sprayed with preservative within 5 seconds.

- The ThinPrep Pap Test is a liquid-based method of preserving cells that reduces blood, mucus, and inflammation. The Pap specimen is obtained in the manner described above except that the cervix is not swabbed before collection of the sample. The collection device (brush, spatula, or broom) is rinsed in a vial of preserving solution that is provided by the laboratory. The sealed vial with solution is sent off to the appropriate laboratory. A special processing device filters the contents, and a thin layer of cervical cells is deposited on a slide, which is then examined microscopically. The AutoPap and Papnet tests are similar to the ThinPrep test. If cytology is abnormal, liquid-based methods allow follow-up testing for HPV DNA with the same sample (Gingrich, 2004).
- Label the slides or vial with the woman's name and site. Include on the form to accompany the specimens the woman's name, age, parity, and chief complaint or reason for taking the cytologic specimens.
- Send specimens to the pathology laboratory promptly for staining, evaluation, and a written report, with special reference to abnormal elements, including cancer cells.
- Advise the woman that repeated tests may be necessary if the specimen is not adequate.
- Instruct the woman concerning routine checkups for cervical and vaginal cancer. The American Cancer Society (2005) advises women who have been sexually active for 3 years or who are 21 years old to have yearly Pap tests (or every 2 years if liquid-based test). At age 30, after three normal Pap results, screening may be every 2 to 3 years. A pelvic examination is recommended every 3 years from age 20 to 40 and every 1 to 3 years thereafter.
- Record the examination date on the woman's record.

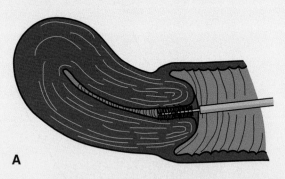 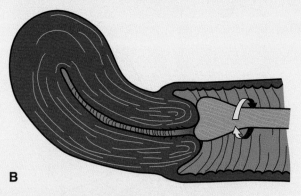

A   B

Pap test. **A,** Collecting cells from endocervix using a cytobrush. **B,** Obtaining cells from the transformation zone using a wooden spatula. (From Stenchever, M., Droegemueller, W., Herbst, A., & Mishell, D. [2001]. *Comprehensive gynecology* [4th ed.]. St. Louis: Mosby.)

Bimanual palpation

The examiner stands for this part of the examination. A small amount of lubricant is placed on the first and second fingers of the gloved hand for the internal examination. To prevent tissue trauma and contamination, the thumb is abducted and the ring and little fingers are flexed into the palm (Fig. 4-14).

The vagina is palpated for distensibility, lesions, and tenderness. The cervix is examined for position, shape, consistency, motility, and lesions. The fornix around the cervix is palpated.

The other hand is placed on the abdomen halfway between the umbilicus and symphysis pubis and exerts pressure downward toward the pelvic hand. Upward pressure

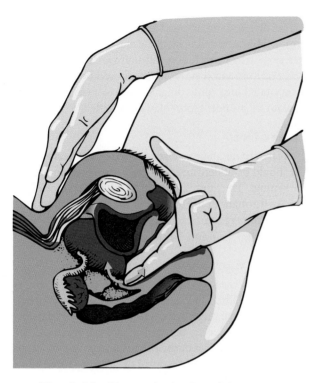

Fig. 4-14 Bimanual palpation of the uterus.

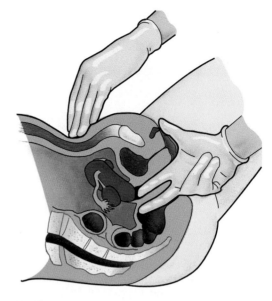

Fig. 4-15 Rectovaginal examination. (From Seidel, H., Ball, J., Dains, J., & Benedict, G. [2003]. *Mosby's guide to physical examination* [5th ed.]. St. Louis: Mosby.)

from the pelvic hand traps reproductive structures for assessment by palpation. The uterus is assessed for position, size, shape, consistency, regularity, motility, masses, and tenderness.

With the abdominal hand moving to the right lower quadrant and the fingers of the pelvic hand in the right lateral fornix, the adnexa is assessed for position, size, tenderness, and masses. The examination is repeated on the woman's left side.

Just before the intravaginal fingers are withdrawn, the woman is asked to tighten her vagina around the fingers as much as she can. If the muscle response is weak, the woman is assessed for her knowledge about Kegel exercises.

Rectovaginal palpation

To prevent contamination of the rectum from organisms in the vagina (e.g., *N. gonorrhoeae*) it is necessary to change gloves, add fresh lubricant, and then reinsert the index finger into the vagina and the middle finger into the rectum (Fig. 4-15). Insertion is facilitated if the woman strains down. The maneuvers of the abdominovaginal examination are repeated. The rectovaginal examination permits assessment of the rectovaginal septum, the posterior surface of the uterus, and the region behind the cervix and the adnexa. The vaginal finger is removed and folded into the palm, leaving the middle finger free to rotate 360 degrees. The rectum is palpated for rectal tenderness and masses.

After the rectal examination, the woman is assisted into a sitting position, given tissues or wipes to cleanse herself, and given privacy to dress. The woman often returns to the

examiner's office for a discussion of findings, prescriptions for therapy, and counseling.

Pelvic examination during pregnancy is discussed in Chapter 9.

Laboratory and Diagnostic Procedures

The following laboratory and diagnostic procedures are ordered at the discretion of the clinician: complete blood count or hemoglobin and hematocrit, total blood cholesterol, fasting plasma glucose, urinalysis for bacteria, syphilis serology (Venereal Disease Research Laboratory [VDRL] test or rapid plasma reagin test [RPR]) and other screening tests for STIs, mammogram, tuberculin skin test, hearing test, electrocardiogram, chest x-ray film, fecal occult blood, and bone mineral density. HIV and drug screening may be offered or encouraged with informed consent, especially in high risk populations. Results of tests usually are reported by phone call or letter.

ANTICIPATORY GUIDANCE FOR HEALTH PROMOTION AND PREVENTION

Knowledge alone is not enough to bring about healthy behaviors. The woman must be convinced that she has some control over her life and that healthy life habits, including periodic health examinations, are a sound investment. She must believe in the efficacy of prevention, early detection, and therapy and in her ability to perform self-care practices, such as BSE. The model illustrated in Fig. 4-16 incorporates the major aspects to be included when counseling women.

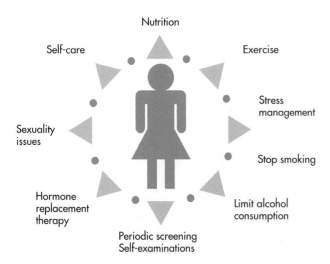

Fig. 4-16 Nursing care model for counseling women about self-care. (Courtesy Design Center, University of North Carolina School of Nursing, Chapel Hill, NC.)

Nutrition

To maintain good nutrition, women should be counseled to eat a variety of foods. Foods low in saturated fat and cholesterol, moderate sodium and sugar intake, whole grain products, and a variety of fruits and vegetables should be selected. At least four to six glasses of water in addition to other fluids such as juices should be included in the diet daily. Coffee, tea, soft drinks, and alcoholic beverages should be used in moderation (U.S. Department of Health and Human Services & Department of Agriculture, 2005). Red meats and processed meats as well as refined grains should be limited (ACS, 2005).

Most women do not recognize the importance of calcium to health, and their diets are insufficient in calcium. Women who are unlikely to get enough calcium in the diet may need calcium supplements in the form of calcium carbonate, which contains more elemental calcium than other preparations.

The diet can be assessed using a standard assessment form—a 24-hour recall is adequate and quick—and then food likes and dislikes, including cultural variations and typical food portions and dietary habits, should be discussed and incorporated into counseling. Referral to a weight reduction program or support group may be beneficial.

Exercise

Physical activity and exercise counseling for persons of all ages should be undertaken at schools, work sites, and primary care settings. The nurse should stress the importance of daily exercise throughout life for weight management and health promotion, suggesting exercises that are enjoyable to the individual (Figs. 4-17 and 4-18).

Kegel exercises

Kegel exercises, or pelvic muscle exercises, were developed to strengthen the supportive pelvic floor muscles to control or reduce incontinent urine loss. These exercises are also beneficial during pregnancy and postpartum. They strengthen the muscles of the pelvic floor, providing support for the pelvic organs and control of the muscles surrounding the vagina and urethra.

The Association of Women's Health, Obstetric and Neonatal Nurses conducted a research utilization project focused on continence for women (Sampselle et al., 2000). Educational strategies for teaching women how to perform Kegel exercises that were compiled by nurse researchers involved in the project are described in the Teaching Guidelines box.

Stress Management

Because it is neither possible nor desirable to avoid all stress, women need to learn how to manage stress. The nurse should assess each woman for signs of stress, using therapeutic communication skills to determine risk factors and the woman's ability to function.

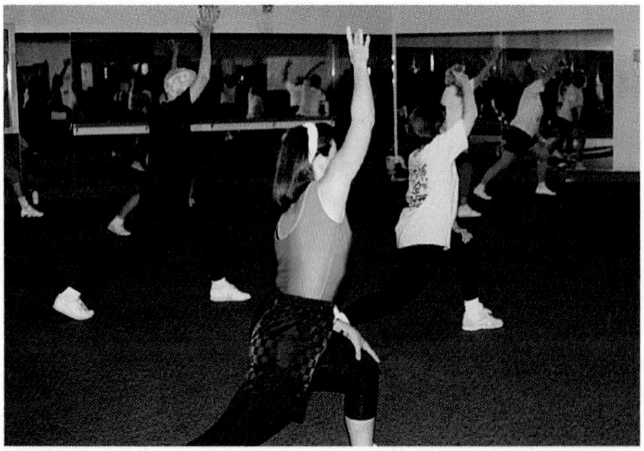

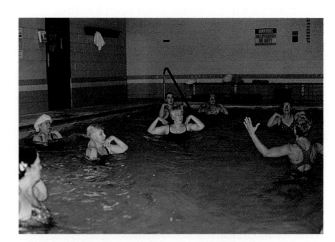

Fig. 4-17 Weight-bearing exercise may delay bone loss and increase bone mass. (Courtesy Jonas McCoy, Raleigh, NC.)

Fig. 4-18 Water aerobics improves cardiovascular function. (Courtesy Jonas McCoy, Raleigh, NC.)

TEACHING GUIDELINES

Kegel Exercises

DESCRIPTION AND RATIONALE

- Kegel exercise, or pelvic muscle exercise, is a technique used to strengthen the muscles that support the pelvic floor. This exercise involves regularly tightening (contracting) and relaxing the muscles that support the bladder and urethra. By strengthening these pelvic muscles, a woman can prevent or reduce accidental urine loss.

TECHNIQUE

- The woman needs to learn how to target the muscles for training and how to contract them correctly. One suggestion for teaching is to have the woman pretend she is trying to prevent the passage of intestinal gas. Have her use this tightening motion on the muscles around her vagina and the upper pelvis. She should feel these muscles drawing inward and upward. Other suggested techniques are to have the woman pretend she is trying to stop the flow of urine in midstream or to have her think about how her vagina is able to contract around and move up the length of the penis during intercourse.

  The woman should avoid straining or bearing-down motions while performing the exercise. She should be taught how bearing down feels by having her take a breath, hold it, and push down with her abdominal muscles as though she were trying to have a bowel movement. Then the woman can be taught how to avoid straining down by exhaling gently and keeping her mouth open each time she contracts her pelvic muscles.

SPECIFIC INSTRUCTIONS

1 Each contraction should be as intense as possible without contracting the abdomen, thighs, or buttocks.
2 Contractions should be held for at least 10 seconds. The woman may have to start with as little as 2 seconds per contraction until her muscles get stronger.
3 The woman should rest for 10 seconds or more between contractions, so that the muscles have time to recover and each contraction can be as strong as the woman can make it.
4 The woman should feel the pulling up over the three muscle layers so that the contraction reaches the highest level of her pelvis.

OTHER SUGGESTIONS FOR IMPLEMENTATION

1 At first the woman should set aside about 15 minutes a day to do the Kegel exercises.
2 The woman may want to put up reminders, such as notes on her bathroom mirror, her refrigerator, her television, or her calendar, to do the exercises.
3 Guidelines for practicing Kegel exercises suggest performing between 24 and 100 contractions a day; however, positive results can be achieved with only 24 to 45 a day.
4 The best position for learning how to do Kegel exercises is to lie supine with the knees bent. Another position to use is on the hands and knees. Once the woman learns the proper technique, she can perform the exercises in other positions such as standing or sitting.

From Sampselle, C. (2000). Behavioral interventions for urinary incontinence in women: Evidence for practice. *Journal of Midwifery & Women's Health, 45*(2), 94-103; Sampselle, C. (2003). Behavior interventions in young and middle-aged women: Simple interventions to combat a complex problem. *American Journal of Nursing, 103* (suppl), 9-19; Sampselle, C. et al. (2000). Continence for women: A test of AWHONN's evidence-based protocol. *Journal of Obstetric, Gynecologic, and Neonatal Nursing, 29*(1), 312-317.

Some women must be referred for counseling or other mental health therapy. Women are almost twice as likely as men to suffer from depression, anxiety, or panic attacks (National Women's Health Resource Center, 2003). Nurses need to be alert to the symptoms of serious mental disorders, such as depression and anxiety, and make referrals to mental health practitioners when necessary. Women experiencing major life changes, such as divorce and separation, bereavement, serious illness, and unemployment, also need special attention.

For many women the nurse is able to provide comfort, reassurance, and advice concerning helping resources, such as support groups. Many centers offer support groups to help women prevent or manage stress. The nurse can help them become more aware of the relationship between good nutrition, rest, relaxation, and exercise or diversion and their ability to deal with stress. In the case of role overload, determining what needs immediate attention and what can wait is important. Practical advice includes regular breaks, taking time for friends, developing interests outside of work or the home, setting realistic goals, and learning self-acceptance. Anticipatory guidance for developmental or expected situational crises can help women plan strategies for dealing with potentially stressful events.

Role-playing, relaxation techniques, biofeedback, meditation, desensitization, imagery, assertiveness training, yoga, diet, exercise, and weight control are techniques nurses can include in their repertoire of helping skills. Insufficient time prevents one-on-one assistance in many situations, but the more nurses know about these resources, the better able they are to intervene, counsel, and direct women to appropriate resources. Careful follow-up of all women experiencing difficulty in dealing with stress is important.

Substance Use Cessation

All women at all ages will receive substantial and immediate benefits from smoking cessation. However, this is not easy, and most people stop several times before they accomplish their goal (Box 4-2). Many are never able to do so. Those who wish to stop smoking can be referred to a smoking cessation program where individualized methods can be implemented. At the very least, individuals should be guided to self-help materials available from the March of Dimes Birth Defects Foundation, American Lung Association, and ACS. During pregnancy, women seem to be highly motivated to stop or at least to limit smoking to 10 or fewer cigarettes per day. Insult to the fetus can be

---

BOX 4-2

Interventions for Smoking Cessation: The Four A's

ASK

- What was her age when she started smoking? How many cigarettes does she smoke a day? When was her last cigarette? Has she tried to quit? Does she want to quit?

ASSESS

- What were her reasons for not being able to quit before, or what made her start again? Does she have anyone who can help her? Does anyone else smoke at home? Does she have friends or family who have quit successfully?

ADVISE

- Give her information about the effects of smoking on pregnancy and her fetus, on her own future health, and on the members of her household.

ASSIST

- Provide support; give self-help materials. Encourage her to set a quit date. Refer to a smoking cessation program or provide information about nicotine replacement products (not recommended during pregnancy) if she is interested. Teach and encourage use of stress reduction activities. Provide for follow-up with a phone call, letter, or clinic visit.

Source: American College of Obstetricians and Gynecologists (ACOG). (1997). *Smoking and women's health. ACOG Technical Bulletin no. 240.* Washington, DC: ACOG.

---

reduced or even avoided if this is done by the end of the first trimester.

Counseling women who appear to be drinking excessively or using drugs may include strategies to increase self-esteem and teaching new coping skills to resist and maintain resistance to alcohol abuse and drug use. Appropriate referrals should be made, with the health care provider arranging the contact and then following up to be sure that appointments are kept. General referral to sources of support should also be provided. National groups that provide information and support for those who are chemically dependent are listed in the Resources section at the end of the chapter. Many of these organizations have local branches or contacts that are listed in the telephone book.

Safer Sexual Practices

Prevention of STIs is predicated on the reduction of high risk behaviors by educating toward a behavioral change. Behaviors of concern include multiple and casual sexual partners and unsafe sexual practices. The abuse of alcohol and drugs is also a high risk behavior resulting in impaired judgment and thoughtless acts. Specific self-care measures for "safer sex" are described in Chapter 5.

In addition to information about the prevention of STIs, women of childbearing years need information regarding contraception and family planning (see Chapter 6).

Health Screening Schedule

Periodic health screening includes history, physical examination, education, counseling, and selected diagnostic and laboratory tests. This regimen provides the basis for overall health promotion, prevention of illness, early diagnosis of problems, and referral for appropriate management. Such screening should be customized according to a woman's age and risk factors. In most instances, it is completed in health care offices, clinics, or hospitals; however,

portions of the screening are now being carried out at events such as Community Health Fairs. An overview of health screening recommendations for women older than 18 years of age is found in Table 4-2.

Health Risk Prevention

Often, simple safety factors are forgotten or perceived not to be important; yet injuries continue to have a major impact on health status among all age groups. Being aware of hazards and implementing safety guidelines will reduce risks. The nurse should frequently reinforce commonsense concepts that will protect the individual, such as wearing seat belts at all times in a moving vehicle and protecting the skin from ultraviolet light with sunscreen and clothing.

Health Protection

Nurses can make a difference in stopping violence against women and preventing further injury. Educating women that abuse is a violation of their rights and facilitating their access to protective and legal services constitute a first step. Also, encouraging health care institutions to implement appropriate IPV assessment and intervention programs is needed (Dienemann, Campbell, Wiederhorn, Laughon, & Jordon, 2003). Other helpful measures for women to discourage their fall into abusive relationships are promoting assertiveness and self-defense courses; suggesting support and self-help groups that encourage positive self-regard, confidence, and empowerment; and recommending educational and skills development classes that will enhance independence or at least the ability to take care of oneself.

Numerous national and local organizations provide information and assistance for women experiencing abusive situations. Nurses and victims may find these resources helpful. National resources and hotlines are listed at the end of this chapter. All nurses who work in women's health care should become familiar with local services and legal options.

TABLE 4-2

Health Screening Recommendations for Women Aged 18 Years and Older

INTERVENTION	RECOMMENDATION*
PHYSICAL EXAMINATION	
Blood pressure	Every visit, but at least every 2 years
Height and weight	Every visit, but at least every 2 years
Pelvic examination	Annually until age 70; recommended for any woman who has ever been sexually active
Breast examination	
Self-examination	Initiated or taught at time of first pelvic examination; done monthly at end of menses
Clinical examination†	Every 3 years, ages 20 to 39; annually after age 40
High risk	Annually after age 18 with history of premenopausal breast cancer in first-degree relative
Risk groups	At least annually:
Skin examination	Family history of skin cancer or increased exposure to sunlight after age 40; every 3 years between ages 20 to 40; monthly self-examinations also recommended
Oral cavity examination	Mouth lesion or exposure to tobacco or excessive alcohol
LABORATORY AND DIAGNOSTIC TESTS	
Blood cholesterol (fasting lipoprotein analysis)	Every 5 years
High risk	More often per clinical judgment with potential for cardiac or lipid abnormalities
Papanicolaou test†	Initially, 3 years after becoming sexually active but no later than age 21; yearly with conventional Pap test or every 2 years with liquid-based Pap tests. After age 30 and after three normal test results in a row, every 2 to 3 years; after age 70 and no abnormal test results in 10 years, screening may be stopped
Mammography‡	Annually over age 50
	Annually over age 40
	Every 1 to 2 years between ages 40 and 49 and annually thereafter
Colon cancer screening	Fecal occult blood test annually and flexible sigmoidoscopy every 5 years after age 50; more often if family history of colon cancer or polyps
Risk groups	
Fasting blood sugar	Annually with family history of diabetes or gestational diabetes or if significantly obese; every 3 to 5 years for all women older than 45 years of age
Hearing screen	Annually with exposure to excessive noise or when loss is suspected
Sexually transmitted infection screen	As needed with multiple sexual partners
Tuberculin skin test	Annually with exposure to persons with tuberculosis or in risk categories for close contact with the disease
Endometrial biopsy	At menopause for women at risk for endometrial cancer
Vision	Every 2 years between ages 40 and 64; annually after age 65
Bone mineral density testing	All women age 65 and older; younger women with risk for osteoporosis may need periodic screenings
IMMUNIZATIONS	
Tetanus-diphtheria	Booster is given every 10 years after primary series
Measles, mumps, rubella	Once if born after 1956 and no evidence of immunity
Hepatitis B	Primary series of three for all who are in risk categories
Influenza	Annually after age 65 or in risk categories, such as chronic diseases, immunosuppression, renal dysfunction

Sources: American Cancer Society (ACS). (2005). *Cancer facts and figures 2005.* New York: ACS; Centers for Disease Control and Prevention (CDC). (2002). *Sexually transmitted diseases treatment guidelines 2002. Morbidity and Mortality Weekly Report, 51*(RR-6), 1-80; Expert Panel on Detection, Evaluation, and Treatment of High Blood Cholesterol in Adults. (2001). Executive summary of the third report of the national education program (NCEP) expert panel on detection, evaluation, and treatment of high blood cholesterol in adults (Adult Treatment Panel III). *Journal of the American Medical Association, 285*(19), 2486-2497; National Women's Health Resource Center. (2001). Screening tests and women's health. *National Women's Health Report, 23*(6), 1-7; U.S. Preventive Services Task Force. (1996). *Guide to clinical preventive services* (2nd ed.). Baltimore: Williams & Wilkins; U.S. Preventive Services Task Force. (2003). *Screening for cervical cancers.* AHRQ Publication 03-535, January, 2003. Rockville, MD: Agency for Healthcare Research and Quality.
*Unless otherwise noted, the recommended intervention should be performed routinely every 1 to 3 years.
†American Cancer Society (ACS). (2005).
‡Note: There is no consensus regarding mammograms for women between 40 and 49 years of age; therefore various recommendations are listed. Women are urged to discuss circumstances with their health care providers.

Identify and visit resources in your community appropriate for referring the following women. Evaluate the resource in terms of access, costs (insurance, health maintenance organization, Medicaid coverage), confidentiality, and follow-up service. Develop a resource file for each woman's needs.

a. A 30-year-old woman who is wheelchair bound who needs a Pap test
b. A Spanish-speaking woman who is a victim of IVP (husband)
c. A 40-year-old woman who is requesting a mammogram

Key Points

- The female reproductive system consists of external and internal structures.
- Normal feedback regulation of the menstrual cycle depends on an intact hypothalamic-pituitary-gonadal mechanism.
- The female's reproductive tract structures and breasts respond predictably to changing levels of sex steroids across her life span.
- The myometrium of the uterus is uniquely designed to expel the fetus and promote hemostasis after birth.
- Prostaglandins play an important role in reproductive functions by their effect on smooth muscle contractility and modulation of hormones.
- Culture, religion, socioeconomic status, personal circumstances, the uniqueness of the individual, and stage of development are among the factors that influence a person's recognition of need for care and response to the health care system and therapy.
- The changing status and roles of women affect their health, needs, and ability to cope with problems.

- Assessment is more comprehensive and learning is best in a safe environment in which the atmosphere is nonjudgmental and sensitive and the interaction is strictly confidential.
- Preconception care allows identification and possible remediation of potentially harmful personal and social conditions, medical and psychologic conditions, and environmental conditions before conception.
- Conditions that increase a woman's health risks also increase risks for her offspring.
- Violence against women is a major social and health care problem in the United States.
- Periodic health screening, including history, physical examination, and diagnostic and laboratory tests, provides the basis for overall health promotion, prevention of illness, early diagnosis of problems, and referral for management.
- Health promotion and prevention assist women to actualize health potential by increasing motivation, providing information, and suggesting how to access specific resources.

Answer Guidelines to Critical Thinking Exercise

Preconception Counseling

1 Yes, there is sufficient evidence that preconception counseling is needed.
2 Assumptions include the following:
   a. Assessing for risk factors that can affect pregnancy is an important component of preconception care. Areas that should be assessed include a medical history including illnesses, medical conditions (e.g., diabetes, hypertension, asthma), medication use; a family history including genetic conditions and birth defects; a reproductive history including contraception use, gynecologic problems, STIs, and obstetric history; psychosocial history including support system, history of depression, victim of IVP; and environmental history including home and work conditions.
   b. Health promotion activities before pregnancy can prevent or decrease the chances of maternal and fetal complications. These include taking folic acid supplements, exercising and getting sufficient rest, maintaining an appropriate weight, not smoking or abusing drugs, engaging in safer sex practices, obtaining immunizations, getting routine physical examinations, and having existing medical conditions well controlled.

   c. The critical period of organogenesis is week 3 to week 8 (days 17 to 56 after conception) when all major organs are being formed. Exposure to teratogens (substances or conditions that can cause abnormal development and birth defects) during this period pose a great risk to the developing embryo and can occur because pregnancy often is not confirmed until after an exposure.
   d. The woman who is over the age of 35 is at risk for certain conditions that can affect pregnancy. For example, the risk for certain genetic anomalies (e.g., Down syndrome) increases with the age of the woman. Chronic diseases such as cardiac disease or hypertension may increase in severity over time. Older women are at risk for certain pregnancy-related conditions, as well (e.g., gestational hypertension, placental problems, infertility).
3 The implication for care is to build on Margo's motivation as evidenced by her questions. Priorities include assessing her health status, particularly in relation to nutrition (e.g., folic acid intake) and exercise, substance use, and stress management; and assessing for risk factors in the medical history, including medications, reproductive history, family history including genetic conditions, psychosocial history, environmental exposure

history, and support system. After assessment and identification of any problem areas, provide anticipatory guidance, treatment for existing conditions, and referrals if needed.

4 Yes, there is evidence to support providing preconception care (e.g., March of Dimes [folic acid], *Healthy People 2010*, Association of Women's Health, Obstetric and Neonatal Nurses).

5 There is a move to provide health promotion and disease prevention information to all women of childbearing age at each health encounter rather than providing preconception care in isolation or as a separate program or clinic. In this case Margo would have holistic care and be better prepared for a desired pregnancy as well as lifelong wellness.

Resources

Alcoholics Anonymous (for individuals who are alcohol dependent)
P.O. Box 459
Grand Central Station
New York, NY 10163
212-870-3400
www.alcoholics-anonymous.org

Al-Anon (for families of alcoholics); Alateen (for teenage children of alcoholics)
www.al-anon.org

Anorexia Nervosa and Related Eating Disorders, Inc.
www.anred.com

COCAINE Hotline
800-COCAINE

Harvard Eating Disorders Center
356 Boylston St.
Boston, MA 02166
888-236-1188
www.hedc.org

Institute for Women's Policy Research
1707 L St., NW, Suite 750
Washington, DC 20036
202-785-5100
www.iwpr.org

Narcotics Anonymous (for drug abusers)
888-336-4066

National Cancer Institute Cancer Information Service
800-4-CANCER
www.nci.nih.gov

National Clearinghouse for Alcohol and Drug Abuse Information
P.O. Box 2345
Rockville, MD 20847
800-729-6686
www.health.org

National Coalition Against Domestic Violence
P.O. Box 34103
Washington, DC 20043-4301
202-638-8638
800-333-SAFE (7223) (hotline)
(Many states have local coalitions against domestic violence.)

National Coalition Against Sexual Assault
912 North 2nd St.
Harrisburg, PA 17102
717-232-6771

National Domestic Violence and Abuse Hotline
800-799-SAFE

National Organization for Women (NOW)
Legal Defense and Education Fund
99 Hudson St.
New York, NY 10013-2871
212-925-6635

National Ovarian Cancer Coalition
2335 East Atlantic Blvd., #401
Pompano Beach, FL 33062
888-682-7426
www.ovarian.org

National Resource Center for Domestic Violence
800-537-2238

National Women's Health Resource Center
120 Albany St., Suite 820
New Brunswick, NJ 08901
877-986-9472
www.healthywomen.org

National Women's Health Information Center
The Office on Women's Health
Department of Health and Human Resources
800-994-9662
www.4woman.gov

National Alcohol and Drug Abuse Hotline
800-252-6465

The National Center on Women and Family Law
799 Broadway, Room 402
New York, NY 10003
212-674-8200
(Legal Information)

Office of Minority Health Resource Center
P.O. Box 37337
Washington, DC 20013-7337
301-587-1938

Society for Women's Health Research
1828 L St., NW, Suite 625
Washington, DC 20036
202-223-8224
www.womens-health.org

Women's Cancer Network
c/o Gynecologic Cancer Foundation
401 N. Michigan Ave.
Chicago, IL 60611
312-644-6610
www.wcn.org

References

American Cancer Society (ACS). (2005). *Cancer facts and figures 2005.* New York: ACS.

American College of Obstetricians and Gynecologists (ACOG). (1997). *Smoking and women's health. ACOG Technical Bulletin no. 240.* Washington, DC: ACOG.

Barkauskas, V., Baumann, L., & Darling-Fisher, C. (2002). *Health and physical assessment* (3rd ed.). St. Louis: Mosby.

Behrman, R., & Shiono, P. (2002). Neonatal risk factors. In A. Fanaroff & R. Martin (Eds.), *Neonatal-perinatal medicine: Diseases of the fetus and infant.* (7th ed.). St. Louis: Mosby.

Bonvicini, K., & Perlin, M. (2003).The same but different: Clinician-patient communication with gay and lesbian patients. *Patient Education and Counseling, 51*(2), 115-122.

Briggs, G., Freeman, R., & Yaffe, S. (2002). *A reference guide to fetal and neonatal risk: Drugs in pregnancy and lactation* (6th ed.). Philadelphia: Lippincott Williams & Wilkins.

Centers for Disease Control and Prevention (CDC). (2002). Sexually transmitted diseases treatment guidelines 2002. *Morbidity and Mortality Weekly Report, 51*(RR-6), 1-80.

Cesario, S. (2003). Obesity in pregnancy. What every nurse needs to know. *AWHONN Lifelines 7*(2), 118-125.

Cnattingius, S. (2000). Caffeine intake and the risk of first-trimester spontaneous abortion. *New England Journal of Medicine, 343*(25), 1839-1845.

Dienemann, J., Campbell, J., Wiederhorn, N., Laughon, K., & Jordon, E. (2003). A critical pathway for intimate partner violence across the continuum of care. *Journal of Obstetric, Gynecologic, and Neonatal Nursing, 32*(5), 594-603.

DiSaia, P., & Creasman, W. (2002). *Clinical gynecologic oncology* (6th ed.). St. Louis: Mosby.

Edge, V., & Miller, M. (1994). *Women's health care.* St. Louis: Mosby.

Eustace, L., Kang, D., & Coombs, D. (2003). Fetal alcohol syndrome: A growing concern for health care professionals. *Journal of Obstetric, Gynecologic, and Neonatal Nursing, 32*(2), 215-221.

Expert Panel on Detection, Evaluation, and Treatment of High Blood Cholesterol in Adults. (2001). Executive summary of the third report of the national education program (NCEP) expert panel on detection, evaluation, and treatment of high blood cholesterol in adults (Adult Treatment Panel III). *Journal of the American Medical Association, 285*(19), 2486-2497.

Flegal, K., Carroll, M., Ogden, C., & Johnson, C. (2002). Prevalence and trends in obesity among U.S. adults, 1999-2000. *Journal of the American Medical Association, 288*(14), 1723-1727.

Gingrich, P. (2004). Management and follow-up of abnormal Papanicolaou tests. *Journal of the American Medical Women's Association, 59*(1), 54-60.

Hauenstein, E. (2003). Depression in adolescence. *Journal of Obstetric, Gynecologic, and Neonatal Nursing, 32*(2), 239-248.

Helton, A. (1987). *A protocol of care for the battered woman.* White Plains, NY: March of Dimes Birth Defects Foundation.

Hobbins, D. (2003). Full circle: The evolution of preconception health promotion in America. *Journal of Obstetric, Gynecologic, and Neonatal Nursing, 32*(4), 516-522.

Hoyert, D., Kung, H., & Smith, B. (2005). Deaths: Preliminary data for 2003. *National Vital Statistics Report, 53*(15), 1-48.

Hutchinson, M., Sosa, D., & Thompson, A. (2001). Sexual protective strategies of late adolescent females: More than just condoms. *Journal of Obstetric, Gynecologic, and Neonatal Nursing, 30*(4), 429-438.

Kealy, M. (2003). Preventing obesity: Exploring the surgeon general's outline for action. *AWHONN Lifelines, 7*(1), 24-27.

Kowal, D. (2004). Expanding perspectives on reproductive health. In R. Hatcher et al., *Contraceptive technology* (18th ed.). New York: Ardent Media Inc.

Martin, J., Kochanek, K., Strobino, D., Guyer, B., & MacDorman, M. (2005). Annual summary of vital statistics—2003. *Pediatrics, 115*(3), 619-634.

Masters, W. (1992). *Human sexuality* (4th ed.). New York: HarperCollins.

Mattson, S. (2000). Striving for cultural competence: Providing care for the changing face of the U.S. *AWHONN Lifelines, 4*(3), 48-52.

Mattson, S. (2003). Caring for Latino women. *AWHONN Lifelines, 7*(3), 258-260.

Miller D., Martin, I., & Herbison, P. (2003). Interventions for relieving the pain and discomfort of screening mammography (Cochrane Review). In *The Cochrane Library,* Issue 2, 2004. Chichester, UK: John Wiley & Sons.

Molnar, B., Buka, S., & Kessler, R. (2001). Child sexual abuse and subsequent psychopathology: Results from the national comorbidity survey. *American Journal of Public Health, 91*(5), 753-760.

Moos, M. (2003). Preconceptional wellness as a routine objective for women's health: An integrated strategy. *Journal of Obstetric, Gynecologic, and Neonatal Nursing, 32*(4), 550-556.

National Center for Chronic Disease Prevention and Health Promotion. (2000). *U.S. obesity trends 1985 to 2000.* Atlanta: Centers for Disease Control and Prevention.

National Women's Health Information Center (NWHIC). (2003). *Violence against women.* Internet document available at http://www.4woman.gov/violence/index.cfm (accessed June 16, 2004).

National Women's Health Resource Center. (2001). Screening tests and women's health. *National Women's Health Report, 23*(6), 1-7.

National Women's Health Resource Center. (2003). Depression and women. *National Women's Health Report, 25*(4), 1-4.

National Women's Law Center. (2000). *Making the grade on women's health: A national and state-by-state report card.* Washington, DC: National Women's Law Center.

Niebyl, J. (2002) Drugs in pregnancy and lactation. In S. Gabbe, J. Niebyl, & J. Simpson (Eds.), *Obstetrics: Normal and problem pregnancies* (4th ed.). New York: Churchill Livingstone.

Postlethwaite, D. (2003). Preconception health counseling for women exposed to teratogens: The role of the nurse. *Journal of Obstetric, Gynecologic, and Neonatal Nursing, 32*(4), 523-532.

Sampselle, C. (2000). Behavioral interventions for urinary incontinence in women: Evidence for practice. *Journal of Midwifery & Women's Health, 45*(2), 94-103.

Sampselle, C. (2003). Behavior interventions in young and middle-aged women: Simple interventions to combat a complex problem. *American Journal of Nursing, 103*(suppl), 9-19.

Sampselle, C., Wyman, J., Thomas, K., Newman, D., Gray, M., Dougherty, M., & Burns, P. (2000). Continence for women: A test of AWHONN's evidence-based protocol. *Journal of Obstetric, Gynecologic, and Neonatal Nursing, 29*(1), 312-317.

Seidel, H., Ball, J., Dains, J., & Benedict, G. (2003). *Mosby's guide to physical examination* (5th ed.). St. Louis: Mosby.

Stenchever, M., Droegemueller, W., Herbst, A., & Mishell, D. (2001). *Comprehensive gynecology* (4th ed.). St. Louis: Mosby.

Stuart, G., & Laraia, M. (2001). *Stuart and Sundeen's principles and practices of psychiatric nursing* (7th ed.). St. Louis: Mosby.

Tjaden, P., & Thoennes, N. (2000). *Extent, nature and consequences of intimate partner violence: Findings from the national violence against women survey.* Washington, DC: U.S. Department of Justice.

U.S. Department of Health and Human Services & U.S. Department of Agriculture. (2005). *Dietary guidelines for Americans 2005.* Hyattsville, MD: U.S. Department of Agriculture.

U.S. Preventive Services Task Force. (1996). *Guide to clinical preventive services* (2nd ed.). Baltimore: Williams & Wilkins.

U.S. Preventive Services Task Force. (2003). *Screening for Cervical Cancers.* AHRQ Publication 03-535, January, 2003, Rockville, MD: Agency for Healthcare Research and Quality.

U.S. Preventive Services Task Force. (2003). *Guide to clinical preventive services: Periodic updates* (3rd ed.). Washington, DC: U.S. Department of Health and Human Services. Office of Disease Prevention and Health Promotion.

Viau, P., Padula, C., & Eddy, B. (2002). An exploration of health concerns and health-promotion behaviors in pregnant women over age 35. *MCN American Journal of Maternal Child Nursing, 27*(6), 328-334.

Walker, L. (1984). *The battered woman syndrome* (Vol. 6). New York: Springer.

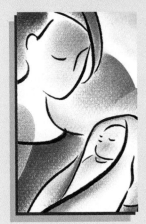

CHAPTER 5

Common Reproductive Concerns

DEITRA LEONARD LOWDERMILK

LEARNING OBJECTIVES

- *Differentiate among the signs and symptoms of common menstrual disorders.*
- *Develop a nursing care plan for the woman with primary dysmenorrhea.*
- *Outline patient teaching about premenstrual syndrome.*
- *Relate the pathophysiology of endometriosis to associated symptoms.*
- *Consider use of alternative therapies for menstrual disorders.*
- *Describe prevention of sexually transmitted infections in women.*
- *Differentiate signs, symptoms, diagnoses, and management of women with bacterial and viral sexually transmitted infections.*

- *Differentiate signs, symptoms, and management of selected vaginal infections.*
- *Review principles of infection control, including Standard Precautions and precautions for invasive procedures.*
- *Discuss the pathophysiology of selected benign breast conditions and malignant neoplasms of the breasts found in women.*
- *Discuss the emotional effects of benign and malignant neoplasms.*
- *Compare alternatives for treatment for the woman with a lump in her breast.*

KEY TERMS AND DEFINITIONS

amenorrhea Absence or cessation of menstruation

dysfunctional uterine bleeding (DUB) Excessive uterine bleeding with no demonstrable organic cause

dysmenorrhea Painful menstruation beginning 2 to 6 months after menarche, related to ovulation or to organic disease such as endometriosis, pelvic inflammatory disease, or uterine neoplasm

endometriosis Tissue closely resembling endometrial tissue located outside the uterus

fibroadenoma Firm, freely movable solitary, solid, benign breast tumor

fibrocystic changes Benign changes in breast tissue

leiomyoma Benign smooth muscle tumor

lumpectomy Removal of a wide margin of normal breast tissue surrounding a breast cancer

menorrhagia Abnormally profuse or excessive menstrual flow

metrorrhagia Abnormal bleeding from the uterus, particularly when it occurs at any time other than the menstrual period

modified radical mastectomy Surgery that includes removal of the breast and fascia over the pectoralis major muscle

oligomenorrhea Abnormally light or infrequent menstruation

pelvic inflammatory disease (PID) Infection of internal reproductive structures and adjacent tissues usually secondary to sexually transmitted infections

premenstrual syndrome (PMS) Syndrome of nervous tension, irritability, weight gain, edema, headache, mastalgia, dysphoria, and lack of coordination occurring during the last few days of the menstrual cycle preceding the onset of menstruation

radical mastectomy Surgery that includes total removal of the breast, as well as underlying pectoralis major and pectoralis minor muscles

simple mastectomy Surgery that includes removal of the breast without underlying muscle or fascial tissue

Throughout her life, the average woman is likely to have some concerns related to her menstrual and gynecologic health and will experience bleeding, pain, or discharge associated with her reproductive organs or functions. In addition, during a woman's life span, she may experience infections associated with her reproductive or sexual life. Many women will seek out nurses as advisors, counselors, and health care providers for these concerns. Nurses must have accurate, up-to-date information to meet these women's needs. This chapter provides information on common menstrual problems, sexually transmitted infections (STIs) and selected other infections that can affect reproductive functions, and benign breast conditions. Breast cancer is also included because it is the most common reproductive cancer occurring in women.

MENSTRUAL PROBLEMS

Women typically have menstrual cycles for approximately 40 years. Once the predictable pattern of monthly bleeding is established, women may worry about any deviation from that pattern, or what they have been told is normal for all menstruating women. A sign such as amenorrhea or excessive menstrual bleeding can be a source of severe distress and concern for a woman as she wonders what is wrong.

Amenorrhea

Amenorrhea, the absence or cessation of menstrual flow, is a clinical sign of a variety of disorders. Although the criteria used to determine when amenorrhea is a clinical problem are not universal, the following circumstances should generally be evaluated: (1) the absence of both menarche and secondary sexual characteristics by age 14; (2) the absence of menses by age 16, regardless of presence of normal growth and development (primary amenorrhea); or (3) a 6-month cessation of menses after a period of menstruation (secondary amenorrhea) (Harlow, 2000).

Amenorrhea is most commonly a result of pregnancy, although it may occur from any defect or interruption in the hypothalamic-pituitary-ovarian-uterine axis (see Chapter 4). It may also result from anatomic abnormalities; other endocrine disorders, such as hypothyroidism or hyperthyroidism; chronic diseases, such as type 1 diabetes; medications, such as phenytoin (Dilantin); eating disorders; strenuous exercise; emotional stress; and oral contraceptive use.

Assessment of amenorrhea begins with a thorough history and physical examination. An important initial step is to confirm that the woman is not pregnant. Specific components of the assessment process depend on a woman's age—adolescent, young adult, or perimenopausal—and whether or not she has previously menstruated.

Hypogonadotropic amenorrhea

Hypogonadotropic amenorrhea reflects a problem in the central hypothalamic-pituitary axis. In rare instances a pituitary lesion or genetic inability to produce follicle-stimulating hormone (FSH) and luteinizing hormone (LH) is at fault. More commonly it results from hypothalamic suppression as a result of two principal influences: stress (in the home, school, or workplace) or a body fat-to-lean ratio that is inappropriate for an individual woman, especially during a normal growth period (Parent-Stevens & Burns, 2000). Research has demonstrated a biologic basis for the relation of stress to physiologic processes. Exercise-associated amenorrhea can occur in women undergoing vigorous physical and athletic training (Sanborn, Horea, Siemers, & Dieringer, 2000) and is thought to be associated with many factors, including body composition (height, weight, and percentage of body fat); type, intensity, and frequency of exercise; nutritional status; and presence of emotional or physical stressors. Amenorrhea is one of the classic signs of anorexia nervosa, and the interrelatedness of disordered eating, amenorrhea, and premature osteoporosis has been described as the female athlete triad (Kleposki, 2002). Calcium loss from bone, comparable to that seen in postmenopausal women, may occur with this type of amenorrhea.

Management. Counseling and education are primary interventions because many of the causes are potentially reversible (e.g., stress, weight loss for nonorganic reasons). When a stressor known to predispose a woman to hypothalamic amenorrhea is identified, initial management involves addressing the stressor. Together the woman and nurse plan how to decrease or discontinue medications known to affect menstruation, correct weight loss, deal more effectively with psychologic stress, and eliminate substance abuse. Deep breathing exercises and relaxation techniques are simple yet effective stress-reduction measures. Referral for biofeedback or massage therapy also may be useful. In some instances, referrals for psychotherapy may be indicated.

If a woman's exercise program is thought to contribute to her amenorrhea, several options exist for management. She may decide to decrease the intensity or duration of her training, if possible, or to gain some weight, if appropriate. Accepting this alternative may be difficult for one who is committed to a strenuous exercise regimen. Many young women athletes may not understand the consequences of low bone density or osteoporosis; nurses can point out the connection between low bone density and stress fractures. If the woman continues to have low estrogen levels, estrogen therapy may be instituted as well as calcium supplementation for osteoporosis prevention (Stenchever, Droegemueller, Herbst, & Mishell, 2001).

Cyclic perimenstrual pain and discomfort

Cyclic perimenstrual pain and discomfort (CPPD) is a new concept developed by a nurse science team for a research project for the Association of Women's Health, Obstetric and Neonatal Nurses (Collins Sharp, Taylor, Thomas, Killeen, & Dawood, 2002). This concept includes dysmenorrhea, premenstrual syndrome (PMS), and premenstrual dysphoric disorder (PDD) as well as symptom clusters that occur before and after the menstrual flow starts. CPPD is a health problem that can have a significant impact on the quality of life for a woman. The following discussion focuses on the three main conditions of CPPD. See the Evidence-Based practice box for further discussion of the clinical guidelines for nursing practice for CPPD.

Dysmenorrhea

Dysmenorrhea, pain during or shortly before menstruation, is one of the most common gynecologic problems in women of all ages. Many adolescents have dysmenorrhea in the first 3 years after menarche. Young adult women ages 17 to 24 years are most likely to report painful menses. Between 30% and 40% of women report some level of discomfort associated with menses, and 7% to 15% report severe dysmenorrhea (Parent-Stevens & Burns, 2000); however, the amount of disruption in women's lives is difficult to determine. It has been estimated that up to 10% of women with dysmenorrhea have severe enough pain to interfere with their functioning for 1 to 3 days a month. Menstrual problems, including dysmenorrhea, are more common in women who smoke and who are obese. Severe dysmenorrhea is also associated with early menarche, nulliparity, and stress (Stenchever et al., 2001). Traditionally dysmenorrhea is differentiated as primary or secondary. Symptoms usually begin with menstruation, although some women have discomfort several hours before onset of flow. The range and severity of symptoms are different from woman to woman and from cycle to cycle in the same woman. Symptoms of dysmenorrhea may last several hours or several days.

Pain is usually located in the suprapubic area or lower abdomen. Women describe the pain as sharp, cramping, or gripping or as a steady dull ache; pain may radiate to the lower back or upper thighs.

Primary dysmenorrhea

Primary dysmenorrhea is a condition associated with ovulatory cycles. Research has shown that primary dysmenorrhea has a biochemical basis and arises from the release of prostaglandins with menses. During the luteal phase and subsequent menstrual flow, prostaglandin F_2 alpha ($PGF_{2\alpha}$) is secreted. Excessive release of $PGF_{2\alpha}$ increases the amplitude and frequency of uterine contractions and causes vasospasm of the uterine arterioles, resulting in ischemia and cyclic lower abdominal cramps. Systemic responses to $PGF_{2\alpha}$ include backache, weakness, sweats, gastrointestinal symptoms (anorexia, nausea, vomiting, and diarrhea), and central nervous system symptoms (dizziness, syncope, headache, and poor concentration). Pain usually begins at the onset of menstruation and lasts 8 to 48 hours (Stenchever et al., 2001).

Primary dysmenorrhea usually appears 6 to 12 months after menarche when ovulation is established. Anovulatory bleeding, common in the few months or years after menarche, is painless. Because both estrogen and progesterone are necessary for primary dysmenorrhea to occur, it is experienced only with ovulatory cycles. This problem is most commonly experienced by women in their late teens and early twenties; the incidence declines with age. Psychogenic factors may influence symptoms, but symptoms are definitely related to ovulation and do not occur when ovulation is suppressed.

Management. Management of primary dysmenorrhea depends on the severity of the problem and the individual woman's response to various treatments. Important components of nursing care are information and support. Because menstruation is so closely linked to reproduction and sexuality, menstrual problems such as dysmenorrhea can have a negative influence on sexuality and self-worth. Nurses can correct myths and misinformation about menstruation and dysmenorrhea by providing facts about what is normal. Nurses must support their patients' feelings of positive sexuality and self-worth.

Often, more than one alternative for alleviating menstrual discomfort and dysmenorrhea can be offered, giving women options to try and decide which works best for them. Heat (heating pad or hot bath) minimizes cramping by increasing vasodilation and muscle relaxation and minimizing uterine ischemia. Massaging the lower back can reduce pain by relaxing paravertebral muscles and increasing pelvic blood supply. Soft, rhythmic rubbing of the abdomen (effleurage) may be useful because it provides distraction and an alternative focal point. Biofeedback, transcutaneous electrical nerve stimulation (TENS), progressive relaxation, Hatha yoga, acupuncture, and meditation also have been used to decrease menstrual discomfort although there is insufficient evidence to determine effectiveness (Proctor, Smith, Farquhar, & Stones, 2002).

EVIDENCE-BASED PRACTICE
AWHONN Research-Based Practice Guidelines for Cyclic Perimenstrual Pain and Discomfort

BACKGROUND

- Most women experience some perimenstrual symptoms, which can cause loss of work or school and extra medical visits and costs. Conventionally, research has focused on discrete aspects of menstrual changes, such as pain or negative affect. However, most women experience several symptoms simultaneously. A more comprehensive and functional concept of cyclic perimenstrual pain and discomfort (CPPD) includes the symptom clusters that occur throughout the luteal phase and menstruation. Up to 100 perimenstrual symptoms have been identified.

OBJECTIVES

- Many women do not seek medical advice about CPPD, and many health care providers are poorly informed about CPPD management. Women often use over-the-counter treatments ineffectively. Nurses are ideally positioned to offer first-line screening and advice about management of CPPD. The Association of Women's Health, Obstetric and Neonatal Nurses (AWHONN) selected CPPD as a focus for its Research-Based Practice project, with the goal of providing guidelines for nursing practice.

METHODS
Search Strategy

- The AWHONN science team researched CINAHL, MEDLINE, and the Cochrane databases, as well as references. Search keywords included *cyclic pain, pelvic pain, comfort, pain guidelines,* and *dysmenorrhea.* Thirty-three relevant research articles, dated 1992 to 1999, were selected, ranging from case studies to clinical trials.

Statistical Analyses

- Because the studies were so varied, the research team analyzed the data holistically. Three nursing diagnoses emerged: perimenstrual cyclic pain, perimenstrual discomfort, and perimenstrual negative affect.

FINDINGS

- Research-based nursing interventions fell into six categories:
  1. Fundamental symptom management: Principles of general pain management and assisting with coping enhancement and mutual goal setting are appropriate for CPPD.
  2. Self-monitoring: Instruction on daily tracking of symptoms and stressors increases self-esteem and efficacy.
  3. Self-regulation:
     a. Pharmacologic agents had the strongest research. Nonsteroidal antiinflammatory drugs (NSAIDs) and low-dose, combined oral contraceptives were very effective.
     b. Nutritional supplements were supported by moderately good evidence.
        i. Calcium, 1200 mg/day, may significantly decrease premenstrual syndrome symptoms by the third cycle.
        ii. Magnesium helps stabilize blood sugar and decreases constipation and bloating.
        iii. Vitamin B$_6$ (pyridoxine) may relieve negative affect symptoms but can be toxic in overdose.
        iv. Essential fatty acids, such as evening primrose oil, borage, and black currant oil, may decrease dysmenorrhea, breast tenderness, and fluid retention.
     c. Topical—cutaneous: The strongest research supported the use of Transcutaneous Electrical Nerve Stimulation (TENS), which may disrupt the sensory perception of pain, combined with NSAIDs. Moderately strong research backed the use of abdominal heat and massage, which may increase blood flow. Weaker evidence showed some pain relief using acupressure points at the abdomen, back, and inner ankle.
     d. Behavioral—cognitive: There was some evidence of symptom relief with daily practice of relaxation, breathing, stretching, meditation, or guided imagery.
  4. Self-Modification:
     a. Nutritional: Eliminating smoking, alcohol, salt, caffeine, and sugars, eating frequent small meals, and drinking six to eight glasses of fluids a day resulted in some improvement in symptoms. Moderate evidence supported a program of multivitamins and minerals, which may be individualized to include vitamin E, essential fatty acids, B-complex vitamins, calcium, and amino acids L-tyrosine and L-tryptophan.
     b. Research was equivocal that exercise may increase blood flow, metabolism, and endorphins.
  5. Environmental: Time management and communication skills helped somewhat to modify the stressors that compound CPPD.
  6. Referral: Chinese herbals, chiropractic treatment, acupuncture, and homeopathy have shown some promise anecdotally, but lack strong evidence yet.

LIMITATIONS

- The complexity of CPPD, combined with the range of qualitative and quantitative studies made synthesis of the literature a Herculean task. Each woman has her own cluster of discomforts each cycle, and the treatment must be as dynamic as the symptoms. No critical pathway or decision tree can be established yet. Treatment is still an art, with some science.

IMPLICATIONS FOR PRACTICE

- CPPD is a quality-of-life issue for women. The authors recommended routine screening for CPPD, specifically pelvic pain and other discomforts, and efficacy of self-treatment. Individualized, multimodal management should produce treatment options based on the strongest evidence.

IMPLICATIONS FOR FURTHER RESEARCH

- Further research, especially randomized, controlled complementary and alternative medicine research is needed to yield more generalizability to the studies. Possible combinations of therapies may show promise for symptom relief.

Reference: Colllins Sharp, B., Taylor, D., Thomas, K., Killeen, M., & Dawood, M. (2002). Cyclic perimenstrual pain and discomfort: The scientific basis for practice. *Journal of Obstetric, Gynecologic, and Neonatal Nursing, 31*(6), 637-649.

Exercise has been found to help relieve menstrual discomfort through increased vasodilation and subsequent decreased ischemia; release of endogenous opiates, specifically beta-endorphins; suppression of prostaglandins; and shunting of blood flow away from the viscera, resulting in less pelvic congestion. Specific exercises that nurses can suggest include pelvic rock and heels-over-the-head yoga position.

In addition to maintaining good nutrition at all times, specific dietary changes may be helpful in decreasing some of the systemic symptoms associated with dysmenorrhea. Decreased salt and refined sugar intake 7 to 10 days before expected menses may reduce fluid retention. Natural diuretics, such as asparagus, cranberry juice, peaches, parsley, or watermelon may help reduce edema and related discomforts. Decreasing red meat intake may also help minimize dysmenorrheal symptoms.

Medications used to treat primary dysmenorrhea include prostaglandin synthesis inhibitors, primarily nonsteroidal antiinflammatory drugs (NSAIDs) (Parent-Stevens & Burns, 2000) (Table 5-1). NSAIDs are most effective if started several days before menses or at least by the onset of bleeding. All NSAIDs have potential gastrointestinal side effects, including nausea, vomiting, and indigestion. All women taking NSAIDs should be warned to report dark-colored stools because this may be an indication of gastrointestinal bleeding.

> **NURSE ALERT** If one NSAID is ineffective, often a different one may be effective. If the second drug is unsuccessful after a 6-month trial, combined oral contraceptive pills (OCPs) may be used. Women with a history of aspirin sensitivity or allergy should avoid all NSAIDs.

Combined OCPs prevent ovulation and can decrease the amount of menstrual flow, which can decrease the amount of prostaglandin, thus decreasing dysmenorrhea. There is evidence that combined OCPs can effectively treat dysmenorrhea (Proctor, Roberts, & Farquhar, 2001). Combined OCPs may be used in place of NSAIDs if the woman wants oral contraception and has primary dysmenorrhea. OCPs have side effects and women who do not need or want them for contraception may not wish to use them for dysmenorrhea. OCPs also may be contraindicated for some women.

Over-the-counter (OTC) preparations that are indicated for primary dysmenorrhea include the same active ingredients (e.g., ibuprofen, naproxen sodium) as prescription preparations. However, the labeled recommended dose may be subtherapeutic. Preparations containing acetaminophen are even less effective because acetaminophen does not have the antiprostaglandin properties of NSAIDs.

Herbal preparations have long been used for management of menstrual problems including dysmenorrhea (Table 5-2). Herbal medicines may be valuable in treating dysmenorrhea; however, it is essential that women understand that these therapies are not without potential toxicity and may cause drug interactions and that research is inconclusive about the effectiveness of use (Wilson & Murphy, 2001).

Secondary dysmenorrhea

Secondary dysmenorrhea is acquired menstrual pain that develops later in life than primary dysmenorrhea, typically after age 25. It is associated with pelvic pathology such as adenomyosis, endometriosis, pelvic inflammatory disease (PID), endometrial polyps, submucous or interstitial myomas (uterine fibroids), or use of an intrauterine device (IUD). Pain often begins a few days before menses, but it can be present at ovulation and continue through the first days of menses or start after menstrual flow has begun. In contrast to primary dysmenorrhea, the pain of secondary dysmenorrhea is often characterized by dull, lower abdominal aching radiating to the back or thighs. Often, women experience feelings of bloating or pelvic fullness. Treatment is directed toward removal of the underlying pathology. Many of the measures described for pain relief of primary dysmenorrhea are also helpful for women with secondary dysmenorrhea.

Premenstrual Syndrome

About 85% of women experience mood and/or somatic symptoms that occur with their menstrual cycles (American College of Obstetricians and Gynecologists [ACOG], 2000). It is difficult to establish a universal definition of premenstrual syndrome (PMS), as so many symptoms have been associated with the condition, and at least two different syndromes have been recognized: PMS and premenstrual dysphoric disorder (PDD). PMS is a complex, poorly understood condition that includes one or more of a large number (more than 100) of physical and psychologic symptoms beginning in the luteal phase of the menstrual cycle, occurring to such a degree that lifestyle or work is affected, and followed by a symptom-free period. Symptoms include fluid retention (abdominal bloating, pelvic fullness, edema of the lower extremities, breast tenderness, and weight gain); behavioral or emotional changes (depression, crying spells, irritability, panic attacks, and impaired ability to concentrate); premenstrual cravings (sweets, salt, increased appetite, and food binges); and headache, fatigue, and backache. PDD is a more severe variant of PMS in which women have marked irritability, dysphoria, mood lability, anxiety, fatigue, appetite changes, and a sense of feeling overwhelmed (Elliot, 2002).

A diagnosis of PMS is made only if the following criteria are met:

- Symptoms occur in the luteal phase and resolve within a few days of menses onset.
- A symptom-free period occurs in the follicular phase.
- Symptoms are recurrent.

The cause of PMS is unknown. It has been theorized that PMS has a significant psychologic component or may result from cultural beliefs that lead to the menstrual cycle being associated with a variety of negative reactions. In reality PMS is most likely not a single disorder but rather a collection of different problems (Pritham, 2002). There is much controversy regarding PMS. The existence, diagnosis, and etiology

TABLE 5-1

Nonsteroidal Antiinflammatory Agents Used to Treat Dysmenorrhea

DRUG	BRAND NAME AND STATUS	RECOMMENDED DOSAGE†	COMMON Side Effects‡	COMMENTS	CONTRAINDICATIONS
Diclofenac	Cataflam Rx	50 mg tid or 100 mg initially then 50 mg tid to 150 mg/day	Nausea, diarrhea, constipation, abdominal distress, dyspepsia, flatulence	Enteric coated: immediate release	For all NSAIDs: Do not give if patient has hemophilia or bleeding ulcers; do not give if patient has had an allergic or anaphylactic reaction to aspirin or another NSAID; do not give if patient is taking anticoagulant medication
Ibuprofen	Motrin Rx Advil OTC, Nuprin OTC, Motrin IB OTC	400 mg q4-6h 200 mg q4-6h to 1200 mg/day	Nausea, dyspepsia, rash, pruritus	If GI upset occurs, take with food, milk, or antacids; avoid alcoholic beverages; do not take with aspirin	
Ketoprofen	Orudis Rx Orudis KT OTC Actron OTC	25-50 mg q6-8h to 300 mg/day 12.5 mg q6-8h to 75 mg/day	Nausea, diarrhea, constipation, abdominal distress, dyspepsia, flatulence	See ibuprofen	
Meclofenamate	Meclomen Rx	100 mg tid to 300 mg	See ketoprofen	See ibuprofen	
Mefenamic acid	Ponstel Rx	50 mg initially; then 250 mg q6-8h to 1000 mg/day	See ketoprofen	Very potent and effective prostaglandin-synthesis inhibitor Antagonizes already formed prostaglandins Increased incidence of adverse GI side effects	
Naproxen	Naprosyn Rx	500 mg initially, then 250 mg q6-8h to 1250 mg/day	See ibuprofen	See ibuprofen	
Naproxen sodium	Anaprox Rx Aleve OTC	550 mg initially, then 275 mg q6-8h to 1375 mg/day 440 mg initially, then 220 mg q6-8h to 660 mg/day	See ibuprofen	See ibuprofen	

Sources: Clinical Pharmacology. (2004). *Drugs used to treat dysmenorrhea.* Gold Standard Multimedia. Internet document available at http://cp.gsm.com (accessed October 1, 2004); Facts and Comparisons. (2002). *Loose-leaf drug information service.* St. Louis: Facts and Comparisons; Parent-Stevens, L., & Burns, E. (2000). Menstrual disorders. In M. Smith & L. Shimp (Eds.), *20 Common problems in women's health care.* New York: McGraw-Hill.

GI, Gastrointestinal; *NSAID,* nonsteroidal antiinflammatory drugs; *OTC,* over the counter; *Rx,* prescription; *tid,* three times a day.
†Dosages are current recommendations and should be verified before use. Recommended dosages for over-the-counter preparations are generally less than recommendations for therapeutic dosages. As needed dosing is recommended by manufacturer; scheduled dosing may be more effective.
‡Risk with all NSAIDs is gastrointestinal ulceration, possible bleeding, and prolonged bleeding time. Incidence of side effects is dose related. Reported incidence, 3% to 9%.

TABLE 5-2

Herbal Therapies for Menstrual Disorders

SYMPTOMS OR INDICATIONS	HERBAL THERAPY	ACTION
Menstrual cramping	Black Haw	Uterine antispasmodic
	Ginger	Antiinflammatory
Premenstrual discomfort	Black cohosh root	Estrogen-like LH suppressant; binds to estrogen receptors
	Chaste tree fruit	Decreases prolactin levels
Tension, breast pain	Bugleweed	Antigonadotropic; decreases prolactin levels
Dysmenorrhea	Potentilla	Uterotonic
	Dong quai	Antiinflammatory; possibly analgesic activity
Menorrhea, metrorrhagia	Shepherd's purse	Uterotonic

Sources: Bascom, A. (2002). *Incorporating herbal medicine into clinical practice.* Philadelphia: FA Davis; Fugh-Berman, A., & Awang, D. (2001). Black co-hosh. *Alternative Therapies in Women's Health, 39*(11), 81-85; Dog, L. (2001). Conventional and alternative treatments for endometriosis. *Alternative Therapies, 7*(6), 50-56; Stevinson, C., & Ernst, E. (2001). Complementary/alternative therapies for premenstrual syndrome: A systemic review of randomized controlled trials. *American Journal of Obstetrics and Gynecology, 185*(1), 227-235.
LH, Luteinizing hormone.

of PMS are hotly and widely debated. Readers are encouraged to explore current feminist, medical, and social science literature for more information on these topics.

Management

There is little agreement on management. A careful, detailed history and daily log of symptoms and mood fluctuations spanning several cycles may give direction to a plan

 ### Critical Thinking Exercise

Premenstrual Syndrome

Joanna is a 22-year-old, single Caucasian woman who works as a manager at a fast food restaurant. She smokes about a half pack of cigarettes per day and drinks one to two beers a day. During her yearly checkup, including a Pap test, she tells you that she is experiencing uncomfortable symptoms—bloating, breast pain, and backache—before her menstrual period begins. She feels so stressed some days that she can't get any work done, and then she gets depressed. She asks you if there is anything she can do to stop having these problems.

1. Evidence—Is there sufficient evidence to draw conclusions about what advice the nurse should give to Joanna?
2. Assumptions—Describe underlying assumptions about the following issues:
   a. Educational self-help strategies (e.g., for PMS)
   b. Cyclic perimenstrual pain and related discomforts (CPPD)
   c. Quality of life issues for women experiencing perimenstrual pain and discomfort
   d. Coping enhancement as a nursing strategy
3. What implications and priorities for nursing care can be drawn at this time?
4. Does the evidence objectively support your conclusion?
5. Are there alternative perspectives to your conclusion?

of management. Any changes that assist a woman with PMS to exert control over her life have a positive impact. For this reason, lifestyle changes are often effective in the treatment of PMS.

Education is an important component of the management of PMS. Nurses can advise women that self-help modalities often result in significant symptom improvement. Women have found a number of complementary and alternative therapies to be useful in managing the symptoms of PMS. Diet and exercise changes are a useful way to begin and provide symptom relief for some women. Nurses can suggest that women not smoke and limit their consumption of refined sugar (less than 5 tbsp/day), salt (less than 3 g/day), red meat (up to 3 oz/day), alcohol (less than 1 oz/day), and caffeinated beverages. They can be encouraged to include whole grains, legumes, seeds, nuts, vegetables, fruits, and vegetable oils in their diet. Three small-to-moderate-sized meals and three small snacks a day that are rich in complex carbohydrates and fiber have been reported to improve symptoms (Jones, 2001). Use of natural diuretics (see section on dysmenorrhea management) may help reduce fluid retention as well. Nutritional supplements may assist in symptom relief. Calcium (1000 to 1200 mg daily), magnesium (300 to 400 mg daily), and vitamin B_6 (100 to 150 mg daily) have been shown to be moderately effective in relieving symptoms, to have few side effects, and to be safe. Daily supplements of evening primrose oil are thought to be useful in relieving breast symptoms with minimal side effects.

Regular exercise (aerobic exercise three to four times a week), especially in the luteal phase, is widely recommended for relief of PMS symptoms (Rapkin, 2003). A monthly program that varies in intensity and type of exercise according to PMS symptoms is best. Women who exercise regularly seem to have less premenstrual anxiety than do nonathletic women. It is thought that aerobic exercise increases beta-endorphin levels to offset symptoms of depression and elevate mood. Yoga, acupuncture, hypnosis, chiropractic therapy, and massage therapy have all been reported to have a beneficial effect on PMS. Herbal therapies have long been used to treat PMS; specific suggestions are found in Table 5-2.

Nurses can explain the relation between cyclic estrogen fluctuation and changes in serotonin levels, that serotonin is one of the brain chemicals that assist in coping with normal life stresses, and how the different management strategies recommended help maintain serotonin levels. Counseling, in the form of support groups or individual or couple counseling, may be helpful. Stress reduction techniques also may assist with symptom management (Rapkin, 2003).

If these strategies do not provide significant symptom relief in 1 to 2 months, medication is often begun. Many medications have been used in treatment of PMS, but no single medication alleviates all PMS symptoms. Medications often used in the treatment of PMS include diuretics, prostaglandin inhibitors (NSAIDs), progesterone, and OCPs. Fluoxetine (Sarafem or Prozac, 20 mg/day), a selective serotonin reuptake inhibitor (SSRI), is the only U.S. Food and Drug Administration (FDA)–approved agent for PMS. Use of this medication results in a decrease in emotional symptoms, especially depression (Jones, 2001; Lin & Thompson, 2001).

Endometriosis

Endometriosis is characterized by the presence and growth of endometrial tissue outside of the uterus. The tissue may be implanted on the ovaries, cul-de-sac, uterine ligaments, rectovaginal septum, sigmoid colon, pelvic peritoneum, cervix, or inguinal area (Fig. 5-1). Endometrial lesions have been found in the vagina and in surgical scars; on the vulva, perineum, and bladder; and in sites far from the pelvic area, such as the thoracic cavity, gallbladder, and heart. A chocolate cyst is a cystic area of endometriosis in the ovary. The dark coloring of the cyst's contents is caused by old blood.

Endometrial tissue contains glands and stoma and responds to cyclic hormonal stimulation in the same way that the uterine endometrium does but often out of phase with it. During the proliferative and secretory phases of the cycle, the endometrial tissue grows. During or immediately after menstruation, the tissue bleeds, resulting in an inflammatory response with subsequent fibrosis and adhesions to adjacent organs.

Endometriosis is a common gynecologic problem, affecting from 5% to 15% of women of reproductive age (Stenchever et al., 2001). Although the condition usually develops in the third or fourth decade of life, endometriosis has been found in 4% to 10% of adolescents with disabling pelvic pain or abnormal vaginal bleeding (Motta, 2004). The condition is found equally in Caucasian and African-American women, is slightly more prevalent in Asian women, and may have a familial tendency for development (Nakad & Isaacson, 2002; Stenchever et al., 2001). Endometriosis may worsen with repeated cycles, or it may remain asymptomatic and undiagnosed, eventually disappearing after menopause.

Several theories to account for the cause of endometriosis have been suggested, yet the etiology and pathology of this condition continue to be poorly understood. One of the most widely accepted, long-debated theories is transtubal migration or retrograde menstruation. According to this theory, endometrial tissue is regurgitated or mechanically transported from the uterus during menstruation to the uterine tubes and into the peritoneal cavity, where it implants on the ovaries and other organs.

Symptoms vary among women, from nonexistent to incapacitating. Severity of symptoms can change over time and may be disconnected from the extent of the disease. The major symptoms of endometriosis are dysmenorrhea and deep pelvic dyspareunia (painful intercourse). Women also experience chronic noncyclic pelvic pain, pelvic heaviness, or pain radiating into the thighs. Many women report bowel symptoms such as diarrhea, pain with defecation, and constipation secondary to avoiding defecation because of the pain. Less common symptoms include abnormal bleeding (hypermenorrhea, menorrhagia, or premenstrual staining) and pain during exercise as a result of adhesions (Lemaire, 2004). Women who have endometriosis may also have other conditions such as chronic fatigue syndrome, fibromyalgia, endocrine disorders, and autoimmune disorders (Conversations with Colleagues, 2002-2003).

Impaired fertility may result from adhesions around the uterus that pull the uterus into a fixed, retroverted position. Adhesions around the uterine tubes may block the fimbriated ends or prevent the spontaneous movement that carries the ovum to the uterus or blocks the fimbriated ends.

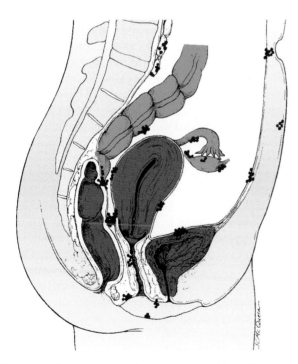

Fig. 5-1 Common sites of endometriosis. (From Stenchever, M., Droegemueller, W., Herbst, A., & Mishell, D. [2001]. *Comprehensive gynecology* [4th ed.]. St. Louis: Mosby.)

Management

Treatment is based on the severity of symptoms and the goals of the woman or couple. Women without pain who do not want to become pregnant need no treatment. Women with mild pain who may desire a future pregnancy may use NSAIDs for pain relief. Women who have severe pain and can postpone pregnancy may be treated with OCPs that have a low estrogen-to-progestin ratio to shrink endometrial tissue. However, when this therapy is stopped, women often experience high rates of recurrence of pain and other symptoms.

Hormonal antagonists that suppress ovulation and reduce endogenous estrogen production and subsequent endometrial lesion growth are currently used to treat mild to severe endometriosis in women who wish to become pregnant at a future time. Gonadotropin-releasing hormone (GnRH) agonist therapy (leuprolide, nafarelin [Synarel], goserelin acetate [Zoladex]) acts by suppressing pituitary gonadotropin secretion. FSH and LH stimulation to the ovary declines noticeably, and ovarian function decreases significantly. The hypoestrogenism results in hot flashes in almost all women. In addition, there may be minor bone loss, most of which is reversible within 12 to 18 months after the medication is stopped. Leuprolide (3.75 mg intramuscular injection given once a month) or nafarelin (200 mg administered twice daily by nasal spray) are both effective and well tolerated. Both medications reduce endometrial lesions and pelvic pain associated with endometriosis and have posttreatment pregnancy rates similar to that of danazol therapy (Stenchever et al., 2001). Common side effects of these drugs are those of natural menopause–hot flashes and vaginal dryness. Some women report headaches and muscle aches.

Danazol (Danocrine), a mildly androgenic synthetic steroid, suppresses FSH and LH secretion, thus producing anovulation with resulting decreased secretion of estrogen and progesterone and regression of endometrial tissue. Bothersome side effects include masculinizing traits in the woman–weight gain, edema, decreased breast size, oily skin, hirsutism, and deepening of the voice–all of which often disappear when treatment is discontinued. Other side effects are amenorrhea, hot flashes, vaginal dryness, insomnia, and decreased libido. Migraine headaches, dizziness, fatigue, and depression are also reported. Further, decreases in bone density have been noted that may be only partially reversible. Danazol should never be prescribed when pregnancy is suspected, and contraception should be used with it because ovulation may not be suppressed. Danazol can produce pseudohermaphroditism in female fetuses. The drug is contraindicated in women with liver disease and should be used with caution in women with cardiac and renal disease.

Surgical intervention is often needed for severe, acute, or incapacitating symptoms. Decisions regarding the extent and type of surgery are influenced by a woman's age, desire for children, and location of the disease. For women who do not want to preserve their ability to have children, the only definite cure is hysterectomy and bilateral salpingo-oophorectomy (BSO) (total abdominal hysterectomy [TAH] with BSO). In women who are in their childbearing years and want children and in whom the disease does not prevent it, reproductive capacity should be retained through careful removal by surgery or laser therapy of all endometrial tissue possible and with retention of ovarian function (Nakad & Isaacson, 2002).

Short of TAH with BSO, endometriosis recurs in approximately 40% of women, regardless of the form of treatment. Therefore for many women, endometriosis is a chronic disease with conditions such as chronic pain or infertility. Counseling and education are critical components of nursing care of women with endometriosis. Women need an honest discussion of treatment options with potential risks and benefits of each option reviewed. Because pelvic pain is a subjective, personal experience that can be frightening, support is important. Sexual dysfunction resulting from painful intercourse (dyspareunia) may be present and may necessitate referral for counseling. Support groups for women with endometriosis may be found in some locations (see Resources at the end of the chapter). The nursing care measures discussed in the section on dysmenorrhea are appropriate for managing chronic pelvic pain associated with endometriosis (see Plan of Care).

Alterations in Cyclic Bleeding

Women often experience changes in amount, duration, interval, or regularity of menstrual cycle bleeding. Commonly, women worry about menstruation that is infrequent or scanty (oligomenorrhea), is excessive (menorrhagia), or occurs between periods (metrorrhagia).

Treatment depends on the cause and may include education and reassurance. For example, women should be told that OCPs can cause scanty menstrual flow and midcycle spotting. Progestin intramuscular injections and implants can also cause midcycle bleeding. A single episode of heavy bleeding may signal an early pregnancy loss such as a miscarriage or ectopic pregnancy. This type of bleeding is often thought to be a period that is heavier than usual, perhaps delayed, and is associated with abdominal pain or pelvic discomfort. When early pregnancy loss is suspected, a hematocrit and pregnancy test should be done.

Uterine leiomyomas (fibroids or myomas) are a common cause of menorrhagia. Fibroids are benign tumors of the smooth muscle of the uterus whose etiology is unknown. Fibroids occur in approximately one fourth of women of reproductive age; the incidence of fibroids is two to three times higher in African-American women than in Caucasian or Hispanic women (Friedman & Carlson, 2002). Other uterine growths ranging from endometrial polyps to adenocarcinoma and endometrial cancer are common causes of heavy menstrual bleeding, as well as intermenstrual bleeding.

Treatment for menorrhagia depends on the cause of the bleeding. If the bleeding is related to contraceptive method, the nurse provides factual information and reassurance and discusses other contraceptive options. If bleeding is

PLAN OF CARE *Endometriosis*

NURSING DIAGNOSIS Acute pain related to menstruation secondary to endometriosis

Expected Outcome *Patient will verbalize a decrease in intensity and frequency of pain during each menstrual cycle.*

Nursing Interventions/*Rationales*

- Assess location, type, and duration of pain and history of discomfort *to determine severity of dysmenorrhea.*
- Administer analgesics *to assist with pain relief.*
- Administer hormone altering medications if ordered *to suppress ovulation.*
- Provide nonpharmacologic methods such as heat *to increase blood flow to the pelvic region.*

NURSING DIAGNOSIS Deficient knowledge related to unfamiliarity with treatment, as evidenced by patient statements

Expected Outcome *Patient will verbalize correct understanding of the use of self-care methods and prescribed therapies.*

Nursing Interventions/*Rationales*

- Assess patient's current understanding of the disorder and related therapies *to validate the accuracy of knowledge base.*
- Give information to patient regarding the disorder and treatment regimen *to empower the patient to become a partner in her own care.*

NURSING DIAGNOSIS Situational low self-esteem related to infertility as evidenced by patient's statements of decreased self-worth

Expected Outcome *Patient will verbalize positive feelings of self-worth.*

Nursing Interventions/*Rationales*

- Provide therapeutic communication *to validate feelings and provide support.*
- Refer to support group *to enhance feelings of self-worth through group communication.*

NURSING DIAGNOSIS Anxiety related to possible invasive surgical procedure as evidenced by patient's verbal report

Expected Outcome *Patient will report a decreased number of anxious feelings.*

Nursing Interventions/*Rationales*

- Provide opportunity to discuss feelings *to identify source of anxiety.*
- Reinforce information provided *to keep expectations realistic and dispel myths or inaccuracies.*
- Provide emotional support *to encourage verbalization of feelings.*

NURSING DIAGNOSIS Risk for injury related to disease progression

Expected Outcome *Woman will report any changes in health status to health care provider.*

Nursing Interventions/*Rationales*

- Teach woman to report any changes in health status *to initiate prompt treatment.*
- Review side effects of medications *to recognize possible rationales for changes in health status.*
- Encourage ongoing communication with health care provider *to promote trust and comfort.*

---

related to presence of fibroids, the degree of disability and discomfort associated with the fibroids and the woman's plans for childbearing will influence treatment decisions. Treatment options include medical and surgical management. Most fibroids can be monitored by frequent examinations to judge growth, if any, and correction of anemia, if present. Women with metrorrhagia should be warned not to use aspirin because of its tendency to increase bleeding. Medical treatment is directed toward temporarily reducing symptoms, shrinking the myoma, and reducing its blood supply (Stenchever et al., 2001). This reduction is often accomplished with the use of a GnRH agonist. If the woman wishes to retain childbearing potential, a myomectomy may be done. Myomectomy, or removal of the tumors only, is particularly difficult if multiple myomas must be removed. If the woman does not want to preserve her childbearing function, or if she has severe symptoms (severe anemia, severe pain, considerable disruption of lifestyle), hysterectomy or endometrial ablation (laser surgery or electrocoagulation) may be done.

Dysfunctional uterine bleeding

Abnormal uterine bleeding (AUB) is any form of uterine bleeding that is irregular in amount, duration, or timing and not related to regular menstrual bleeding. Box 5-1 lists possible causes of AUB. Although often used interchangeably, the terms AUB and dysfunctional uterine bleeding (DUB) are not synonymous. Dysfunctional uterine bleeding is a subset of AUB defined as "excessive uterine bleeding with no demonstrable organic cause, genital or extragenital" (Stenchever et al., 2001). DUB is most commonly caused by anovulation. When there is no surge of LH or if insufficient progesterone is produced by the corpus luteum to support the endometrium, it will begin to involute and shed. This most often occurs at the extremes of a woman's reproductive years—when the menstrual cycle is just becoming established at menarche or when it draws to a close at menopause. DUB can also be found with any condition that gives rise to chronic anovulation associated with continuous estrogen production. Such conditions include obesity, hyperthyroidism and hypothyroidism, polycystic ovarian syndrome, and any of the endocrine conditions discussed in the sections on amenorrhea and oligomenorrhea. A diagnosis of DUB is made only after all other causes of abnormal menstrual bleeding have been ruled out (American College of Nurse-Midwives [ACNM], 2002).

The most effective medical treatment of acute bleeding episodes of DUB is administration of oral or intravenous estrogen. A dilation and curettage may be done if the bleeding

BOX 5-1

Possible Causes of Abnormal Uterine Bleeding

ANOVULATION
- Hypothalamic dysfunction
- Polycystic ovary syndrome

PREGNANCY-RELATED CONDITIONS
- Threatened or spontaneous miscarriage
- Retained products of conception after elective abortion
- Ectopic pregnancy

LOWER REPRODUCTIVE TRACT INFECTIONS
- Chlamydial cervicitis
- Pelvic inflammatory disease

NEOPLASMS
- Endometrial hyperplasia
- Cancer of cervix and endometrium
- Endometrial polyps
- Hormonally active tumors (rare)

- Leiomyomata
- Vaginal tumors (rare)

TRAUMA
- Genital injury (accidental, coital trauma, sexual abuse)
- Foreign body
- Primary coagulation disorders

SYSTEMIC DISEASES
- Diabetes mellitus
- Thyroid dysfunction (hypothyroidism, hyperthyroidism)
- Severe organ disease (renal or liver failure)

IATROGENIC CAUSES
- Exogenous hormone use (oral contraceptives, menopausal hormone therapy)
- Medications with estrogenic activity
- Herbal preparation (ginseng)

Sources: American College of Nurse-Midwives (ACNM). (2002). Abnormal and dysfunctional uterine bleeding. ACNM Clinical Bulletin No. 6. *Journal of Midwifery and Women's Health, 47*(3), 207-213; Stenchever, M., et al. (2001). *Comprehensive gynecology* (4th ed.). St. Louis: Mosby.

has not stopped in 12 to 24 hours. An oral conjugated estrogen and progestin regimen is usually given for at least 3 months. If the woman wants contraception, she should continue to take OCPs. If she has no need for contraception, the treatment may be stopped to assess the woman's bleeding pattern. If her menses does not resume, a progestin regimen (e.g., medoxyprogesterone, 10 mg each day for 10 days before the expected date of her menstrual period) may be prescribed after ruling out pregnancy. This is done to prevent persistent anovulation with chronic unopposed endogenous estrogen hyperstimulation of the endometrium, which can result in eventual atypical tissue changes.

If the recurrent, heavy bleeding is not controlled by hormonal therapy, ablation of the endometrium through laser treatment may be performed (Stenchever et al., 2001). Nursing roles include informing women of their options, counseling and education as indicated, and referring to the appropriate specialists and health care services.

CARE MANAGEMENT ■

Assessment and Nursing Diagnoses

In addition to taking a careful menstrual, obstetric, sexual, and contraceptive history, the nurse should explore the woman's perceptions of her condition, cultural or ethnic influences, experiences with other caregivers, lifestyle, and patterns of coping (see Guidelines/Guías box). The amount of pain or bleeding experienced and its effect on daily activities should be evaluated. Home remedies and prescriptions to relieve discomfort are noted. A symptom diary, in which the woman records emotions, behaviors,

physical symptoms, diet, and exercise and rest patterns, is a useful diagnostic tool.

Nursing diagnoses for the woman experiencing menstrual disorders include the following:

- *Risk for ineffective individual coping related to*
  - insufficient knowledge of the cause of the disorder
  - emotional and physiologic effects of the disorder
- *Deficient knowledge related to*
  - self-care
  - available therapy for the disorder
- *Risk for disturbed body image related to*
  - menstrual disorder
  - sexual dysfunction
- *Risk for situational low self-esteem related to*
  - others' perception of her discomfort
  - inability to conceive
- *Acute or chronic pain related to*
  - menstrual disorder

Expected Outcomes of Care

After data collection and review, mutual expected outcomes are established and a plan of care is developed. Expected outcomes for the woman are that she will do the following:
- Verbalize her understanding of reproductive anatomy, etiology of her disorder, medication regimen, and diary use
- Verbalize understanding and accept her emotional and physical responses to her menstrual cycle
- Develop personal goals that benefit her emotionally and physically

GUIDELINES/GUÍAS

Menstruation

- At what age did you begin to menstruate?
- *¿A qué edad empezó a menstruar?*

- When was your last menstrual cycle?
- *¿Cuándo fue su última menstruación (regla)?*

- Was it normal?
- *¿Fue normal?*

- Do you have pains with your period?
- *¿Tiene algún dolor con la menstruación (regla)?*

- How many days does your period last?
- *¿Por cuántos días dura su menstruación (regla)?*

- Is the flow light or heavy?
- *¿Tiene mucha o poquita hemorragia durante su menstruación (regla)?*

- Choose appropriate therapeutic measures for her menstrual problems
- Adapt successfully to the condition, if cure is not possible

Plan of Care and Interventions

During the history and diagnostic workup, the clinician's concern and acceptance of the woman's symptoms as valid are in themselves therapeutic. Data from the daily diary of emotional status, subjective feelings, and physical state are correlated with physiologic changes. If the woman has a partner, both the woman and her partner keep separate diaries that include how each perceives the other's responses day by day. Through the diaries, feelings are vented, problems are identified and clarified, insights occur, and possible solutions begin to develop. The clinician facilitates insights and suggests therapeutic options. The woman (couple) makes choices considered best for her (them). Nurses need to discuss the options available to women with menstrual disorders. They must understand basic information about the anatomy and physiology, pathophysiology, psychologic impact, and treatment for the condition.

Support groups are an important resource. Nurses can use a local women's center or clinic to bring together women who want to learn more about their condition and support each other (see Resources at end of this chapter).

Evaluation

The nurse can be assured that care has been effective when the woman reports improvement in the quality of her life, skill in self-care, and a positive self-concept and body image.

INFECTIONS

Infections of the reproductive tract can occur throughout a woman's life and are often the cause of significant reproductive morbidity including ectopic pregnancy and tubal factor infertility (Centers for Disease Control and Prevention [CDC], 2002b). The direct economic costs of these infections can be substantial, and the indirect cost equally overwhelming. Some consequences of maternal infection, such as infertility, last a lifetime. The emotional costs may include damaged relationships and lowered self-esteem.

Sexually Transmitted Infections

Sexually transmitted infections (STIs) are infections or infectious disease syndromes primarily transmitted by sexual contact (Box 5-2). The term *sexually transmitted infection* includes more than 25 infectious organisms that are transmitted through sexual activity and the dozens of clinical syndromes that they cause. Despite the U.S. Surgeon General targeting STIs as a priority for prevention and control efforts, STIs are among the most common health problems in the United States today, with an estimated 15 million people in the United States being infected with STIs every year (Workowski, Levine, & Wasserheit, 2002). The most common STIs in women are discussed in this chapter. Effects on pregnancy and the fetus are discussed in Chapter 23. Neonatal effects are discussed in Chapter 27.

Prevention

Preventing infection (primary prevention) is the most effective way of reducing the adverse consequences of STIs for women. Prompt diagnosis and treatment of current infections (secondary prevention) also can prevent personal complications and transmission to others. Preventing the spread

---

BOX 5-2

Sexually Transmitted Infections

BACTERIA
- Chlamydia
- Gonorrhea
- Syphilis
- Chancroid
- Lymphogranuloma venereum
- Genital mycoplasmas
- Group B streptococci

VIRUSES
- Human immunodeficiency virus
- Herpes simplex virus, types 1 and 2
- Cytomegalovirus
- Viral hepatitis A and B
- Human papillomavirus

PROTOZOA
- Trichomoniasis

PARASITES
- Pediculosis (may or may not be sexually transmitted)
- Scabies (may or may not be sexually transmitted)

BOX 5-3

Essential Areas of Assessment for a Woman at Risk for or Who Has a Sexually Transmitted Infection

CURRENT PROBLEM
What symptoms are present?
- Vaginal discharge
- Lesions
- Rash
- Dysuria
- Fever
- Itching, burning
- Dyspareunia
- Malaise

MEDICAL HISTORY
- History of STIs
- Allergies, especially to medications

MENSTRUAL HISTORY
- Last menstrual period (possibility of pregnancy)

PERSONAL AND SOCIAL HISTORY
Sexual History
- Sexual preference
- Number of partners (past, present)
- Types of sexual activity
- Frequency of sexual activity

LIFESTYLE BEHAVIORS
- Intravenous drug use (or use by partner)
- Smoking
- Alcohol use
- Inadequate or poor nutrition
- High levels of stress, fatigue

STI, Sexually transmitted infection.

of STIs requires that women at risk for transmitting or acquiring infections change their behavior. A critical first step is for the nurse to include questions about a woman's sexual history, sexual risk behaviors, and drug-related risky behaviors as a part of her assessment (Box 5-3). When risk factors or risky behaviors are identified, the nurse has an opportunity to provide prevention counseling. Techniques that are effective in providing prevention counseling include using open-ended questions, using understandable language, and reassuring the woman that treatment will be provided regardless of consideration such as ability to pay, language spoken, or lifestyle (CDC, 2002a). Prevention messages should include descriptions of specific actions to be taken to prevent contracting or transmitting STIs (e.g., refraining from sexual activity when STI-related symptoms are present) and should be tailored to the individual woman, with attention given to her specific risk factors.

To be motivated to take preventive actions, a woman must believe that catching a disease will be serious for her and that she is at risk for infection. Unfortunately, most individuals tend to underestimate their personal risk of infection in a given situation. Therefore many women may not perceive themselves as being at risk for contracting an STI. Although levels of awareness of STIs are generally high, widespread misconceptions or specific gaps in knowledge also exist. Therefore nurses have a responsibility to ensure that their patients have accurate, complete knowledge about transmission and symptoms of STIs and risky behaviors that place them at risk for contracting an infection.

Primary preventive measures are individual activities aimed at deterring infection. Risk-free options include complete abstinence from sexual activities that transmit semen, blood, or other body fluids or that allow for skin-to-skin contact (Hatcher et al., 2004). Alternatively, involvement in a mutually monogamous relationship with an uninfected partner also eliminates the risk of contracting STIs.

Safer sex practices. An essential component of primary prevention is counseling women regarding safer sex practices, including knowledge of her partner, reduction of number of partners, low risk sex, and avoiding the exchange of body fluids.

No aspect of prevention is more important than knowing one's partner. Reducing the number of partners and avoiding partners who have had many previous sexual partners decreases a woman's chance of contracting an STI. Deciding not to have sexual contact with casual acquaintances also may be helpful. Discussing each new partner's previous sexual history and exposure to STIs will augment other efforts to reduce risk; however sexual partners are not always truthful about their sexual history. Critically important is whether or not male partners resist wearing condoms. Counseling on ways to negotiate with the partner about condom use may be helpful. For example, talking about condom use at a time removed from sexual activity may make it easier to bring up the subject

Women should be taught low risk sexual practices and which sexual practices to avoid. Mutual masturbation is low risk as long as bodily fluids come in contact only with intact skin. Caressing, hugging, body rubbing, massage, and hand-to-genital touching are low risk behaviors. Anal-genital intercourse, anal-oral contact, and anal digital activity are high risk sexual behaviors and should be avoided.

Currently, the sole physical barrier promoted for the prevention of sexual transmission of STI infections is the condom. Nurses can encourage women to have sexual partners use condoms by first discussing the subject with them. Such a discussion gives women permission to discuss any concerns, misconceptions, or hesitations they may have about using condoms. Women need to know how to purchase and use condoms. Information to be discussed includes importance of using latex rather than natural skin condoms. The nurse should remind women that only condoms with a current expiration date should be used and that they should be stored away from high heat. Women may choose to safely carry condoms in wallets, in shoes, or inside a bra. Women can be taught the differences among condoms, price ranges, sizes, and where they can be purchased. Instructions for how to apply a condom are found in Chapter 6. Women should be reminded to use a condom only one time and with every sexual encounter.

The female condom–a lubricated polyurethane sheath with a ring on each end that is inserted into the vagina–has been shown in laboratory studies to be an effective mechanical barrier to viruses, including human immunodeficiency virus (HIV). Although no clinical studies have been completed to evaluate the efficacy of female condoms in protecting against STIs, the CDC (2002a) states that, when used correctly and consistently, the female condom may substantially reduce STI risk and recommends its use when a male condom cannot be used properly. What is important and should be stressed by nurses is the consistent use of condoms for every act of sexual intimacy when there is the possibility of transmission of disease.

Evidence has shown that vaginal spermicides do not protect against certain STIs (e.g., chlamydia, cervical gonorrhea) and that frequent use of spermicides containing nonoxynol-9 has been associated with genital lesions and may increase HIV transmission (Wilkinson, Ramjee, Tholandi, & Rutherord, 2002). Condoms lubricated with nonoxynol-9 are not recommended (CDC, 2002a).

Women should be counseled to watch out for situations that make it hard to talk about and practice safer sex. These include romantic times when condoms are not available and when alcohol or drugs make it difficult to make wise decisions about safer sex.

Bacterial Sexually Transmitted Infections
Chlamydial infection

Chlamydia trachomatis is the most common and fastest spreading STI in U.S. women (CDC, 2002b). These infections are often silent and highly destructive; their sequelae and complications can be very serious. In women, chlamydial infections are difficult to diagnose; the symptoms, if present, are nonspecific, and the organism is expensive to culture.

Acute salpingitis, or PID, is the most serious complication of chlamydial infections. Past chlamydial infections are associated with an increased risk of ectopic pregnancy and tubal factor infertility. Furthermore, chlamydial infection of the cervix causes inflammation, resulting in microscopic cervical ulcerations that may increase risk of acquiring HIV infection.

Sexually active women younger than 20 years of age are the most likely to become infected with chlamydia. Women older than age 30 have the lowest rate of infection. Risky behaviors, including multiple partners and not using barrier methods of birth control, increase a woman's risk of chlamydial infection.

Screening and diagnosis. In addition to obtaining information regarding the presence of risk factors (e.g., women younger than 20 years old, women who do not use barrier contraceptives, women with new or multiple partners), the nurse should inquire about the presence of any symptoms (CDC, 2002a). Although infection is usually asymptomatic, some women may experience spotting or postcoital bleeding, mucoid or purulent cervical discharge, or dysuria. Bleeding results from inflammation and erosion of the cervical columnar epithelium.

Diagnosis of chlamydia is by culture (expensive and labor intensive), DNA probe (less expensive but less sensitive), enzyme immunoassay (less expensive but less sensitive), and nucleic acid amplification (expensive but has sensitivity of about 90%) (Rawlins, 2001). Special culture media and proper handling of specimens are important, so nurses should always know what is required in their individual practice sites.

Management. The CDC recommendations for treatment of chlamydial infections are doxycycline (100 mg orally twice a day for 7 days) or azithromycin (1 g orally in a single dose) (CDC, 2002a). Azithromycin is often prescribed when compliance may be a problem, because only one dose is needed; however, expense is a concern with this medication. Because chlamydia is often asymptomatic, the woman should be cautioned to take all medication prescribed. All exposed sexual partners should be treated. Woman treated with doxycycline or azithromycin do not need to be retested unless symptoms continue. Women treated with erythromycin may be retested 3 weeks after completing the medication, although the validity of this practice has not been established (CDC, 2002a).

Gonorrhea

Gonorrhea is caused by the aerobic, gram-negative diplococci *Neisseria gonorrhoeae*. Gonorrhea is almost exclusively transmitted by the contact of sexual activity. The principal means of communication is genital-to-genital contact; however, it is also spread by oral-to-genital and anal-to-genital contact. Gonorrhea also can be transmitted to the newborn in the form of ophthalmia neonatorum during birth by direct contact with gonococcal organisms in the cervix.

Age is probably the most important risk factor associated with gonorrhea. The majority of those contracting gonorrhea are younger than age 20 years. Other risk factors include early onset of sexual activity and multiple sexual partners.

Women are often asymptomatic, but when symptomatic they may have a greenish-yellow purulent endocervical discharge or may experience menstrual irregularities. Women may complain of pain; chronic or acute severe pelvic or lower abdominal pain; or longer, more painful menses. Gonococcal rectal infection may occur in women after anal intercourse. Individuals with rectal gonorrhea may be completely asymptomatic or, conversely, may experience severe symptoms with profuse purulent anal discharge, rectal pain, and blood in the stool. Rectal itching, fullness, pressure, and pain also are common symptoms, as is diarrhea. A diffuse vaginitis with vulvitis is the most common form of gonococcal infection in prepubertal girls. There may be few signs of infection, or vaginal discharge, dysuria, and swollen, reddened labia may be present.

Screening and diagnosis. Gonococcal infection cannot be diagnosed reliably by clinical signs and symptoms alone. Cultures are considered the gold standard for diagnosis of gonorrhea. Cultures should be obtained from the endocervix, rectum, and, when indicated, the pharynx. Thayer-Martin cultures are recommended to diagnose gonorrhea in women. Because STIs tend to coexist, any woman suspected of having gonorrhea should have a chlamydial culture and serologic test for syphilis if one has not been done in the past 2 months.

Management. Management of gonorrhea is straightforward, and the cure is usually rapid with appropriate antibiotic therapy. Single-dose efficacy is a major consideration in selecting an antibiotic regimen for women with gonorrhea. Another important consideration is the high percentage (45%) of women with coexisting chlamydial infections. The recommended treatment is one dose of the following medications: ceftriaxone 125 mg intramuscularly, cefixime 400 mg orally, ciprofloxacin 500 mg orally, ofloxacin 400 mg orally, or levofloxacin 250 mg orally (CDC, 2002a). The CDC also suggests concomitant treatment for chlamydia because coinfection is common.

Gonorrhea is a highly communicable disease. Recent (past 30 days) sexual partners should be examined, cultured, and treated with appropriate regimens. Most treatment failures result from reinfection; the woman needs to be informed of this, as well as of the consequences of reinfection in terms of chronicity, complications, and potential infertility. Women are counseled to have their partners use condoms. All patients with gonorrhea should be offered confidential counseling and testing for HIV infection.

LEGAL TIP Reporting a Communicable Disease

Gonorrhea is a reportable communicable disease. Health care providers are legally responsible for reporting all cases to the health authorities, usually the local health department in the woman's county of residence. Women should be informed that the case will be reported, told why, and informed of the possibility of being contacted by a health department epidemiologist.

Syphilis

Syphilis is caused by *Treponema pallidum*, a motile spirochete. Transmission is thought to be by entry in the subcutaneous tissue through microscopic abrasions that can occur during sexual intercourse. The disease can also be transmitted through kissing, biting, or oral-genital sex. Transplacental transmission may occur at any time during pregnancy; the degree of risk is related to the quantity of spirochetes in the maternal bloodstream.

Rates of syphilis have declined among women and African-Americans, although rates continue to be high in southern states (CDC, 2003).

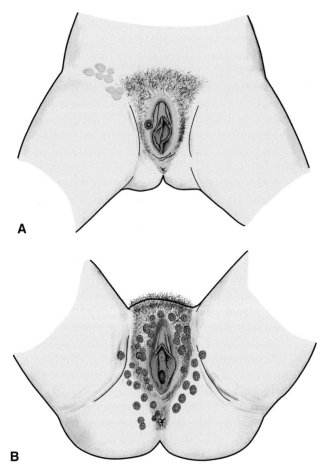

Fig. 5-2 Syphilis. **A,** Primary stage: chancre with inguinal adenopathy. **B,** Secondary stage: condyloma lata.

Syphilis is a complex disease that can lead to serious systemic disease and even death if untreated. Infection manifests itself in distinct stages with different symptoms and clinical manifestations. Primary syphilis is characterized by a primary lesion, the chancre, that appears 5 to 90 days after infection; this lesion often begins as a painless papule at the site of inoculation and then erodes to form a nontender, shallow, indurated, clean ulcer several millimeters to centimeters in size (Fig. 5-2, *A*). Secondary syphilis, occurring 6 weeks to 6 months after the appearance of the chancre, is characterized by a widespread, symmetric maculopapular rash on the palms and soles and generalized lymphadenopathy. The infected individual also may experience fever, headache, and malaise. Condyloma lata (wartlike infectious lesions) may develop on the vulva, perineum, or anus (Fig. 5-2, *B*). If the woman is untreated, she enters a latent phase that is asymptomatic for most individuals. If left untreated, approximately one third of patients will develop tertiary syphilis. Neurologic and cardiovascular, musculoskeletal, or multiorgan system complications can develop in this third stage.

Screening and diagnosis. Diagnosis is dependent on microscopic examination of primary and secondary lesion tissue and serology during latency and late infection. Any test for antibodies may not be reactive in the presence of active infection because it takes time for the body's immune system to develop antibodies to any antigens. Two types of serologic tests are used: nontreponemal and treponemal. Nontreponemal antibody tests such as the Venereal Disease Research Laboratory (VDRL) or rapid plasma reagin (RPR) are used as screening tests. False-positive results are not unusual, particularly when conditions such as acute infection, autoimmune disorders, malignancy, pregnancy, and drug addiction exist and after immunization or vaccination. The treponemal tests, fluorescent treponemal antibody absorbed (FTA-ABS) and microhemagglutination assays for antibody to *T. pallidum* (MHA-TP), are used to confirm positive results. Test results in patients with early primary or incubating syphilis may be negative. Seroconversion usually takes place 6 to 8 weeks after exposure, so testing should be repeated in 1 to 2 months when a suspicious genital lesion exists. Positive nontreponemal tests usually become nonreactive after treatment, but most patients with positive treponemal antibody test results will remain positive for life, regardless of treatment or disease activity (CDC, 2002a). Tests for chlamydia and gonorrhea should be done, and HIV testing offered.

Management. Penicillin is the preferred medication for treating patients with all stages of syphilis (CDC, 2002a). One intramuscular injection of penicillin G benzathine (2.4 million units) is the recommended dose.

NURSE ALERT *Patients treated for syphilis may experience a Jarisch-Herxheimer reaction after antibiotic therapy, an acute febrile reaction often accompanied by headache, myalgias, and arthralgias that develop within the first 24 hours of treatment. This reaction may be treated symptomatically with analgesics and antipyretics.*

Monthly follow-up is mandatory so that retreatment may be given if needed. The nurse should emphasize the necessity of long-term serologic testing even in the absence of symptoms. The patient should be advised to practice sexual abstinence until treatment is completed, all evidence of primary and secondary syphilis is gone, and serologic evidence of a cure is demonstrated. Women should be told to notify all partners who may have been exposed. They should be informed that the disease is reportable. Preventive measures should be discussed.

Pelvic inflammatory disease

Pelvic inflammatory disease (PID) is an infectious process that most commonly involves the uterine tubes (salpingitis), uterus (endometritis), and, more rarely, the ovaries and peritoneal surfaces. Multiple organisms have been found to cause PID, and most cases are associated with more than one organism. *C. trachomatis* is estimated to cause one half of all cases of PID. In addition to gonorrhea and chlamydia, a wide variety of anaerobic and aerobic bacteria are recognized to cause PID. Because PID may be caused by a wide variety of infectious agents and encompasses a wide variety of pathologic processes, the infection can be acute, subacute, or chronic and has a wide range of symptoms.

Most PID results from ascending spread of microorganisms from the vagina and endocervix to the upper genital tract. This spread most frequently happens at the end of or just after menses following reception of an infectious agent. PID also may develop after an elective abortion, pelvic surgery, or childbirth.

Risk factors for acquiring PID are those associated with the risk of contracting an STI–a history of PID or STIs, intercourse with a partner who has untreated urethritis, recent IUD insertion, and nulliparity.

Women who have had PID are at increased risk for ectopic pregnancy, infertility, and chronic pelvic pain. Other problems associated with PID include dyspareunia (painful intercourse), pyosalpinx (pus in the uterine tubes), tubo-ovarian abscess, and pelvic adhesions.

The symptoms of PID vary, depending on whether the infection is acute, subacute, or chronic; however, pain is common to all types of infection. It may be dull, cramping, and intermittent (subacute) or severe, persistent, and incapacitating (acute). Women may also report one or more of the following: fever, chills, nausea and vomiting, increased vaginal discharge, symptoms of a urinary tract infection, and irregular bleeding. Abdominal pain is usually present; upper abdominal pain may result from liver capsule inflammation (Fitz-Hugh-Curtis syndrome) (Stenchever et al., 2001).

Screening and diagnosis. PID is difficult to diagnose because of the accompanying wide variety of symptoms. The CDC (2002a) recommends treatment for PID in all sexually active young women and others at risk for STIs, if the following criteria are present and no other cause(s) of the illness can be found: lower abdominal tenderness, bilateral adnexal tenderness, and cervical motion tenderness. Other criteria for diagnosing PID include oral temperature 38.3° C or above, abnormal cervical or vaginal discharge, elevated erythrocyte sedimentation rate, elevated C-reactive protein, and laboratory documentation of cervical infection with *N. gonorrhoeae* or *C. trachomatis*.

Management. Perhaps the most important nursing intervention is prevention. Primary prevention includes education in preventing the acquisition of STIs, and secondary prevention involves preventing a lower genital tract infection from ascending to the upper genital tract. Instructing women in self-protective behaviors such as practicing safer sex and using barrier methods is critical. Also important is the detection of asymptomatic gonorrheal and chlamydial infections through routine screening of women with risky behaviors or specific risk factors such as age.

Although treatment regimens vary with the infecting organism, a broad-spectrum antibiotic generally is used (CDC, 2002b). Treatment may be oral (ofloxacin plus metronidazole) or parenteral (e.g., cefotetan plus doxycycline [oral]), and regimens can be administered in inpatient or outpatient settings. The woman with acute PID should be on bed rest in a semi-Fowler's position. Comfort measures include analgesics for pain and all other nursing measures applicable to a patient confined to bed. As few pelvic examinations as possible should be done during the acute phase of the disease. During the recovery phase, the woman should restrict her activity and make every effort to get adequate rest and a nutritionally sound diet. Follow-up laboratory work after treatment should include endocervical cultures for a test of cure.

Health education is central to effective management of PID. Nurses should explain to women the nature of their disease and should encourage them to comply with all therapy and prevention recommendations, emphasizing the necessity of taking all medication, even if symptoms disappear. Women should be counseled to refrain from sexual intercourse until their treatment is completed. Contraceptive counseling should be provided. The nurse can suggest the woman select barrier methods such as condoms or a diaphragm. A woman with a history of PID should not choose an IUD as her contraceptive method (Stenchever et al., 2001).

The potential or actual loss of reproductive capabilities can be devastating and can adversely affect a woman's self-concept. Because PID is so closely tied to sexuality, body image, and self-concept, the woman diagnosed with it will need supportive care. Referral to a support group or for counseling may be appropriate.

Viral Sexually Transmitted Infections
Human papillomavirus

Human papillomavirus (HPV) infections, also known as *condylomata acuminata*, or *genital warts*, is the most common viral STI seen in ambulatory health care settings. An estimated 20 million Americans are infected with HPV, and about 6.2 million new infections occur every year (CDC, 2005). HPV, a double-stranded DNA virus, has more than 30 serotypes that can be sexually transmitted, five of which are known to cause genital wart formation and eight of which are currently thought to have oncogenic potential (CDC, 2002a). HPV is the primary cause of cervical neoplasia (ACS, 2005).

Genital warts in women are most commonly seen in the posterior part of the introitus (Fig. 5-3). However, lesions also are found on the buttocks, vulva, vagina, anus, and cervix. Typically warts are small, 2 to 3 mm in diameter and 10 to 15 mm in height, soft, papillary swellings occurring singularly or in clusters on the genital and anal-rectal region. Infections of long duration may appear as a cauliflower-like mass. In moist areas such as the vaginal introitus, the lesions may appear to have multiple, fine, fingerlike projections.

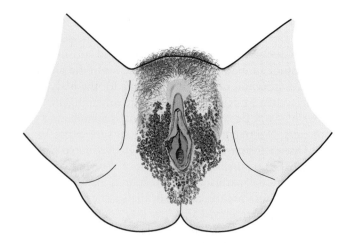

Fig. 5-3 Human papillomavirus infection.

Vaginal lesions are often multiple. Flat-topped papules, 1 to 4 mm in diameter, are seen most often on the cervix. Often, these lesions are visualized only under magnification. Warts are usually flesh colored or slightly darker on Caucasian women, black on African-American women, and brownish on Asian women. Condylomata acuminata are often painless but may also be uncomfortable, particularly when very large. They can become inflamed and ulcerated.

Screening and diagnosis. Viral screening and typing for HPV is available but not standard practice. History, evaluation of signs and symptoms, Papanicolaou (Pap) test, and physical examination are used in making a diagnosis. The HPV-DNA test can be used in women over the age of 30 in combination with the Pap test to test for types of HPV that are likely to cause cancer or in women with abnormal Pap test results (ACS, 2005) (see Chapter 4). The only definitive diagnostic test for presence of HPV is histologic evaluation of a biopsy specimen.

Management. Untreated warts may resolve on their own in young women, as their immune system may be strong enough to fight the HPV infection. If treatment is needed, a topical application of podofilox 0.5% solution or gel may be applied to the warts (CDC, 2002a). Cryotherapy, electrocautery, and laser therapy may also be used. No one treatment is best, and no therapy has been shown to eradicate HPV. The goal of treatment is removal of warts and relief of signs and symptoms. The woman often must make multiple office visits; frequently, many different treatments are tried.

Women who are experiencing discomfort associated with genital warts may find that bathing with an oatmeal solution and drying the area with a cool hair dryer will provide some relief. Keeping the area clean and dry will also decrease growth of the warts. Cotton underwear and loose-fitting clothes that decrease friction and irritation also may decrease discomfort. Women should be advised to maintain a healthy lifestyle to aid the immune system; women can be counseled regarding diet, rest, stress reduction, and exercise.

Patient counseling is essential. Women must understand the virus, how it is transmitted, that no immunity is conferred with infection, and that reinfection is likely with repeated contact. Women need to know that their partners should be checked, even if they are asymptomatic. All sexually active women with multiple partners or a history of HPV should be encouraged to use latex condoms and a vaginal spermicide for intercourse to decrease acquisition or transmission of the infection. Semiannual or annual health examinations are recommended to assess disease recurrence and screening for cervical cancer. At least annual Pap tests should be done on women who have been treated for HPV infections (CDC, 2002a).

Genital herpes simplex virus

Unknown until the middle of the twentieth century, genital herpes simplex virus (HSV) is now one of the most common STIs in the United States, especially in women. HSV is a painful vesicular eruption of the skin and mucosa of the genitals caused by two different antigen subtypes of HSV: herpes simplex virus 1 (HSV-1) and herpes simplex virus 2 (HSV-2). HSV-2 is usually transmitted sexually, and HSV-1 nonsexually. Although HSV-1 is more commonly associated with gingivostomatitis and oral labial ulcers (fever blisters) and HSV-2 with genital lesions, neither type is exclusively associated with the respective sites.

It is estimated that at least one in every five people in the United States is infected with herpes (CDC, 2002a). Women between ages 15 and 34 are most likely to become infected. Recurrent HSV infections are common. Prevalence is higher in women with multiple sex partners.

An initial herpetic infection characteristically has both systemic and local symptoms and lasts about 3 weeks. Women generally have a more severe clinical course than do men. Often, the first symptoms after incubation are genital discomfort and neuralgic pain. Systemic symptoms appear early, peak 3 to 4 days after lesions appear, and then subside over 3 to 4 days (Fig. 5-4). Ulcerative lesions last 4 to 15 days before crusting over. New lesions may develop up to the tenth day of the course of the infection. Viral shedding and therefore infectivity may last 6 or 8 weeks.

Common systemic symptoms with the primary infection include fever, malaise, headache, and photophobia. Women with primary genital herpes have many lesions that progress from macules to papules, then vesicles, pustules, and ulcers that crust and heal without scarring. These ulcers are extremely tender, and primary infections may be bilateral. Women also may have itching, inguinal tenderness, and lymphadenopathy. Severe vulvar edema may develop, and women may have difficulty sitting. Cervicitis also is common with initial infections, and a heavy, watery to purulent vaginal discharge is common. Extragenital lesions may be present because of autoinoculation. Urinary retention and dysuria may occur secondary to autonomic involvement of the sacral nerve root.

Women experiencing recurrent episodes of HSV infections often will have only local symptoms, which are usually less severe than those associated with the initial infection. Systemic symptoms are usually absent, although the characteristic prodromal genital tingling is common. Recurrent lesions are unilateral, are less severe, and usually last 7 to 10 days without prolonged viral shedding. Lesions begin as vesicles and progress rapidly to ulcers. Very few women with recurrent disease have cervicitis.

Screening and diagnosis. Although a diagnosis of herpes infection may be suspected from the history and physical examination, it is confirmed by viral tissue cultures.

Management. Genital herpes is a chronic and recurring disease for which there is no known cure. Oral medications used for treating HSV infections include acyclovir, famciclovir, and valacyclovir. Intravenous acyclovir may be used for women with severe disease (CDC, 2002a; Hatcher et al., 2004). Management is directed toward specific treatment during primary and recurrent infections, prevention, self-help measures, and psychologic support.

Cleaning lesions twice a day with saline will help prevent secondary infection. Bacterial infection must be treated with appropriate antibiotics. Measures that may increase comfort for women when lesions are active include warm sitz baths with baking soda; keeping lesions warm and dry by blowing the area dry using a hair dryer set on cool or patting dry with a soft towel; wearing cotton underwear and loose clothing; using drying aids such as hydrogen peroxide, Burrow's solution, or oatmeal baths; applying cool, wet black tea bags to lesions; and applying compresses with an infusion of cloves or peppermint oil and clove oil to lesions.

Analgesics such as aspirin or ibuprofen may be used to relieve pain and systemic symptoms associated with initial infections. Because the mucous membranes affected by herpes are very sensitive, any topical agents should be used with caution. Nonantiviral ointments, especially those containing cortisone, should be avoided. A thin layer of lidocaine ointment or an antiseptic spray may be applied to decrease discomfort, especially if walking is difficult.

Counseling and education are critical components of the nursing care of women with herpes infections. Information

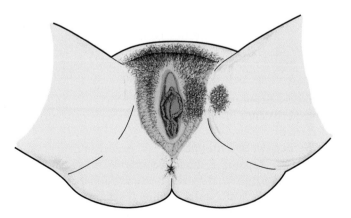

Fig. 5-4 Herpes genitalis.

regarding the etiology, signs and symptoms, transmission, and treatment should be provided. Women should be helped to understand when viral shedding and therefore transmission to a partner is most likely, and that they should refrain from sexual contact from the onset of prodrome until complete healing of lesions. Condoms may not prevent transmission, particularly male-to-female transmission; however, this does not mean that the partners should avoid all intimacy. Women can be encouraged to maintain close contact with their partners while avoiding contact with lesions. Women should be taught how to look for herpetic lesions using a mirror and good light source to aid vision and a wet cloth or finger covered with a finger cot to rub lightly over the labia. The nurse should ensure that women understand that when lesions are active, sharing intimate articles (e.g., washcloth, wet towel) that come into contact with the lesions should be avoided. Plain soap and water are all that is needed to clean hands that have come in contact with herpetic lesions.

Stress, menstruation, trauma, febrile illnesses, chronic illness, and ultraviolet light have all been found to trigger recurrences of genital herpes (Fraley, 2002). Women may wish to keep a diary to identify which stressors seem to be associated with recurrent herpes attacks so that they can then avoid those stressors when possible. Referral for stress reduction therapy, yoga, or meditation classes may be done when indicated. The role of exercise in reducing stress can be discussed. Avoiding excessive heat and sun and hot baths and using a lubricant during sexual intercourse to reduce friction also may be helpful.

The emotional effect of contracting an incurable STI such as herpes is considerable. At diagnosis many emotions may surface—helplessness, anger, denial, guilt, anxiety, shame, or inadequacy. Women need the opportunity to discuss their feelings and help in learning to live with the disease. Herpes can affect a woman's sexuality, her sexual practices, and her current and future relationships. She may need help in raising the issue with her partner or with future partners.

Hepatitis

Hepatitis A, B, and C viruses are discussed; hepatitis D and E viruses, most common among users of intravenous drugs and recipients of multiple blood transfusions, are not included in this discussion.

Hepatitis A. Hepatitis A virus (HAV) infection is acquired primarily through a fecal-oral route by ingestion of contaminated food, particularly milk, shellfish, or polluted water, or person-to-person contact. HAV infection is characterized by flulike symptoms with malaise, fatigue, anorexia, nausea, pruritus, fever, and upper right quadrant pain. Serologic testing to detect the immunoglobulin M (IgM) antibody is done to confirm acute infections. Because HAV infection is self-limited and does not result in chronic infection or chronic liver disease, treatment is usually supportive. Women who become dehydrated from nausea and vomiting or who have fulminating hepatitis A may need to be hospitalized. Medications that might cause liver damage or that are metabolized in the liver should be used with caution. No specific diet or activity restrictions are necessary. Hepatitis A vaccine and immune globulin (IG) for intramuscular administration are effective in preventing most hepatitis A infections (CDC, 2002a).

Hepatitis B. Hepatitis B virus (HBV), a common STI, is much more contagious than HIV. It is caused by a large DNA virus and is associated with three antigens and their antibodies: hepatitis B surface antigen (HBsAg), HBV antigen (HBeAg), HBV core antigen (HBcAg), antibody to HBsAg (anti-HBs), antibody to HBeAg (anti-HBe), and antibody to HBcAg (anti-HBc). Screening for active or chronic disease or disease immunity is based on testing for these antigens and their antibodies.

Populations at risk include women of Asian, Pacific Island (Polynesian, Micronesian, Melanesian), or Alaskan Eskimo descent and women born in Haiti or sub-Saharan Africa. Women with a history of acute or chronic liver disease, who work or receive treatment in a dialysis unit, or who have household or sexual contact with a hemodialysis patient are at greater risk. Women who work or live in institutions for the mentally retarded are considered to be at risk, as are women with a history of multiple blood transfusions. Health care workers and public safety workers exposed to blood in the workplace are at risk. Behaviors such as multiple sexual partners and a history of intravenous drug use increase the risk of contracting HBV infections.

HBsAg has been found in blood, saliva, sweat, tears, vaginal secretions, and semen. Drug abusers who share needles are at risk, as are health care workers who are exposed to blood and needlesticks. Perinatal transmission most often occurs in mothers who have acute hepatitis infection late in the third trimester or during the intrapartum or postpartum periods from exposure to HBsAg-positive vaginal secretions, blood, amniotic fluid, saliva, and breast milk. HBV has also been transmitted by artificial insemination. Although HBV can be transmitted via blood transfusion, the incidence of such infections has decreased significantly since testing of blood for HBsAg became routine.

Hepatitis B (HB) is a disease of the liver and is often a silent infection. In the adult, the course of the infection can be fulminating and the outcome fatal. Early symptoms include skin eruptions, urticaria, arthralgias, arthritis, lassitude, anorexia, nausea, vomiting, headache, fever, and mild abdominal pain. Later the patient may have clay-colored stools, dark urine, increased abdominal pain, and jaundice. Between 5% and 10% of individuals with HB have persistence of HBsAg and become chronic hepatitis B carriers.

Screening and diagnosis. All women at high risk for contracting hepatitis B should be screened on a regular basis. The HBsAg screening test is usually done, as a rise in HBsAg occurs at the onset of clinical symptoms and usually indicates an active infection. If HBsAg persists in the blood, the woman is identified as a carrier. If the HBsAg test result is positive, further laboratory studies may be ordered: anti-HBe, anti-HBc, serum glutamic-oxaloacetic transaminase (SGOT), alkaline phosphatase, and liver panel.

Management. There is no specific treatment for hepatitis B. Recovery is usually spontaneous in 3 to 16 weeks. Women should be advised to increase bed rest; eat a high-protein, low-fat diet; and increase their fluid intake. They should avoid drugs and alcohol and medications metabolized in the liver. Women with a definite exposure to hepatitis B should be given hepatitis B immune globulin (HBIG) and begin the hepatitis B vaccine series within 14 days of the most recent contact to prevent infection (CDC, 2002a).

Hepatitis B vaccination is the most effective means of preventing HBV infections. Vaccination is also recommended for all nonimmune women who have had multiple sex partners within the past 6 months, intravenous drug users, residents of correctional or long-term care facilities, persons seeking care for an STI, sex workers, women whose partners are intravenous drug users or bisexual, and women who work in high risk occupations. The vaccine is given in a series of three (some authorities recommend four) doses over a 6-month period, with the first two doses given at least 1 month apart and the first and third doses at least 4 months apart (CDC, 2002b). The vaccine may be given in the deltoid muscle or gluteal muscle in adults.

Patient education includes explaining the meaning of hepatitis B infection, including transmission, state of infectivity, and sequelae. The nurse should also explain the need for immunoprophylaxis for household members and sexual contacts. To decrease transmission of the virus, women with hepatitis B or who test positive for HBV should be advised to maintain a high level of personal hygiene: wash hands after using the toilet; carefully dispose of tampons, pads, and Band-Aids in plastic bags; do not share razor blades, toothbrushes, needles, and manicure implements; have male partner use a condom if unvaccinated and without hepatitis; avoid sharing saliva through kissing, or sharing of silverware or dishes; and wipe up blood spills immediately with soap and water. They should inform all health care providers of their carrier state.

Hepatitis C. Hepatitis C virus (HCV) infection has become an important health problem as increasing numbers of persons acquire the disease. Hepatitis C is responsible for nearly 50% of the cases of chronic viral hepatitis. Risk factors include having STIs such as hepatitis B and HIV, multiple sexual partners, history of blood transmissions, and history of intravenous drug use. HCV is readily transmitted through exposure to blood and much less efficiently via semen, saliva, or urine.

Most patients with hepatitis C are asymptomatic or have general flulike symptoms similar to those of hepatitis A. HCV infection is confirmed by the presence of anti-C antibody during laboratory testing. Interferon-alpha alone or with ribavirin for 6 to 12 months is the main therapy for HCV-related liver disease, although effectiveness of this treatment varies. Currently there is no vaccine for hepatitis C.

Human immunodeficiency virus

About 40,000 new HIV infections occur in the United States each year (CDC, 2004). An estimated 30% of these new infections occur in women. African-American women are estimated to have 64% of these infections, whereas Hispanic and Caucasian women are estimated to have 18% each (CDC, 2004).

Transmission of HIV, a retrovirus, occurs primarily through exchange of body fluids (semen, blood, vaginal secretions). Severe depression of the cellular immune system associated with HIV infection characterizes acquired immunodeficiency syndrome (AIDS). Although behaviors that place women at risk have been well documented, all women should be assessed for the possibility of HIV exposure. The most commonly reported opportunistic diseases are *Pneumocystis carinii* pneumonia (PCP), *Candida* esophagitis, and wasting syndrome. Other viral infections such as HSV and cytomegalovirus infections seem to be more prevalent in women than men (Williams, 2003). PID may be more severe in HIV-infected women, and rates of HPV and cervical dysplasia may be higher. The clinical course of HPV infection in women with HIV infection is accelerated, and recurrence is more frequent.

Once HIV enters the body, seroconversion to HIV positivity usually occurs within 6 to 12 weeks. Although HIV seroconversion may be totally asymptomatic, it usually is accompanied by a viremic, influenza-like response. Symptoms include fever, headache, night sweats, malaise, generalized lymphadenopathy, myalgias, nausea, diarrhea, weight loss, sore throat, and rash.

Laboratory studies may reveal leukopenia, thrombocytopenia, anemia, and an elevated erythrocyte sedimentation rate. HIV has a strong affinity for surface-marker proteins on T lymphocytes. This affinity leads to significant T-cell destruction. Both clinical and epidemiologic studies have shown that declining CD_4 levels are strongly associated with increased incidence of AIDS-related diseases and death in many different groups of HIV-infected persons.

HIV testing and counseling. Screening, teaching, and counseling regarding HIV risk factors, indications for being tested, and testing are major roles for nurses caring for women today. A number of behaviors place women at risk for HIV infection, including intravenous drug use, high risk sex partners, multiple sex partners, and a previous history of multiple STIs. HIV infection is usually diagnosed by using HIV-1 and HIV-2 antibody tests. Antibody testing is first done with a sensitive screening test such as the enzyme immunoassay (EIA). Reactive screening tests must be confirmed by an additional test, such as the Western blot or an immunofluorescence assay. If a positive antibody test is confirmed by a supplemental test, it means that a woman is infected with HIV and is capable of infecting others. HIV antibodies are detectable in at least 95% of patients within 3 months after infection. Although a negative antibody test usually indicates that a person is not infected, antibody tests cannot exclude recent infection. Because HIV antibody crosses the placenta, definite diagnosis of HIV in children younger than 18 months is based on laboratory evidence of HIV in blood or tissues by culture, nucleic acid, or antigen detection (CDC, 2002a).

The FDA has approved two methods of rapid testing for HIV. OraQuick Rapid HIV Antibody tests can use a blood sample obtained by fingerstick or venipuncture or an oral fluid sample to provide test results within 20 minutes with an accuracy rate over 99%. If the results are reactive, further testing is done (Centers for Disease Control and Prevention, Divisions of HIV/AIDS Prevention, 2004; FDA, 2004). Quicker results mean that patients don't have to make extra visits for follow-up standard tests, and the oral test provides an option for patients who do not want to have a blood test.

The CDC (2002a) guidelines recommend offering HIV testing to all women whose behavior places them at risk for HIV infection. On entry into the health care system a woman can be handed written information about the risk factors for the AIDS virus and asked to inform the nurse if she believes she is at risk. She should be told that she does not have to say why she may be at risk, only that she thinks she might be.

Counseling before and after HIV testing is standard nursing practice today. It is a nursing responsibility to assess a woman's understanding of the information such a test would provide and to be sure the woman thoroughly understands the emotional, legal, and medical implications of a positive or negative test result before she is ready to take an HIV test.

> **LEGAL TIP**   **HIV Testing**
>
> - *If HIV test results are placed in the patient's chart—the appropriate place for all health information—they are available to all who have access to the chart. The woman must be informed of this before testing. Informed consent must be obtained before an HIV test is performed. In some states written consent is mandated.*
> - *Counseling associated with HIV testing has two components: pretest and posttest counseling. During pretest counseling, nurses conduct a personalized risk assessment, explain the meaning of positive and negative test results, obtain informed consent for HIV testing, and help women develop a realistic plan for reducing risk and preventing infection. Posttest counseling includes informing the patient of the test results, reviewing the meaning of the results, and reinforcing prevention messages. All pretest and posttest counseling should be documented.*

Unless rapid testing is done, there is generally a 1- to 3-week waiting period after testing for HIV, which can be an anxious time for the woman. It is helpful if the nurse informs her that this time period between blood drawing and test results is routine. Test results, whatever they are, always must be communicated in person and women informed in advance that such is the procedure. Whenever possible the person who provided the pretest counseling should also tell the woman her test results. Women's reactions to a negative test should be explored with the question "How do you feel?" HIV-negative result counseling sessions are another opportunity to provide education. Emphasis can be placed on ways in which a woman can remain HIV free and encouraged to stay negative. She should be reminded that if she has been exposed to HIV in the past 6 months she should be retested, and that if she continues high risk behaviors she should have ongoing testing.

When providing posttest counseling to an HIV-positive woman, privacy with no interruptions is essential. The nurse should make sure that the woman understands what a positive test means and review the reliability of the test results. Safer sex guidelines must be reemphasized. Referral for appropriate medical evaluation and follow-up should be made, and the need or desire for psychosocial or psychiatric referrals should be assessed. The importance of early medical evaluation so that a baseline assessment can be made and prophylactic medication begun should be stressed.

Management. During the initial contact with an HIV-infected woman, the nurse should establish what the woman knows about HIV infection. The nurse should ensure that the woman is being cared for by a medical practitioner or at a facility with expertise in caring for persons with HIV infections, including AIDS. Psychologic referral also may be indicated. Resources such as counseling for financial assistance, legal advocacy, suicide prevention, and death and dying may be appropriate. All women who are drug users should be referred to a substance abuse program. A major focus of counseling is prevention of transmission of HIV to partners.

Nurses counseling seropositive women wishing contraceptive information may recommend oral contraceptives and latex condoms or tubal sterilization or vasectomy and latex condoms. The IUD is not an ideal choice for the HIV-infected woman because of increased risk of infection. Insertion in a woman who is immunocompromised should be avoided (World Health Organization, 2000). Female condoms or abstinence can be offered to women whose partners refuse to use condoms.

No cure is available for HIV infections at this time. Rare and unusual diseases are characteristic of HIV infections. Opportunistic infections and concurrent diseases should be managed vigorously with treatment specific to the infection or disease. Routine gynecologic care for HIV-positive women should include a pelvic examination every 6 months. Careful Pap screening is essential because of the greatly increased incidence of abnormal findings on examination (Williams, 2003). In addition, HIV-positive women should be screened for syphilis, gonorrhea, chlamydia, and other vaginal infections and treated if infections are present. Discussion of the medical care of HIV-positive women or women with AIDS is beyond the scope of this chapter. HIV in pregnancy is discussed in Chapter 22 (see Resources at end of chapter for current information and recommendations).

Vaginal Infections

Vaginal discharge and itching of the vulva and vagina are among the most common reasons a woman seeks help from a health care provider. Indeed, more women complain of vaginal discharge than of any other gynecologic symptom. Vaginal discharge resulting from infection must be distinguished from normal secretions. Normal vaginal secretion or leukorrhea is clear to cloudy in appearance and may turn yellow after drying; the discharge is slightly slimy, is non-irritating, and has a mild inoffensive odor. Normal vaginal secretions are acidic, with a pH range of 4 to 5. The amount of leukorrhea present differs with phases of the menstrual cycle, with greater amounts occurring at ovulation and just before menses. Leukorrhea is also increased during pregnancy. Normal vaginal secretions contain lactobacilli and epithelial cells. Women who have adequate endogenous or exogenous estrogen will have vaginal secretions.

The most common vaginal infections are bacterial vaginosis (BV), candidiasis, and trichomoniasis. Vulvovaginitis, or inflammation of the vulva and vagina, may be caused by vaginal infection; copious amounts of leukorrhea, which can cause maceration of tissues; and chemical irritants, allergens, and foreign bodies, which may produce inflammatory reactions.

Bacterial vaginosis

BV, formerly called *nonspecific vaginitis, Haemophilus vaginitis,* or *Gardnerella,* is the most common type of vaginitis today (Schwebke, 2000). BV is associated with preterm labor and birth. The exact etiology of BV is unknown. It is a syndrome in which normal, H_2O_2-producing lactobacilli are replaced with high concentrations of anaerobic bacteria (e.g., *Gardnerella, Mobiluncus*). With the proliferation of anaerobes, the level of vaginal amines is raised and the normal acidic pH of the vagina is altered. Epithelial cells slough, and numerous bacteria attach to their surfaces (clue cells). When the amines are volatilized, the characteristic odor of BV occurs.

Many women with BV complain of a characteristic "fishy odor." The odor may be noticed by the woman or her partner after heterosexual intercourse because semen releases the vaginal amines. When present, the BV discharge is usually profuse, thin, and white or gray, or milky, in appearance. Some women also may experience mild irritation or pruritus.

Screening and diagnosis. A careful history may help distinguish BV from other vaginal infections if the woman is symptomatic. Reports of fishy odor and increased thin vaginal discharge are most significant, and a report of increased odor after intercourse is also suggestive of BV. Women with previous occurrence of similar symptoms, diagnosis, and treatment should be queried, because women with BV often have been treated incorrectly because of misdiagnosis.

Microscopic examination of vaginal secretions is always done (Table 5-3). Both normal saline and 10% potassium hydroxide (KOH) smears should be made. The presence of clue cells (vaginal epithelial cells coated with bacteria) on wet saline smear is highly diagnostic because the phenomenon is specific to BV. Vaginal secretions should be tested for pH and amine odor. Nitrazine paper is sensitive enough to detect a pH of 4.5 or greater. The fishy odor of BV will be released when KOH is added to vaginal secretions on the lip of the withdrawn speculum.

Management. Treatment of BV with oral metronidazole (Flagyl) is most effective (CDC, 2002a). Side effects of metronidazole are numerous, including sharp, unpleasant metallic taste in the mouth, furry tongue, central nervous system reactions, and urinary tract disturbances. When oral metronidazole is taken, the woman is advised not to drink alcoholic beverages, or she will experience the severe side effects of abdominal distress, nausea, vomiting, and headache. Gastrointestinal symptoms are common whether alcohol is consumed or not. Treatment of sexual partners is not routinely recommended (CDC, 2002a).

TABLE 5-3

Wet Smear Tests for Vaginal Infections

INFECTION	TEST	POSITIVE FINDINGS
Trichomoniasis	Saline wet smear (vaginal secretions mixed with normal saline on a glass slide)	Presence of many white blood cell protozoa
Candidiasis	Potassium hydroxide (KOH) preparation (vaginal secretions mixed with KOH on a glass slide)	Presence of hyphae and pseudohyphae (buds and branches of yeast cells)
Bacterial vaginosis	Normal saline smear	Presence of clue cells (vaginal epithelial cells coated with bacteria)
	Whiff test (vaginal secretions mixed with KOH)	Release of fishy odor

Candidiasis

Vulvovaginal candidiasis, or yeast infection, is the second most common type of vaginal infection in the United States. Although vaginal candidiasis infections are common in healthy women, those seen in women with HIV infection are often more severe and persistent. Genital candidiasis lesions may be painful, coalescing ulcerations necessitating continuous prophylactic therapy.

The most common organism is *Candida albicans;* it is estimated that 80% to 95% of the yeast infections in women are caused by this organism. However, in the past 10 years, the incidence of non–*C. albicans* infections has risen steadily. Women with chronic or recurrent infections often are infected with these organisms.

Numerous factors have been identified as predisposing a woman to yeast infections, including antibiotic therapy, particularly broad-spectrum antibiotics such as ampicillin, tetracycline, cephalosporins, and metronidazole; diabetes, especially when uncontrolled; pregnancy; obesity; diets high in refined sugars or artificial sweeteners; use of corticosteroids and exogenous hormones; and immunosuppressed states. Clinical observations and research have suggested that tight-fitting clothing and underwear or pantyhose made of nonabsorbent materials create an environment in which vaginal fungus can grow.

The most common symptom of yeast infections is vulvar and possibly vaginal pruritus. The itching may be mild or intense, may interfere with rest and activities, and may occur during or after intercourse. Some women report a feeling of dryness. Others may experience painful urination as the urine flows over the vulva; this usually occurs in women who have excoriations resulting from scratching. Most often the discharge is thick, white, lumpy, and cottage cheese–like. The discharge may be found in patches on the vaginal walls, cervix, and labia. Commonly, the vulva is red and swollen, as are the labial folds, vagina, and cervix. Although there is not a characteristic odor with yeast infections, sometimes a yeasty or musty smell occurs.

Screening and diagnosis.   In addition to a careful history of the woman's symptoms, their onset, and their course, the history is a valuable screening tool for identifying predisposing risk factors. Physical examination should include a thorough inspection of the vulva and vagina. A speculum examination is always done. Commonly, saline and KOH wet smear and vaginal pH are obtained (see Table 5-3). Vaginal pH is normal with a yeast infection; if the pH is greater than 4.5 one should suspect trichomoniasis or BV. The characteristic pseudohyphae (bud or branching of a fungus) may be seen on a wet smear done with normal saline; however, they may be confused with other cells and artifacts.

Management.   A number of antifungal preparations are available for the treatment of *C. albicans* infection. Intravaginal agents include miconazole, clotrimazole, butoconazole, and terconazole; fluconazole is an effective oral agent (CDC, 2002a). Many of these medications (e.g., Monistat, Gyne-Lotrimin) are available OTC. Exogenous lactobacillus

(in the form of dairy products or powder, tablet, capsule or suppository supplements) has been suggested for prevention and treatment of vulvovaginal candidiasis, but research is inconclusive and no recommendation for use in practice has been made (Jeavons, 2003). The first time a woman suspects that she may have a yeast infection, she should see a health care provider for confirmation of the diagnosis and treatment recommendation. If she experiences another infection, she may wish to purchase an OTC preparation and self-treat; if she elects to do this, she should always be counseled regarding seeking care for numerous recurrent or chronic yeast infections. If vaginal discharge is extremely thick and copious, vaginal debridement with a cotton swab followed by application of vaginal medication may be useful.

Women who have extensive irritation, swelling, and discomfort of the labia and vulva may find sitz baths helpful in decreasing inflammation and increasing comfort. Adding Aveeno powder to the bath may also increase the woman's comfort. Not wearing underpants to bed may help decrease symptoms and prevent recurrences. Completing the full course of treatment prescribed is essential to removing the pathogen, and women are instructed to continue medication even during menstruation. They should be counseled not to use tampons during menses because the medication will be absorbed by the tampon. If possible, intercourse is avoided during treatment; if this is not feasible, the woman's partner should use a condom to prevent introduction of more organisms (see Patient Instructions for Self-Care box).

Trichomoniasis

Trichomonas vaginalis is almost always an STI. It is also a common cause of vaginal infection (up to 25% of all vaginitis) and discharge and therefore is discussed in this section.

Trichomoniasis is caused by *T. vaginalis,* an anaerobic, one-celled protozoan with characteristic flagella. Although

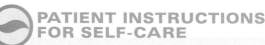

PATIENT INSTRUCTIONS FOR SELF-CARE

Prevention of Genital Tract Infections

- Practice genital hygiene.
- Choose underwear or hosiery with a cotton crotch.
- Avoid tight-fitting clothing (especially tight jeans).
- Select cloth car seat covers instead of vinyl.
- Limit time spent in damp exercise clothes (especially swimsuits, leotards, and tights).
- Limit exposure to bath salts or bubble bath.
- Avoid colored or scented toilet tissue.
- If sensitive, discontinue use of feminine hygiene deodorant sprays.
- Use condoms.
- Void before and after intercourse.
- Decrease dietary sugar.
- Drink yeast-active milk and eat yogurt (with lactobacilli).
- Do not douche.

trichomoniasis may be asymptomatic, commonly women experience characteristically yellowish to greenish, frothy, mucopurulent, copious, malodorous discharge. Inflammation of the vulva, vagina, or both may be present, and the woman may complain of irritation and pruritus. Dysuria and dyspareunia are often present. Typically, the discharge worsens during and after menstruation. Often, the cervix and vaginal walls demonstrate characteristic "strawberry spots," or tiny petechiae, and the cervix may bleed on contact. In severe infections the vaginal walls, the cervix, and occasionally the vulva may be acutely inflamed.

Screening and diagnosis. In addition to obtaining a history of current symptoms, a careful sexual history should be obtained. Any history of similar symptoms in the past and treatment used should be noted. The nurse should determine whether the woman's partner or partners were treated and if she has had subsequent relations with new partners.

A speculum examination is always done, even though it may be uncomfortable for the woman; relaxation techniques and breathing exercises may help the woman with the procedure. Any of the classic signs may or may not be seen on physical examination. The typical one-celled flagellate trichomonads are easily distinguished on a normal saline wet preparation (see Table 5-3). Trichomoniasis also may be identified on Pap smears. Because trichomoniasis is an STI, once diagnosis is confirmed the appropriate laboratory studies for other STIs should be carried out.

Management. The recommended treatment is metronidazole, 2 g orally in a single dose (CDC, 2002a) Although the male partner is usually asymptomatic, it is recommended that he receive treatment also because he often harbors the trichomonads in the urethra or prostate. It is important that nurses discuss the importance of partner treatment with their patients. If partners are not treated, it is likely that the infection will recur.

Women with trichomoniasis need to understand the sexual transmission of this disease. It is important that the woman know the organism may be present without symptoms, perhaps for several months, and that it is not possible to determine when she became infected.

Group B streptococci

Group B streptococci (GBS) may be considered normal vaginal flora in a woman who is not pregnant and therefore no treatment is needed. GBS is a concern in pregnancy because of increased risk for problems such as preterm labor and transmission to the newborn. For further discussion, see Chapters 23 and 27.

Infection Control

Infection control measures are essential to protect care providers and to prevent nosocomial infection of patients, regardless of the infectious agent. The risk for occupational transmission varies with the disease. Even when the risk is low, as with HIV, the existence of any risk warrants reasonable precautions. Precautions against airborne disease transmission are available in all health care agencies. Standard Precautions (precautions to use in care of all persons for infection control) and additional precautions for labor and birth settings are listed in Box 5-4.

PROBLEMS OF THE BREASTS ■

Benign Problems
Fibrocystic changes

Approximately 50% of women experience a breast problem at some point in their adult life. The most common benign breast problem is fibrocystic changes. Fibrocystic changes are found in varying degrees in breasts of healthy women. There is no known etiologic agent responsible for these changes. One theory is that estrogen excess and progesterone deficiency in the luteal phase of the menstrual cycle may cause changes in breast tissue.

Fibrocystic changes are characterized by lumpiness, with or without tenderness in both breasts (Stenchever et al., 2001). Single simple cysts may also occur. Symptoms usually develop about a week before menstruation begins and subside about a week after menstruation ends. Symptoms include dull heavy pain and a sense of fullness and tenderness often in the upper outer quadrants of the breasts. On physical examination there may be excessive nodularity that is described as feeling like a "plate of peas." Larger cysts may be described as feeling like water-filled balloons. Women in their twenties report the most severe pain. Women in their thirties have premenstrual pain and tenderness; small multiple nodules are usually present. Women in their forties usually do not report severe pain, but cysts will be tender; cysts often regress in size.

Steps in the workup of a breast lump may begin with ultrasonography to determine whether it is fluid filled or solid. Fluid-filled cysts are aspirated, and the woman is followed on a routine basis for development of other cysts (Lucas & Cone, 2003). If the lump is solid, mammography is obtained if the woman is older than 50 years of age. A fine-needle aspiration (FNA) is performed, regardless of the woman's age, to determine the nature of the lump. In some cases a core biopsy may need to follow FNA to harvest adequate amounts of tissue for pathologic examination (Stenchever et al., 2001).

Management depends on the severity of the symptoms. Diet changes and vitamin supplements are one management approach. Although research findings are contradictory, some practitioners advocate reducing consumption or eliminating methylxanthines (e.g., colas, coffee, tea, chocolate) and tobacco (Friedenreich et al., 2000).

Women may report decreased symptoms with such measures as taking vitamin E supplements and decreasing sodium intake or taking mild diuretics shortly before menses. Other pain relief measures include taking analgesics or NSAIDs, wearing a supportive bra, and applying heat to the breasts. Oral contraceptives, danazol, bromocriptine, and tamoxifen

Standard Precautions

- Medical history and examination cannot reliably identify all persons infected with human immunodeficiency virus (HIV) or other blood-borne pathogens. Standard Precautions should therefore be used consistently in the care of all persons. These precautions apply to blood, body fluids, and all secretions and excretions, except sweat, nonintact skin, and mucous membranes. Standard Precautions are recommended to reduce the risk of transmission of microorganisms from known and unknown sources of infection (Bolyard et al., 1998; CDC, 2001).

  1 Prompt and thorough handwashing is recommended between patient contacts. Hands and other skin surfaces should be washed immediately and thoroughly if contaminated with blood or other body fluids. Hands should be washed immediately after gloves are removed.

  2 In addition to handwashing, all health care workers should routinely use appropriate barrier precautions to prevent skin and mucous membrane exposure when contact with blood or other body fluids of any person is anticipated. Latex gloves should be worn for touching blood and body fluids, mucous membranes, or nonintact skin of all persons; for handling items or surfaces soiled with blood or body fluids; and for performing venipuncture and other vascular access procedures. Gloves should be changed after contact with each patient. Masks and protective eyewear or face shields should be worn during procedures that are likely to generate droplets of blood or other body fluids to prevent exposure of mucous membranes of the mouth, nose, and eyes. Gowns or aprons should be worn during procedures that are likely to generate splashes of blood or other body fluids.

    Leg coverings, boots, or shoe covers also can be worn to provide protection against splashes and may be recommended for certain procedures such as surgery.

  3 All health care workers should take precautions to prevent injuries caused by needles, scalpels, and other sharp instruments or devices during procedures; when cleaning used instruments; during disposal of used needles; and when handling sharp instruments after procedures. To prevent needlestick injuries, needles should not be recapped, purposely bent or broken by hand, removed from disposable syringes, or otherwise manipulated by hand. After they are used, disposable syringes and needles, scalpel blades, and other sharp items should be immediately placed in a puncture-resistant container for disposal; puncture-resistant containers should be located as close as is practical to the use area.

  4 Although saliva has not been implicated in HIV transmission, mouthpieces, resuscitation bags, or other ventilation devices should be available for use in areas in which the need for resuscitation is predictable, thus minimizing the chance for emergency mouth-to-mouth resuscitation.

  5 Health care workers who have exudative lesions or weeping dermatitis should refrain from all direct patient care and from handling patient care equipment until the condition resolves.

PRECAUTIONS FOR INVASIVE PROCEDURES

- An invasive procedure is surgical entry into tissues, cavities, or organs, for (1) repair of major traumatic injuries in an operating or birthing room, emergency department, or out-of-hospital setting, including both physicians' and dentists' offices, or (2) a vaginal or cesarean birth or other invasive obstetric procedure during which bleeding may occur. Standard Precautions, combined with the following precautions, should serve as minimum precautions for all such invasive procedures:

  1 All health care workers who participate in invasive procedures must routinely use appropriate barrier precautions to prevent skin and mucous membrane contact with blood and other body fluids of all patients. Gloves and surgical masks must be worn for all invasive procedures. Protective eyewear or face shields should be worn for procedures that commonly result in the generation of droplets, splashing of blood or other body fluids, or the generation of bone chips. Gowns or aprons made of materials that provide an effective barrier should be worn during invasive procedures that are likely to result in the splashing of blood or other body fluids. All health care workers who perform or assist in vaginal or cesarean births should wear gloves and gowns when handling the placenta or the infant until blood and amniotic fluid have been removed from the infant's skin. Gloves should be worn during infant eye prophylaxis, care of the umbilical cord, circumcision site, parenteral procedures, diaper changes, contact with colostrum, and postpartum assessments.

  2 If a glove is torn or a needlestick or other injury occurs, the glove should be removed and a new glove used as promptly as patient safety permits; the needle or instrument involved in the incident also should be removed from the sterile field.

  3 Any needlestick or other injury should be reported and appropriate treatment obtained as specified by the health care facility.

have also been used with varying degrees of success (Stenchever et al., 2001).

Surgical removal of nodules is done only in rare cases. In the presence of multiple nodules, the surgical approach would involve multiple incisions and tissue manipulation and may not prevent the development of more nodules.

Fibroadenoma

The next most common benign condition of the breast is a fibroadenoma. It is the single most common type of tumor seen in the adolescent population, although it can also occur in women in their thirties. Fibroadenomas are characterized by discrete, usually solitary lumps less than 3 cm in diameter (Stenchever et al., 2001). Occasionally the woman with a fibroadenoma will experience tenderness in the tumor during the menstrual cycle. Fibroadenomas increase in size during pregnancy and decrease in size as the woman ages. The cause of fibroadenomas is unknown.

Diagnosis is made by reviewing patient history and physical examination. Mammography, ultrasound, or magnetic resonance imaging may be used to determine the cause of the lesion. FNA may be used to determine underlying pathology. Surgical excision may be necessary if the lump is suspicious or if the symptoms are severe. Periodic observation of masses by professional physical examination or mammography may be all that is necessary for those masses not needing surgical intervention. Women should be instructed to perform monthly breast self-examinations (see Chapter 4).

Nipple discharge

Nipple discharge is a common occurrence that concerns many women. Although most nipple discharge is physiologic, each woman who has this problem must be evaluated carefully, because a small percentage will be found to have a serious endocrine disorder or malignancy.

Another form of breast discharge not related to malignancy is galactorrhea, which manifests as a bilaterally spontaneous, milky, sticky discharge. It is a normal finding in pregnancy. It can also occur as the result of elevated prolactin levels occurring as a result of a thyroid disorder, pituitary tumor, or chest wall surgery or trauma. It is essential to obtain a complete medication history on each woman. Oral contraceptives and neuroleptic drugs are known to precipitate galactorrhea in some women (Leung & Pacaud, 2004; Perese & Perese, 2003).

Diagnostic tests that may be indicated include a prolactin level, a microscopic analysis of the discharge from each breast, a thyroid profile, a pregnancy test, and a mammogram (Leung & Pacaud, 2004).

Mammary duct ectasia is an inflammation of the ducts behind the nipple. It occurs most often in perimenopausal women. It is characterized by a nipple discharge that is thick, sticky, and colored white, brown, green, or purple. Frequently the woman experiences a burning pain, an itching, or a palpable mass behind the nipple. The workup includes a mammogram and aspiration and culture of fluid. Treatment is usually symptomatic; warm compresses applied to the breast may provide relief. If a mass is present or an abscess occurs, treatment may include a local excision of the affected duct(s), provided the woman has no future plans to breastfeed.

Intraductal papilloma

Intraductal papilloma is a rare, benign condition that develops within the terminal nipple ducts. The cause is unknown. It usually occurs in women between ages 30 and 50. The papilloma is usually too small to be palpated, and the characteristic sign is nipple discharge that is serous, serosanguineous, or bloody. After the possibility of malignancy is eliminated, the affected segments of the ducts and breasts are surgically excised (Stenchever et al., 2001). Table 5-4 compares manifestations of benign breast diseases.

Cancer of the Breast

The United States has one of the highest rates of carcinoma in the world. One in eight American women will develop breast cancer in her lifetime (National Cancer Institute [NCI], 2002). There is no clear method for prevention. Prognosis for and survival of the woman are improved with early detection. Therefore the woman must be educated about risk factors, early detection, and screening.

Although the exact cause of breast cancer continues to elude investigators, certain risk factors that increase a

---

TABLE 5-4

Comparison of Common Manifestations of Benign Breast Masses

FIBROCYSTIC CHANGES	FIBROADENOMA	LIPOMA	INTRADUCTAL PAPILLOMA	MAMMARY DUCT ECTASIA
Multiple lumps	Single lump	Single lump	Single or multiple	Mass behind nipple
Nodular	Well delineated	Well delineated	Not well delineated	Not well delineated
Palpable	Palpable	Palpable	Nonpalpable	Palpable
Movable	Movable	Movable	Nonmobile	Nonmobile
Round, smooth	Round, lobular	Round, lobular	Small, ball-like	Irregular
Firm or soft	Firm	Soft	Firm or soft	Firm
Tenderness influenced by menstrual cycle	Usually asymptomatic	Nontender	Usually nontender	Painful, burning, itching
Bilateral	Unilateral	Unilateral	Unilateral	Unilateral
May or may not have nipple discharge	No nipple discharge	No nipple discharge	Serous or bloody nipple discharge	Thick, sticky nipple discharge

---

BOX 5-5

Risk Factors for Breast Cancer*

- Age
- Previous history of breast cancer
- Family history of breast cancer, especially a mother or sister (particularly significant if premenopausal)
- Previous history of ovarian, endometrial, colon, or thyroid cancer
- Early menarche (before age 12)
- Late menopause (after age 55)
- Nulliparity or first pregnancy after age 30
- Use of estrogen replacement therapy
- Obesity after menopause
- Previous history of benign breast disease with epithelial hyperplasia
- Race (Caucasian women have highest incidence)
- High socioeconomic status
- Sedentary lifestyle

*Risk factors are cumulative—the more risk factors present, the greater the likelihood of breast cancer occurring.

---

woman's risk for developing a malignancy have been identified. These factors are listed in Box 5-5. The most important predictor for breast cancer is age; the risk increases as the woman ages.

There has been much discussion about possible links between breast cancer and hormonal therapy; several large research studies including the Women's Health Initiative have found that there is an increased risk of breast cancer when a woman is taking combined estrogen and progesterone. However, estrogen alone does not appear to increase the risk (Furniss, 2000; Rossouw et al., 2002).

In a long-term study of breast implant patients implemented by the National Cancer Institute, silicone breast implants did not increase the risk of breast cancer (Nelson, 2000).

Although most breast cancers are not related to genetic factors, the identification of the BRCA-1 and BRCA-2 genes has demonstrated the role of heredity and genetic mutations in this disease. Only about 10% of all breast cancers are attributed to heredity. Women who have abnormalities in the BRCA-1 and BRCA-2 genes have a 35% to 85% chance of developing breast cancer (ACS, 2004). Other genetic mutations that can cause breast cancer include mutations of the ATM gene, the p53 tumor suppressor gene, and the CHEC-2 gene (ACS, 2004) (Box 5-6).

Although the clinical applicability of risk factors has limits, women at increased risk should be screened at more frequent intervals and should consider changing risk factors that can be changed, such as losing weight if obese and limiting alcohol intake (ACS, 2004).

Screening and diagnosis

It is estimated that 90% of all breast lumps are detected by the woman. Of this 90%, only 20% to 25% are malignant. More than half of all lumps are discovered in the upper outer quadrant of the breast. The most common presenting symptom is a lump or thickening of the breast. The lump may feel hard and fixed or soft and spongy. It may have well-defined or irregular borders. It may be fixed to the skin, thereby causing dimpling to occur. A nipple discharge that is bloody or clear also may be present.

Early detection and diagnosis reduce risk of mortality because cancer is found when it is smaller, lesions are more localized, and there tends to be a lower percentage of positive nodes. However, cultural factors may influence a woman's decision to participate in breast cancer screening. Knowledge of these factors and use of culturally sensitive tailored messages and materials that appeal to the unique concerns, beliefs, and reading abilities of target groups of underutilizers may assist the nurse in helping women overcome barriers to seeking care. For example, the ACS (2004) reported that women who were African-American, Hispanic, or Native American were less likely to get mammograms than Caucasian or Asian-American women.

Regular breast self-examination from midadolescence on, a clinical examination by a qualified health care provider, and screening mammography (x-ray examination of the breast) (Fig. 5-5) may aid in the early detection of breast cancers (Table 5-5).

When a suspicious finding on a mammogram is noted or a lump is detected, diagnosis is confirmed by needle aspiration, a core needle biopsy, or surgical excision (Fig. 5-6). Ultrasound may also be used to assess a specific area of abnormality found during a mammogram procedure (ACS, 2004). Patients need specific information regarding advantages and disadvantages of these procedures in making a decision about which is most appropriate for them.

BOX 5-6

Ethical Considerations for Genetic Testing

The ability to test for BRCA-1 and BRCA-2 has generated heated ethical debate within the health care community. Testing is expensive (approximately $2500 for the first person in the family to be tested [National Women's Health Resource Center, 2000]) and often not covered by insurance. Who should be tested (usually not recommended for women without family history of breast or ovarian cancer) and who should pay for it have not been addressed adequately. What to do when a positive result is discovered is not universally agreed on. Women and their families will most likely have increased anxiety after a positive finding. How often should screening be performed? Should prophylactic mastectomies be recommended? Will there be employment discrimination if this information is in a woman's medical record? Women requesting testing must be fully informed of the possible risks and benefits of testing before consenting to the procedure. Genetic counseling should include helping the woman determine how to inform other family members (Cummings, 2001; National Women's Health Resource Center, 2000).

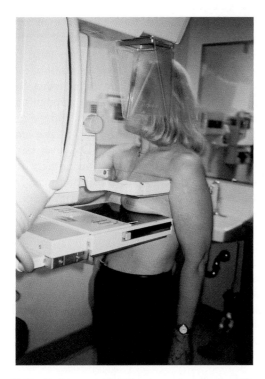

Fig. 5-5 Patient undergoing mammography. (Courtesy Shannon Perry, Phoenix, AZ.)

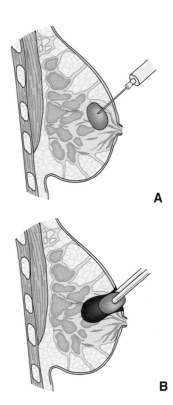

Fig. 5-6 Diagnosis. **A,** Needle aspiration. **B,** Open biopsy. (Redrawn from National Women's Health Resource Center. [1995]. Breast health. *National Women's Health Report,* 13[5], 3.)

Laboratory diagnosis of breast cancer and possible metastases includes complete blood count, liver enzyme levels, serum calcium, and alkaline phosphatase level. Elevated liver enzyme levels indicate possible liver metastases, and increased serum calcium and alkaline phosphatase levels suggest bone metastases. A HER2/neu test may be done on the biopsied breast tissue. HER2/neu is a growth-promoting hormone and in about 50% of breast cancers excessive amounts of the hormone are present, causing the cancer to be more aggressive in spreading than other types of breast cancer. Treatment can be more effective if HER2/neu testing is done (ACS, 2004).

Other tests to determine the spread of the cancer include chest x-ray examination, bone scan, computed tomography (CT), magnetic resonance imaging (MRI), and positron emission tomography (PET scan). Once the stage or spread of cancer is determined, treatment options can be identified.

Nodal involvement and tumor size are the most significant prognostic criteria for long-term survival. One factor that has been helpful in predicting response to therapy and survival is whether the tumor is estrogen- or progesterone-receptor positive or hormone-receptor (HR) positive. Women with HR-positive tumors tend to respond better to treatment and have higher survival rates (ACS, 2004).

Management

Controversy continues regarding the best treatment of breast cancer. The women is faced with difficult decisions about the various treatment options. Questions that must be addressed in decision making are listed in Box 5-7. Most health care providers recommend that the malignant mass be removed, as well as the axillary nodes for staging purposes (DiSaia & Creasman, 2002). The treatment can be

TABLE 5-5

Detection in Asymptomatic Women Recommended by the American Cancer Society

AGE (YR)	EXAMINATION	FREQUENCY
20-39	Breast self-examination (BSE)	Monthly
	Clinical breast examination	Every 3 yr
40 and older	BSE	Monthly
	Clinical breast examination	Yearly
	Mammography	Yearly

Source: American Cancer Society. (2005). *Cancer facts and figures, 2005.* New York: American Cancer Society.

Decision-Making Questions to Ask

1 What kind of breast cancer is it (invasive or noninvasive)?
2 What is the stage of the cancer (i.e., how extensive is the spread)?
3 Did the cancer test positive for hormone (estrogen)? (May be slower growing.)
4 What further tests are recommended?
5 What are the treatment options? (Pros and cons of each, including side effects.)
6 If surgery is recommended, what will the scar look like?
7 If a mastectomy is done, can breast reconstruction be done (at the time of surgery or later)?
8 How long will the patient be in the hospital? What kind of postoperative care will the patient need?
9 How long will treatment last if radiation or chemotherapy is recommended? What effects can the patient expect from these treatments?
10 What community resources are available for support?

Source: National Women's Health Resource Center. (1999). Breast health. *National Women's Health Report, 17*(5), 1-11.

conservative or more radical. The most frequently recommended surgical approaches for the treatment of breast cancer are lumpectomy and modified radical mastectomy. Breast-conserving surgery, such as a **lumpectomy** (Fig. 5-7, *A*) or quadrectomy (Fig 5-7, *B*) is the removal of the breast tumor and a small amount of surrounding tissue. Sampling of axillary lymph nodes is usually done through a separate incision at the time of these procedures, and the surgery is usually followed by radiation therapy to the remaining breast tissue (Crane-Okada, 2001; DiSaia & Creasman, 2002). These procedures are used for the primary treatment of women with early-stage (I or II) breast cancer. Lumpectomy offers survival equivalent to that with modified radical mastectomy (DiSaia & Creasman, 2002).

A **simple mastectomy** (Fig. 5-7, *C*) is the removal of the breast containing the tumor. A **modified radical mastectomy** is the removal of the breast tissue, skin, and fascia of the pectoralis muscle and dissection of the axillary nodes. A **radical mastectomy,** although rarely performed, is the removal of the breast and underlying pectoralis muscles and complete axillary node dissection (Fig. 5-7, *D*). After surgery, follow-up treatment may include radiation, chemotherapy,

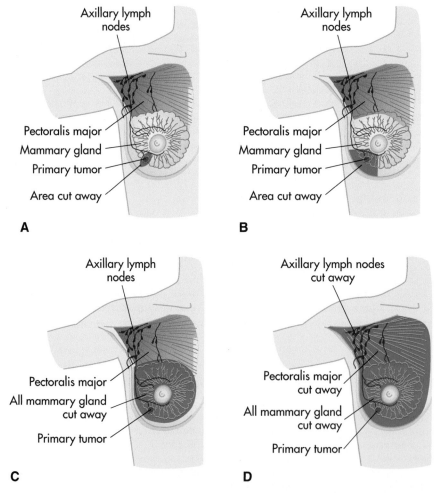

Fig. 5-7 Surgical alternatives for breast cancer. **A,** Lumpectomy (tylectomy). **B,** Quadrectomy (segmental resection). **C,** Total (simple) mastectomy. **D,** Radical mastectomy.

Medication Guide

Tamoxifen (Nolvadex)

ACTION

- Antiestrogenic effects; attaches to hormone receptors on cancer cells and prevents natural hormones from attaching to the receptors.

INDICATION

- For treatment of metastatic breast cancer; for treatment of breast cancer in postmenopausal women after breast cancer surgery and radiation therapy; to reduce the incidence of breast cancer in women at high risk.

DOSAGE

- 20 to 40 mg orally, daily. Doses greater than 20 mg should be given in divided doses (AM and PM).

ADVERSE REACTIONS

- Common side effects include hot flashes, nausea, vomiting, vaginal bleeding or discharge, menstrual irregularities, and rash. Hair loss is an uncommon effect. Serious side effects include deep vein thrombosis, increased risk of endometrial cancer, and stroke.

NURSING CONSIDERATIONS

- The medication may be taken on an empty stomach or with food. Missed doses should be taken as soon as possible, but taking two doses at once is not recommended. A barrier or nonhormonal form of contraception is recommended in premenopausal women because tamoxifen may be harmful to the fetus.

---

or hormonal therapy (ACS, 2004). The decision to include follow-up therapy is based on the stage of disease, age and menopausal status of the woman, the woman's preference, and her hormonal receptor status. Follow-up treatment is usually used to decrease the risk of recurrence in women who have no evidence of metastasis.

Radiation is usually recommended as follow-up therapy for women who have stage I or II cancer. Hormone therapy with tamoxifen, an estrogen agonist, is recommended for women over the age of 50 for at least 5 years (DiSaia & Creasman, 2002) (see Medication Guide). Chemotherapy is often given to premenopausal women who have positive nodes. Therapy for more advanced tumors usually includes surgery followed by chemotherapy, radiation, or both (Stenchever et al., 2001).

Surgery may be performed in an outpatient surgical setting or as an inpatient procedure, depending on what type of surgery is being done. Nursing care and teaching are

PATIENT INSTRUCTIONS FOR SELF-CARE

Mastectomy

- Wash hands well before and after touching incision area or drains.
- Empty surgical drains twice a day and as needed, recording the date, time, drain site (if more than one drain is present), and amount of drainage in milliliters in diary you will take to each surgical checkup until your drains are removed. (Before discharge, you may receive a graduated container for emptying drains and measuring drainage.)
- Avoid driving, lifting more than 10 pounds, or reaching above your head until given permission by surgeon.
- Take medications for pain as soon as pain begins.
- Perform arm exercises as directed.
- Call physician if inflammation of incision or swelling of the incision or the arm occurs.
- Avoid tight clothing, tight jewelry, and other causes of decreased circulation in the affected arm.
- Until drains are removed, wear loose-fitting underwear (camisole or half-slip) and clothes, pinning surgical drains inside of clothing. (You will be taught how to do this safely.)
- After drains are removed and surgical sites are healing and still tender, wear a mastectomy bra or camisole with a cotton-filled, muslin temporary prosthesis. Temporary prostheses of this type are often available from Reach to Recovery.
- Avoid depilatory creams, strong deodorants, and shaving of affected chest area, axilla, and arm.

- Sponge bathe until drains are removed.
- Return to the surgeon's office for incision check, drain inspection, and possible drain removal as directed.
- Contact Reach to Recovery for assistance in obtaining external prosthesis and lingerie when dressings, drains, and staples are removed and wound is healing and nontender.
- Contact insurance company for information about coverage of prosthesis and wig if needed. Obtain prescriptions for prosthesis and wig to submit with receipts of purchase for these items to the insurance company. If insurance does not pay for these items, contact hospital or agency social worker or local American Cancer Society for assistance.
- Continue with monthly breast self-examination (BSE) of unaffected side and affected surgical site and axilla.
- Encourage mother, sisters, and daughters (if applicable) to learn and practice monthly BSE and to have annual professional breast examinations and mammography (if appropriate).
- Keep follow-up visits for professional examination, mammography, and testing to detect recurrent breast cancer.
- Expect decreased sensation and tingling at incision sites and in the affected arm for weeks to months after surgery.
- Resume sexual activities as desired.

focused on the perioperative period. Preoperatively, women need to be assessed for psychologic preparation and specific teaching needs related to the procedure to be performed and what to expect after surgery. A visit from a woman who has had a similar experience may be beneficial preoperatively, as well as postoperatively.

Postoperative nursing care focuses on recovery. Women who had surgery in an outpatient setting usually go home within a few hours after surgery. A 24- to 48-hour stay is usual after modified radical mastectomy. Precautions should be taken to avoid taking the blood pressure, giving injections, or taking blood from the arm on the affected side. The woman may have drainage tubes from the incision site that will need to be assessed and drained. Incision care may include dressing changes. If postoperative arm exercises are appropriate, these may be initiated during the early postoperative period. The woman is usually discharged to home after being given self-care instructions. Since teaching time is short, providing printed information gives the woman and her family something to refer to at home (see Patient Instructions for Self-Care box).

Information about reconstruction surgery should be given before surgery, although not all women will be candidates for the procedure or are interested in it. Available options include grafts of muscle and skin from the woman's back, abdomen, or hip, and saline-filled prostheses (Resnick & Belcher, 2002). Use of silicone gel implants is restricted by the FDA to women in safety studies (Zuckerman, 2002).

Concerns about appearance after breast surgery may affect the woman's self-concept (Sammarco, 2001). Before surgery the woman and her partner need information about what the woman's postoperative appearance will be like. Both the woman and her partner need to be able to discuss feelings and concerns about accepting the changes. Nurses can assist the couple to communicate these feelings and concerns. Information about community resources and support groups such as Reach to Recovery may be beneficial (see Resources at end of the chapter).

COMMUNITY ACTIVITY

Investigate the resources in your community for one of the following situations. Your investigation should include where services are provided, ease of access, cost of services, information (e.g., pamphlets, newspaper, flyers) that advertises the services, appropriateness of information (e.g., age, culture, language). Evaluate whether the resources are adequate, and if not, suggest what is needed.

1 A 34-year-old African-American woman who has found a lump in her breast
2 A teenage girl who is sexually active at risk for STIs
3 A 25-year-old Latino woman (non-English speaking) who needs a Pap test

Key Points

- Menstrual disorders diminish the quality of life for affected women and their families.
- PMS is a disorder that begins in the luteal phase of the menstrual cycle and resolves with the onset of menses.
- PMS is a disorder with both psychologic and physiologic characteristics.
- Endometriosis is characterized by dysmenorrhea, infertility, and, less often, alterations in menstrual cycle bleeding and dyspareunia.
- Safer sex practices are key STI prevention strategies.
- HIV is transmitted through body fluids, primarily blood, semen, and vaginal secretions.
- HPV is the most common viral STI.
- Syphilis has reemerged as a common STI.
- Chlamydia is the most common cause of PID.
- Young sexually active women who do not practice safer sex behaviors and have multiple partners are at greatest risk for STIs and HIV.
- STIs are responsible for substantial morbidity and mortality, personal suffering, and a heavy economic burden in the United States.

- STIs and vaginitis are biologic events for which all individuals have a right to expect objective, compassionate, and effective health care.
- The development of breast neoplasms, whether benign or malignant, can have a significant physical and emotional effect on the woman and her family.
- The risk of U.S. women developing breast cancer is 1 in 8.
- An estimated 90% of all breast lumps are detected by women during monthly breast self-examination (BSE).
- Monthly BSE, yearly clinical breast examinations by a health care provider, and routine screening mammograms are recommended for early detection of breast cancer.
- The primary therapy for most women with stage I or II breast cancer is breast-conserving surgery with axillary lymph node sampling followed by radiation therapy.
- Tamoxifen is a common adjuvant therapy for breast cancers that are estrogen-receptor positive.

Answer Guidelines to Critical Thinking Exercise

Premenstrual Syndrome

1 No, there is not sufficient evidence for the nurse to draw conclusions and give advice to Joanna. The nurse needs more information regarding Joanna's menstrual cycle and when the symptoms occur. Joanna may have PMS or PDD or another cyclic perimenstrual problem. Even if Joanna's diagnosis is PMS, there is no agreement on the best management of PMS. However, there are strategies that might be effective for Joanna.

2 a. Most women use self-management interventions before seeking medical management for menstrual pain and discomforts. However, many women lack information they could use to adequately self-manage their symptoms. They may take subtherapeutic doses of effective medications or have misconceptions about their symptoms. Therefore nurses can educate women about potentially relevant treatments. These include over-the-counter NSAIDs, heat therapy, exercise, massage, acupressure, relaxation therapy, stress management, and nutritional counseling.

b. CPPD is a concept developed by AWHONN (see Collins Sharp et al., 2002). It encompasses the individual concepts of dysmenorrhea, PMS, and PDD as well as symptom clusters occurring during the time period both before and after the menstrual flow begins. The cyclic pain experience is usually coupled with other discomforts such as moodiness and irritability. The combination of pain and related discomforts increases the impact on the woman's functional status and quality of life. Although research is still needed on effectiveness of interventions for CPPD, AWHONN has developed a clinical guideline for practice that is based on the available research.

c. Quality-of-life issues for women with perimenstrual pain and discomforts include loss of work or school time because of symptoms, financial costs for seeking relief from symptoms, and increased stress because of strained relationships with family, friends, and co-workers or time demands of work or home. Emotional and life stressors may increase the severity of symptoms. Women need to be assessed for their perceptions of how their quality of life is affected. Nurses can then provide counseling and education about how to manage and change these stressors.

d. Coping enhancement is a strategy that nurses can use to help a patient adapt to perceived stressors that interfere with her ability to meet life and role expectations. Nursing care is directed at providing an accepting atmosphere and empowering the patient to be more aware and sensitive to her own needs. Self-monitoring of symptoms can promote self awareness and enhance the woman's coping abilities. For example, monitoring symptoms can prompt women to make changes that reduce the severity of symptoms.

3 The nurse needs to assess for pain and discomfort. AWHONN (Collins Sharp et al., 2002)] suggests using four questions: Do you have pelvic pain or cramps during or around the time of your period? Are you able to treat the pain so it doesn't bother you? Do you have other discomforts during or around the time of your period? Are you able to treat these discomforts so they don't bother you?

Based on this assessment, symptom management strategies can be planned. Joanna can be educated about pain management, coping enhancement, and self-help strategies (Collins Sharp et al., 2002). For example, she can quit smoking, take NSAIDS, use heat therapy, and/or use herbal remedies.

4 Because there is no agreement on management, many strategies could be suggested (Collins Sharp et al., 2002). Multiple strategies may be more effective than single treatment strategies. Some interventions have a strong research base for practice (e.g., NSAIDs) whereas others have a moderate base (e.g., heat therapy). However, interventions with only moderate or minimal science support may still be appropriate, but the science base is still in development. In suggesting management strategies, the nurse should look at the desired patient outcome, the research associated with the intervention, the acceptance of the intervention to Joanna, and the feasibility for implementing the intervention.

5 Yes, there are alternatives as identified in number 4. AWHONN suggests that if the nurse can identify more than four appropriate interventions, she or he should consider the strength of the evidence in making recommendations to women.

Resources

American Cancer Society
1599 Clifton Rd., NE
Atlanta, GA 30329
800-ACS-2345
www.cancer.org

American Social Health Association (ASHA)
P.O. Box 13827
Research Triangle Park, NC 27709
919-361-8400
www.ashastd.org

Association of Women's Health, Obstetric and Neonatal Nurses (AWHONN)
2000 L St., NW, Suite 740
Washington, DC 20036
800-673-8499 (United States)
800-245-0231 (Canada)
www.awhonn.org

Centers for Disease Control and Prevention
1600 Clifton Rd., NE
Atlanta, GA 30333
404-329-1819; 404-329-3286
www.cdc.gov

Endometriosis Association
8585 N. 76th Place
Milwaukee, WI 53223
414-355-2200
800-992-3636
www.ivf.com/endohtml.html

Endometriosis Research Center (ERC)
630 Ibis Dr.
Delray Beach, FL 33444
561-274-7442
www.endocenter.org

Food and Drug Administration (FDA)
Office of Consumer Affairs
Public Inquiries
5600 Fishers Ln. (HFE-88)
Rockville, MD 20857
301-443-3170
www.fda.gov

Hysterectomy Educational Resource and Services (HERS)
 Foundation
422 Bryn Mawr Ave.
Bala Cynwyd, PA 19004
1-888-750-HERS
www.hersfoundation.com

Myriad Genetics, Inc.
320 Wakara Way
Salt Lake City, UT 84108
800-469-7423
www.myriad.com

National AIDS Hotline
800-342-2437
800-344-7432 (Spanish)
800-243-7889 (hearing impaired)

National AIDS Information Clearing House
P.O. Box 6003
Rockville, MD 20850
800-458-5231

National Alliance of Breast Cancer Organizations
9 E. 37th St., 10th Floor
New York, NY 10016
800-719-0154
www.nabco.org

National Breast Cancer Coalition
P.O. Box 66373
Washington, DC 20035
202-296-7477
800-935-0434
www.natbec.org

National Cancer Institute Cancer Information Service
800-4-CANCER
www.nci.nih.gov

National Herpes Resource Center
www.ashastd.org/hrc
herpesnet@ashastd.org

National Women's Health Resource Center
120 Albany St., Suite 820
New Brunswick, NJ 08901
877-986-9472
www.healthywomen.org

Reach to Recovery *(breast cancer)*
(see American Cancer Society)

Resolve, Inc. *(impaired fertility)*
1310 Broadway, Dept. GM
Summerville, MA 02144-1713
617-623-0744
888-299-1585
www.resolve.org

Y-ME National Breast Cancer Organization
www.y-me.org

References

American Cancer Society (ACS). (2004). *Breast cancer.* Internet document available at http://www.cancer.org. (accessed September 19, 2004).

American Cancer Society (ACS). (2005). *Cancer facts and figures, 2005.* New York: ACS.

American College of Nurse-Midwives (ACNM). (2002). Abnormal and dysfunctional uterine bleeding. ACNM Clinical Bulletin No. 6. *Journal of Midwifery and Women's Health, 47*(3), 207-213.

American College of Obstetricians and Gynecologists (ACOG). (2000). *ACOG issues guidelines on diagnosis and treatment of PMS.* Internet document available at http://www.acog.org/from_home publication/press-release/nr03-31-00-1.html. (accessed September 1, 2004).

Bascom, A. (2002). *Incorporating herbal medicine into clinical practice.* Philadelphia: FA Davis.

Bolyard, E. et al. (1998). Guidelines for infection control in health care personnel, 1998. Hospital Infection Control Practices Advisory Committee. *Infection Control Hospital Epidemiology,19*(7), 493.

Centers for Disease Control and Prevention (CDC). (2001). Updated U.S. Public Health Service guidelines for the management of occupational exposures to HBV, HCV, and HIV and recommendations for postexposure prophylaxis. *Morbidity and Mortality Weekly Report, 50*(RR-11), 1-52.

Centers for Disease Control and Prevention (CDC). (2002a). Sexually transmitted diseases treatment guidelines 2002. *Morbidity and Mortality Weekly Report, 51*(RR-6), 1-82.

Centers for Disease Control and Prevention (CDC). (2002b). *STD Surveillance 2002: STDs in women and infants.* Internet document available at http://www.cdc.gov/std/stats/women&inf.htm (accessed August 24, 2004).

Centers for Disease Control and Prevention (CDC). (2003). Primary and secondary syphilis—United States, 2002. *Morbidity and Mortality Weekly Report, 52,* 1117-1120.

Centers for Disease Control and Prevention (CDC). (2004). *HIV/AIDS update: A glance at the HIV epidemic.* Internet document available at http://www.cdc.gov. (accessed August 24, 2004).

Centers for Disease Control and Prevention (CDC). (2005). *Genital HPV Infection-CDC Fact Sheet.* Internet document available at www.cdc.gov/std/HPV/STDfact-HPV.htm#common (accessed June 20, 2005).

Centers for Disease Control and Prevention, Divisions of HIV/AIDS Prevention. (2004). *Frequently asked questions about the OraQuick Rapid HIV-1 Antibody Test.* Internet document available at www.cdc.gov/hiv/PUBS/faq/oraqckfaq.htm (accessed August 24, 2004).

Clinical Pharmacology. (2004). Drugs used to treat dysmenorrhea. *Gold Standard Multimedia.* Internet document available at http://cp.gsm.com (accessed October 1, 2004).

Collins Sharp, B., Taylor, D., Thomas, K., Killeen, M., & Dawood, M. (2002). Cyclic perimenstrual pain and discomfort: The scientific basis for practice. *Journal of Obstetric, Gynecologic, and Neonatal Nursing, 31*(6), 637-649.

Conversations with Colleagues. (2002-2003). Endometriosis sufferers risk other diseases. *AWHONN Lifelines, 6*(6), 502-504.

Crane-Okada, R. (2001). Breast cancers. In S. Otto (Ed.), *Oncology nursing* (4th ed.). St. Louis: Mosby.

Cummings, S. (2001). Weighing the risks: Genetic counseling for hereditary breast and ovarian cancer. Perspective. *Cancer Nursing, 23*(4), 258-267.

DiSaia, P., & Creasman, W. (2002). *Clinical gynecologic oncology* (6th ed.). St. Louis: Mosby.

Dog, L. (2001). Conventional and alternative treatments for endometriosis. *Alternative Therapies, 7*(6), 50-56.

Elliot, H. (2002). Premenstrual dysphoric disorder. *North Carolina Medical Journal, 63*(2), 72-75.

Facts and Comparisons. (2002). *Loose-leaf drug information service.* St. Louis: Facts and Comparisons.

Fraley, S. (2002). Psychosocial outcomes in individuals living with genital herpes. *Journal of Obstetric, Gynecologic, and Neonatal Nursing, 31*(5), 508-513.

Friedenreich, C., Bryant, H., Alexander, F., Hugh, J., Danyluk, J., & Page, D. (2000). Risk factors for benign breast disease. *International Journal of Epidemiology, 29*(4), 637-644.

Friedman, A., & Carlson, K. (2002). Uterine fibroids. In K. Carlson, et al. (Ed.), *Primary care of women* (2nd ed.). St. Louis: Mosby.

Fugh-Berman, A., & Awang, D. (2001). Black cohosh. *Alternative Therapies in Women's Health, 39*(11), 81-85.

Furniss, K. (2000). Tomatoes, Pap smears and tea? Adopting behaviors that may prevent reproductive cancers and improve health. *Journal of Obstetric, Gynecologic, and Neonatal Nursing, 29*(6), 641-652.

Harlow, S. (2000). Menstruation and menstrual disorders. In M. Goldman & M. Hatch (Eds.), *Women and health.* San Diego: Academic Press.

Hatcher, R., Zienan, M., Cwiak, C., Darney, P., Creinin, M., & Stosur, H. (2004). *A pocket guide to managing contraception.* Tiger, GA: Bridging the Gap Foundation, 2004.

Jeavons, H. (2003). Prevention and treatment of vulvovaginal candidiasis using exogenous lactobacillus. *Journal of Obstetric, Gynecologic, and Neonatal Nursing, 32*(3), 287-296.

Jones, C. (2001). Premenstrual dysphoric disorder. *Advances for Nurse Practitioners,* (2001, March), 87-90.

Kleposki, R. (2002). The female athlete triad: A terrible trio implications for primary care. *Journal of the American Academy of Nurse Practitioners, 14*(10), 26-31.

Lemaire, G. (2004). More than just menstrual cramps: Symptoms and uncertainty among women with endometriosis. *Journal of Obstetric, Gynecologic, and Neonatal Nursing, 33*(10):71-79.

Leung, A., & Pacaud, D. (2004). Diagnosis and management of galactorrhea. *American Family Physician, 70*(3), 543-550.

Lin, J., & Thompson, D. (2001). Treating premenstrual dysphoric disorder using serotonin agents. *Journal of Women's Health & Gender-Based Medicine, 10*(6), 745-750.

Lucas, J., & Cone, D. (2003). Breast cyst aspiration. *American Family Physician, 68*(10), 1983-1986.

Motta, G. (2004). Teenage endometriosis. *Advance for Nurses Southwestern States, 6*(9):32-34.

Nakad, T., & Isaacson, K. (2002). Endometriosis. In K. Carlson et al. (Eds.), *Primary care of women* (2nd ed.). St. Louis: Mosby.

National Cancer Institute (NCI). (2002). Cancer facts: *Lifetime probability of breast cancer in American women.* Internet document available at http://cis.nci.nih.gov/fact/5_6.htm (accessed 9/30/05).

National Women's Health Resource Center. (1999). Breast health. *National Women's Health Report, 17*(5), 1-11.

National Women's Health Resource Center. (2000). Genetic testing and women's health. *National Women's Health Report, 22*(6), 1-8.

Nelson, N. (2000). Silicone breast implants not linked to breast cancer risk. *Journal of the National Cancer Institute, 92*(21), 1714-1715.

Parent-Stevens, L., & Burns, E. (2000). Menstrual disorders. In M. Smith & L. Shimp (Eds.), *20 Common problems in women's health care* (pp. 381-414). New York: McGraw-Hill.

Perese, E., & Perese, K. (2003). Health problems of women with severe mental illness. *Journal of the American Academy of Nurse Practitioners, 15*(5), 212-219.

Pritham, U. (2002). Managing PMS and PMDD. *AWHONN Lifelines, 6*(5), 431-437.

Proctor, M., Roberts, H., & Farquhar, C. (2001). Combined oral contraceptive pills (OCP) as treatment for primary dysmenorrhoea. *Cochrane Database of Systematic Reviews,* 2001, Issue 4, CD002120.

Proctor, M., Smith, C., Farquhar, C., & Stones, R. (2002). Transcutaneous electrical nerve stimulation and acupuncturefor primary dysmenorrhoea. *Cochrane Database of Systematic Reviews,* 2002, Issue 1, CD002123.

Rapkin, Q. (2003). A review of treatment of premenstrual syndrome and premenstrual dysphoric disorder. *Psychoneuroendocrinology, 28*(suppl 3), 39-53.

Rawlins, S. (2001). Nonviral sexually transmitted infections. *Journal of Obstetric, Gynecologic, and Neonatal Nursing, 30*(3), 324-331.

Resnick, B., & Belcher, A. (2002). Breast reconstruction. *American Journal of Nursing, 102*(4), 26-33.

Rossouw, J., et al. (2002). Risks and benefits of estrogen plus progestin in health postmenopausal women: Principal results from the Women's Health Initiative randomized controlled trial. *Journal of the American Medical Association, 288*(3), 321-333.

Sammarco, A. (2001). Perceived social support, uncertainty, and quality of life of younger breast cancer survivors. *Cancer Nursing, 24*(3), 212-218.

Sanborn, C., Horea, M., Siemers, B., & Dieringer, K. (2000). Disorders of eating and the female athlete triad. *Clinics in Sports Medicine, 19*(2), 199-213.

Schwebke, J. (2000). Bacterial vaginosis. *Current Infectious Disease Reports, 2*(1), 14-17.

Stenchever, M., Droegemueller, W., Herbst, A., & Mishell, D. (2001). *Comprehensive gynecology* (4th ed.). St. Louis: Mosby.

Stevinson, C., & Ernst, E. (2001). Complementary/alternative therapies for premenstrual syndrome: A systematic review of randomized controlled trials. *American Journal of Obstetrics and Gynecology, 185*(1), 227-235.

U.S. Food and Drug Administration (FDA). (2004). FDA approves first oral fluid based rapid HIV test kit. *News release,* March 26, 2004.

Wilkinson, D., Ramjee, G., Tholandi, M., & Rutherford, G. (2002). Nonoxynol-9 spermicide for prevention of vaginally acquired HIV and other sexually transmitted infections: Systematic review and meta-analysis of randomised controlled trials including more than 5000 women. *Lancet Infectious Diseases, 2*(10), 613-617.

Williams, A. (2003). Gynecologic care for women with HIV infection. *Journal of Obstetric, Gynecologic, and Neonatal Nursing, 32*(1), 87-93.

Wilson, M., & Murphy, P. (2001). Herbal and dietary therapies for primary and secondary dysmenorrhoea. *Cochrane Database of Systematic Reviews,* 2001, Issue 3, CD002124.

Workowski, K., Levine, W., & Wasserheit, J. (2002). U.S. Centers for Disease Control and Prevention guidelines for the treatment of sexually transmitted diseases: An opportunity to unify clinical and public health practice. *Annals of Internal Medicine, 137*(4), 255-262.

World Health Organization (WHO), Department of Reproductive Health and Research. (2000). *Improving access to quality care in family planning: Medical eligibility criteria for contraceptive use* (2nd ed.). Geneva: WHO.

Zuckerman, D. (2002). The breast cancer information gap. *RN, 65*(2), 39-41.

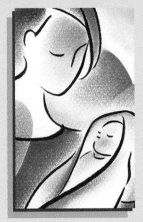

CHAPTER 6

Contraception, Abortion, and Infertility

DONNA ROWE ● DEITRA LEONARD LOWDERMILK

LEARNING OBJECTIVES

- *Compare the various methods of contraception.*
- *State the advantages and disadvantages of commonly used methods of contraception.*
- *Explain the common nursing interventions that facilitate contraceptive use.*
- *Recognize the various ethical, legal, cultural, and religious considerations of contraception.*
- *Describe the techniques used for medical and surgical interruption of pregnancy.*
- *Recognize the various ethical and legal considerations of elective abortion.*
- *List common causes of infertility.*
- *Discuss the psychologic impact of infertility.*
- *Identify common diagnoses and treatments for infertility.*
- *Examine the various ethical and legal considerations of assisted reproductive therapies for infertility.*

KEY TERMS AND DEFINITIONS

assisted reproductive therapies (ARTs) Treatments for infertility, including in vitro fertilization procedures, embryo adoption, embryo hosting, and therapeutic insemination

basal body temperature (BBT) Lowest body temperature of a healthy person taken immediately after awakening and before getting out of bed

fertility awareness methods (FAMs) Methods of family planning that identify the beginning and end of the fertile period of the menstrual cycle

induced abortion Intentionally produced termination of pregnancy

in vitro fertilization Fertilization in a culture dish or test tube

periodic abstinence Contraceptive methods in which a woman abstains from sexual intercourse during the fertile period of her menstrual cycle; also referred to as *natural family planning* (NFP) because no other form of birth control is used during this period

semen analysis Examination of semen specimen to determine liquefaction, volume, pH, sperm density, and normal morphology

sterilization Surgical contraceptive procedures intended to be permanent contraception

therapeutic donor insemination (TDI) Introduction of donor semen by instrument injection into the vagina or uterus for impregnation

ELECTRONIC RESOURCES

Additional information related to the content in Chapter 6 can be found on

the companion website at **evolve**
http://evolve.elsevier.com/Lowdermilk/Maternity/
- NCLEX Review Questions
- WebLinks

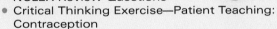
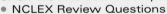

or on the interactive companion CD
- NCLEX Review Questions
- Critical Thinking Exercise—Patient Teaching: Contraception
- Plan of Care—Infertility

The reproductive spectrum is the focus of this chapter, covering voluntary control of fertility, interruption of pregnancy, and impaired fertility. The nursing role in the care of women varies, depending on whether management of these fertility-related concerns is associated with assessment of needs, investigation of problems, or implementation of interventions.

CONTRACEPTION

Contraception is the intentional prevention of pregnancy during sexual intercourse. Birth control is the device and/or practice to decrease the risk of conceiving, or bearing, offspring. Family planning is the conscious decision on when to conceive, or avoid pregnancy, throughout the reproductive years. With the wide assortment of birth control options available, it is possible for a woman to use several different contraceptive methods at various stages throughout her fertile years. Nurses interact with the woman to compare and contrast available options, reliability, relative cost, protection from sexually transmitted infections (STIs), the individual's comfort level, and partner's willingness to use a particular birth control method. Those who use contraception may still be at risk for pregnancy simply because their choice of contraceptive method is not perfect or is used inconsistently and/or incorrectly. Providing adequate instruction about how to use a contraceptive method, when to use a backup method, and when to use emergency contraception could decrease the risk of an unintended pregnancy (Stewart, Trussell, & Van Look, 2004).

Critical Thinking Exercise

Contraception

Arleta is a 25-year-old African-American woman who has three children ages 5 years, 3 years, and 18 months. She is at the family planning clinic today because she wants a new form of birth control. She says she has used condoms and foams and birth control pills and had contraceptive failures with both methods. She says she really does not want to get pregnant now but she doesn't want to have to deal with birth control every time she has sex. What advice should the nurse give Arleta?

1 Evidence—Is there sufficient evidence to draw conclusions about what response the nurse should give?
2 Assumptions—What are the underlying assumptions about the following issues:
  a. Personal considerations for choosing a birth control method
  b. Efficacy of methods of birth control
  c. Education for informed consent
3 What implications and priorities for nursing care can be drawn at this time?
4 Does the evidence objectively support your conclusion?
5 Are there alternative perspectives to your conclusion?

CARE MANAGEMENT

Family, friends, media, partner(s), religious affiliation, and health care professionals all influence a woman's perception of contraceptive choices. Because of these external influences, a woman formulates her unique view. The nurse assists in supporting the woman's decision which is based on the woman's individual situation.

Assessment and Nursing Diagnoses

The woman's knowledge about contraception and her sexual partner's commitment to any particular method are determined. Data are required about the frequency of coitus, the number of sexual partners, the level of contraceptive involvement, and her or his partner's objections to any methods (see Guidelines/Guías box). The woman's level of comfort and willingness to touch her genitals and cervical mucus are assessed. Myths are identified, and religious and cultural factors are determined. The woman's verbal and nonverbal responses to hearing about the various available methods are carefully

GUIDELINES/GUÍAS

Contraception

- Do you plan to have more children?
- *¿Piensa tener más hijos?*

- Are you sexually active?
- *¿Tiene relaciones sexuales?*

- Do you have many partners?
- *¿Tiene muchas parejas sexuales?*

- Have you had many partners in the past?
- *¿Ha tenido muchas parejas sexuales en el pasado?*

- Do you presently use contraception or birth control?
- *¿Usa anticonceptivos/control de natalidad actualmente?*

- The Pill? Condoms? The diaphragm? The IUD?
- *¿La píldora anticonceptiva? ¿Los condones (preservativos)? ¿El diafragma? ¿El dispositivo intrauterino (DIU)?*

- Spermicides? The rhythm method? Injection (Depo-Provera)?
- *¿Los espermaticidas? ¿El método del ritmo? ¿La inyección (Depo-Provera)?*

- How long have you used this method?
- *¿Por cuánto tiempo ha usado este método?*

- Do you like this method?
- *¿Le gusta este método?*

- Why did you stop using it?
- *¿Por qué dejó de usarlo?*

- Do you want to change to a different method?
- *¿Quiere cambiar a otro método?*

- Have you had a tubal ligation?
- *¿Ha tenido una ligadura de trompas?*

- Has he had a vasectomy?
- *¿Tuvo él una vasectomía?*

noted. An individual's reproductive life plan must be considered. A history (including menstrual, contraceptive, and obstetric), physical examination (including pelvic examination), and laboratory tests are usually completed.

Informed consent is a vital component in the education of the patient concerning contraception or sterilization. The nurse has the responsibility of documenting information provided and the understanding of that information by the patient. Using the acronym *BRAIDED* may be useful (see Legal Tip).

CD: Critical Thinking Exercise—Patient Teaching: Contraception

---

LEGAL TIP **Informed Consent**

B — *Benefits: information about advantages and success rates*

R — *Risks: information about disadvantages and failure rates*

A — *Alternatives: information about other available methods*

I — *Inquiries: opportunity to ask questions*

D — *Decisions: opportunity to decide or to change mind*

E — *Explanations: information about method and how it is used*

D — *Documentation: information given and patient's understanding*

Nursing diagnoses reflect analysis of the assessment findings. Examples of nursing diagnoses that may emerge regarding contraception include those listed.

- *Decisional conflict related to*
  - –contraceptive alternatives
  - –partner's willingness to agree on contraceptive method
- *Fear related to*
  - –contraceptive method side effects
- *Risk for infection related to*
  - –unprotected sexual intercourse
  - –use of contraceptive method
  - –broken skin or mucous membrane after surgery or intrauterine device (IUD) insertion
- *Ineffective sexuality patterns related to*
  - –fear of pregnancy
- *Acute pain related to*
  - –postoperative recovery after sterilization
- *Risk for spiritual distress related to*
  - –discrepancy between religious or cultural beliefs and choice of contraception

Expected Outcomes of Care

Planning is a collaborative effort among the woman, her sexual partner (when appropriate), the primary health care provider, and the nurse. The expected outcomes are determined and stated in patient-centered terms and may include that the woman or couple will do the following:

- Verbalize understanding about contraceptive methods
- Verbalize understanding of all information necessary to give informed consent

- State comfort and satisfaction with the chosen method
- Use the contraceptive method correctly and consistently
- Experience no adverse sequelae as a result of the chosen method of contraception
- Prevent unplanned pregnancy or plan a pregnancy

Plan of Care and Interventions

To foster a safe environment for consultation, a private setting should be provided in which the patient can openly interact. Distractions should be minimized, and samples of birth control devices for interactive teaching should be available (Fig. 6-1). The ideal contraceptive should be safe, easily available, economical, acceptable, simple to use, and promptly reversible. Although no method may ever achieve all these objectives, significant advances in the development of new contraceptive technologies have occurred over the past 30 years (World Health Organization [WHO], 2004).

Contraceptive failure rate refers to the percentage of contraceptive users expected to have an accidental pregnancy during the first year, even when they use a method consistently and correctly. Contraceptive effectiveness varies from couple to couple and depends on both the properties of the method and the characteristics of the user (WHO, 2004). Failure rates decrease over time, either because a user gains experience by using a method more appropriately or because those for whom a method is less effective stop using it.

NURSE ALERT *A backup method of birth control and emergency contraceptive pills (ECPs) should be readily available during the initial learning phase when a woman uses a new method of contraception to help avoid an unintentional conception.*

Safety of a method depends on the woman's medical history. Barrier methods offer some protection from STIs, and oral contraceptives may reduce the incidence of breast, ovarian, and endometrial cancer but increase the risk of thromboembolic problems.

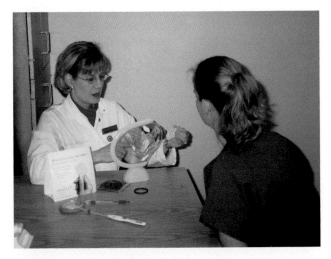

Fig. 6-1 Nurse counseling woman about contraceptive methods. (Courtesy Dee Lowdermilk, Chapel Hill, NC.)

Methods of Contraception

The following discussion of contraceptive methods provides the nurse with information needed for patient teaching. After implementing the appropriate teaching for contraceptive use, the nurse supervises return demonstrations to assess patient understanding. The woman is given written instructions and telephone numbers for questions. If the woman has difficulty understanding written instructions, she (and her partner, if available) is offered graphic material and a telephone number to call as necessary. She may also be offered an opportunity to return for further instruction.

Coitus interruptus

Coitus interruptus (withdrawal or "pulling out") involves the male partner withdrawing the entire penis from the woman's vagina and moving away from her external genitalia before he ejaculates. In theory, the spermatozoa are unlikely to reach the ovum to cause fertilization. Although the effectiveness of coitus interruptus depends mostly on the man's disciplined capability to consistently ignore the powerful urge to continue thrusting, it has some concrete advantages over using no method. Adolescents and men with premature ejaculation may find this method difficult to use. This method is immediately available, costs nothing, and involves no hormonal alterations or chemicals; the effectiveness of this birth control technique is similar to that of barrier methods (Kowal, 2004). The percentage of women who will experience an unintended pregnancy within the first year of typical use (failure rate) of withdrawal is about 27% (Trussell, 2004). Some religions and cultures prohibit this technique. Coitus interruptus does not adequately protect against STIs or human immunodeficiency virus (HIV) infection.

Fertility awareness methods

Fertility awareness methods (FAMs) of contraception depend on identifying the beginning and end of the fertile period of the menstrual cycle. When women who want to use FAMs are educated about the menstrual cycle, three phases are identified:

1. Infertile phase: before ovulation
2. Fertile phase: about 5 to 7 days around the middle of the cycle, including several days before, during, and the day after ovulation
3. Infertile phase: after ovulation

Although ovulation can be unpredictable in many women, teaching the woman about how she can directly observe her fertility patterns is an empowering tool. There are nearly a dozen categories of FAMs. Each one uses a combination of charts, records, calculations, tools, observations, and either abstinence (natural family planning) or barrier methods of birth control during the fertile period in the menstrual cycle to prevent pregnancy (Jennings, Arevalo, & Kowal, 2004). The charts and calculations associated with these methods can also be used to increase the likelihood of detecting the optimal timing of intercourse to achieve conception.

BOX 6-1

Potential Pitfalls of Using Fertility Awareness Methods of Contraception

Potential pitfalls of using fertility awareness methods include the five Rs:
- **R**estriction on sexual spontaneity
- **R**igorous daily monitoring
- **R**equired training
- **R**isk of pregnancy during prolonged training period
- **R**isk of pregnancy high on unsafe days

Source: Hatcher, R. et al. (2004). *A pocket guide to managing contraception.* Tiger, GA: Bridging the Gap Foundation.

Advantages of these methods include low to no cost, absence of chemicals and hormones, and lack of alteration in the menstrual flow pattern. Disadvantages of FAM include adherence to strict record-keeping, unintentional interference from external influences that may alter the woman's core body temperature and vaginal secretions, decreased effectiveness in women with irregular cycles (particularly adolescents who have not established regular ovulatory patterns), decreased spontaneity of coitus, and attending possibly time-consuming training sessions by qualified instructors (Jennings, Arevalo, & Kowal, 2004) (Box 6-1). The typical failure rate for most FAMs is 25% during the first year of use (Trussell, 2004). FAMs do not protect against STIs or HIV infection.

FAMs involve several techniques to identify high risk fertile days. The following discussion includes the most common techniques as well as some promising techniques for the future.

Periodic abstinence. Periodic abstinence, or natural family planning (NFP), provides contraception by using methods that rely on avoidance of intercourse during fertile periods. NFP methods are the only contraceptive practices acceptable to the Roman Catholic Church. Fertility awareness is the combination of charting signs and symptoms of the menstrual cycle with the use of abstinence during fertile periods. Signs and symptoms most commonly used are menstrual bleeding, cervical mucus, and basal body temperature (see later discussions) (Jennings, Arevalo, & Kowal, 2004).

The human ovum can be fertilized no later than 16 to 24 hours after ovulation. Motile sperm have been recovered from the uterus and the oviducts as long as 60 hours after coitus. However, their ability to fertilize the ovum probably lasts no longer than 24 to 48 hours. Pregnancy is unlikely to occur if a couple abstains from intercourse for 4 days before and for 3 or 4 days after ovulation (fertile period). Unprotected intercourse on the other days of the cycle (safe period) should not result in pregnancy. However, there are two principal problems with this method: the exact time of ovulation cannot be predicted accurately, and couples may find it difficult to exercise restraint for several days before and after ovulation. Women with irregular menstrual periods have the greatest risk of failure with this form of contraception. The typical failure rate is 25% during the first year of use.

Calendar rhythm method. Practice of the calendar rhythm method is based on the number of days in each cycle counting from the first day of menses. With this method the fertile period is determined after accurately recording the lengths of menstrual cycles for 6 months. The beginning of the fertile period is estimated by subtracting 18 days from the length of the shortest cycle. The end of the fertile period is determined by subtracting 11 days from the length of the longest cycle (Jennings, Arevalo, & Kowal, 2004). If the shortest cycle is 24 days and longest is 30 days, application of the formula is as follows:

Shortest cycle: 24 − 18 = sixth day
Longest cycle: 30 − 11 = nineteenth day

To avoid conception the couple would abstain during the fertile period–days 6 through 19. If the woman has very regular cycles of 28 days each, the formula indicates the fertile days to be as follows:

Shortest cycle: 28 − 18 = tenth day
Longest cycle: 28 − 11 = seventeenth day

To avoid pregnancy, the couple abstains from day 10 through 17 because ovulation occurs on day 14 plus or minus 2 days.

Standard days method. The Standard Days Method (SDM) is essentially a modified form of the calendar rhythm method that has a "fixed" number of days of fertility for each cycle–that is, days 8 to 19 (Institute of Reproductive Health, 2003). A CycleBeads necklace–a color-coded string of beads–can be purchased as a concrete tool to track fertility (Fig. 6-2). Day 1 of the menstrual flow is counted as the first day to begin the counting. Women who use this device are taught to avoid unprotected intercourse on days 8 to 19 (white beads on CycleBeads necklace). Although this method is useful to women whose cycles are 26 to 32 days long, it is unreliable to those who have longer or shorter cycles (CycleBeads, 2003). The typical failure rate for the SDM is 12% during the first year of use (Sinai, Jennings, and Arevalo, 2004).

Ovulation method. The cervical mucus ovulation-detection method (also called the Billings method and the Creighton model ovulation method) requires that the woman recognize and interpret the cyclic changes in the amount and consistency of cervical mucus that characterize her own unique pattern of changes (see Patient Instructions for Self-Care box). The cervical mucus that accompanies ovulation is necessary for viability and motility of sperm. It alters the pH environment, neutralizing the acidity, to be more compatible for sperm survival. Without adequate cervical mucus, coitus does not result in conception. Women check quantity and character of mucus on the vulva or introitus with fingers or tissue paper each day for several months to learn cycle. To ensure an accurate assessment of changes, the cervical mucus should be free from semen, contraceptive gels or foams, and blood or discharge from vaginal infections for at least one full cycle. Other factors that create difficulty in identifying mucus changes include douches and vaginal deodorants, being in the sexually aroused state (which thins the mucus), and taking medications such as antihistamines (which dry up the mucus). Intercourse is considered safe without restriction beginning the fourth day after the last day of wet, clear, slippery mucus (postovulation) (Hatcher et al., 2004).

Some women may find this method unacceptable if they are uncomfortable touching their genitals. Whether or not the individual wants to use this method for contraception, it is to the woman's advantage to learn to recognize mucus characteristics at ovulation (Barron & Daly, 2001).

Basal body temperature method. The basal body temperature (BBT) is the lowest body temperature of a healthy person, taken immediately after waking and before getting out of bed. The BBT usually varies from 36.2° C to 36.3° C during menses and for about 5 to 7 days afterward (Fig. 6-3). At about the time of ovulation, a slight decrease in temperature (approximately 0.05° C) may occur in some women, but others may have no decrease at all. After ovulation, in concert with the increasing progesterone levels of the early luteal phase of the cycle, the BBT increases slightly (approximately 0.4° C to 0.8° C). The temperature remains on an elevated plateau until 2 to 4 days before menstruation, and then it decreases to the low levels recorded during the previous cycle, unless pregnancy has occurred, and the temperature remains elevated. If ovulation fails to occur, the pattern of lower body temperature continues throughout the cycle.

To use this method, the fertile period is defined as the day of first temperature drop, or first elevation through 3 consecutive days of elevated temperature. Abstinence begins the

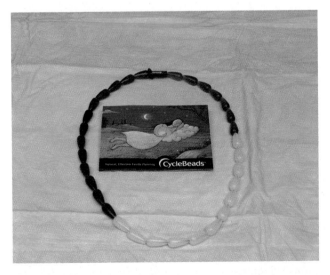

Fig. 6-2 Cyclebeads. Red bead marks the first day of the menstrual cycle. White beads mark days that are likely to be fertile days; therefore unprotected intercourse should be avoided. Brown beads are days when pregnancy is unlikely and unprotected intercourse is permitted. (Courtesy Dee Lowdermilk, Chapel Hill, NC.)

PATIENT INSTRUCTIONS FOR SELF-CARE
Cervical Mucus Characteristics

SETTING THE STAGE

- Show charts of menstrual cycle along with changes in the cervical mucus.
- Have woman practice with raw egg white.
- Supply her with a basal body temperature (BBT) log and graph if she does not already have one.
- Explain that assessment of cervical mucus characteristics is best when mucus is not mixed with semen, contraceptive jellies or foams, or discharge from infections. Douching should not be done before assessment.

CONTENT RELATED TO CERVICAL MUCUS

- Explain to woman (couple) how cervical mucus changes throughout the menstrual cycle.
  a. Postmenstrual mucus: scant.
  b. Preovulation mucus: cloudy, yellow or white, sticky
  c. Ovulation mucus: clear, wet, sticky, slippery
  d. Postovulation fertile mucus: thick, cloudy, sticky
  e. Postovulation, postfertile mucus: scant

- Right before ovulation, the watery, thin, clear mucus becomes more abundant and thick (Fig. A). It feels like a lubricant and can be stretched 5+ cm between the thumb and forefinger; this is called *spinnbarkeit* (Fig. B). This indicates the period of maximal fertility. Sperm deposited in this type of mucus can survive until ovulation occurs.

ASSESSMENT TECHNIQUE

- Stress that good handwashing is imperative to begin and end all self-assessment.
- Start observation from last day of menstrual flow.
- Assess cervical mucus several times a day for several cycles. Mucus can be obtained from vaginal introitus; no need to reach into vagina to cervix.
- Record findings on the same record on which BBT is entered.

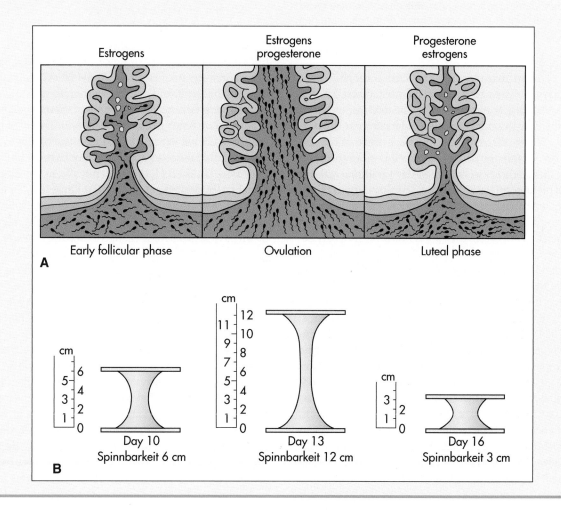

Estrogens | Estrogens progesterone | Progesterone estrogens

Early follicular phase | Ovulation | Luteal phase

A

Day 10 Spinnbarkeit 6 cm | Day 13 Spinnbarkeit 12 cm | Day 16 Spinnbarkeit 3 cm

B

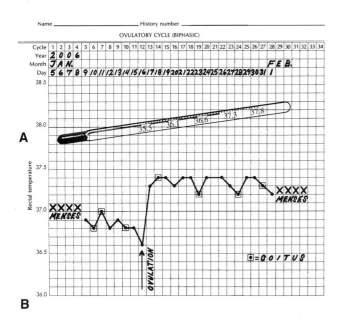

Fig. 6-3 **A,** Special thermometer for recording basal body temperature, marked in tenths to enable person to read more easily. **B,** Basal temperature record shows drop and sharp rise at time of ovulation. Biphasic curve indicates ovulatory cycle.

first day of menstrual bleeding and lasts through 3 consecutive days of sustained temperature rise (at least 0.2° C). (Jennings, Arevalo, & Kowal, 2004). The decrease and subsequent increase in temperature are referred to as the *thermal shift.* When the entire month's temperatures are recorded on a graph, the pattern described is more apparent. It is more difficult to perceive day-to-day variations without the entire picture. Infection, fatigue, less than 3 hours sleep per night, awakening late, and anxiety may cause temperature fluctuations, altering the expected pattern. If a new BBT thermometer is purchased, this fact is noted on the chart because the readings may vary slightly. Jet lag, alcohol and antipyretic medications taken the evening before, or sleeping in a heated waterbed also must be noted on the chart because each affects the BBT. Therefore the BBT alone is not a reliable method of predicting ovulation (Jennings, Arevalo, & Kowal, 2004). To determine whether an increase in temperature is indeed the thermal shift, the woman must be aware of other signs of approaching ovulation while she continues to assess the BBT (see later discussion of symptothermal method for other indicators of ovulation).

Postovulation method. The postovulation method permits unprotected intercourse only after signs of ovulation (BBT, cervical mucus alterations, etc) have subsided. If a woman experiences an anovulatory cycle, this demands great self-control, as complete abstinence is the only way to assure that pregnancy will not occur. This method is difficult for those in early adolescence, when the woman approaches menopause, and in postpartum women when cycles are irregular (or absent). The typical failure rate for the postovulation method is 25% during the first year of use (Trussell, 2004).

Symptothermal method. The symptothermal method is a tool that the woman learns to gain fertility awareness as she tracks the physiologic and psychologic symptoms that mark the phases of her cycle. This method combines at least two methods, usually cervical mucus changes with BBT, in addition to heightened awareness of secondary, cycle phase-related symptoms. Secondary symptoms may include increased libido, midcycle spotting, mittelschmerz, pelvic fullness or tenderness, and vulvar fullness. The woman is taught to palpate her cervix to assess for changes in texture, position, and dilation, which indicate ovulation. During the preovulatory and ovulatory periods, the cervix softens, opens, rises in the vagina, and is more moist. During the postovulatory period the cervix drops, becomes firm, and closes. The woman notes days on which coitus, changes in routine, illness, and so on have occurred (Fig. 6-4). Calendar calculations and cervical mucus changes are used to estimate the onset of the fertile period; changes in cervical mucus or the BBT are used to estimate its end.

Home predictor test kits for ovulation

All of the preceding methods discussed are indicative of but do not prove the occurrence and exact timing of ovulation. The urine predictor test for ovulation is a major addition to the NFP and fertility-awareness methods to help women who want to plan the time of their pregnancies and those who are trying to conceive (Fig. 6-5). The urine predictor test for ovulation detects the sudden surge of luteinizing hormone (LH) that occurs approximately 12 to 24 hours before ovulation. Unlike BBT, the test is not affected by illness, emotional upset, or physical activity. For home use, a test kit contains sufficient material for several days of testing during each cycle. A positive response indicative of an LH surge is noted by an easy-to-read color change. Directions for use of urine predictor test kits vary with the manufacturer. Saliva predictor tests for ovulation use dried, nonfoamy saliva as a tool to show fertility patterns. More research is needed to determine the efficacy of use of these tests for pregnancy prevention.

The Marquette Model (MM) is a natural family planning method that was developed through the Marquette University College of Nursing Institute for Natural Family Planning. The MM uses cervical monitoring along with the ClearPlan Easy Fertility Monitor. The ClearPlan Monitor is a handheld device that uses test strips to measure urinary metabolites of estrogen and LH. The monitor provides the user with "Low," "High," and "Peak" fertility readings. The MM incorporates the use of the monitor as an aid to learning NFP and fertility awareness. The MM is currently being tested at different sites in the United States for its effectiveness in helping couples avoid pregnancy (Institute for Natural Family Planning Services, 2005).

TwoDay method of family planning. Based on monitoring and the recording of cervical secretions, a new algorithm for identifying the fertile window has been developed by the Institute for Reproductive Health, Georgetown

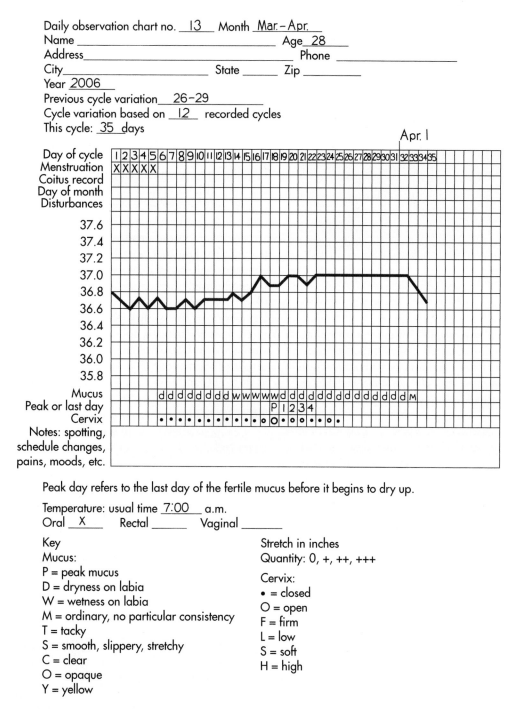

Daily observation chart no. __13__ Month _Mar.-Apr._
Name _____ Age_28_
Address_____ Phone _____
City_____ State _____ Zip _____
Year _2006_
Previous cycle variation__26-29_____
Cycle variation based on _12_ recorded cycles
This cycle: _35_ days

Fig. 6-4 Example of a completed symptothermal chart.

Peak day refers to the last day of the fertile mucus before it begins to dry up.

Temperature: usual time _7:00_ a.m.
Oral _X_   Rectal _____   Vaginal _____

Key
Mucus:
P = peak mucus
D = dryness on labia
W = wetness on labia
M = ordinary, no particular consistency
T = tacky
S = smooth, slippery, stretchy
C = clear
O = opaque
Y = yellow

Stretch in inches
Quantity: 0, +, ++, +++

Cervix:
• = closed
O = open
F = firm
L = low
S = soft
H = high

University (Arevalo, Jennings, Nikula, & Sinai, 2004). The TwoDay Algorithm appears to be simpler to teach, learn, and use than current natural methods. Results suggest that the algorithm can be an effective alternative for low literacy populations or for programs that find current Natural Family Planning methods too time consuming or otherwise not feasible to incorporate into their services. Two questions are posed. Each day, the woman is to ask herself, (1) "Did I note secretions today?" and (2) "Did I note secretions yesterday?" If the answer is yes to either question, she should avoid coitus or use a backup method of birth control. If the answer is no to both questions, her probability of getting pregnant is very low. Further studies are needed to determine the efficacy of the TwoDay Algorithm in avoiding pregnancy and to assess its acceptability to users and providers.

Barrier methods

Barrier contraceptives have gained in popularity not only as a contraceptive method but also as a protective measure against the spread of STI, such as human papilloma virus

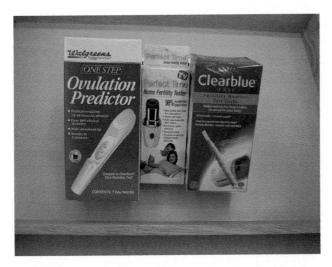

Fig. 6-5 Examples of ovulation prediction tests. (Courtesy Shannon Perry, Phoenix, AZ.)

(HPV) and herpes simplex virus (HSV). Some male condoms and female vaginal methods provide a physical barrier to several STIs, and some male condoms provide protection against HIV (Cates & Stewart, 2004; Warner, Hatcher, & Steiner, 2004). Spermicides serve as chemical barriers against the sperm.

Spermicides. Spermicides, such as nonoxynol-9, work by reducing the sperm's mobility, as the chemicals attack the sperm flagella and body, thereby preventing the sperm from reaching the cervical os. Nonoxynol-9, the most commonly used spermicidal chemical in the United States, is a surfactant that destroys the sperm cell membrane; however, recent data suggest that frequent use (more than two times a day) of nonoxynol-9, or use as a lubricant during anal intercourse, may increase the transmission of HIV and can cause lesions. (Cates & Raymond, 2004). Women with high risk behaviors that increase their likelihood of contracting HIV and other STIs are advised to avoid the use of spermicidal products containing nonoxynol-9, including those lubricated condoms, diaphragms, and cervical caps to which nonoxynol-9 is added (WHO, 2004). Intravaginal spermicides are marketed and sold without a prescription as foams, tablets, suppositories, creams, films, and gels (Fig. 6-6). Preloaded, single-dose applicators small enough to be carried in a small purse are available. Effectiveness of spermicides depends on consistent and accurate use. Caution patients against misunderstanding terms: contraceptive gel differs from fruit jelly, and cosmetics or hair products containing the nonspermicidal forms of nonoxynol are not adequate substitutes. The spermicide should be inserted high into the vagina so that it makes contact with the cervix. Some spermicide should be inserted at least 15 minutes before, and no longer than 1 hour before, sexual intercourse. Spermicide needs to be reapplied for each additional act of intercourse, even if a barrier method is used. Studies have shown varying effectiveness rates for spermicidal use alone. Typical failure rates for spermicide use alone range between 20% and 50% (U.S. Food and Drug Administration [FDA], 2003).

Condoms. The male condom is a thin, stretchable sheath that covers the penis before genital, oral, or anal contact and is removed after the penis is withdrawn from the partner's orifice after ejaculation (Fig. 6-7, *A*). When condoms are used as a primary contraceptive, it is helpful to have ECPs available, as couples may experience condom breakage or slippage in 3% to 5% of acts of coitus (Hatcher et al., 2004). Condoms are made of latex rubber, polyurethane (strong, thin plastic), or natural membranes (animal tissue). In addition to providing a physical barrier for sperm, nonspermicidal latex condoms also provide a barrier for STIs (particularly gonorrhea, chlamydia, and trichomonas) and HIV transmission. Condoms lubricated with nonoxynol-9 are no longer recommended for preventing STIs or HIV (Centers for Disease Control and Prevention, 2002). Latex condoms will break down with oil-based lubricants and should be used only with water-based or silicone lubricants (Warner, Hatcher, & Steiner, 2004). Because of the growing number of people with latex allergies, condom manufacturers have begun using polyurethane, which is thinner and stronger than latex. Research is being conducted to determine the effectiveness of polyurethane condoms to protect against STIs and HIV.

NURSE ALERT *All persons should be questioned about the potential for latex allergy. Latex condom use is contraindicated for people with latex sensitivity.*

A small percentage of condoms are made from the lamb cecum (natural skin). Natural skin condoms do not provide the same protection against STIs and HIV infection as latex condoms. Natural skin condoms contain small pores that could allow passage of viruses such as hepatitis B, HSV, and HIV. Condoms need to be discarded after each single use. They are available without a prescription.

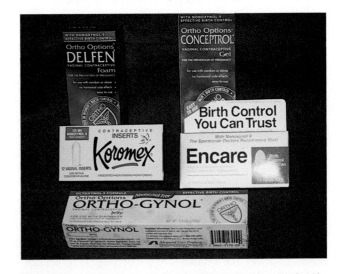

Fig. 6-6 Spermicides. (Courtesy Marjorie Pyle, RNC, Lifecircle, Costa Mesa, CA.)

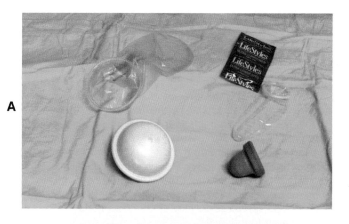

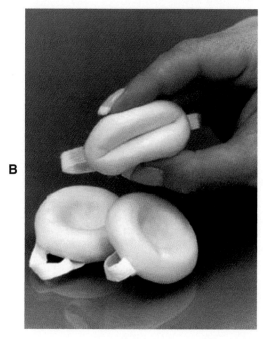

Fig. 6-7 **A,** Mechanical barriers. From the top left corner clockwise: female condom, male condom, cervical cap, diaphragm. (Courtesy Dee Lowdermilk, Chapel Hill, NC.) **B,** Contraceptive sponge. (Courtesy Allendale Pharmaceuticals, Inc., Allendale, NJ.)

A functional difference in condom shape is the presence or absence of a sperm-reservoir tip (see Fig. 6-7, *A*). To enhance vaginal stimulation, some condoms are contoured and rippled or have ribbed or roughened surfaces. Thinner construction increases heat transmission and sensitivity; a variety of colors and flavors increase condoms' acceptability and attractiveness (Hatcher et al., 2004). A wet jelly or dry powder lubricates some condoms. Typical failure rate in the first year of male condom use is 15% (Trussell, 2004). To prevent unintended pregnancy and the spread of STIs, it is essential that condoms be used consistently and correctly. Instructions, such as those listed in Box 6-2, can be used for patient teaching.

The female condom is a lubricated vaginal sheath made of polyurethane and has flexible rings at both ends (see Fig. 6-7, *A*). The closed end of the pouch is inserted into the vagina and is anchored around the cervix, and the open ring covers the labia. Women whose partner will not wear a male condom can use this as a protective mechanical barrier. Rewetting drops or oil- or water-based lubricants can be used to help decrease the distracting noise that is produced while penile thrusting occurs. The female condom is available in one size, intended for single use only, and is sold over the counter. Male condoms should not be used concurrently, because the friction from both sheaths can increase the likelihood of either or both tearing (Female Condom, 2004). Typical failure rate in the first year of female condom use is 21% (Trussell, 2004).

Diaphragms, cervical caps, shields, and sponges. Diaphragms, cervical caps, and shields are soft latex or silicone barriers that cover the cervix and prevent the sperm from migrating to fertilize the ovum. They are washable and reusable and need inspection for holes, tears, or other problems before each use. Each needs to be filled with spermicidal jelly or cream before vaginal insertion. These mechanical barriers are nonhormonal but still require a prescription from a licensed health care provider. It is essential the patient undergo proper fitting of the device. Women who choose to use these methods need to be willing to touch their genitalia and be capable of providing accurate return demonstrations of proper insertion and removal techniques.

Diaphragms. The contraceptive diaphragm is a shallow, dome-shaped latex or silicone device with a flexible rim that covers the cervix (see Fig. 6-7, *A*). There are three types of diaphragms available: coil spring, arcing spring, and wide seal rim. Available in many sizes, the diaphragm should be the largest size the woman can wear without her being aware of its presence. Typical failure rate of the diaphragm combined with spermicide is 16% in the first year of use (Trussell, 2004). Effectiveness of the diaphragm is less when used without spermicide (Trussell, 2004). Women at high risk for HIV should avoid use of nonoxynol-9 spermicides with the diaphragm (Cates & Raymond, 2004).

The woman is informed that she needs an annual gynecologic examination to assess the fit of the diaphragm. The device should be inspected before every use, replaced every 2 years, and may need to be refitted for a 20% weight fluctuation, after any abdominal or pelvic surgery, and after every pregnancy (Planned Parenthood, 2004). Because various types of diaphragms are on the market, the nurse uses the package insert for teaching the woman how to use and care for the diaphragm (see Patient Instructions for Self-Care).

Disadvantages of diaphragm use include the reluctance of some women to insert and remove the diaphragm. Although it can be inserted up to 6 hours before intercourse, a cold diaphragm and a cold gel temporarily reduce vaginal response to sexual stimulation if insertion of the diaphragm occurs immediately before intercourse. Some women or couples object to the messiness of the spermicide. These annoyances of diaphragm use, along with failure to insert the

PATIENT INSTRUCTIONS FOR SELF-CARE
Use and Care of the Diaphragm

POSITIONS FOR INSERTION OF DIAPHRAGM
Squatting

Squatting is the most commonly used position, and most women find it satisfactory.

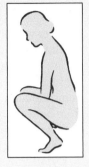

Leg-up Method

Another position is to raise the left foot (if right hand is used for insertion) on a low stool and, while in a bending position, insert the diaphragm.

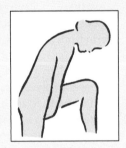

Chair Method

Another practical method for diaphragm insertion is to sit far forward on the edge of a chair.

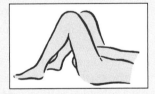

Reclining

You may prefer to insert the diaphragm while in a semi-reclining position in bed.

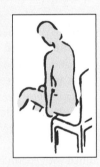

INSPECTION OF DIAPHRAGM

Your diaphragm must be inspected carefully before each use. The best way to do this is as follows:

- Hold the diaphragm up to a light source. Carefully stretch the diaphragm at the area of the rim, on all sides, to make sure there are no holes. Remember, it is possible to puncture the diaphragm with sharp fingernails.
- Another way to check for pinholes is to carefully fill the diaphragm with water. If there is any problem, it will be seen immediately.
- If your diaphragm is puckered, especially near the rim, this could mean thin spots.
- The diaphragm should not be used if you see any of these; consult your health care provider.

PREPARATION OF DIAPHRAGM

Rinse off cornstarch. Your diaphragm must always be used with a spermicidal lubricant to be effective. Pregnancy cannot be prevented effectively by the diaphragm alone.

Always empty your bladder before inserting the diaphragm. Place about 2 teaspoonfuls of contraceptive jelly or contraceptive cream on the side of the diaphragm that will rest against the cervix (or whichever way you have been instructed). Spread it around to coat the surface and the rim. This aids in insertion and offers a more complete seal. Many women also spread some jelly or cream on the other side of the diaphragm (Fig. A).

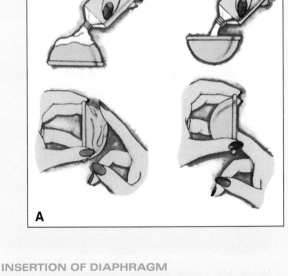

A

INSERTION OF DIAPHRAGM

The diaphragm can be inserted as long as 6 hours before intercourse. Hold the diaphragm between your thumb and fingers. The dome can either be up or down, as directed by your health care provider. Place your index finger on the outer rim of the compressed diaphragm (Fig. B).

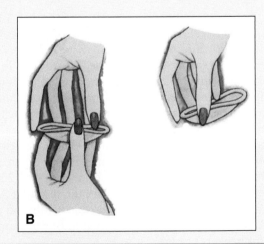

B

PATIENT INSTRUCTIONS FOR SELF-CARE
Use and Care of the Diaphragm—cont'd

Use the fingers of the other hand to spread the labia (lips of the vagina). This will assist in guiding the diaphragm into place.

Insert the diaphragm into the vagina. Direct it inward and downward as far as it will go to the space behind and below the cervix (Fig. C).

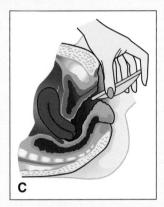

Tuck the front of the rim of the diaphragm behind the pubic bone so that the rubber hugs the front wall of the vagina (Fig. D).

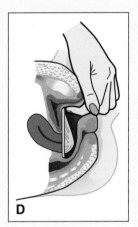

Feel for your cervix through the diaphragm to be certain it is properly placed and securely covered by the rubber dome (Fig. E).

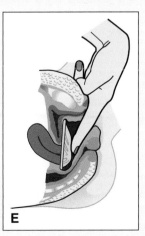

GENERAL INFORMATION

Regardless of the time of the month, you must use your diaphragm every time intercourse takes place. Your diaphragm must be left in place for at least 6 hours after the last intercourse. If you remove your diaphragm before the 6-hour period, your chance of becoming pregnant could be greatly increased. If you have repeated acts of intercourse, you must add more spermicide for each act of intercourse.

REMOVAL OF DIAPHRAGM

The only proper way to remove the diaphragm is to insert your forefinger up and over the top side of the diaphragm and slightly to the side.

Next, turn the palm of your hand downward and backward, hooking the forefinger firmly on top of the inside of the upper rim of the diaphragm, breaking the suction.

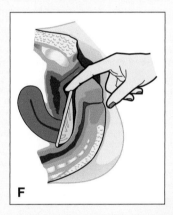

Pull the diaphragm down and out. This avoids the possibility of tearing the diaphragm with the fingernails. You should not remove the diaphragm by trying to catch the rim from below the dome (Fig. F).

CARE OF DIAPHRAGM

When using a vaginal diaphragm, avoid using oil-based products, such as certain body lubricants, mineral oil, baby oil, vaginal lubricants, or vaginitis preparations. These products can weaken the rubber.

A little care means longer wear for your diaphragm. After each use, wash the diaphragm in warm water and mild soap. Do not use detergent soaps, cold-cream soaps, deodorant soaps, and soaps containing oil products, because they can weaken the rubber.

After washing, dry the diaphragm thoroughly. All water and moisture should be removed with a towel. Then dust the diaphragm with cornstarch. Scented talc, body powder, baby powder, and the like should not be used because they can weaken the rubber.

To clean the introducer (if one is used), wash with mild soap and warm water, rinse, and dry thoroughly.

Place the diaphragm back in the plastic case for storage. Do not store it near a radiator or heat source or exposed to light for an extended period.

BOX 6-2

Male Condoms

MECHANISM OF ACTION
- Sheath is applied over the erect penis before insertion or loss of preejaculatory drops of semen. Used correctly, condoms prevent sperm from entering the cervix. Spermicide-coated condoms cause ejaculated sperm to be immobilized rapidly, thus increasing contraceptive effectiveness.

FAILURE RATE
- Typical users, 15%
- Correct and consistent users, 2%

ADVANTAGES
- Safe.
- No side effects.
- Readily available.
- Premalignant changes in cervix can be prevented or ameliorated in women whose partners use condoms.
- Method of male nonsurgical contraception.

DISADVANTAGES
- Must interrupt lovemaking to apply sheath.
- Sensation may be altered.
- If condom is used improperly, spillage of sperm can result in pregnancy.
- Condoms occasionally may tear during intercourse.

PROTECTION AGAINST STIs
If a condom is used throughout the act of intercourse and there is no unprotected contact with female genitals, a latex rubber condom, which is impermeable to viruses, can act as a protective measure against STIs.

NURSING CONSIDERATIONS
Teach man to do the following:
- Use a new condom (check expiration date) for each act of sexual intercourse or other acts between partners that involve contact with the penis.
- Place condom after penis is erect and before intimate contact.
- Place condom on head of penis (Fig. A) and unroll it all the way to the base (Fig. B).

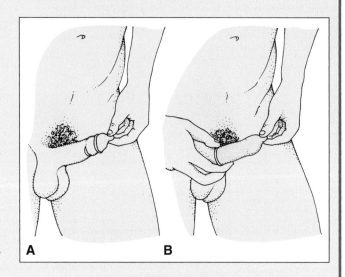

- Leave an empty space at the tip (Fig. A); remove any air remaining in the tip by gently pressing air out toward the base of the penis.
- If a lubricant is desired, use water-based products such as K-Y lubricating jelly. Do not use petroleum-based products because they can cause the condom to break.
- After ejaculation, carefully withdraw the still-erect penis from the vagina, holding onto condom rim; remove and discard the condom.
- Store unused condoms in cool, dry place.
- Do not use condoms that are sticky, brittle, or obviously damaged.

STIs, Sexually transmitted infections.

---

device once foreplay has begun, are the most common reasons for failures of this method. Side effects may include irritation of tissues related to contact with spermicides. The diaphragm is not a good option for women with poor vaginal muscle tone or recurrent urinary tract infections. For proper placement, the diaphragm must rest behind the pubic symphysis and completely cover the cervix. To decrease the chance of exerting urethral pressure, the woman should be reminded to empty her bladder before diaphragm insertion and immediately after intercourse. Diaphragms are contraindicated for women with pelvic relaxation (uterine prolapse) or a large cystocele. Women with a latex allergy should not use latex diaphragms.

Toxic shock syndrome (TSS), although reported in very small numbers, can occur in association with the use of the contraceptive diaphragm and cervical caps (Cates & Stewart, 2004). The nurse should instruct the woman about ways to reduce her risk for TSS. These measures include prompt removal 6 to 8 hours after intercourse, not using the diaphragm or cervical caps during menses, and learning and watching for danger signs of TSS.

NURSE ALERT *The nurse should be alert for signs of TSS in women who use a diaphragm or cervical cap as a contraceptive method. The most common signs include a sunburn-type rash, diarrhea, dizziness, faintness, weakness, sore throat, aching muscles and joints, sudden high fever, and vomiting (Planned Parenthood, 2004).*

Cervical caps. Three types of cervical caps are available; two come in varying sizes and one is one size fits all. They are made of rubber or latex-free silicone and have soft domes and firm brims (see Fig. 6-7, *A*). The cap fits snugly around

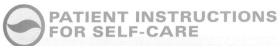

PATIENT INSTRUCTIONS FOR SELF-CARE

Use of the Cervical Cap

- Push cap up into vagina until it covers cervix.

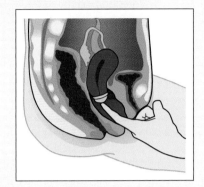

- Press rim against cervix to create a seal.

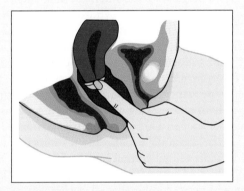

- To remove, push rim toward right or left hip to loosen from cervix, and then withdraw.

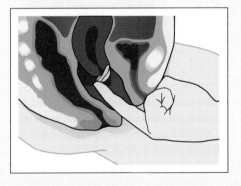

- The woman can assume several positions to insert the cervical cap. See the four positions shown for inserting the diaphragm.

the base of the cervix close to the junction of the cervix and vaginal fornices. It is recommended that the cap remain in place no less than 6 hours and not more than 48 hours at a time. It is left in place at least 6 hours after the last act of intercourse. The seal provides a physical barrier to sperm: spermicide inside the cap adds a chemical barrier. The extended period of wear may be an added convenience for women.

Instructions for the actual insertion and use of the cervical cap closely resemble the instructions for the use of the contraceptive diaphragm. Some of the differences are that the cervical cap can be inserted hours before sexual intercourse without a need for additional spermicide later, no additional spermicide is required for repeated acts of intercourse when the cap is used, and the cervical cap requires less spermicide than the diaphragm when initially inserted. The angle of the uterus, the vaginal muscle tone, and the shape of the cervix may interfere with the cervical cap's ease of fitting and use. Correct fitting requires time, effort, and skill from both the woman and the clinician. The woman must check the cap's position before and after each act of intercourse (see Patient Instructions for Self-Care box).

Because of the potential risk of TSS associated with the use of the cervical cap, another form of birth control is recommended for use during menstrual bleeding and up to at least 6 weeks postpartum. The cap should be refitted after any gynecologic surgery or birth and after major weight losses or gains. Otherwise, the size should be checked at least once a year.

Women who are not good candidates for wearing the cervical cap include those with abnormal Papanicolaou (Pap) test results, those who cannot be fitted properly with the existing cap sizes, those who find the insertion and removal of the device too difficult, those with a history of TSS, those with vaginal or cervical infections, and those who experience allergic responses to the latex cap or spermicide. Failure rates the first year of use are 16% in nulliparas and 32% in multiparous women (Trussell, 2004).

Contraceptive sponge. The vaginal sponge is a small, round, polyurethane sponge that contains nonoxynol-9 spermicide (see Fig. 6-7, *B*). It is designed to fit over the cervix (one size fits all). The side that is placed next to the cervix is concave for better fit. The opposite side has a woven polyester loop to be used for removal of the sponge.

The sponge must be moistened with water before it is inserted. It provides protection for up to 24 hours and for repeated instances of sexual intercourse. The sponge should be left in place for at least 6 hours after the last act of intercourse. Wearing longer than 24 to 30 hours may put the woman at risk for TSS (Cates & Stewart, 2004). A vaginal contraceptive sponge that had been unavailable in the U.S. since 1994 is once again marketed in the United States, as well as in Canada and Europe.

Hormonal methods

More than 30 different contraceptive formulations are available in the United States today. General classes are described in Table 6-1. Because of the wide variety of preparations available, the woman and nurse must read the package insert for information about specific products prescribed. Formulations include combined estrogen-progestin medications and progestational agents. The formulations are administered orally, transdermally, vaginally, by implantation, by injection, or via the intrauterine route.

Hormonal Contraception

COMPOSITION	ROUTE OF ADMINISTRATION	DURATION OF EFFECT
Combination estrogen and progestin	Oral	24 hours; extended cycle- 12 weeks
(synthetic estrogens and progestins	Transdermal	7 days
in varying doses and formulations)	Vaginal ring insertion	3 weeks
Progestin only		
Norethindrone, norgestrel	Oral	24 hours
Medroxyprogesterone acetate	Intramuscular injection	3 months
Progestin etongestrel	Subdermal	Up to 3 years
Levonorgestrel	Intrauterine device	Up to 5 years

Combined estrogen-progestin contraceptives

Oral contraceptives. The normal menstrual cycle is maintained by a feedback mechanism. Follicle-stimulating hormone (FSH) and LH are secreted in response to fluctuating levels of ovarian estrogen and progesterone. Regular ingestion of combined oral contraceptive pills (COCs) suppresses the action of the hypothalamus and anterior pituitary, leading to inappropriate secretion of FSH and LH; therefore, follicles do not mature and ovulation is inhibited.

Other contraceptive effects are induced by the combined steroids. Maturation of the endometrium is altered, making it a less favorable site for implantation. COCs also have a direct effect on the endometrium, so that from 1 to 4 days after the last COC is taken, the endometrium sloughs and bleeds as a result of hormone withdrawal. The withdrawal bleeding usually is less profuse than that of normal menstruation and may last only 2 to 3 days. Some women have no bleeding at all. The cervical mucus remains thick from the effect of the progestin (Hatcher & Nelson, 2004).

Cervical mucus under the effect of progesterone does not provide as suitable an environment for sperm penetration as does the thin, watery mucus at ovulation. The possible effect, if any, of altered tubal and uterine motility induced by COCs is not clear.

Monophasic pills provide fixed dosages of estrogen and progestin. Multiphasic pills (e.g., biphasic and triphasic oral contraceptives) alter the amount of progestin and sometimes the amount of estrogen within each cycle. These preparations reduce the total dosage of hormones in a single cycle without sacrificing contraceptive efficacy (Hatcher & Nelson, 2004). To maintain adequate hormonal levels for contraception and enhance compliance, COCs should be taken at the same time each day.

Advantages. Because taking the pill does not relate directly to the sexual act, its acceptability may be increased. Improvement in sexual response may occur once the possibility of pregnancy is not an issue. For some women, it is convenient to know when to expect the next menstrual flow.

Evidence of noncontraceptive benefits of oral contraceptives is based on studies of high-dose pills (50 mg of estrogen). Few data exist on noncontraceptive benefits of low-dose oral contraceptives (less than 35 mg of estrogen)

(Hatcher & Nelson, 2004). The noncontraceptive health benefits of COCs include decreased menstrual blood loss and decreased iron-deficiency anemia, regulation of menorrhagia and irregular cycles, and reduced incidence of dysmenorrhea and premenstrual syndrome (PMS). Oral contraceptives also offer protection against endometrial cancer and ovarian cancer, reduce the incidence of benign breast disease, improve acne, protect against the development of functional ovarian cysts and salpingitis, and decrease the risk of ectopic pregnancy. Oral contraceptives are considered a safe option for nonsmoking women until menopause. Perimenopausal women can benefit from regular bleeding cycles, a regular hormonal pattern, and the noncontraceptive health benefits of oral contraceptives (Hatcher & Nelson, 2004).

Women taking combined oral contraceptives are examined before the medication is prescribed and yearly thereafter. The examination includes medical and family history, weight, blood pressure, general physical and pelvic examinations, and screening cervical cytologic analysis (Pap test). Consistent monitoring by the health care provider is valuable in the detection of non–contraception-related disorders as well, so that timely treatment can be initiated. Most health care providers assess the woman 3 months after she begins COCs to detect any complications.

Use of oral hormonal contraceptives is initiated on one of the first days of the menstrual cycle (day 1 of the cycle is the first day of menses). With a "Sunday start," women begin taking pills on the first Sunday after the start of their menstrual period. If contraceptives are to be started at any time other than during normal menses, or within 3 weeks after birth, miscarriage, or induced abortion, another method of contraception should be used throughout the first week to avoid the risk of pregnancy (Hatcher & Nelson, 2004). Taken exactly as directed, oral contraceptives prevent ovulation, and pregnancy cannot occur; the overall effectiveness rate is almost 100%. Almost all failures (i.e., occurrence of pregnancy) are caused by omission of one or more pills during the regimen. The typical failure rate of COCs resulting from omission is 8% (Trussell, 2004).

Disadvantages and Side Effects. Since hormonal contraceptives have come into use, the amount of estrogen and progestational agent contained in each tablet has been reduced considerably. This is important because adverse effects are, to a degree, dose related.

Women must be screened for medical conditions that preclude the use of oral contraceptives. Contraindications for COC use include a history of thromboembolic disorders, cerebrovascular or coronary artery disease, breast cancer or other estrogen-dependent tumors, impaired liver function, liver tumor, smoking if woman is older than 35 years of age (more than 15 cigarettes per day), headaches with focal neurologic symptoms, surgery with prolonged immobilization or any surgery on the legs, hypertension (160/100), and diabetes mellitus (of more than 20 years' duration) with vascular disease (Hatcher & Nelson, 2004).

Certain side effects of COCs are attributable to estrogen, progestin, or both. Serious adverse effects documented with high doses of estrogen and progesterone include stroke, myocardial infarction, thromboembolism, hypertension, gallbladder disease, and liver tumors. Common side effects of estrogen excess include nausea, breast tenderness, fluid retention, and chloasma. Side effects of estrogen deficiency include early spotting (days 1 to 14), hypomenorrhea, nervousness, and atrophic vaginitis leading to painful intercourse (dyspareunia). Side effects of progestin excess include increased appetite, tiredness, depression, breast tenderness, vaginal yeast infection, oily skin and scalp, hirsutism, and postpill amenorrhea. Side effects of progestin deficiency include late spotting and breakthrough bleeding (days 15 to 21), heavy flow with clots, and decreased breast size. One of the most common side effects of combined COCs is bleeding irregularities (Hatcher & Nelson, 2004).

In the presence of side effects, especially those that are bothersome to the woman, a different product, different drug content, or another method of contraception may be required. The "right" product for a woman contains the lowest dose of hormones that prevents ovulation and that has the fewest and least harmful side effects. There is no way to predict the right dosage for any particular woman. Issues to consider in prescribing oral contraceptives include history of oral contraceptive use, side effects during past use, menstrual history, and drug interactions (Hatcher & Nelson, 2004).

The effectiveness of oral contraceptives can be negatively influenced when the following medications are taken simultaneously (Hatcher & Nelson, 2004).

- Anticonvulsants: barbiturates, oxcarbazepine, phenytoin, phenobarbital, felbamate, carbamazepine, primidone, and topiramate
- Systemic antifungals: griseofulvin
- Antituberculosis drugs: rifampicin and rifabutin
- Anti-HIV protease inhibitors

NURSE ALERT *Over-the-counter medications, as well as some herbal supplements (such as St John's wort) can alter the effectiveness of COCs. Women should be asked about their use when COCs are being considered for contraception.*

No strong pharmacokinetic evidence exists that shows a relationship between broad-spectrum antibiotic use and altered hormonal levels among oral contraceptive users, although potential antibiotic interaction can occur (Hatcher & Nelson, 2004). Metaanalysis of studies on the incidence of breast cancer in COC users has not found a significant increase of breast cancer in women who use COCs (Marchbanks et al., 2002).

After discontinuation of oral contraception, return to fertility usually happens quickly, but fertility rates are slightly lower the first 3 to 12 months after discontinuation (Hatcher & Nelson, 2004). Many women ovulate the next month after stopping oral contraceptives. Women who discontinue oral contraception for a planned pregnancy commonly ask whether they should wait before attempting to conceive. Studies indicate that these infants have no greater chance of being born with any type of birth defect than do infants born to women in the general population, even if conception occurred in the first month after the medication was discontinued (Hatcher & Nelson, 2004). Little evidence suggests that oral contraceptives cause postpill amenorrhea. Amenorrhea after oral contraceptive use is probably related to the woman's menstrual cycle before taking the pill (Hatcher & Nelson, 2004).

Nursing Considerations. Many different preparations of oral hormonal contraceptives are available. The nurse reviews the prescribing information in the package insert with the woman. Because of the wide variations, each woman must be clear about the unique dosage regimen for the preparation prescribed for her. Directions for care after missing one or two tablets also vary (Fig. 6-8).

Withdrawal bleeding tends to be short and scanty when some combination pills are taken. A woman may see no fresh blood at all. A drop of blood or a brown smudge on a tampon or the underwear counts as a menstrual period.

About 68% of women who start taking oral contraceptives are still taking them after 1 year (Trussell, 2004). It therefore is important that nurses recommend that all women choosing to use oral contraceptives be provided with a second method of birth control and be instructed and comfortable with this backup method. Most women stop taking oral contraceptives for nonmedical reasons.

The nurse also reviews the signs of potential complications associated with the use of oral contraceptives (see Signs of Potential Complications box). Oral contraceptives do not protect a woman against STIs or HIV. A barrier method such as condoms and spermicide should be used for protection.

Oral contraceptives 91-day regimen. An extended-cycle oral contraceptive was approved by the FDA in 2003. Levonorgestrel–ethinyl estradiol (Seasonale) contains both estrogen and progestin, taken in 3-month cycles of 12 weeks of active pills followed by one week of inactive pills. Menstrual periods occur during the thirteenth week of the cycle. There is no protection from STIs, and risks are similar to those of COCs. Available only by prescription, Seasonale must be taken on a daily schedule, regardless of

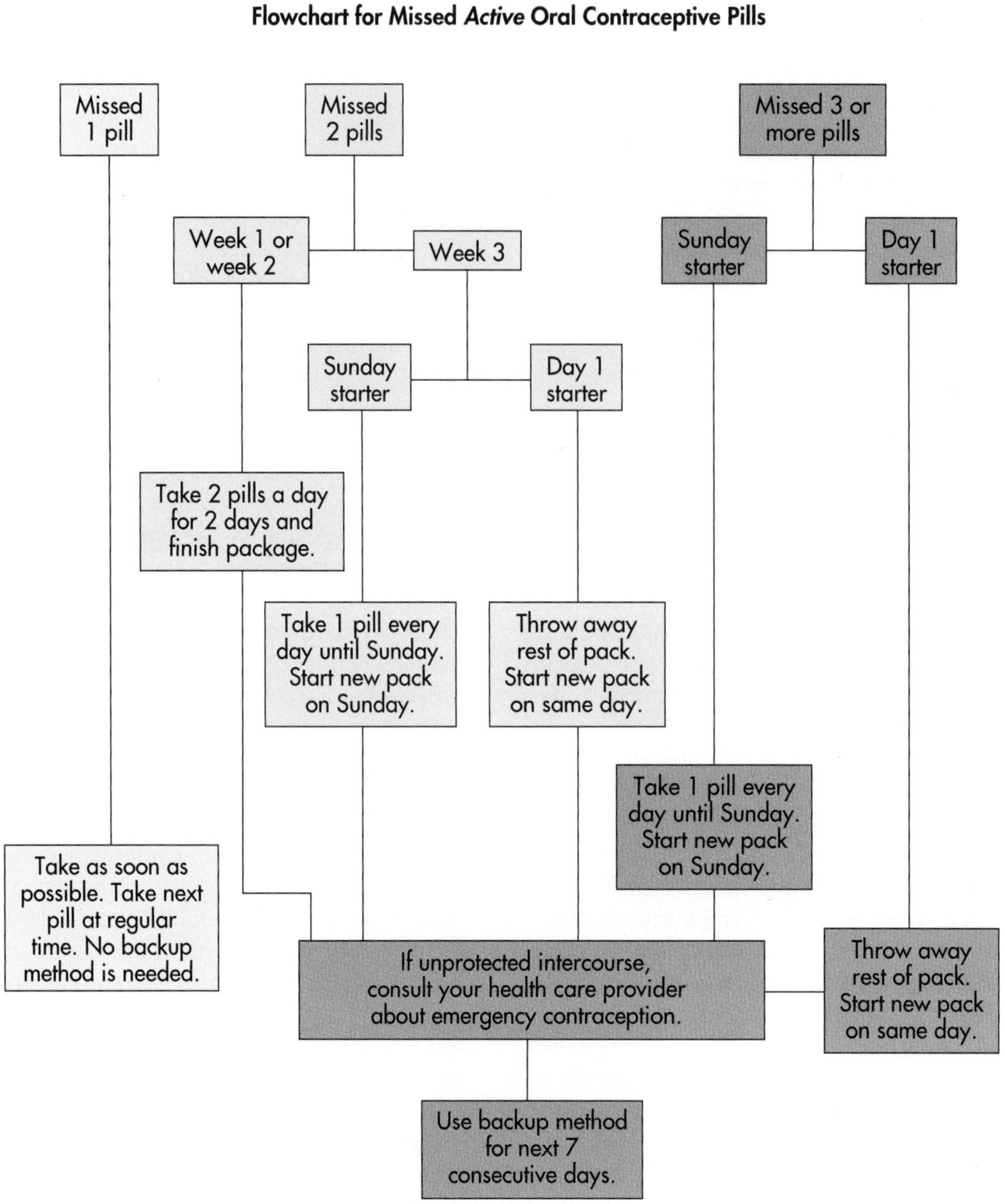

Flowchart for Missed *Active* Oral Contraceptive Pills

```
Missed          Missed                          Missed 3 or
1 pill          2 pills                         more pills

                Week 1 or ──── Week 3           Sunday ──── Day 1
                week 2                          starter     starter

                Sunday ──── Day 1
                starter     starter

        Take 2 pills a day
        for 2 days and
        finish package.

                Take 1 pill every   Throw away
                day until Sunday.   rest of pack.
                Start new pack      Start new pack
                on Sunday.          on same day.

                                            Take 1 pill every
                                            day until Sunday.
                                            Start new pack
                                            on Sunday.

Take as soon as
possible. Take next                                    Throw away
pill at regular          If unprotected intercourse,   rest of pack.
time. No backup          consult your health care provider   Start new pack
method is needed.        about emergency contraception.      on same day.

                        Use backup method
                        for next 7
                        consecutive days.
```

Fig. 6-8 Flowchart for missed contraceptive pills. (Courtesy Patsy Huff, PharmD, Chapel Hill, NC.)

the frequency of intercourse. Because users will have fewer menstrual flows, they should consider the possibility of pregnancy if they do not experience their thirteenth-week flow. Typical failure rate in the first year of Seasonale use is less than 2% (FDA, 2003).

Transdermal contraceptive system. Available by prescription only, the contraceptive transdermal patch delivers continuous levels of norelgestromin (progesterone) and ethinyl estradiol. The patch can be applied to intact skin of the upper outer arm, upper torso (front and back, excluding the breasts), lower abdomen, or buttocks (Fig. 6-9). Application is on the same day once a week for 3 weeks, followed by a week without the patch. Withdrawal bleeding occurs during the "no patch" week. Mechanism of action, efficacy,

contraindications, skin reactions, and side effects are similar to those of COCs. The typical failure rate during the first year of use is under 2% in women weighing less than 198 pounds (FDA, 2003).

Vaginal contraceptive ring. Available only with a prescription, the vaginal contraceptive ring is a flexible ring (made of ethylene vinyl acetate copolymer) worn in the vagina to deliver continuous levels of etonorgestrel (progesterone) and ethinyl estradiol (see Fig. 6-9). One vaginal ring is worn for 3 weeks, followed by a week without the ring. The ring is inserted by the woman and does not have to be fitted. Some wearers may experience vaginitis, leukorrhea, and vaginal discomfort (Hatcher & Nelson, 2004). Withdrawal bleeding occurs during the "no ring" week. If the woman or partner notices discomfort during coitus, the ring should not be removed from the vagina for any longer than 3 hours for it to still be effective for the rest of the 3 week period. Mechanism of action, efficacy, contraindications, and side effects are similar to those of COCs. The typical failure rate of the vaginal contraceptive ring is reportedly under 2% during the first year of use (FDA, 2003).

Progestin-only contraceptives. Progestin-only methods impair fertility by inhibiting ovulation, thickening and decreasing the amount of cervical mucus, thinning the endometrium, and altering cilia in the uterine tubes (Hatcher, 2004).

Oral progestins (minipill). Failure rate of progestin-only pills for typical users is about 8% in the first year of use (Trussell, 2004). Effectiveness is increased if minipills are taken correctly. Because minipills contain such a low dose of progestin, the minipill must be taken at the same time

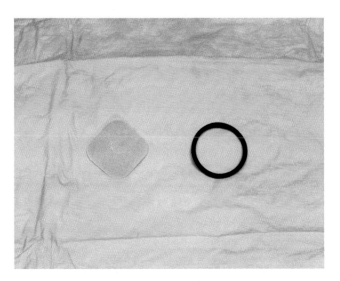

Fig. 6-9 Hormonal contraceptive transdermal patch and vaginal ring. (Courtesy Dee Lowdermilk, Chapel Hill, NC.)

every day (Hatcher, 2004). Users often complain of irregular vaginal bleeding.

Injectable progestins. Depot medroxyprogesterone acetate (DMPA or Depo-Provera), 150 mg, is given intramuscularly in the deltoid or gluteus maximus muscle. A 21- to 23-gauge needle, 2.5 to 4 cm long, should be used. DMPA should be initiated during the first 5 days of the menstrual cycle and administered every 11 to 13 weeks.

NURSE ALERT *When administering an intramuscular injection of progestin (e.g., Depo-Provera), do not massage the site after the injection, because this action can hasten the absorption and shorten the period of effectiveness.*

Advantages of DMPA include a contraceptive effectiveness comparable to that of combined oral contraceptives, long-lasting effects, requirement of injections only four times a year, and unlikelihood that lactation will be impaired (Hatcher, 2004). Side effects at the end of a year include decreased bone mineral density, weight gain, lipid changes, increased risk of venous thrombosis and thromboembolism, irregular vaginal spotting, decreased libido, and breast changes (Contraception Online, 2003). Other disadvantages include a lack of protection against STIs (including HIV). A delay in return to fertility may be as long as 18 months after discontinuing DMPA. Typical failure rate is 3% in the first year of use (Trussell, 2004).

NURSE ALERT *Women who use DMPA may lose significant bone mineral density with increasing duration of use. It is unknown if this effect is reversible. It is unknown if use of DMPA during adolescence or early adulthood, a critical period of bone accretion, will reduce peak bone mass and increase the risk of osteoporotic fracture in later life. DMPA should be used as a long-term birth control method (e.g., longer than 2 years) only if other birth control methods are inadequate. Women who receive DMPA should be counseled about calcium intake and exercise (Hatcher, 2004).*

Implantable progestins. The Norplant system consists of six flexible, nonbiodegradable polymeric silicone (Silastic) capsules. The Silastic capsules contain levonorgestrel, providing up to 5 to 7 years of contraception, dependent on the patient's weight and age. Insertion and removal of the capsules are minor surgical procedures involving a local anesthetic, a small incision, and no sutures. The capsules are placed subdermally in the inner aspect of the nondominant upper arm. The progestin prevents some, but not all, ovulatory cycles and thickens cervical mucus. Other advantages include reversibility and long-term continuous contraception that is not related to frequency of coitus. Irregular menstrual bleeding is the most common side effect. Less common side effects include headaches, nervousness, nausea, skin changes, and vertigo. No STI protection is provided with the Norplant method, so condoms should be used for protection.

Since July 2002 the Norplant system has been unavailable in the United States because of questions about effectiveness (FDA, 2003). A single rod implant (Implanon) is available in Europe and Australia and is expected to be available in the United States by the time this text is published (Hatcher, 2004).

Emergency contraception

Emergency contraception is available in over 100 countries, and in about one third of those countries it is available without a prescription. Although there is much support for making emergency contraception available over-the-counter in the United States, it is currently only available without a prescription in limited pharmacies and clinics in six states: Alaska, California, Hawaii, Maine, New Mexico, and Washington.

In the United States only one product is approved and marketed as emergency contraception. This product is Plan B, which contains 2 doses of levonorgestrel. Other options that the FDA has determined to be safe for emergency contraception include high doses of oral progestins or COCs and insertion of the copper IUD (Stewart, Trussell, & Van Look, 2004).

Emergency contraception should be taken by a woman as soon as possible but within 120 hours (Ellertson et al., 2003) of unprotected intercourse or birth control mishap (e.g., broken condom, dislodged ring or cervical cap, missed OCPs, late for injection) to prevent unintended pregnancy. If taken before ovulation, emergency contraception prevents ovulation by inhibiting follicular development. If taken after ovulation occurs, there is little effect on ovarian hormone production or the endometrium. Recommended oral medication regimens with progestin only and estrogen-progestin pills for emergency contraception are presented in Table 6-2. To minimize the side effect of nausea that occurs with high doses of estrogen and progestin, the woman can be advised to take an over-the-counter antiemetic 1 hour before each dose. Women with contraindications for estrogen use should use progestin-only emergency contraception. No medical contraindications for emergency contraception exist, except pregnancy and undiagnosed abnormal vaginal bleeding (Stewart, Trussell, & Van Look, 2004). If the woman does not begin menstruation within 21 days after taking the pills, she should be evaluated for pregnancy (Stewart, Trussell, & Van Look, 2004). Emergency contraception is ineffective if the woman is pregnant, as the pills do not disturb an implanted pregnancy. Risk of pregnancy is reduced by as much as 75% and 89% if the woman takes oral ECPs (Stewart, Trussell, & Van Look, 2004).

NURSE ALERT *Emergency contraception will not protect the woman against pregnancy if she engages in unprotected intercourse in the days or weeks that follow treatment. Because ingestion of ECPs may delay ovulation, caution the woman that she needs to establish a reliable form of birth control in order to prevent unintended pregnancy (Stewart, Trussell, & Van Look, 2004). Information about emergency contraception method options and access to providers are available on the web at http//www.NOT-2-LATE.com or by calling 1-888-NOT-2-LATE.*

TABLE 6-2

Emergency Contraceptive Pills Dosages

BRAND NAMES	FIRST DOSE (WITHIN 120 HR)	SECOND DOSE (12 HR LATER)
COMBINED ORAL CONTRACEPTIVES*		
Ovral	2 white tablets	2 white tablets
Orgestrel	2 white tablets	2 white tablets
Lo/Ovral	4 white tablets	4 white tablets
Low-Orgestrel	4 white tablets	4 white tablets
Nordette tablets	4 light orange	4 light orange tablets
Levlen tablets	4 light orange	4 light orange tablets
Trivora	4 yellow tablets	4 yellow tablets
Levora	4 white tablets	4 white tablets
Triphasil	4 yellow tablets	4 yellow tablets
Tri-Levlen	4 yellow tablets	4 yellow tablets
Alesse	5 pink tablets	5 pink tablets
Levlite	5 pink tablets	5 pink tablets
Aviane	5 orange tablets	5 orange tablets
PROGESTIN ONLY		
Ovrette	20 yellow tablets	20 yellow tablets
Plan B†	1 white tablet	1 white tablet

Sources: American College of Obstetricians and Gynecologists (ACOG). (2001). *Emergency oral contraception. ACOG Practice Bulletin no. 25.* Washington, DC: ACOG; Stewart, F., Trussell, J., & Van Look, P. (2004). Emergency contraception. In R. Hatcher et al. (Eds.). *Contraceptive technology* (18th ed.). New York: Ardent Media Inc.
*Antinausea medications needed for any of the combined oral contraceptives.
†May take both pills at same time.

IUDs containing copper (see later discussion) provide another emergency contraception option. The IUD should be inserted within 8 days of unprotected intercourse (Stewart, Trussell, & Van Look, 2004). This method is suggested only for women who wish to have the benefit of long-term contraception. The risk of pregnancy is reduced by as much as 99% with emergency insertion of the copper-releasing IUD.

Contraceptive counseling should be provided to all women requesting emergency contraception, including a discussion of modification of risky sexual behaviors to prevent STIs and unwanted pregnancy (Kettyle & Klima, 2002).

Intrauterine devices

An IUD is a small, T-shaped device with bendable arms for insertion through the cervix (Fig. 6-10). Once the trained health care provider inserts the IUD against the uterine fundus, the arms open near the fallopian tubes to maintain position of the device and to adversely affect the sperm motility and irritate the lining of the uterus. Two strings hang from the base of the stem through the cervix and protrude into the vagina for the woman to feel to assure that the device has not been dislodged (Grimes, 2004). The patient should have had a negative pregnancy test, treatment for dysplasia, cervical cultures to rule out STIs, and a consent form signed before IUD insertion. Advantages to choosing this method of contraception include long-term protection from pregnancy and immediate return to fertility when removed. Disadvantages include increased risk of pelvic inflammatory disease (PID) shortly after placement, unintentional expulsion of the device, infection, and possible uterine perforation. IUDs offer no protection against HIV or other STIs. Therefore, women who are in mutually monogamous relationships are the best candidates for this device.

There are two FDA-approved IUDs. The ParaGard T-380A (copper IUD) is made of radiopaque polyethylene and fine solid copper and is approved for 10 years of use. The copper primarily serves as a spermicide and inflames the endometrium, preventing fertilization (Grimes, 2004). Sometimes women experience more bleeding and cramping within the first year after insertion, but nonsteroidal antiinflammatory drugs (NSAIDs) may be taken for pain relief. The

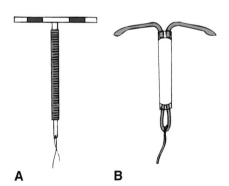

Fig. 6-10 Intrauterine devices (IUDs). **A,** Copper T-380A. **B,** Levonorgestrel-releasing IUD.

typical failure rate in the first year of use of the copper IUD is less than 1% (Trussell, 2004).

Mirena is a hormonal intrauterine system that releases levonorgestrel from its vertical reservoir. Effective for up to 5 years, it impairs sperm motility, irritates the lining of the uterus, and has some anovulatory effects (Grimes, 2004). Uterine cramping and uterine bleeding is usually improved with this device, although irregular spotting is common in the first few months after insertion. The typical failure rate in the first year of use is less than 1% (Trussell, 2004).

Nursing considerations. The woman should be taught to check for the presence of the IUD strings after menstruation to rule out expulsion of the device. If pregnancy occurs with the IUD in place, an ultrasound should confirm that it is not ectopic. Early removal of the IUD helps decrease the risk of spontaneous miscarriage or preterm labor. The woman should report any signs of flulike illness, as this may indicate a septic miscarriage (Grimes, 2004). In some women who are allergic to copper, a rash develops, necessitating the removal of the copper-bearing IUD. Signs of potential complications to be taught to the woman are listed in the accompanying box (Signs of Potential Complications Box).

Sterilization

Sterilization refers to surgical procedures intended to render a person infertile. Most procedures involve the occlusion of the passageways for the ova and sperm (Fig. 6-11). For the woman, the uterine tubes are occluded; for the man, the vas deferens are occluded. Only surgical removal of the ovaries (oophorectomy) and/or the uterus (hysterectomy) will result in absolute sterility for the woman. Most other sterilization procedures have a less than 1% failure rate (Trussell, 2004).

Female sterilization. Female sterilization *(bilateral tubal ligation [BTL])* (see Fig. 6-11, *A*) may be done immediately after childbirth (within 48 hours), concomitant with abortion, or as an interval procedure (during any phase of the menstrual cycle). If sterilization is performed as an interval procedure, the health care provider must be certain that the woman is not pregnant. Half of all female sterilization procedures in the United States are performed immediately after a pregnancy (Hatcher et al., 2004). Sterilization procedures can be safely done on an outpatient basis.

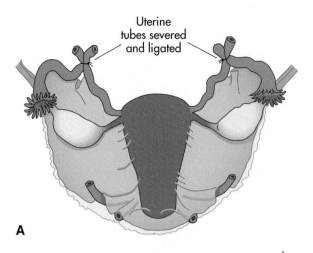

Uterine tubes severed and ligated

A

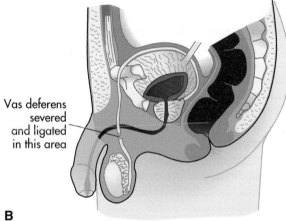

Vas deferens severed and ligated in this area

B

Fig. 6-11 Sterilization. **A,** Uterine tubes severed and ligated (tubal ligation). **B,** Sperm duct severed and ligated (vasectomy).

Tubal occlusion. A laparoscopic approach or a minilaparotomy may be used for tubal ligation (salpingectomy), tubal electrocoagulation (bipolar cautery), or the application of bands (Silastic: Fallope ring or Yoon Band) or clips (Hulka-Clemens spring clip or Filshie clip). Electrocoagulation and ligation are considered to be permanent methods. Use of the bands or clips has the theoretic advantage of possible removal and return of tubal patency (Pollack, Carignan, & Jacobstein, 2004).

For the mini-laparotomy, the woman is admitted the morning of surgery, having taken nothing by mouth since midnight. Preoperative sedation is given. The procedure may be carried out with a local anesthetic, but general anesthetic also may be used. A small incision is made in the abdominal wall below the umbilicus. The woman may experience sensations of tugging, but no pain, and the operation is completed within 20 minutes. She may be discharged several hours later after she has recovered from anesthesia. Any abdominal discomfort usually can be controlled with a mild analgesic (e.g., acetaminophen). Within days the scar is almost invisible (see Patient Instructions for Self-Care box). As with any surgery, there is always a possibility of complications of anesthesia, infection, hemorrhage, and trauma to other organs.

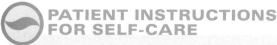

PATIENT INSTRUCTIONS FOR SELF-CARE

What to Expect after Tubal Ligation

- You should expect no change in hormones and their influence.
- Your menstrual period will be about the same as before the sterilization.
- You may feel pain at ovulation.
- The ovum disintegrates within the abdominal cavity.
- It is highly unlikely that you will become pregnant.
- You should not have a change in sexual functioning; you may enjoy sexual relations more because you will not be concerned about becoming pregnant.
- Sterilization offers no protection against STIs; therefore, you may need to use condoms.

Transcervical sterilization. Still considered experimental, hysteroscopic techniques can be used to inject occlusion agents into the uterine tubes. One FDA-approved device is the Essure System, an interval sterilization method (not intended for the postpartum period). A trained health care professional inserts a small catheter holding the polyester fibers through the vagina and cervix and places the small metallic implants into each uterine tube. The device works by stimulating the woman's own scar tissue formation to occlude the uterine tubes and prevent conception (FDA, 2003). Advantages include the nonhormonal nature of the contraception and the ability to insert the device during an office procedure without anesthesia. Analgesia is recommended to decrease mild to moderate discomfort associated with tubal spasm. Particularly convenient for obese women or those with abdominal adhesions, the transcervical approach eliminates the need for abdominal surgery. Because the procedure is not immediately effective, it is essential that the woman and her partner use another form of contraception until tubal blockage is proven. It may take up to 3 months for tubal occlusion to fully occur, and success must be confirmed by hysterosalpingogram. Other disadvantages include expulsion and perforation (Essure, 2004). Typical failure rate during the first year of use of the Essure System is less than 1% (FDA, 2003). Long-term efficacy and safety rates are unknown (Pollack, Carignan, & Jacobstein, 2004).

Tubal reconstruction. Restoration of tubal continuity (reanastomosis) and function is technically feasible except after laparoscopic tubal electrocoagulation. Sterilization reversal, however, is costly, difficult (requiring microsurgery), and uncertain. The success rate varies with the extent of tubal destruction and removal. The risk of ectopic pregnancy after tubal reanastomosis is increased between 2% and 12.5% (Pollack, Carignan, & Jacobstein, 2004).

Male sterilization. *Vasectomy* is the sealing, tying, or cutting of a man's vas deferens so that the sperm cannot travel from the testes to the penis (FDA, 2003). It is considered the easiest and most commonly used operation for male sterilization. Vasectomy can be carried out with local anesthesia on an outpatient basis. Pain, bleeding, infection, and other postsurgical complications are considered the disadvantages to the surgical procedure (FDA, 2003). It is considered a permanent method of sterilization because reversal is generally unsuccessful.

Two methods are used for scrotal entry: conventional and no-scalpel vasectomy. The surgeon identifies and immobilizes the vas deferens through the scrotum. Then the vas is ligated or cauterized (see Fig. 6-11, *B*). Surgeons vary in their techniques to occlude the vas deferens: ligation with sutures, division, cautery, application of clips, excision of a segment of the vas, fascial interposition, or some combination of these methods (Pollack, Carignan, & Jacobstein, 2004).

The man is instructed in self-care to promote a safe return to routine activities. To reduce swelling and relieve discomfort, ice packs are applied to the scrotum intermittently for a few hours after surgery. A scrotal support may be applied to decrease discomfort. Moderate inactivity for about 2 days is advisable because of local scrotal tenderness. Sexual intercourse may be resumed as desired; however, sterility is not immediate. Some sperm will remain in the proximal portions of the sperm ducts after vasectomy. One week to several months are required to clear the ducts of sperm (i.e., after approximately 20 ejaculations); therefore, some form of contraception is needed until the sperm count in the ejaculate on two consecutive tests is down to zero (Pollack, Carignan, & Jacobstein, 2004).

Vasectomy has no effect on potency (ability to achieve and maintain erection) or volume of ejaculate. Endocrine production of testosterone continues so that secondary sex characteristics are not affected. Sperm production continues, but sperm are unable to leave the epididymis and are lysed by the immune system. Complications after vasectomy are uncommon and usually not serious. They include hematoma, bruising, wound infection, epididymitis, or adverse reaction to anesthetic agent (Pollack, Carignan, & Jacobstein, 2004). Less common are painful granulomas from accumulation of sperm. Typical failure rate in the first year for male sterilization is 0.15% (Trussell, 2004).

Vasectomy reversal. Microsurgery to reanastomose (restore tubal continuity) the sperm ducts can be accomplished successfully (i.e., sperm in the ejaculate) in more than 90% of cases; however, the fertility rate is only about 50% (Hatcher et al., 2004). The rate of success decreases as the time since the procedure increases. The vasectomy may result in permanent changes in the testes that leave men unable to initiate a pregnancy. The skill of the surgeon, presence of antisperm antibodies in the man, and his partner's fertility influence the likelihood for procreation after vasectomy reversal (Hatcher et al., 2004).

Laws and regulations. All states have strict regulations for informed consent. Many states permit voluntary sterilization of any mature, rational woman without reference to her marital or pregnancy status. Although the law does not require the partner's consent, the woman is encouraged to discuss the situation with the partner, and health care providers may request the partner's consent. Sterilization of minors or mentally incompetent individuals is restricted by most states and often requires the approval of a board of eugenicists or other court-appointed individuals (see Legal Tip).

LEGAL TIP   Sterilization

- *If federal funds are used for sterilization, the person must be aged 21 years or older.*
- *Informed consent must include an explanation of the risks, benefits, and alternatives; a statement that describes sterilization as a permanent, irreversible method of birth control; and a statement that mandates a 30-day waiting period between giving consent and the sterilization.*
- *Informed consent must be in the person's native language, or a translator must be provided to read the consent form to the person.*

Nursing considerations. The nurse plays an important role in assisting people with decision making so that all requirements for informed consent are met. The nurse also provides information about alternatives to sterilization, such as contraception. The nurse acts as a "sounding board" for people who are exploring the possibility of choosing sterilization and their feelings about and motivation for this choice. The nurse records this information, which may be the basis for referral to a family-planning clinic, a psychiatric social worker, or another professional health care provider.

Information must be given about what is entailed in various procedures, how much discomfort or pain can be expected, and what type of care is needed. Many individuals fear sterilization procedures because of the imagined effect on their sex life. They need reassurance concerning the hormonal and psychologic basis for sexual function and that uterine tube occlusion or vasectomy has no biologic sequelae in terms of sexual adequacy (Hatcher et al., 2004).

Preoperative care includes health assessment, which includes a psychologic assessment, physical examination, and laboratory tests. The nurse assists with the health assessment, answers questions, and confirms the patient's understanding of printed instructions (e.g., nothing by mouth after midnight). Ambivalence and extreme fear of the procedure are reported to the physician.

Postoperative care depends on the procedure performed (e.g., laparoscopy, laparotomy, or vasectomy). General care includes recovery after anesthesia, vital signs, fluid and electrolyte balance (intake and output, laboratory values), prevention of or early identification and treatment for infection or hemorrhage, control of discomfort, and assessment of emotional response to the procedure and recovery.

Discharge planning depends on the type of procedure performed. In general, the patient is given written instructions about observing for and reporting symptoms and signs of complications, the type of recovery to be expected, and the date and time for a follow-up appointment.

Breastfeeding: Lactational Amenorrhea Method

Lactational Amenorrhea Method (LAM) can be a highly effective, *temporary* method of birth control. It is more popular in underdeveloped countries and traditional societies where breastfeeding is used to prolong birth intervals. The method has seen limited use in the United States, because only about half of new mothers initiate breastfeeding and most American women do not establish breastfeeding patterns that provide maximum protection against pregnancy (Kennedy & Trussell, 2004).

When the infant suckles at the mother's breast, a surge of prolactin hormone is released, which inhibits estrogen production and suppresses ovulation and the return of menses. LAM works best if the mother is exclusively or almost exclusively breastfeeding, if the woman has not had a menstrual flow since giving birth, and if the infant is under 6 months of age. Effectiveness is enhanced by frequent feedings at intervals of less than 4 hours during the day and no more than 6 hours during the night, long duration of each feeding, and no bottle supplementation or limited supplementation by spoon or cup. The typical failure rate is 2% (Kennedy & Trussell, 2004).

NURSE ALERT *The woman should be counseled that disruption of the breastfeeding pattern or supplementation can increase the risk of pregnancy.*

Future trends

Contraceptive options are more limited in the United States and Canada than in some other industrialized countries. Lack of funding for research, governmental regulations, conflicting values about contraception, and high costs of liability coverage for contraception have been cited as blocks to new and improved methods. Existing methods of contraception are being improved, however, and a variety of new methods are being developed.

Lower-dose COCs (15 mcg of ethinyl estradiol) are available in Europe. Female barrier methods (new female condoms, patient-fitted diaphragms, and new vaginal sponges) are being tested. Vaginal hormonal methods including progestin-only vaginal rings and progesterone daily suppositories are under investigation. Two new IUDs and spermicidal microbicides are being evaluated. Male hormonal methods also are being investigated, including hormonal injections (testosterone), gonadotropin-releasing hormone (GnRH) antagonists, antisperm compounds, immunologic methods, and contraceptive vaccines (Hatcher et al., 2004; Hutti, 2003).

Evaluation

The nurse can be reasonably assured that care was effective when the patient-centered expected outcomes have been achieved: the woman and her partner learn about the various methods of contraception; the couple achieve pregnancy only when planned; and they have no adverse sequelae as a result of the chosen method of contraception.

INDUCED ABORTION

Induced abortion is the purposeful interruption of a pregnancy before 20 weeks of gestation. (Spontaneous abortion [miscarriage] is discussed in Chapter 23.) If the abortion is performed at the woman's request, the term *elective abortion* is used; if performed for reasons of maternal or fetal health or disease, the term *therapeutic abortion* applies. Many factors contribute to a woman's decision to have an abortion. Indications include (1) preservation of the life or health of the mother, (2) genetic disorders of the fetus, (3) rape or incest, and (4) the pregnant woman's request. The control of birth, dealing as it does with human sexuality and the question of life and death, is one of the most emotional components of health care and has been a controversial social issue since the mid-twentieth century. Regulations exist to protect the mother from the complications of abortion.

Abortion is regulated in most countries, including the United States. Before 1970 legal abortion was not widely available in the United States. However, in January, 1973, the U.S. Supreme Court set aside previous antiabortion laws and legalized abortion. This decision established a trimester approach to abortion. In the first trimester, abortion is permissible, the decision is between the woman and her health care provider, and a state has little right to interfere (Stewart, Ellertson, & Cates, 2004). In the second trimester, abortion was left to the discretion of the individual states to regulate procedures as long as they are reasonably related to the woman's health. In the third trimester, abortions may be limited or even prohibited by state regulation unless the

Critical Thinking Exercise

Abortion

Meghan is a 21-year-old college senior who engaged in unprotected intercourse with her date after attending a party where she admits to drinking too many beers. She has missed a period and at the clinic today learns that she is 7 weeks pregnant. She has requested an appointment for an abortion. She has many questions about the choices she has and what she can expect during the procedure and afterward. How should the nurse respond?

1 Evidence—Is there sufficient evidence to draw conclusions about what response the nurse should give?
2 Assumptions—Describe underlying assumptions about the following issues:
  a. Physical response related to termination of pregnancy with vacuum aspiration
  b. Psychologic and emotional response
  c. Future childbearing
3 What implications and priorities for nursing care can be drawn at this time?
4 Does the evidence objectively support your conclusion?
5 Are there alternative perspectives to your conclusion?

restriction interferes with the life or health of the pregnant woman (Stewart, Ellertson, & Cates, 2004).

In 1992 the U.S. Supreme Court made another landmark ruling, this time allowing states to restrict early abortion services as long as the restrictions did not place an "undue burden" on the woman's ability to choose abortion. Since then many bills have been introduced to limit access to and funds for women seeking abortion.

The laws for abortion in Canada have changed over the last 35 years as well. Before 1969, abortion was permitted only to save the life of the woman. Between 1969 and 1988 the laws became more liberal in interpretation of the health of the life of the woman. In 1988 this law was struck down and Canada is now one of the only countries in the world without abortion regulation. Abortion is available throughout pregnancy (Santoro, 2004).

LEGAL TIP	Induced Abortion

It is important for nurses to know the laws regarding abortion in their state of practice before they offer abortion counseling or nursing care to a woman choosing an abortion. Many states enforce a mandatory delay or state-directed counseling before a woman may legally obtain an abortion.

Incidence

The reported number of abortions performed in the United States in 2001 was 853,485 (Strauss et al., 2004). About 88% of all abortions are performed in the first trimester, with about 60% of these in the first 9 weeks after the last menstrual period. Most women who are having an elective abortion are Caucasian, younger than 24 years of age, and unmarried. Over 60% have had at least one previous live birth (Strauss et al., 2004). In 2002, 105,154 abortions were reportedly performed in Canada (National Campus Life Network, 2005).

Decision to Have an Abortion

A woman who is deciding whether or not to have an abortion is often ambivalent. She needs information and an opportunity to discuss her feelings about pregnancy, abortion, and the impact of either choice on her future. She needs to make her decision without feeling coercion about her choice (Robinson, Dollins, & McConlogue-O'Shaughnessy, 2000).

Nurses and other health care providers often struggle with the same values and moral convictions as those of the pregnant woman. The conflicts and doubts of the nurse can be readily communicated to women who are already anxious and overly sensitive. Regardless of personal views on abortion, nurses who provide care to women seeking abortion have a responsibility to counsel women about their options or to make appropriate referrals (Goss, 2002).

AWHONN (1999) continues to support a nurse's right to choose to participate in abortion procedures in keeping with his or her "personal, moral, ethical, or religious beliefs." AWHONN also advocates that "nurses have a professional obligation to inform their employers, at the time of employment, of any attitudes and beliefs that may interfere with essential job functions."

LEGAL TIP	Refusal to Give Care Based on Moral, Religious, and Ethical Reasons

Nurses' rights and responsibilities related to abortion as described by AWHONN (1999) should be protected through institutional policies that are written to address how the institution will make "reasonable accommodations" for the nurse's moral or ethical beliefs and what the nurse should do to give notice in such situations to avoid patient abandonment. Nurses should know what policies are in place in their institutions and encourage such policies to be written if they are not available (JCAHO, 2000).

First-Trimester Abortion

Methods for performing early abortion (less than 9 weeks of gestation) include surgical (aspiration) and medical methods (mifepristone with misoprostol) and methotrexate with misoprostol.

Aspiration

Aspiration (vacuum or suction curettage) is the most common procedure in the first trimester, with about 95% of all procedures being performed by this method (Strauss et al., 2004). Aspiration abortion is usually performed using local anesthesia in the physician's office, the clinic, or the hospital. The suction procedure for performing an early elective abortion (ideal time is 8 to 12 weeks since the last menstrual period) usually requires less than 5 minutes.

A bimanual examination is done before the procedure to assess uterine size and position. A speculum is inserted and the cervix is anesthetized with a local anesthetic agent. The cervix is dilated if necessary and a cannula connected to suction is inserted into the uterine cavity. The products of conception are evacuated from the uterus.

During the procedure the nurse or physician keeps the woman informed about what to expect next (e.g., menstrual-like cramping, sounds of the suction machine). The nurse assesses the woman's vital signs. The aspirated uterine contents must be carefully inspected to ascertain whether all fetal parts and adequate placental tissue have been evacuated. After the abortion the woman rests on the table until she is ready to stand. Then she remains in the recovery area or waiting room for 1 to 3 hours for detection of excessive cramping or bleeding; then she is discharged.

Bleeding after the operation is normally about the equivalent of a heavy menstrual period, and cramps are rarely severe. Excessive vaginal bleeding and infection, such as endometritis or salpingitis, are the most common complications of elective abortion. Retained products of conception are the primary cause of vaginal bleeding. Evacuation of the uterus, uterine massage, and administration of oxytocin or methylergonovine (Methergine) or both may be necessary. Prophylactic antibiotics to decrease the risk

EVIDENCE-BASED PRACTICE
Comparing Medical and Surgical Abortions

BACKGROUND

- Abortion has been practiced for millennia. Approximately 53 million abortions are performed each year. An estimated one third of these are performed in unsafe circumstances, mostly in developing countries, and account for one out of eight maternal deaths worldwide. Surgical abortion in safe settings has the lowest complication rates. Complications are 2.3 times higher for dilation and curettage (D&C) as compared with vacuum aspiration. Complications of surgical abortion include infection, incomplete evacuation, cervical trauma, uterine perforation, hemorrhage, complications with anesthesia, and possible associations with infertility, miscarriages, and low birth weight in subsequent pregnancies. Medical abortions use pharmaceuticals to terminate pregnancy growth or stimulate expulsion of uterine contents. Four protocols are commonly used: misoprostol (prostaglandin E_1), mifepristone, mifepristone with misoprostol, and methotrexate with misoprostol. Methotrexate stops rapid cell replication. Misoprostol causes uterine contractions. Both methotrexate and misoprostol are teratogenic. Side effects of medical abortion are moderate to heavy bleeding, pain, nausea, vomiting, diarrhea, and more observed blood loss and passage of tissue.

OBJECTIVES

- The reviewers compared medical versus surgical methods of first trimester abortion.
- Outcomes were efficacy, side effects, and acceptability of the procedure. Primary outcomes included incomplete abortion, pelvic infection, blood transfusion, blood loss or hemoglobin drop, uterine perforation, cervical injury, and readmission. Secondary outcomes included hospital stay exceeding 24 hours, duration of bleeding, use of uterotonic or antibiotic drugs not routinely given, pain or analgesia use, vomiting, diarrhea, and dissatisfaction.

METHODS
Search Strategy

- The authors searched Cochrane, MEDLINE, and POPLINE, and contacted experts at the World Health Organization (WHO). Search keywords included *abortion, pregnancy termination, first trimester, vacuum aspiration, suction, dilation and curettage, D&C, mifepristone, misoprostol, prostaglandin, methotrexate,* and *RU 486.*
- Five randomized trials comparing medical versus surgical abortion were chosen. The trials represented 989 women from Sweden, Denmark, the United Kingdom, the United States, and a WHO multicenter trial from India, Vietnam, Slovenia, Zambia, China, Sweden, and Hungary. The trials were published from 1984 to 2000.

Statistical Analyses

- Outcomes of each medical abortion protocol were compared with outcomes of vacuum aspiration, the surgical treatment of choice for first trimester abortion.

FINDINGS

- *Misoprostol alone, versus vacuum aspiration:* The misoprostol group resulted in significantly more incomplete abortions and increased bleeding and pain, compared with vacuum aspiration. No significant differences were found between groups in infection rates.
- *Mifepristone alone, versus vacuum aspiration:* No significant differences were found between groups in infection rates, incomplete abortions, or perforations.
- *Mifepristone plus misoprostol, versus vacuum aspiration:* No difference in blood loss occurred, but the medical group had significantly longer duration of bleeding.
- *Methotrexate plus misoprostol, versus vacuum aspiration:* Duration of bleeding and use of analgesia for pain were both significantly greater in the medical abortion group. No differences between groups were found in incomplete abortion rates.
- Overall efficacy rate for medical abortions was 76% to 97% and for surgical abortions was 94% to 100%. Mifepristone alone had the lowest efficacy, at 76%. One perforation occurred in the surgical groups. Medical intervention groups experienced more days of bleeding than surgical patients. The medical group also experienced more pain, which may reflect the use of analgesia during the surgical procedure. The longer the gestation, the less acceptable the medical procedure was to the women. In one study, 63% of the medical group would choose that method again, whereas 92% of the surgical group would opt to repeat the surgical procedure, should the need arise. Overall, vacuum aspiration may be more effective than misoprostol alone and seems to be associated with less pain and bleeding.

LIMITATIONS

- The small number of trials and small sample sizes limit the generalizability of the results to the larger population. Many patients were lost to follow-up.

CONCLUSIONS

- Both medical and surgical abortions are effective and safe; vacuum extraction was more effective than medical abortion and was associated with less pain and bleeding.

IMPLICATIONS FOR PRACTICE

- The decision between a medical or a surgical abortion carries trade-offs. Careful counseling is necessary to prepare the woman for realistic expectations of each protocol, with careful attention to the attitude toward pregnancy and abortion. The setting may dictate one procedure over another, depending on whether a safe surgical procedure is available, or the proximity of a woman to a health facility for the duration of the medical abortion.

IMPLICATIONS FOR FURTHER RESEARCH

- Larger studies about women's preferences for methods of abortion, and the efficacy of the methods, are needed. More information about the pain experienced in abortion, preparation techniques, precounseling, alternative therapies, and presence of a support person would be useful.

Reference: Say, L. et al. (2002). Medical versus surgical methods for first trimester termination of pregnancy (Cochrane Review). In *The Cochrane Library,* Issue 4, 2005. Chichester, UK: John Wiley & Sons.

signs of
POTENTIAL COMPLICATIONS

Induced Abortion

Call your health care provider if you have any of the following signs:

- Fever greater than 38° C (100.4° F)
- Chills
- Bleeding greater than two saturated pads in 2 hours or heavy bleeding lasting a few days
- Foul-smelling vaginal discharge
- Severe abdominal pain, cramping, or backache
- Abdominal tenderness (when pressure applied)
- No return of menstrual period within 6 weeks

Reference: Stewart, F., Ellertson, C., & Cates, W. (2004). Abortion. In R. Hatcher et al. (Eds.), *Contraceptive technology* (18th ed.). New York: Ardent Media Inc.

of infection are commonly prescribed (Stewart, Ellertson, & Cates, 2004). Postabortion pain may be relieved with NSAIDs such as ibuprofen.

Postabortion instructions differ among health care providers (e.g., tampons should not be used for at least 3 days or should be avoided for up to 3 weeks, and resumption of sexual intercourse may be permitted within 1 week or discouraged for 2 weeks). The woman may shower daily. Instruction is given to watch for excessive bleeding and other signs of complications (see Signs of Potential Complications Box) and to avoid douches of any type. The woman may expect her menstrual period to resume 4 to 6 weeks from the day of the procedure. Information about the birth control method the woman prefers is offered if this has not been done previously during the counseling interview that usually precedes the decision to have an abortion. Some methods, such as an IUD insertion, can be initiated immediately. Hormonal methods may be started immediately or within a week (Stewart, Ellertson, & Cates, 2004). The woman must be strongly encouraged to return for her follow-up visit so that complications can be detected. A pregnancy test may also be performed to determine whether the pregnancy was successfully terminated (Stenchever, Droegemueller, Herbst, & Mishell, 2001).

Medical abortion

Early medical abortion has been popular in Canada and Europe for more than 15 years, but it is a relatively new procedure in the United States. Medical abortions are available for use in the United States for up to 9 weeks after the last menstrual period. Methotrexate, misoprostol, and mifepristone are the drugs used in the current regimens to induce early abortion. About 3% of all reported abortion procedures in 2001 were medical procedures (Strauss et al., 2004).

Methotrexate is a cytotoxic drug that causes early abortion by blocking folic acid in fetal cells so that they cannot divide. Misoprostol (Cytotec) is a prostaglandin analog that acts directly on the cervix to soften and dilate and on the uterine muscle to stimulate contractions. Mifepristone, formerly known as RU 486, was approved by the FDA in 2000.

It works by binding to progesterone receptors and blocking the action of progesterone, which is necessary for maintaining pregnancy (Kahn et al., 2000; Taylor & Hwang, 2003-2004).

Methotrexate and misoprostol. There is no standard protocol, but methotrexate is given intramuscularly or orally (usually mixed with orange juice). Vaginal placement of misoprostol follows in 3 to 7 days. The woman returns for a follow-up visit to confirm the abortion is complete. If not, the woman is offered an additional dose of misoprostol or vacuum aspiration is performed (Kahn et al., 2000).

Mifepristone and misoprostol. Mifepristone can be taken up to 7 weeks after the last menstrual period. The FDA-approved regimen is that the woman takes 600 mg of mifepristone orally; 48 hours later she returns to the office and takes 400 mcg of misoprostol orally (unless abortion has already occurred and been confirmed). Two weeks after the administration of mifepristone, the woman must return to the office for a clinical examination or ultrasound to confirm that the pregnancy has been terminated. In about 1% to 5% of cases, the drugs do not work, and surgical abortion (aspiration) is needed (Kahn et al., 2000).

Research has demonstrated a more effective regimen that has fewer side effects. This regimen can be given up to 9 weeks after the last menstrual period and includes administration of 200 mg mifepristone orally followed by misoprostol 800 mcg vaginally in 24 to 48 hours. This vaginal insertion can be done at home by the woman. A follow-up visit occurs in 4 to 8 days (National Abortion Federation, 2003).

With any medical abortion regimen, the woman usually will experience bleeding and cramping. Side effects of the medications include nausea, vomiting, diarrhea, headache, dizziness, fever, and chills. These are attributed to misoprostol and usually subside in a few hours after administration (Taylor & Hwang, 2003-2004).

Second-Trimester Abortion

Second-trimester abortion is associated with more complications and costs than first-trimester abortion. Dilation and evacuation (D&E) accounts for almost all procedures performed in the United States. Induction of uterine contractions with hypertonic solutions (e.g., saline, urea) injected directly into the uterus, and uterotonic agents (e.g., misoprostol, dinoprostone) account for only about 0.5% of all reported abortions (Strauss et al., 2004).

Dilation and evacuation

D&E can be performed at up to 20 weeks of gestation, although it is most commonly performed between 13 and 16 weeks of gestation (Stewart, Ellertson, & Cates, 2004). The cervix requires more dilation because the products of conception are larger. Often, osmotic dilators (e.g., laminaria) are inserted several hours or several days before the procedure, or misoprostol can be applied to the cervix. The procedure is similar to vaginal aspiration except a larger cannula is used and other instruments may be needed to remove the fetus and placenta. Nursing care includes monitoring vital signs, providing emotional support, administering analgesics, and using postoperative monitoring. Disadvantages of D&E may include possible long-term harmful effects on the cervix.

Nursing Considerations

The woman will need help exploring the meaning of the various alternatives and consequences to herself and her significant others. It is often difficult for a woman to express her true feelings (e.g., what abortion means to her now and in the future and what support or regret her friends and peers may demonstrate). A calm, matter-of-fact approach on the part of the nurse can be helpful (e.g., "Yes, I know you are pregnant. I am here to help. Let's talk about alternatives."). Listening to what the woman has to say and encouraging her to speak are essential. Neutral responses such as "Oh," "Uh-huh," and "Umm" and nonverbal encouragement such as nodding, maintaining eye contact, and use of touch are helpful in setting an open, accepting environment. Clarifying, restating, and reflecting statements; open-ended questions; and feedback are communication techniques that can be used to maintain a realistic focus on the situation and bring the woman's problems into the open. Once a decision has been made, the woman must be assured of continued support. Information about what is entailed in various procedures, how much discomfort or pain can be expected, and what type of care is needed must be given. A discussion of the various feelings including depression, guilt, regret, and relief that the woman might experience after the abortion is needed. Information about community resources for postabortion counseling may be needed (Goss, 2002). If family or friends cannot be involved, scheduling time for nursing personnel to give the necessary support is an essential component of the care plan.

After the abortion, studies have indicated that most women report relief, but some have temporary distress or mixed emotions. Guilt and anxiety may occur more with young women, women with poor social support, multiparous women, and women with a history of psychiatric illness. Women having second-trimester abortions may have more emotional distress than do women having abortions in the first trimester (Williams, 2000). Also, women feeling pressure to have an abortion had symptoms of short-term grief in the study reported by Williams (2000). Because symptoms can vary among women who have had abortions, nurses must assess women for grief reactions and facilitate the grieving process through active listening and nonjudgmental support and care.

INFERTILITY

Infertility is a serious medical concern that affects quality of life and is a problem for 10% to 15% of reproductive-age couples (American Society for Reproductive Medicine [ASRM], 2005; Nelson & Marshall, 2004). The term *infertility* implies subfertility, a prolonged time to conceive,

as opposed to *sterility*, which means inability to conceive. Normally, a fertile couple has approximately a 20% chance of conception in each ovulatory cycle. Primary infertility applies to a woman who has never been pregnant; secondary infertility applies to a woman who has been pregnant in the past.

The prevalence of infertility is relatively stable among the overall population but increases with the age of the woman, particularly in those older than 40 years (Stenchever et al., 2001). Probable causes include the trend toward delaying pregnancy until later in life, when fertility decreases naturally and the prevalence of diseases such as endometriosis and ovulatory dysfunction increases. There is some controversy regarding whether there has been an increase in male infertility, or whether male infertility is being more readily identified because of improvements in diagnosis.

Diagnosis and treatment of infertility require considerable physical, emotional, and financial investment over an extended period. Men and women often perceive infertility differently, with women having more stress from tests and treatments, placing greater importance on having children, being more accepting of indicated treatments, and wanting children more than men (King, 2003; Sherrod, 2004). The attitude, sensitivity and caring nature of those who are involved in the assessment and treatment of infertility lay the foundation for the patients' ability to cope with the many tests and treatments they must undergo.

Factors Associated with Infertility

Many factors, in both men and women, contribute to normal fertility. A normally developed reproductive tract in both the male and female partner is essential. Normal functioning of an intact hypothalamic-pituitary-gonadal axis supports

Critical Thinking Exercise

Infertility

Bob, 37, and Shirley, 36, have been married for 5 years and have been unsuccessful in their attempts to achieve a pregnancy. They have come to the Center for Reproductive Medicine for an infertility workup. Shirley tells the nurse that she is sure that in vitro fertilization is the answer to their problem and is asking questions about the procedure. How should the nurse respond to Shirley's comments and questions?

1 Evidence—Is there sufficient evidence to draw conclusions about what response the nurse should give?
2 Assumptions—Describe underlying assumptions about the following issues:
   a. Age and fertility
   b. Infertility as a major life stressor
3 What implications and priorities for nursing care can be drawn at this time?
4 Does the evidence objectively support your conclusion?
5 Are there alternative perspectives to your conclusion?

gametogenesis—the formation of sperm and ova. Although sperm remain viable in the female's reproductive tract for 48 hours or more, probably only a few retain fertilization potential for more than 24 hours. Ova remain viable for approximately 24 hours, but the optimal time for fertilization may be no more than 1 to 2 hours (Cunningham et al., 2001). Therefore the timing of intercourse is critical.

After fertilization the conceptus must travel down the patent uterine tube to the uterus and implant within 7 to 10 days in a hormone-prepared endometrium. The conceptus must develop normally, reach viability, and be born in good condition for extrauterine life.

An alteration in one or more of these structures, functions, or processes results in some degree of impaired fertility. In general, about 20% of couples will have unexplained or idiopathic causes of infertility. Among the 80% of couples who have an identifiable cause of infertility, about 40% are related to factors in the female partner, 40% are related to factors in the male partner, and 20% are related to factors in both partners (Nelson & Marshall, 2004; Stenchever et al., 2001). Boxes 6-3 and 6-4 list factors affecting female and male infertility.

CARE MANAGEMENT ■

Assessment and Nursing Diagnoses

The nurse assists in the assessment by obtaining data relevant to fertility through interview and physical examination. The database must include information to determine whether infertility is primary or secondary. Religious, cultural, and ethnic data are noted because they may place restrictions on tests and treatments (see Box 6-5).

Some of the data needed to investigate impaired fertility are of a sensitive, personal nature. Obtaining these data may be viewed as an invasion of privacy. The tests and examinations are occasionally painful and intrusive and can take the romance out of lovemaking. A high level of motivation is needed to endure the investigation.

Because multiple factors involving both partners are common, the investigation of impaired fertility is conducted systematically and simultaneously for both male and female partners. Both partners must be interested in the solution to the problem. The medical investigation requires time (3 to 4 months) and considerable financial expense, and it causes emotional distress and strain on the couple's interpersonal relationship (Angard, 2000).

Assessment of female infertility. Investigation of impaired fertility begins for the woman with a complete history and physical examination. The history explores the duration of infertility and past obstetric events and contains a detailed menstrual and sexual history. Medical and surgical conditions are evaluated. Exposure to reproductive hazards in the home (e.g., mutagens such as vinyl chlorides, teratogens such as alcohol, and emotional stresses) and workplace are explored.

BOX 6-3

Factors Affecting Female Fertility

OVARIAN FACTORS
- Developmental anomalies
- Anovulation, primary
  - Pituitary or hypothalamic hormone disorder
  - Adrenal gland disorder
  - Congenital adrenal hyperplasia
- Anovulation, secondary
  - Disruption of hypothalamic-pituitary-ovarian axis
  - Amenorrhea after discontinuing oral contraceptive pills
  - Premature ovarian failure
  - Increased prolactin levels

UTERINE, TUBAL, AND PERITONEAL FACTORS
- Developmental anomalies
- Tubal motility reduced
- Inflammation within the tube
- Tubal adhesions
- Endometrial and myometrial tumors
- Asherman syndrome (uterine adhesions or scar tissue)
- Endometriosis
- Chronic cervicitis
- Hostile or inadequate cervical mucus

OTHER FACTORS
- Nutritional deficiencies (e.g., anemia)
- Thyroid dysfunction
- Idiopathic condition

BOX 6-4

Factors Affecting Male Fertility

STRUCTURAL OR HORMONAL DISORDERS
- Undescended testes
- Hypospadias
- Varicocele
- Obstructive lesions of the vas deferens or epididymis
- Low testosterone levels
- Hypopituitarism
- Endocrine disorders
- Testicular damage caused by mumps
- Retrograde ejaculation

OTHER FACTORS
- Sexually transmitted infections
- Exposure to workplace hazards such as radiation or toxic substances
- Exposure of scrotum to high temperatures
- Nutritional deficiencies
- Antisperm antibodies
- Substance abuse
  - Changes in sperm—cigarette smoking, heroin, marijuana, amyl nitrate, butyl nitrate, ethyl chloride, methaqualone
  - Decrease in libido—heroin, methadone, selective serotonin reuptake inhibitors, and barbiturates
  - Impotence—alcohol, antihypertensive medications
- Idiopathic condition

Religious and Cultural Considerations of Fertility

RELIGIOUS CONSIDERATIONS

Civil laws and religious proscriptions about sex must always be kept in mind by the health care provider.

Conservative and reform Jewish couples are accepting of most infertility treatment; however, the Orthodox Jewish husband and wife may face infertility investigation and management problems because of religious laws that govern marital relations. For example, according to Jewish law, the Orthodox couple may not engage in marital relations during menstruation and through the following 7 "preparatory days." The wife then is immersed in a ritual bath *(mikvah)* before relations can resume. Fertility problems can arise when the woman has a short cycle (i.e., a cycle of 24 days or fewer; when ovulation would occur on day 10 or earlier).

The Roman Catholic Church regards the embryo as a human being from the first moment of existence and regards as unacceptable technical procedures such as in vitro fertilization, therapeutic donor insemination, and freezing of embryos.

Other religious groups may have ethical concerns about infertility tests and treatments. For example, most Protestant denominations and Muslims usually support infertility management as long as in vitro fertilization (IVF) is done with the husband's sperm, there is no reduction of fetuses, and insemination is done with the husband's sperm. These groups are less supportive of surrogacy and use of donor sperm and eggs. Christian Scientists do not permit surgical procedures or IVF but do permit insemination with husband and donor sperm.

Care providers should seek to understand the woman's spirituality and how it affects her perception of health care, especially in relation to infertility. Women may wish to seek infertility treatment but have questions about proposed diagnostic and therapeutic procedures because of religious proscriptions. These women are encouraged to consult their minister, rabbi, priest, or other spiritual leader for advice.

CULTURAL CONSIDERATIONS

Worldwide cultures continue to use symbols and rites that celebrate fertility. One fertility rite that persists today is the custom of throwing rice at the bride and groom. Other fertility symbols and rites include passing out of congratulatory cigars, candy, or pencils by a new father and baby showers held in anticipation of a child's birth.

In many cultures, the responsibility for infertility is usually attributed to the woman. A woman's inability to conceive may be a result of her sins, of evil spirits, or of the fact that she is an inadequate person. The virility of a man in some cultures remains in question until he demonstrates his ability to reproduce by having at least one child (D'Avanzo & Geissler, 2003).

A complete general physical examination is followed by a specific assessment of the reproductive tract. Evidence of endocrine system abnormalities is sought. Inadequate development of secondary sex characteristics (e.g., inappropriate distribution of body fat and hair) may point to problems with the hypothalamic-pituitary-ovarian axis or genetic aberrations (e.g., polycystic ovarian syndrome, Turner syndrome).

A woman may have an abnormal uterus and tubes as a result of exposure to diethylstilbestrol (DES) in utero. Evidence of past infection of the genitourinary system or endometriosis is sought. Bimanual examination of internal organs may reveal lack of mobility of the uterus or abnormal contours of the uterus and adnexa. Data from routine urine and blood tests are obtained along with results of other diagnostic tests.

Diagnosis. The basic infertility survey of the woman involves evaluation of the cervix, uterus, tubes, and peritoneum (Figs. 6-12, 6-13, and 6-14); detection of ovulation; assessment of immunologic compatibility; and evaluation of psychogenic factors (Nelson & Marshall, 2004). The nurse can alleviate some of the anxiety associated with diagnostic testing by explaining to patients the timing and rationale for each test (Table 6-3). Test findings that are favorable to fertility are summarized in Box 6-6.

Assessment of male infertility. The systematic investigation of infertility in the male patient begins with a thorough history and physical examination. Assessment of the male patient starts with noninvasive tests.

Semen analysis. The basic test for male infertility is the semen analysis. A complete semen analysis, study of the effects of cervical mucus on sperm forward motility and survival, and evaluation of the sperm's ability to penetrate an ovum provide basic information. Semen is collected by ejaculation into a clean container or a plastic sheath that does not contain

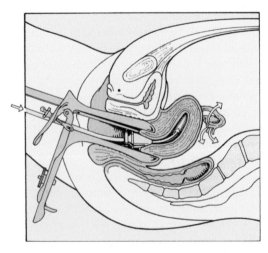

Fig. 6-12 Hysterosalpingography. Note that contrast medium flows through intrauterine cannula and out through the uterine tubes.

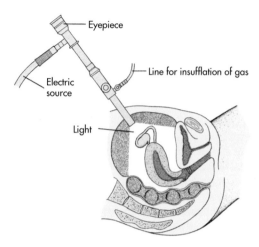

Fig. 6-13 Laparoscopy.

a spermicidal agent. The specimen is usually collected by masturbation after 2 to 5 days of abstinence from ejaculation. The semen is taken to the laboratory in a sealed container within 2 hours of ejaculation. Exposure to excessive heat or cold is avoided. Commonly accepted values based on the WHO criteria for semen characteristics are given in Box 6-7. If results are in the fertile range, no further sperm evaluation is necessary. If not within this range, the test is repeated. If results are still in the subfertile range, further evaluation is needed to identify the problem (Nelson & Marshall, 2004).

Seminal deficiency may be attributable to one or more of a variety of factors. The male is assessed for these factors: hypopituitarism; nutritional deficiency; debilitating or chronic disease; trauma; exposure to environmental hazards such as radiation and toxic substances; use of tobacco, alcohol, and

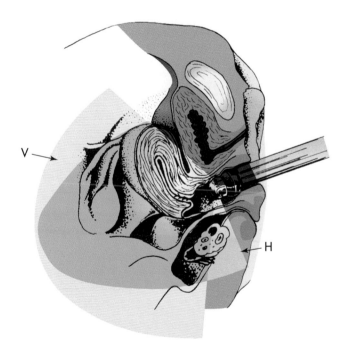

Fig. 6-14 Vaginal ultrasonography. Major scanning planes of transducer. *H,* horizontal; *V,* vertical.

marijuana; gonadotropic inadequacy; and obstructive lesions of the epididymis and vas deferens. Congenital absence of the vas deferens can occur more frequently in men with the gene for cystic fibrosis. If this abnormality is found, genetic counseling would be helpful before any fertility treatments (Keye, 2000). Hormone analyses are done for testosterone, gonadotropin, FSH, and LH. The sperm penetration assay may be used to evaluate the ability of sperm to penetrate an egg. Because human oocytes are not readily available, hamster eggs have been used as a substitute to evaluate sperm penetration abilities (no actual fertilization occurs). Testicular biopsy may be warranted.

Assessment of the couple

Postcoital test. The postcoital test (PCT) is one method used to test for adequacy of coital technique, cervical mucus, sperm, and degree of sperm penetration through cervical mucus. Intercourse is synchronized with the expected time of ovulation (as determined from evaluation of BBT, cervical mucus changes, and usual length of menstrual cycle or use of an LH detection kit to determine LH surge). The test is performed in the clinic or physician's office within several hours after ejaculation of semen into the vagina. A specimen of cervical mucus is obtained from the cervical os and examined under a microscope. The quality of mucus and the number of forward-moving sperm are noted. A PCT with good mucus and motile sperm is associated with fertility.

Examples of nursing diagnoses related to impaired fertility include the following:

- *Anxiety related to*
  −unknown outcome of diagnostic workup
- *Disturbed body image or situational low self-esteem related to*
  −impaired fertility
- *Risk for ineffective individual coping related to*
  −methods used in the investigation of impaired fertility
  −alternatives to therapy: child-free living or adoption
- *Interrupted family processes related to*
  −unmet expectations for pregnancy
- *Acute pain related to*
  −effects of diagnostic tests (or surgery)
- *Ineffective sexuality patterns related to*
  −loss of libido secondary to medically imposed restrictions
- *Deficient knowledge related to*
  −preconception risk factors
  −factors surrounding ovulation
  −factors surrounding fertility

Expected Outcomes of Care

The expected outcomes are phrased in patient-centered terms and may include that the couple will do the following:

- Verbalize understanding of the anatomy and physiology of the reproductive system

TABLE 6-3

Tests for Impaired Fertility

TEST OR EXAMINATION	TIMING (MENSTRUAL CYCLE DAYS)	RATIONALE
Hysterosalpingogram	7-10	Late follicular, early proliferative phase; will not disrupt a fertilized ovum; may open uterine tubes before time of ovulation
Postcoital test	1-2 days before ovulation	Ovulatory late proliferative phase; look for normal motile sperm in cervical mucus
Sperm immobilization antigen-antibody reaction	Variable, ovulation	Immunologic test to determine sperm and cervical mucus interaction
Assessment of cervical mucus	Variable, ovulation	Cervical mucus should have low viscosity, high spinnbarkeit
Ultrasound diagnosis of follicular collapse	Ovulation	Collapsed follicle is seen after ovulation
Serum assay of plasma progesterone	20-25	Midluteal midsecretory phase; check adequacy of corpus luteal production of progesterone
Basal body temperature	Chart entire cycle	Elevation occurs in response to progesterone, documents ovulation
Endometrial biopsy	21-27	Late luteal, late secretory phase; check endometrial response to progesterone and adequacy of luteal phase
Sperm penetration assay	After 2 days but no more than 1 week of abstinence	Evaluation of ability of sperm to penetrate an egg

BOX 6-6

Summary of Findings Favorable to Fertility

1 Follicular development, ovulation, and luteal development are supportive of pregnancy:
 a. Basal body temperature (BBT) (presumptive evidence of ovulatory cycles) is biphasic, with temperature elevation that persists for 12 to 14 days before menstruation
 b. Cervical mucus characteristics change appropriately during phases of menstrual cycle
 c. Laparoscopic visualization of pelvic organs verifies follicular and luteal development
2 The luteal phase is supportive of pregnancy:
 a. Levels of plasma progesterone are adequate
 b. Findings from endometrial biopsy samples are consistent with day of cycle
3 Cervical factors are receptive to sperm during expected time of ovulation:
 a. Cervical os is open
 b. Cervical mucus is clear, watery, abundant, and slippery and demonstrates good spinnbarkeit and arborization (fern pattern)
 c. Cervical examination does not reveal lesions or infections
 d. Postcoital test findings are satisfactory (adequate number of live, motile, normal sperm present in cervical mucus)
 e. No immunity to sperm demonstrated

4 The uterus and uterine tubes are supportive of pregnancy:
 a. Uterine and tubal patency are documented by:
  (1) Spillage of dye into peritoneal cavity
  (2) Outlines of uterine and tubal cavities of adequate size and shape, with no abnormalities
 b. Laparoscopic examination verifies normal development of internal genitals and absence of adhesions, infections, endometriosis, and other lesions
5 The male partner's reproductive structures are normal:
 a. No evidence of developmental anomalies of penis, testicular atrophy, or varicocele (varicose veins on the spermatic vein)
 b. No evidence of infection in prostate, seminal vesicles, and urethra
 c. Testes are >4 cm in largest diameter
6 Semen is supportive of pregnancy:
 a. Sperm (number per milliliter) are adequate in ejaculate
 b. Most sperm show normal morphology
 c. Most sperm are motile, forward moving
 d. No autoimmunity exists
 e. Seminal fluid is normal

BOX 6-7

Semen Analysis

- Liquefaction usually complete within 10 to 20 min
- Semen volume 2 ml to 6 ml
- Semen pH 7.2 to 8.0
- Sperm density 20 million to 200 million per milliliter
- Total sperm count 40 million per milliliter
- Normal morphology 30% (normal oval)
- Motility (important consideration in sperm evaluation)—percentage of forward-moving sperm estimated with respect to abnormally motile and nonmotile sperm, 50%
- White cell count 1 million per milliliter
- Ovum penetration test (may be done if further evaluation necessary)

Note: These values are not absolute but are only relative to final evaluation of the couple as a single reproductive unit. Values also differ according to source used as a reference. These values are based on WHO (1992).

- Verbalize understanding of treatment for any abnormalities identified through various tests and examinations (e.g., infections, blocked uterine tubes, sperm allergy, varicocele) and be able to make an informed decision about treatment
- Verbalize understanding of their potential to conceive
- Resolve guilt feelings and not need to focus blame
- Conceive or, failing to conceive, decide on an alternative acceptable to both of them (e.g., child-free living, adoption)

Plan of Care and Interventions

Psychosocial.   Within the United States, feelings connected to impaired fertility are numerous and complex. The origins of some of these feelings are myths, superstitions, and misinformation about the causes of infertility. Other feelings arise from the need to undergo many tests and examinations and from being different from others.

Infertility is recognized as a major life stressor that can affect self-esteem; relations with the spouse, family, and friends; and careers. Couples often need assistance in separating their concepts of success and failure related to treatment for infertility from personal success and failure. Recognizing the significance of infertility as a loss and resolving these feelings are crucial to putting infertility into perspective, even if treatment is successful (Nelson & Marshall, 2004).

Psychologic responses to a diagnosis of infertility may tax a couple's giving and receiving of physical and sexual closeness. The prescriptions and proscriptions for achieving conception may add tension to a couple's sexual functioning. Couples may report decreased desire for intercourse, orgasmic dysfunction, or midcycle erectile disorders.

To be able to deal comfortably with a couple's sexuality, nurses must be comfortable with their own sexuality so that they can better help couples understand why the private act of lovemaking must be shared with health care profession-

als. Nurses need up-to-date factual knowledge about human sexual practices and must be able to accept the preferences and activities of others without being judgmental. They must be skilled in interviewing and in therapeutic use of self, sensitive to the nonverbal cues of others, and knowledgeable regarding each couple's sociocultural and religious beliefs.

The support systems of the couple with impaired fertility must be explored. This exploration should include persons available to assist, their relationship to the couple, their ages, their availability, and the cultural or religious support that is available.

If the couple conceives, nurses need to be aware that the concerns and problems of the previously infertile couple may not be over. Many couples are overjoyed with the pregnancy; however, some are not. Some couples rearrange their lives, sense of self, and personal goals within their acceptance of their infertile state. The couple may feel that those who worked with them to identify and treat impaired fertility expect them to be happy with the pregnancy. The couple may be shocked to find that they themselves feel resentment because the pregnancy, once a cherished dream, now necessitates another change in goals, aspirations, and identities. The normal ambivalence toward pregnancy may be perceived as reneging on the original choice to become parents. The couple might choose to abort the pregnancy at this time. Other couples worry about miscarriage. If the couple wishes to continue with the pregnancy, they will need the care other expectant couples need. A history of impaired fertility is considered to be a risk factor for pregnancy.

If the couple does not conceive, they are assessed regarding their desire to be referred for help with adoption, therapeutic intrauterine insemination, other reproductive alternatives, or with choosing a child-free state. The couple may find a list of agencies, support groups, and other resources in their community helpful (see Resources at end of chapter).

Nonmedical.   Simple changes in lifestyle may be effective in the treatment of subfertile men. Only water-soluble lubricants should be used during intercourse because many commonly used lubricants contain spermicides or have spermicidal properties. High scrotal temperatures may be caused by daily hot tub bathing or saunas in which the testes are kept at temperatures too high for efficient spermatogenesis.

Treatment is available for women who have immunologic reactions to sperm. The use of condoms during genital intercourse for 6 to 12 months will reduce female antibody production in most women who have elevated antisperm antibody titers. After the serum reaction subsides, condoms are used at all times except at the expected time of ovulation. Approximately one third of couples with this problem conceive by following this course of action.

Changes in nutrition and habits may increase fertility for both men and women. For example, a well-balanced diet, exercise, decreased alcohol intake, not smoking or abusing drugs, and stress management may be effective.

Herbal alternative measures. Most herbal remedies have not been proven clinically to promote fertility or to be safe in early pregnancy and should be taken by the woman only as prescribed by a physician or nurse-midwife who has expertise in herbology. Relaxation, osteopathy, stress management (e.g., aromatherapy, yoga), and nutritional and exercise counseling have been reported to increase pregnancy rates in some women (Tiran & Mack, 2000). Herbal remedies that promote fertility in general include red clover flowers, nettle leaves, dong quai, St. John's wort, chastenberry, and false unicorn root (Weed, 1986). Vitamin E, calcium, and magnesium may promote fertility and conception (Tiran & Mack, 2000). Herbs to avoid while trying to conceive include licorice root, yarrow, wormwood, ephedra, fennel, goldenseal, lavender, juniper, flaxseed, pennyroyal, passionflower, wild cherry, cascara, sage, thyme, and periwinkle (Kennedy, Griffin, & Frishman, 1998; Sampey, Bourque, & Wren, 2004).

Medical. Pharmacologic therapy for female infertility is often directed at treating ovulatory dysfunction either by stimulating ovulation or by enhancing ovulation so that more oocytes mature. The most common medications include clomiphene citrate, human menopausal gonadotropin (HMG), FSH, recombinant FSH, and human chorionic gonadotropin. GnRH agonists, progesterone, and bromocriptine are also used (Leibowitz & Hoffman, 2000; Nelson & Marshall, 2004). Table 6-4 describes common medications used for treating infertility. Thyroid-stimulating hormone is indicated if the woman has hypothyroidism. Combined oral contraceptives, GnRH agonists, or danazol may be used to treat endometriosis; progesterone may be used to treat luteal phase defects (Nelson & Marshall, 2004).

Drug therapy may be indicated for male infertility. Problems with the thyroid or adrenal glands are corrected with appropriate medications. Infections are identified and treated

---

TABLE 6-4

Medications Used in the Treatment of Infertility

DRUG	INDICATION	MECHANISM OF ACTION	DOSE	SELECTED SIDE EFFECTS
Clomiphene citrate	Ovulation induction, treatment of luteal-phase inadequacy	Thought to bind to estrogen receptors in the pituitary, blocking them from detecting estrogen	Tablets, starting with 50 mg/day for 5 days beginning on fifth day of menses; if ovulation does not occur, may increase dose next cycle-variable dosage	Vasomotor flushes, abdominal discomfort, nausea and vomiting, breast tenderness, ovarian enlargement
Menotropins (human menopausal gonadotropins)	Ovarian follicular growth and maturation	LH and FSH in 1:1 ratio, direct stimulation of ovarian follicle; given sequentially with hCG to induce ovulation	Intramuscular injections, dosage regimen variable based on ovarian response. Initial dose is 75 international units of FSH and 75 international units of LH (1 ampule) daily for 7-12 days followed by 10,000 international units hCG	Ovarian enlargement, ovarian hyperstimulation, local irritation at injection site, multifetal gestations
Follitropins (purified FSH)	Treatment of polycystic ovarian disease; follicle stimulation for assisted reproductive techiques	Direct action on ovarian follicle	Subcutaneous or intramuscular injections, dosage regimen variable	Ovarian enlargement, ovarian hyperstimulation, local irritation at injection site, multifetal gestations
Human chorionic gonadotropin (hCG)	Ovulation induction	Direct action on ovarian follicle to stimulate meiosis and rupture of the follicle	5000-10,000 international units intramuscularly 1 day after last dose of menotropins; dosage regimen variable	Local irritation at injection site; headaches, irritability, edema, depression, fatigue

TABLE 6-4

Medications Used in the Treatment of Infertility—cont'd

DRUG	INDICATION	MECHANISM OF ACTION	DOSE	SELECTED SIDE EFFECTS
Androgens (danazol)	Treatment of endometriosis	Combination of estrogen and androgen suppresses ovarian activity, eliminating stimulation to endometrial glands and stroma, with resultant shrinkage and disappearance	200-800 mg/day for 3 to 6 mo	Mild hirsutism, acne, edema and weight gain, increase of liver enzyme levels
GnRH agonists (nafarelin acetate, leuprolide acetate)	Treatment of endometriosis, uterine fibroids	Desensitization and downward regulation of GnRH receptors of pituitary, resulting in suppression of LH, FSH, and ovarian function	Nafarelin, 200 mcg (1 spray) intranasally twice daily for 6 mo; leuprolide acetate- depot 3.75 mg IM every 28 days for 6 mo	Nafarelin irritation, nosebleeds; both Nafarelin and leuprolide–hot flashes, vaginal dryness, myalgia and arthralgia, headaches, mild bone loss (usually reversible within 12-18 mo after treatment)
Progesterone (progesterone in oil, Progestoral)	Treatment of luteal-phase inadequacy	Direct stimulation of endometrium	Vaginal suppositories, 25-50 mg twice daily or 50 mg every night; rectal suppositories, 12.25 mg every 12 hr; progesterone capsules, 100 mg by mouth three times daily	Breast tenderness, local irritation, headaches
GnRH antagonists (ganirelix acetate, cetrorelix acetate)	Controlled ovarian stimulation for infertility treatment	Suppresses gonadotropin secretion; inhibits premature LH surges in women undergoing ovarian hyperstimulation	250 mcg daily subcutaneously usually in the early to mid-follicular phase of the menstrual cycle; usually followed by hCG administration	Abdominal pain, headache, vaginal bleeding, irritation at the injection site

References. Clinical Pharmacology (2005). *Nafarelin and Leuprolide.* Gold Standard Multimedia. Internet document available at http://cp.gsm.com (assessed June 24, 2005); Leibowitz, D., & Hoffman, J. (2000). Fertility drug therapies: Past, present, and future. *Journal of Obstetric, Gynecologic, and Neonatal Nursing, 29*(2), 201-210; Weiner, C., & Buhimschi, C. (2004). *Drugs for pregnant and lactating women.* Philadelphia: Churchill Livingstone. *FSH,* follicle-stimulating hormone; *GnRH,* gonadotropin-releasing hormone; *LH,* luteinizing hormone.

promptly with antimicrobials. FSH, HMG, and clomiphene may be used to stimulate spermatogenesis in males with hypogonadism (Leibowitz & Hoffman, 2000).

The primary care provider is responsible for informing patients fully about the prescribed medications. However, the nurse must be ready to answer patients' questions and to confirm their understanding of the drug, its administration, potential side effects, and expected outcomes. Because information varies with each drug, the nurse needs to consult the medication package inserts, pharmacology references, physician, and pharmacist as necessary.

Surgical.   A number of surgical procedures can be used to treat problems causing female infertility. Ovarian tumors must be excised. When possible, functional ovarian tissue is left intact. Scar tissue adhesions caused by chronic infections may cover much or all of the ovary. These adhesions usually necessitate surgery to free and expose the ovary so that ovulation can occur.

Hysterosalpingography is useful for identification of tubal obstruction and also for the release of blockage (see Fig. 6-12). During laparoscopy, delicate adhesions may be divided and removed and endometrial implants may be destroyed by electrocoagulation or laser (see Fig. 6-13). Laparotomy and even microsurgery may be required to do extensive repair of the damaged tube. Prognosis depends on the degree to which tubal patency and function can be restored.

Issues to Be Addressed by Infertile Couples before Treatment

- Risks of multiple gestation
- Possible need for multifetal reduction
- Possible need for donor oocytes, sperm, or embryos or gestational carrier (surrogate mother)
- Freezing of embryos for later use
- Possible risks of long-term effects of medications and treatment on women, children, and families

Surgical removal of tumors or fibroids involving the endometrium or uterus often improves the woman's chance of conceiving and maintaining the pregnancy to viability. Surgical treatment of uterine tumors or maldevelopment that results in successful pregnancy usually requires birth by cesarean surgery near term gestation to prevent uterine rupture as a result of weakness of the area of surgical healing.

Surgical procedures may also be used for problems causing male infertility. Surgical repair of varicocele has been relatively successful in increasing sperm counts but not fertility rates.

Reproductive alternatives

Assisted reproductive therapies. There have been remarkable developments in reproductive medicine. **Assisted reproductive therapies (ARTs)** have created ethical and legal issues (Box 6-8). The lack of information or misleading information about success rates and the risks and benefits of treatment alternatives prevents couples from making informed decisions. Nurses can provide information so that couples have an accurate understanding of their chances for a successful pregnancy and live birth. Some of the ARTs for treatment of infertility include **in vitro fertilization** procedures including in vitro fertilization-embryo transfer (IVF-ET), gamete intrafallopian transfer (GIFT) (Fig. 6-15), zygote intrafallopian transfer (ZIFT), ovum transfer (oocyte donation), embryo adoption, embryo hosting, surrogate mothering, **therapeutic donor insemination (TDI),** intracytoplasmic sperm injection, and assisted hatching. Table 6-5 describes these procedures and the possible indications for the ARTs.

LEGAL TIP **Cryopreservation of Human Embryos**

Couples who have excess embryos frozen for later transfer must be fully informed before consenting to the procedure, to make decisions regarding the disposal of embryos in the event of (1) death, (2) divorce, or (3) the decision that the couple no longer wants the embryos at a later time.

Complications. Other than the established risks associated with laparoscopy and general anesthesia, few risks are associated with IVF-ET, GIFT, and ZIFT. The more common transvaginal needle aspiration requires only local or

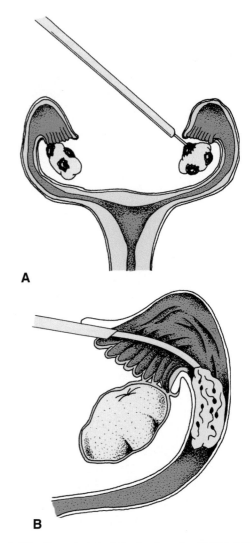

A

B

Fig. 6-15 Gamete intrafallopian transfer (GIFT). **A,** Through laparoscopy, a ripe follicle is located and fluid containing the egg is removed. **B,** The sperm and egg are placed separately in the uterine tube, where fertilization occurs.

intravenous analgesia. Congenital anomalies occur no more frequently than among naturally conceived embryos. Multiple gestations are more likely and are associated with increased risks for both the mother and infants (Wright, Schieve, Reynolds, Jeng, & Kissin, 2004). Ectopic pregnancies occur more often as well, and these carry a significant maternal risk. There is no increase in maternal or perinatal complications with TDI; the same frequencies of anomalies (approximately 5%) and obstetric complications (between 5% and 10%) that accompany natural insemination (through sexual intercourse) apply also to TDI.

Preimplantation Genetic Diagnosis. Preimplantation genetic diagnosis (PGD) is a form of early genetic testing designed to eliminate embryos with serious genetic defects before implantation through one of the ARTs and to prevent later termination of the pregnancy for genetic reasons. There are over 20 centers worldwide where PGD

TABLE 6-5

Assisted Reproductive Therapies

PROCEDURE	DEFINITION	INDICATIONS
In vitro fertilization–embryo transfer (IVF-ET)	A woman's eggs are collected from her ovaries, fertilized in the laboratory with sperm, and transferred to her uterus after normal embryo development has occurred.	Tubal disease or blockage; severe male infertility; endometriosis; unexplained infertility; cervical factor; immunologic infertility
Gamete intrafallopian transfer (GIFT)	Oocytes are retrieved from the ovary, placed in a catheter with washed motile sperm, and immediately transferred into the fimbriated end of the uterine tube. Fertilization occurs in the uterine tube.	Same as for IVF-ET, except there must be normal tubal anatomy, patency, and absence of previous tubal disease in at least one uterine tube
IVF-ET and GIFT with donor sperm	This process is the same as described above except in cases where the male partner's fertility is severely compromised and donor sperm can be used; if donor sperm are used, the woman must have indications for IVF and GIFT.	Severe male infertility; azoospermia; indications for IVF-ET or GIFT
Zygote intrafallopian transfer (ZIFT)	This process is similar to IVF-ET; after in vitro fertilization the ova are placed in one uterine tube during the zygote stage.	Same as for GIFT
Donor oocyte	Eggs are donated by an IVF procedure, and the donated eggs are inseminated. The embryos are transferred into the recipient's uterus, which is hormonally prepared with estrogen/progesterone therapy.	Early menopause; surgical removal of ovaries; congenitally absent ovaries; autosomal or sex-linked disorders; lack of fertilization in repeated IVF attempts because of subtle oocyte abnormalities or defects in oocyte-spermatozoa interaction
Donor embryo (embryo adoption)	A donated embryo is transferred to the uterus of an infertile woman at the appropriate time (normal or induced) of the menstrual cycle.	Infertility not resolved by less aggressive forms of therapy; absence of ovaries; male partner is azoospermic or is severely compromised
Gestational carrier (embryo host); surrogate mother	A couple undertakes an IVF cycle, and the embryo(s) is transferred to the uterus of another woman (the carrier) who has contracted with the couple to carry the baby to term. The carrier has no genetic investment in the child. Surrogate motherhood is a process by which a woman is inseminated with semen from the infertile woman's partner and then carries the baby until birth.	Congenital absence or surgical removal of uterus; a reproductively impaired uterus, myomas, uterine adhesions, or other congenital abnormalities; a medical condition that might be life-threatening during pregnancy, such as diabetes, immunologic problems, or severe heart, kidney, or liver disease
Therapeutic donor insemination (TDI)	Donor sperm are used to inseminate the female partner.	Male partner is azoospermic or has a very low sperm count; couple has a genetic defect; male partner has antisperm antibodies
Intracytoplasmic sperm injection	Selection of one sperm cell that is injected directly into the egg to achieve fertilization. Used with IVF.	Same as TDI
Assisted hatching	The zona pellucida is penetrated chemically or manually to create an opening for the dividing embryo to hatch and implant into uterine wall.	Recurrent miscarriages; to improve implantation rate in women with previously unsuccessful IVF attempts; advanced age

Data from American Society for Reproductive Medicine (ASRM). (2005). *Frequently asked questions about infertility.* Internet document available at www.asrm.org (accessed June 27, 2005); Angard, N. (1999). Diagnosis infertility. *AWHONN Lifelines, 3*(3), 22-29; Kennedy, H., Griffin, M., & Frishman, G. (1998). Enabling conception and pregnancy: Midwifery care of women experiencing infertility. *Journal of Nurse-Midwifery, 43*(3), 190-207; Stenchever, M., Droegemueller, W., Herbst, A., & Mishell, D. (2001). *Comprehensive gynecology* (4th ed.). St. Louis: Mosby; Van Voorhis, B. et al. (1998). Cost effective treatment of the infertile couple. *Fertility and Sterility, 70*(6), 995-1005.

PLAN OF CARE   *Infertility*

NURSING DIAGNOSIS Deficient knowledge related to lack of understanding of the reproductive process with regard to conception as evidenced by patient questions

Expected Outcome *Patient and partner will verbalize understanding of the components of the reproductive process, common problems leading to infertility, usual infertility testing, and the importance of completing testing in a timely manner.*

Nursing Interventions/*Rationales*

- Assess patient's current level of understanding of the factors promoting conception *to identify gaps or misconceptions in knowledge base.*
- Provide information in a supportive manner regarding factors promoting conception including common factors leading to infertility of either partner *to raise patient's awareness and promote trust in caregiver.*
- Identify and describe the basic infertility tests and the rationale for precise scheduling *to enhance completion of the diagnostic phase of the infertility workup.*

NURSING DIAGNOSIS Risk for ineffective individual coping related to inability to conceive as evidenced by patient and partner statements

Expected Outcome *Patient and partner will identify situational stressors and positive coping* methods to deal with testing and unknown outcomes.

Nursing Interventions/*Rationales*

- Provide opportunities through therapeutic communication to discuss feelings and concerns *to identify common feelings and perceived stressors.*
- Evaluate couple's support system, including support of each other during this process, *to identify any barriers to effective coping.*
- Identify support groups and refer as needed *to enhance coping by sharing experiences with other couples experiencing similar problems.*

NURSING DIAGNOSIS Hopelessness related to inability to conceive as evidenced by woman's and partner's statements

Expected Outcome *Woman and partner will verbalize a realistic plan to decrease feelings of hopelessness.*

Nursing Interventions/*Rationales*

- Provide support for couple while grieving for loss of fertility *to allow couple to work through feelings.*
- Assess for behaviors indicating possible depression, anger, and frustration *to prevent impending crisis.*
- Refer to support groups *to promote a common bond with other couples during expression of feelings and concerns*

---

is being used clinically. Couples must be counseled about their options and choices, as well as the implications of their choices, when genetic analysis is considered (Jones, 2000).

Adoption. Couples may choose to build their family by adopting children who are not their own biologically. However, with increased availability of birth control and abortion and increasing numbers of single mothers keeping their babies, the adoption of Caucasian infants is extremely limited. Minority infants, infants with special needs, older children, and foreign adoptions are other options.

Couples who decide to adopt a child have decided that being a parent and having a child is more important than the actual process of birthing the child. The birth process is a small aspect of having a baby and becoming a parent. So much emphasis is placed on being pregnant and having a child composed of one's own genetic makeup that the focus of the reason to have a child becomes cloudy. The question to be answered by couples who are considering adoption is, "What is important to you—that you become parents or that you go through the experience of pregnancy and birth?" Nurses should have information on options for adoption available for couples or refer them to community resources for further assistance (ASRM, 2003; Salzer, 2000) (see Resources at end of chapter).

Evaluation

Evaluation of the effectiveness of care of the couple experiencing impaired fertility is based on the previously stated outcomes (see Plan of Care).

COMMUNITY ACTIVITY

Contraception

Visit a clinic that provides family planning services in your community. What are the fee schedules for women with and without insurance? Are local state or federal funds available? What are the hours of the clinic? Is the clinic location easily accessed by public and private transportation? How long is a typical wait for a scheduled appointment? What methods of contraception are available? How are women taught how to use a method?

Abortion

What are the laws in your state related to abortion, informed consent, and treatment of minors who request an abortion? What methods of abortion are available in your community? How easily is emergency contraception obtained in your community?

Infertility

What adoption options are available in your community? What are the services provided by each option and what are the costs? What are the procedures for adoption associated with each option? How well are the options publicized in the community? Is there a support network and, if so, how do prospective adopting parents gain access?

Key Points

- A variety of contraceptive methods is available with various effectiveness rates, advantages, and disadvantages.
- Nurses need to help couples choose the contraceptive method or methods best suited to them.
- Effective contraceptives are available through both prescription and nonprescription sources.
- A variety of techniques are available to enhance the effectiveness of periodic abstinence in motivated couples who prefer this natural method.
- Hormonal contraception includes both precoital and postcoital prevention through various modalities and requires thorough patient education.
- Emergency contraceptive methods should be initiated as soon as possible after unprotected intercourse, but no later than 120 hours.
- The barrier methods of diaphragm and cervical cap provide safe and effective contraception for women or couples motivated to use them consistently and correctly.
- Proper use of latex condoms provides protection against STIs.
- Tubal ligations and vasectomies are permanent sterilization methods that have become two of the most widely used methods of contraception.

- Elective abortion performed in the first trimester is safer than an abortion performed in the second trimester.
- The most common complications of elective abortion include infection, retained products of conception, and excessive vaginal bleeding.
- Major psychologic sequelae of elective abortion are rare.
- Infertility is the inability to conceive and carry a child to term gestation at a time the couple has chosen to do so.
- Infertility affects between 10% and 15% of otherwise healthy adults. Infertility increases in women older than 40 years.
- In the United States, 80% of infertility has an identified cause related to factors involving the man and the woman and 20% of infertility is related to unexplained causes.
- Common etiologic factors of infertility include decreased sperm production, ovulation disorders, tubal occlusion, and endometriosis.
- Reproductive alternatives for family building include IVF-ET, GIFT, ZIFT, oocyte donation, embryo donation, TDI, surrogate motherhood, and adoption.

Answer Guidelines to Critical Thinking Exercises

Contraception

1 Yes, there is sufficient evidence for the nurse to discuss methods of birth control that are effective but also not directly related to sexual activity.

2 a. A method that does not fit the woman's personal lifestyle is likely not to be used correctly or consistently. Personal considerations for a 25-year-old woman with three children may reflect the desire to prevent further pregnancies or to space her pregnancies. Questions the woman may ask herself when deciding on a method include (Trussell, 2004): Have I had problems with this method before? Does this method affect my menstrual periods? Could this method cause me serious complications? Will I have trouble remembering how to use this method? Will I have trouble remembering to use this method?

b. Efficacy or contraceptive effectiveness is the most frequently asked question about methods of birth control. Pregnancy rates for typical use (actual use including inconsistent and incorrect use) and perfect use (consistently following directions for use) are often used to describe efficacy. Factors that influence efficacy include inherent efficacy (methods such as sterilization and injectable hormones allow little room for user error) and characteristics of the user (age, frequency of intercourse, imperfect use, menstrual cycle regularity).

c. Arleta should be fully informed about the contraceptive method she chooses. Informed consent includes information about risks and benefits, information about alternatives, an opportunity to ask questions, an opportunity to make her decision or to change her mind, and information about how to use the method.

3 The nursing priority at this time is to provide information about the methods that are effective but low maintenance, such as an IUD or Depo-Provera injections.

4 Yes, there is evidence that both of these methods provide effective contraception with low failure rates. The failure rate for typical use for the IUD is less than 1%, whereas the rate for the Depo-Provera injections is 3%.

5 Arleta may decide that she would like to try oral contraception again, or she may decide that she would like a sterilization procedure. Both would provide protection (typical failure rate for OCPs is 8% and for sterilization is less than 1%), and neither would be a method that has to be used at time of sexual activity.

Abortion

1 Yes, at this stage of pregnancy vacuum aspiration is the most common procedure done. Although medical abortion can be done in the first trimester, its use is usually up to 49 days after the first day of the last menstrual period. Second-trimester abortions are associated with more complications.

2 a. The procedure is performed using local anesthesia in the clinic office. Meghan's cervix will be dilated and the products of conception will be evacuated from the uterus. Meghan may feel cramping during the procedure. She will likely have vaginal bleeding and mild cramping afterward. Excessive bleeding and infections are the most common complications. Menses should return within 4 to 6 weeks.

b. Meghan may experience some fear or anxiety during the procedure. Various feelings may be experienced after the abortion and include depression, guilt, regret, and relief.

Information about postabortion counseling may be needed. Support by the nurse and friends and family if possible will help Meghan cope with any of these reactions

c. The abortion is unlikely to affect future childbearing; however Meghan needs counseling about contraception. If she had unprotected intercourse because she did not like the method she was using, she may need to make another choice. She may need some counseling on how to say no or how to recognize situations that could lead to risky behaviors.

3 Nursing priorities at this time are to ensure that Meghan knows the options available and then to support her in her decision. Patient teaching about the procedure, self-care after the procedure, and contraception are needed.

4 Yes, there are excellent data about the safety of the procedure and about a woman's response to the procedure (Goss, 2002; Stewart, Ellertson, & Cates, 2004).

5 Meghan does have other options. After learning about the abortion procedures, she may decide not to have an abortion at all, to have a second-trimester abortion, or to continue the pregnancy and either keep the baby or give it up for adoption. Meghan should be given the opportunity to discuss her feelings about pregnancy, abortion, and the impact of her choice on her future and to make her decision without feeling coerced by anyone.

Infertility

1 No. Since a cause of infertility has not been determined, the type of procedure that can be used cannot be identified. The prognosis is determined by the cause and by the therapy.

2 a. Infertility increases with the age of the woman, especially in those over age 40. Fertility naturally decreases with age, and the woman may develop problems that affect fertility such as endometriosis and ovulatory dysfunction.

b. Feelings about infertility are numerous and complex. Infertility can affect the man or woman's self-esteem, their careers, and their relationships with each other, family members, and friends. Frustration, isolation, depression, and stress are common reactions. Infertility is seen as a loss, and couples must work through their grief to some resolution, whether it is choosing to try reproductive therapies or to deal with not having a child.

3 It is essential that an assessment be made first to collect data about both Bob and Shirley. This assessment should include a history and physical examination and laboratory evaluation. Critical elements for Shirley include menstrual history, STIs, reproductive problems, coital activity, and endocrinologic factors. A semen analysis is the initial test for Bob. If a course is identified, information should then be provided about options for treatment including risks, costs, and the likelihood of being successful.

4 Yes, there is evidence to support the conclusion of correcting Shirley's understanding about what an infertility workup is and why a treatment is not implemented until after a cause has been identified.

5 Bob and Shirley may decide not to pursue infertility treatment; they may decide to try for adoption or to live a child-free life.

Resources

American College of Obstetricians and Gynecologists (ACOG)
409 12th St., SW
Washington, DC 20024
800-762-2264
www.acog.com

American Society for Reproductive Medicine (ASRM)
1209 Montgomery Hwy.
Birmingham, AL 35316
205-978-5000
www.asrm.com

Association of Reproductive Health Professionals
2401 Pennsylvania Ave., NW, Suite 350
Washington, DC 20037
202-466-3825
www.arhp.org

Contraception Online
www.contraceptiononline.org

Emergency Contraception Hotline
P.O. Box 33344
Washington, DC 20033
888-668-2528
www.not-2-late.com

Endometriosis Association
8585 N. 76th Place
Milwaukee, WI 53223
414-355-2200
800-992-3636
www.endometriosisassn.org

Georgia Reproductive Services
5445 Meridian Mark Dr., Suite 270
Atlanta, GA 30342
404-843-2229
www.ivf.com

International Council on Infertility
Information Dissemination
703-379-9178
www.inciid.org

Internet Health Resources–Infertility
Resources for Consumers
www.ihr.com/infertility/

National Abortion Federation
1755 Massachusetts Ave., NW, Suite 600
Washington, DC 20036
800-772-9100 Consumer Hotline
www.prochoice.org

National Clearinghouse for Family
Planning Information
P.O. Box 10716
Rockville, MD 20850
703-558-4990

National Women's Health
Resource Center
120 Albany St., Suite 820
New Brunswick, NJ 08901
877-986-9472
www.healthywomen.org

Office of Population Research
Princeton University
21 Prospect Ave.
Princeton, NJ 08544
609-258-4870
www.ec.princeton.edu

Planned Parenthood Federation of America, Inc.
810 Seventh Ave.
New York, NY 10019
800-669-0156
www.plannedparenthood.org

Resolve–The National Fertility Association
7910 Woodmont Ave, Suite 1350
Bethesda MD 20814
301-652-8585
888-623-0744 (Helpline)
www.resolve.org

References

American College of Obstetricians and Gynecologists (ACOG). (2001). *Emergency oral contraception: ACOG Practice Bulletin no. 25.* Washington, DC: ACOG.

American Society for Reproductive Medicine (ASRM). (2003). *Patient's fact sheet: Adoption.* Internet document available at http://www.asrm.org (accessed December 23, 2004).

American Society for Reproductive Medicine (ASRM). (2005). *Frequently asked questions about infertility.* Internet document available at http://www.asrm.org (accessed June 27, 2005).

Angard, N. (1999). Diagnosis infertility. *AWHONN Lifelines, 3*(3), 22-29.

Angard, N. (2000). Seeking coverage for infertility. *AWHONN Lifelines, 4*(3), 22-24.

Arevalo, M., Jennings, V., Nikula, M., & Sinai, I. (2004). Efficacy of the new TwoDay method of family planning. *Fertility and Sterility, 82*(4), 885-892.

Association of Women's Health, Obstetric and Neonatal Nurses. (1999). *Nurses' rights and responsibilities related to abortion and sterilization. Policy Position Statement.* Internet Document available at http://www.awhonn.org. (accessed June 26, 2005).

Barron, M., & Daly, K. (2001). Expert in fertility appreciation: The Creighton model practitioner. *Journal of Obstetric, Gynecologic, and Neonatal Nursing, 30*(4), 386-391.

Cates, W., & Raymond, E. (2004). Vaginal spermicides. In R. Hatcher et al. (Eds.), *Contraceptive technology* (18th ed.). New York: Ardent Media.

Cates, W., & Stewart, F. (2004). Vaginal barriers: The female condom, diaphragm, contraceptive sponge, cervical cap, Lea's Shield and FemCap. In R. Hatcher et al. (Eds.), *Contraceptive technology* (18th ed.). New York: Ardent Media.

Centers for Disease Control and Prevention. (2002). Sexually transmitted disease treatment guidelines, 2002. *Morbidity and Mortality Weekly Report, 51*(RR-6), 1-80.

Clinical Pharmacology. (2005). *Nafarelin and Leuprolide.* Gold Standard Multimedia. Internet document available at http://cp.gsm.com (accessed June 24, 2005.

Contraception Online. (2003). Facts about injectable contraception. *The Contraception Report, 14*(3). Internet document available at http://www.contraceptiononline.org/contrareport/article01.cfm?art=256 (accessed October 27, 2004).

CycleBeads. (2003). *Frequently asked questions.* Internet document available at http://cyclebeads.com/ (accessed December 28, 2004).

Cunningham, F., Leveno, K., Blooms, S., Hauth, J., Gilstrap, L., & Wenstrom, K. (2001). *Williams obstetrics* (22nd ed.). New York: McGraw-Hill.

D'Avanzo, C., & Geissler, E. (2003). *Pocket guide to cultural health assessment* (3rd ed.). St. Louis: Mosby.

Ellertson, C., Evans, M., Ferden, S., Leadbetter, C., Spears, A., Johnstone, K, & Trusell, J. (2003). Extending the time limit for stating the Yuzpe regimen of emergency contraception to 120 hours. *Obstetrics & Gynecology, 101,* 1165-1171.

Essure. (2004). *Patient Information Booklet.* Internet document available at http://www.essure.com/Patient_Information_Booklet.pdf (accessed December 5, 2004).

Female Condom: The Product. Internet document available at http://www.femalehealth.com/theproduct.html (accessed November 28, 2004).

Goss, G. (2002). Pregnancy termination: Understanding and supporting women who undergo medical abortion. *AWHONN Lifelines, 6*(1), 46-50.

Grimes, D. (2004). Intrauterine devices (IUDs). In R. Hatcher et al. (Eds.). *Contraceptive technology* (18th ed.). New York: Ardent Media.

Hatcher, R. (2004). Depo-Provera injections, implants, and progestin-only pills (minipills). In R. Hatcher et al. (Eds.), *Contraceptive technology* (18th ed.). New York: Ardent Media.

Hatcher, R., & Nelson, A. (2004). Combined hormonal contraceptive methods. In R. Hatcher et al. (Eds.), *Contraceptive technology* (18th ed.). New York: Ardent Media.

Hatcher, R., Zieman, M., Cwiak, C., Darney, P., Creinin, M., & Stosur, H. (2004). *A pocket guide to managing contraception.* Tiger, GA: Bridging the Gap Foundation.

Hutti, M. (2003). New and emerging contraceptive methods: Nurses can help women make wise choices. *AWHONN Lifelines, 6*(1), 32-39.

Institute for Natural Family Planning Services. (2005). *Definition of natural family planning. Marquette method.* Internet document available at http://www.marquette.edu/nursing/nfp. (accessed June 26, 2005).

Institute of Reproductive Health. (March 2003). *Standard Days Method.* Internet document available at http://www.irh.org (accessed December 4, 2004).

Jennings, V., Arevalo, M., & Kowal, D. (2004). Fertility awareness-based methods. In R. Hatcher et al. (Eds.), *Contraceptive technology* (18th ed.). New York: Ardent Media.

Joint Commission on Accreditation of Healthcare Organizations. (2000). Standards, infants, and examples for managing staff requests. In *Comprehension accreditation manual for hospitals: the official handbook.* Oakbrook Terrace, IL: Author.

Jones, S. (2000). Reproductive genetic technologies. Exploring ethical and policy implications. *AWHONN Lifelines, 4*(5), 33-36.

Kahn, J., Becker, B., MacIsaa, L., Amor, J., Neuhaus, J., Olkin, I., et al. (2000). The efficacy of medical abortion: A meta-analysis. *Contraception, 61*(1), 29-40.

Kennedy, H., Griffin, M., & Frishman, G. (1998). Enabling conception and pregnancy: Midwifery care of women experiencing infertility, *Journal of Nurse-Midwifery, 43*(3), 190-207.

Kennedy, K., & Trussell, J. (2004). Postpartum contraception and lactation. In R. Hatcher et al. (Eds.), *Contraceptive technology* (18th ed.). New York: Ardent Media.

Kettyle, E., & Klima, C. (2002). Adolescent emergency contraception: Attitudes and practices of certified nurse-midwives. *Journal of Midwifery & Women's Health, 47*(2), 68-73.

Keye, W. (2000). Medical aspects of infertility for the counselor. In H. Burns & S. Covington (Eds.), *Infertility counseling: A comprehensive handbook for clinicians.* New York: Parthenon Publishing Group.

King, R. (2003). Subfecundity and anxiety in a nationally representative sample. *Social Science Medicine, 56*(4), 739-751.

Kowal, D. (2004). Coitus interruptus (withdrawal). In R. Hatcher et al. (Eds.), *Contraceptive technology* (18th ed.). New York: Ardent Media.

Leibowitz, D., & Hoffman, J. (2000). Fertility drug therapies: Past, present, and future. *Journal of Obstetric, Gynecologic, and Neonatal Nursing, 29*(2), 201-210.

Marchbanks, P., McDonald, J., Wilson, H., Folger, S., Mandel, M., Daling, J., et al. (2002). Oral contraceptives and the risk of breast cancer. *New England Journal of Medicine, 346*(26), 2025-2032.

National Abortion Federation. (2003). *Clinical policy guidelines.* Washington, DC: National Abortion Federation.

National Campus Life Network. (2005). *Frequently Asked Questions. How many abortions are performed in Canada?* Internet document available at http://www.ncln.ca/resources (accessed June 26, 2005).

Nelson, A., & Marshall, J. (2004). Impaired fertility. In R. Hatcher et al. (Eds.), *Contraceptive technology* (18th ed.). New York: Ardent Media.

Planned Parenthood. (2004). *Diaphragms* (updated July, 2004). Internet document available at http://www.plannedparenthood.org/bc/diaphragms.htm (accessed November 27, 2004).

Pollack, A., Carignan, C., & Jacobstein, R. (2004). Female and male sterilization. In R. Hatcher et al. (Eds.), *Contraceptive technology* (18th ed.). New York: Ardent Media.

Robinson, D., Dollins, A., & McConlogue-O'Shaughnessy, L. (2000). Care of the woman before and after an elective abortion. *American Journal of Nurse Practitioners, 4*(3), 17-29.

Salzer, L. (2000). Adoption after infertility. In H. Burns & S. Covington (Eds.), *Infertility counseling: A comprehensive handbook for clinicians.* New York: Parthenon Publishing Group.

Sampey, A., Bourque, J., & Wren, K. (2004). Learning scope: Herbal medicines. *Advance for Nurses, 6*(25), 13-19.

Santoro, D. (2004). *A short summary of the criminal law surrounding abortion.* Internet document available at http://www.ncln.ca/articles (accessed June 26, 2005).

Say, L., Kulier, R., Gülmezoglu, M., & Campana, A. (2002). Medical versus surgical methods for first trimester termination of pregnancy (Cochrane Review). In *The Cochrane Library,* Issue 4, 2005. Chichester, UK: John Wiley & Sons.

Sherrod, R. (2004). Understanding the emotional aspects of infertility: Implications for nursing practice. *Journal of Psychosocial Nursing and Mental Health Services, 42*(3), 40-49.

Sinai, I., Jennings, V., & Arevalo, M. (2004). The importance of screening and monitoring the standard day method and cycle regularity. *Contraception, 69*(3)201-206.

Stenchever, M., Droegemueller, W., Herbst, A., & Mishell, D. (2001). *Comprehensive gynecology* (4th ed.). St. Louis: Mosby.

Stewart, F., Ellertson, C., & Cates, W. (2004). Abortion. In R. Hatcher et al. (Eds.), *Contraceptive technology* (18th ed.). New York: Ardent Media.

Stewart, F., Trussell, J., & Van Look, P. (2004). Emergency contraception. In R. Hatcher et al. (Eds.), *Contraceptive technology* (18th ed.). New York: Ardent Media Inc.

Strauss, L., Herdon, J., Chang, J., Parker, W., Levy, D., Bowens, S., Berg, C., CDC. (2004). Abortion surveillance–United States, 2001. *Morbidity and Mortality Weekly Report Surveillance Summaries, 53*(9), 1-32.

Taylor, D., & Hwang, A. (2003-2004). Mifepristone for medical abortion: Exploring new options for nurse practitioners. *AWHONN Lifelines, 7*(6), 524-529.

Tiran, D., & Mack, S. (2000). *Complementary therapies for pregnancy and childbirth.* Edinburgh: Baillière Tindall.

Trussell, J. (2004). Contraceptive efficacy. In R. Hatcher et al. (Eds.), *Contraceptive technology* (18th ed.). New York: Ardent Media.

U.S. Food and Drug Administration (FDA). (2003). *Birth control guide.* Internet document available at http://www.fda.gov/fdac/features/1997/babyguide2.pdf (accessed November 15, 2004).

Van Voorhis, B., et al. (1998). Cost-effective treatment of the infertile couple. *Fertility and Sterility, 70*(6), 995-1005.

Warner, L., Hatcher, R., & Steiner M. (2004). Male condoms. In R. Hatcher et al. (Eds.), *Contraceptive technology* (18th ed.). New York: Ardent Media.

Weed, S. (1986). *Wise woman herbal for the childbearing years.* Woodstock, NY: Ash Tree Publishing.

Weiner, C., & Buhimschi, C. (2004). *Drugs for pregnant and lactating women.* Philadelphia: Churchill Livingstone.

Williams, G. (2000). Grief after elective abortion: Exploring nursing interventions for another kind of perinatal loss. *AWHONN Lifelines, 4*(2), 37-40.

World Health Organization (WHO). (1992). *Laboratory manual for the examination of semen and sperm-cervical mucus interaction.* Geneva: WHO.

World Health Organization (WHO) Department of Reproductive Health and Research. (2004). *Medical criteria for contraceptive use* (3rd ed.). Geneva: WHO.

Wright, V., Schieve, L., Reynolds, M., Jeng, G., and Kissin, D. (2004). Assisted reproductive technology surveillance–United States, 2000. *Morbidity and Mortality Weekly Report Surveillance Summaries, 53*(1), 1-20.

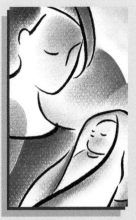

CHAPTER

7

Genetics, Conception, and Fetal Development

SHANNON E. PERRY

LEARNING OBJECTIVES

- Explain the key concepts of basic human genetics.
- Discuss the purpose, key findings, and potential outcomes of the Human Genome Project.
- Describe expanded roles for nurses in genetics and genetic counseling.
- Examine ethical dimensions of genetic screening.
- Discuss the current status of gene therapy (gene transfer).
- Summarize the process of fertilization.
- Describe the development, structure, and functions of the placenta.
- Describe the composition and functions of the amniotic fluid.
- Identify three organs or tissues arising from each of the three primary germ layers.
- Summarize the significant changes in growth and development of the embryo and fetus.
- Identify the potential effects of teratogens during vulnerable periods of embryonic and fetal development.

KEY TERMS AND DEFINITIONS

blastocyst Stage in development of a mammalian embryo, occurring after the morula stage, that consists of an outer layer, or trophoblast, and a hollow sphere of cells enclosing a cavity

chorionic villi Tiny vascular protrusions on the chorionic surface that project into the maternal blood sinuses of the uterus and that help form the placenta and secrete human chorionic gonadotropin

chromosomes Elements within the cell nucleus carrying genes and composed of DNA and proteins

conception Union of the sperm and ovum resulting in fertilization; formation of the one-celled zygote

decidua basalis Maternal aspect of the placenta made up of uterine blood vessels, endometrial stroma, and glands; shed in lochial discharge after birth

embryo Conceptus from day 15 of development until approximately the eighth week after conception

fertilization Union of an ovum and a sperm

fetal membranes Amnion and chorion surrounding the fetus

fetus Child in utero from approximately the ninth week after conception until birth

gamete Mature male or female germ cell; the mature sperm or ovum

genetics Study of single gene or gene sequences and their effects on living organism

genome Complete copy of genetic material in an organism

genomics Study of the entire deoxyribonucleic acid (DNA) structure of all of an organism's genes including functions and interactions of genes

implantation Embedding of the fertilized ovum in the uterine mucosa; nidation

karyotype Schematic arrangements of the chromosomes within a cell to demonstrate their numbers and morphology

meiosis Process by which germ cells divide and decrease their chromosomal numbers by one half

mitosis Process of somatic cell division in which a single cell divides, but both of the new cells have the same number of chromosomes as the first

monosomy Chromosomal aberration characterized by the absence of one chromosome from the normal diploid complement

morula Developmental stage of the fertilized ovum in which there is a solid mass of cells resembling a mulberry

mosaicism Condition in which some somatic cells are normal, whereas others show chromosomal aberrations

sex chromosomes Chromosomes associated with determination of sex: the X (female) and Y (male) chromosomes; the normal female has two X chromosomes, and the normal male has one X and one Y chromosome

teratogens Environmental substances or exposures that result in functional or structural disability

zygote Cell formed by the union of two reproductive cells or gametes; the fertilized ovum resulting from the union of a sperm and an ovum

175

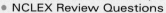

ELECTRONIC RESOURCES

Additional information related to the content in Chapter 7 can be found on

the companion website at **evolve**
http://evolve.elsevier.com/Lowdermilk/Maternity/
● NCLEX Review Questions
● WebLinks

or on the interactive companion CD
● NCLEX Review Questions
● Anatomy Review—Fetal Circulation
● Critical Thinking Exercise—Genetic Counseling
● Plan of Care—The Family with an Infant Who Has Down Syndrome

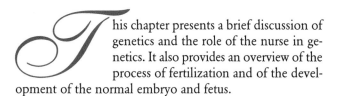

his chapter presents a brief discussion of genetics and the role of the nurse in genetics. It also provides an overview of the process of fertilization and of the development of the normal embryo and fetus.

GENETICS

Genetics is currently recognized as a contributing factor in virtually all human illnesses. In maternity care, genetics issues occur before, during, and after pregnancy (Hamilton & Wynshaw-Boris, 2004). With growing public interest in genetics, increasing commercial pressures, and Web-based opportunities for individuals, families, and communities to participate in the direction and design of their genetic health care, genetic services are rapidly becoming an integral part of routine health care (see Resources at end of this chapter).

For most genetic conditions, therapeutic or preventive measures do not exist or are very limited. Consequently, the most useful means of reducing the incidence of these disorders is by preventing their transmission. It is standard practice to assess all pregnant women for heritable disorders to identify potential problems.

Genetic disease affects people of all ages, from all socioeconomic levels, and from all racial and ethnic backgrounds. Genetic disease affects not only individuals, but also families, communities, and society. Advances in genetic testing and genetically based treatments have altered the care provided to affected individuals. Improvements in diagnostic capability have resulted in earlier diagnosis and enabled individuals who previously would have died in childhood to survive into adulthood. The genetic aberrations that lead to disease are present at birth but may not be manifested for many years, or possibly never manifested.

Some disorders appear more often in ethnic groups. Examples include Tay-Sachs disease in Ashkenazi Jews, French Canadians of the Eastern St. Laurence River valley area of Quebec, Cajuns from Louisiana, and the Amish in Pennsylvania; beta thalassemia in Mediterranean, Middle Eastern, Transcaucasus, Central Asian, Indian, and Far Eastern groups, as well as those of African heritage; sickle cell anemia in African-Americans; alpha thalassemia in those from Southeast Asia, South China, the Philippine Islands, Thailand, Greece, and Cyprus; lactase deficiency in adult

Chinese and Thailanders; neural tube defects in Irish, Scots, and Welsh; phenylketonuria (PKU) in Irish, Scots, Scandinavians, Icelanders, and Polish; cystic fibrosis (CF) in Caucasians, Ashkenazi Jews, and Hispanics; and Niemann-Pick disease, type A, in Ashkenazi Jews (Hamilton & Wynshaw-Boris, 2004; Jenkins & Wapner, 2004).

Genomics

Genomics address the functions and interactions of all the genes in an organism. It is the study of the entire DNA structure. New fields incorporating genomic knowledge are emerging, for example, nutrigenomics and pharmacogenomics (Horner, 2004). Genomic health care incorporates assessment, diagnosis, and treatment that use information about gene function. It is highly individualized because treatment options are based on the phenotypic responses of an individual. Genetic information includes personal data as well as information about blood relatives (Horner, 2004).

Relevance of Genetics to Nursing

Genetic disorders span every clinical practice specialty and site, including school, clinic, office, hospital, mental health agency, and community health settings. Because the potential impact on families and the community is significant (Box 7-1), genetics must be integrated into nursing education and practice. A genetic paradigm must be embraced; that is, genetic information, technology, and testing must be incorporated into health care services.

Although many of the roles for nurses in genetics are being expanded or developed, all nurses should be prepared to collaborate in interdisciplinary clinical partnerships and provide five main genetics-related nursing activities (International Society of Nurses in Genetics [ISONG], 1998; Lea, Feetham, & Monsen, 2002). The five main activities are as follows:

● Collecting, reporting, and recording genetics information
● Offering genetics information and resources to patients and families
● Participating in the informed consent process and facilitating informed decision making
● Participating in management of patients and families affected by genetic conditions

BOX 7-1

Potential Impact of Genetic Disease on Family and Community

- Financial cost to family
- Decrease in planned family size
- Loss of geographic mobility
- Decreased opportunities for siblings
- Loss of family integrity
- Loss of career opportunities and job flexibility
- Social isolation
- Lifestyle alterations
- Reduction in contributions to their community by families
- Disruption of husband-wife or partner relationship
- Threatened family self-concept
- Coping with intolerant public attitudes
- Psychologic effects
- Stresses and uncertainty of treatment
- Physical health problems
- Loss of dreams and aspirations
- Cost to society of institutionalization or home or community care
- Cost to society because of additional problems and needs of other family members
- Cost of long-term care
- Housing and living arrangement changes

From Lashley, F. (1998). *Clinical genetics in nursing practice* (2nd ed.). New York: Springer.

- Evaluating and monitoring the impact of genetics information, testing, and treatment on patients and their families

These activities are not limited to particular practice settings, nor are they limited to specific specialty areas.

Genetics-related activities that all nurses should be able to provide are further delineated in the *Statement on the Scope and Standards of Genetics Clinical Nursing Practice* (ISONG, 1998). This document includes standards and levels of practice for genetics nursing that were established cooperatively by ISONG and the American Nurses Association (ANA).

Although diagnosis and treatment of genetic disorders requires medical skills, nurses with advanced preparation are assuming important roles in counseling people about genetically transmitted or genetically influenced conditions. Nurses are usually the ones who provide follow-up care and maintain contact with the patients. Community health nurses can identify groups within populations that are at high risk for illness, as well as provide care to individuals, families, and groups. They are a vital link in follow-up for newborns who may need newborn screening.

Referral to appropriate agencies is an essential part of the follow-up management. Many organizations and foundations (e.g., the Cystic Fibrosis Foundation and the Muscular Dystrophy Association) help provide services and equipment for affected children. There are also numerous parent groups in which the family can share experiences and derive mutual support from other families with similar problems.

Probably the most important of all nursing functions is providing emotional support to the family during all aspects of the counseling process. Feelings that are generated under the real or imagined threat posed by a genetic disorder are as varied as the people being counseled. Responses may include a variety of stress reactions such as apathy, denial, anger, hostility, fear, embarrassment, grief, and loss of self-esteem.

Genetic History-Taking and Genetic Counseling Services

It is standard practice in obstetrics to determine whether a heritable disorder exists in a couple or in anyone in either of their families. The goal of screening is to detect or define risk for disease in low risk populations and identify those for whom diagnostic testing may be appropriate. A nurse can obtain a genetics history using a questionnaire or checklist such as the one in Fig. 7-1.

Genetic counseling that follows may occur in the office, or referral to a geneticist may be necessary. The most efficient counseling services are associated with the larger universities and major medical centers. This is also where support services are available (e.g., biochemistry and cytology laboratories), usually from a group of specialists under the leadership of a physician trained in medical genetics. Health professionals should become familiar with people who provide genetic counseling and the places that offer counseling services in their area of practice. See Resources at the end of this chapter for information on genetics resources.

Ethical Considerations

Researchers have proposed using fetal neurologic, liver, and pancreatic tissues to treat adults with Parkinson disease, metabolic disorders, or head and spinal cord injury. The use of fetal tissue in research was banned in the United States for several years, but the ban was lifted in 1993.

Most genetic testing is offered prenatally in order to identify genetic disorders in fetuses (Jenkins & Wapner, 2004). When an affected fetus is identified, termination of the pregnancy is an option. Other requests for genetic testing occur for sex selection or for late-onset disorders. An ethic of social responsibility should guide genetic counselors in their interactions with patients while recognizing that people make their choices by integrating personal values and beliefs with their new knowledge of genetic risk and medical treatments.

Other ethical issues relate to autonomy, privacy, and confidentiality. Should genetic testing be done when there is no treatment available for the disease? When is it appropriate to warn family members at risk for inherited diseases? When should presymptomatic testing be done? Some who might benefit from genetic testing choose not to have it, fearing discrimination based on the risk of a genetic disorder. Several states have prohibitions against insurance discrimination; other states are expected to follow their lead. Until guidelines for genetic testing are created, caution should be exercised. The benefits of testing should be weighed carefully

CD: Critical Thinking Excercise—Genetic Counseling

Risk Factors for Genetic Disorders

Review the following list of risk factors and place a check next to the "yes" responses.

_____ Will you be age 35 or older when your baby is due?

_____ If you or your partner are of Mediterranean or Asian descent, do either of you or anyone in your families have thalassemia?

_____ Is there a family history of neural tube defects?

_____ Have you ever had a child with a neural tube defect?

_____ Is there a family history of congenital heart defects?

_____ Is there a family history of Down syndrome?

_____ Have you ever had a child with Down syndrome?

_____ If you or your partner are of Eastern European Jewish or French Canadian descent, is there a family history of Tay-Sachs?

_____ If you or your partner are of Eastern European Jewish descent, is there a family history of Canavan disease?

_____ If you or your partner are African-American, is there a family history of sickle cell disease or trait?

_____ Is there a family history of hemophilia?

_____ Is there a family history of muscular dystrophy?

_____ Is there a family history of cystic fibrosis?

_____ Is there a family history of Huntington disease?

_____ Is anyone in your or your partner's family mentally retarded?

_____ If so, was that person tested for Fragile X syndrome?

_____ Do you, your partner, anyone in your families, or any of your children have any other genetic diseases, chromosomal disorders, or birth defects?

_____ Do you have a metabolic disorder such as diabetes or phenylketonuria?

_____ Have you had more than two miscarriages in a row?

_____ Have you ever had a baby who was stillborn?

Fig. 7-1 Questionnaire for identifying couples having increased risk for offspring with genetic disorders.

against the potential for harm. The American Academy of Pediatrics (2001) recommends that children not have genetic testing for disorders that have a late-onset and for which there is no treatment.

Preimplantation genetic diagnosis (PGD) is available in a limited number of centers. In this procedure, embryos are tested before implantation by in vitro fertilization (IVF) (Jones & Fallon, 2002). PGD has the potential to eliminate specific disorders in pregnancies conceived by IVF.

The Human Genome Project

The Human Genome Project began in 1990 as an international effort to map and sequence the genetic makeup of humans; it is funded by the National Institutes of Health (NIH) and the Department of Energy. Initial sequencing of the human genome (the copy of genetic material) was completed in June 2000, well ahead of schedule. A substantially complete version of the human genome was announced in April 2002. The map will facilitate study of hereditary diseases and will provide the potential for making changes at the gene level to treat or prevent hereditary diseases.

Two key findings from initial efforts to sequence and analyze the human genome are that (1) all human beings are 99.9% identical at the DNA level, and (2) approximately 30,000 to 40,000 genes (pieces or sequences of DNA that contain information needed to make proteins) make up the human genome (International Human Genome Sequencing Consortium, 2001). The finding that human beings are 99.9% identical at the DNA level should help to discourage the use of science as a justification for drawing precise racial boundaries around certain groups of people (Collins & Mansoura, 2001). The vast majority of the 0.1% genetic variations are found within and not among populations. The finding that humans have 30,000 to 40,000 genes, which is only twice as many as roundworms (18,000) and flies (13,000), was unexpected. Scientists had estimated that there were 80,000 to 150,000 genes in the human genome. It had been assumed that the main reason that humans are more evolved and more highly sophisticated than other species is that they have more genes.

Initial efforts to sequence and analyze the human genome have proven invaluable in the identification of genes involved in disease and in the development of genetic tests. More than 100 genes involved in diseases such as Huntington disease (HD), breast cancer, colon cancer, Alzheimer disease, achondroplasia, and cystic fibrosis have been identified. Genetic tests for more than 1446 inherited conditions are commercially available (see Chapter 21); of these, 836 are clinical tests and 310 are research tests (Gene Tests website, www.genetics.org [accessed July 1, 2005]).

Genetic testing

Most of the genetic tests now being offered in clinical practice are tests for single-gene disorders in patients with clinical symptoms or who have a family history of a genetic disease (Yoon et al., 2001). Some of these genetic tests are prenatal tests or tests used to identify the genetic status of a pregnancy at risk for a genetic condition. Current prenatal testing options include maternal serum screening (a blood test used to see if a pregnant woman is at increased risk for carrying a fetus with a neural tube defect or a chromosomal abnormality such as Down syndrome) and invasive procedures (amniocentesis and chorionic villus sampling). Other tests are carrier screening tests, which are used to identify individuals who have a gene mutation for a genetic condition but do not show symptoms of the condition because it is a condition that is inherited in an autosomal recessive form (e.g., CF, sickle cell disease, and Tay-Sachs disease). Another type of genetic testing is predictive testing, which is used to clarify the genetic status of asymptomatic family members. The two types of predictive testing are presymptomatic and predispositional. Mutation analysis for HD, a neurodegenerative disorder, is an example of presymptomatic testing. If the gene mutation for HD is present, symptoms of HD are certain to appear if the individual lives long enough. Testing for a BRCA-1 gene

mutation to determine breast cancer susceptibility is an example of predispositional testing. Predispositional testing differs from presymptomatic testing in that a positive result (indicating that a BRCA-1 mutation is present) does not indicate a 100% risk of developing the condition (breast cancer).

Pharmacogenomics

One of the most immediate clinical applications of the Human Genome Project may be pharmacogenomics, or the use of genetic information to individualize drug therapy (Phillips, Veenstra, Oren, Lee, & Sadee, 2001). There has been speculation that pharmacogenomics may become part of standard practice for a large number of disorders and drugs by 2020 (Collins & McKusick, 2001). The expectation is that by identifying common variants in genes that are associated with the likelihood of a good or bad response to a specific drug, drug prescriptions can be individualized based on the individual's unique genetic makeup (Roses, 2000). A primary benefit of pharmacogenomics is the potential to reduce adverse drug reactions.

Gene therapy (gene transfer)

In the early 1990s a great deal of optimism was felt about the possibility of using genetic information to provide quick solutions to a long list of health problems (Collins & McKusick, 2001). However, the field of gene therapy, also known as *gene transfer,* has sustained a number of major disappointments during the past few years. Although the early optimism about gene therapy was probably never fully justified, it is likely that the development of safer and more effective methods for gene delivery will ensure a significant role for gene therapy in the treatment of some diseases (Collins & McKusick, 2001). Major challenges include targeting the right gene to the right location in the right cells, expressing the transferred gene at the right time, and minimizing adverse reactions (Brower, 2001). Some reports detail exciting possibilities regarding the application of gene therapy for hemophilia B (Kay et al., 2000) and severe combined immunodeficiency (Anderson, 2000; Cavazzana-Calvo et al., 2000). According to a scientist who is very active in the field of gene therapy, "Gene therapy will succeed with time. And it is important that it does, because no other area of medicine holds as much promise for providing cures for the many devastating diseases that ravage humankind" (Anderson, 2000).

Ethical, legal, and social implications

An integral part of the Human Genome Project is the Ethical, Legal, and Social Implications (ELSI) program; 5% of the Human Genome Project budget was designated for the study of the ELSI of human genome research. This program addresses the potential that genetic information may be used to discriminate against individuals or for eugenic purposes. Continued awareness of and vigilance against such misuse of information is the collective responsibility of health care providers, ethicists, and society.

Management of Genetic Disorders

At this time, no cures exist for genetic disorders, although remedies can be implemented to prevent or reduce the harmful effects of a few disorders. Structural defects can sometimes be modified to produce normal or near-normal function. Surgical therapy is employed for congenital heart defects and cosmetic defects such as cleft lip. Advances in fetal surgery are occurring. Other conditions are treated with product replacement (e.g., thyroid for hereditary cretinism), diet modification (e.g., low-phenylalanine diet for PKU), and corrective devices for missing limbs. Research is being conducted on methods to influence or change genes directly by placing substitute DNA in the cells of those with a genetic mutation, thereby preventing or curing the disease process or relieving symptoms.

The possibility exists that understanding embryonic stem cells (primitive cells that can develop into all types of body tissue, including muscles, nerves, and bones) will lead to new medical discoveries (Box 7-2). The successful cloning of sheep, cattle, mice, and pigs; the production of rhesus monkeys through nuclear transfer of embryonic cells; and the isolation of stem cells constitute breakthroughs in technology. They also raise other ethical questions. On August 25, 2000, the NIH published guidelines for research using human stem cells (NIH, 2000). The nurse involved in genetics must keep abreast of new developments and be prepared to discuss ethical implications with patients and other health care providers.

BOX 7-2

Stem Cells

Stem cells are able to divide for indefinite periods and can differentiate into the many different types of cells that make up an organism. Embryonic stem cells are derived from the blastocyst before it implants in the uterine wall. A zygote is described as *totipotent* because it has the potential to produce all the cells and tissues that compose an embryo and to support its in utero development. The term *pluripotent* is used to describe stem cells that generate cells derived from the three embryonic germ layers (endoderm, mesoderm, and ectoderm). The embryonic stem cell is pluripotent. Human stem cells were derived and maintained for the first time in 1998 by Thomson and colleagues by using blastocysts donated by couples undergoing in vitro fertilization. Potential uses of human embryonic stem cells include transplant therapy, in which tissues damaged by disease or injury (e.g., as in diabetes, Parkinson disease, heart disease, and multiple sclerosis) are replaced or restored. Stem cell research engenders ethical concerns related to the source of human embryonic stem cells (embryos left over from in vitro fertilization and aborted fetuses). Currently federal support for research is restricted to existing cell lines.

From National Institutes of Health. *Stem cells: Scientific progress and future research directions.* Department of Health and Human Services, June, 2001. Internet document available at http://stemcells.nih.gov/info/ scireport (accessed June 28, 2005).

Estimation of risk

The risks of recurrence of a genetic disorder are determined by the mode of inheritance. The risk of recurrence for disorders caused by a factor that segregates during cell division (i.e., genes and chromosomes) can be estimated with a high degree of accuracy by application of mendelian principles. In a dominant disorder the risk is 50%, or one in two, that a subsequent offspring will be affected; an autosomal recessive disease carries a one-in-four risk of recurrence; and an X-linked disorder is related to the child's sex, as described in the section related to X-linked inheritance. Translocation chromosomes have a high risk of recurrence.

Disorders in which a subsequent pregnancy would carry no more risk than there is for pregnancy alone (estimated at 1 in 30) include those resulting from isolated incidences not likely to be present in another pregnancy. These disorders include maternal infections (e.g., rubella and toxoplasmosis), maternal ingestion of drugs, most chromosomal abnormalities, and a disorder determined to be the result of a fresh mutation.

Interpretation of risk

Counselors explain the risk estimates to patients without making recommendations or decisions and without allowing their own biases to interfere. The counselor provides appropriate information about the nature of the disorder, the extent of the risks in the specific case, the probable consequences, and (if appropriate) alternative options available; however, the final decision to become pregnant or to continue a pregnancy must be left to the family. An important nursing role is reinforcing the information the families are given and continuing to interpret this information at their level of understanding.

The most important concept that must be emphasized to families is that *each pregnancy is an independent event.* For example, in monogenic disorders, in which the risk factor is one in four that the child will be affected, the risk remains the same no matter how many affected children are already in the family. Families may make the erroneous assumption that the presence of one affected child ensures that the next three will be free of the disorder. However, "chance has no memory." The risk is one in four for *each* pregnancy. On the other hand, in a family with a child who has a disorder with multifactorial causes, the risk increases with each subsequent child born with the disorder.

Genes and Chromosomes

The hereditary material carried in the nucleus of each somatic (body) cell determines an individual's physical characteristics. This material—DNA—forms threadlike strands known as **chromosomes.** Each chromosome is composed of many smaller segments of DNA referred to as genes. Genes or combinations of genes contain coded information that determines an individual's unique characteristics. The code consists of the specific linear order of the molecules that combine to form the strands of DNA. Genes never act in isolation; they always interact with other genes and the environment.

All normal human somatic cells contain 46 chromosomes arranged as 23 pairs of homologous (matched) chromosomes; one chromosome of each pair is inherited from each parent. There are 22 pairs of autosomes, which control most traits in the body, and one pair of sex chromosomes, which determines sex and some other traits. The large female chromosome is called the X; the tiny male chromosome is the Y. When one X chromosome and one Y chromosome are present, the embryo develops as a male. When two X chromosomes are present, the embryo develops as a female.

Because each gene occupies a specific chromosome location, and because chromosomes are inherited as homologous pairs, each person has two genes for every trait. In other words, if an autosome has a gene for hair color, its partner also has a gene for hair color at the same location on the chromosome. Although both genes code for hair color, they may not code for the same hair color. Different genes coding for different variations of the same trait are called *alleles*. An individual with two copies of the same allele for a given trait is said to be *homozygous* for that trait. With two different alleles, the person is said to be *heterozygous* for the trait.

The term *genotype* typically is used to refer to the genetic makeup of an individual when discussing a specific gene pair, but at times, *genotype* is used to refer to an individual's entire genetic makeup or all the genes that the individual can pass on to future generations. *Phenotype* refers to the observable expression of an individual's genotype, such as physical features, a biochemical or molecular trait, and even a psychologic trait. A trait or disorder is considered dominant if it is expressed or phenotypically apparent when only one copy of the gene is present. It is considered recessive if it is expressed only when two copies of the gene are present.

The pictorial analysis of the number, form, and size of an individual's chromosomes is known as a karyotype. Cells from any nucleated, replicating body tissue (not red blood cells, nerves, or muscles) can be used (Scheuerle, 2001). The most commonly used tissues are white blood cells and fetal cells in amniotic fluid. The cells are grown in a culture and arrested when they are in metaphase, and then the cells are dropped onto a slide. This breaks the cell membranes and spreads the chromosomes, making them easier to visualize. The cells are stained with special stains (e.g., Giemsa stain) that create striping or "banding" patterns. Once the chromosome spreads are photographed or scanned by a computer, they are cut out and arranged in a specific numeric order according to their length and shape. The chromosomes are numbered from largest to smallest, 1 to 22, and the sex chromosomes are designated by the letter X or Y. Each chromosome is divided into two "arms" designated by p (short arm) and q (long arm). A female karyotype is designated as 46,XX and a male karyotype is designated as 46,XY. Fig. 7-2 illustrates the chromosomes in a body cell and a karyotype. Karyotypes can be used to determine the sex of a child and the presence of any gross chromosomal abnormalities.

Chromosomal Abnormalities

Chromosomal abnormalities occur in 0.5% to 0.6% of newborn infants; most of these have no significant physical abnormality associated with the defect. The incidence of

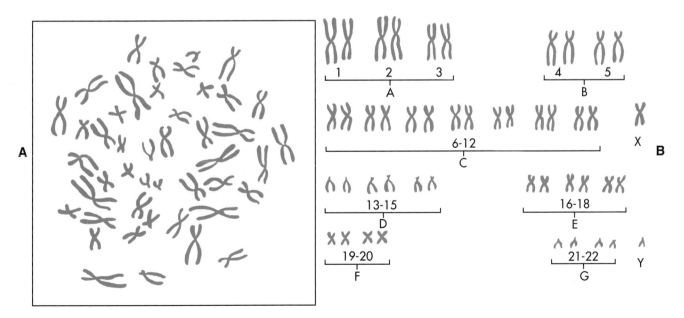

Fig. 7-2 Chromosomes during cell division. **A,** Example of photomicrograph. **B,** Chromosomes arranged in karyotype; female and male sex-determining chromosomes.

chromosomal abnormalities in fetuses spontaneously miscarried is as high as 61.5%. Chromosomal abnormalities account for approximately 10% of neonatal deaths (Hamilton & Wynshaw-Boris, 2004). Errors resulting in chromosomal abnormalities can occur in mitosis or meiosis. These occur in either the autosomes or the sex chromosomes. Even without the presence of obvious structural malformations, small deviations in chromosomes can cause problems in fetal development.

Autosomal abnormalities

Autosomal abnormalities involve differences in the number or structure of chromosomes resulting from unequal distribution of the genetic material during gamete (egg and sperm) formation.

Abnormalities of chromosome number. Euploidy denotes the correct number of chromosomes. Deviations from the correct number of chromosomes can be one of two types: (1) polyploidy, in which the deviation is an exact multiple of the haploid number of chromosomes or one chromosome set (23 chromosomes); or (2) aneuploidy, in which the numerical deviation is not an exact multiple of the haploid set (Hamilton & Wynshaw-Boris, 2004).

Aneuploidy is the most commonly identified chromosome abnormality in humans. Aneuploidy occurs in at least 5% of all clinically recognized pregnancies, and it is the leading known cause of pregnancy loss (Hassold & Hunt, 2001). Aneuploidy also is the leading genetic cause of mental retardation. The two most common aneuploid conditions are monosomies and trisomies. A monosomy is the product of the union between a normal gamete and a gamete that is missing a chromosome. Monosomic individuals only have 45 chromosomes in each of their cells. Limited data are available concerning the origin of monosomies because when an embryo is missing an autosomal chromosome, the embryo never survives.

The product of the union of a normal gamete with a gamete containing an extra chromosome is a trisomy. Trisomies are more common than monosomies. Trisomic individuals have 47 chromosomes in each of their cells. Most trisomies are caused by nondisjunction during the first meiotic division. That is, one pair of chromosomes fails to separate. One of the resulting cells contains two chromosomes, and the other contains none.

The most common trisomal abnormality is Down syndrome, or trisomy 21 (see discussion in Chapter 27; Nursing Plan of Care). Other autosomal trisomies that have been identified are trisomy 18 (Edwards syndrome) and trisomy 13 (Patau syndrome). Both conditions have a very poor prognosis, and most affected children die from cardiac or respiratory complications within 6 months of birth.

Nondisjunction can also occur during mitosis. If this occurs early in development, when cell lines are forming, the individual has a mixture of cells, some with a normal number of chromosomes and others either missing a chromosome or containing an extra chromosome. This condition is known as mosaicism.

Abnormalities of chromosome structure. Abnormalities of chromosome structure involve chromosome breakage, usually resulting from one of two events: (1) translocation and (2) additions or deletions (or both). Translocation occurs when genetic material is transferred from one chromosome to a different chromosome. Thus instead of two normal pairs of chromosomes, the individual has one normal chromosome of each pair and a third chromosome that is a fusion of the other two chromosomes. As long as all genetic material is retained in the cell, the individual is unaffected but is a carrier of a balanced translocation.

If a gamete receives the two normal chromosomes or the fused chromosome, the resulting offspring will be clinically normal. If the gamete receives one of the two normal chromosomes and the fused version, the resulting offspring will have an extra copy of one of the chromosomes. This condition is called an *unbalanced translocation* and often has serious clinical effects.

Whenever a portion of a chromosome is deleted from one chromosome and added to another, the gamete produced may have either extra copies of genes or too few copies. The clinical effects produced may be mild or severe depending on the amount of genetic material involved.

Sex chromosome abnormalities

Several sex chromosome abnormalities are caused by nondisjunction during gametogenesis in either parent. The most common deviation in females is Turner syndrome, or monosomy X (having only one X chromosome); the affected female exhibits juvenile external genitalia with undeveloped ovaries. She is usually short in stature with webbing of the neck. Intelligence may be impaired. Most affected embryos miscarry spontaneously.

The most common deviation in males is Klinefelter syndrome, or trisomy XXY. The affected male has poorly developed secondary sexual characteristics and small testes. He is infertile, usually tall, and effeminate. Males who are mosaic for Klinefelter syndrome may be fertile. Subnormal intelligence is usually present.

Patterns of Genetic Transmission

Heritable characteristics are those that can be passed on to offspring. The patterns by which genetic material is transmitted to the next generation are affected by the number of genes involved in the expression of the trait. Many phenotypic characteristics result from two or more genes on different chromosomes acting together (referred to as *multifactorial inheritance*); others are controlled by a single gene (*unifactorial inheritance).*

Defects at the gene level cannot be determined by conventional laboratory methods such as karyotyping. Instead, genetic specialists predict the probability of the presence of an abnormal gene from the known occurrence of the trait in the individual's family and the known patterns by which the trait is inherited.

Multifactorial inheritance

Most common congenital malformations, such as cleft lip and palate and neural tube defects, result from multifactorial inheritance, a combination of genetic and environmental factors. Each malformation may range from mild to severe, depending on the number of genes for the defect present or the amount of environmental influence. Multifactorial disorders tend to occur in families. Some malformations occur more often in one sex than the other. For example, pyloric stenosis and cleft lip are more common in males, and cleft palate is more common in females.

Unifactorial inheritance

If a single gene controls a particular trait, disorder, or defect, its pattern of inheritance is referred to as *unifactorial mendelian* or *single-gene inheritance*. The number of unifactorial abnormalities far exceeds the number of chromosomal abnormalities. This is understandable, considering that 30,000 to 40,000 genes in the haploid number (23) of chromosomes are passed on to an offspring from each parent.

Unifactorial or single-gene disorders follow the inheritance patterns of dominance, segregation, and independent assortment described by Mendel and include autosomal dominant, autosomal recessive, and X-linked dominant and recessive modes of inheritance (Fig. 7-3).

Autosomal dominant inheritance. Autosomal dominant inheritance disorders are those in which the abnormal gene for the trait is expressed even when the other member of the pair is normal. The abnormal gene may appear as a result of a mutation, a spontaneous and permanent change in the normal gene structure. In this case the disor-

der occurs for the first time in the family. Usually an affected individual comes from multiple generations having the disorder (see Fig. 7-3, *B* and *C*). Males and females are equally affected.

Examples of common autosomal dominantly inherited disorders are Marfan syndrome (a disorder of connective tissue resulting in skeletal, ocular, and cardiovascular abnormalities), achondroplasia (dwarfism), polydactyly (extra digits), Huntington disease, and polycystic kidney disease.

Neurofibromatosis (NF) is a progressive disorder of the nervous system that causes tumors to form on nerves anywhere in the body. NF affects all races, all ethnic groups, and both sexes equally. Half of the cases of NF result from spontaneous genetic mutation, whereas the other half are inherited in an autosomal dominant manner. Two genetically distinct forms of NF are NF1, the most common type, with an incidence of 1 in 3000 (Mueller & Young, 2001), and NF2, with an incidence of 1 in 35,000. The most notable features of NF1 are the small pigmented skin lesions known as *café-au-lait spots* and the neurofibromata (small, soft, fleshy growths). Individuals with NF1 generally are able to live a normal, healthy life. Café-au-lait spots and neurofibromata can occur with NF2, but they are far less common than with NF1.

Autosomal recessive inheritance. Autosomal recessive inheritance disorders are those in which both genes of a pair must be abnormal for the disorder to be expressed. Heterozygous individuals have only one abnormal gene and are unaffected clinically because their normal gene overshadows the abnormal gene. They are known as carriers of the recessive trait. For the trait to be expressed, two carriers must each contribute the abnormal gene to the offspring (Fig. 7-3, *C*). Males and females are equally affected. Most inborn errors of metabolism, such as PKU, galactosemia, maple syrup urine disease, Tay-Sachs disease, sickle cell anemia, and CF, are autosomal recessive inherited disorders.

X-linked dominant inheritance. X-linked dominant inheritance disorders occur in males and heterozygous females. Because the females also have a normal gene, the effects are less severe than in affected males. Affected males transmit the abnormal gene only to their daughters, on the X chromosome. Fragile X syndrome and vitamin D–resistant rickets are examples of X-linked dominant inherited disorders.

X-linked recessive inheritance. Abnormal genes for X-linked recessive inheritance disorders are carried on the X chromosome. Females may be heterozygous or homozygous for traits carried on the X chromosome because they have two X chromosomes. Males are hemizygous because they have only one X chromosome carrying genes, with no alleles on the Y chromosome. Therefore X-linked recessive disorders are most often manifested in the male with the abnormal gene on his single X chromosome. Hemophilia, color blindness, and Duchenne muscular dystrophy are all X-linked recessive disorders.

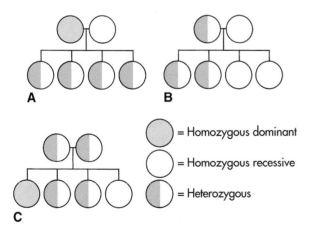

Fig. 7-3 Possible offspring in three types of matings. **A,** Homozygous-dominant parent and homozygous-recessive parent. Children: all heterozygous, displaying dominant trait. **B,** Heterozygous parent and homozygous-recessive parent. Children: 50% heterozygous, displaying dominant trait; 50% homozygous, displaying recessive trait. **C,** Both parents heterozygous. Children: 25% homozygous, displaying dominant trait; 25% homozygous, displaying recessive trait; 50% heterozygous, displaying dominant trait.

EVIDENCE-BASED PRACTICE
Folate Supplements to Prevent Neural Tube Defects

BACKGROUND

- Within 3 weeks of implantation, the embryonic neural groove is formed on the dorsum and will give rise to the brain and spinal cord. The groove folds into a tube by 1 month postfertilization (6 weeks from last menstrual period [LMP]). Defects in this closure can lead to anencephaly (absence of brain, cranial vault, and covering skin), which is incompatible with survival, and spina bifida (herniation of the spinal cord and/or meninges), which has a high mortality rate and mild to extreme neural damage. Neural tube defects (NTDs) may be attributed to both genetic and environmental causes. Screening during the second trimester, using maternal serum alpha-fetoprotein estimation or fetal ultrasound, can identify NTDs while the pregnancy can still be terminated. This has led to a decrease in birth rates of infants with NTDs, but it does not address primary prevention.

    Higher dietary folate, taken periconceptionally (before conception and during the first 2 months of pregnancy), seems to greatly decrease the incidence of NTDs.

OBJECTIVES

- The reviewers' primary objective was to inquire as to whether periconceptional folate or multivitamins can decrease the prevalence of NTDs.
- Interventions were the folate supplements or multivitamins. Outcomes, aside from NTDs, might include other defects, miscarriage, multiple pregnancy, preterm birth, perinatal and infant mortality, length of supplementation before conception, blood and tissue levels of folate, and attitudes toward and knowledge of NTDs in the population and among practitioners.

METHODS
Search Strategy

- The reviewers searched Cochrane, MEDLINE, and Zetoc, using the search keywords *neural tube defects.*
- Four randomized or quasi-randomized, controlled trials, representing 6425 women, were selected. One dissemination trial looked at the impact of printed materials on six communities. The trials took place in Hungary, the Republic of Ireland, the United Kingdom, Israel, Australia, Canada, the former USSR, and France, from 1981 to 1994.

Statistical Analyses

- Statistical analyses of homogeneous data were performed, using relative risks with 95% confidence intervals.

FINDINGS

- NTDs were significantly decreased by periconceptional folate supplementation. There was a consistent increase in multiple pregnancies across three trials, though it did not reach statistical significance. There were no associations of folate supplementation with other birth defects, ectopic pregnancies, stillbirths, miscarriages, or increase in conception. The doses of folate ranged from 0.36 to 4 mg/day. In one trial the folate group experienced less nausea and vomiting of pregnancy in the first trimester than the controls.
- Multivitamins alone did not decrease the rate of NTDs.

    In the literature dissemination trial, there was a significant increase in knowledge and intervention in the sample studied. Many women were not aware that folate was required periconceptionally for effective prevention of NTDs.

LIMITATIONS

- Randomization was not clear, nor was the dropout rate discussed in the review. These studies did not reach those whose pregnancy was unplanned, which can number half of all pregnancies in some areas. There was little information about the effects of folate on other drugs. None of the trials looked at dietary folate, which may be more practical in certain developing countries than supplementation.

CONCLUSIONS

- There is evidence that folate supplementation reduces the incidence of NTDs.

IMPLICATIONS FOR PRACTICE

- Most national policy statements call for 0.4 mg/day for all women of childbearing age, especially if they are contemplating pregnancy. For women with a history of an affected prior pregnancy, the recommended dose is 4 mg/day. Printed materials are a cost-effective way to educate and reinforce the message about folate supplementation. Most prenatal multivitamins now include the recommended dose of folate. Certain drugs may alter folate metabolism, such as antiseizure medication, which causes higher risk of NTD.

IMPLICATIONS FOR FURTHER RESEARCH

- New trials on cost-effective information dissemination can identify the most effective methods to educate childbearing-age women so that they can take folate before pregnancy. Large randomized, controlled trials can determine any side effects of folate, such as multiple births, which could change the relative risks and benefits of folate supplementation substantially. Trials involving food products that contain added folate would be informative. Folate deficiency recently has been tied to cardiovascular disease. Some trials in the future may establish the need for increased folate throughout life.

Reference: Lumley, J., Watson, L., Watson, M., & Bower, C. (2001). Periconceptional supplementation with folate and/or multivitamins for preventing neural tube defects. *The Cochrane Database of Systematic Reviews,* Issue 3, 2001, Art. No.: CD00156.

Inborn errors of metabolism

Disorders of protein, fat, or carbohydrate metabolism that reflect absent or defective enzymes generally follow a recessive pattern of inheritance. Enzymes, the actions of which are ge-netically determined, are essential for all the physical and chemical processes that sustain body systems. Defective enzyme action interrupts the normal series of chemical reactions from the affected point onward. The result may be an accumulation of

PLAN OF CARE *The Family with an Infant Who Has Down Syndrome*

NURSING DIAGNOSIS Risk for interrupted family processes related to birth of a neonate with an inherited disorder
Expected Outcome *The couple will verbalize accurate information about Down syndrome, including implications for future pregnancies.*

Nursing Interventions/Rationales

- Assess knowledge base of couple regarding the clinical signs and symptoms of Down syndrome and inheritance patterns *to correct any misconceptions and establish basis for teaching plan.*
- Provide information throughout the genetics evaluation regarding risk status and clinical signs and symptoms of Down syndrome *to give couple a realistic picture of neonate's defects and assist with decision making for future pregnancies.*
- Use therapeutic communication during discussions with the couple *to provide opportunity for expression of concern.*
- Refer to support groups, social services, or counseling *to assist with family cohesive actions and decision making.*
- Refer to child development specialist *to provide family with realistic expectations regarding cognitive and behavioral differences of child with Down syndrome.*

NURSING DIAGNOSIS Situational low self-esteem related to diagnosis of inherited disorder as evidenced by parents' statements of guilt and shame
Expected Outcome *The parents will express an increased number of positive statements regarding the birth of a neonate with Down syndrome.*

Nursing Interventions/Rationales

- Assist parents to list strengths and coping strategies that have been helpful in past situations *to promote use of appropriate strategies during this situational crisis.*
- Encourage expression of feelings using therapeutic communication *to provide clarification and emotional support.*
- Clarify and provide information regarding Down syndrome *to decrease feelings of guilt and gradually increase feelings of positive self-esteem.*
- Refer for further counseling as needed *to provide more in-depth and ongoing support.*

NURSING DIAGNOSIS Risk for impaired parenting related to birth of neonate with Down syndrome
Expected Outcome *Parents demonstrate competent skills in parenting a child with Down syndrome and willingness to care for neonate.*

Nursing Interventions/Rationales

- Assist parents to see and describe normal aspects of infant *to promote bonding.*
- Encourage and assist with breastfeeding if that is parents' choice of feeding method *to facilitate closeness with infant and provide benefits of breast milk.*

- Assure parents that information regarding the neonate will remain confidential *to assist the parents to maintain some situational control and allow for time to work through their feelings.*
- Discuss and role play with parents ways of informing family and friends of infant's diagnosis and prognosis *to promote positive aspects of infant and decrease potential isolation from social interactions.*
- Provide anticipatory guidance about what to expect as infant develops *to assist family to be prepared for behavior problems or mental deficits.*

NURSING DIAGNOSIS Spiritual distress related to situational crisis of child born with Down syndrome
Expected Outcome *Parents seek appropriate support persons (family members, priest, minister, rabbi) for assistance.*

Nursing Interventions/Rationales

- Listen for cues indicative of parents' feelings ("Why did God do this to us?") *to identify messages indicating spiritual distress.*
- Acknowledge parents' spiritual concerns and encourage expression of feelings *to help build a therapeutic relationship.*
- Facilitate visits from clergy and provide privacy during visits *to demonstrate respect for parents' relationship with clergy.*
- Encourage parents to discuss concerns with clergy *to use expert spiritual care resources to help the parents.*
- Facilitate interaction with family members and other support persons *to encourage expressions of concern and seeking comfort.*

NURSING DIAGNOSIS Risk for social isolation related to full-time caretaking responsibilities for a neonate with Down syndrome
Expected Outcome *Parents will describe a plan to use resources to prevent social isolation.*

Nursing Interventions/Rationales

- Provide opportunity for parents to express feelings about caring for a neonate with Down syndrome *to facilitate effective communication and trust.*
- Discuss with parents their expectations about caring for the neonate *to identify potential areas of concern.*
- Assist parents to identify potential caregiving resources *to permit parents to return to a routine at home.*
- Identify appropriate referrals for home care *to provide continuity of care.*
- Refer to support groups of parents of children with Down Syndrome *to enlist support, understanding, and strategies for coping.*

a damaging product such as phenylalanine or the absence of a necessary product such as thyroxin or melanin.

Phenylketonuria (PKU) is an uncommon disorder caused by autosomal recessive genes. A deficiency in the liver enzyme phenylalanine hydroxylase results in failure to metabolize the amino acid phenylalanine, allowing its metabolites to accumulate in the blood. The incidence of this disorder is 1 in every 10,000 to 20,000 births. The highest incidence is found in Caucasians (from northern Europe and the United States). It is rarely seen in Jewish, African, or Japanese populations. Screening for PKU is routinely performed on all infants through a blood test.

Tay-Sachs disease, inherited as an autosomal recessive trait, results from a deficiency in hexosaminidase. It occurs more commonly in Ashkenazi Jews and French-Canadians from Quebec. Infants appear normal until 4 to 6 months of age, then the clinical symptoms appear: apathy and regression in motor and social development, and decreased vision. Death occurs between ages 3 and 4 years. No treatment exists.

CF (mucoviscidosis or fibrocystic disease of the pancreas) is inherited as an autosomal recessive trait and is characterized by generalized involvement of exocrine glands. Clinical features are related to the altered viscosity of mucus-secreting glands throughout the body. Overall incidence is 1 per every 2000 births. Advances in diagnosis and treatment have improved the prognosis; many affected individuals live to adulthood. Some affected women have borne children, but men generally are sterile.

Meconium ileus occurs in about 10% of newborns with CF. Although an initial stool may be passed from the rectum with none thereafter, usually no meconium is passed during the first 24 to 48 hours. The abdomen becomes increasingly distended, and eventually the newborn requires a laparotomy for diagnosis and treatment of the condition. (See discussion in Chapter 27.)

Nongenetic Factors Influencing Development

Not all congenital disorders are inherited. Congenital means that the condition was present at birth. Some congenital malformations may be the result of teratogens, that is, environmental substances or exposures that result in functional or structural disability. In contrast to other forms of developmental disabilities, disabilities caused by teratogens are, in theory, totally preventable. Known human teratogens are drugs and chemicals, infections, exposure to radiation, and certain maternal conditions such as diabetes and PKU (Box 7-3). A teratogen has the greatest effect on the organs and parts of an embryo during its periods of rapid differentiation. This occurs during the embryonic period, specifically from days 15 to 60. Brain growth and development continue during the fetal period, and teratogens can severely affect mental development throughout gestation (Fig. 7-4).

In addition to genetic makeup and the influence of teratogens, the adequacy of maternal nutrition influences development. The embryo and fetus must obtain the nutrients they need from the mother's diet; they cannot tap the maternal reserves. Malnutrition during pregnancy produces low-birth-weight newborns who are susceptible to infection. Malnutrition also affects brain development during the latter half of gestation and may result in learning disabilities in the child. Inadequate folic acid is associated with neural tube defects.

The field of human behavioral genetics seeks to understand genetic and environmental influences on variations in human behavior (McInerney, 2004). Behavior involves multiple genes. Study of behavior and genes requires analysis of families and populations to compare those who have the trait with those who do not. The result is an estimate of the amount of variation in the population attributable to genetic factors. The findings of this research have significant political and social implications. For example, what are the social consequences of determining a genetic diagnosis of traits such as intelligence, criminality, or homosexuality? Caution must be exercised in accepting discoveries in behavioral genetics until there is substantial scientific corroboration (McInerney & Rothstein, 2004).

BOX 7-3

Etiology of Human Malformations

ETIOLOGY	MALFORMED LIVE BIRTHS (%)
Environmental	10
Maternal conditions	4
Alcoholism, diabetes, endocrinopathies, phenylketonuria, smoking, nutritional problems	
Infectious agents	3
Rubella, toxoplasmosis, syphilis, herpes simplex, cytomegalic inclusion disease, varicella, Venezuelan equine encephalitis	
Mechanical problems (deformations)	2
Amniotic band constrictions, umbilical cord constraint, disparity in uterine size and uterine contents	
Chemicals, drugs, radiation, hyperthermia	1
Genetic	20-25
Single-gene disorders	
Chromosomal abnormalities	
Unknown	65-70
Polygenic or multifactorial (gene-environment interactions)	
"Spontaneous" errors of development	
Other unknowns	

From Hudgins, L., & Cassidy, S. (2002). Congenital anomalies. In A. Fanaroff & R. Martin (Eds.), *Neonatal-perinatal medicine: Diseases of the fetus and infant* (7th ed.). St. Louis: Mosby.

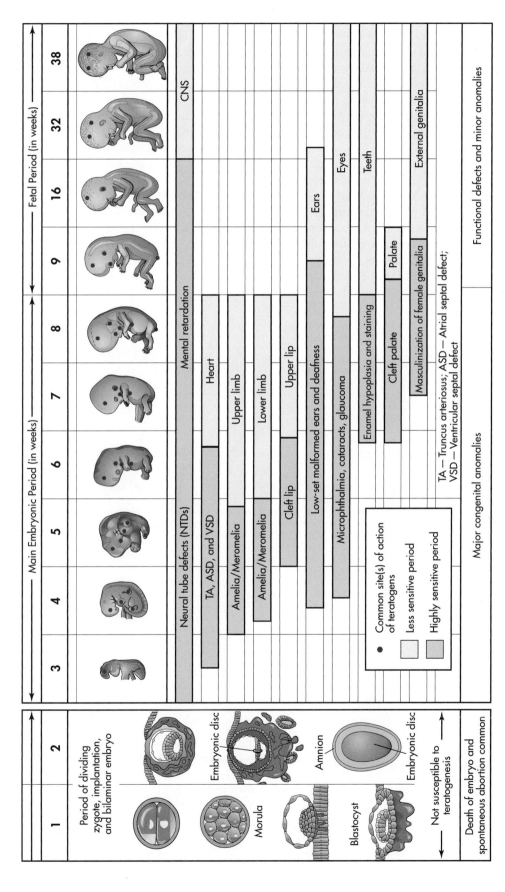

Fig. 7-4 Sensitive, or critical, periods in human development. Dark color denotes highly sensitive periods; light color indicates stages that are less sensitive to teratogens. (From Moore, K., & Persaud, T. [2003]. *Before we are born: Essentials of embryology and birth defects* [6th ed.]. Philadelphia: Saunders.)

CONCEPTION

Cell Division

Cells are reproduced by two different methods: mitosis and meiosis. In *mitosis* the body cells replicate to yield two cells with the same genetic makeup as the parent cell. First the cell makes a copy of its DNA; then it divides, with each daughter cell receiving one copy of the genetic material. Mitotic division facilitates growth and development or cell replacement.

Meiosis, the process by which germ cells divide and decrease their chromosomal number by half, produces gametes (eggs and sperm). Each homologous pair of chromosomes contains one chromosome received from the mother and one from the father; thus meiosis results in cells that contain one of each of the 23 pairs of chromosomes. Because these germ cells contain 23 single chromosomes, half of the genetic material of a normal somatic cell, they are called *haploid.* When the female gamete (egg or ovum) and the male gamete (spermatozoon) unite to form the zygote, the diploid number of human chromosomes (46, or 23 pairs) is restored.

The process of DNA replication and cell division in meiosis allows different alleles for genes to be distributed at random by each parent and then rearranged on the paired chromosomes. The chromosomes then separate and proceed to different gametes. Because the two parents have genotypes derived from four different grandparents, many combinations of genes on each chromosome are possible. This random mixing of alleles accounts for the variation of traits seen in the offspring of the same two parents.

Gametogenesis

When a male reaches puberty, his testes begin the process of spermatogenesis. The cells that undergo meiosis in the male are called *spermatocytes.* The primary spermatocyte, which undergoes the first meiotic division, contains the diploid number of chromosomes. The cell has already copied its DNA before division, so four alleles for each gene are

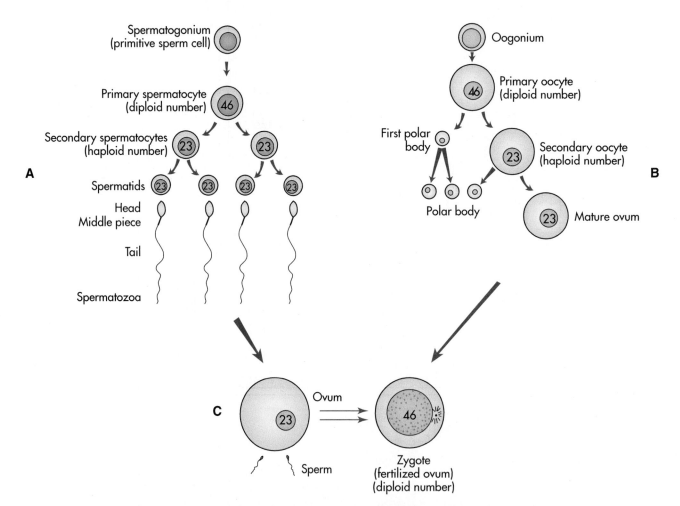

Fig. 7-5 Spermatogenesis. **A,** Gametogenesis in the male produces four mature gametes, the sperm. **B,** Oogenesis. Gametogenesis in the female produces one mature ovum and three polar bodies. Note relative difference in overall size between ovum and sperm. **C,** Fertilization results in the single-cell zygote and restoration of the diploid number of chromosomes.

present. Because the copies are bound together (i.e., one allele plus its copy on each chromosome), the cell is still considered diploid.

During the first meiotic division, two haploid secondary spermatocytes are formed. Each secondary spermatocyte contains 22 autosomes and one sex chromosome; one contains the X chromosome (plus its copy) and the other the Y chromosome (plus its copy). During the second meiotic division the male produces two gametes with an X chromosome and two gametes with a Y chromosome, all of which will develop into viable sperm (Fig. 7-5, *A*).

Oogenesis, the process of ovum formation, begins during fetal life of the female. All the cells that may undergo meiosis in a woman's lifetime are contained in her ovaries at birth. The majority of the estimated 2 million primary oocytes (the cells that undergo the first meiotic division) degenerate spontaneously. Only 400 to 500 ova will mature during the approximately 35 years of a woman's reproductive life. The primary oocytes begin the first meiotic division (i.e., they replicate their DNA) during fetal life but remain suspended at this stage until puberty (Fig. 7-5, *B*). Then, usually monthly, one primary oocyte matures and completes the first meiotic division, yielding two unequal cells: the secondary oocyte and a small polar body. Both contain 22 autosomes and one X sex chromosome.

At ovulation the second meiotic division begins. However, the ovum does not complete the second meiotic division unless fertilization occurs. At fertilization, a second polar body and the zygote (the united egg and sperm) are produced (Fig. 7-5, *C*). The three polar bodies degenerate. If fertilization does not occur, the ovum also degenerates.

Conception

Conception, defined as the union of a single egg and sperm, marks the beginning of a pregnancy. Conception occurs not as an isolated event but as part of a sequential process. This sequential process includes gamete (egg and sperm) formation, ovulation (release of the egg), union of the gametes (which results in an embryo), and implantation in the uterus.

Ovum

Each month, one ovum matures with a host of surrounding supportive cells. At ovulation the ovum is released from the ruptured ovarian follicle. High estrogen levels increase the motility of the uterine tubes so that their cilia are able to capture the ovum and propel it through the tube toward the uterine cavity. An ovum cannot move by itself.

Two protective layers surround the ovum (Fig. 7-6). The inner layer is a thick, acellular layer called the zona pellucida. The outer layer, called the corona radiata, is composed of elongated cells.

Ova are considered fertile for about 24 hours after ovulation. If unfertilized by a sperm, the ovum degenerates and is reabsorbed.

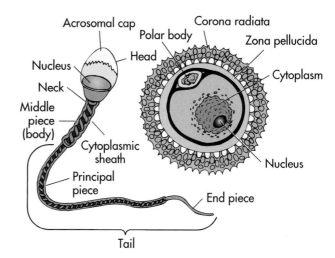

Fig. 7-6 Sperm and ovum.

Sperm

Ejaculation during sexual intercourse normally propels almost a teaspoon of semen containing as many as 200 to 500 million sperm into the vagina. The sperm swim by means of the flagellar movement of their tails. Some sperm can reach the site of fertilization within 5 minutes, but average transit time is 4 to 6 hours. Sperm remain viable within the woman's reproductive system for an average of 2 to 3 days. Most sperm are lost in the vagina, within the cervical mucus, or in the endometrium; or they enter the tube that contains no ovum.

As sperm travel through the female reproductive tract, enzymes are produced to aid in their capacitation. Capacitation is a physiologic change that removes the protective coating from the heads of the sperm. Small perforations then form in the acrosome (a cap on the sperm) and allow enzymes (e.g., hyaluronidase) to escape. These enzymes are necessary for the sperm to penetrate the protective layers of the ovum before fertilization.

Fertilization

Fertilization takes place in the ampulla (the outer third) of the uterine tube. When a sperm successfully penetrates the membrane surrounding the ovum, both sperm and ovum are enclosed within the membrane, and the membrane becomes impenetrable to other sperm; this process is termed the *zona reaction*. The second meiotic division of the oocyte is then completed, and the ovum nucleus becomes the female pronucleus. The head of the sperm enlarges to become the male pronucleus, and the tail degenerates. The nuclei fuse and the chromosomes combine, restoring the diploid number (46) (Fig. 7-7). Conception, the formation of the zygote (the first cell of the new individual), has been achieved.

Mitotic cellular replication, called cleavage, begins as the zygote travels the length of the uterine tube into the uterus. This voyage takes 3 to 4 days. Because the fertilized egg divides rapidly with no increase in size, successively smaller cells,

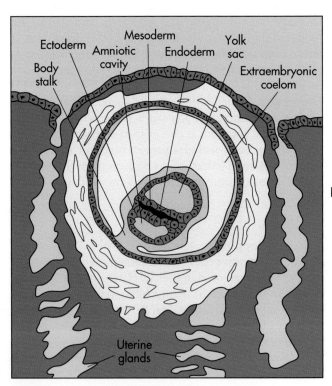

Fig. 7-7 Fertilization. **A,** Ovum fertilized by X-bearing sperm to form female zygote. **B,** Ovum fertilized by Y-bearing sperm to form male zygote.

called blastomeres, are formed with each division. A 16-cell **morula,** a solid ball of cells, is produced within 3 days and is still surrounded by the protective zona pellucida (Fig. 7-8, *A*). Further development occurs as the morula floats freely within the uterus. Fluid passes through the zona pellucida into the intercellular spaces between the blastomeres, separating them into two parts: the trophoblast (which gives rise to the placenta) and the embryoblast (which gives rise to the embryo). A cavity forms within the cell mass as the spaces come together, forming a structure called the **blastocyst** cavity. When the cavity becomes recognizable, the whole structure of the developing embryo is known as the blastocyst. Stem cells are derived from the inner cell mass of the blastocyst. The outer layer of cells surrounding the cavity is the trophoblast.

Implantation

The zona pellucida degenerates, and the trophoblast attaches itself to the uterine endometrium, usually in the anterior or posterior fundal region. Between 6 and 10 days after conception, the trophoblast secretes enzymes that enable it to burrow into the endometrium until the entire blastocyst is covered. This is known as **implantation.** Endometrial blood vessels erode, and some women experience slight implantation bleeding (slight spotting and bleeding during the time of the first missed menstrual period). **Chorionic villi,** or fingerlike projections, develop out of the trophoblast and extend into the blood-filled spaces of the endometrium. These villi are vascular processes that obtain oxygen and nutrients from the maternal bloodstream and dispose of carbon dioxide and waste products into the maternal blood.

After implantation the endometrium is called the *decidua.* The portion directly under the blastocyst, where the chorionic villi tap into the maternal blood vessels, is the **decidua basalis.** The portion covering the blastocyst is the decidua capsularis, and the portion lining the rest of the uterus is the decidua vera (Fig. 7-9).

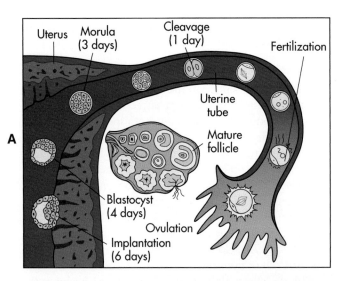

Fig. 7-8 **A,** First weeks of human development. Follicular development in ovary, ovulation, fertilization, and transport of early embryo down uterine tube and into uterus, where implantation occurs. **B,** Blastocyst embedded in endometrium. Germ layers forming. (**A,** From Carlson, B. [2004]. *Human embryology and developmental biology.* [3rd ed.] St. Louis: Mosby. **B,** Adapted from Langley, L. et al. [1980]. *Dynamic human anatomy and physiology* [5th ed.]. New York: McGraw-Hill.)

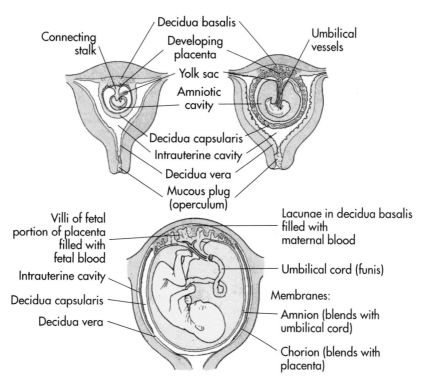

Fig. 7-9   Development of fetal membranes. Note gradual obliteration of intrauterine cavity as decidua capsularis and decidua vera meet. Also note thinning of uterine wall. Chorionic and amnionic membranes are in apposition to each other but may be peeled apart.

THE EMBRYO AND FETUS

Pregnancy lasts approximately 10 lunar months, 9 calendar months, 40 weeks, or 280 days. Length of pregnancy is computed from the first day of the last menstrual period (LMP) until the day of birth. However, conception occurs approximately 2 weeks after the first day of the LMP. Thus the postconception age of the fetus is 2 weeks less, for a total of 266 days or 38 weeks. Postconception age is used in the discussion of fetal development.

Intrauterine development is divided into three stages: ovum or preembryonic, embryo, and fetus (see Fig. 7-4). The stage of the ovum lasts from conception until day 14. This period covers cellular replication, blastocyst formation, initial development of the embryonic membranes, and establishment of the primary germ layers.

Primary Germ Layers

During the third week after conception the embryonic disk differentiates into three primary germ layers: the *ectoderm*, *mesoderm*, and *endoderm* (or *entoderm*) (see Fig. 7-8, *B*). All tissues and organs of the embryo develop from these three layers.

The ectoderm, or upper layer of the embryonic disk, gives rise to the epidermis, glands (anterior pituitary, cutaneous, and mammary), nails and hair, central and peripheral nervous systems, lens of the eye, tooth enamel, and floor of the amniotic cavity.

The mesoderm, or middle layer, develops into the bones and teeth, muscles (skeletal, smooth, and cardiac), dermis and connective tissue, cardiovascular system and spleen, and urogenital system.

The endoderm, or lower layer, gives rise to the epithelium lining the respiratory tract and digestive tract, including the oropharynx, liver and pancreas, urethra, bladder, and vagina. The endoderm forms the roof of the yolk sac.

Development of the Embryo

The stage of the embryo lasts from day 15 until approximately 8 weeks after conception, when the embryo measures approximately 3 cm from crown to rump. The embryonic stage is the most critical time in the development of the organ systems and the main external features. Developing areas with rapid cell division are the most vulnerable to malformation by environmental teratogens. At the end of the eighth week, all organ systems and external structures are present, and the embryo is unmistakably human (see Fig. 7-4).

Membranes

At the time of implantation, two fetal membranes that will surround the developing embryo begin to form. The chorion develops from the trophoblast and contains the chorionic villi on its surface. The villi burrow into the decidua basalis and increase in size and complexity as the vascular processes develop into the placenta. The chorion becomes the covering

Critical Thinking Exercise

Ultrasound Dating of Pregnancy

Adrienne believes she is 8 weeks pregnant, but her obstetrician believes she is closer to 12 weeks of gestation. Adrienne has come to the clinic for an ultrasound examination for dating. She has many questions for the nurse: How can they tell the length of gestation? What would the fetus look like at this time if she is at 8 weeks of gestation? If she is at 12 weeks of gestation? What fetal structures would be apparent on ultrasound if she is 8 weeks pregnant? If she is 12 weeks pregnant? Would any structural anomalies be apparent at 8 weeks? At 12 weeks? Why is it important to date a pregnancy accurately?

What information should the nurse provide Adrienne?

1 Evidence—Is there sufficient evidence to draw conclusions about what information the nurse should provide Adrienne?
2 Assumptions—What assumptions can be made about the following factors:
  a. Adrienne's motivation to learn about fetal development
  b. Adrienne's understanding of fetal development
  c. Adrienne's knowledge about ultrasound examinations?
  d. Why dating the pregnancy is important
3 What implications and priorities for nursing care can be drawn at this time?
4 Does the evidence objectively support your conclusion?
5 Are there alternative perspectives to your conclusion?

---

of the fetal side of the placenta. It contains the major umbilical blood vessels that branch out over the surface of the placenta. As the embryo grows, the decidua capsularis stretches. The chorionic villi on this side atrophy and degenerate, leaving a smooth chorionic membrane.

The inner cell membrane, the amnion, develops from the interior cells of the blastocyst. The cavity that develops between this inner cell mass and the outer layer of cells (trophoblast) is the amniotic cavity (see Fig. 7-8, *B*). As it grows larger, the amnion forms on the side opposite the developing blastocyst (see Fig. 7-8, *B*, and Fig. 7-9). The developing embryo draws the amnion around itself to form a fluid-filled sac. The amnion becomes the covering of the umbilical cord and covers the chorion on the fetal surface of the placenta. As the embryo grows larger, the amnion enlarges to accommodate the embryo/fetus and the surrounding amniotic fluid. The amnion eventually comes in contact with the chorion surrounding the fetus.

Amniotic Fluid

At first the amniotic cavity derives its fluid by diffusion from the maternal blood. The amount of fluid increases weekly, and 800 to 1200 ml of transparent liquid are normally present at term. The volume of amniotic fluid changes constantly. The fetus swallows fluid, and fluid flows into and out of the fetal lungs. The fetus urinates into the fluid, greatly increasing its volume.

The amniotic fluid serves many functions for the embryo/fetus. Amniotic fluid helps maintain a constant body temperature. It serves as a source of oral fluid and as a repository for waste. It cushions the fetus from trauma by blunting and dispersing outside forces. It allows freedom of movement for musculoskeletal development. The fluid keeps the embryo from tangling with the membranes, facilitating symmetric growth of the fetus. If the embryo does become tangled with the membranes, amputations of extremities or other deformities can occur from constricting amniotic bands.

The volume of amniotic fluid is an important factor in assessing fetal well-being. Having less than 300 ml of amniotic fluid (oligohydramnios) is associated with fetal renal abnormalities. Having more than 2 L of amniotic fluid (hydramnios) is associated with gastrointestinal and other malformations.

Amniotic fluid contains albumin, urea, uric acid, creatinine, lecithin, sphingomyelin, bilirubin, fructose, fat, leukocytes, proteins, epithelial cells, enzymes, and lanugo hair. Study of fetal cells in amniotic fluid through amniocentesis yields much information about the fetus. Genetic studies (karyotyping) provide knowledge about the sex of the fetus and the number and structure of chromosomes. Other studies such as the lecithin/sphingomyelin (L/S) ratio determine the health or maturity of the fetus.

Yolk Sac

At the same time the amniotic cavity and amnion are forming, another blastocyst cavity forms on the other side of the developing embryonic disk (see Fig. 7-8, *B*). This cavity becomes surrounded by a membrane, forming the yolk sac. The yolk sac aids in transferring maternal nutrients and oxygen, which have diffused through the chorion, to the embryo. Blood vessels form to aid transport. Blood cells and plasma are manufactured in the yolk sac during the second and third weeks. At the end of the third week, the primitive heart begins to beat and circulate the blood through the embryo, connecting stalk, chorion, and yolk sac.

The folding in of the embryo during the fourth week results in incorporation of part of the yolk sac into the embryo's body as the primitive digestive system. Primordial germ cells arise in the yolk sac and move into the embryo. The shrinking remains of the yolk sac degenerate (see Fig. 7-8, *B*), and by the fifth or sixth week, the remnant has separated from the embryo.

Umbilical Cord

By day 14 after conception the embryonic disk, amniotic sac, and yolk sac are attached to the chorionic villi by the connecting stalk. During the third week the blood vessels develop to supply the embryo with maternal nutrients and oxygen. During the fifth week, the embryo has curved inward on itself from both ends (bringing the connecting stalk to the ventral side of the embryo). The connecting stalk becomes compressed from both sides by the amnion and forms the narrower umbilical cord (see Fig. 7-9). Two arteries carry blood to the chorionic villi from the embryo, and one vein returns blood to the embryo. Approximately 1% of umbilical cords contain only two vessels: one artery and one vein. This occurrence is sometimes associated with congenital malformations.

The cord rapidly increases in length. At term the cord is 2 cm in diameter and ranges from 30 to 90 cm in length (with an average of 55 cm). It twists spirally on itself and loops around the embryo and fetus. A true knot is rare, but false knots occur as folds or kinks in the cord and may jeopardize circulation to the fetus. Connective tissue called *Wharton's jelly* prevents compression of the blood vessels and ensures continued nourishment of the embryo and fetus. Compression can occur if the cord lies between the fetal head and the pelvis or is twisted around the fetal body. When the cord is wrapped around the fetal neck, it is called a *nuchal cord*.

Because the placenta develops from the chorionic villi, the umbilical cord is usually located centrally. A peripheral location is less common and is known as a *battledore placenta*. The blood vessels are arrayed out from the center to all parts of the placenta.

Placenta

Structure

The placenta begins to form at implantation. During the third week after conception the trophoblast cells of the chorionic villi continue to invade the decidua basalis. As the uterine capillaries are tapped, the endometrial spiral arteries fill with maternal blood. The chorionic villi grow into the spaces with two layers of cells: the outer syncytium and the inner cytotrophoblast. A third layer develops into anchoring septa, dividing the projecting decidua into separate areas called *cotyledons*. In each of the 15 to 20 cotyledons, the chorionic villi branch out, and a complex system of fetal blood vessels forms. Each cotyledon is a functional unit. The whole structure is the placenta (Fig. 7-10).

The maternal-placental-embryonic circulation is in place by day 17, when the embryonic heart starts beating. By the end of the third week, embryonic blood is circulating between the embryo and the chorionic villi. In the intervillous spaces, maternal blood supplies oxygen and nutrients to the embryonic capillaries in the villi (Fig. 7-11). Waste products and carbon dioxide diffuse into the maternal blood.

The placenta functions as a means of metabolic exchange. Exchange is minimal at this time because the two cell layers of the villous membrane are too thick. Permeability increases as the cytotrophoblast thins and disappears; by the fifth month, only the single layer of syncytium is left between the maternal blood and the fetal capillaries. The syncytium is the functional layer of the placenta. By the eighth week, genetic testing may be done on a sample of chorionic villi obtained by aspiration biopsy; however, limb defects have been associated with chorionic villus sampling done

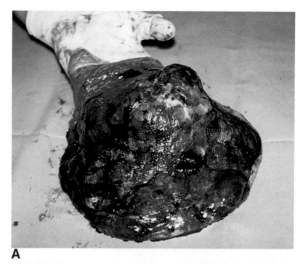

A

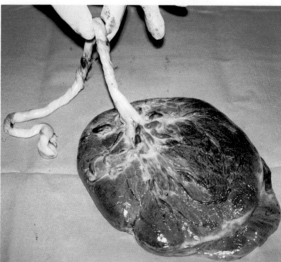

B

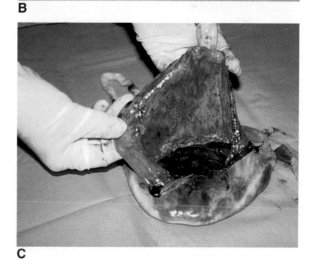

C

Fig. 7-10 Full-term placenta. **A,** Maternal (or uterine) surface, showing cotyledons and grooves. **B,** Fetal (or amniotic) surface, showing blood vessels running under amnion and converging to form umbilical vessels at attachment of umbilical cord. **C,** Amnion and smooth chorion are arranged to show that they are (1) fused and (2) continuous with margins of placenta. (Courtesy Marjorie Pyle, RNC, Lifecircle, Costa Mesa, CA.)

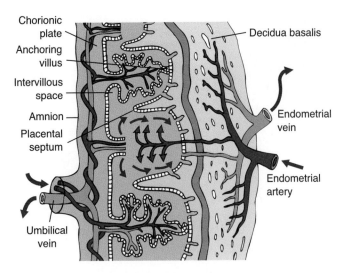

Chorionic plate
Anchoring villus
Intervillous space
Amnion
Placental septum
Umbilical vein
Decidua basalis
Endometrial vein
Endometrial artery

Fig. 7-11 Schematic drawing of the placenta illustrating how it supplies oxygen and nutrition to the embryo and removes its waste products. Deoxygenated blood leaves the fetus through the umbilical arteries and enters the placenta, where it is oxygenated. Oxygenated blood leaves the placenta through the umbilical vein, which enters the fetus via the umbilical cord.

before 10 weeks. The structure of the placenta is complete by the twelfth week. The placenta continues to grow wider until 20 weeks, when it covers about half of the uterine surface. It then continues to grow thicker. The branching villi continue to develop within the body of the placenta, increasing the functional surface area.

Functions

One of the early functions of the placenta is as an endocrine gland that produces four hormones necessary to maintain the pregnancy and support the embryo/fetus. The hormones are produced in the syncytium.

The protein hormone human chorionic gonadotropin (hCG) can be detected in the maternal serum by 7 to 10 days after conception, shortly after implantation. This hormone is the basis for pregnancy tests. The hCG preserves the function of the ovarian corpus luteum, ensuring a continued supply of estrogen and progesterone needed to maintain the pregnancy. Miscarriage occurs if the corpus luteum stops functioning before the placenta can produce sufficient estrogen and progesterone. The hCG reaches its maximum level at 50 to 70 days, then begins to decrease.

The other protein hormone produced by the placenta is human chorionic somatomammotropin (hCS) or human placental lactogen (hPL). This substance is similar to a growth hormone and stimulates maternal metabolism to supply needed nutrients for fetal growth. This hormone increases the resistance to insulin, facilitates glucose transport across the placental membrane, and stimulates breast development to prepare for lactation.

The placenta eventually produces more of the steroid hormone progesterone than the corpus luteum does during the first few months of pregnancy. Progesterone maintains the endometrium, decreases the contractility of the uterus, and stimulates development of breast alveoli and maternal metabolism.

By 7 weeks after fertilization, the placenta is producing most of the maternal estrogens, which are steroid hormones. The major estrogen secreted by the placenta is estriol, whereas the ovaries produce mostly estradiol. Measuring estriol levels is a clinical assay for placental functioning. Estrogen stimulates uterine growth and uteroplacental blood flow. It causes a proliferation of the breast glandular tissue and stimulates myometrial contractility. Placental estrogen production increases greatly toward the end of pregnancy. One theory for the cause of the onset of labor is the decrease in circulating levels of progesterone and the increased levels of estrogen.

The metabolic functions of the placenta are respiration, nutrition, excretion, and storage. Oxygen diffuses from the maternal blood across the placental membrane into the fetal blood, and carbon dioxide diffuses in the opposite direction. In this way the placenta functions as a lung for the fetus.

Carbohydrates, proteins, calcium, and iron are stored in the placenta for ready access to meet fetal needs. Water, inorganic salts, carbohydrates, proteins, fats, and vitamins pass from the maternal blood supply across the placental membrane into the fetal blood, supplying nutrition. Water and most electrolytes with a molecular weight less than 500 readily diffuse through the membrane. Hydrostatic and osmotic pressures aid in the flow of water and some solutions. Facilitated and active transport assists in the transfer of glucose, amino acids, calcium, iron, and substances with higher molecular weights. Amino acids and calcium are transported against the concentration gradient between the maternal blood and fetal blood.

The fetal concentration of glucose is lower than the glucose level in the maternal blood because of its rapid metabolism by the fetus. This fetal requirement demands larger concentrations of glucose than simple diffusion can provide. Therefore maternal glucose moves into the fetal circulation by active transport.

Pinocytosis is a mechanism used for transferring large molecules such as albumin and gamma globulins across the placental membrane. This mechanism conveys the maternal immunoglobulins that provide early passive immunity to the fetus.

Metabolic waste products of the fetus cross the placental membrane from the fetal blood into the maternal blood. The maternal kidneys then excrete them. Many viruses can cross the placental membrane and infect the fetus. Some bacteria and protozoa first infect the placenta and then infect the fetus. Drugs can also cross the placental membrane and may harm the fetus. Caffeine, alcohol, nicotine, carbon monoxide and other toxic substances in cigarette smoke, and prescription and recreational drugs (such as marijuana and cocaine) readily cross the placenta (Box 7-4).

BOX 7-4

Developmentally Toxic Exposures in Humans

Aminopterin	Lead
Androgens	Lithium
Angiotensin-converting enzyme inhibitors	Methimazole
	Methyl mercury
Carbamazepine	Parvovirus B19
Cigarette smoke	Penicillamine
Cocaine	Phenytoin
Coumarin anticoagulants	Radioiodine
Cytomegalovirus	Rubella
Diethylstilbestrol	Syphilis
Ethanol (>1 drink/day)	Tetracycline
Etretinate	Thalidomide
Hyperthermia	Toxoplasmosis
Iodides	Trimethadione
Ionizing radiation (>10 rad)	Valproic acid
	Varicella
Isotretinoin	

Although no direct link exists between the fetal blood in the vessels of the chorionic villi and the maternal blood in the intervillous spaces, only one cell layer separates them. Breaks occasionally occur in the placental membrane. Fetal erythrocytes then leak into the maternal circulation, and the mother may develop antibodies to the fetal red blood cells. This is often the way the Rh-negative mother becomes sensitized to the erythrocytes of her Rh-positive fetus (see the discussion of isoimmunization in Chapter 27).

Though the placenta and fetus are living tissue transplants, they are not destroyed by the host mother (Silver, Peltier, & Branch, 2004). Either the placental hormones suppress the immunologic response, or the tissue evokes no response.

Placental function depends on the maternal blood pressure supplying the circulation. Maternal arterial blood, under pressure in the small uterine spiral arteries, spurts into the intervillous spaces (see Fig. 7-11). As long as rich arterial blood continues to be supplied, pressure is exerted on the blood already in the intervillous spaces, pushing it toward drainage by the low-pressure uterine veins. At term gestation, 10% of the maternal cardiac output goes to the uterus.

If there is interference with the circulation to the placenta, the placenta cannot supply the embryo or fetus. Vasoconstriction, such as that caused by hypertension or cocaine use, diminishes uterine blood flow. Decreased maternal blood pressure or decreased cardiac output also diminishes uterine blood flow.

When a woman lies on her back with the pressure of the uterus compressing the vena cava, blood return to the right atrium is diminished (see the discussion of supine hypotension in Chapter 8 and Fig. 14-5). Excessive maternal exercise that diverts blood to the muscles away from the uterus compromises placental circulation. Optimum circulation is achieved when the woman is lying at rest on her

side. Decreased uterine circulation may lead to intrauterine growth restriction of the fetus and infants who are small for gestational age.

Braxton Hicks contractions seem to enhance the movement of blood through the intervillous spaces, aiding placental circulation. However, prolonged contractions or too-short intervals between contractions during labor can reduce the blood flow to the placenta.

Fetal Maturation

The stage of the fetus lasts from 9 weeks (when the embryo becomes recognizable as a human being) until the pregnancy ends. Changes during the fetal period are not as dramatic, because refinement of structure and function is taking place. The fetus is less vulnerable to teratogens, except for those that affect central nervous system functioning.

Viability refers to the capability of the fetus to survive outside the uterus. In the past the earliest age at which fetal survival could be expected was 28 weeks after conception. With modern technology and advances in maternal and neonatal care, viability is now possible about 20 weeks after conception (22 weeks since LMP; fetal weight of 500 g or more). The limitations on survival outside the uterus are based on central nervous system function and oxygenation capability of the lungs.

Respiratory system

The respiratory system begins development during embryonic life and continues through fetal life and into childhood. The development of the respiratory tract begins in week 4 and continues through week 17 with formation of the trachea, bronchi, and lung buds. Between 16 and 24 weeks the bronchi and terminal bronchioles enlarge, and vascular structures and primitive alveoli are formed. Between 24 weeks and term birth, more alveoli form. Specialized alveolar cells, type I and type II cells, secrete pulmonary surfactants to line the interior of the alveoli. After 32 weeks, sufficient surfactant is present in developed alveoli to provide infants with a good chance of survival.

Pulmonary surfactants. The detection of the presence of pulmonary surfactants (surface-active phospholipids) in amniotic fluid has been used to determine the degree of fetal lung maturity, or the ability of the lungs to function after birth. Lecithin (L) is the most critical alveolar surfactant required for postnatal lung expansion. It is detectable at approximately 21 weeks and increases in amount after week 24. Another pulmonary phospholipid, sphingomyelin (S), remains constant in amount. Therefore the measure of lecithin in relation to sphingomyelin, or the L/S ratio, is used to determine fetal lung maturity. When the L/S ratio reaches 2:1, the infant's lungs are considered to be mature. This occurs at approximately 35 weeks of gestation (Mercer, 2004).

Certain maternal conditions that cause decreased maternal placental blood flow, such as maternal hypertension, placental dysfunction, infection, or corticosteroid use, accelerate lung maturity. This apparently is caused by the resulting fetal hypoxia, which stresses the fetus and increases the blood levels of corticosteroids that accelerate alveolar and surfactant development.

Conditions such as gestational diabetes and chronic glomerulonephritis can retard fetal lung maturity. The use of intrabronchial synthetic surfactant in the treatment of respiratory distress syndrome in the newborn has greatly improved the chances of survival for preterm infants.

Fetal respiratory movements have been seen on ultrasound as early as the eleventh week. These fetal respiratory movements may aid in development of the chest wall muscles and regulate lung fluid volume. The fetal lungs produce fluid that expands the air spaces in the lungs. The fluid drains into the amniotic fluid or is swallowed by the fetus.

Before birth, secretion of lung fluid decreases. The normal birth process squeezes out approximately one third of the fluid. Infants of cesarean births do not benefit from this squeezing process; therefore they may have more respiratory difficulty at birth. The fluid remaining in the lungs at birth is usually reabsorbed into the infant's bloodstream within 2 hours of birth.

Fetal circulatory system

The cardiovascular system is the first organ system to function in the developing human. Blood vessel and blood cell formation begins in the third week and supplies the embryo with oxygen and nutrients from the mother. By the end of the third week the tubular heart begins to beat, and the primitive cardiovascular system links the embryo, connecting stalk, chorion, and yolk sac. During the fourth and fifth weeks the heart develops into a four-chambered organ. By the end of the embryonic stage, the heart is developmentally complete.

The fetal lungs do not function for respiratory gas exchange, so a special circulatory pathway, the ductus arteriosus, bypasses the lungs. Oxygen-rich blood from the placenta flows rapidly through the umbilical vein into the fetal abdomen (Fig. 7-12). When the umbilical vein reaches the liver, it divides into two branches. One branch circulates some oxygenated blood through the liver. Most of the blood passes through the ductus venosus into the inferior vena cava. There it mixes with the deoxygenated blood from the fetal legs and abdomen on its way to the right atrium. Most of this blood passes straight through the right atrium and

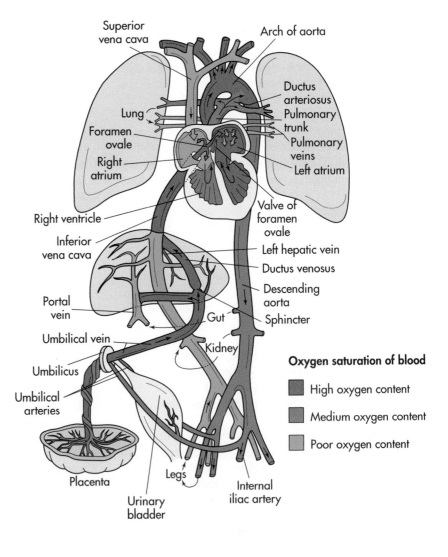

Fig. 7-12 Schematic illustration of the fetal circulation. The colors indicate the oxygen saturation of the blood, and the arrows show the course of the blood from the placenta to the heart. The organs are not drawn to scale. Observe that three shunts permit most of the blood to bypass the liver and lungs: (1) ductus venosus, (2) foramen ovale, and (3) ductus arteriosus. The poorly oxygenated blood returns to the placenta for oxygen and nutrients through the umbilical arteries. (From Moore, K., & Persaud, T. [2003]. *Before we are born: Essentials of embryology and birth defects* [6th ed.]. Philadelphia: Saunders.)

The mother also becomes aware of the sleep and wake cycles of the fetus.

Sensory awareness. Purposeful movements of the fetus have been demonstrated in response to a firm touch transmitted through the mother's abdomen. Because it can feel, the fetus requires anesthesia when invasive procedures are done.

Fetuses respond to sound by 24 weeks. Different types of music evoke different movements. The fetus can be soothed by the sound of the mother's voice. Acoustic stimulation can be used to evoke an FHR response. The fetus becomes accustomed (habituates) to noises heard repeatedly. Hearing is fully developed at birth.

The fetus is able to distinguish taste. By the fifth month, when the fetus is swallowing amniotic fluid, a sweetener added to the fluid causes the fetus to swallow faster. The fetus also reacts to temperature changes. A cold solution placed into the amniotic fluid can cause fetal hiccups.

The fetus can see. Eyes have both rods and cones in the retina by the seventh month. A bright light shone on the mother's abdomen in late pregnancy causes abrupt fetal movements. During sleep time, rapid eye movements (REMs) have been observed similar to those occurring in children and adults while dreaming.

At term the fetal brain is approximately one fourth the size of an adult brain. Neurologic development continues. Stressors on the fetus and neonate (e.g., chronic poor nutrition or hypoxia, drugs, environmental toxins, trauma, or disease) cause damage to the central nervous system long after the vulnerable embryonic time for malformations in other organ systems. Neurologic insult can result in cerebral palsy, neuromuscular impairment, mental retardation, and learning disabilities.

Endocrine system

The thyroid gland develops along with structures in the head and neck during the third and fourth weeks. The secretion of thyroxine begins during the eighth week. Maternal thyroxine does not readily cross the placenta; therefore the fetus that does not produce thyroid hormones will be born with congenital hypothyroidism. If untreated, hypothyroidism can result in severe mental retardation. Screening for hypothyroidism is typically included in the testing when screening for PKU after birth.

The adrenal cortex is formed during the sixth week and produces hormones by the eighth or ninth week. As term approaches, the fetus produces more cortisol. This is believed to aid in initiation of labor by decreasing the maternal progesterone and stimulating production of prostaglandins.

The pancreas forms from the foregut during the fifth through eighth weeks. The islets of Langerhans develop during the twelfth week. Insulin is produced by the twentieth week. In infants of mothers with uncontrolled diabetes, maternal hyperglycemia produces fetal hyperglycemia, stimulating hyperinsulinemia and islet cell hyperplasia. This results

in a macrosomatic (large-sized) fetus. The hyperinsulinemia also blocks lung maturation, placing the neonate at risk for respiratory distress and hypoglycemia when the maternal glucose source is lost at birth. Control of the maternal glucose level before and during pregnancy minimizes problems for the fetus and infant.

Reproductive system

Sex differentiation begins in the embryo during the seventh week. Distinguishing characteristics appear around the ninth week and are fully differentiated by the twelfth week. When a Y chromosome is present, testes are formed. By the end of the embryonic period, testosterone is being secreted and causes formation of the male genitalia. By week 28 the testes begin descending into the scrotum. After birth, low levels of testosterone continue to be secreted until the pubertal surge.

The female, with two X chromosomes, forms ovaries and female external genitalia. By the sixteenth week, oogenesis has been established. At birth the ovaries contain the female's lifetime supply of ova. Most female hormone production is delayed until puberty. However, the fetal endometrium responds to maternal hormones, and withdrawal bleeding or vaginal discharge (pseudomenstruation) may occur at birth when these hormones are lost. The high level of maternal estrogen also stimulates mammary engorgement and secretion of fluid ("witch's milk") in newborn infants of both sexes.

Musculoskeletal system

Bones and muscles develop from the mesoderm by the fourth week of embryonic development. At that time the cardiac muscle is already beating. The mesoderm next to the neural tube forms the vertebral column and ribs. The parts of the vertebral column grow toward each other to enclose the developing spinal cord. Ossification, or bone formation, begins. If there is a defect in the bony fusion, various forms of spina bifida may occur. A large defect affecting several vertebrae may allow the membranes and spinal cord to pouch out from the back, producing neurologic deficits and skeletal deformity.

The flat bones of the skull develop during the embryonic period, and ossification continues throughout childhood. At birth, connective tissue sutures exist where the bones of the skull meet. The areas where more than two bones meet (called *fontanels*) are especially prominent. The sutures and fontanels allow the bones of the skull to mold, or move during birth, enabling the head to pass through the birth canal.

The bones of the shoulders, arms, hips, and legs appear in the sixth week as a continuous skeleton with no joints. Differentiation occurs, producing separate bones and joints. Ossification will continue through childhood to allow growth. Beginning in the seventh week, muscles contract spontaneously. Arm and leg movements are visible on ultrasound, although the mother does not perceive them until sometime between 16 and 20 weeks.

Integumentary system

The epidermis begins as a single layer of cells derived from the ectoderm at 4 weeks. By the seventh week, there are two layers of cells. The cells of the superficial layer are sloughed and become mixed with the sebaceous gland secretions to form the white, cheesy vernix caseosa, the material that protects the skin of the fetus. The vernix is thick at 24 weeks but becomes scant by term.

The basal layer of the epidermis is the germinal layer, which replaces lost cells. Until 17 weeks the skin is thin and wrinkled, with blood vessels visible underneath. The skin thickens, and all layers are present at term. After 32 weeks, as subcutaneous fat is deposited under the dermis, the skin becomes less wrinkled and red in appearance.

By 16 weeks the epidermal ridges are present on the palms of the hands, the fingers, the bottom of the feet, and the toes. These handprints and footprints are unique to that infant.

Hairs form from hair bulbs in the epidermis that project into the dermis. Cells in the hair bulb keratinize to form the hair shaft. As the cells at the base of the hair shaft proliferate, the hair grows to the surface of the epithelium. Very fine hairs, called lanugo, appear first at 12 weeks on the eyebrows and upper lip. By 20 weeks they cover the entire body. At this time the eyelashes, eyebrows, and scalp hair are beginning to grow. By 28 weeks the scalp hair is longer than the lanugo, which thins and may disappear by term gestation.

Fingernails and toenails develop from thickened epidermis at the tips of the digits beginning during the tenth week. They grow slowly. Fingernails usually reach the fingertips by 32 weeks, and toenails reach toetips by 36 weeks.

Immunologic system

During the third trimester, albumin and globulin are present in the fetus. The only immunoglobulin (Ig) that crosses the placenta, IgG, provides passive acquired immunity to specific bacterial toxins. The fetus produces IgM immunoglobulins by the end of the first trimester. These are produced in response to blood group antigens, gram-negative enteric organisms, and some viruses. IgA immunoglobulins are not produced by the fetus; however, colostrum, the precursor to breast milk, contains large amounts of IgA and can provide passive immunity to the neonate who is breastfed (Table 7-1).

The normal term neonate can fight infection, but not as effectively as an older child. The preterm infant is at much greater risk for infection.

Table 7-2 summarizes embryonic and fetal development.

Multifetal Pregnancy

Twins

The incidence of twinning is 1 in 43 pregnancies (Benirschke, 2004). There has been a steady rise in multiple births since 1973. This is partly attributed to delayed childbearing. The use of ovulation-enhancing drugs is also a factor.

Dizygotic twins. When two mature ova are produced in one ovarian cycle, both have the potential to be fertilized by separate sperm. This results in two zygotes, or dizygotic twins (Fig. 7-13). There are always two amnions, two chorions, and two placentas that may be fused together. These dizygotic or fraternal twins may be the same sex or different sexes and are genetically no more alike than siblings born at different times. Dizygotic twinning occurs in families, is more common among African-American women than Caucasian women, and is least common among Asian-American women. Dizygotic twinning increases in frequency with maternal age up to 35 years, with parity, and with the use of fertility drugs.

Monozygotic twins. Identical or monozygotic twins develop from one fertilized ovum, which then divides (Fig. 7-14). They are the same sex and have the same genotype. If division occurs soon after fertilization, two embryos, two amnions, two chorions, and two placentas that may be fused will develop. Most often, division occurs between 4 and 8 days after fertilization, and there are two embryos,

---

TABLE 7-1

Characteristics of Immunoglobulins

CLASS	LOCATION	CHARACTERISTICS
IgG	Plasma, interstitial fluid	Is only immunoglobulin that crosses placenta Is responsible for secondary immune response
IgA	Body secretions, including tears, saliva, breast milk, colostrum	Lines mucous membranes and protects body surfaces
IgM	Plasma	Is responsible for primary immune response Forms antibodies to ABO blood antigens
IgD	Plasma	Is present on lymphocyte surface Assists in the differentiation of B lymphocytes
IgE	Plasma, interstitial fluids	Causes symptoms of allergic reactions Fixes to mast cells and basophils Assists in defense against parasitic infections

Modified from Lewis, S., Heitkemper, M., & Dirksen, S. (2004). *Medical-surgical nursing: Assessment and management of clinical problems* (6th ed.). St. Louis: Mosby.

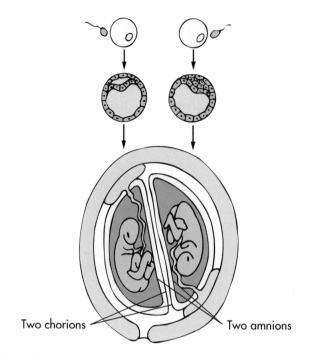

Fig. 7-13   Formation of dizygotic twins. There is fertilization of two ova, two implantations, two placentas, two chorions, and two amnions.

Two chorions

Two amnions

two amnions, one chorion, and one placenta. Rarely, division occurs after the eighth day following fertilization. In this case there are two embryos within a common amnion and a common chorion with one placenta. This often causes circulatory problems because the umbilical cords may tangle together, and one or both fetuses may die. If division occurs very late, cleavage may not be complete, and conjoined or "Siamese" twins could result. Monozygotic twinning occurs in approximately 1 of 250 births (Benirschke, 2004). There is no association with race, heredity, maternal age, or parity. Fertility drugs increase the incidence of monozygotic twinning.

Other multifetal pregnancies

The occurrence of multifetal pregnancies with three or more fetuses has increased with the use of fertility drugs and IVF. Triplets occur in about 1 of 1341 pregnancies (Benirschke, 2004). They can occur from the division of one zygote into two, with one of the two dividing again, producing identical triplets. Triplets can also be produced from two zygotes, one dividing into a set of identical twins and the second zygote a single fraternal sibling, or from three zygotes. Quadruplets, quintuplets, sextuplets, and so on have similar possible derivations.

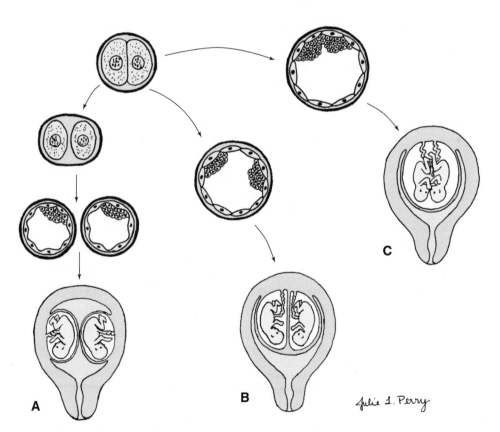

Fig. 7-14   Formation of monozygotic twins. **A,** One fertilization: blastomeres separate, resulting in two implantations, two placentas, and two sets of membranes. **B,** One blastomere with two inner cell masses, one fused placenta, one chorion, and separate amnions. **C,** One blastomere with incomplete separation of cell mass resulting in conjoined twins.

TABLE 7-2

Milestones in Human Development before Birth since Last Menstrual Period

4 WEEKS	8 WEEKS	12 WEEKS
EXTERNAL APPEARANCE		
Body flexed, C shaped; arm and leg buds present; head at right angles to body	Body fairly well formed; nose flat, eyes far apart; digits well formed; head elevating; tail almost disappeared; eyes, ears, nose, and mouth recognizable	Nails appearing; resembles a human; head erect but disproportionately large; skin pink, delicate
CROWN-TO-RUMP MEASUREMENT; WEIGHT		
0.4-0.5 cm; 0.4 g	2.5-3 cm; 2 g	6-9 cm; 19 g
GASTROINTESTINAL SYSTEM		
Stomach at midline and fusiform; conspicuous liver; esophagus short; intestine a short tube	Intestinal villi developing; small intestines coil within umbilical cord; palatal folds present; liver very large	Bile secreted; palatal fusion complete; intestines have withdrawn from cord and assume characteristic positions
MUSCULOSKELETAL SYSTEM		
All somites present	First indication of ossification—occiput, mandible, and humerus; fetus capable of some movement; definitive muscles of trunk, limbs, and head well represented	Some bones well outlined, ossification spreading; upper cervical to lower sacral arches and bodies ossify; smooth muscle layers indicated in hollow viscera
CIRCULATORY SYSTEM		
Heart develops, double chambers visible, begins to beat; aortic arch and major veins completed	Main blood vessels assume final plan; enucleated red cells predominate in blood	Blood forming in marrow
RESPIRATORY SYSTEM		
Primary lung buds appear	Pleural and pericardial cavities forming; branching bronchioles; nostrils closed by epithelial plugs	Lungs acquire definite shape; vocal cords appear
RENAL SYSTEM		
Rudimentary ureteral buds appear	Earliest secretory tubules differentiating; bladder-urethra separates from rectum	Kidney able to secrete urine; bladder expands as a sac
NERVOUS SYSTEM		
Well-marked midbrain flexure; no hindbrain or cervical flexures; neural groove closed	Cerebral cortex begins to acquire typical cells; differentiation of cerebral cortex, meninges, ventricular foramina, cerebrospinal fluid circulation; spinal cord extends entire length of spine	Brain structural configuration almost complete; cord shows cervical and lumbar enlargements; fourth ventricle foramina are developed; sucking present
SENSORY ORGANS		
Eye and ear appearing as optic vessel and otocyst	Primordial choroid plexuses develop; ventricles large relative to cortex; development progressing; eyes converging rapidly; internal ear developing; eyelids fuse	Earliest taste buds indicated; characteristic organization of eye attained
GENITAL SYSTEM		
Genital ridge appears (fifth week)	Testes and ovaries distinguishable; external genitalia sexless but begin to differentiate	Sex recognizable; internal and external sex organs specific

TABLE 7-2

Milestones in Human Development before Birth since Last Menstrual Period—cont'd

16 WEEKS	20 WEEKS	24 WEEKS
EXTERNAL APPEARANCE		
Head still dominant; face looks human; eyes, ears, and nose approach typical appearance on gross examination; arm/leg ratio proportionate; scalp hair appears	Vernix caseosa appears; lanugo appears; legs lengthen considerably; sebaceous glands appear	Body lean but fairly well proportioned; skin red and wrinkled; vernix caseosa present; sweat glands forming
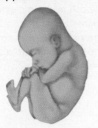	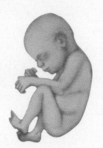	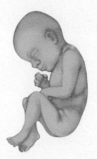
CROWN-TO-RUMP MEASUREMENT; WEIGHT		
11.5-13.5 cm; 100 g	16-18.5 cm; 300 g	23 cm; 600 g
GASTROINTESTINAL SYSTEM		
Meconium in bowel; some enzyme secretion; anus open	Enamel and dentine depositing; ascending colon recognizable	
MUSCULOSKELETAL SYSTEM		
Most bones distinctly indicated throughout body; joint cavities appear; muscular movements can be detected	Sternum ossifies; fetal movements strong enough for mother to feel	
CIRCULATORY SYSTEM		
Heart muscle well developed; blood formation active in spleen		Blood formation increases in bone marrow and decreases in liver
RESPIRATORY SYSTEM		
Elastic fibers appears in lungs; terminal and respiratory bronchioles appear	Nostrils reopen; primitive respiratory-like movements begin	Alveolar ducts and sacs present; lecithin begins to appear in amniotic fluid (weeks 26 to 27)
RENAL SYSTEM		
Kidney in position; attains typical shape and plan		
NERVOUS SYSTEM		
Cerebral lobes delineated; cerebellum assumes some prominence	Brain grossly formed; cord myelination begins; spinal cord ends at level of first sacral vertebra (S1)	Cerebral cortex layered typically; neuronal proliferation in cerebral cortex ends
SENSORY ORGANS		
General sense organs differentiated	Nose and ears ossify	Can hear
GENITAL SYSTEM		
Testes in position for descent into scrotum: vagina open		Testes at inguinal ring in descent to scrotum

Continued

TABLE 7-2

Milestones in Human Development before Birth since Last Menstrual Period—cont'd

28 WEEKS	30-31 WEEKS	36 AND 40 WEEKS
EXTERNAL APPEARANCE		
Lean body, less wrinkled and red; nails appear	Subcutaneous fat beginning to collect; more rounded appearance; skin pink and smooth; has assumed birth position	**36 Weeks** Skin pink, body rounded; general lanugo disappearing; body usually plump **40 Weeks** Skin smooth and pink; scant vernix caseosa; moderate to profuse hair; lanugo on shoulders and upper body only; nasal and alar cartilage apparent
CROWN-TO-RUMP MEASUREMENT; WEIGHT		
27 cm; 1100 g	31 cm; 1800-2100 g	**36 Weeks** 35 cm; 2200-2900 g **40 Weeks** 40 cm; 3200+ g
MUSCULOSKELETAL SYSTEM		
Astragalus (talus, ankle bone) ossifies; weak, fleeting movements, minimum tone	Middle fourth phalanxes ossify; permanent teeth primordia seen; can turn head to side	**36 Weeks** Distal femoral ossification centers present; sustained, definite movements; fair tone; can turn and elevate head **40 Weeks** Active, sustained movement; good tone; may lift head
RESPIRATORY SYSTEM		
Lecithin forming on alveolar surfaces	L/S ratio = 1.2:1	**36 Weeks** L/S ratio $\geq$ 2:1 **40 Weeks** Pulmonary branching only two thirds complete
RENAL SYSTEM		
		36 Weeks Formation of new nephrons ceases
NERVOUS SYSTEM		
Appearance of cerebral fissures, convolutions rapidly appearing; indefinite sleep-wake cycle; cry weak or absent; weak suck reflex		**36 Weeks** End of spinal cord at level of third lumbar vertebra (L3); definite sleep-wake cycle **40 Weeks** Myelination of brain begins; patterned sleep-wake cycle with alert periods; cries when hungry or uncomfortable; strong suck reflex
SENSORY ORGANS		
Eyelids reopen; retinal layers completed, light receptive; pupils capable of reacting to light	Sense of taste present; aware of sounds outside mother's body	
GENITAL SYSTEM		
	Testes descending to scrotum	**40 Weeks** Testes in scrotum; labia majora well developed

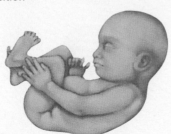

Select two Web addresses for resources on genetics for parents from the Resource list provided in this chapter. Access the sites.

Compare and contrast the appearance, the readability, and the information contained in the sites.

To whom would you recommend these sites?
Is the information culturally relevant?
What information would parents need?
How could you as a nurse use this information?

Key Points

- Genetic disease affects people of all ages, from all socioeconomic levels, and from all racial and ethnic backgrounds.
- Genetic disorders span every clinical practice specialty.
- Nurses with advanced preparation are assuming important roles in genetic counseling.
- Genes are the basic units of heredity, responsible for all human characteristics. They make up 23 pairs of chromosomes: 22 pairs of autosomes and one pair of sex chromosomes.
- Genetic disorders follow mendelian inheritance patterns of dominance, segregation, and independent assortment of normal genetic transmission.

- Multifactorial inheritance includes both genetic and environmental contributions.
- Human gestation is approximately 280 days after the LMP, or 266 days after conception.
- Fertilization occurs in the uterine tube within 24 hours of ovulation. The zygote undergoes mitotic divisions, creating a 16-cell morula.
- Critical periods occur in human development during which the embryo or fetus is vulnerable to environmental teratogens.

Answer Guidelines to Critical Thinking Exercise

Ultrasound Dating of Pregnancy

1 Yes, ultrasound dating of pregnancies is well established. The nurse can use photographs or drawings of a fetus to educate Adrienne about the appearance of a fetus at different gestational ages. In addition, charts of embryonic development including critical periods of development can be used.
2 The nurse can assume the following:
   a. Adrienne wants to learn about fetal development.
   b. Depending on prior education, Adrienne may know little about embryonic and fetal development.
   c. Adrienne has the right to know the risks and benefits of ultrasound examination and to give informed consent for the procedure.
   d. Dating the pregnancy is important to identify and prepare for variations from normal.

3 Priorities for nursing care include educating Adrienne about fetal development, ensuring that she is aware of the risks and benefits of ultrasound testing, obtaining a signature for the procedure on a consent form (if her physician has not already done so), informing Adrienne what ultrasound testing entails, and providing support as necessary during the procedure.
4 Yes, ultrasound testing can provide accurate dating of a pregnancy and allow detection of structural anomalies in a fetus.
5 Adrienne has the right to refuse to learn about fetal development and to refuse ultrasound testing. She may or may not want to learn the sex of the fetus; her wishes should be respected in this regard.

Resources

Alliance of Genetic Support Groups
www.geneticalliance.org

Ask NOAH About: Pregnancy
www.noah.cuny.edu/pregnancy/pregnancy.html

Family Guide to Cystic Fibrosis Genetic Testing
www.phd.msu.edu/cf/fam.html

GeneClinics
www.geneclinics.org

Gene Tests
www.hslib.washington.edu/helix

Genetics & Ethics
www.genethics.ca/

Genetics Education for Nurses
www.cincinnatichildrens.org/ed/clinical/gpnf/default.htm

Genetics Home Reference
www.ghr.nlm.nih.gov/

Information for Genetic Professionals
www.kumc.edu/gec/geneinfo.html

International Society of Nurses in Genetics (ISONG)
www.nursing.creighton.edu/isong

MEDLINE: PubMed and Internet Grateful Med
www.nlm.nih.gov/databases/databases-medline.html

National Center for Human Genome Research
www.nhgri.nih.gov

National Down Syndrome Society
www.ndss.org

National Fragile X Foundation
www.nfxf.org

National Information Resource on Ethics and Human Genetics
www.georgetown.edu/research/nrcbl/nirehg/

National Marfan Foundation
www.marfan.org

National Society of Genetic Counselors
http://members.aol.com/nsgcweb/nsgchome.htm

Neurofibromatosis
www.nf.org/

Online Mendelian Inheritance in Man (OMIM)
www.ncbi.nlm.nih.gov/Omim

Organization of Teratogen Information Services
www.otispregnancy.org

Osteogenesis Imperfecta Foundation
www.oif.org

Stem Cell Information
http://stemcells.nih.gov

Understanding Gene Testing
www.gene.com/ae/AE/AEPC/NIH/index.html

Visible Embryo
http://visembryo.ucsf.edu

Webget
http://med.upenn.edu/bioethic/webget

World of Genetics Societies
http://faseb.org/genetics/mainmenu.htm

References

American Academy of Pediatrics. (2001). Ethical issues with genetic testing in pediatrics. *Pediatrics, 107*(6), 1451-1455.

Anderson, W. (2000). Gene therapy: The best of times, the worst of times. *Science, 288*(5466), 627-628.

Benirschke, K. (2004). Multiple gestation. The biology of twinning. In R. Creasy, R. Resnik, & J. Iams (Eds.), *Maternal-fetal medicine: Principles and practice* (5th ed.). Philadelphia: Saunders.

Brower, V. (2001). Gene therapy revisited: In spite of problems and drawbacks, gene therapy moves forward. *EMBO Reports, 2*(12), 1064-1065.

Burke, W., Pinsky, L., & Press, N. (2001). Categorizing genetic tests to identify their ethical, legal, and social implications. *American Journal of Medical Genetics, 106*(3), 233-240.

Carlson, B. (2004). *Human embryology and developmental biology* (3rd ed.). St. Louis: Mosby.

Cavazzana-Calvo, M. et al. (2000). Gene therapy of human severe combined immunodeficiency (SCID)-X1 disease. *Science, 288*(5466), 669-672.

Collins, F., & Mansoura, M. (2001). The Human Genome Project: Revealing the shared inheritance of all humankind. *Cancer Supplement, 91,* 221-225.

Collins, F., & McKusick, V. (2001). Implications of the Human Genome Project for medical science. *Journal of the American Medical Association, 285*(5), 540-544.

Hamilton, B., & Wynshaw-Boris, A. (2004). Basic genetics and patterns of inheritance. In R. Creasy, R. Resnik, & J. Iams (Eds.), *Maternal-fetal medicine: Principles and practice* (5th ed.). Philadelphia: Saunders.

Hassold, T., & Hunt, P. (2001). To err (meiotically) is human: The genesis of human aneuploidy. *Nature Reviews Genetics, 2*(4), 280-291.

Horner, S. (2004). Ethics and genetics. *Clinical Nurse Specialist, 18*(5), 228-231.

Hudgins, L., & Cassidy, S. (2002). Congenital anomalies. In A. Fanaroff & R. Martin (Eds.), *Neonatal-perinatal medicine: Diseases of the fetus and infant* (7th ed.). St. Louis: Mosby.

International Human Genome Sequencing Consortium. (2001). Initial sequencing and analysis of the human genome. *Nature, 409* (6822), 860-921.

International Society of Nurses in Genetics (ISONG). (1998). *Statement on the scope and standards of genetics clinical nursing practice.* Washington, DC: American Nurses Association.

Jenkins, T., & Wapner, R. (2004). Prenatal diagnosis of congenital disorders. In R. Creasy, R. Resnik, & J. Iams (Eds.), *Maternal-fetal medicine: Principles and practice* (5th ed.). Philadelphia: Saunders.

Jones, S., & Fallon, L. (2002). Reproductive options for individuals at risk for transmission of a genetic disorder. *Journal of Obstetric, Gynecologic, and Neonatal Nursing, 31*(2), 193-199.

Kay, M., et al. (2000). Evidence for gene transfer and expression of factor IX in haemophilia B patients treated with an AAV vector. *Nature Genetics, 24*(3), 257-261.

Langley, L. et al. (1980). *Dynamic human anatomy and physiology* (5th ed.). New York: McGraw-Hill.

Lashley, F. (1998). *Clinical genetics in nursing practice* (2nd ed.). New York: Springer.

Lea, D., Feetham, S., & Monsen, R. (2002). Genomic-based health care in nursing: A bi-directional approach to bringing genetics into nursing's body of knowledge. *Journal of Professional Nursing, 18*(3), 120-129.

Lewis, S., Heitkemper, M., & Dirksen, S. (2004). *Medical-surgical nursing: Assessment and management of clinical problems* (6th ed.). St. Louis: Mosby.

Lumley, J., Watson, L., Watson, M., & Bower, C. (2001). Periconceptional supplementation with folate and/or multivitamins for preventing neural tube defects. *The Cochrane Database of Systematic Reviews* Issue 3, 2001, Art. No.: CD00156.

McInerney, J. (2004). *What is behavioral genetics? Human Genome Project Information.* Internet document available at www.ornl.bov/sci/techresources/Human_Genome/elsi/behavior.shtml (accessed August 12, 2004).

McInerney, J., & Rothstein, M. (2004). *What implications does behavioral genetics research have for society? Human Genome Project Information.* Internet document available at www.ornl.bov/sci/techresources/Human_Genome/elsi/behavior.shtml (accessed August 12, 2004).

Mercer, B. (2004). Assessment and induction of fetal pulmonary maturity. In R. Creasy, R. Resnik, & J. Iams (Eds.), *Maternal-fetal medicine: Principles and practice* (5th ed.). Philadelphia: Saunders.

Moore, K., & Persaud, T. (2003). *Before we are born: Essentials of embryology and birth defects* (6th ed.). Philadelphia: Saunders.

Mueller, R., & Young, I. (2001). *Emery's elements of medical genetics* (11th ed.). New York: Churchill Livingstone.

National Institutes of Health (NIH). (2000). *NIH publishes final guidelines for stem cell research.* News release. Internet document available at www.nih.gov/news/pr/aug2000 (accessed December 13, 2004).

National Institutes of Health. *Stem cells: Scientific progress and future research directions, 2001.* Internet document available at http:// stemcells.nih.gov/info/scireport (accessed June 28, 2005).

Phillips, K., Veenstra, D., Oren, E., Lee, J., & Sadee, W. (2001). Potential role of pharmacogenomics in reducing adverse drug reactions: A systematic review. *Journal of the American Medical Association, 286*(18), 2270-2279.

Roses, A. (2000). Pharmacogenetics and the practice of medicine. *Nature, 405*(6788), 857-865.

Scheuerle, A. (2001). Diagnosis of genetic disease. In M. Mahowald et al. (Eds.), *Genetics in the clinic: Clinical, ethical, and social implications for primary care.* St. Louis: Mosby.

Silver, R., Peltier, M., & Branch, E. (2004). The immunology of pregnancy. In R. Creasy, R. Resnik, & J. Iams (Eds.), *Maternal-fetal medicine: Principles and practice* (5th ed.). Philadelphia: Saunders.

Thompson, J. et al. (1998). Embryonic stem cell lines derived from human blastocysts. *Science, 282,* 1145-1147.

Yoon, P., et al. (2001). Public health impact of genetic tests at the end of the 20th century. *Genetic Medicine, 3*(6), 405-410.

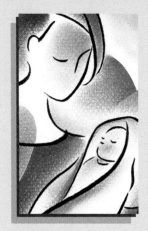

 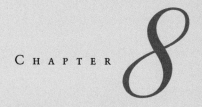

Anatomy and Physiology of Pregnancy

DEITRA LEONARD LOWDERMILK

LEARNING OBJECTIVES

- *Determine gravidity and parity by using the five- and four-digit systems.*
- *Describe the various types of pregnancy tests including the timing of tests and interpretation of results.*
- *Explain the expected maternal anatomic and physiologic adaptations to pregnancy for each body system.*
- *Differentiate among presumptive, probable, and positive signs of pregnancy.*
- *Compare normal adult laboratory values with values for pregnant women.*
- *Identify the maternal hormones produced during pregnancy, their target organs, and their major effects on pregnancy.*
- *Compare the characteristics of the abdomen, vulva, and cervix of the nullipara and multipara.*

KEY TERMS AND DEFINITIONS

ballottement Diagnostic technique using palpation: a floating fetus, when tapped or pushed, moves away and then returns to touch the examiner's hand

Braxton Hicks sign Mild, intermittent, painless uterine contractions that occur during pregnancy; occur more frequently as pregnancy advances but do not represent true labor; however, they should be distinguished from preterm labor

carpal tunnel syndrome Pressure on the median nerve at the point at which it goes through the carpal tunnel of the wrist; causes soreness, tenderness, and weakness of the muscles of the thumb

Chadwick sign Violet color of vaginal mucous membrane that is visible from approximately the fourth week of pregnancy; caused by increased vascularity

chloasma Increased pigmentation over bridge of nose and cheeks of pregnant women and some women taking oral contraceptives; also known as "mask of pregnancy"

colostrum Fluid in the acini cells of the breasts present from early pregnancy into the early postpartal period; rich in antibodies, which provide protection to the breastfed newborn from many diseases; high in protein, which binds bilirubin; and laxative acting, which speeds the elimination of meconium and helps loosen mucus

diastasis recti abdominis Separation of the two rectus muscles along the median line of the abdominal wall; often seen in women with repeated childbirths or with a multiple gestation (e.g., triplets)

epulis Tumorlike benign lesion of the gingiva seen in pregnant women

funic souffle Soft, muffled, blowing sound produced by blood rushing through the umbilical vessels and synchronous with the fetal heart sounds

Goodell sign Softening of the cervix, a probable sign of pregnancy, occurring during the second month

Hegar sign Softening of the lower uterine segment that is classified as a probable sign of pregnancy, may be present during the second and third months of pregnancy, and is palpated during bimanual examination

human chorionic gonadotropin (hCG) Hormone that is produced by chorionic villi; the biologic marker in pregnancy tests

leukorrhea White or yellowish mucus discharge from the cervical canal or the vagina that may be normal physiologically or caused by pathologic states of the vagina and endocervix

lightening Sensation of decreased abdominal distention produced by uterine descent into the pelvic cavity as the fetal presenting part settles into the pelvis; usually occurs 2 weeks before the onset of labor in nulliparas

KEY TERMS AND DEFINITIONS—cont'd

linea nigra Line of darker pigmentation seen in some women during the latter part of pregnancy that appears on the middle of the abdomen and extends from the symphysis pubis toward the umbilicus

Montgomery tubercles Small, nodular prominences (sebaceous glands) on the areolas around the nipples of the breasts that enlarge during pregnancy and lactation

operculum Plug of mucus that fills the cervical canal during pregnancy

palmar erythema Rash on the surface of the palms sometimes seen in pregnancy

ptyalism Excessive salivation

pyrosis Burning sensation in the epigastric and sternal region from stomach acid (heartburn)

quickening Maternal perception of fetal movement; usually occurs between weeks 16 and 20 of gestation

striae gravidarum "Stretch marks"; shining reddish lines caused by stretching of the skin, often found on the abdomen, thighs, and breasts during pregnancy; these streaks turn to a fine pinkish white or silver tone in time in fair-skinned women and brownish in darker-skinned women

uterine souffle Soft, blowing sound made by the blood in the arteries of the pregnant uterus and synchronous with the maternal pulse

ELECTRONIC RESOURCES

Additional information related to the content in Chapter 8 can be found on

the companion website at **evolve**
http://evolve.elsevier.com/Lowdermilk/Maternity/
• NCLEX Review Questions
• WebLinks

or on the interactive companion CD
• NCLEX Review Questions

The goal of maternity care is a healthy pregnancy with a physically safe and emotionally satisfying outcome for mother, infant, and family. Consistent health supervision and surveillance are of utmost importance in achieving this outcome. However, many maternal adaptations are unfamiliar to pregnant women and their families. Helping the pregnant woman recognize the relation between her physical status and the plan for her care assists her in making decisions and encourages her to participate in her own care.

GRAVIDITY AND PARITY

An understanding of the following terms used to describe pregnancy and the pregnant woman is essential to the study of maternity care.

• **gravida:** a woman who is pregnant
• **gravidity:** pregnancy
• **multigravida:** a woman who has had two or more pregnancies
• **multipara:** a woman who has completed two or more pregnancies to the stage of fetal viability
• **nulligravida:** a woman who has never been pregnant
• **nullipara:** a woman who has not completed a pregnancy with a fetus or fetuses who have reached the stage of fetal viability

• **parity:** the number of pregnancies in which the fetus or fetuses have reached viability when they are born, not the number of fetuses (e.g., twins) born. Whether the fetus is born alive or is stillborn (fetus who shows no signs of life at birth) after viability is reached does not affect parity
• **postdate or postterm:** a pregnancy that goes beyond 42 weeks of gestation
• **preterm:** a pregnancy that has reached 20 weeks of gestation but before completion of 37 weeks of gestation
• **primigravida:** a woman who is pregnant for the first time
• **primipara:** a woman who has completed one pregnancy with a fetus or fetuses who have reached the stage of fetal viability
• **term:** a pregnancy from the beginning of week 38 of gestation to the end of week 42 of gestation
• **viability:** capacity to live outside the uterus; about 22 to 24 weeks since last menstrual period, or fetal weight greater than 500 g

Gravidity and parity information is obtained during history-taking interviews and may be recorded in patient records in several ways. One way is to describe gravidity and parity with two numbers. For example 1/0 means that a woman is pregnant for the first time and has not yet carried a pregnancy to viability. Another system commonly used in maternity centers consists of five digits separated with hyphens.

TABLE 8-1

Gravidity and Parity Using Five-Digit (GTPAL) System

CONDITION	PREGNANCIES	TERM BIRTHS	PRETERM BIRTHS	ABORTIONS AND MISCARRIAGES	LIVING CHILDREN
Jamilla is pregnant for the first time.	1	0	0	0	0
She carries the pregnancy to 35 weeks, and the neonate survives.	1	0	1	0	1
She becomes pregnant again.	2	0	1	0	1
Her second pregnancy ends in miscarriage at 10 weeks.	2	0	1	1	1
During her third pregnancy, she gives birth at 38 weeks.	3	1	1	1	2

This system provides more specific information about parity. The first digit represents the total number of pregnancies, including the present one (gravidity); the second digit represents the total number of term births; the third indicates the number of preterm births; the fourth identifies the number of abortions (miscarriage or elective termination of pregnancy before viability); and the fifth is the number of children currently living. The acronym *GTPAL* (gravidity, term, preterm, abortions, living children) may be helpful in remembering this system of notation. For example, if a woman pregnant only once gives birth at week 34 and the infant survives, the abbreviation that represents this information is "1-0-1-0-1." During her next pregnancy, the abbreviation is "2-0-1-0-1." Additional examples are given in Table 8-1.

PREGNANCY TESTS

Early detection of pregnancy allows early initiation of care. Human chorionic gonadotropin (hCG) is the earliest biochemical marker for pregnancy, and pregnancy tests are based on the recognition of hCG or a beta (β) subunit of hCG. Production of β-hCG begins as early as the day of implantation and can be detected as early as 7 to 10 days after conception (Stewart, 2004). The level of hCG increases until it peaks at about 60 to 70 days of gestation and then declines until about 80 days of pregnancy. It remains stable until about 30 weeks and then gradually increases until term. Higher than normal levels of hCG may indicate ectopic pregnancy, abnormal gestation (e.g., fetus with Down syndrome), or multiple gestation; abnormally slow increase or a decrease in hCG levels may indicate impending miscarriage (Buster & Carson, 2002).

Serum and urine pregnancy tests are performed in clinics, offices, women's health centers, and laboratory settings, and urine pregnancy tests may be performed at home. Both serum and urine tests can provide accurate results. A 7- to 10-ml sample of venous blood is collected for serum testing. Most urine tests require a first-voided morning urine specimen because it contains levels of hCG approximately the same as those in serum. Random urine samples usually have lower levels. Urine tests are less expensive and provide more immediate results than do serum tests (Stewart, 2004).

Many different pregnancy tests are available. The wide variety of tests precludes discussion of each; however, several categories of tests are described here. The nurse should read the manufacturer's directions for the test to be used.

Radioimmunoassay (RIA) pregnancy tests for the beta subunit of hCG in serum or urine samples use radioactively

Critical Thinking Exercise

Home Pregnancy Testing

Sylvia and her partner want to have a baby and have not been using any contraception for 3 months. Sylvia's period is now a week late. She uses a home pregnancy test kit and the results are negative. She is disappointed and has called the health line at the local women's health clinic for advice about having another test.

1 Evidence—Is there sufficient evidence to draw conclusions about what advice the nurse should give to Sylvia?
2 Assumptions—What assumptions can be made about home pregnancy testing?
3 What implications and priorities for giving advice to Sylvia can be made at this time?
4 Does the evidence objectively support your conclusion?
5 Are there alternative perspectives to your conclusion?

labeled markers and are usually performed in a laboratory. These tests are accurate with low hCG levels (5 milli-international units/ml) and can confirm pregnancy as soon as 1 week after conception. Results are available within a few hours (Stewart, 2004).

Radioreceptor assay (RRA) is a serum test that measures the ability of a blood sample to inhibit the binding of radio-labeled hCG to receptors. The test is 90% to 95% accurate from 6 to 8 days after conception (Pagana & Pagana, 2003).

Enzyme-linked immunosorbent assay (ELISA) testing is the most popular method of testing for pregnancy. It uses a specific monoclonal antibody (anti-hCG) with enzymes to bond with hCG in urine. Depending on the specific test, levels of hCG as low as 25 milli-international units/ml can be detected as early as 7 days after conception (Stewart, 2004). As an office or home procedure, it requires minimal time and offers results in less than 5 minutes. A positive test result is indicated by a simple color change reaction.

ELISA technology is the basis for most over-the-counter home pregnancy tests. With these one-step tests, the woman usually applies urine to a strip and reads the results. The test kits come with directions for collection of the specimen, the testing procedure, and reading of the results. Most manufacturers of the kits provide a toll-free telephone number to call if users have concerns and questions about test procedures or results (see Teaching Guidelines). The most common error in performing home pregnancy tests is performing the test too early in pregnancy (Stewart, 2004).

Interpreting the results of pregnancy tests requires some judgment. The type of pregnancy test and its degree of sensitivity (ability to detect low levels of a substance) and specificity (ability to discern the absence of a substance) must be considered in conjunction with the woman's history. This includes the date of her last normal menstrual period (LNMP), her usual cycle length, and results of previous pregnancy tests. It is important to know if the woman is a substance abuser and what medications she is taking, because medications such as anticonvulsants and tranquilizers can cause false-positive results, whereas diuretics and

promethazine can cause false-negative results (Pagana & Pagana, 2003). Improper collection of the specimen, hormone-producing tumors, and laboratory errors also may cause false results. Whenever there is any question, further evaluation or retesting may be appropriate.

ADAPTATIONS TO PREGNANCY

Maternal physiologic adaptations are attributed to the hormones of pregnancy and to mechanical pressures arising from the enlarging uterus and other tissues. These adaptations protect the woman's normal physiologic functioning, meet the metabolic demands pregnancy imposes on her body, and provide a nurturing environment for fetal development and growth. Although pregnancy is a normal phenomenon, problems can occur.

Signs of Pregnancy

Some of the physiologic adaptations are recognized as signs and symptoms of pregnancy. Three commonly used categories of signs and symptoms of pregnancy are presumptive (those changes felt by the woman—e.g., amenorrhea, fatigue, nausea and vomiting, breast changes); probable (those changes observed by an examiner—e.g., Hegar sign, ballottement, pregnancy tests); and positive (those signs that are attributable only to the presence of the fetus—e.g., hearing fetal heart tones, visualization of the fetus, and palpating fetal movements). Table 8-2 summarizes these signs of pregnancy in relation to when they might occur and other causes for their occurrence.

Reproductive System and Breasts
Uterus
Changes in size, shape, and position. The phenomenal uterine growth in the first trimester is stimulated by high levels of estrogen and progesterone. Early uterine enlargement results from increased vascularity and dilation of blood vessels, hyperplasia (production of new muscle fibers and fibroelastic tissue) and hypertrophy (enlargement of preexisting muscle fibers and fibroelastic tissue), and development of the decidua. By 7 weeks of gestation, the uterus is the size of a large hen's egg; by 10 weeks of gestation, it is the size of an orange (twice its nonpregnant size); and by 12 weeks of gestation, it is the size of a grapefruit. After the third month, uterine enlargement is primarily the result of mechanical pressure of the growing fetus.

As the uterus enlarges, it also changes in shape and position. At conception the uterus is shaped like an upside-down pear. During the second trimester, as the muscular walls strengthen and become more elastic, the uterus becomes spherical or globular. Later, as the fetus lengthens, the uterus becomes larger and more ovoid and rises out of the pelvis into the abdominal cavity.

The pregnancy may "show" after the fourteenth week, although this depends to some degree on the woman's height

TEACHING GUIDELINES
Home Pregnancy Testing

- Follow the manufacturer's instructions carefully. Do not omit steps.
- Review the manufacturer's list of foods, medications, and other substances that can affect the test results.
- Use a first-voided morning urine specimen.
- If the test done at the time of your missed period is negative, repeat the test in 1 week if you still have not had a period.
- If you have questions about the test, contact the manufacturer.
- Contact your health care provider for follow-up if the test result is positive or if the test result is negative and you still have not had a period.

TABLE 8-2

Signs of Pregnancy

TIME OF OCCURRENCE (GESTATIONAL AGE)	SIGN	OTHER POSSIBLE CAUSE
PRESUMPTIVE SIGNS		
3-4 wk	Breast changes	Premenstrual changes, oral contraceptives
4 wk	Amenorrhea	Stress, vigorous exercise, early menopause, endocrine problems, malnutrition
4-14 wk	Nausea, vomiting	Gastrointestinal virus, food poisoning
6-12 wk	Urinary frequency	Infection, pelvic tumors
12 wk	Fatigue	Stress, illness
16-20 wk	Quickening	Gas, peristalsis
PROBABLE SIGNS		
5 wk	Goodell sign	Pelvic congestion
6-8 wk	Chadwick sign	Pelvic congestion
6-12 wk	Hegar sign	Pelvic congestion
4-12 wk	Positive result of pregnancy test (serum)	Hydatidiform mole, choriocarcinoma
6-12 wk	Positive result of pregnancy test (urine)	False-positive results may be caused by pelvic infection, tumors
16 wk	Braxton Hicks contractions	Myomas, other tumors
16-28 wk	Ballottement	Tumors, cervical polyps
POSITIVE SIGNS		
5-6 wk	Visualization of fetus by real-time ultrasound examination	No other causes
6 wk	Fetal heart tones detected by ultrasound examination	No other causes
16 wk	Visualization of fetus by radiographic study	No other causes
8-17 wk	Fetal heart tones detected by Doppler ultrasound stethoscope	No other causes
17-19 wk	Fetal heart tones detected by fetal stethoscope	No other causes
19-22 wk	Fetal movements palpated	No other causes
Late pregnancy	Fetal movements visible	No other causes

and weight. Abdominal enlargement may be less apparent in the nullipara with good abdominal muscle tone (Fig. 8-1). Posture also influences the type and degree of abdominal enlargement that occurs. In normal pregnancies, the uterus enlarges at a predictable rate. As the uterus grows, it may be palpated above the symphysis pubis some time between the twelfth and fourteenth weeks of pregnancy (Fig. 8-2). The uterus rises gradually to the level of the umbilicus at 22 to 24 weeks of gestation and nearly reaches the xiphoid process at term. Between weeks 38 and 40, fundal height drops as the fetus begins to descend and engage in the pelvis (lightening) (see Fig. 8-2, *dashed line*). Generally, lightening occurs in the nullipara about 2 weeks before the onset of labor and at the start of labor in the multipara.

Uterine enlargement is determined by measuring fundal height, a measurement commonly used to estimate the duration of pregnancy. However, variation in the position of the fundus or the fetus, variations in the amount of amniotic fluid present, the presence of more than one fetus, ma-

ternal obesity, and variation in examiner techniques can reduce the accuracy of this estimation of the duration of pregnancy.

The uterus normally rotates to the right as it elevates, probably because of the presence of the rectosigmoid colon on the left side, but the extensive hypertrophy (enlargement) of the round ligaments keeps the uterus in the midline. Eventually the growing uterus touches the anterior abdominal wall and displaces the intestines to either side of the abdomen (Fig. 8-3). Whenever a pregnant woman is standing, most of her uterus rests against the anterior abdominal wall, and this contributes to altering her center of gravity.

At approximately 6 weeks of gestation, softening and compressibility of the lower uterine segment (the uterine isthmus) occur (Hegar sign) (Fig. 8-4). This results in exaggerated uterine anteflexion during the first 3 months of pregnancy. In this position, the uterine fundus presses on the urinary bladder, causing the woman to have urinary frequency.

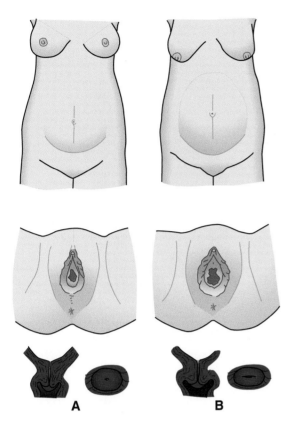

Fig. 8-1 Comparison of abdomen, vulva, and cervix in **A,** nullipara, and **B,** multipara, at the same stage of pregnancy.

Changes in contractility. Soon after the fourth month of pregnancy, uterine contractions can be felt through the abdominal wall. These contractions are referred to as the Braxton Hicks sign. Braxton Hicks contractions are irregular and painless and occur intermittently throughout pregnancy. These contractions facilitate uterine blood flow through the intervillous spaces of the placenta and thereby promote oxygen delivery to the fetus. Although Braxton Hicks contractions are not painful, some women complain that they are annoying. After the twenty-eighth week, these contractions become much more definite, but they usually cease with walking or exercise. Braxton Hicks contractions can be mistaken for true labor; however, they do not increase in intensity or frequency or cause cervical dilation.

Uteroplacental blood flow. Placental perfusion depends on the maternal blood flow to the uterus. Blood flow increases rapidly as the uterus increases in size. Although uterine blood flow increases twentyfold, the fetoplacental unit grows more rapidly. Consequently, more oxygen is extracted from the uterine blood during the latter part of pregnancy (Cunningham et al., 2005). In a normal term pregnancy, one sixth of the total maternal blood volume is within the uterine vascular system. The rate of blood flow through the uterus averages 500 ml/min, and oxygen consumption of the gravid uterus increases to meet fetal needs.

A low maternal arterial pressure, contractions of the uterus, and maternal supine position are three factors known to decrease blood flow. Estrogen stimulation may increase uterine blood flow. Doppler ultrasound examination can be used to measure uterine blood flow velocity, especially in pregnancies at risk because of conditions associated with decreased placental perfusion such as hypertension, intrauterine growth restriction, diabetes mellitus, and multiple gestation (Harman, 2004). By using an ultrasound device or a fetal stethoscope, the health care provider may hear the uterine souffle (sound made by blood in the uterine arteries that is synchronous with the maternal pulse) or the funic souffle (sound made by blood rushing through the umbilical vessels and synchronous with the fetal heart rate).

Cervical changes. A softening of the cervical tip called Goodell sign may be observed about the beginning of the sixth week in a normal, unscarred cervix. This sign is brought about by increased vascularity, slight hypertrophy, and hyperplasia (increase in number of cells) of the muscle and its collagen-rich connective tissue, which becomes loose, edematous, highly elastic, and increased in volume. The glands near the external os proliferate beneath the stratified squamous epithelium, giving the cervix the velvety appearance characteristic of pregnancy. *Friability* is increased and may cause slight bleeding after coitus with deep penetration or after vaginal examination. Pregnancy also can cause the squamocolumnar junction, the site for obtaining cells for cervical cancer screening, to be located away from the cervix. Because of all these changes, evaluation of abnormal Papanicolaou (Pap) tests during pregnancy can be complicated. Careful assessment of all pregnant women is important, however, because about 3% of

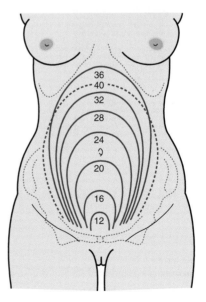

Fig. 8-2 Height of fundus by weeks of normal gestation with a single fetus. Dashed line, height after lightening. (From Seidel, H., Ball, J., Dains, J., & Benedict, G. [2003]. *Mosby's guide to physical examination* [5th ed.]. St. Louis: Mosby.)

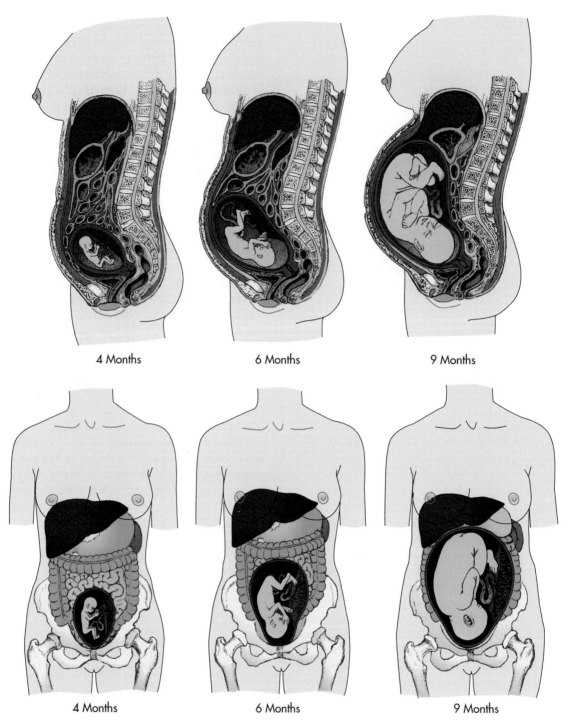

4 Months   6 Months   9 Months

4 Months   6 Months   9 Months

Fig. 8-3 Displacement of internal abdominal structures and diaphragm by the enlarging uterus at 4, 6, and 9 months of gestation.

all cervical cancers are diagnosed during pregnancy (Berman, DiSaia, & Tewari, 2004).

The cervix of the nullipara is rounded. Lacerations of the cervix almost always occur during the birth process. With or without lacerations, however, after childbirth, the cervix becomes more oval in the horizontal plane, and the external os appears as a transverse slit (see Fig. 8-1).

Changes related to the presence of the fetus. Passive movement of the unengaged fetus is called **ballottement** and can be identified generally between the sixteenth and eighteenth week. Ballottement is a technique of palpating a floating structure by bouncing it gently and feeling it rebound. In the technique used to palpate the fetus, the examiner places a finger in the vagina and taps gently

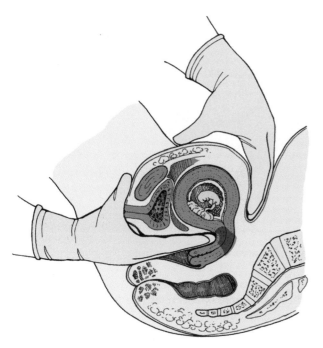

Fig. 8-4 Hegar sign. Bimanual examination for assessing compressibility and softening of the isthmus (lower uterine segment) while the cervix is still firm.

upward, causing the fetus to rise. The fetus then sinks, and a gentle tap is felt on the finger (Fig. 8-5).

The first recognition of fetal movements, or "feeling life," by the multiparous woman may occur as early as the fourteenth to sixteenth week. The nulliparous woman may not notice these sensations until the eighteenth week or later. Quickening is commonly described as a flutter and is difficult to distinguish from peristalsis. Fetal movements gradually increase in intensity and frequency. The week when quickening occurs provides a tentative clue in dating the duration of gestation.

Vagina and vulva

Pregnancy hormones prepare the vagina for stretching during labor and birth by causing the vaginal mucosa to thicken, the connective tissue to loosen, the smooth muscle to

hypertrophy, and the vaginal vault to lengthen. Increased vascularity results in a violet-bluish color of the vaginal mucosa and cervix. The deepened color, termed the Chadwick sign, may be evident as early as the sixth week but is easily noted at the eighth week of pregnancy (Monga & Sanborn, 2004).

Leukorrhea is a white or slightly gray mucoid discharge with a faint musty odor. This copious mucoid fluid occurs in response to cervical stimulation by estrogen and progesterone. The fluid is whitish because of the presence of many exfoliated vaginal epithelial cells caused by the hyperplasia of normal pregnancy. This vaginal discharge is never pruritic or blood stained. Because of the progesterone effect, ferning usually does not occur in the dried cervical mucus smear, as it would in a smear of amniotic fluid. Instead, a beaded or cellular crystallizing pattern formed in the dried mucus is seen (Gibbs, Sweet, & Duff, 2004). The mucus fills the endocervical canal, resulting in the formation of the mucous plug (operculum) (Fig. 8-6). The operculum acts as a barrier against bacterial invasion during pregnancy.

During pregnancy, the pH of vaginal secretions is more acidic (ranging from about 3.5 to 6 [normal 4 to 7]) because of increased production of lactic acid caused by *Lactobacillus acidophilus* action on glycogen in the vaginal epithelium, probably resulting from increased estrogen levels (Cunningham et al., 2005). While this acidic environment provides more protection from some organisms, the pregnant woman is more vulnerable to other infections, especially yeast infections because the glycogen-rich environment is more susceptible to *Candida albicans* (Gibbs, Sweet, & Duff, 2004).

The increased vascularity of the vagina and other pelvic viscera results in a marked increase in sensitivity. The increased sensitivity may lead to a high degree of sexual interest and arousal, especially during the second trimester of pregnancy. The increased congestion plus the relaxed walls of the blood vessels and the heavy uterus may result in edema and varicosities of the vulva. The edema and varicosities usually resolve during the postpartum period.

External structures of the perineum are enlarged during pregnancy because of an increase in vasculature, hypertrophy of the perineal body, and deposition of fat (Fig. 8-7).

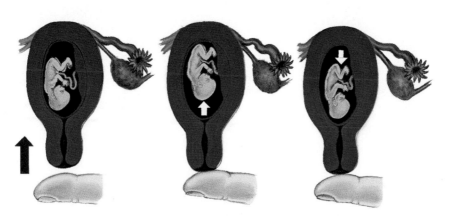

Fig. 8-5 Internal ballottement (18 weeks).

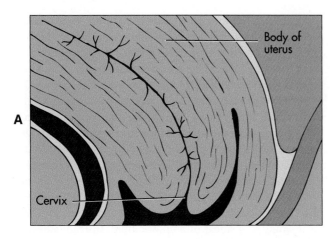
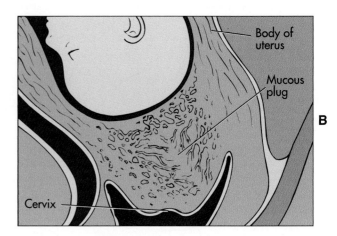

Fig. 8-6   A, Cervix in nonpregnant woman. **B,** Cervix during pregnancy.

The labia majora of the nullipara approximate and obscure the vaginal introitus; those of the parous woman separate and gape after childbirth and perineal or vaginal injury. Fig. 8-1 compares the perineum of the nullipara and the multipara in relation to the pregnant abdomen, vulva, and cervix.

Breasts

Fullness, heightened sensitivity, tingling, and heaviness of the breasts begin in the early weeks of gestation in response to increased levels of estrogen and progesterone. Breast sensitivity varies from mild tingling to sharp pain. Nipples and areolae become more pigmented, secondary pinkish areolae develop, extending beyond the primary areolae, and nipples become more erectile. Hypertrophy of the sebaceous (oil) glands embedded in the primary areolae,

called **Montgomery tubercles** (see Fig. 4-6), may be seen around the nipples. These sebaceous glands may have a protective role in that they keep the nipples lubricated for breast-feeding.

The richer blood supply causes the vessels beneath the skin to dilate. Once barely noticeable, the blood vessels become visible, often appearing in an intertwining blue network beneath the surface of the skin. Venous congestion in the breasts is more obvious in primigravidas. Striae gravidarum may appear at the outer aspects of the breasts.

During the second and third trimesters, growth of the mammary glands accounts for the progressive breast enlargement. The high levels of luteal and placental hormones in pregnancy promote proliferation of the lactiferous ducts and lobule-alveolar tissue, so that palpation of the breasts reveals a generalized, coarse nodularity. Glandular tissue

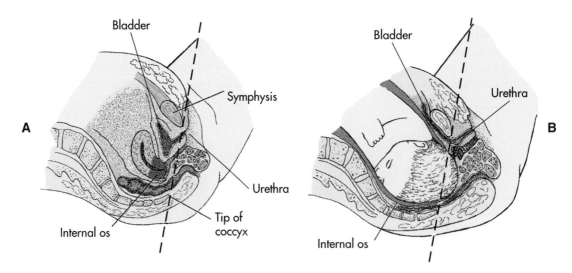

Fig. 8-7   A, Pelvic floor in nonpregnant woman. **B,** Pelvic floor at end of pregnancy. Note marked hypertrophy and hyperplasia below dotted line joining tip of coccyx and inferior margin of symphysis. Note elongation of bladder and urethra as a result of compression. Fat deposits are increased.

displaces connective tissue, and as a result, the tissue becomes softer and looser.

Although development of the mammary glands is functionally complete by midpregnancy, lactation is inhibited until a decrease in estrogen level occurs after the birth. A thin, clear, viscous secretory material (precolostrum) can be found in the acini cells by the third month of gestation. **Colostrum,** the creamy, white-to-yellowish to orange premilk fluid, may be expressed from the nipples as early as 16 weeks of gestation (Lawrence & Lawrence, 2004). See Chapter 20 for discussion of lactation.

General Body Systems
Cardiovascular system

Maternal adjustments to pregnancy involve extensive changes in the cardiovascular system, both anatomic and physiologic. Cardiovascular adaptations protect the woman's normal physiologic functioning, meet the metabolic demands pregnancy imposes on her body, and provide for fetal developmental and growth needs.

Slight cardiac hypertrophy (enlargement) is probably secondary to the increased blood volume and cardiac output that occurs. The heart returns to its normal size after childbirth. As the diaphragm is displaced upward by the enlarging uterus, the heart is elevated upward and rotated forward to the left (Fig. 8-8). The apical impulse, a point of maximal intensity (PMI), is shifted upward and laterally about 1 to

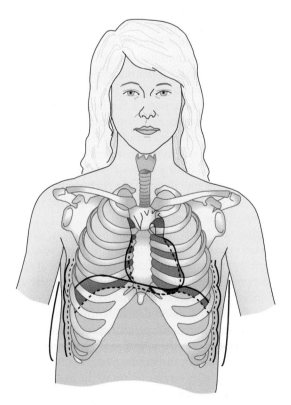

Fig. 8-8 Changes in position of heart, lungs, and thoracic cage in pregnancy. *Broken line,* nonpregnant; *solid line,* change that occurs in pregnancy.

1.5 cm. The degree of shift depends on the duration of pregnancy and the size and position of the uterus.

The changes in heart size and position and increases in blood volume and cardiac output contribute to auscultatory changes common in pregnancy. There is more audible splitting of S_1 and S_2, and S_3 may be readily heard after 20 weeks of gestation. In addition, systolic and diastolic murmurs may be heard over the pulmonic area. These are transient and disappear shortly after the woman gives birth (Cunningham et al., 2005).

Between 14 and 20 weeks of gestation, the pulse increases about 10 to 15 beats/min, which then persists to term. Palpitations may occur. In twin gestations the maternal heart rate increases significantly in the third trimester (Malone & D'Alton, 2004).

The cardiac rhythm may be disturbed. The pregnant woman may experience sinus arrhythmia, premature atrial contractions, and premature ventricular systole. In the healthy woman with no underlying heart disease, no therapy is needed; however, women with preexisting heart disease will need close medical and obstetric supervision during pregnancy (see Chapter 22).

Blood pressure. Arterial blood pressure (brachial artery) is affected by age, activity level, presence of health problems, and circadian rhythm (Hermida, Ayala, Mojon, & Fernandez, 2001). Additional factors must be considered during pregnancy. These factors include maternal anxiety, maternal position, and size and type of blood pressure apparatus.

Maternal anxiety can elevate readings. If an elevated reading is found, the woman is given time to rest, and the reading is repeated.

Maternal position affects readings. Brachial blood pressure is highest when the woman is sitting, lowest when she is lying in the lateral recumbent position, and intermediate when she is supine, except for some women who experience supine hypotensive syndrome (see discussion later). Therefore at each prenatal visit, the reading should be obtained in the same arm and with the woman in the same position. The position and arm used should be recorded along with the reading (Gonik & Foley, 2004).

The proper-size cuff is absolutely necessary for accurate readings. The cuff should be 20% wider than the diameter of the arm around which it is wrapped, or about 12 to 14 cm for average-sized individuals and 18 to 20 cm for obese persons. Too small a cuff yields a false high reading; too large a cuff yields a false low reading. Caution also should be used when comparing auscultatory and oscillatory blood pressure readings, because discrepancies can occur (Pickering, 2002).

Systolic blood pressure usually remains the same as the prepregnancy level but may decrease slightly as pregnancy advances. Diastolic blood pressure begins to decrease in the first trimester, continues to drop until 24 to 32 weeks, then gradually increases and returns to prepregnancy levels by term (Blackburn, 2003; Monga, 2004).

Calculating the *mean arterial pressure (MAP)* (mean of the blood pressure in the arterial circulation) can increase the diagnostic value of the findings. Normal MAP readings in the nonpregnant woman are 86.4 mm Hg ± 7.5 mm Hg. MAP readings for a pregnant woman are slightly higher (Gonik & Foley, 2004). One way to calculate an MAP is illustrated in Box 8-1.

Some degree of compression of the vena cava occurs in all women who lie flat on their backs during the second half of pregnancy (see Fig. 14-5). Some women experience a decrease in their systolic blood pressure of more than 30 mm Hg. After 4 to 5 minutes a reflex bradycardia is noted, cardiac output is reduced by half, and the woman feels faint. This condition is referred to as *supine hypotensive syndrome* (Cunningham et al., 2005).

Compression of the iliac veins and inferior vena cava by the uterus causes increased venous pressure and reduced blood flow in the legs (except when the woman is in the lateral position). These alterations contribute to the dependent edema, varicose veins in the legs and vulva, and hemorrhoids that develop in the latter part of term pregnancy (Fig. 8-9).

Blood volume and composition. The degree of blood volume expansion varies considerably. Blood volume increases by approximately 1500 ml, or 40% to 45% above nonpregnancy levels (Cunningham et al., 2005). This increase consists of 1000 ml plasma plus 450 ml red blood cells (RBCs). The blood volume starts to increase at about the tenth to twelfth week, peaks at about the thirty-second to thirty-fourth week, and then decreases slightly at the fortieth week. The increase in volume of a multiple gestation is greater than that for a pregnancy with a single fetus (Malone & D'Alton, 2004). Increased volume is a protective mechanism. It is essential for meeting the blood volume needs of the hypertrophied vascular system of the enlarged uterus, for adequately hydrating fetal and maternal tissues when the woman assumes an erect or supine position, and for providing a fluid reserve to compensate for blood loss during birth and the puerperium. Peripheral vasodilation maintains a normal blood pressure despite the increased blood volume in pregnancy.

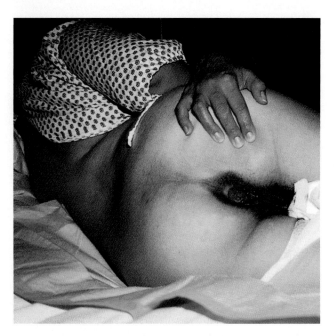

Fig. 8-9 Hemorrhoids. (Courtesy Marjorie Pyle, RNC, Lifecircle, Costa Mesa, CA.)

During pregnancy there is an accelerated production of RBCs (normal, 4.2 to 5.4 million/mm³). The percentage of increase depends on the amount of iron available. The RBC mass increases by about 20% to 30% (Monga, 2004).

Because the plasma increase exceeds the increase in RBC production, there is a decrease in normal hemoglobin values (12 to 16 g/dl blood) and hematocrit values (37% to 47%). This state of hemodilution is referred to as *physiologic anemia.* The decrease is more noticeable during the second trimester, when rapid expansion of blood volume takes place faster than RBC production. If the hemoglobin value decreases to 10 g/dl or less or if the hematocrit decreases to 35% or less, the woman is considered anemic.

The total white cell count increases during the second trimester and peaks during the third trimester. This increase is primarily in the granulocytes; the lymphocyte count stays about the same throughout pregnancy. See Table 8-3 for laboratory values during pregnancy.

Cardiac output. Cardiac output increases from 30% to 50% over the nonpregnant rate by the thirty-second week of pregnancy; it declines to about a 20% increase at 40 weeks of gestation. This elevated cardiac output is largely a result of increased stroke volume and heart rate and occurs in response to increased tissue demands for oxygen (Monga, 2004). Cardiac output in late pregnancy is appreciably higher when the woman is in the lateral recumbent position than when she is supine. In the supine position the large, heavy uterus often impedes venous return to the heart and affects blood pressure. Cardiac output increases with any exertion, such as labor and birth. Table 8-4 summarizes cardiovascular changes in pregnancy.

BOX 8-1

Calculation of Mean Arterial Pressure

Blood pressure: 106/70 mm Hg

Formula:
$$\frac{(systolic) + 2(diastolic)}{3}$$

$$\frac{(106) + 2(70)}{3}$$

$$\frac{106 + 140}{3}$$

$$246/3 = 82 \text{ mm Hg}$$

TABLE 8-3

Laboratory Values for Pregnant and Nonpregnant Women

VALUES	NONPREGNANT	PREGNANT
HEMATOLOGIC		
Complete Blood Count (CBC)		
Hemoglobin, g/dl	12-16*	>11*
Hematocrit, PCV, %	37-47	>33*
Red blood cell (RBC) volume, per ml	1600	1500-1900
Plasma volume, per ml	2400	3700
RBC count, million per mm^3	4.2-5.4	5.0-6.25
White blood cells, total per mm^3	5000-10,000	5000-15,000
Neutrophils, %	55-70	60-85
Lymphocytes, %	20-40	15-40
Erythrocyte sedimentation rate, mm/hr	20	Elevated in second and third trimesters
Mean corpuscular hemoglobin concentration (MCHC), g/dl packed RBCs	32-36	No change in hemoglobin concentration
Mean corpuscular hemoglobin (MCH), pg	27-31	No change per pg (less than 1 ng)
Mean corpuscular volume (MCV), μm^3	80-95	No change per μm^3
Blood Coagulation and Fibrinolytic Activity†		
Factor VII	65-140	Increase in pregnancy, return to normal in early puerperium
Factor VIII	55-145	Increases during pregnancy and immediately after birth
Factor IX	60-140	Increase in pregnancy returns to normal in early puerperium
Factor X	45-155	
Factor XI	65-135	Decrease in pregnancy
Factor XII	50-150	Increase in pregnancy, returns to normal in early puerperium
Prothrombin time (PT), sec	11-12.5	Slight decrease in pregnancy
Partial thromboplastin time (PTT), sec	60-70	Slight decrease in pregnancy and decrease during second and third stage of labor (indicates clotting at placental site)
Bleeding time, min	1-9 (Ivy)	No appreciable change
Coagulation time, min	6-10 (Lee/White)	No appreciable change
Platelets, per mm^3	150,000-400,000	No significant change until 3-5 days after birth and then a rapid increase (may predispose woman to thrombosis) and gradual return to normal
Fibrinolytic activity	Normal	Decreases in pregnancy and then abruptly returns to normal (protection against thromboembolism)
Fibrinogen, mg/dl	200-400	Increased levels late in pregnancy
Mineral and Vitamin Concentrations		
Vitamin B$_{12}$, folic acid, ascorbic acid	Normal	Moderate decrease
Serum Proteins		
Total, g/dl	6.4-8.3	5.5-7.5
Albumin, g/dl	3.5-5	Slight increase
Globulin, total, g/dl	2.3-3.4	3.0-4.0
Blood glucose		
Fasting, mg/dl	70-105	Decreases
2-hr postprandial, mg/dl	<140	<140 after a 100-g carbohydrate meal is considered normal

*At sea level. Permanent residents of higher altitudes (e.g., Denver) require higher levels of hemoglobin.
†Pregnancy represents a hypercoagulable state.
pg, picogram; *μm^3*, cubic micrometer; *mm^3*, cubic millimeter; *dl*, deciliter; *ng*, nanogram; *PVC*, packed cell volume.

Continued

TABLE 8-3

Laboratory Values for Pregnant and Nonpregnant Women—cont'd

VALUES	NONPREGNANT	PREGNANT
HEMATOLOGIC—cont'd		
Acid-base Values in Arterial Blood		
P_{O_2}, mm Hg	80-100	104-108 (increased)
P_{CO_2}, mm Hg	35-45	27-32 (decreased)
Sodium bicarbonate (HCO_3), mEq/L	21-28	18-31 (decreased)
Blood pH	7.35-7.45	7.40-7.45 (slightly increased, more alkaline)
HEPATIC		
Bilirubin, total, mg/dl	≤1	Unchanged
Serum cholesterol, mg/dl	120-200	Increases from 16 to 32 weeks of pregnancy; remains at this level until after birth
Serum alkaline phosphatase, units/L	30-120	Increases from week 12 of pregnancy to 6 weeks after birth
Serum albumin, g/dl	3.5-5.0	Slight increase
RENAL		
Bladder capacity, ml	1300	1500
Renal plasma flow (RPF), ml/min	490-700	Increase by 25%-30%
Glomerular filtration rate (GFR), ml/min	88-128	Increase by 30%-50%
Nonprotein nitrogen (NPN), mg/dl	25-40	Decreases
Blood urea nitrogen (BUN), mg/dl	10-20	Decreases
Serum creatinine, mg/dl	0.5-1.1	Decreases
Serum uric acid, mg/dl	2.7-7.3	Decreases
Urine glucose	Negative	Present in 20% of pregnant women
Intravenous pyelogram (IVP)	Normal	Slight-to-moderate hydroureter and hydronephrosis; right kidney larger than left kidney

From Gordon, M. (2002). Maternal physiology in pregnancy. In S. Gabbe, J. Niebyl, & J. Simpson (Eds.), *Obstetrics: Normal and problem pregnancies* (4th ed.). New York: Churchill Livingstone; Pagana, K., & Pagana, T. (2003). *Mosby's diagnostic and laboratory test reference* (6th ed.). St. Louis: Mosby.

TABLE 8-4

Cardiovascular Changes in Pregnancy

Heart rate	Increases 10-15 beats/min
Blood pressure	Remains at prepregnancy levels in first trimester
	Slight decrease in second trimester
	Returns to prepregnancy levels in third trimester
Blood volume	Increases by 1500 ml or 40%-50% above prepregnancy level
Red blood cell mass	Increases 17%
Hemoglobin	Decreases
Hematocrit	Decreases
White blood cell count	Increases in second and third trimesters
Cardiac output	Increases 30%-50%

Circulation and coagulation times. The circulation time decreases slightly by week 32. It returns to near normal by near term. There is a greater tendency for blood to coagulate (clot) during pregnancy because of increases in various clotting factors (factors VII, VIII, IX, X, and fibrinogen). This, combined with the fact that fibrinolytic activity (the splitting up or the dissolving of a clot) is depressed during pregnancy and the postpartum period, provides a protective function to decrease the chance of bleeding but also makes the woman more vulnerable to thrombosis, especially after cesarean birth.

Respiratory system

Structural and ventilatory adaptations occur during pregnancy to provide for maternal and fetal needs. Maternal oxygen requirements increase in response to the acceleration in the metabolic rate and the need to add to the tissue mass in the uterus and breasts. In addition, the fetus requires oxygen and a way to eliminate carbon dioxide.

Elevated levels of estrogen cause the ligaments of the rib cage to relax, permitting increased chest expansion (see Fig. 8-8). The transverse diameter of the thoracic cage increases by about 2 cm, and the circumference increases by 6 cm (Cunningham et al., 2005). The costal angle increases, and the lower rib cage appears to flare out. The chest may not return to its prepregnant state after birth (Seidel, Ball, Dains, & Benedict, 2003).

The diaphragm is displaced by as much as 4 cm during pregnancy. As pregnancy advances, thoracic (costal) breathing replaces abdominal breathing, and it becomes less possible for the diaphragm to descend with inspiration. Thoracic breathing is accomplished primarily by the diaphragm rather than by the costal muscles (Whitty & Dombrowski, 2004).

The upper respiratory tract becomes more vascular in response to elevated levels of estrogen. As the capillaries become engorged, edema and hyperemia develop within the nose, pharynx, larynx, trachea, and bronchi. This congestion within the tissues of the respiratory tract gives rise to several conditions commonly seen during pregnancy, including nasal and sinus stuffiness, epistaxis (nosebleed), changes in the voice, and a marked inflammatory response that can develop into a mild upper respiratory infection.

Increased vascularity of the upper respiratory tract also can cause the tympanic membranes and eustachian tubes to swell, giving rise to symptoms of impaired hearing, earaches, or a sense of fullness in the ears.

Pulmonary function.   Respiratory changes in pregnancy are related to the elevation of the diaphragm and to chest wall changes. Changes in the respiratory center result in a lowered threshold for carbon dioxide. The actions of progesterone and estrogen are presumed responsible for the increased sensitivity of the respiratory center to carbon dioxide. In addition, pregnant women become more aware of the need to breathe; some may even complain of dyspnea at rest, especially in the third trimester (Blackburn, 2003) (see Table 8-5 for respiratory changes in pregnancy). Although pulmonary function is not impaired by pregnancy, diseases of the respiratory tract may be more serious during this time (Cunningham et al., 2005). One important factor responsible for this may be the increased oxygen requirement.

Basal metabolic rate.   The basal metabolic rate (BMR) increases during pregnancy. This increase varies considerably depending on the prepregnancy nutritional status of the woman and fetal growth (Blackburn, 2003). The BMR returns to nonpregnant levels by 5 to 6 days after birth. The elevation in BMR during pregnancy reflects increased oxygen demands of the uterine-placental-fetal unit

and greater oxygen consumption because of increased maternal cardiac work. Peripheral vasodilation and acceleration of sweat gland activity help dissipate the excess heat resulting from the increased BMR during pregnancy. Pregnant women may experience heat intolerance, which is annoying to some women. Lassitude and fatigability after only slight exertion are experienced by many women in early pregnancy. These feelings, along with a greater need for sleep, may persist and may be caused in part by the increased metabolic activity.

Acid-base balance.   By about the tenth week of pregnancy, there is a decrease of about 5 mm Hg in the partial pressure of carbon dioxide (Pco_2). Progesterone may be responsible for increasing the sensitivity of the respiratory center receptors, so that tidal volume is increased, Pco_2 decreases, the base excess (HCO_3 or bicarbonate) decreases, and pH increases slightly. These alterations in acid-base balance indicate that pregnancy is a state of compensatory respiratory alkalosis (Blackburn, 2003). These changes also facilitate the transport of CO_2 from the fetus and O_2 release from the mother to the fetus (see Table 8-3).

Renal system

The kidneys are responsible for maintaining electrolyte and acid-base balance, regulating extracellular fluid volume, excreting waste products, and conserving essential nutrients.

Anatomic changes.   Changes in renal structure during pregnancy result from hormonal activity (estrogen and progesterone), pressure from an enlarging uterus, and an increase in blood volume. As early as the tenth week of pregnancy, the renal pelves and the ureters dilate. Dilation of the ureters is more pronounced above the pelvic brim, in part because they are compressed between the uterus and the pelvic brim. In most women, the ureters below the pelvic brim are of normal size. The smooth-muscle walls of the ureters undergo hyperplasia, hypertrophy, and muscle tone relaxation. The ureters elongate, become tortuous, and form single or double curves. In the latter part of pregnancy, the renal pelvis and ureter are dilated more on the right side than on the left because the heavy uterus is displaced to the right by the sigmoid colon.

Because of these changes, a larger volume of urine is held in the pelves and ureters, and urine flow rate is slowed. The resulting urinary stasis or stagnation has the following consequences:

- A lag occurs between the time urine is formed and when it reaches the bladder. Therefore clearance test results may reflect substances contained in glomerular filtrate several hours before.
- Stagnated urine is an excellent medium for the growth of microorganisms. In addition, the urine of pregnant women contains more nutrients, including glucose, thereby increasing the pH (making the urine more alkaline). This makes pregnant women more susceptible to urinary tract infection.

TABLE 8-5

Respiratory Changes in Pregnancy

Respiratory rate	Unchanged or slightly increased
Tidal volume	Increased 30%-40%
Vital capacity	Unchanged
Inspiratory capacity	Increased
Expiratory volume	Decreased
Total lung capacity	Unchanged to slightly decreased
Oxygen consumption	Increased 15%-20%

Bladder irritability, nocturia, and urinary frequency and urgency (without dysuria) are commonly reported in early pregnancy. Near term, bladder symptoms may return, especially after lightening occurs.

Urinary frequency results initially from increased bladder sensitivity and later from compression of the bladder (see Fig. 8-7). In the second trimester, the bladder is pulled up out of the true pelvis into the abdomen. The urethra lengthens to 7.5 cm as the bladder is displaced upward. The pelvic congestion that occurs in pregnancy is reflected in hyperemia of the bladder and urethra. This increased vascularity causes the bladder mucosa to be traumatized and bleed easily. Bladder tone may decrease, which increases the bladder capacity to 1500 ml. At the same time, the bladder is compressed by the enlarging uterus, resulting in the urge to void even if the bladder contains only a small amount of urine.

Functional changes. In normal pregnancy, renal function is altered considerably. Glomerular filtration rate (GFR) and renal plasma flow (RPF) increase early in pregnancy (Cunningham et al., 2005). These changes are caused by pregnancy hormones, an increase in blood volume, the woman's posture, physical activity, and nutritional intake. The woman's kidneys must manage the increased metabolic and circulatory demands of the maternal body and the excretion of fetal waste products. Renal function is most efficient when the woman lies in the lateral recumbent position and least efficient when the woman assumes a supine position. A side-lying position increases renal perfusion, which increases urinary output and decreases edema. When the pregnant woman is lying supine, the heavy uterus compresses the vena cava and the aorta, and cardiac output decreases. As a result, blood flow to the brain and heart is continued at the expense of other organs, including the kidneys and uterus.

Fluid and electrolyte balance. Selective renal tubular reabsorption maintains sodium and water balance regardless of changes in dietary intake and losses through sweat, vomitus, or diarrhea. From 500 to 900 mEq of sodium is normally retained during pregnancy to meet fetal needs. To prevent excessive sodium depletion, the maternal kidneys undergo a significant adaptation by increasing tubular reabsorption. Because of the need for increased maternal intravascular and extracellular fluid volume, additional sodium is needed to expand fluid volume and to maintain an isotonic state. As efficient as the renal system is, it can be overstressed by excessive dietary sodium intake or restriction or by use of diuretics. Severe hypovolemia and reduced placental perfusion are two consequences of using diuretics during pregnancy.

The capacity of the kidneys to excrete water during the early weeks of pregnancy is more efficient than it is later in pregnancy. As a result, some women feel thirsty in early pregnancy because of the greater amount of water loss. The pooling of fluid in the legs in the latter part of pregnancy decreases renal blood flow and GFR. This pooling of blood in the lower legs is sometimes referred to as *physiologic edema*

or dependent edema and requires no treatment. The normal diuretic response to the water load is triggered when the woman lies down, preferably on her side, and the pooled fluid reenters general circulation.

Normally the kidney reabsorbs almost all of the glucose and other nutrients from the plasma filtrate. In pregnant women, however, tubular reabsorption of glucose is impaired, so that glucosuria occurs at varying times and to varying degrees. Normal values range from 0 to 20 mg/dl, meaning that during any day, the urine is sometimes positive and sometimes negative. In nonpregnant women, blood glucose levels must be at 160 to 180 mg/dl before glucose is "spilled" into the urine (not reabsorbed). During pregnancy, glucosuria (glycosuria) occurs when maternal glucose levels are lower than 160 mg/dl. Why glucose, as well as other nutrients such as amino acids, is wasted during pregnancy is not understood, nor has the exact mechanism been discovered. Although glucosuria may be found in normal pregnancies (2+ levels may be seen with increased anxiety states), the possibility of diabetes mellitus and gestational diabetes must be kept in mind.

Proteinuria usually does not occur in normal pregnancy except during labor or after birth (Cunningham et al., 2005). However, the increased amount of amino acids that must be filtered may exceed the capacity of the renal tubules to absorb it, so that small amounts of protein are then lost in the urine. Values of trace to 1+ protein (dipstick assessment) or less than 300 mg per 24 hours are acceptable during pregnancy (Gordon, 2002). The amount of protein excreted is not an indication of the severity of renal disease, nor does an increase in protein excretion in a pregnant woman with known renal disease necessarily indicate a progression in her disease. However, a pregnant woman with hypertension and proteinuria must be carefully evaluated because she may be at greater risk for an adverse pregnancy outcome (see Table 8-3).

Integumentary system

Alterations in hormonal balance and mechanical stretching are responsible for several changes in the integumentary system during pregnancy. Hyperpigmentation is stimulated by the anterior pituitary hormone melanotropin, which is increased during pregnancy. Darkening of the nipples, areolae, axillae, and vulva occurs about the sixteenth week of gestation. Facial melasma, also called **chloasma** or mask of pregnancy, is a blotchy, brownish hyperpigmentation of the skin over the cheeks, nose, and forehead, especially in dark-complexioned pregnant women. Chloasma appears in 50% to 70% of pregnant women, beginning after the sixteenth week and increasing gradually until term. The sun intensifies this pigmentation in susceptible women. Chloasma caused by normal pregnancy usually fades after birth.

The **linea nigra** (Fig. 8-10) is a pigmented line extending from the symphysis pubis to the top of the fundus in the midline; this line is known as the *linea alba* before

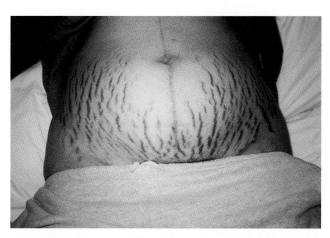

Fig. 8-10 Striae gravidarum and linea nigra in a dark-skinned person. (Courtesy Shannon Perry, Phoenix, AZ.)

hormone-induced pigmentation. In primigravidas the extension of the linea nigra, beginning in the third month, keeps pace with the rising height of the fundus; in multigravidas, the entire line often appears earlier than the third month. Not all pregnant women develop linea nigra, and some women notice hair growth along the line with or without the change in pigmentation.

Striae gravidarum, or stretch marks (seen over lower abdomen in Fig. 8-10), which appear in 50% to 90% of pregnant women during the second half of pregnancy, may be caused by action of adrenocorticosteroids. Striae reflect separation within the underlying connective (collagen) tissue of the skin. These slightly depressed streaks tend to occur over areas of maximal stretch (i.e., abdomen, thighs, and breasts). The stretching sometimes causes a sensation that resembles itching. The tendency to develop striae may be familial. After birth they usually fade, although they never disappear completely. Color of striae varies depending on the pregnant woman's skin color. The striae appear pinkish on a woman with light skin and are lighter than surrounding skin in dark-skinned women. In the multipara, in addition to the striae of the present pregnancy, glistening silvery lines (in light-skinned women) or purplish lines (in dark-skinned women) are commonly seen. These represent the scars of striae from previous pregnancies.

Angiomas are commonly referred to as *vascular spiders.* They are tiny, star-shaped or branched, slightly raised and pulsating end-arterioles usually found on the neck, thorax, face, and arms. They occur as a result of elevated levels of circulating estrogen. The spiders are bluish in color and do not blanch with pressure. Vascular spiders appear during the second to the fifth month of pregnancy in almost 65% of Caucasian women and 10% of African-American women. The spiders usually disappear after birth (Blackburn, 2003).

Pinkish-red, diffuse mottling or well-defined blotches are seen over the palmar surfaces of the hands in about 60% of Caucasian women and 35% of African-American women

during pregnancy (Blackburn, 2003). These color changes, called palmar erythema, are related primarily to increased estrogen levels.

NURSE ALERT *Because integumentary system changes vary greatly among women of different racial backgrounds, the color of a woman's skin should be noted along with any changes that may be attributed to pregnancy when performing physical assessments.*

Some dermatologic conditions have been identified as unique to pregnancy or as having an increased incidence during pregnancy. Pruritus is a relatively common dermatologic symptom in pregnancy, with *cholestasis of pregnancy* being the most common cause of pruritic rash. Other forms are uncommon or rare (Rapini, 2004) (Box 8-2). The goal of management is to relieve the itching. Topical steroids are the usual treatment, although systemic steroids may be needed. The problem usually resolves in the postpartum period (Stambuk & Colven, 2002). Preexisting skin diseases may complicate pregnancy or be improved.

NURSE ALERT *Women with severe acne taking isotretinoin (Accutane) should avoid pregnancy while receiving the treatment because it is teratogenic and is associated with major malformations.*

Gum hypertrophy may occur. An epulis (gingival granuloma gravidarum) is a red, raised nodule on the gums that bleeds easily. This lesion may develop around the third month and usually continues to enlarge as pregnancy progresses. It is usually managed by avoiding trauma to the gums (e.g., using a soft toothbrush). An epulis usually regresses spontaneously after birth.

Nail growth may be accelerated. Some women may notice thinning and softening of the nails. Oily skin and acne vulgaris may occur during pregnancy. For some women, the skin clears and looks radiant. Hirsutism, the excessive growth of hair or growth of hair in unusual places, is commonly reported. An increase in fine hair growth may occur but tends to disappear after pregnancy; however, growth of coarse or

BOX 8-2

Frequency of Dermatologic Disorders of Pregnancy

Cholestasis of pregnancy: 1.5%-2%
Pruritic urticarial papules and plaques of pregnancy: 0.6%
Prurigo of pregnancy: 0.3%
Herpes gestationis: 0.002%
Impetigo herpetiformis: very rare

Source: Rapini, R. (2004). The skin and pregnancy. In R. Creasy, R. Resnik, & J. Iams (Eds.), *Maternal-fetal medicine: Principles and practice* (5th ed.). Philadelphia: Saunders.

bristly hair does not usually disappear. The rate of scalp hair loss slows during pregnancy, and increased hair loss may be noted in the postpartum period.

Increased blood supply to the skin leads to increased perspiration. Women feel hotter during pregnancy, a condition possibly related to a progesterone-induced increase in body temperature and the increased BMR.

Musculoskeletal system

The gradually changing body and increasing weight of the pregnant woman cause noticeable alterations in her posture (Fig. 8-11) and the way she walks. The great abdominal distention that gives the pelvis a forward tilt, decreased abdominal muscle tone, and increased weight bearing require a realignment of the spinal curvature late in pregnancy. The woman's center of gravity shifts forward. An increase in the normal lumbosacral curve (lordosis) develops, and a compensatory curvature in the cervicodorsal region (exaggerated anterior flexion of the head) develops to help her maintain her balance. Aching, numbness, and weakness of the upper extremities may result. Large breasts and a stoop-shouldered stance will further accentuate the lumbar and dorsal curves. Walking is more difficult, and the waddling gait of the pregnant woman, called "the proud walk of pregnancy" by Shakespeare, is well known. The ligamentous and muscular structures of the middle and lower spine may be severely stressed. These and related changes often cause

musculoskeletal discomfort, especially in older women or those with a back disorder or a faulty sense of balance.

Slight relaxation and increased mobility of the pelvic joints are normal during pregnancy. They are secondary to the exaggerated elasticity and softening of connective and collagen tissue caused by increased circulating steroid sex hormones, especially estrogen. Relaxin, an ovarian hormone, assists in this relaxation and softening. These adaptations permit enlargement of pelvic dimensions to facilitate labor and birth. The degree of relaxation varies, but considerable separation of the symphysis pubis and the instability of the sacroiliac joints may cause pain and difficulty in walking. Obesity and multifetal pregnancy tend to increase the pelvic instability. Peripheral joint laxity also increases as pregnancy progresses, but the cause is not known (Cunningham et al., 2005).

The muscles of the abdominal wall stretch and ultimately lose some tone. During the third trimester, the rectus abdominis muscles may separate (Fig. 8-12), allowing abdominal contents to protrude at the midline. The umbilicus flattens or protrudes. After birth, the muscles gradually regain tone; however, separation of the muscles (**diastasis recti abdominis**) may persist.

Neurologic system

Little is known regarding specific alterations in function of the neurologic system during pregnancy, aside from hypothalamic-pituitary neurohormonal changes. Specific

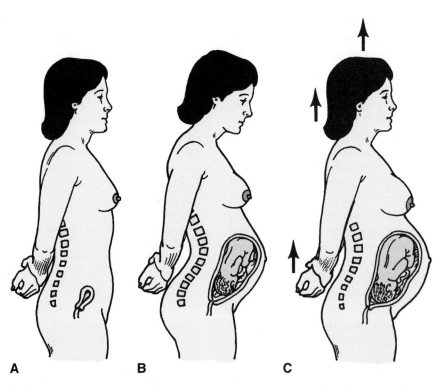

Fig. 8-11 Postural changes during pregnancy. **A,** Nonpregnant. **B,** Incorrect posture. **C,** Correct posture during pregnancy.

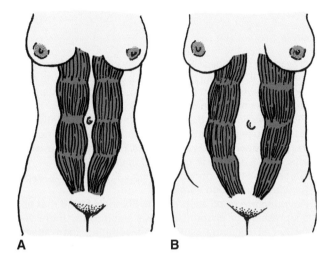

Fig. 8-12 Possible change in rectus abdominis muscles during pregnancy. **A,** Normal position in nonpregnant woman. **B,** Diastasis recti abdominis in pregnant woman.

physiologic alterations resulting from pregnancy may cause the following neurologic or neuromuscular symptoms:

- Compression of pelvic nerves or vascular stasis caused by enlargement of the uterus may result in sensory changes in the legs.
- Dorsolumbar lordosis may cause pain because of traction on nerves or compression of nerve roots.
- Edema involving the peripheral nerves may result in carpal tunnel syndrome during the last trimester (Padua et al., 2001). The syndrome is characterized by paresthesia (abnormal sensation such as burning or tingling) and pain in the hand, radiating to the elbow. The sensations are caused by edema that compresses the median nerve beneath the carpal ligament of the wrist. Smoking and alcohol consumption can impair the microcirculation and may worsen the symptoms (Padua et al., 2001). The dominant hand is usually affected most, although as many as 80% of women experience symptoms in both hands. Symptoms usually regress after pregnancy. In some cases, surgical treatment may be necessary (Aminoff, 2004).
- Acroesthesia (numbness and tingling of the hands) is caused by the stoop-shouldered stance (see Fig. 8-11, *B*) assumed by some women during pregnancy. The condition is associated with traction on segments of the brachial plexus.
- Tension headache is common when anxiety or uncertainty complicates pregnancy. However, vision problems, sinusitis, or migraine also may be responsible for headaches.
- "Light-headedness," faintness, and even syncope (fainting) are common during early pregnancy. Vasomotor instability, postural hypotension, or hypoglycemia may be responsible.
- Hypocalcemia may cause neuromuscular problems such as muscle cramps or tetany.

Gastrointestinal system

Appetite. During pregnancy, the woman's appetite and food intake fluctuate. Early in pregnancy, some women have nausea with or without vomiting (morning sickness), possibly in response to increasing levels of hCG and altered carbohydrate metabolism (Gordon, 2002). Morning sickness or nausea and vomiting of pregnancy (NVP) appears at about 4 to 6 weeks of gestation and usually subsides by the end of the third month (first trimester) of pregnancy. Severity varies from mild distaste for certain foods to more severe vomiting. The condition may be triggered by the sight or odor of various foods. By the end of the second trimester, the appetite increases in response to increasing metabolic needs. Rarely does NVP have harmful effects on the embryo, fetus, or the woman; some beneficial effects may be that these pregnancies may be less likely to result in miscarriage, preterm labor, or intrauterine growth restriction (Furneaux, Langley-Evans, & Langley-Evans, 2001). Whenever the vomiting is severe or persists beyond the first trimester, or when it is accompanied by fever, pain, or weight loss, further evaluation is necessary, and medical intervention is likely.

Women also may have changes in their sense of taste, leading to cravings and changes in dietary intake. Some women have nonfood cravings (called *pica*), such as for ice, clay, and laundry starch. Usually the subjects of these cravings, if consumed in moderation, are not harmful to the pregnancy if the woman has adequate nutrition with appropriate weight gain (Gordon, 2002).

Mouth. The gums become hyperemic, spongy, and swollen during pregnancy. They tend to bleed easily because the increasing levels of estrogen cause selective increased vascularity and connective tissue proliferation (a nonspecific gingivitis). Epulis (discussed in the section on the integumentary system) may develop at the gumline. Some pregnant women complain of ptyalism (excessive salivation), which may be caused by the decrease in unconscious swallowing by the woman when nauseated or from stimulation of salivary glands by eating starch (Cunningham et al., 2005).

Esophagus, stomach, and intestines. Herniation of the upper portion of the stomach (hiatal hernia) occurs after the seventh or eighth month of pregnancy in about 15% to 20% of pregnant women. This condition results from upward displacement of the stomach, which causes the hiatus of the diaphragm to widen. It occurs more often in multiparas and older or obese women.

Increased estrogen production causes decreased secretion of hydrochloric acid; therefore peptic ulcer formation or flare-up of existing peptic ulcers is uncommon during pregnancy and may improve (Winbery & Blaho, 2001).

Increased progesterone production causes decreased tone and motility of smooth muscles, resulting in esophageal regurgitation, slower emptying time of the stomach, and reverse peristalsis. As a result, the woman may experience "acid indigestion" or heartburn (pyrosis) beginning as early as the first trimester and intensifying through the third trimester.

EVIDENCE-BASED PRACTICE
Relief for First-Trimester Nausea and Vomiting

BACKGROUND

- In the first trimester of pregnancy, nausea affects 70% to 85% of all women, and vomiting affects 50%. The discomfort can last all day, and, for 13% of affected women, can persist beyond the twentieth week. About one pregnant woman in three loses some time from work or home duties. In its most severe form, hyperemesis gravidarum can cause dehydration and starvation, and even death. Before the current era of easy replacement with intravenous fluids, hyperemesis was a major reason for pregnancy termination. It has been speculated that nausea and vomiting of pregnancy is attributable to the level of human chorionic gonadotropin. The occurrence of nausea and vomiting is low in women who eventually have a miscarriage and high in women with multiple pregnancies.

OBJECTIVES

- The authors of this review wished to discover any effective interventions for relief of nausea and vomiting of early pregnancy.
- Intervention for nausea and vomiting of pregnancy could include antihistamine or antiemetic medications, pyridoxine (vitamin B$_6$), acupuncture, or acupressure at the p6 point, which is the inner aspect of the wrist, between the two tendons, about three fingerbreadths proximal from the wrist. For hyperemesis gravidarum, interventions could include ginger, corticosteroid or adrenocorticotropic hormone (ACTH) injections, intravenous diazepam, oral ondansetron, and acupuncture. Outcome measures included nausea, vomiting, retching, side effects of medications, and fetal outcomes.

METHODS

Search Strategy

- Search strategy included Cochrane, MEDLINE, manual searches of 30 journals, and weekly awareness service of 37 journals. Search keywords included *nausea and vomiting* and *pregnancy*.
- Twenty-eight trials met the inclusion criteria, representing 3577 women. Publication dates ranged from 1958 to 2000. Countries were not noted in the review.

Statistical Analyses

- Statistical analyses of homogeneous data enabled pooling. All data were assigned an odds ratio with a 95% confidence interval. Analysis revealed whether the differences between groups were possibly a result of chance alone (insignificant).

FINDINGS

- *Antiemetic drugs (12 trials):* Nausea is significantly reduced by use of antiemetic drugs, but the medications may cause sleepiness. Bendectin was withdrawn from the market in 1983 owing to fears that it could cause birth defects, but subsequent large, randomized, controlled trials showed no evidence of teratogenicity.
- *Pyridoxine (vitamin B$_6$):* Two trials found significantly reduced nausea but no effect on vomiting in the pyridoxine groups compared with controls. There may be greater effect of 75 mg/day than with 30 mg/day.
- *Ginger:* One trial reported that ginger is significantly helpful with nausea and vomiting.
- *Acupuncture or p6 acupressure:* Six trials found that p6 acupressure or acupuncture was significantly more effective at relieving nausea and vomiting than sham acupuncture or sham acupressure at incorrect sites.
- No intervention helped hyperemesis gravidarum, but oral methylprednisone and intravenous diazepam were associated with lower readmission rates. Ginger showed some promise, but not significantly.
- There was no evidence of birth defects caused by the interventions in these trials.

LIMITATIONS

- The challenges in reviewing such a large pool of studies are the diverse protocols, variable periods of observation, and diverse sample criteria. Several trials did not report how they randomized, or what happened to their dropouts, which limits generalizability. Most of the trials were small. The long time span (42 years) in which the trials occurred makes comparisons problematic, because technology has solved some problems (such as ease of intravenous hydration) and created others (such as side effects of antiemetic drugs).

CONCLUSIONS

- Several therapies are effective in reducing nausea and vomiting of early pregnancy. These therapies include pyridoxine, fresh ginger root, Sea-Bands, and antiemetic drugs.

IMPLICATIONS FOR PRACTICE

- Women may benefit from taking 10 to 25 mg of pyridoxine three times a day for nausea and vomiting of early pregnancy. Fresh ginger root may be beneficial. Women can try Sea-Bands, which are elastic wristbands with a plastic knob, to be applied to the p6 acupressure site. Remedies may not work consistently. Antiemetic drugs are available, if necessary.

IMPLICATIONS FOR FURTHER RESEARCH

- More information about hyperemesis gravidarum is necessary to identify interventions for this intractable disease. More information about the fetal outcomes of antiemetic medications is essential.

Reference: Jewell, D., & Young, G. (2003). Interventions for nausea and vomiting in early pregnancy (Cochrane Review). In *The Cochrane Library,* Issue 2, 2004. Chichester, UK: John Wiley & Sons.

Iron is absorbed more readily in the small intestine in response to increased needs during pregnancy. Even when the woman is deficient in iron, it will continue to be absorbed in sufficient amounts for the fetus to have a normal hemoglobin level.

Increased progesterone (causing loss of muscle tone and decreased peristalsis) results in an increase in water absorption from the colon and may cause constipation. Constipation also may result from hypoperistalsis (sluggishness of the bowel), food choices, lack of fluids, iron supplementation, decreased activity level, abdominal distention by the pregnant uterus, and displacement and compression of the intestines. If the pregnant woman has hemorrhoids (see Fig. 8-9) and is constipated, the hemorrhoids may become everted or may bleed during straining at stool.

Gallbladder and liver. The gallbladder is quite often distended because of its decreased muscle tone during pregnancy. Increased emptying time and thickening of bile caused by prolonged retention are typical changes. These features, together with slight hypercholesterolemia from increased progesterone levels, may account for the development of gallstones during pregnancy.

Hepatic function is difficult to appraise during pregnancy; however, only minor changes in liver function develop. Occasionally, intrahepatic cholestasis (retention and accumulation of bile in the liver, caused by factors within the liver) occurs late in pregnancy in response to placental steroids and may result in pruritus gravidarum (severe itching) with or without jaundice. These distressing symptoms subside soon after birth.

Abdominal discomfort. Intraabdominal alterations that can cause discomfort include pelvic heaviness or pressure, round ligament tension, flatulence, distention and bowel cramping, and uterine contractions. In addition to displacement of intestines, pressure from the expanding uterus causes an increase in venous pressure in the pelvic organs. Although most abdominal discomfort is a consequence of normal maternal alterations, the health care provider must be constantly alert to the possibility of disorders such as bowel obstruction or an inflammatory process.

Appendicitis may be difficult to diagnose in pregnancy because the appendix is displaced upward and laterally, high and to the right, away from McBurney's point (Fig. 8-13).

Endocrine system

Profound endocrine changes are essential for pregnancy maintenance, normal fetal growth, and postpartum recovery.

Pituitary and placental hormones. During pregnancy, the elevated levels of estrogen and progesterone (produced first by the corpus luteum in the ovary until about 14 weeks of gestation and then by the placenta) suppress secretion of follicle-stimulating hormone (FSH) and luteinizing hormone (LH) by the anterior pituitary. The maturation of a follicle and ovulation do not occur. Although the majority of women have amenorrhea (absence of menses), at least 20% have some slight, painless spotting

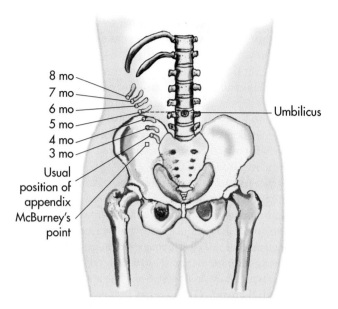

Fig. 8-13 Change in position of appendix in pregnancy. Note McBurney's point.

during early gestation. Implantation bleeding and bleeding after intercourse related to cervical friability can occur. Most of the women experiencing slight gestational bleeding continue to term and have normal infants; however, all instances of bleeding should be reported and evaluated.

After implantation, the fertilized ovum and the chorionic villi produce hCG, which maintains the production by the corpus luteum of estrogen and progesterone until the placenta takes over production (Buster & Carson, 2002).

Progesterone is essential for maintaining pregnancy by relaxing smooth muscles, resulting in decreased uterine contractility and prevention of miscarriage. Progesterone and estrogen cause fat to deposit in subcutaneous tissues over the maternal abdomen, back, and upper thighs. This fat serves as an energy reserve for both pregnancy and lactation. Estrogen also promotes the enlargement of the genitals, uterus, and breasts and increases vascularity, causing vasodilation. Estrogen causes relaxation of pelvic ligaments and joints. It also alters metabolism of nutrients by interfering with folic acid metabolism, increasing the level of total body proteins, and promoting retention of sodium and water by kidney tubules. Estrogen may decrease secretion of hydrochloric acid and pepsin, which may be responsible for digestive upsets such as nausea.

Serum prolactin produced by the anterior pituitary begins to increase early in the first trimester and increases progressively to term. It is responsible for initial lactation; however, the high levels of estrogen and progesterone inhibit lactation by blocking the binding of prolactin to breast tissue until after birth (Liu, 2004).

Oxytocin is produced by the posterior pituitary in increasing amounts as the fetus matures. This hormone can stimulate uterine contractions during pregnancy, but high levels of progesterone prevent contractions until near term.

Oxytocin also stimulates the let-down or milk-ejection reflex after birth in response to the infant's sucking at the mother's breast.

Human chorionic somatomammotropin (hCS), previously called human placental lactogen and produced by the placenta has been suggested to act as a growth hormone and contribute to breast development. It also may decrease the maternal metabolism of glucose and increase the amount of fatty acids for metabolic needs; however, its function is poorly understood (Liu, 2004).

Thyroid gland. During pregnancy, gland activity and hormone production increase. The increased activity is reflected in a moderate enlargement of the thyroid gland caused by hyperplasia of the glandular tissue and increased vascularity (Cunningham et al., 2005). Thyroxine-binding globulin (TBG) increases as a result of increased estrogen levels. This increase begins at about 20 weeks of gestation. The level of total (free and bound) thyroxine (T_4) increases between 6 and 9 weeks of gestation and plateaus at 18 weeks of gestation. Free thyroxine (T_4) and free triiodothyronine (T_3) return to nonpregnant levels after the first trimester. Despite these changes in hormone production, hyperthyroidism usually does not develop in the pregnant woman (Cunningham et al., 2005).

Parathyroid gland. Parathyroid hormone controls calcium and magnesium metabolism. Pregnancy induces a slight hyperparathyroidism, a reflection of increased fetal requirements for calcium and vitamin D. The peak level of parathyroid hormone occurs between 15 and 35 weeks of gestation, when the needs for growth of the fetal skeleton are greatest. Levels return to normal after birth.

Pancreas. The fetus requires significant amounts of glucose for its growth and development. To meet its need for fuel, the fetus not only depletes the store of maternal glucose but also decreases the mother's ability to synthesize glucose by siphoning off her amino acids. Maternal blood glucose levels decrease. Maternal insulin does not cross the placenta to the fetus. As a result, in early pregnancy the pancreas decreases its production of insulin.

As pregnancy continues, the placenta grows and produces progressively greater amounts of hormones (i.e., hCS, estrogen, and progesterone). Cortisol production by the adrenals also increases. Estrogen, progesterone, hCS, and cortisol collectively decrease the mother's ability to use insulin. Cortisol stimulates increased production of insulin but also increases the mother's peripheral resistance to insulin (i.e., the tissues cannot use the insulin). Decreasing the mother's ability to use her own insulin is a protective mechanism that ensures an ample supply of glucose for the needs of the fetoplacental unit. The result is an added demand for insulin by the mother that continues to increase at a steady rate until term. The normal beta cells of the islets of Langerhans in the pancreas can meet this demand for insulin.

Adrenal glands. The adrenal glands change little during pregnancy. Secretion of aldosterone is increased, resulting in reabsorption of excess sodium from the renal tubules. Cortisol levels also are increased (Blackburn, 2003).

COMMUNITY ACTIVITY

Go to a local pharmacy and get information on at least three different home pregnancy test kits. (The pharmacist may be able to provide product information.)

1 Compare the directions for use, interpretation of test results, and the costs. Do any of the kits have directions in languages other than English?
2 During a conference with others in your clinical group, discuss the pros and cons of using the different types of kits.
3 Develop a poster presentation to guide women in decisions about use of home pregnancy tests for display in a family planning clinic.

Key Points

- The biochemical, physiologic, and anatomic adaptations that occur during pregnancy are profound and revert to the nonpregnant state after birth and lactation.
- Maternal adaptations are attributed to the hormones of pregnancy and to mechanical pressures exerted by the enlarging uterus and other tissues.
- ELISA testing, with monoclonal antibody technology, is the most popular method of pregnancy testing and is the basis for most over-the-counter home pregnancy tests.
- Presumptive, probable, and positive signs of pregnancy aid in the diagnosis of pregnancy; only positive signs (identification of a fetal heartbeat, verification of fetal movements, and visualization of the fetus) can establish the diagnosis of pregnancy.

- Adaptations to pregnancy protect the woman's normal physiologic functioning, meet the metabolic demands pregnancy imposes, and provide for fetal development and growth needs.
- Although the pH of the pregnant woman's vaginal secretions is more acidic, she is more vulnerable to some vaginal infections, especially yeast infections.
- Increased vascularity and sensitivity of the vagina and other pelvic viscera may lead to a high degree of sexual interest and arousal.
- Some adaptations to pregnancy result in discomforts such as fatigue, urinary frequency, nausea, and breast sensitivity.
- As pregnancy progresses, balance and coordination are affected by changes in the woman's joints and her center of gravity.

Answer Guidelines to Critical Thinking Exercise

Home Pregnancy Testing

1 No. More information is needed about Sylvia's menstrual cycle history to determine regularity and possible ovulation time and what if any medications she may be taking that could affect the results of the test. More information is also needed about the test used, what time of day the test was taken, and how the test was performed in relation to the directions.

2 a. Home pregnancy tests are based on presence of hCG in urine sample as early as 7 days after conception.

b. False-negative results are more common than false positive results.

c. All tests do not have the same degree of sensitivity or specificity.

3 The priority is to help Sylvia become aware of timing and events that could have affected the result of her test and to assist her in making a decision to retest or come in for a serum test.

4 Yes. The test may have been performed too soon—the most common mistake in home testing. Suggesting that retesting with a home urine test be done in 1 week or having a serum test done is the appropriate intervention.

5 Other conditions can cause a woman to miss a menstrual period. If a second test is negative, further assessment would be appropriate.

Resources

Alexian Brothers Medical Center
Elk Grove, IL
www.alexian.org/progserv/babies/ babytoo.html

Ovulation calculation and other information
www.ovulation.com

Babies Online
(information on pregnancy and baby care)
www.babiesonline.com

Childbirth.org (source of links to other sites related to pregnancy and birth)
www.childbirth.org

New York Online Access to Health (consumer-level information site, includes information on tests, fetal development, postnatal topics, etc., in English and Spanish)
www.noah-health.org/en/pregnancy

Perinatal Education Associates, Inc. (source of information on physiologic and emotional aspects of pregnancy)
www.birthsource.com

References

Aminoff, M. (2004). Neurologic disorders. In R. Creasy, R. Resnik, & J. Iams (Eds.), *Maternal-fetal medicine: Principles and practice* (5th ed.). Philadelphia: Saunders.

Berman, M., DiSaia, P., & Tewari, K. (2004). Pelvic malignancies, gestational trophoblastic neoplasia, and nonpelvic malignancies. In R. Creasy, R. Resnik, & J. Iams (Eds.), *Maternal-fetal medicine: Principles and practice* (5th ed.). Philadelphia: Saunders.

Blackburn, S. (2003). *Maternal, fetal, & neonatal physiology: A clinical perspective* (2nd ed.). St Louis: Saunders.

Buster, J., & Carson, S. (2002). Endocrinology and diagnosis of pregnancy. In S. Gabbe, J. Niebyl, & J. Simpson (Eds.), *Obstetrics: Normal and problem pregnancies* (4th ed.). New York: Churchill Livingstone.

Cole, K. et al. (2004). Accuracy of home pregnancy tests at time of missed menses. *American Journal of Obstetrics and Gynecology, 190*(1), 100-105.

Cunningham, F., Leveno, K., Bloom, S., Hauth, J., Gilstrap, L., & Wenstrom, K. (2005). *Williams obstetrics* (22nd ed.). New York: McGraw-Hill.

Furneaux, E., Langley-Evans, A., & Langley-Evans, S. (2001). Nausea and vomiting of pregnancy: Endocrine basis and contribution to pregnancy outcome. *Obstetrical and Gynecological Survey, 56*(12): 775-782.

Gibbs, R, Sweet, R., & Duff, W. (2004). Maternal and fetal infectious disorders. In R. Creasy, R. Resnik, & J. Iams (Eds.), *Maternal-fetal medicine: Principles and practice* (5th ed.). Philadelphia: Saunders.

Gonik, B., & Foley, M. (2004). Intensive care monitoring of the critically ill pregnant patient. In R. Creasy, R. Resnik, & J. Iams (Eds.), *Maternal-fetal medicine: Principles and practice* (5th ed.). Philadelphia: Saunders.

Gordon, M. (2002). Maternal physiology in pregnancy. In S. Gabbe, J. Niebyl, & J. Simpson (Eds.), *Obstetrics: Normal and problem pregnancies* (4th ed.). New York: Churchill Livingstone.

Harman, C. (2004). Assessment of fetal health. In R. Creasy, R. Resnik, & J. Iams (Eds.), *Maternal-fetal medicine: Principles and practice* (5th ed.). Philadelphia: Saunders.

Hermida, R., Ayala, D., Mojon, A., & Fernandez, J. (2001). Time-qualified reference values for ambulatory blood pressure monitoring in pregnancy. *Hypertension, 38*(3 Pt 2), 746-752.

Jewell, D., & Young, G. (2003). Interventions for nausea and vomiting in early pregnancy. (Cochrane Review). In *The Cochrane Library*, Issue 2, 2004. Chichester, UK: John Wiley & Sons.

Lawrence, R., & Lawrence, R. (2004). The breast and the physiology of lactation. In R. Creasy, R. Resnik, & J. Iams (Eds.), *Maternal-fetal medicine: Principles and practice* (5th ed.). Philadelphia: Saunders.

Liu, J. (2004). Endocrinology of pregnancy. In R. Creasy, R. Resnik, & J. Iams (Eds.), *Maternal-fetal medicine: Principles and practice* (5th ed.). Philadelphia: Saunders.

Malone, F., & D'Alton, M. (2004). Multiple gestation: Clinical characteristics and management. In R. Creasy, R. Resnik, & J. Iams (Eds.), *Maternal-fetal medicine: Principles and practice* (5th ed.). Philadelphia: Saunders.

Monga, M. (2004). Maternal cardiovascular and renal adaptation to pregnancy. In R. Creasy, R. Resnik, & J. Iams (Eds.), *Maternal-fetal medicine: Principles and practice* (5th ed.). Philadelphia: Saunders.

Monga, M., & Sanborn, M. (2004). Biology and physiology of the reproductive tract and control of myometrial contraction. In R. Creasy, R. Resnik, & J. Iams (Eds.), *Maternal-fetal medicine: Principles and practice* (5th ed.). Philadelphia: Saunders.

Padua, L., Aprile, I., Caliandro, P., Carboni, T., Meloni, A., Massi, S. et al. (2001). Symptoms and neurophysical picture of carpal tunnel syndrome in pregnancy. *Clinical Neurophysiology, 112*(10), 1946-1951.

Pagana, K., & Pagana, T. (2003). *Mosby's diagnostic and laboratory test reference* (6th ed.). St. Louis: Mosby.

Pickering, T. (2002). Principles and techniques of blood pressure measurement. *Cardiology Clinics, 20*(2), 207-223.

Rapini, R. (2004). The skin and pregnancy. In R. Creasy, R. Resnik, & J. Iams (Eds.), *Maternal-fetal medicine: Principles and practice* (5th ed.). Philadelphia: Saunders.

Seidel, H., Ball, J., Dains, J., & Benedict, G. (2003). *Mosby's guide to physical examination* (5th ed.). St. Louis: Mosby.

Stambuk, R., & Colven, R. (2002). Dermatologic disorders. In S. Gabbe, J. Niebyl, & J. Simpson (Eds.), *Obstetrics: Normal and problem pregnancies* (4th ed.). New York: Churchill Livingstone.

Stewart, F. (2004). Pregnancy testing and management of early pregnancy. In R. Hatcher et al (Eds.), *Contraceptive technology* (18th ed.). New York: Ardent Media.

Whitty, J., & Dombrowski, M. (2004). Respiratory diseases in pregnancy. In R. Creasy, R. Resnik, & J. Iams (Eds.), *Maternal-fetal medicine: Principles and practice* (5th ed.). Philadelphia: Saunders.

Winbery, S., & Blaho, K. (2001). Dyspepsia in pregnancy. *Obstetrics and Gynecology Clinics of North America, 28*(2), 333-350.

CHAPTER 9

Nursing Care during Pregnancy

ROBIN WEBB CORBETT

LEARNING OBJECTIVES

- Describe the process of confirming pregnancy and estimating the date of birth.
- Summarize the physical, psychosocial, and behavioral changes that usually occur as the mother and other family members adapt to pregnancy.
- Discuss the benefits of prenatal care and problems of accessibility for some women.
- Outline the patterns of health care used to assess maternal and fetal health status at the initial and follow-up visits during pregnancy.

- Identify the typical nursing assessments, diagnoses, interventions, and methods of evaluation in providing care for the pregnant woman.
- Discuss education needed by pregnant women to understand physical discomforts related to pregnancy and to recognize signs and symptoms of potential complications.
- Examine the impact of culture, age, parity, and number of fetuses on the response of the family to the pregnancy and on the prenatal care provided.

KEY TERMS AND DEFINITIONS

birth plan A tool by which parents can explore their childbirth options and choose those that are most important to them

couvade syndrome The phenomenon of expectant fathers' experiencing pregnancy-like symptoms

cultural prescriptions Practices that are expected or acceptable

cultural proscriptions Forbidden; taboo practices

doula Trained assistant hired to give the woman support during pregnancy, labor and birth, and/or postpartum

home birth Planned birth of the child at home, usually done under the supervision of a midwife

morning sickness Nausea and vomiting that affect some women during the first few months of their pregnancy; may occur at any time of day

multifetal pregnancy Pregnancy in which there is more than one fetus in the uterus at the same time; multiple pregnancy

Nägele's rule One method for calculating the estimated date of birth, or "due date"

pelvic tilt (rock) Exercise used to help relieve low back discomfort during menstruation and pregnancy

pinch test Determines whether nipples are everted or inverted by placing thumb and forefinger on areola and pressing inward; the nipple will stand erect or will invert

supine hypotension Shock; fall in blood pressure caused by impaired venous return when gravid uterus presses on ascending vena cava, when woman is lying flat on her back; vena cava syndrome

trimesters One of three periods of approximately 3 months each into which pregnancy is divided

The prenatal period is a time of physical and psychologic preparation for birth and parenthood. Becoming a parent is considered one of the maturational milestones of adult life, and as such, it is a time of intense learning for both parents and those close to them. The prenatal period provides a unique opportunity for nurses and other members of the health care team to influence family health. During this period, essentially healthy women seek regular care and guidance. The nurse's health promotion interventions can affect the well-being of the woman, her unborn child, and the rest of her family for many years.

Regular prenatal visits, ideally beginning soon after the first missed menstrual period, offer opportunities to ensure the health of the expectant mother and her fetus. Prenatal health care permits diagnosis and treatment of maternal disorders that may have preexisted or may develop during the pregnancy. Care is designed to monitor the growth and development of the fetus and to identify abnormalities that may interfere with the course of normal labor. Education and support for self-care and parenting can be provided.

Pregnancy spans 9 months, but health care providers, in contrast to using the familiar monthly calendar to ascertain fetal age or discuss the pregnancy, use the concept of lunar months, which last 28 days, or 4 weeks. Normal pregnancy, then, lasts about 10 lunar months, which is the same as 40 weeks or 280 days. Health care providers also refer to early, middle, and late pregnancy as trimesters. The first trimester lasts from weeks 1 through 13; the second, from weeks 14 through 26; and the third, from weeks 27 through 40. A pregnancy is considered to be at term if it advances to 38 to 40 weeks.

The focus of this chapter is on meeting the health needs of the expectant family over the course of pregnancy, which is known as the *prenatal period*.

DIAGNOSIS OF PREGNANCY

Women may suspect pregnancy when they miss a menstrual period. Many women come to the first prenatal visit after a positive home pregnancy test; however, the clinical diagnosis of pregnancy before the second missed period may be difficult in some women. Physical variations, obesity, or tumors, for example, may confound even the experienced examiner. Accuracy is important, however, because emotional, social, medical, or legal consequences of an inaccurate diagnosis, either positive or negative, can be extremely serious. A correct date for the *last (normal) menstrual period* (*LMP* or *LNMP*) and for the date of intercourse and a basal body temperature (BBT) record may be of great value in the accurate diagnosis of pregnancy (see Chapter 6).

Signs and Symptoms

Great variability is possible in the subjective and objective signs and symptoms of pregnancy; therefore the diagnosis of pregnancy may be uncertain for a time. Many of the indicators of pregnancy are clinically useful in the diagnosis of pregnancy, and they are classified as presumptive, probable, or positive (see Table 8-2).

The presumptive indicators of pregnancy can be caused by conditions other than gestation. For example, amenorrhea may be caused by illness or excessive exercise; fatigue may signify anemia or infection; a tumor may cause enlargement of the abdomen; and nausea or vomiting may be caused by a gastrointestinal (GI) upset or food allergy. Therefore these signs alone are not reliable for diagnosis.

Estimating Date of Birth

After the diagnosis of pregnancy, the woman's first question usually concerns when she will give birth. This date has traditionally been termed the *estimated date of confinement (EDC)*, although *estimated date of delivery (EDD)* also has been used. To promote a more positive perception of both pregnancy and birth, however, the term *estimated date of birth (EDB)* is suggested. Because the precise date of conception generally is unknown, several formulas have been suggested for calculating the EDB. None of these guides is infallible, but Nägele's rule is reasonably accurate and is usually used.

Nägele's rule is as follows: After determining the first day of the LMP, subtract 3 calendar months, add 7 days and

---

BOX 9-1

Use of Nägele's Rule

July 10, 2006, is the first day of the last menstrual period.

$$
\begin{array}{cccc}
 & 7 & 10 & 2006 \\
 & -3 & +7 & \\
\text{EDB} = & 4 & 17 & 2007 \\
\end{array}
$$

The estimated date of birth (EDB) is April 17, 2007.

---

1 year; or alternatively, add 7 days to the LMP and count forward 9 calendar months. Box 9-1 demonstrates use of Nägele's rule.

Nägele's rule assumes that the woman has a 28-day menstrual cycle and that pregnancy occurred on the fourteenth day. An adjustment is in order if the woman's cycle is longer or shorter than 28 days. With the use of Nägele's rule, only about 5% of pregnant women give birth spontaneously on the EDB (Katz, Farmer, Tufariello, & Carpenter, 2001). Most women give birth during the period extending from 7 days before to 7 days after the EDB.

ADAPTATION TO PREGNANCY ▪

Pregnancy affects all family members, and each family member must adapt to the pregnancy and interpret its meaning in light of his or her own needs. This process of family adaptation to pregnancy takes place within a cultural environment influenced by societal trends. Dramatic changes have occurred in Western society in recent years, and the nurse must be prepared to support single-parent families, reconstituted families, dual-career families, and alternative families, as well as traditional families, in the childbirth experience.

Much of the investigation of family dynamics in pregnancy by scholars in the United States and Canada has been done with Caucasian, middle-class nuclear families, and findings may not apply to families who do not fit the traditional North American model. Adaptation of terms is appropriate to avoid embarrassment to the nurse and offense to the family. Additional research is needed on a variety of families to determine if study findings generated in traditional families are applicable to others.

Maternal Adaptation

Women of all ages use the months of pregnancy to adapt to the maternal role, a complex process of social and cognitive learning. Early in pregnancy, nothing seems to be happening, and a woman may spend much time sleeping. With the perception of fetal movement in the second trimester, the woman turns her attention inward to her pregnancy and to relationships with her mother and other women who have been or who are pregnant.

Pregnancy is a maturational milestone that can be stressful but also rewarding as the woman prepares for a new level of caring and responsibility. Her self-concept changes in readiness for parenthood as she prepares for her new role. She moves gradually from being self-contained and independent to being committed to a lifelong concern for another human being. This growth requires mastery of certain developmental tasks: accepting the pregnancy, identifying with the role of mother, reordering the relationships between herself and her mother and between herself and her partner, establishing a relationship with the unborn child, and preparing for the birth experience (Lederman, 1996). The partner's emotional support is an important factor in the successful accomplishment of these developmental tasks. Single women with limited support may have difficulty making this adaptation.

Accepting the pregnancy

The first step in adapting to the maternal role is accepting the idea of pregnancy and assimilating the pregnant state into the woman's way of life. Mercer (1995) described this process as *cognitive restructuring* and credited Reva Rubin (1984) as the nurse theorist who pioneered our understanding of maternal role attainment. The degree of acceptance is reflected in the woman's emotional responses. Many women are dismayed initially at finding themselves pregnant, especially if the pregnancy is unintended. Eventual acceptance of pregnancy parallels the growing acceptance of the reality of a child. Nonacceptance of the pregnancy, however, should not be equated with rejection of the child, for a woman may dislike being pregnant but feel love for the child to be born.

Women who are happy and pleased about their pregnancy often view it as biologic fulfillment and part of their life plan. They have high self-esteem and tend to be confident about outcomes for themselves, their babies, and other family members. Despite a general feeling of well-being, many women are surprised to experience emotional lability, that is, rapid and unpredictable changes in mood. These swings in emotions and increased sensitivity to others are disconcerting to the expectant mother and those around her. Increased irritability, explosions of tears and anger, and feelings of great joy and cheerfulness alternate, apparently with little or no provocation.

Profound hormonal changes that are part of the maternal response to pregnancy may be responsible for mood changes. Other reasons such as concerns about finances and changed lifestyle contribute to this seemingly erratic behavior.

Most women have ambivalent feelings during pregnancy whether the pregnancy was intended or not. Ambivalence—having conflicting feelings simultaneously—is considered a normal response for people preparing for a new role. During pregnancy, women may, for example, feel great pleasure that they are fulfilling a lifelong dream, but they also may feel great regret that life as they now know it is ending.

Even women who are pleased to be pregnant may experience feelings of hostility toward the pregnancy or unborn child from time to time. Such incidents as a partner's chance remark about the attractiveness of a slim, nonpregnant woman or news of a colleague's promotion can give rise to ambivalent feelings. Body sensations, feelings of dependence, or the realization of the responsibilities of child care also can generate such feelings.

Intense feelings of ambivalence that persist through the third trimester may indicate an unresolved conflict with the motherhood role (Mercer, 1995). After the birth of a healthy child, memories of these ambivalent feelings usually are dismissed. If the child is born with a defect, however, a woman may look back at the times when she did not want the pregnancy and feel intensely guilty. She may believe that her ambivalence caused the birth defect. She then will need assurance that her feelings were not responsible for the problem.

Identifying with the mother role

The process of identifying with the mother role begins early in each woman's life when she is being mothered as a child. Her social group's perception of what constitutes the feminine role can subsequently influence her toward choosing between motherhood or a career, being married or single, being independent rather than interdependent, or being able to manage multiple roles. Practice roles, such as playing with dolls, baby-sitting, and taking care of siblings, may increase her understanding of what being a mother entails.

Many women have always wanted a baby, liked children, and looked forward to motherhood. Their high motivation to become a parent promotes acceptance of pregnancy and eventual prenatal and parental adaptation. Other women apparently have not considered in any detail what motherhood means to them. During pregnancy, conflicts such as not wanting the pregnancy and child-related or career-related decisions must be resolved.

Reordering personal relationships

Close relationships of the pregnant woman undergo change during pregnancy as she prepares emotionally for the new role of mother. As family members learn their new roles, periods of tension and conflict may occur. An understanding of the typical patterns of adjustment can help the nurse to reassure the pregnant woman and explore issues related to social support. Promoting effective communication patterns between the expectant mother and her own mother and between the expectant mother and her partner are common nursing interventions provided during the prenatal visits.

The woman's own relationship with her mother is significant in adaptation to pregnancy and motherhood. Important components in the pregnant woman's relationship with her mother are the mother's availability (past and present), her reactions to the daughter's pregnancy, respect for her daughter's autonomy, and the willingness to reminisce (Mercer, 1995).

The mother's reaction to the daughter's pregnancy signifies her acceptance of the grandchild and of her daughter. If the mother is supportive, the daughter has an opportunity to discuss pregnancy and labor and her feelings of joy or ambivalence with a knowledgeable and accepting

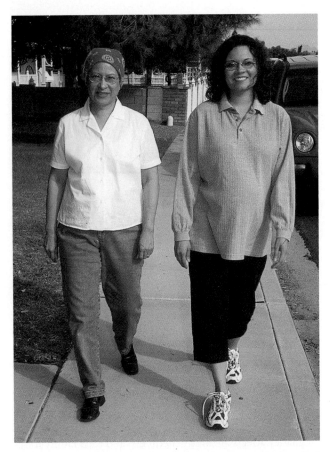

Fig. 9-1 A pregnant woman and her mother enjoying their walk together. (Courtesy Michael S. Clement, MD, Mesa, AZ.)

woman (Fig. 9-1). Reminiscing about the pregnant woman's early childhood and sharing the prospective grandmother's account of her childbirth experience help the daughter to anticipate and prepare for labor and birth.

Although the woman's relationship with her mother is significant in considering her adaptation in pregnancy, the most important person to the pregnant woman is usually the father of her child. The support and concern of a partner during pregnancy have positive consequences for a woman's desire to carry out the pregnancy (Kroelinger & Oths, 2000), and she has fewer emotional and physical symptoms, fewer labor and childbirth complications, and an easier postpartum adjustment. Women express two major needs within this relationship during pregnancy: feeling loved and valued and having the child accepted by the partner.

The marital or committed relationship is not static but evolves over time. The addition of a child changes forever the nature of the bond between partners. This may be a time when couples grow closer, and the pregnancy has a maturing effect on the partners' relationship as they assume new roles and discover new aspects of one another. Partners who trust and support each other are able to share mutual-dependency needs (Mercer, 1995).

Sexual expression during pregnancy is highly individual. The sexual relationship is affected by physical, emotional, and interactional factors, including myths about sex during pregnancy, sexual dysfunction, and physical changes in the woman. Myths about body functions and fantasies about the influence of the fetus as a third party in lovemaking are commonly expressed. An individual may also inaccurately attribute anomalies, mental retardation, and other injuries to the fetus and mother to sexual relations during pregnancy. Some couples fear that the woman's genitals will be drastically changed by the birth process. Couples may not express their concerns to the health care provider because of embarrassment or because they do not want to appear foolish.

As pregnancy progresses, changes in body shape, body image, and levels of discomfort influence both partners' desire for sexual expression. During the first trimester, the woman's sexual desire may decrease, especially if she has breast tenderness, nausea, fatigue, or sleepiness. As she progresses into the second trimester, however, her sense of well-being combined with the increased pelvic congestion that occurs at this time may increase her desire for sexual release. In the third trimester, somatic complaints and physical bulkiness may increase her physical discomfort and again diminish her interest in sex. As a woman's pregnancy progresses, her enlarging gravid abdomen may limit the use of the man-on-top position for intercourse. Therefore other positions (e.g., side to side or the woman on top) may allow intercourse and minimize pressure on the woman's abdomen (Westheimer & Lopater, 2005).

Partners need to feel free to discuss their sexual responses during pregnancy with each other and with their health care provider. Their sensitivity to each other and willingness to share concerns can strengthen their sexual relationship. Partners who do not understand the rapid physiologic and emotional changes of pregnancy can become confused by the other's behavior. By talking to each other about the changes they are experiencing, couples can define problems and then offer the needed support. Nurses can facilitate communication between partners by talking to expectant couples about possible changes in feelings and behaviors they may experience as pregnancy progresses (see later discussion).

Establishing a relationship with the fetus

Emotional attachment—feelings of being tied by affection or love—begins during the prenatal period as women use fantasizing and daydreaming to prepare themselves for motherhood (Rubin, 1975). They think of themselves as mothers and imagine maternal qualities they would like to possess. Expectant parents desire to be warm, loving, and close to their child. They try to anticipate changes that the child will bring in their lives and wonder how they will react to noise, disorder, reduced freedom, and caregiving activities. The mother-child relationship progresses through pregnancy as a developmental process that unfolds in three phases.

In phase 1 the woman accepts the biologic fact of pregnancy. She needs to be able to state, "I am pregnant" and incorporate the idea of a child into her body and self-image. The woman's thoughts center around herself and the reality of her pregnancy. The child is viewed as part of herself, not a separate and unique person.

In phase 2 the woman accepts the growing fetus as distinct from herself, usually accomplished by the fifth month. She can now say, "I am going to have a baby." This differentiation of the child from the woman's self permits the beginning of the mother-child relationship that involves not only caring but also responsibility. Attachment of a mother to her child is enhanced by experiencing a planned pregnancy, and it increases when ultrasound examination and quickening confirm the reality of the fetus.

With acceptance of the reality of the child (hearing the heart beat and feeling the child move) and an overall feeling of well-being, the woman enters a quiet period and becomes more introspective. A fantasy child becomes precious to the woman. As the woman seems to withdraw and to concentrate her interest on the unborn child, her partner sometimes feels left out. If there are other children in the family, they may become more demanding in their efforts to redirect the mother's attention to themselves.

During phase 3 of the attachment process, the woman prepares realistically for the birth and parenting of the child. She expresses the thought, "I am going to be a mother" and defines the nature and characteristics of the child. She may, for example, speculate about the child's sex and personality traits based on patterns of fetal activity.

Although the mother alone experiences the child within, both parents and siblings believe the unborn child responds in a very individualized, personal manner. Family members may interact a great deal with the unborn child by talking to the fetus and stroking the mother's abdomen, especially when the fetus shifts position (Fig. 9-2). The fetus may even have a nickname used by family members.

Preparing for childbirth

Many women actively prepare for birth by reading books, viewing films, attending parenting classes, and talking to other women. They seek the best caregiver possible for advice, monitoring, and caring. The multigender has her own history of labor and birth, which influences her approach to preparation for this childbirth experience.

Anxiety can arise from concern about a safe passage for herself and her child during the birth process (Mercer, 1995; Rubin, 1975). This concern may not be expressed overtly, but cues are given as the nurse listens to plans women make for care of the new baby and other children in case "anything should happen." These feelings persist despite statistical evidence about the safe outcome of pregnancy for mothers and their infants. Many women fear the pain of childbirth or mutilation because they do not understand anatomy and the birth process. Education by the nurse can alleviate many of these fears. Women also express concern over what behaviors are appropriate during the birth process and whether caregivers will accept them and their actions.

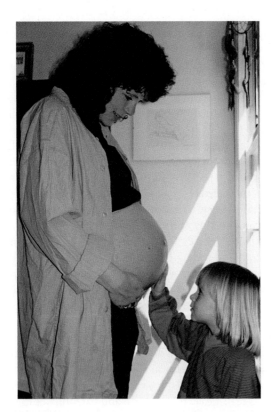

Fig. 9-2 Sibling feeling movement of fetus. (Courtesy Kim Molloy, Knoxville, IA.)

Toward the end of the third trimester, breathing is difficult, and fetal movements become vigorous enough to disturb the woman's sleep. Backaches, frequency and urgency of urination, constipation, and varicose veins can become troublesome. The bulkiness and awkwardness of her body interfere with the woman's ability to care for other children, perform routine work-related duties, and assume a comfortable position for sleep and rest. By this time, most women become impatient for labor to begin, whether the birth is anticipated with joy, dread, or a mixture of both. A strong desire to see the end of pregnancy, to be over and done with it, makes women at this stage ready to move on to childbirth.

Paternal Adaptation

The father's beliefs and feelings about the ideal mother and father and his cultural expectation of appropriate behavior during pregnancy affect his response to his partner's need for him. One man may engage in nurturing behavior. Another may feel lonely and alienated as the woman becomes physically and emotionally engrossed in the unborn child. He may seek comfort and understanding outside the home or become interested in a new hobby or involved with his work. Some men view pregnancy as proof of their masculinity and their dominant role. To others, pregnancy has no meaning in terms of responsibility to either mother or child. However, for most men, pregnancy can be a time of preparation for the parental role with intense learning.

Accepting the pregnancy

The ways fathers adjust to the parental role has been the subject of considerable research. In older societies the man enacted the ritual couvade; that is, he behaved in specific ways and respected taboos associated with pregnancy and giving birth so the man's new status was recognized and endorsed. Now, some men experience pregnancy-like symptoms, such as nausea, weight gain, and other physical symptoms. This phenomenon is known as the couvade syndrome. Changing cultural and professional attitudes have encouraged fathers' participation in the birth experience in the past 30 years (Fig. 9-3).

The man's emotional responses to becoming a father, his concerns, and his informational needs change during the course of pregnancy. Phases of the developmental pattern become apparent. May (1982) described three phases characterizing the developmental tasks experienced by the expectant father:

- The announcement phase may last from a few hours to a few weeks. The developmental task is to accept the biologic fact of pregnancy. Men react to the confirmation of pregnancy with joy or dismay, depending on whether the pregnancy is desired or unplanned or unwanted. Ambivalence in the early stages of pregnancy is common.

  If pregnancy is unplanned or unwanted, some men find the alterations in life plans and lifestyles difficult to accept. Some men engage in extramarital affairs for the first time during their partner's pregnancy. Others batter their wives for the first time or escalate the frequency of battering episodes (Martin et al., 2001). Chapter 4 provides information about violence against women and offers guidance on assessment and intervention.

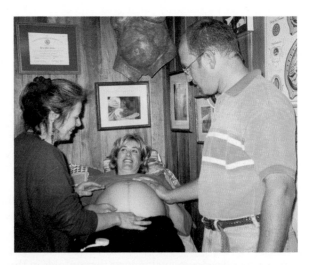

Fig. 9-3 Father participating in prenatal visit. Nurse-midwife discusses feeling fetal movement while father puts hand on mother's abdomen. (Courtesy Shannon Perry, Phoenix, AZ.)

- The second phase, the moratorium phase, is the period when he adjusts to the reality of pregnancy. The developmental task is to accept the pregnancy. Men appear to put conscious thought of the pregnancy aside for a time. They become more introspective and engage in many discussions about their philosophy of life, religion, childbearing, and childrearing practices and their relationships with family members, particularly with their father. Depending on the man's readiness for the pregnancy, this phase may be relatively short or persist until the last trimester.
- The third phase, the focusing phase, begins in the last trimester and is characterized by the father's active involvement in both the pregnancy and his relationship with his child. The developmental task is to negotiate with his partner the role he is to play in labor and to prepare for parenthood. In this phase the man concentrates on his experience of the pregnancy and begins to think of himself as a father.

Identifying with the father role

Each man brings to pregnancy attitudes that affect the way in which he adjusts to the pregnancy and parental role. His memories of the fathering he received from his own father, the experiences he has had with child care, and the perceptions of the male and father roles within his social group will guide his selection of the tasks and responsibilities he will assume. Some men are highly motivated to nurture and love a child. They may be excited and pleased about the anticipated role of father. Others may be more detached or even hostile to the idea of fatherhood.

Reordering personal relationships

The partner's main role in pregnancy is to nurture and respond to the pregnant woman's feelings of vulnerability. The partner also must deal with the reality of the pregnancy. The partner's support indicates involvement in the pregnancy and preparation for attachment to the child.

Some aspects of a partner's behavior may indicate rivalry, and it may be especially evident during sexual activity. For example, men may protest that fetal movements prevent sexual gratification or that they are being watched by the fetus during sexual activity. However, feelings of rivalry may be unconscious and not verbalized, but expressed in subtle behaviors.

The woman's increased introspection may cause her partner to feel uneasy as she becomes preoccupied with thoughts of the child and of her motherhood, with her growing dependence on her physician or midwife, and with her reevaluation of the couple's relationship.

Establishing a relationship with the fetus

The father-child attachment can be as strong as the mother-child relationship, and fathers can be as competent as mothers in nurturing their infants. The father-child attachment also begins during pregnancy. A father may rub or kiss the maternal abdomen, try to listen, talk, or sing to the fetus, or play with the fetus as he notes movement. Calling the unborn child by name or nickname helps to confirm the reality of pregnancy and promote attachment.

Men prepare for fatherhood in many of the same ways as women do for motherhood—by reading and by fantasizing about the baby. Daydreaming about their role as father is common in the last weeks before the birth; men rarely describe their thoughts unless they are reassured that such daydreams are normal.

Preparing for childbirth

The days and weeks immediately before the expected day of birth are characterized by anticipation and anxiety. Boredom and restlessness are common as the couple focuses on the birth process; however, during the last 2 months of pregnancy, many expectant fathers experience a surge of creative energy at home and on the job. They may become dissatisfied with their present living space. If possible, they tend to act on the need to alter the environment (remodeling, painting, etc.). This activity may be overt evidence of their sharing in the childbearing experience. They are able to channel the anxiety and other feelings experienced during the final weeks before birth into productive activities. This behavior earns recognition and compliments from friends, relatives, and their partners.

Major concerns for the man are getting the woman to a medical facility in time for the birth and not appearing ignorant. Many men want to be able to recognize labor and determine when it is appropriate to leave for the hospital or call the physician or nurse-midwife. They may fantasize different situations and plan what they will do in response to them, or they may rehearse taking various routes to the hospital, timing each route at different times of the day.

Some prospective fathers have questions about the labor suite's furniture, nursing staff, and location, as well as the availability of the physician and anesthesiologist. Others want to know what is expected of them when their partners are in labor. The man also may have fears concerning safe passage of his child and partner and the possible death or complications of his partner and child. It is important he verbalize these fears, otherwise he cannot help his mate deal with her own unspoken or overt apprehension.

With the exception of childbirth preparation classes, a man has few opportunities to learn ways to be an involved and active partner in this rite of passage into parenthood. The tensions and apprehensions of the unprepared, unsupportive father are readily transmitted to the mother and may increase her fears.

The same fears, questions, and concerns may affect birth partners who are not the biologic fathers. Birth partners need to be kept informed, supported, and included in all activities in which the mother desires their participation. The nurse can do much to promote pregnancy and birth as a family experience.

Sibling Adaptation

Sharing the spotlight with a new brother or sister may be the first major crisis for a child. The older child often experiences a sense of loss or feels jealous at being "replaced" by the new sibling. Some of the factors that influence the child's response are age, the parents' attitudes, the role of the father, the length of separation from the mother, the hospital's visitation policy, and the way the child has been prepared for the change.

A mother with other children must devote time and effort to reorganizing her relationships with them. She needs to prepare siblings for the birth of the child (Fig. 9-4 and Box 9-2) and begin the process of role transition in the family by including the children in the pregnancy and being sympathetic to older children's concerns about losing their places in the family hierarchy. No child willingly gives up a familiar position.

Siblings' responses to pregnancy vary with their age and dependency needs. The 1-year-old infant seems largely unaware of the process, but the 2-year-old child notices the change in his or her mother's appearance and may comment that "Mommy's fat." The toddlers' need for sameness in the environment makes the children aware of any change. They may exhibit more clinging behavior and revert to dependent behaviors in toilet training or eating.

By age 3 or 4 years, children like to be told the story of their own beginning and accept its being compared with the present pregnancy. They like to listen to the fetal heart beat and feel the baby moving in utero (see Fig. 9-2). Sometimes they worry about how the baby is being fed and what it wears.

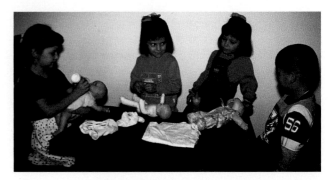

Fig. 9-4 A sibling class of preschoolers learns infant care using dolls. (Courtesy Marjorie Pyle, RNC, Lifecircle, Costa Mesa, CA.)

School-age children take a more clinical interest in their mother's pregnancy. They may want to know in more detail, "How did the baby get in there?" and "How will it get out?" Children in this age group notice pregnant women in stores, churches, and schools and sometimes seem shy if they need to approach a pregnant woman directly. On the whole, they look forward to the new baby, see themselves as "mothers" or "fathers," and enjoy buying baby supplies and readying a place for the baby. Because they still think in concrete terms and base judgments on the here and now, they respond positively to their mother's current good health.

Early and middle adolescents preoccupied with the establishment of their own sexual identity may have difficulty accepting the overwhelming evidence of the sexual activity of their parents. They reason that if they are too young for

---

BOX 9-2

Tips for Sibling Preparation

PRENATAL

- Take your child on a prenatal visit. Let the child listen to the fetal heart beat and feel the baby move.
- Involve the child in preparations for the baby, such as helping decorate the baby's room.
- Move the child to a bed (if still sleeping in a crib) at least 2 months before the baby is due.
- Read books, show videos, and/or take child to sibling preparation classes, including a hospital tour.
- Answer your child's questions about the coming birth, what babies are like, and any other questions.
- Take your child to the homes of friends who have babies so that the child has realistic expectations of what babies are like.

DURING THE HOSPITAL STAY

- Have someone bring the child to the hospital to visit you and the baby (unless you plan to have the child attend the birth).
- Do not force interactions between the child and the baby. Often the child will be more interested in seeing you and being reassured of your love.

- Help the child explore the infant by showing how and where to touch the baby.
- Give the child a gift (from you or you, the father, and baby).

GOING HOME

- Leave the child at home with a relative or baby-sitter.
- Have someone else carry the baby from the car so that you can hug the child first.

ADJUSTMENT AFTER THE BABY IS HOME

- Arrange for a special time with the child alone with each parent.
- Do not exclude the child during infant feeding times. The child can sit with you and the baby and feed a doll or drink juice or milk with you or sit quietly with a game.
- Prepare small gifts for the child so that when the baby gets gifts, the sibling won't feel left out. The child can also help open the baby gifts.
- Praise the child for acting age appropriately (so that being a baby does not seem better than being older).

such activity, certainly their parents are too old. They seem to take on a critical parental role and may ask, "What will people think?" or "How can you let yourself get so fat?" or "How can you let yourself get pregnant?" Many pregnant women with teenage children will confess that the attitudes of their teenagers are the most difficult aspect of their current pregnancy.

Late adolescents do not appear to be unduly disturbed. They are busy making plans for their own lives and realize that they soon will be gone from home. Parents usually report they are comforting and act more as other adults than as children.

Grandparent Adaptation

Every pregnancy affects all family relationships. For expectant grandparents, a first pregnancy in a child is undeniable evidence that they are growing older. Many think of a grandparent as old, white-haired, and becoming feeble of mind and body; however, some people face grandparenthood while still in their 30s or 40s. Parents-to-be announcing their pregnancy to their parents may be greeted by a negative response, indicating that they are not ready to be grandparents. Both the parents-to-be and their parents may be hurt by this initial response. Daughter and mother both may be startled and hurt by the response.

In some family units some expectant grandparents are nonsupportive and may also inadvertently decrease the self-esteem of the parents-to-be. Mothers may talk about their terrible pregnancies; fathers may discuss the endless cost of rearing children; and mothers-in-law may complain that their sons are neglecting them because their concern is now directed toward the pregnant daughters-in-law.

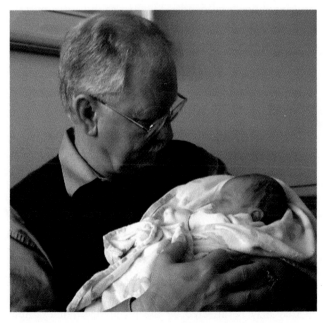

Fig. 9-5 Grandfather getting to know his grandson. (Courtesy Sharon Johnson, Petaluma, CA.)

However, most grandparents are delighted at the prospect of a new baby in the family. It reawakens the feelings of their own youth, the excitement of giving birth, and their delight in the behavior of the parents-to-be when they were infants. They set up a memory store of the child's first smiles, first words, and first steps, which they can use later for "claiming" the newborn as a member of the family. These behaviors provide a link between the past and present for the parents- and grandparents-to-be.

In addition, the grandparent is the historian who transmits the family history, a resource person who shares knowledge based on experience; a role model; and a support person. The grandparent's presence and support can strengthen family systems by widening the circle of support and nurturance (Fig. 9-5).

CARE MANAGEMENT ■

The purpose of prenatal care is to identify existing risk factors and other deviations from normal so that pregnancy outcomes may be enhanced (Johnson & Niebyl, 2002). Major emphasis is placed on preventive aspects of care, primarily to motivate the pregnant woman to practice optimal self-care and to report unusual changes early so that problems can be minimized or prevented. If health behaviors must be modified in early pregnancy, nurses need to understand psychosocial factors that may have influence on the woman (Walker, Cooney, & Riggs, 1999). In holistic care, nurses provide information and guidance about not only the physical changes but also the psychosocial impact of pregnancy on the woman and members of her family. The goals of prenatal nursing care, therefore, are to foster a safe birth for the infant and to promote satisfaction of the mother and family with the pregnancy and birth experience.

Advances have been made in the number of women in the United States who receive adequate prenatal care. In 2003, 84.1% of all women received care in the first trimester and 3.5% had late or no prenatal care. There is disparity in use of prenatal care in the first trimester by race and ethnicity: non-Hispanic Caucasians (89%), non-Hispanic blacks (76%), and Hispanic (77.4%) (Martin, Kochanek, Strobino, Guyer, & MacDorman, 2005). Although prenatal care is sought routinely by women of middle or high socioeconomic status, women living in poverty or who lack health insurance may not be able to use public medical services or gain access to private care. Lack of culturally sensitive care providers and barriers in communication resulting from differences in language also interfere with access to care (Shaffer, 2002). Likewise, immigrant women who come from cultures in which prenatal care is not emphasized may not know to seek routine prenatal care. Birth outcomes in these populations are therefore less positive, with higher rates of maternal and fetal or newborn complications. Problems with low birth weight (LBW; less than 2500 g) and infant mortality have in particular been associated with lack of adequate prenatal care.

BOX 9-3

Traditional Prenatal Visit Schedule*

- First visit within the first trimester
- Monthly visits through week 28
- Every two weeks from week 29 to week 36
- Weekly visits week 36 to birth

*Frequency of visits may be decreased in low risk women and increased in women with high risk pregnancies.

Barriers to obtaining health care during pregnancy include lack of transportation, unpleasant clinic facilities or procedures, inconvenient clinic hours, and personal attitudes (Boyle, Banks, Petrizzi, & Larimore, 2003; Chandler, 2002; Handler, Rosenberg, Raube, & Lyons, 2003; Sword, 2003). The availability and accessibility of prenatal care may be improved by the increasing use of advanced practice nurses in collaborative practice with physicians (Boyle et al., 2003). The effectiveness of a regular schedule of home visiting by nurses during pregnancy also has been validated (Fetrick, Christensen, & Mitchell, 2003).

The current model for provision of prenatal care has been used for more than a century. The initial visit usually occurs in the first trimester, with monthly visits through week 28 of pregnancy. Thereafter, visits are scheduled every 2 weeks until week 36, and then every week until birth (see Box 9-3). This model is currently being questioned, and in some practices there is a growing tendency to have fewer visits with women who are at low risk for complications (Villar, Carroli, Khan-Neelofur, Piaggio, & Gulmezoglu, 2001).

Prenatal care is ideally a multidisciplinary activity in which nurses work with physicians or midwives, nutritionists, social workers, and others. Collaboration among these individuals is necessary to provide holistic care. The case management model, which makes use of care maps and critical pathways, is one system that promotes comprehensive care with limited overlap in services. To emphasize the nursing role, care management here is organized around the central elements of the nursing process: assessment, nursing diagnoses, expected outcomes, plan of care and interventions, and evaluation.

Assessment and Nursing Diagnoses

Once the presence of pregnancy has been confirmed and the woman's desire to continue the pregnancy has been validated, prenatal care is begun. The assessment process begins at the initial prenatal visit and is continued throughout the pregnancy. Assessment techniques include the interview, physical examination, and laboratory tests. Because the initial visit and follow-up visits are distinctly different in content and process, they are described separately.

Initial visit

The pregnant woman and family members who may be present should be told that the first prenatal visit is more lengthy and detailed than are future visits. The initial evaluation includes a comprehensive health history emphasizing the current pregnancy, previous pregnancies, the family, a psychosocial profile, a physical assessment, diagnostic testing, and an overall risk assessment. A prenatal history form (Fig. 9-6) is the best way to document information obtained.

Interview.   The therapeutic relationship between the nurse and the woman is established during the initial assessment interview. It is a time for planned, purposeful communication that focuses on specific content. The data collected are of two types: the woman's subjective appraisal of her health status and the nurse's objective observations. During the interview the nurse observes the woman's affect, posture, body language, skin color, and other physical and emotional signs.

Often the pregnant woman is accompanied by one or more family members. The nurse needs to build a relationship with these people as part of the social context of the patient. With her permission, those accompanying the woman can be included in the initial prenatal interview, and the observations and information about the woman's family form part of the database. For example, if the woman is accompanied by small children, the nurse can ask about her plans for child care during the time of labor and birth. Special needs are noted at this time (e.g., wheelchair access, assistance in getting on and off the examining table, and cognitive deficits).

Reason for seeking care.   Although pregnant women are scheduled for "routine" prenatal visits, they often come to the health care provider seeking information or reassurance about a particular concern. When the patient is asked a broad, open-ended question such as, "How have you been feeling?," she may reveal problems that could otherwise be overlooked. The woman's chief concerns should be recorded in her own words to alert other personnel to the priority of needs as identified by her. At the initial visit the desire for information about what is normal in the course of pregnancy is typical.

Current pregnancy.   The presumptive signs of pregnancy may be of great concern to the woman. A review of symptoms she is experiencing and how she is coping with them helps to establish a database to develop a plan of care. Some early teaching may be provided at this time.

Obstetric and gynecologic history.   Data are gathered on the woman's age at menarche, menstrual history, and contraceptive history; the nature of any infertility or gynecologic conditions; her history of any sexually transmitted infections (STIs); her sexual history; and a detailed history of all her pregnancies, including the present pregnancy, and their outcomes. The date of the last Papanicolaou (Pap) test and the result are noted. The date of her LMP is obtained to establish the EDB (see Guidelines/Guías box).

Medical history.   The medical history includes those medical or surgical conditions that may affect the pregnancy or that may be affected by the pregnancy. For example, a pregnant woman who has diabetes, hypertension, or epilepsy requires special care. Because most women are anxious

GUIDELINES/GUÍAS
Prenatal Interview

- Have you had a pregnancy test?
- *¿Ha tenido una prueba del embarazo?*

- When was your last menstrual period?
- *¿Cuándo fue su última menstruación (regla)?*

- Have you been pregnant before?
- *¿Ha quedado embarazada antes?*

- How many times?
- *¿Cuántas veces?*

- How many children do you have?
- *¿Cuántos hijos tiene usted?*

- Have you ever had a miscarriage (spontaneous abortion)?
- *¿Ha perdido un bebé alguna vez? (¿Ha tenido un aborto espontáneo?)*

- Have you ever had a therapeutic abortion?
- *¿Ha tenido un aborto provocado?*

- Have you ever had a stillborn?
- *¿Ha tenido un niño que nació sin vida?*

- Have you ever had a cesarean?
- *¿Ha tenido una operación cesárea?*

- Have you had any problems with past pregnancies?
- *¿Ha tenido problemas durante sus embarazos anteriores?*

- Do you take drugs? Prescription medicine?
- *¿Usa drogas? ¿Medicina recetada?*

- If so, which type of medicine do you use and for what?
- *Qué clases de medicina toma? ¿Para qué las toma?*

- Do you drink alcohol? Do you smoke?
- *¿Toma bebidas alcohólicas? ¿Fuma?*

during the initial interview, the nurse's reference to cues, such as a MedicAlert bracelet, prompts the woman to explain allergies, chronic diseases, or medications being taken (e.g., cortisone, insulin, or anticonvulsants).

The nature of previous surgical procedures also should be described. If a woman has undergone uterine surgery or extensive repair of the pelvic floor, a cesarean birth may be necessary; appendectomy rules out appendicitis as a cause of right lower quadrant pain in pregnancy; and spinal surgery may contraindicate the use of spinal or epidural anesthesia. Any injury involving the pelvis is noted.

Often women who have chronic or handicapping conditions forget to mention them during the initial assessment because they have become so adapted to them. Special shoes or a limp may indicate the existence of a pelvic structural defect, which is an important consideration in pregnant women. The nurse who observes these special characteristics and inquires about them sensitively can obtain individualized data that will provide the basis for a comprehensive nursing care plan. Observations are vital components of the interview process because they prompt the nurse and woman to focus on the specific needs of the woman and her family.

Nutritional history. The woman's nutritional history is an important component of the prenatal history because her nutritional status has a direct effect on the growth and development of the fetus. A dietary assessment can reveal special diet practices, food allergies, eating behaviors, the practice of pica (Corbett, Ryan, & Weinrich, 2003), and other factors related to her nutritional status. Pregnant women are usually motivated to learn about good nutrition and respond well to nutritional advice generated by this assessment.

History of drug and herbal preparations use. A woman's past and present use of legal (over-the-counter [OTC] and prescription medications; herbal preparations; caffeine; alcohol; nicotine) and illegal (marijuana, cocaine, heroin) drugs must be assessed because many substances cross the placenta and may therefore harm the developing fetus. Periodic urine toxicology screening tests are often recommended during the pregnancies of women who have a history of illegal drug use. Results of such tests have been used for criminal prosecution, which results in a breach in patient-provider relationship and in ethical responsibilities to the patient (Foley, 2002; Harris & Paltrow, 2003). Nurses may have ethical concerns if pregnant women are not informed of the possibility of random urine testing for presence of drugs. The other side of this concern is the unborn child and whether the mother has a duty not to harm him or her.

LEGAL TIP Informed Consent for Drug Therapy

Hospitals must obtain informed consent from a pregnant woman before she can be tested for drug use (Kehringer, 2003).

Family history. The family history provides information about the woman's immediate family, including parents, siblings, and children. These data help identify familial or genetic disorders or conditions that could affect the present health status of the woman or her fetus.

Social, experiential, and occupational history. Situational factors such as the family's ethnic and cultural background and socioeconomic status are assessed while the history is obtained. The following information may be obtained in several encounters. The woman's perception of this pregnancy is explored by asking her such questions as the following: Is this pregnancy planned or not, wanted or not? Is the woman pleased, displeased, accepting, or nonaccepting? What problems related to finances, career, or living accommodations may arise as a result of the pregnancy? The family support system is determined by asking her such questions as the following: What primary support is available to her? Are changes needed to promote adequate support? What are the existing relationships among the mother, father or partner, siblings, and in-laws? What preparations are being made for her care and that of dependent family members during labor and for the care of the infant after birth? Is financial, educational, or other support needed from the community? What are the woman's ideas about

Text continued on p. 246.

DATE _____

NAME _____
        LAST   FIRST   MIDDLE

ID # _____ HOSPITAL OF DELIVERY _____

NEWBORN'S PHYSICIAN _____ REFERRED BY _____

| FINAL EDD _____ | PRIMARY PROVIDER/GROUP _____ |

BIRTH DATE AGE RACE MARITAL STATUS MONTH DAY YEAR S M W D SEP	ADDRESS
OCCUPATION EDUCATION (LAST GRADE COMPLETED)	ZIP PHONE (H) (O)
LANGUAGE	INSURANCE CARRIER/MEDICAID #
HUSBAND/DOMESTIC PARTNER PHONE	POLICY #
FATHER OF BABY PHONE	EMERGENCY CONTACT PHONE

TOTAL PREG	FULL TERM	PREMATURE	AB. INDUCED	AB. SPONTANEOUS	ECTOPICS	MULTIPLE BIRTHS	LIVING

MENSTRUAL HISTORY

LMP ☐ DEFINITE   ☐ APPROXIMATE (MONTH KNOWN)   MENSES MONTHLY ☐ YES ☐ NO   FREQUENCY: Q _____ DAYS   MENARCHE _____ (AGE ONSET)

     ☐ UNKNOWN   ☐ NORMAL AMOUNT/DURATION   PRIOR MENSES _____ DATE   ON BCP AT CONCEPT ☐ YES ☐ NO   hCG + ___/___/___

     ☐ FINAL _____

PAST PREGNANCIES (LAST SIX)

DATE MONTH/ YEAR	GA WEEKS	LENGTH OF LABOR	BIRTH WEIGHT	SEX M/F	TYPE DELIVERY	ANES.	PLACE OF DELIVERY	PRETERM LABOR YES/NO	COMMENTS/ COMPLICATIONS

MEDICAL HISTORY

	O Neg. + Pos.	DETAIL POSITIVE REMARKS INCLUDE DATE & TREATMENT		O Neg. + Pos.	DETAIL POSITIVE REMARKS INCLUDE DATE & TREATMENT
1. DIABETES			17. D (Rh) SENSITIZED		
2. HYPERTENSION			18. PULMONARY (TB, ASTHMA)		
3. HEART DISEASE			19. SEASONAL ALLERGIES		
4. AUTOIMMUNE DISORDER			20. DRUG/LATEX ALLERGIES/ REACTIONS		
5. KIDNEY DISEASE/UTI					
6. NEUROLOGIC/EPILEPSY			21. BREAST		
7. PSYCHIATRIC			22. GYN SURGERY		
8. DEPRESSION/POSTPARTUM DEPRESSION					
9. HEPATITIS/LIVER DISEASE			23. OPERATIONS/ HOSPITALIZATIONS (YEAR & REASON)		
10. VARICOSITIES/PHLEBITIS					
11. THYROID DYSFUNCTION			24. ANESTHETIC COMPLICATIONS		
12. TRAUMA/VIOLENCE			25. HISTORY OF ABNORMAL PAP		
13. HISTORY OF BLOOD TRANSFUS.			26. UTERINE ANOMALY/DES		

	AMT/DAY PREPREG	AMT/DAY PREG	# YEARS USE	27. INFERTILITY	
14. TOBACCO				28. RELEVANT FAMILY HISTORY	
15. ALCOHOL					
16. ILLICIT/RECREATIONAL DRUGS				29. OTHER	

COMMENTS _____

ACOG ANTEPARTUM RECORD (FORM A)

Version 5. Copyright © 2003 The American College of Obstetricians and Gynecologists, 409 12th Street, SW, PO Box 96920, Washington, DC 20090-6920   AA129   12345/76543

Fig. 9-6 A sample prenatal history form. (Copyright © 2003 The American College of Obstetricians and Gynecologists, 409 12th Street, SW, P.O. Box 96920, Washington, DC, 20090-6920.)

Patient Addressograph

SYMPTOMS SINCE LMP

GENETIC SCREENING/TERATOLOGY COUNSELING INCLUDES PATIENT, BABY'S FATHER, OR ANYONE IN EITHER FAMILY WITH:					
	YES	NO		YES	NO
1. PATIENT'S AGE ≥35 YEARS AS OF ESTIMATED DATE OF DELIVERY			12. HUNTINGTON'S CHOREA		
2. THALASSEMIA (ITALIAN, GREEK, MEDITERRANEAN, OR ASIAN BACKGROUND): MCV <80			13. MENTAL RETARDATION/AUTISM		
			IF YES, WAS PERSON TESTED FOR FRAGILE X?		
3. NEURAL TUBE DEFECT (MENINGOMYELOCELE, SPINA BIFIDA, OR ANENCEPHALY)			14. OTHER INHERITED GENETIC OR CHROMOSOMAL DISORDER		
4. CONGENITAL HEART DEFECT			15. MATERNAL METABOLIC DISORDER (EG, TYPE 1 DIABETES, PKU)		
5. DOWN SYNDROME			16. PATIENT OR BABY'S FATHER HAD A CHILD WITH BIRTH DEFECTS NOT LISTED ABOVE		
6. TAY-SACHS (EG, JEWISH, CAJUN, FRENCH CANADIAN)			17. RECURRENT PREGNANCY LOSS, OR A STILLBIRTH		
7. CANAVAN DISEASE			18. MEDICATIONS (INCLUDING SUPPLEMENTS, VITAMINS, HERBS OR OTC DRUGS)/ILLICIT/RECREATIONAL DRUGS/ALCOHOL SINCE LAST MENSTRUAL PERIOD		
8. SICKLE CELL DISEASE OR TRAIT (AFRICAN)					
9. HEMOPHILIA OR OTHER BLOOD DISORDERS			IF YES, AGENT(S) AND STRENGTH/DOSAGE		
10. MUSCULAR DYSTROPHY					
11. CYSTIC FIBROSIS			19. ANY OTHER		

COMMENTS/COUNSELING _____

_____

INFECTION HISTORY	YES	NO		YES	NO
1. LIVE WITH SOMEONE WITH TB OR EXPOSED TO TB			4. HISTORY OF STD, GONORRHEA, CHLAMYDIA, HPV, SYPHILIS		
2. PATIENT OR PARTNER HAS HISTORY OF GENITAL HERPES					
3. RASH OR VIRAL ILLNESS SINCE LAST MENSTRUAL PERIOD			5. OTHER (See Comments)		

COMMENTS _____

_____

_____ **INTERVIEWER'S SIGNATURE** _____

INITIAL PHYSICAL EXAMINATION					
DATE ____/____/____ HEIGHT _____ BP _____					
1. HEENT	☐ NORMAL	☐ ABNORMAL	12. VULVA	☐ NORMAL	☐ CONDYLOMA	☐ LESIONS
2. FUNDI	☐ NORMAL	☐ ABNORMAL	13. VAGINA	☐ NORMAL	☐ INFLAMMATION	☐ DISCHARGE
3. TEETH	☐ NORMAL	☐ ABNORMAL	14. CERVIX	☐ NORMAL	☐ INFLAMMATION	☐ LESIONS
4. THYROID	☐ NORMAL	☐ ABNORMAL	15. UTERUS SIZE	_____ WEEKS		☐ FIBROIDS
5. BREASTS	☐ NORMAL	☐ ABNORMAL	16. ADNEXA	☐ NORMAL	☐ MASS	
6. LUNGS	☐ NORMAL	☐ ABNORMAL	17. RECTUM	☐ NORMAL	☐ ABNORMAL	
7. HEART	☐ NORMAL	☐ ABNORMAL	18. DIAGONAL CONJUGATE	☐ REACHED	☐ NO	_____ CM
8. ABDOMEN	☐ NORMAL	☐ ABNORMAL	19. SPINES	☐ AVERAGE	☐ PROMINENT	☐ BLUNT
9. EXTREMITIES	☐ NORMAL	☐ ABNORMAL	20. SACRUM	☐ CONCAVE	☐ STRAIGHT	☐ ANTERIOR
10. SKIN	☐ NORMAL	☐ ABNORMAL	21. SUBPUBIC ARCH	☐ NORMAL	☐ WIDE	☐ NARROW
11. LYMPH NODES	☐ NORMAL	☐ ABNORMAL	22. GYNECOID PELVIC TYPE	☐ YES	☐ NO	

COMMENTS (Number and explain abnormals) _____

_____

_____ **EXAM BY** _____

ACOG ANTEPARTUM RECORD (FORM B)

Fig. 9-6, cont'd

Patient Addressograph

NAME _____
      LAST   FIRST   MIDDLE

DRUG ALLERGY	LATEX ALLERGY

IS BLOOD TRANSFUSION ACCEPTABLE IN AN EMERGENCY? ☐ YES ☐ NO | ANESTHESIA CONSULT PLANNED ☐ YES ☐ NO

PROBLEMS/PLANS

1. _____
2. _____
3. _____
4. _____
5. _____
6. _____

MEDICATION LIST   Start date   Stop date

1. _____ ___/___/___   ___/___/___
2. _____ ___/___/___   ___/___/___
3. _____ ___/___/___   ___/___/___
4. _____ ___/___/___   ___/___/___
5. _____ ___/___/___   ___/___/___
6. _____ ___/___/___   ___/___/___

EDD CONFIRMATION

INITIAL EDD

LMP	___/___/___ =	EDD ___/___/___
INITIAL EXAM	___/___/___ = ___ WKS =	EDD ___/___/___
ULTRASOUND	___/___/___ = ___ WKS =	EDD ___/___/___
INITIAL EDD	___/___/___	INITIALED BY _____

18–20-WEEK EDD UPDATE

QUICKENING	___/___/___	+22 WKS = ___/___/___
FUNDAL HT. AT UMBIL.	___/___/___	+20 WKS = ___/___/___
ULTRASOUND	___/___/___ =	___ WKS = ___/___/___
FINAL EDD	___/___/___	INITIALED BY _____

PREPREGNANCY WEIGHT _____

WEEKS GEST. (BEST EST.)	FUNDAL HEIGHT (CM)	PRESENTATION	FHR	FETAL MOVEMENT	PRETERM LABOR SIGNS/SYMPTOMS + = PRESENT o = ABSENT	CERVIX EXAM (DIL/EFF/STA.) ULTRASOUND LENGTH	BLOOD PRESSURE	WEIGHT	URINE (ALBUMIN/GLUCOSE)	NEXT APPOINTMENT	PROVIDER (INITIALS)

COMMENTS

_____
_____
_____
_____
_____
_____
_____
_____
_____
_____
_____
_____

PROBLEMS _____

COMMENTS _____

ACOG ANTEPARTUM RECORD (FORM C)

Fig. 9-6, cont'd   A sample prenatal history form. (Copyright © 2003 The American College of Obstetricians and Gynecologists, 409 12th Street, SW, P.O. Box 96920, Washington, DC, 20090-6920.)

LABORATORY AND EDUCATION

INITIAL LABS	DATE	RESULT	REVIEWED
BLOOD TYPE	/ /	A B AB O	
D (Rh) TYPE	/ /		
ANTIBODY SCREEN	/ /		
HCT/HGB	/ /	_____ % _____ g/dL	
PAP TEST	/ /	NORMAL/ABNORMAL _____	
RUBELLA	/ /		
VDRL	/ /		
URINE CULTURE/SCREEN	/ /		
HBsAg	/ /		
HIV COUNSELING/TESTING*	/ /	POS. NEG. DECLINED	

OPTIONAL LABS	DATE	RESULT	REVIEWED
HGB ELECTROPHORESIS	/ /	AA AS SS AC SC AF ↑A$_2$	
PPD	/ /		
CHLAMYDIA	/ /		
GONORRHEA	/ /		
GENETIC SCREENING TESTS (SEE FORM B)	/ /		
OTHER			

8–18-WEEK LABS (WHEN INDICATED/ELECTED)	DATE	RESULT	
ULTRASOUND	/ /		
MSAFP/MULTIPLE MARKERS	/ /		
AMNIO/CVS	/ /		
KARYOTYPE	/ /	46,XX OR 46,XY/OTHER _____	
AMNIOTIC FLUID (AFP)	/ /	NORMAL _____ ABNORMAL _____	

24–28-WEEK LABS (WHEN INDICATED)	DATE	RESULT	
HCT/HGB	/ /	_____ % _____ g/dL	
DIABETES SCREEN	/ /	1 HOUR _____	
GTT (IF SCREEN ABNORMAL)	/ /	_____ FBS _____ 1 HOUR _____ 2 HOUR _____ 3 HOUR	
D (Rh) ANTIBODY SCREEN	/ /		
ANTI-D IMMUNE GLOBULIN (RhIG) GIVEN (28 WKS)	/ /	SIGNATURE _____	

32–36-WEEK LABS	DATE	RESULT	
HCT/HGB	/ /	_____ % _____ g/dL	
ULTRASOUND (WHEN INDICATED)	/ /		
VDRL (WHEN INDICATED)	/ /		
GONORRHEA (WHEN INDICATED)	/ /		
CHLAMYDIA (WHEN INDICATED)	/ /		
GROUP B STREP	/ /		

COMMENTS/ADDITIONAL LABS

*Check state requirements before recording results.

PROVIDER SIGNATURE (AS REQUIRED) _____

ACOG ANTEPARTUM RECORD (FORM D)

Fig. 9-6, cont'd

childbearing, her expectations of the infant's behavior, and her outlook on life and the female role?

Other such questions that should be asked include the following: What does the woman think it will be like to have a baby in the home? How is her life going to change by having a baby? What plans does having a baby interrupt? During interviews throughout the pregnancy the nurse should remain alert to the appearance of potential parenting problems, such as depression, lack of family support, and inadequate living conditions. The nurse needs to assess the woman's attitude toward health care, particularly during childbearing, her expectations of health care providers, and her view of the relationship between herself and the nurse.

Coping mechanisms and patterns of interacting also are identified. Early in the pregnancy the nurse should determine the woman's knowledge of pregnancy; maternal changes; fetal growth; self-care; and care of the newborn, including feeding. Asking about attitudes toward unmedicated or medicated childbirth and about her knowledge of the availability of parenting skills classes is important. Before planning for nursing care, the nurse needs information about the woman's decision-making abilities and living habits (e.g., exercise, sleep, diet, diversional interests, personal hygiene, clothing). Common stressors during childbearing include the baby's welfare, labor and birth process, behaviors of the newborn, woman's relationship with the baby's father and her family, changes in body image, and physical symptoms.

Attitudes concerning the range of acceptable sexual behavior during pregnancy also should be explored by asking questions such as the following: What has your family (partner, friends) told you about sex during pregnancy? The woman's sexual self-concept is given more emphasis by asking questions such as the following: How do you feel about the changes in your appearance? How does your partner feel about your body now? How do you feel about wearing maternity clothes?

History of physical abuse.   All women should be assessed for a history or risk of physical abuse, particularly because the likelihood of abuse increases during pregnancy (see Guidelines/Guías box). Although visual cues from the woman's appearance or behavior may suggest the possibility, if questioning is limited to those women who fit the supposed profile of the battered woman, many women will be missed. Identification of abuse and immediate clinical intervention that includes information about safety can result in behaviors that may prevent future abuse and increase the safety and well-being of the woman and her infant (McFarlane, Parker, & Cross, 2001).

GUIDELINES/GUÍAS
Recognizing Violence in a Relationship

ARE YOU IN A RELATIONSHIP IN WHICH YOU ARE . . .

¿TIENE UNA RELACIÓN CON SU PAREJA EN LA QUE . . .

- afraid of your partner's temper?
- *tiene miedo de que él pierda los estribos?*

- afraid to break up because your partner has threatened to hurt someone?
- *tiene miedo de dejarlo porque él ha amenazado con pegar o lastimar a alguien?*

- constantly apologizing for or defending your partner's behavior?
- *constantemente tiene que disculparse por o defender el comportamiento de su pareja?*

- afraid to disagree with your partner?
- *tiene miedo de discutir con su pareja?*

- isolated from your family or friends?
- *está aislada de su familia o sus amigos?*

- embarrassed in front of others because of your partner's words or actions?
- *las palabras o acciones de su pareja delante de otra gente le dan vergüenza?*

- intimidated by your partner and forced into having sex?
- *su pareja le intimida a usted y le obliga a tener relaciones sexuales con él?*

- depressed and jumpy?
- *está deprimida y/o nerviosa?*

A PERSON WHO IS VIOLENT IN A RELATIONSHIP OFTEN . . .

UNA PERSONA QUE TIENE UN CARÁCTER VIOLENTO EN UNA RELACIÓN A MENUDO . . .

- has an explosive temper.
- *pierde los estribos.*

- is possessive or jealous of his partner's time, friends, or family.
- *es posesivo o tiene celos de que su pareja pase tiempo con la familia o los amigos.*

- constantly criticizes his partner's thoughts, feelings, or appearance.
- *critica constantemente los sentimientos, ideas, o apariencia física de su pareja.*

- pinches, slaps, grabs, shoves, or throws things at his partner.
- *pellizca, pega, agarra, empuja, o lanza objetos que pueden lastimar a su pareja.*

- forces his partner into having sex.
- *obliga a su pareja a tener relaciones sexuales.*

- causes his partner to be afraid.
- *causa que su pareja tenga miedo.*

During pregnancy, the target body parts change during abusive episodes. Women report physical blows directed to the head, breasts, abdomen, and genitalia. Sexual assault is common.

Battering and pregnancy in teenagers constitute a particularly difficult situation. Adolescents may be trapped in the abusive relationship because of their inexperience. Many professionals and the adolescents themselves ignore the violence because it may not be believable, because relationships are transient, and because the jealous and controlling behavior is interpreted as love and devotion. Routine screening for abuse and sexual assault is recommended for pregnant adolescents. Because pregnancy in young adolescent girls is commonly the result of sexual abuse, the nurse should assess the desire to maintain the pregnancy (see Chapter 4 for further discussion).

Review of systems. During this portion of the interview, the woman is asked to identify and describe preexisting or concurrent problems in any of the body systems, and her mental status is assessed. The woman is questioned about physical symptoms she has experienced, such as shortness of breath or pain. Pregnancy affects and is affected by all body systems; therefore information on the present status of the body systems is important in planning care. For each sign or symptom described, the following additional data should be obtained: body location, quality, quantity, chronology, aggravating or alleviating factors, and associated manifestations (onset, character, course) (Seidel, Ball, Dains, & Benedict, 2003).

Physical examination. The initial physical examination provides the baseline for assessing subsequent changes. The examiner should determine the woman's needs for basic information regarding reproductive anatomy and provide this information, along with a demonstration of the equipment that may be used and an explanation of the procedure itself. The interaction requires an unhurried, sensitive, and gentle approach with a matter-of-fact attitude.

The physical examination begins with assessment of vital signs including height and weight (for calculation of body mass index [BMI]) and blood pressure (BP) (see Guidelines/Guías box). The bladder should be empty before pelvic examination. A urine specimen may be obtained to test for protein, glucose, or leukocytes or for other urine tests.

Each examiner develops a routine for proceeding with the physical examination; most choose the head-to-toe progression. Heart and lung sounds are evaluated, and extremities are examined. Distribution, amount, and quality of body hair are of particular importance because the findings reflect nutritional status, endocrine function, and attention to hygiene. The thyroid gland is assessed carefully. The height of the fundus is noted if the first examination is done after the first trimester of pregnancy. During the examination the examiner needs to remain alert to the woman's cues that give direction to the remainder of the assessment and that indicate imminent untoward response

GUIDELINES/GUÍAS
Prenatal Physical Examination

- Get up on the scale, please.
- *Súbase a la balanza, por favor.*

- I need a urine sample.
- *Necesito una muestra de orina.*

- Go to the bathroom, please.
- *Vaya al baño, por favor.*

- I need to take your blood pressure.
- *Necesito verificar su presión sanguínea.*

- I am going to listen to the baby's heart beat.
- *Voy a escuchar el latido del corazón del bebé.*

- The doctor is going to examine you.
- *El doctor le va a examinar.*

- Don't be afraid.
- *No tenga miedo.*

- Lie down, please.
- *Acuéstese, por favor.*

- Separate your legs, please.
- *Sepárese las piernas, por favor.*

- Relax.
- *Afloje los músculos.*

- Go to the laboratory for a blood test, please.
- *Vaya al laboratorio para un análisis de sangre, por favor.*

- Go to this office for your ultrasound, please.
- *Vaya a esta oficina para que se le haga el ultrasonido, por favor.*

such as **supine hypotension**—low BP that occurs while the woman is lying on her back, causing feelings of faintness. See Chapter 4 for a detailed description of the physical examination.

Whenever a pelvic examination is performed, the tone of the pelvic musculature and the woman's knowledge of Kegel exercises are assessed. Particular attention is paid to the size of the uterus because this is an indication of the duration of gestation. The nurse present during the examination can coach the woman in breathing and relaxation techniques at this time, as needed. One vaginal examination during early pregnancy is recommended, but another is usually not done unless medically indicated.

Laboratory tests. The laboratory data yielded by the analysis of the specimens obtained during the examination provide important information concerning the symptoms of pregnancy and the woman's health status.

Specimens are collected at the initial visit so that the cause of any abnormal findings can be treated. Blood is drawn for a variety of tests (Table 9-1). A sickle cell screen is recommended for women of African, Asian, or Middle Eastern descent, and testing for antibody to the human immunodeficiency virus (HIV) is strongly recommended for all pregnant women (Box 9-4). In addition, pregnant women and fathers with a family history of cystic fibrosis

EVOLVE/CD: Case Study—First Trimester

TABLE 9-1

Laboratory Tests in Prenatal Period

LABORATORY TEST	PURPOSE
Hemoglobin, hematocrit, WBC, differential	Detects anemia; detects infection
Hemoglobin electrophoresis	Identifies women with hemoglobinopathies (e.g., sickle cell anemia, thalassemia)
Blood type, Rh, and irregular antibody	Identifies those fetuses at risk for developing erythroblastosis fetalis or hyperbilirubinemia in neonatal period
Rubella titer	Determines immunity to rubella
Tuberculin skin testing; chest film after 20 weeks of gestation in women with reactive tuberculin tests	Screens for exposure to tuberculosis
Urinalysis, including microscopic examination of urinary sediment; pH, specific gravity, color, glucose, albumin, protein, RBCs, WBCs, casts, acetone; hCG	Identifies women with unsuspected diabetes mellitus, renal disease, hypertensive disease of pregnancy; infection; occult hematuria
Urine culture	Identifies women with asymptomatic bacteriuria
Renal function tests: BUN, creatinine, electrolytes, creatinine clearance, total protein excretion	Evaluates level of possible renal compromise in women with a history of diabetes, hypertension, or renal disease
Pap test	Screens for cervical intraepithelial neoplasia, herpes simplex type 2, and HPV
Vaginal or rectal smear for *Neisseria gonorrhoeae*, *Chlamydia*, HPV, GBS	Screens high risk population for asymptomatic infection; GBS done at 35-37 weeks
RPR, VDRL, or FTA-ABS	Identifies women with untreated syphilis
HIV* antibody, hepatitis B surface antigen, toxoplasmosis	Screens for infection
1-hr glucose tolerance	Screens for gestational diabetes; done at initial visit for women with risk factors; done at 24-28 weeks for all pregnant women
3-hr glucose tolerance	Screens for diabetes in women with elevated glucose level after 1-hr test; must have two elevated readings for diagnosis
Cardiac evaluation: ECG, chest x-ray film, and echocardiogram	Evaluates cardiac function in women with a history of hypertension or cardiac disease

BUN, Blood urea nitrogen; *ECG,* electrocardiogram; *FTA-ABS,* fluorescent treponemal antibody absorption test; *GBS,* group B streptococcus; *hCG,* human chorionic gonadotropin; *HIV,* human immunodeficiency virus; *HPV,* human papillomavirus; *RBC,* red blood cell; *RPR,* rapid plasma reagin; *VDRL,* Venereal Disease Research Laboratory; *WBC,* white blood cell.
*With patient permission.

and of Caucasian ethnicity may elect to have blood drawn for testing to ascertain if they are a cystic fibrosis carrier (Fries, Bashford, & Nunes (2005). Urine specimens are usually tested by dipstick; culture and sensitivity tests are ordered as necessary. During the pelvic examination, cervical and vaginal smears may be obtained for cytologic studies and for diagnosis of infection (e.g., *Chlamydia*, gonorrhea, group B streptococcus [GBS]).

The finding of risk factors during pregnancy may indicate the need to repeat some tests at other times. For example, exposure to tuberculosis or an STI would necessitate repeat testing. STIs are common in pregnancy and may have negative effects on mother and fetus. Careful assessment and screening are essential.

Follow-up visits

Monthly visits are scheduled routinely during the first and second trimesters, although additional appointments may be made as the need arises. During the third trimester, however, the possibility for complications increases, and closer monitoring is warranted. Starting with week 28, maternity visits are scheduled every 2 weeks until week 36, and then every week until birth, unless the health care provider individualizes the schedule. Individual needs, complications, and risks of the pregnant woman may warrant visits more or less often. The pattern of interviewing the woman first and then assessing physical changes and performing laboratory tests is maintained.

Interview. Follow-up visits are less intensive than the initial prenatal visit. At each of these follow-up visits, the woman is asked to summarize relevant events that have occurred since the previous visit (Fig. 9-7). She is asked about her general emotional and physiologic well-being, complaints or problems, and questions she may have. Personal and family needs also are identified and explored.

Emotional changes are common during pregnancy, and therefore it is reasonable for the nurse to ask whether the woman has experienced any mood swings, reactions to changes in her body image, bad dreams, or worries. Positive feelings (her own and those of her family) are also noted. The reactions of family members to the pregnancy and the woman's emotional changes are recorded.

HIV Screening

Pregnant women are ethically obligated to seek reasonable care during pregnancy and to avoid causing harm to the fetus. Maternity nurses should be advocates for the fetus while accepting of the pregnant woman's decision regarding testing and/or treatment for HIV.

The incidence of perinatal transmission from an HIV-positive mother to her fetus ranges from 25% to 35%. Zidovudine decreases perinatal transmission and the risk of infant death (Brocklehurst & Volmink, 2002). Elective cesarean birth significantly reduces the risk of transmission from the mother to the child (Brocklehurst, 2002). Testing has the potential to identify HIV-positive women who can then be treated. Health care providers have an obligation to ensure that pregnant women are well informed about HIV symptoms, testing, and methods of decreasing maternal-fetal transmission. However, mandatory HIV screening involves ethical issues related to privacy invasion, discrimination, social stigma, and reproductive risks to the pregnant woman. Although some professional groups advocate mandatory testing, the Association of Women's Health, Obstetric and Neonatal Nurses (AWHONN) does not support either mandatory or universal HIV testing of pregnant women because these models do not have the same standards of confidentiality and counseling that are present with voluntary, confidential testing with counseling (AWHONN, 1999).

During the third trimester, current family situations and their effect on the woman are assessed, for example, siblings' and grandparents' responses to the pregnancy and the coming child. In addition, the following assessments of the woman and her family are made: warning signs of emergencies; signs of preterm and term labor; the labor process and concerns about labor; and fetal development and methods to assess fetal well-being. The nurse should ask if the woman is planning to attend childbirth preparation classes and what she knows about pain management during labor.

A review of the woman's physical systems is appropriate at each prenatal visit, and any suspicious signs or symptoms are assessed in depth. Discomforts reflecting adaptations to pregnancy are identified.

Physical examination. Reevaluation is a constant aspect of a pregnant woman's care. Each woman reacts differently to pregnancy. As a result, careful monitoring of the pregnancy and her reactions to care is vital. The database is updated at each time of contact with the pregnant woman. Physiologic changes are documented as the pregnancy progresses and reviewed for possible deviations from normal progress.

At each visit, physical parameters are measured. Ideally, BP is taken by using the same arm at every visit, with the woman sitting, using a cuff of appropriate size (which is noted on her chart). Her weight is assessed, and the appropriateness of the gestational weight gain is evaluated in relationship to her BMI. Urine may be checked by dipstick, and the presence and degree of edema are noted. For examination of the abdomen, the woman lies on her back with her arms by her side and head supported by a pillow. The bladder should be empty. Abdominal inspection is followed by measurement of the height of the fundus. While the woman lies on her back, the nurse should be alert for the occurrence of supine hypotension (see Emergency box). When a woman is lying in this position, the weight of abdominal contents may compress the vena cava and aorta, causing a decrease in BP and a feeling of faintness.

The findings revealed during the interview and physical examination reflect the status of maternal adaptations. When any of the findings is suspicious, an in-depth examination is performed. For example, careful interpretation of BP is important in the risk factor analysis of all pregnant women. BP is evaluated on the basis of absolute values and the length of gestation and is interpreted in light of modifying factors.

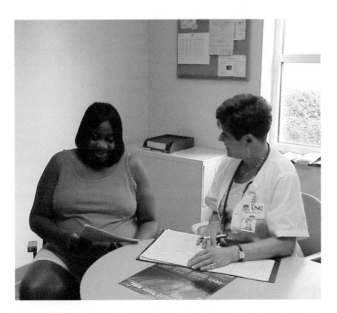

Fig. 9-7 Prenatal interview. (Courtesy Dee Lowdermilk, Chapel Hill, NC.)

EMERGENCY

Supine Hypotension

SIGNS AND SYMPTOMS

Pallor
Dizziness, faintness, breathlessness
Tachycardia
Nausea
Clammy (damp, cool) skin; sweating

INTERVENTIONS

Position woman on her side until her signs and symptoms subside and vital signs stabilize within normal limits (WNL).

NURSE ALERT *Individuals whose systolic BP (SBP) is 120 to 139 mm Hg or whose diastolic BP (DBP) is 80 to 89 mm Hg should be viewed as prehypertensive. To prevent cardiovascular disease, they require health-promoting lifestyle modifications (National High Blood Pressure Education Program, 2003).*

An absolute SBP of 140 mm Hg or more and a DBP of 90 mm Hg or more suggests the presence of hypertension. An SBP ≥125 mm Hg or a DBP ≥75 mm Hg in midpregnancy or an SBP ≥ 130 mm Hg or DBP ≥85 in later pregnancy are indicative of problems and should be reported to the primary health care provider immediately (Peters & Flack, 2004).

A rise in SBP of 30 mm Hg or more than the baseline pressure, or rise in the DBP of 15 mm Hg more than the baseline pressure, is also a significant finding regardless of the absolute values. An increase of 20 mm Hg or more in the mean arterial pressure (MAP) is also an indicator of hypertension (Gilbert & Harmon, 2003). See Chapter 23 for an in-depth discussion of problems associated with hypertension.

The pregnant woman is monitored continuously for a range of signs and symptoms that indicate potential complications in addition to hypertension. For example, persistent and excessive vomiting and ketonuria may indicate the development of hyperemesis gravidarum. Uterine cramping and vaginal bleeding are signs of threatened miscarriage. Chills and fever are symptoms of infection. Discharge from the vagina may be amniotic fluid or may be associated with infection (see Signs of Potential Complications box).

Fetal assessment. Toward the end of the first trimester, before the uterus is an abdominal organ, the fetal heart tones (FHTs) can be heard with an ultrasound fetoscope or an ultrasound stethoscope. To hear the FHTs, place the instrument in the midline, just above the symphysis pubis, and apply firm pressure. The woman and her family should be offered the opportunity to listen to the FHTs (see Fig. 9-9, *A*). The health status of the fetus is assessed at each visit for the remainder of the pregnancy.

Fundal height. During the second trimester, the uterus becomes an abdominal organ. The fundal height, measurement of the height of the uterus above the symphysis pubis, is used as one indicator of fetal growth. The measurement also provides a gross estimate of the duration of pregnancy. From approximately gestational weeks (GW) 18 to 32, the height of the fundus in centimeters is approximately the same as the number of weeks of gestation, (± 2 GW) with an empty bladder at the time of measurement (Cunningham et al., 2005). For example, a woman of 28 gestational weeks, with an empty bladder would measure from 26 to 30 cm. In addition, it may aid in the identification of high risk factors. A stable or decreased fundal height may indicate the presence of intrauterine growth restriction (IUGR); an excessive increase could indicate the presence of multifetal gestation (more than one fetus) or hydramnios.

signs of
POTENTIAL COMPLICATIONS

First, Second, and Third Trimesters

FIRST TRIMESTER

Signs and Symptoms	Possible Causes
Severe vomiting	Hyperemesis gravidarum
Chills, fever	Infection
Burning on urination	Infection
Diarrhea	Infection
Abdominal cramping; vaginal bleeding	Miscarriage, ectopic pregnancy

SECOND AND THIRD TRIMESTERS

Signs and Symptoms	Possible Causes
Persistent, severe vomiting	Hyperemesis gravidarum, hypertension, preeclampsia
Sudden discharge of fluid from vagina before 37 wk	Premature rupture of membranes (PROM)
Vaginal bleeding, severe abdominal pain	Miscarriage, placenta previa, abruptio placentae
Chills, fever, burning on urination, diarrhea	Infection
Severe backache or flank pain	Kidney infection or stones; preterm labor
Change in fetal movements: absence of fetal movements after quickening, any unusual change in pattern or amount	Fetal jeopardy or intrauterine fetal death
Uterine contractions; pressure; cramping before 37 wk	Preterm labor
Visual disturbances: blurring, double vision, or spots	Hypertensive conditions, preeclampsia
Swelling of face or fingers and over sacrum	Hypertensive conditions, preeclampsia
Headaches: severe, frequent, or continuous	Hypertensive conditions, preeclampsia
Muscular irritability or convulsions	Hypertensive conditions, preeclampsia
Epigastric or abdominal pain (perceived as severe stomachache)	Hypertensive conditions, preeclampsia, abruptio placentae
Glycosuria, positive glucose tolerance test reaction	Gestational diabetes mellitus

A paper tape typically is used to measure fundal height. To increase the reliability of the measurement, the same person examines the pregnant woman at each of her prenatal visits, but often this is not possible. All clinicians who examine a particular pregnant woman should be consistent in their measurement technique. Ideally, a protocol should be established for the health care setting in which the measurement technique is explicitly set forth, and the woman's position on the examining table, the measuring device, and method of measurement used are specified. Conditions under which the measurements are taken also can be described in the woman's records, including whether the bladder was empty and whether the uterus was relaxed or contracted at the time of measurement.

Various positions for measuring fundal height have been described. The woman can be supine, have her head elevated, have her knees flexed, or have both her head elevated and knees flexed. Measurements obtained with the woman in the various positions differ, making it even more important to standardize the fundal height measurement technique. The bladder must be empty before the measurement is taken. As much as 3-cm variation is possible if the bladder is full (Cunningham et al., 2005).

Placement of the tape measure also can vary. The tape can be placed in the middle of the woman's abdomen, and the measurement made from the upper border of the symphysis pubis to the upper border of the fundus with the tape measure held in contact with the skin for the entire length of the uterus (Fig. 9-8, *A*). In another measurement technique, the upper curve of the fundus is not included in the measurement. Instead, one end of the tape measure is held at the upper border of the symphysis pubis with one hand, and the other hand is placed at the upper border of the fundus. The tape is placed between the middle and index fingers of the other hand, and the point where these fingers intercept the tape measure is taken as the measurement (Fig. 9-8, *B*).

Gestational age.   In an uncomplicated pregnancy, fetal gestational age is estimated after the duration of pregnancy and the EDB are determined. Fetal gestational age is determined from the menstrual history, contraceptive history, pregnancy test result, and the following findings obtained during the clinical evaluation:

- First uterine evaluation: date, size
- Fetal heart (FH) first heard: date, method (Doppler stethoscope, fetoscope)
- Date of quickening
- Current fundal height, estimated fetal weight (EFW)
- Current week of gestation by history of LMP and/or ultrasound examination
- Ultrasound examination: date, week of gestation, biparietal diameter (BPD)
- Reliability of dates

Quickening ("feeling of life") refers to the mother's first perception of fetal movement. It usually occurs between weeks 16 and 20 of gestation and is initially experienced as a fluttering sensation. The mother's report should be recorded. Multiparas often perceive fetal movement earlier than primigravidas.

Routine use of ultrasound examination (also called a *sonogram*) in early pregnancy has been recommended, and many health care providers have this equipment available in the office. This procedure may be used to establish the duration of pregnancy if the woman cannot give a precise date for her LMP or if the size of the uterus does not conform to the EDB as calculated by Nägele's rule. Ultrasound also provides information about the well-being of the fetus. However, the routine use of ultrasound has not been found to substantively improve fetal outcome (Bricker & Neilson, 2000).

Health status.   The assessment of fetal health status includes consideration of fetal movement. The mother is instructed to note the extent and timing of fetal movements and to report immediately if the pattern changes or if movement ceases. Regular movement has been found to

CD: Assessment Video

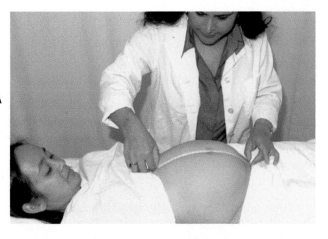
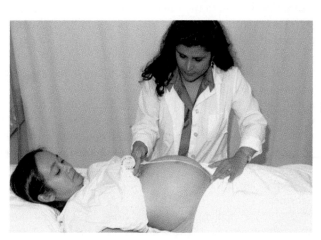

A   **B**

Fig. 9-8   Measurement of fundal height from symphysis that **(A)** includes the upper curve of the fundus and **(B)** does not include the upper curve of the fundus. Note position of hands and measuring tape. (Courtesy Chris Rozales, San Francisco, CA.)

be a reliable indicator of fetal health (Cunningham et al., 2005). One method is for the woman to count fetal movements after a meal. Four or more kick counts in an hour is reassuring.

The fetal heart rate (FHR) is checked on routine visits once it has been heard (Fig. 9-9). Early in the second trimester, the heart beat may be heard with the Doppler stethoscope (Fig. 9-9, *B*). To detect the heart beat before the fetus can be palpated by Leopold maneuvers (see procedure, p. 412), the scope is moved around the abdomen until the heart beat is heard. Each nurse develops a set pattern for searching the abdomen for the heart beat—for example, starting first in the midline about 2 to 3 cm above the symphysis, then moving to the left lower quadrant, and so on. The heart beat is counted for 1 minute, and the quality and rhythm noted. Later in the second trimester, the FHR can be determined with the fetoscope or Pinard fetoscope (Fig. 9-9, *A* and *C*). A normal rate and rhythm are other good indicators of fetal health. Once the heart beat is noted, its absence is cause for immediate investigation.

Fetal health status is investigated intensively if any maternal or fetal complications arise (e.g., gestational hypertension, IUGR, premature rupture of membranes [PROM], irregular or absent FHR, or absence of fetal movements after quickening). Careful, precise, and concise recording of patient responses and laboratory results contributes to the continuous supervision vital to ensuring the well-being of the mother and fetus.

Laboratory tests. The number of routine laboratory tests done during follow-up visits in pregnancy is limited. A clean-catch urine specimen is obtained to test for glucose, protein, nitrites, and leukocytes at each visit. Urine specimens for culture and sensitivity, as well as blood samples, are obtained only if signs and symptoms warrant.

It is recommended that the maternal serum alpha-fetoprotein (MSAFP) screening be done between 15 and 22 GW, ideally between 16 and 18 GW (Jenkins & Wapner, 2004). Elevated levels are associated with open neural tube defects and multiple gestations, whereas low levels are associated with Down syndrome. Abnormal levels are followed by second trimester ultrasonography for more in-depth investigation (Benn, Egan, Fang, & Smith-Bindman, 2004). The multiple-marker, or triple-screen, blood test is also recommended (Graves, Miller, & Sellers, 2002). Done between 16 and 18 weeks of gestation, it measures the MSAFP, human chorionic gonadotropin (hCG), and unconjugated estriol, the levels of which are combined to yield one value. Low levels may be associated with Down syndrome and other chromosomal abnormalities (Cunningham et al., 2005). Other blood tests are repeated as necessary, as are cervical and vaginal smears.

A glucose challenge is usually done between 24 and 28 weeks of gestation. GBS testing is done between 35 and 37 weeks of gestation; cultures collected earlier will not accurately predict GBS status at time of birth (Himmelberger, 2002). GBS testing may be done also at the initial physical

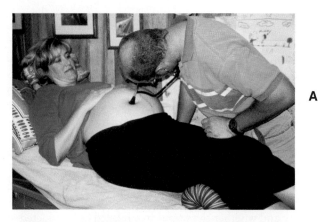

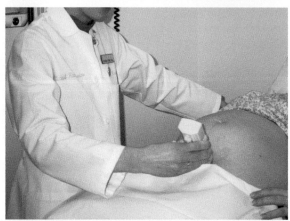

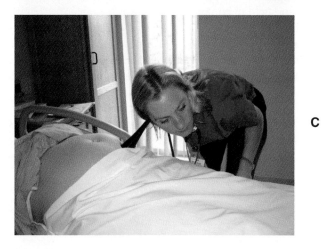

Fig. 9-9 Detecting fetal heart rate. **A,** Father can listen to the fetal heart with a fetoscope (first detectable around 18 to 20 weeks). **B,** Doppler ultrasound stethoscope (fetal heart beat detectable at 12 weeks). **C,** Pinard fetoscope. Note: Hands should not touch fetoscope while listening. (**A,** Courtesy Shannon Perry, Phoenix, AZ. **B,** Courtesy Dee Lowdermilk, Chapel Hill, NC. **C,** Courtesy Julie Perry Nelson, Gilbert, AZ.)

to identify and treat women who are GBS positive who may give birth before 35 GW.

Other tests. Other diagnostic tests are available to assess the health status of both the pregnant woman and the fetus. Ultrasonography, for example, may be performed to determine the status of the pregnancy and to confirm gestational age of the fetus. Amniocentesis, a procedure used to obtain amniotic fluid for analysis, may be needed to evaluate the fetus for genetic disorders or gestational maturity. These and other tests that are used to determine health risks for the mother and infant are described in Chapter 21.

After obtaining information through the assessment process, the data are analyzed to identify deviations from the norm and unique needs of the pregnant woman and her family. Although comprehensive health care requires collaboration among professionals from several disciplines, nurses are in an excellent position to formulate diagnoses that can be used to guide independent interventions. The following are examples of the nursing diagnoses that may be appropriate in the prenatal period

- *Anxiety related to*
  - –physical discomforts of pregnancy
  - –ambivalent and labile emotions
  - –changes in family dynamics
  - –fetal well-being
  - –ability to manage anticipated labor
- *Constipation related to*
  - –progesterone relaxation of gastrointestinal smooth muscle
  - –dietary behaviors
- *Imbalanced nutrition: less than body requirements related to*
  - –morning sickness (nausea and vomiting)
  - –fatigue
- *Disturbed body image related to*
  - –anatomic and physiologic changes of pregnancy
  - –changes in the couple relationship
- *Disturbed sleep patterns related to*
  - –discomforts of late pregnancy
  - –anxiety about approaching labor

Expected Outcomes of Care

The plan of nursing care for women and their families during pregnancy is guided by the diagnoses that have been formulated during prenatal visits. Individualized plans that are developed mutually with the pregnant woman or couple are more likely to result in desirable outcomes than are those developed by the nurse for the woman. Measured outcomes of prenatal care include not only physical outcomes but also developmental and psychosocial outcomes.

The following are examples of outcomes that may be expected. The pregnant woman will achieve the following:

- Verbalize decreased anxiety about the health of her fetus and herself
- Verbalize improved family dynamics
- Show appropriate weight gain patterns per trimester
- Report increasing acceptance of changes in body image
- Demonstrate knowledge for self-care
- Seek clarification of information about pregnancy and birth

- Report signs and symptoms of complications
- Describe appropriate measures taken to relieve physical discomforts
- Develop a realistic birth plan

Plan of Care and Interventions

The nurse-patient relationship is critical in setting the tone for further interaction. The techniques of listening with an attentive expression, touching, and using eye contact have their place, as does recognizing the woman's feelings and her right to express these feelings. The interaction may occur in various formal or informal settings. The clinic, home visits, or telephone conversations all provide opportunities for contact and can be used effectively.

Care Paths

Because a large number of health care professionals can be involved in care of the expectant mother, unintentional gaps or overlaps in care may occur. Care paths can be used to improve the consistency of care and to reduce costs. Although the Care Path on p. 254 focuses only on prenatal education, it is one example of the type of form that might be developed to guide health care providers in carrying out the appropriate assessments and interventions in a timely way. Use of care paths also may contribute to improved satisfaction of families with the prenatal care provided, and members of the health care team may function more efficiently and effectively.

Education about maternal and fetal changes

Expectant parents are typically curious about the growth and development of the fetus and the subsequent changes that occur in the mother's body. Mothers in particular are sometimes more tolerant of the discomforts related to the continuing pregnancy if they understand the underlying causes. Educational literature that describes the fetal and maternal changes is available and can be used in explaining changes as they occur. The nurse's familiarity with any material shared with pregnant families is essential to effective patient education. Educational material may include electronic and written materials appropriate to the pregnant woman's or couple's literacy level and experience and the agency's resources. It is important that available educational materials reflect the pregnant woman's or couple's ethnicity, culture, and literacy level to be most effective.

Education for self-care

The expectant mother needs information about many subjects. The nurse who is observant, listens, and knows typical concerns of expectant parents can anticipate questions that will be asked and prompt mothers and partners to discuss what is on their minds. Many times, printed literature can be given to supplement the individualized teaching the nurse provides, and women often avidly read books and pamphlets related to their own experience. When nurses read

CARE PATH *Prenatal Care Pathway*

PRENATAL EDUCATION CLINICAL PATHWAY

INITIAL VISIT AND ORIENTATION: _____   SOCIAL SERVICE: _____   DIETITIAN: _____

I. EARLY PREGNANCY (WEEKS 1-20) (INITIAL AND DATE AFTER EDUCATION GIVEN)

Fetal growth and development _____   Testing: Labs _____   Ultrasound _____

Maternal changes _____   Possible complications:
    a. Threatened miscarriage _____

Lifestyle: exercise/stress/nutrition _____   b. Diabetes _____
  Drugs, OTC, tobacco, alcohol _____   c. _____ _____
  STIs _____

Introduction to breastfeeding _____

Psychologic/social adjustments: _____   Acceptance of pregnancy
  FOB involved/accepts _____   and childbirth preparation _____
  Baby for adoption _____

Dietary follow-up _____

II. MIDPREGNANCY (WEEKS 21-27) (INITIAL AND DATE AFTER EDUCATION GIVEN)

Fetal growth and development _____   Breastfeeding or bottle feeding _____

Maternal changes _____   Birth plan initiated _____

Daily fetal movement _____   Childbirth preparation _____

Possible complications:
  a. Preterm labor prevention _____   _____
  b. Preeclampsia symptoms _____   Dietary follow-up _____
  c. _____ _____

III. LATE PREGNANCY (WEEKS 28-40) (INITIAL AND DATE AFTER EDUCATION GIVEN)

Fetal growth and development _____   Childbirth preparation:
    S/S of labor; labor process _____

Fetal evaluation: Pain management: natural childbirth, _____
      medications, epidural

  Daily movement _____   NSTs _____   Cesarean; VBAC _____
    Birth plan complete _____
  Kick counts _____   BPPs _____   Review hospital policies _____

Maternal changes _____   Parenting preparation:
    Pediatrician _____   Childcare _____

Possible complications: Siblings _____   Immunizations _____
  a. Preterm labor prevention _____   Car seat/safety _____
  b. Precclampsia symptoms _____
  c. _____ _____   Postpartum:
    PP care and checkup _____

Breastfeeding preparation: Emotional changes _____
    BC options _____
  Nipple assessment _____   Safer sex and STIs _____

Dietary follow-up _____

Signature: _____

BC, Birth control; *BPP,* biophysical profile; *FOB,* father of baby; *NST,* nonstress test; *OTC,* over-the-counter preparations; *PP,* postpartum; *S/S,* signs and symptoms; *STI,* sexually transmitted infection; *VBAC,* vaginal birth after cesarean.

the literature before they distribute it, they have an opportunity to point out areas that may not correspond with local health care practices. As family members are common sources for health information it is also important to include them in the health education endeavors (Lewallen, 2004). In addition, as more individuals use the computer for information, the pregnant woman or couple may have questions from their Internet reviews. Nurses may also share recommended electronic sites from reliable sources.

Patients who receive conflicting advice or instruction are likely to grow increasingly frustrated with members of the health care team and the care provided. Several topics that may cause concerns in pregnant women are discussed in the following sections.

Nutrition. Good nutrition is important for the maintenance of maternal health during pregnancy and the provision of adequate nutrients for embryonic and fetal development (American Dietetic Association [ADA], 2002). Assessing a woman's nutritional status and providing information on nutrition are part of the nurse's responsibilities in providing prenatal care. This includes assessment of weight gain during pregnancy as well as prenatal nutrition. Teaching may include discussion about foods high in iron, encouragement to take prenatal vitamins, and recommendations to moderate or limit caffeine intake. In some settings a registered dietitian conducts classes for pregnant women on the topics of nutritional status and nutrition during pregnancy or interviews them to assess their knowledge of these topics. Nurses can refer women to a registered dietitian if a need is revealed during the nursing assessment. (For detailed information concerning maternal and fetal nutritional needs and related nursing care, see Chapter 10).

Personal hygiene. During pregnancy, the sebaceous (sweat) glands are highly active because of hormonal influences, and women often perspire freely. They may be reassured that the increase is normal and that their previous patterns of perspiration will return after the postpartum period. Baths and warm showers can be therapeutic because they relax tense, tired muscles; help counter insomnia; and make the pregnant woman feel fresh. Tub bathing is permitted even in late pregnancy because little water enters the vagina unless under pressure. However, late in pregnancy, when the woman's center of gravity lowers, she is at risk for falling. Tub bathing is contraindicated after rupture of the membranes.

Prevention of urinary tract infections. Because of physiologic changes that occur in the renal system during pregnancy (see Chapter 8), urinary tract infections are common, but they may be asymptomatic. Women should be instructed to inform their health care provider if blood or pain occurs with urination. These infections pose a risk to the mother and fetus; therefore the prevention or early treatment of these infections is essential.

The nurse can assess the woman's understanding and use of good handwashing techniques before and after urinating and of the importance of wiping the perineum from front to back. Soft, absorbent toilet tissue, preferably white and unscented, should be used; harsh, scented, or printed toilet paper may cause irritation. Bubble bath or other bath oils should be avoided because these may irritate the urethra. Women should wear cotton crotch underpants and panty hose and avoid wearing tight-fitting slacks or jeans for long periods; anything that allows a buildup of heat and moisture in the genital area may foster the growth of bacteria.

Some women do not consume enough fluid and food. After discovering her food preferences, the nurse should advise the woman to drink at least 2 L (eight glasses) of liquid, preferably water, a day to maintain an adequate fluid intake that ensures frequent urination. Pregnant women should not limit fluids in an effort to reduce the frequency of urination. Women need to know that if urine looks dark (concentrated), they must increase their fluid intake. The consumption of yogurt and acidophilus milk also may help prevent urinary tract and vaginal infections. The nurse should review healthy urination practices with the woman. Women are told not to ignore the urge to urinate because holding urine lengthens the time bacteria are in the bladder and allows them to multiply. Women should plan ahead when they are faced with situations that may normally require them to delay urination (e.g., a long car ride). They always should urinate before going to bed at night. Bacteria can be introduced during intercourse; therefore, women are advised to urinate before and after intercourse, and then drink a large glass of water to promote additional urination. Although frequently recommended, there is conflicting evidence regarding the effectiveness of cranberry juice and in particular the effective dosage in the prevention of urinary tract infections (Jepson, Mihaljevic, & Craig, 2005; Kiel, Nashelsky, Robbins, & Bondi, 2003; Raz, Chazan, & Dan, 2004).

Kegel exercises. Kegel exercises, deliberate contraction and relaxation of the pubococcygeus muscle, strengthen the muscles around the reproductive organs and improve muscle tone. Many women are not aware of the muscles of the pelvic floor until it is pointed out that these are the muscles used during urination and sexual intercourse that can be consciously controlled. The muscles of the pelvic floor encircle the vaginal outlet, and they need to be exercised, because an exercised muscle can then stretch and contract readily at the time of birth. Practice of pelvic muscle exercises during pregnancy also results in fewer complaints of urinary incontinence in late pregnancy and postpartum (Sampselle, 2003).

Several ways of performing Kegel exercises have been described. The method described in the Teaching Guidelines in Chapter 4 (see p. 93) demonstrates evidence-based nursing care. This method was developed by nurses involved in a research utilization project for continence in women. Teaching has been effective if the woman reports an increased ability to control urine flow and greater muscular control during sexual intercourse.

Preparation for breastfeeding. Pregnant women are usually eager to discuss their plans for feeding the newborn. Breast milk is the food of choice, in part

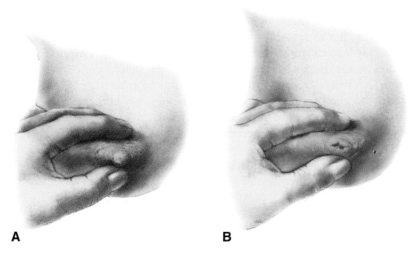

A

B

Fig. 9-10 **A,** Normal nipple everts with gentle pressure. **B,** Inverted nipple inverts with gentle pressure. (Modified from Lawrence, R., and Lawrence, R. [2005]. *Breastfeeding: A guide for the medical profession* [6th ed.]. St. Louis: Mosby.)

because breastfeeding is associated with a decreased incidence of perinatal morbidity and mortality. The American Academy of Pediatrics recommends breastfeeding for at least a year. However, a deep-seated aversion to breastfeeding on the part of the woman or partner, the woman's need for certain medications or use of street drugs, and certain life-threatening illnesses and medical complications, such as HIV infection, are contraindications to breastfeeding (Lawrence & Lawrence, 2005). Although hepatitis B antigen has not been shown to be transmitted through breast milk, as an added precaution, it is recommended that infants born to hepatis B surface antigen (HBsAg)-positive women receive the hepatitis B vaccine and hepatitis B immune globulin (HBIg) immediately after birth. Women who are HIV positive are discouraged from nursing because the risk of HIV transmission outweighs the risk of the infant dying from another cause (Lawrence & Lawrence, 2005).

A woman's decision about the method of infant feeding often is made before pregnancy; therefore the education of women of childbearing age about the benefits of breastfeeding is essential. If undecided, the pregnant woman and her partner are encouraged to choose which method of feeding is suitable for them (Pavill, 2002). Once the couple has been given information about the advantages and disadvantages of bottle feeding and breastfeeding, they can make an informed choice. Health care providers support their decisions and provide any needed assistance.

Women with inverted nipples need special consideration if they are planning to breastfeed. The pinch test is done to determine whether the nipple is everted or inverted (Fig. 9-10). The nurse shows the woman the way to perform the pinch test. It involves having the woman place her thumb and forefinger on her areola and gently press inward. This action will cause her nipple either to stand erect or to invert. Most nipples will stand erect.

Exercises to break the adhesions that cause the nipple to invert do not work and may precipitate uterine contractions (Lawrence & Lawrence, 2005). The use of breast shells, small plastic devices that fit over the nipples, is suggested for women who have flat or inverted nipples (Fig. 9-11). Breast shells work by exerting a continuous, gentle pressure around the areola that pushes the nipple through a central opening in the inner shield. Breast shells should be worn for 1 to 2 hours daily during the last trimester of pregnancy. They should be worn for gradually increasing lengths of time (Lawrence & Lawrence, 2005). Breast stimulation is contraindicated in women at risk for preterm labor; therefore the decision to suggest the use of breast shells to women with flat or inverted nipples must be made judiciously. Continuous support and guidance must be given to the woman as part of the nursing plan of care.

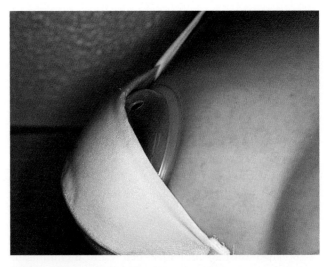

Fig. 9-11 Breast shell in place inside bra to evert nipple. (Courtesy Michael S. Clement, MD, Mesa, AZ.)

The woman is taught to cleanse the nipples with warm water to keep the ducts from being blocked with dried colostrum. Soap, ointments, alcohol, and tinctures should not be applied because they remove protective oils that keep the nipples supple. The use of these substances may cause the nipples to crack during early lactation (Lawrence & Lawrence, 2005).

The woman who plans to breastfeed should purchase a nursing bra that will accommodate her increased breast size during the last few months of pregnancy and during lactation. If her breasts are very heavy, or if the woman feels uncomfortable with the weight unsupported, the bra can be worn day and night.

Dental care. Dental care during pregnancy is especially important because nausea during pregnancy may lead to poor oral hygiene, allowing dental caries to develop. A fluoride toothpaste should be used daily. Inflammation and infection of the gingival and periodontal tissues may occur (Carl, Roux, & Matacale, 2000). Research links periodontal disease with preterm births and LBW (Jared et al., 1999) and an increased risk for preeclampsia (Boggess et al., 2003).

Because calcium and phosphorus in the teeth are fixed in enamel, the old adage "for every child a tooth" is not true. There is no scientific evidence to support the belief that filling teeth or even dental extraction involving the administration of local or nitrous oxide–oxygen anesthesia precipitates miscarriage or premature labor. Antibacterial therapy should be considered for sepsis, however, especially in pregnant women who have had rheumatic heart disease or nephritis. Emergency dental surgery is not contraindicated during pregnancy. However, the risks and benefits of dental surgery must be explained. If dental treatment is necessary, the woman will be most comfortable during the second trimester because the uterus is now outside the pelvis but not so large as to cause discomfort while she sits in a dental chair (Carl, Roux, & Matacale, 2000).

Physical activity. Physical activity promotes a feeling of well-being in the pregnant woman. It improves circulation, promotes relaxation and rest, and counteracts boredom, as it does in the nonpregnant woman (American College of Obstetricians and Gynecologists, [ACOG], 2002). Detailed exercise tips for pregnancy are presented in the Patient Instructions for Self-Care box. Exercises that help relieve the low back pain that often arises during the second trimester because of the increased weight of the fetus are demonstrated in Fig. 9-12.

Posture and body mechanics. Skeletal and musculature changes and hormonal changes (relaxin) in pregnancy may predispose the woman to backache and possible injury. As pregnancy progresses, the pregnant woman's center of

PATIENT INSTRUCTIONS FOR SELF-CARE
Exercise Tips for Pregnant Women

Consult your health care provider when you know or suspect you are pregnant. Discuss your medical and obstetric history, your current exercise regimen, and the exercises you would like to continue throughout pregnancy.

Seek help in determining an exercise routine that is well within your limit of tolerance, especially if you have not been exercising regularly.

Consider decreasing weight-bearing exercises (jogging, running) and concentrating on non–weight-bearing activities such as swimming, cycling, or stretching. If you are a runner, starting in your seventh month, you may wish to walk instead.

Avoid risky activities such as surfing, mountain climbing, skydiving, and racquetball because such activities that require precise balance and coordination may be dangerous. Avoid activities that require holding your breath and bearing down (Valsalva maneuver). Jerky, bouncy motions also should be avoided.

Exercise regularly every day if possible, as long as you are healthy, to improve muscle tone and increase or maintain your stamina. Exercising sporadically may put undue strain on your muscles. Thirty minutes of moderate physical exercise is recommended. This activity can be broken up into shorter segments with rest in between. For example, exercise for 10 to 15 minutes, rest for 2 to 3 minutes, then exercise for another 10 to 15 minutes.

Decrease your exercise level as your pregnancy progresses. The normal alterations of advancing pregnancy, such as decreased cardiac reserve and increased respiratory effort, may produce physiologic stress if you exercise strenuously for a long time.

Take your pulse every 10 to 15 minutes while you are exercising. If it is more than 140 beats/min, slow down until it returns to a maximum of 90 beats/min. You should be able to converse easily while exercising. If you cannot, you need to slow down.

Avoid becoming overheated for extended periods. It is best not to exercise for more than 35 minutes, especially in hot, humid weather. As your body temperature rises, the heat is transmitted to your fetus. Prolonged or repeated elevation of fetal temperature may result in birth defects, especially during the first 3 months. Your temperature should not exceed 38° C.

Avoid the use of hot tubs and saunas.

Warm-up and stretching exercises prepare your joints for more strenuous exercise and lessen the likelihood of strain or injury to your joints. After the fourth month of gestation, you should not perform exercises flat on your back.

A cool-down period of mild activity involving your legs after an exercise period will help bring your respiration, heart, and metabolic rates back to normal and prevent the pooling of blood in the exercised muscles.

Continued

PATIENT INSTRUCTIONS FOR SELF-CARE—cont'd

Exercise Tips for Pregnant Women

Rest for 10 minutes after exercising, lying on your side. As the uterus grows, it puts pressure on a major vein in your abdomen, which carries blood to your heart. Lying on your side removes the pressure and promotes return circulation from your extremities and muscles to your heart, thereby increasing blood flow to your placenta and fetus. You should rise gradually from the floor to prevent dizziness or fainting (orthostatic hypotension).

Drink two or three 8-oz glasses of water after you exercise to replace the body fluids lost through perspiration. While exercising, drink water whenever you feel the need.

Increase your caloric intake to replace the calories burned during exercise and provide the extra energy needs of pregnancy. (Pregnancy alone requires an additional 300 kcal/day.) Choose such high-protein foods as fish, milk, cheese, eggs, and meat.

Take your time. This is not the time to be competitive or train for activities requiring speed or long endurance.

Wear a supportive bra. Your increased breast weight may cause changes in posture and put pressure on the ulnar nerve.

Wear supportive shoes. As your uterus grows, your center of gravity shifts and you compensate for this by arching your back. These natural changes may make you feel off balance and more likely to fall.

Stop exercising immediately if you experience shortness of breath, dizziness, numbness, tingling, pain of any kind, more than four uterine contractions per hour, decreased fetal activity, or vaginal bleeding, and consult your health care provider.

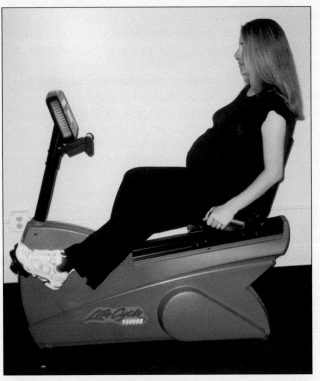

Riding a recumbent bicycle provides exercise while supplying back support. (Courtesy Shannon Perry, Phoenix, AZ.)

Sources: American College of Obstetricians and Gynecologists (ACOG). (2002). Exercise during pregnancy and the postpartum period. ACOG Committee Opinion #267. *Obstetrics & Gynecology, 99*(1), 171-173. Artal, R., & Subak-Sharpe, G. (1998). *Pregnancy and exercise.* New York: Delacorte Press; Kramer, M. (2001). Regular aerobic exercise during pregnancy (Cochrane Review). In *The Cochrane Library,* Issue 1. Oxford: Update Software; Morris, S., & Johnson, N. (2005). Exercise in pregnancy: A critical appraisal of the literature. *Journal of Reproductive Medicine, 50*(3), 181-188.

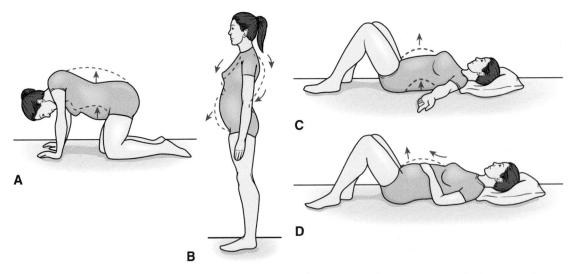

Fig. 9-12 Exercises. **A-C,** Pelvic rocking relieves low backache (excellent for relief of menstrual cramps as well). **D,** Abdominal breathing aids relaxation and lifts abdominal wall off uterus.

gravity changes, pelvic joints soften and relax, and stress is placed on abdominal musculature. Poor posture and body mechanics contribute to the discomfort and potential for injury. To minimize these problems, women can learn good body posture and body mechanics (Fig. 9-13). Strategies to prevent or relieve backache are presented in the Patient Instructions for Self-Care box on p. 260.

Rest and relaxation. The pregnant woman is encouraged to plan regular rest periods, particularly as pregnancy advances. The side-lying position is recommended because it promotes uterine perfusion and fetoplacental oxygenation by eliminating pressure on the ascending vena cava and descending aorta, which can lead to supine hypotension (Fig. 9-14). The mother also should be shown the way to rise slowly from a side-lying position to prevent placing strain on the back and to minimize the orthostatic hypotension caused by changes in position common in the latter part of pregnancy. To stretch and rest back muscles at home or work, the nurse can show the woman the way to do the following exercises:

- Stand behind a chair. Support and balance self by using the back of the chair (Fig. 9-15). Squat for 30 seconds; stand for 15 seconds. Repeat six times, several times per day, as needed.
- While sitting in a chair, lower head to knees for 30 seconds. Raise head. Repeat six times, several times per day, as needed.

Conscious relaxation is the process of releasing tension from the mind and body through deliberate effort and practice. The ability to relax consciously and intentionally can be beneficial for the following reasons:

- To relieve the normal discomforts related to pregnancy
- To reduce stress and therefore diminish pain perception during the childbearing cycle
- To heighten self-awareness and trust in one's own ability to control responses and functions
- To help cope with stress in everyday life situations, whether the woman is pregnant or not

The techniques for conscious relaxation are numerous and varied. Guidelines are given in Box 9-5.

Employment. Employment of pregnant women usually has no adverse effects on pregnancy outcomes. Job discrimination that is based strictly on pregnancy is illegal. However, some job environments pose potential risk to the fetus (e.g., dry-cleaning plants, chemistry laboratories, parking garages). Excessive fatigue is usually the deciding factor in the termination of employment. Strategies to improve safety during pregnancy are described in the Patient Instructions for Self-Care Box on p. 261.

Women with sedentary jobs need to walk around at intervals to counter the usual sluggish circulation in the legs. They also should neither sit nor stand in one position for long periods, and they should avoid crossing their legs at

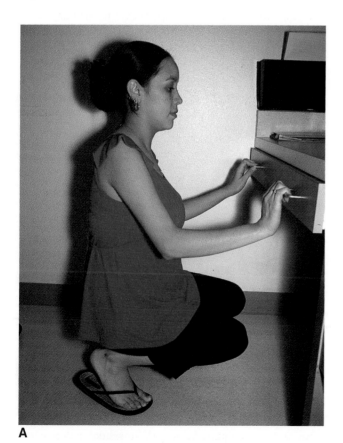

A

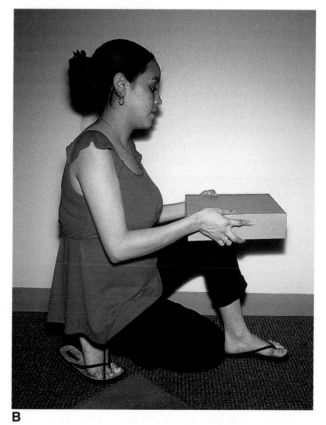

B

Fig. 9-13 Correct body mechanics. **A,** Squatting. **B,** Lifting. (Courtesy Michael S. Clement, MD, Mesa, AZ.)

PATIENT INSTRUCTIONS FOR SELF-CARE
Posture and Body Mechanics

TO PREVENT OR RELIEVE BACKACHE
Do pelvic tilt:
- **Pelvic tilt** (rock) on hands and knees (see Fig. 9-12, *A*) and while sitting in straight-back chair.
- Pelvic tilt (rock) in standing position against a wall, or lying on floor (see Fig. 9-12, *B* and *C*).
- Perform abdominal muscle contractions during pelvic tilt while standing, lying, or sitting to help strengthen rectus abdominis muscle (see Fig. 9-12, *D*).
- Use good body mechanics.
- Use leg muscles to reach objects on or near floor. Bend at the knees, not from the back. Knees are bent to lower body to squatting position. Feet are kept 12 to 18 inches apart to provide a solid base to maintain balance (see Fig. 9-13, *A*).
- Lift with the legs. To lift heavy object (e.g., young child), one foot is placed slightly in front of the other and kept flat as woman lowers herself onto one knee. She lifts the weight holding it close to her body and never higher than the chest. To stand up or sit down, she places one leg slightly behind the other as she raises or lowers herself (see Fig. 9-13, *B*).

TO RESTRICT THE LUMBAR CURVE
- For prolonged standing (e.g., ironing, employment), place one foot on low footstool or box; change positions often.
- Move car seat forward so that knees are bent and higher than hips. If needed, use a small pillow to support low back area.
- Sit in chairs low enough to allow both feet to be placed on floor, preferably with knees higher than hips.

TO PREVENT ROUND LIGAMENT PAIN AND STRAIN ON ABDOMINAL MUSCLES
Implement suggestions given in Table 9-2.

---

the knees, because all these activities can foster the development of varices and thrombophlebitis. Standing for long periods also increases the risk of preterm labor. The pregnant woman's chair should provide adequate back support. Use of a footstool can prevent pressure on veins, relieve strain on varicosities, minimize edema of feet, and prevent backache.

Clothing. Some women continue to wear their usual clothes during pregnancy as long as they fit and feel comfortable. If maternity clothing is needed, outfits may be purchased new or found at thrift shops or garage sales in good condition. Comfortable, loose clothing is recommended. Tight bras and belts, stretch pants, garters, tight-top knee socks, panty girdles, and other constrictive clothing should be avoided because tight clothing over the perineum encourages vaginitis and miliaria (heat rash), and impaired circulation in the legs can cause varicosities.

Maternity bras are constructed to accommodate the increased breast weight, chest circumference, and the size of breast tail tissue (under the arm). These bras also have drop-flaps over the nipples to facilitate breastfeeding. A good bra can help prevent neckache and backache.

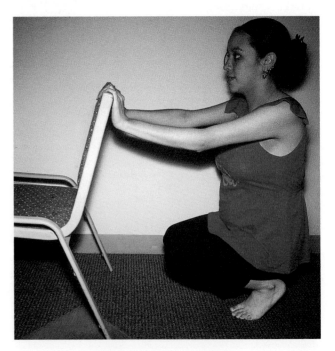

Fig. 9-15 Squatting for muscle relaxation and strengthening and for keeping leg and hip joints flexible. (Courtesy Michael S. Clement, MD, Mesa, AZ.)

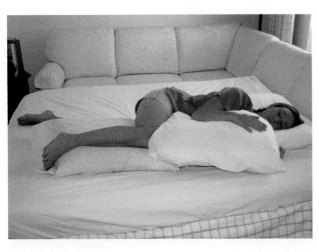

Fig. 9-14 Side-lying position for rest and relaxation. Some women prefer to support upper part of leg with pillows. (Courtesy Julie Perry Nelson, Gilbert, AZ.)

BOX 9-5

Conscious Relaxation Tips

Preparation: Loosen clothing, assume a comfortable sitting or side-lying position with all parts of body well supported with pillows.

Beginning: Allow yourself to feel warm and comfortable. Inhale and exhale slowly, and imagine peaceful relaxation coming over each part of the body, starting with the neck and working down to the toes. Often people who learn conscious relaxation speak of feeling relaxed even if some discomfort is present.

Maintenance: Use imagery (fantasy or daydream) to maintain the state of relaxation. Using active imagery, imagine yourself moving or doing some activity and experiencing its sensations. Using passive imagery, imagine yourself watching a scene, such as a lovely sunset.

Awakening: Return to the wakeful state gradually. Slowly begin to take in stimuli from the surrounding environment.

Further retention and development of the skill: Practice regularly for some periods each day, for example, at the same hour for 10 to 15 minutes each day, to feel refreshed, revitalized, and invigorated.

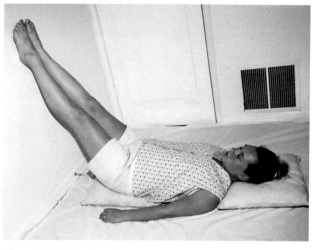

Fig. 9-16 Position for resting legs and for reducing edema and varicosities. Encourage woman with vulvar varicosities to include pillow under her hips. (Courtesy Dale Ikuta, San Jose, CA.)

Maternal support hose give considerable comfort and promote greater venous emptying in women with large varicose veins. Ideally, support stockings should be put on before the woman gets out of bed in the morning. Fig. 9-16 demonstrates a position for resting the legs and reducing swelling and varicosities.

Comfortable shoes that provide firm support and promote good posture and balance also are advisable. Very high heels and platform shoes are not recommended because of the changes in the pregnant woman's center of gravity, and the hormone relaxin, which softens pelvic joints in later pregnancy, all of which can cause her to lose her balance. In addition, in the third trimester, the woman's pelvis tilts forward, and her lumbar curve increases. The resulting leg aches and cramps are aggravated by nonsupportive shoes (Fig. 9-17).

Travel. Travel is not contraindicated in low risk pregnant women. However, women with high risk pregnancies are advised to avoid long-distance travel after fetal viability has been reached to avert possible economic and psychologic consequences of giving birth to a preterm infant far from home. Travel to areas in which medical care is poor, water is untreated, or malaria is prevalent should be avoided if possible. Women who contemplate foreign travel should be aware that many health insurance carriers do not cover a birth in a foreign setting or even hospitalization for preterm labor. In addition, vaccinations for foreign travel may be contraindicated during pregnancy.

Pregnant women who travel for long distances should schedule periods of activity and rest. While sitting, the woman can practice deep breathing, foot circling, and alternately contracting and relaxing different muscle groups.

PATIENT INSTRUCTIONS FOR SELF-CARE

Safety during Pregnancy

Changes in the body resulting from pregnancy include relaxation of joints, alteration to center of gravity, faintness, and discomforts. Problems with coordination and balance are common. Therefore, the woman should follow these guidelines:

- Use good body mechanics.
- Use safety features on tools and vehicles (safety seat belts, shoulder harnesses, headrests, goggles, helmets) as specified.
- Avoid activities requiring coordination, balance, and concentration.
- Take rest periods; reschedule daily activities to meet rest and relaxation needs.

Embryonic and fetal development is vulnerable to environmental teratogens. Many potentially dangerous chemicals are present in the home, yard, and workplace: cleaning agents, paints, sprays, herbicides, and pesticides. The soil and water supply may be unsafe. Therefore the woman should follow these guidelines:

- Read all labels for ingredients and proper use of product.
- Ensure adequate ventilation with clean air.
- Dispose of wastes appropriately.
- Wear gloves when handling chemicals.
- Change job assignments or workplace as necessary.
- Avoid high altitudes (not in pressurized aircraft), which could jeopardize oxygen intake.

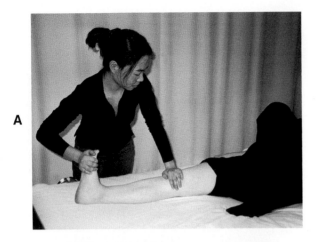

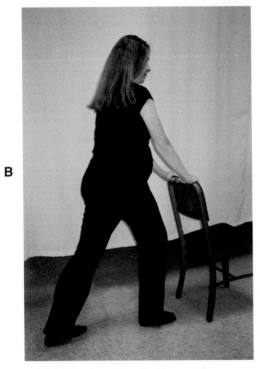

Fig. 9-17 Relief of muscle spasm (leg cramps). **A,** Another person dorsiflexes foot with knee extended. **B,** Woman stands and leans forward, thereby dorsiflexing foot of affected leg. (Courtesy Shannon Perry, Phoenix, AZ.)

She should avoid becoming fatigued. Although travel in itself is not a cause of adverse outcomes such as miscarriage or preterm labor, certain precautions are recommended while traveling in a car. For example, women riding in a car should wear automobile restraints and stop and walk every hour.

Maternal death as a result of injury is the most common cause of fetal death. The next most common cause is placental separation that occurs because body contours change in reaction to the force of a collision. The uterus as a muscular organ can adapt its shape to that of the body, but the placenta is not resilient. At the impact of collision, pla-

cental separation can occur. A combination lap belt and shoulder harness is the most effective automobile restraint, and both should be used (Fig. 9-18). The lap belt should be worn low across the pelvic bones and as snug as is comfortable. The shoulder harness should be worn above the gravid uterus and below the neck to prevent chafing. The pregnant woman should sit upright. The headrest should be used to prevent a whiplash injury.

Pregnant women traveling in high-altitude regions have lowered oxygen levels that may cause fetal hypoxia, especially if the pregnant woman is anemic. However, the current information on this condition is limited, and recommendations are not standardized.

Airline travel in large commercial jets usually poses little risk to the pregnant woman, but policies vary from airline to airline. The pregnant woman is advised to inquire about restrictions or recommendations from her carrier. Most health care providers allow air travel up to 36 weeks gestation in women without medical or pregnancy complications. The 8% humidity at which the cabins of commercial airlines are maintained may result in some water loss; hydration (with water) should therefore be maintained under these conditions. Sitting in the cramped seat of an airliner for prolonged

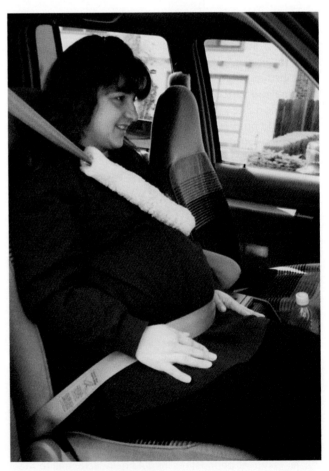

Fig. 9-18 Proper use of seat belt and headrest. (Courtesy Tammie McGee, Millbrae, CA.)

periods may increase the risk of superficial and deep thrombophlebitis; therefore a pregnant woman is encouraged to take a 15-minute walk around the aircraft during each hour of travel to minimize this risk. Metal detectors used at airport security checkpoints are not harmful to the fetus. However, women who are pilots, flight attendants, or frequent flyers expose themselves to in-flight radiation that exceeds recommended levels (Barish, 2004). Resources from the U.S. Federal Aviation Administration will assist the health care provider in determining safe levels for those women at high risk for radiation exposure.

Medications and herbal preparations. Although much has been learned in recent years about fetal drug toxicity, the possible teratogenicity of many medications, both prescription and OTC, is still unknown. This fact is especially true for new medications and combinations of drugs. Moreover, certain subclinical errors or deficiencies in intermediate metabolism in the fetus may cause an otherwise harmless drug to be converted into a hazardous one. The greatest danger of drug-caused developmental defects in the fetus extends from the time of fertilization through the first trimester, a time when the woman may not realize she is pregnant. Self-treatment must be discouraged. The use of all drugs, including OTC medications, herbs, and vitamins, should be limited and a careful record kept of all therapeutic and nontherapeutic agents used.

Immunizations. Some concern has been raised over the safety of various immunization practices during pregnancy. Immunization with live or attenuated live viruses is contraindicated during pregnancy because of its potential teratogenicity but should be part of postpartum care (ACOG, 2003). Live-virus vaccines include those for measles (rubeola and rubella), chickenpox, and mumps, as well as the Sabin (oral) poliomyelitis vaccine (no longer used in the United States) (ACOG). Vaccines consisting of killed viruses may be used. Those that may be administered during pregnancy include tetanus, diphtheria, recombinant hepatitis B, and rabies vaccines.

Alcohol, cigarette smoke, caffeine, and drugs. A safe level of alcohol consumption during pregnancy has not yet been established. Although the consumption of occasional alcoholic beverages may not be harmful to the mother or her developing embryo or fetus, complete abstinence is strongly advised. Maternal alcoholism is associated with high rates of miscarriage and fetal alcohol syndrome; the risk for miscarriage in the first trimester is dose related (three or more drinks per day). Growing evidence indicates that the pattern of drinking (frequency, timing, and duration), especially in the first trimester, is more predictive of fetal damage than is the amount (Wagner, Katikaneni, Cox, & Ryan, 1998). Considerably less alcohol use is reported among pregnant women than in nonpregnant women, but a high prevalence of some alcohol use among pregnant women still exists. Such a finding underscores the need for more systematic public health efforts to educate women about the hazards of alcohol consumption during pregnancy.

Cigarette smoking or continued exposure to secondhand smoke (even if the mother does not smoke) is associated with intrauterine fetal growth restriction (IUGR) and an increase in perinatal and infant morbidity and mortality. Smoking is associated with an increased frequency of preterm labor, PROM, abruptio placentae, placenta previa, and fetal death, possibly resulting from decreased placental perfusion. Smoking cessation activities should be incorporated into routine prenatal care (Todd, LaSala, & Neil-Urban, 2001; Yu, Park, & Schwalberg, 2002).

All women who smoke should be strongly encouraged to quit or at least reduce the number of cigarettes they smoke. Pregnant women need to be told about the negative effects of even secondhand smoke on the fetus and encouraged to avoid such environments (Andres, 2004). Efforts focused on preventing girls and women from beginning to smoke should be intensified.

Most studies of human pregnancy have revealed no association between caffeine consumption and birth defects or LBW (Andres, 2004). In contrast, some studies have documented an increased risk for miscarriage with caffeine intake greater than 300 mg/day (Giannelli, Doyle, Roman, Pelerin, & Hermon, 2003) or intrauterine fetal growth restriction with caffeine intake greater than 223 mg/day (Torstein, Bakketeig, Trygg, Lund-Larsen, & Jacobsen, 2003). Because other effects are unknown, however, pregnant women are advised to limit their caffeine intake, particularly coffee intake, as it has a high caffeine content per unit of measure. Therefore health care providers often encourage pregnant women to limit caffeine intake to no more than 3 cups of coffee or cola per day (ADA, 2002).

Any drug or environmental agent that enters the pregnant woman's bloodstream has the potential to cross the placenta and harm the fetus. Marijuana, heroin, and cocaine are common examples of such substances. Although the problem of substance abuse in pregnancy is considered a major public health concern, comprehensive care of drug-addicted women improves maternal and neonatal outcomes (see Chapter 27).

Normal discomforts. Pregnant women have physical symptoms that would be considered abnormal in the nonpregnant state. Women pregnant for the first time have an increased need for explanations of the causes of the discomforts and for advice on ways to relieve the discomforts. The discomforts of the first trimester are fairly specific. Information about the physiology and prevention of and self-care for discomforts experienced during the three trimesters is given in Table 9-2. Box 9-6 lists alternative and complementary therapies and why they might be used in pregnancy (Fig. 9-19). Nurses can do much to allay a first-time mother's anxiety about such symptoms by telling her about them in advance and using terminology that the woman (or couple) can understand. Understanding the rationale for treatment promotes their participation in their care. Interventions should be individualized, with attention given to the woman's lifestyle and culture.

Text continued on p. 269.

BACKGROUND

- Smoking during pregnancy is linked with low birth weight (<2500 g), very preterm birth (<32 weeks), perinatal death, low rates of breastfeeding, and shorter duration of breastfeeding. Characteristics of women likely to smoke during pregnancy include being of significantly higher parity and lower socioeconomic status, experiencing depression and job strain, and being more likely to be without a partner or practical support system. Even when they have these characteristics, however, certain groups still have lower smoking prevalence rates in pregnancy than the general population, as a result of cultural influences. For example, Mexican-American and African-American women have lower smoking rates in pregnancy, although the rate is rising. Widespread campaigns to discourage smoking during pregnancy may have decreased the incidence, but the women who continue to smoke experience guilt, anxiety, and stress on their relationships with families and health care providers. Smokers are notoriously unreliable in self-reporting how much they smoke, and this is exacerbated in pregnancy, leading to measurement errors in research. Some women erroneously believe that low birth weight is desirable for an easy delivery.

OBJECTIVES

- The reviewers searched for studies comparing the efficacy of smoking cessation interventions in pregnancy. Interventions included information on the risks of smoking, advice to quit, individual counseling, group counseling, feedback of the pathophysiologic effects of smoking on mother or fetus, pictures of the fetus, nicotine replacement therapy, self-help manuals on strategies for quitting, and rewards and incentives. Outcomes included birth weight, gestation at birth, perinatal mortality, method of delivery, breastfeeding initiation and duration, maternal anxiety, depression, family functioning, duration of smoking cessation, and knowledge, attitudes and behavior of health professionals regarding smoking in pregnancy.

METHODS
Search Strategy

- The authors searched the Cochrane database and the Cochrane Tobacco Addiction Group trials register. Search keywords were not reported. Thirty-seven trials, representing 16,916 women, were selected, dated 1976 to 1999. Most of the trials (27) took place in the United States, but other countries represented included the United Kingdom, Argentina, Brazil, Cuba, Mexico, New Zealand, Sweden, Australia, Canada, and Norway.

Statistical Analyses

- The trials were grouped by type and intensity of the intervention. Similar data were pooled. Secondary analysis looked at some outcomes separately.

FINDINGS

- There was a significant decrease in smoking during late pregnancy in the intervention groups. The absolute difference between groups was 6.4%: of 100 women smokers, ten will stop smoking as a result of "usual care," and a further 6 to 7 will stop as a result of intervention. Smoking cessation interventions were associated with significantly fewer low-birth-weight babies and preterm birth and increased mean birth weight. There was no difference detected in very low birth weight (<1500 g) or perinatal mortality.

  Five trials had a smoking relapse prevention intervention, with even fewer women in late pregnancy smoking. About 25% of women who quit smoking during pregnancy relapse while still pregnant. Some data suggested that the stages of change (precontemplation, contemplation, preparation, and action) may be different in pregnancy, and that changes made in early pregnancy may not be sustained.

LIMITATIONS

- A number of trials did not offer informed consent. Many trials did not discuss the method of randomization, and many were quasi-randomized. Because the interventions were not concealed, outside influence may have skewed the results. Intervention protocols varied quite a bit, as did duration of intervention and follow-up. Interventions may not have been culturally appropriate for every setting. The amount of smoking cessation intervention that occurs in the "usual care" control group more recently may exceed the intervention groups of decades ago. Health providers may find it difficult to treat women differently according to their randomized group allocation. Many withdrawals and dropouts in the trials leave gaps in the data. Women who had a fetal death or a preterm infant may not have been counted as late-pregnancy smokers, as they never reached 36 weeks. Self-report inaccuracies may be replaced with biochemical results.

CONCLUSIONS

- Intervention is effective in assisting women to decrease smoking during late pregnancy. The women who quit smoking had fewer low-birth-weight babies and preterm births, but the interventions made no difference in incidence of very low-birth-weight (<1500 g) babies or perinatal mortality.

IMPLICATIONS FOR PRACTICE

- All maternity settings need smoking cessation programs. This review makes it clear that smoking cessation groups perform poorly. Further education can be fostered with programs that take into account the concerns of women who smoke, the staff who counsel them, and cognitive-behavioral strategies and relapse prevention. Health care providers need to team with other community educators to prevent smoking onset in young people and address socioeconomic inequities and stresses.

IMPLICATIONS FOR FURTHER RESEARCH

- Standardization of intervention and outcome measures would strengthen the ability to determine which smoking cessation interventions are successful in pregnancy. Biochemical markers are better indicators of smoking behavior than self-report. Targeting teens would benefit a subset of the population already at risk for low-birth-weight babies. These trials did not measure methods of delivery, breast feeding, or maternal or family psychologic well-being.

Reference: Lumley J., Oliver S., & Waters, E. (1999). Interventions for promoting smoking cessation during pregnancy (Cochrane Review). In *The Cochrane Library*, Issue 2, 2004. Chichester, UK: John Wiley & Sons.

TABLE 9-2

Discomforts Related to Pregnancy

DISCOMFORT	PHYSIOLOGY	EDUCATION FOR SELF-CARE
FIRST TRIMESTER		
Breast changes, new sensation: pain, tingling, tenderness	Hypertrophy of mammary glandular tissue and increased vascularization, pigmentation, and size and prominence of nipples and areolae caused by hormonal stimulation	Wear supportive maternity bras with pads to absorb discharge, may be worn at night; wash with warm water and keep dry; breast tenderness may interfere with sexual expression or foreplay but is temporary
Urgency and frequency of urination	Vascular engorgement and altered bladder function caused by hormones; bladder capacity reduced by enlarging uterus and fetal presenting part	Empty bladder regularly; perform Kegel exercises; limit fluid intake before bedtime; wear perineal pad; report pain or burning sensation to primary health care provider
Languor and malaise; fatigue (early pregnancy, most commonly)	Unexplained; may be caused by increasing levels of estrogen, progesterone, and hCG or by elevated BBT; psychologic response to pregnancy and its required physical and psychologic adaptations	Rest as needed; eat well-balanced diet to prevent anemia
Nausea and vomiting, morning sickness—occurs in 50%-75% of pregnant women; starts between first and second missed periods and lasts until about fourth missed period; may occur any time during day; fathers also may have symptoms	Cause unknown; may result from hormonal changes, possibly hCG; may be partly emotional, reflecting pride in, ambivalence about, or rejection of pregnant state	Avoid empty or overloaded stomach; maintain good posture—give stomach ample room; stop smoking; eat dry carbohydrate on awakening; remain in bed until feeling subsides, or alternate dry carbohydrate every other hour with fluids such as hot herbal decaffeinated tea, milk, or clear coffee until feeling subsides; eat five to six small meals per day; avoid fried, odorous, spicy, greasy, or gas-forming foods; consult primary health care provider if intractable vomiting occurs
Ptyalism (excessive salivation) may occur starting 2 to 3 weeks after first missed period	Possibly caused by elevated estrogen levels; may be related to reluctance to swallow because of nausea	Use astringent mouth wash, chew gum, eat hard candy as comfort measures
Gingivitis and epulis (hyperemia, hypertrophy, bleeding, tenderness of the gums); condition will disappear spontaneously 1 to 2 months after birth	Increased vascularity and proliferation of connective tissue from estrogen stimulation	Eat well-balanced diet with adequate protein and fresh fruits and vegetables; brush teeth gently and observe good dental hygiene; avoid infection; see dentist
Nasal stuffiness; epistaxis (nosebleed)	Hyperemia of mucous membranes related to high estrogen levels	Use humidifier; avoid trauma; normal saline nose drops or spray may be used
Leukorrhea: often noted throughout pregnancy	Hormonally stimulated cervix becomes hypertrophic and hyperactive, producing abundant amount of mucus	Not preventable; do not douche; wear perineal pads; perform hygienic practices such as wiping front to back; report to primary health care provider if accompanied by pruritus, foul odor, or change in character or color
Psychosocial dynamics, mood swings, mixed feelings	Hormonal and metabolic adaptations; feelings about female role, sexuality, timing of pregnancy, and resultant changes in life and lifestyle	Participate in pregnancy support group; communicate concerns to partner, family, and health care provider; request referral for supportive services if needed (financial assistance)

Continued

TABLE 9-2

Discomforts Related to Pregnancy—cont'd

DISCOMFORT	PHYSIOLOGY	EDUCATION FOR SELF-CARE
SECOND TRIMESTER		
Pigmentation deepens; acne, oily skin	Melanocyte-stimulating hormone (from anterior pituitary)	Not preventable; usually resolves during puerperium
Spider nevi (angiomas) appear over neck, thorax, face, and arms during second or third trimester	Focal networks of dilated arterioles (end arteries) from increased concentration of estrogens	Not preventable; they fade slowly during late puerperium; rarely disappear completely
Palmar erythema occurs in 50% of pregnant women; may accompany spider nevi	Diffuse reddish mottling over palms and suffused skin over thenar eminences and fingertips; may be caused by genetic predisposition or hyperestrogenism	Not preventable; condition will fade within 1 wk after giving birth
Pruritus (noninflammatory)	Unknown cause; various types as follows: nonpapular; closely aggregated pruritic papules	Keep fingernails short and clean; contact primary health care provider for diagnosis of cause
	Increased excretory function of skin and stretching of skin possible factors	Not preventable; use comfort measures for symptoms such as Keri baths; distraction; tepid baths with sodium bicarbonate or oatmeal added to water; lotions and oils; change of soaps or reduction in use of soap; loose clothing; see health care provider if mild sedation is needed
Palpitations	Unknown; should not be accompanied by persistent cardiac irregularity	Not preventable; contact primary health care provider if accompanied by symptoms of cardiac decompensation
Supine hypotension (vena cava syndrome) and bradycardia	Induced by pressure of gravid uterus on ascending vena cava when woman is supine; reduces uteroplacental and renal perfusion	Side-lying position or semisitting posture, with knees slightly flexed (see supine hypotension, p. 249)
Faintness and, rarely, syncope (orthostatic hypotension) may persist throughout pregnancy	Vasomotor lability or postural hypotension from hormones; in late pregnancy may be caused by venous stasis in lower extremities	Moderate exercise, deep breathing, vigorous leg movement; avoid sudden changes in position and warm crowded areas; move slowly and deliberately; keep environment cool; avoid hypoglycemia by eating five or six small meals per day; wear elastic hose; sit as necessary; if symptoms are serious, contact primary health care provider
Food cravings	Cause unknown; craving influenced by culture or geographic area	Not preventable; satisfy craving unless it interferes with well-balanced diet; report unusual cravings to primary health care provider
Heartburn (pyrosis or acid indigestion): burning sensation, occasionally with burping and regurgitation of a little sour-tasting fluid	Progesterone slows GI tract motility and digestion, reverses peristalsis, relaxes cardiac sphincter, and delays emptying time of stomach; stomach displaced upward and compressed by enlarging uterus	Limit or avoid gas-producing or fatty foods and large meals; maintain good posture; sip milk for temporary relief; hot herbal tea; primary health care provider may prescribe antacid between meals; contact primary health care provider for persistent symptoms

BBT, Basal body temperature; *GI,* gastrointestinal; *hCG,* human chorionic gonadotropin.

TABLE 9-2

Discomforts Related to Pregnancy—cont'd

DISCOMFORT	PHYSIOLOGY	EDUCATION FOR SELF-CARE
SECOND TRIMESTER—cont'd		
Constipation	GI tract motility slowed because of progesterone, resulting in increased resorption of water and drying of stool; intestines compressed by enlarging uterus; predisposition to constipation because of oral iron supplementation	Drink six to eight glasses of water per day; include roughage in diet; moderate exercise; maintain regular schedule for bowel movements; use relaxation techniques and deep breathing; do not take stool softener, laxatives, mineral oil, other drugs, or enemas without first consulting primary health care provider
Flatulence with bloating and belching	Reduced GI motility because of hormones, allowing time for bacterial action that produces gas; swallowing air	Chew foods slowly and thoroughly; avoid gas-producing foods, fatty foods, large meals; exercise; maintain regular bowel habits
Varicose veins (varicosities): may be associated with aching legs and tenderness; may be present in legs and vulva; hemorrhoids are varicosities in perianal area	Hereditary predisposition; relaxation of smooth muscle walls of veins because of hormones causing tortuous dilated veins in legs and pelvic vasocongestion; condition aggravated by enlarging uterus, gravity, and bearing down for bowel movements; thrombi from leg varices rare but may occur in hemorrhoids	Avoid obesity, lengthy standing or sitting, constrictive clothing, and constipation and bearing down with bowel movements; moderate exercise; rest with legs and hips elevated (see Fig. 9-16); wear support stockings; thrombosed hemorrhoid may be evacuated; relieve swelling and pain with warm sitz baths, local application of astringent compresses
Leukorrhea: often noted throughout pregnancy	Hormonally stimulated cervix becomes hypertrophic and hyperactive, producing abundant amount of mucus	Not preventable; do not douche; maintain good hygiene; wear perineal pads; report to primary health care provider if accompanied by pruritus, foul odor, or change in character or color
Headaches (through week 26)	Emotional tension (more common than vascular migraine headache); eye strain (refractory errors); vascular engorgement and congestion of sinuses resulting from hormone stimulation	Conscious relaxation; contact primary health care provider for constant "splitting" headache, to assess for preeclampsia
Carpal tunnel syndrome (involves thumb, second, and third fingers, lateral side of little finger)	Compression of median nerve resulting from changes in surrounding tissues; pain, numbness, tingling, burning; loss of skilled movements (typing); dropping of objects	Not preventable; elevate affected arms; splinting of affected hand may help; regressive after pregnancy; surgery is curative
Periodic numbness, tingling of fingers (acrodysesthesia) occurs in 5% of pregnant women	Brachial plexus traction syndrome resulting from drooping of shoulders during pregnancy (occurs especially at night and early morning)	Maintain good posture; wear supportive maternity bra; condition will disappear if lifting and carrying baby does not aggravate it
Round ligament pain (tenderness)	Stretching of ligament caused by enlarging uterus	Not preventable; rest, maintain good body mechanics to avoid overstretching ligament; relieve cramping by squatting or bringing knees to chest; sometimes heat helps

Continued

TABLE 9-2

Discomforts Related to Pregnancy—cont'd

DISCOMFORT	PHYSIOLOGY	EDUCATION FOR SELF-CARE
SECOND TRIMESTER—cont'd		
Joint pain, backache, and pelvic pressure; hypermobility of joints	Relaxation of symphyseal and sacroiliac joints because of hormones, resulting in unstable pelvis; exaggerated lumbar and cervicothoracic curves caused by change in center of gravity resulting from enlarging abdomen	Maintain good posture and body mechanics; avoid fatigue; wear low-heeled shoes; abdominal supports may be useful; conscious relaxation; sleep on firm mattress; apply local heat or ice; get back rubs; do pelvic tilt exercises; rest; condition will disappear 6 to 8 wk after birth
THIRD TRIMESTER		
Shortness of breath and dyspnea occur in 60% of pregnant women	Expansion of diaphragm limited by enlarging uterus; diaphragm is elevated about 4 cm; some relief after lightening	Good posture; sleep with extra pillows; avoid overloading stomach; stop smoking; contact health care provider if symptoms worsen to rule out anemia, emphysema, and asthma
Insomnia (later weeks of pregnancy)	Fetal movements, muscle cramping, urinary frequency, shortness of breath, or other discomforts	Reassurance; conscious relaxation; back massage or effleurage; support of body parts with pillows; warm milk or warm shower before retiring
Psychosocial responses: mood swings, mixed feelings, increased anxiety	Hormonal and metabolic adaptations; feelings about impending labor, birth, and parenthood	Reassurance and support from significant other and health care providers; improved communication with partner, family, and others
Urinary frequency and urgency return	Vascular engorgement and altered bladder function caused by hormones; bladder capacity reduced by enlarging uterus and fetal presenting part	Empty bladder regularly, Kegel exercises; limit fluid intake before bedtime; reassurance; wear perineal pad; contact health care provider for pain or burning sensation
Perineal discomfort and pressure	Pressure from enlarging uterus, especially when standing or walking; multifetal gestation	Rest, conscious relaxation, and good posture; contact health care provider for assessment and treatment if pain is present
Braxton Hicks contractions	Intensification of uterine contractions in preparation for work of labor	Reassurance; rest; change of position; practice breathing techniques when contractions are bothersome; effleurage; differentiate from preterm labor
Leg cramps (gastrocnemius spasm), especially when reclining	Compression of nerves supplying lower extremities because of enlarging uterus; reduced level of diffusible serum calcium or elevation of serum phosphorus; aggravating factors: fatigue, poor peripheral circulation, pointing toes when stretching legs or when walking, drinking more than 1 L (1 qt) of milk per day	Check for Homans' sign; if negative, use massage and heat over affected muscle; dorsiflex foot until spasm relaxes (see Fig. 9-17, *A*); stand on cold surface; oral supplementation with calcium carbonate or calcium lactate tablets; aluminum hydroxide gel, 30 ml, with each meal removes phosphorus by absorbing it (consult primary health care provider before taking these remedies)
Ankle edema (nonpitting) to lower extremities	Edema aggravated by prolonged standing, sitting, poor posture, lack of exercise, constrictive clothing, or hot weather	Ample fluid intake for natural diuretic effect; put on support stockings before arising; rest periodically with legs and hips elevated (see Fig. 9-16), exercise moderately; contact health care provider if generalized edema develops; *diuretics are contraindicated*

BOX 9-6

Complementary and Alternative Therapies Used in Pregnancy

MORNING SICKNESS AND HYPEREMESIS
- Acupuncture
- Acupressure (see Fig. 9-19)
- Shiatzu
- Herbal remedies*
  - Lemon balm
  - Peppermint
  - Spearmint
  - Ginger root
  - Raspberry leaf
  - Fennel
  - Chamomile
  - Hops
  - Meadowsweet
  - Wild yam root

RELAXATION AND MUSCLE-ACHE RELIEF
- Yoga
- Biofeedback
- Reflexology
- Therapeutic touch
- Massage

From Beal, M. (1998). Women's use of complementary and alternative therapies in reproductive health. *Journal of Nurse-Midwifery, 43*(3), 224-233; Schirmer, G. (1998). *Herbal medicine.* Bedford, TX: MED2000, Inc; Tiran, D., & Mack, S. (2000). *Complementary therapies for pregnancy and childbirth* (2nd ed.). Edinburgh: Baillière Tindall; Smith, C., Crowther, C., Willson, K,. Hotham, N., & McMillian, V. (2004). A randomized controlled trial of ginger to treat nausea and vomiting in pregnancy. *Obstetrics & Gynecology 103*(4), 639-645.
*Some herbs can cause miscarriage, preterm labor, or fetal or maternal injury. Pregnant women should discuss use with pregnancy health care provider, as well as an expert qualified in the use of the herb.

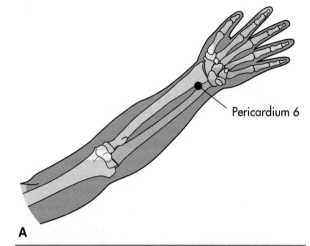

A

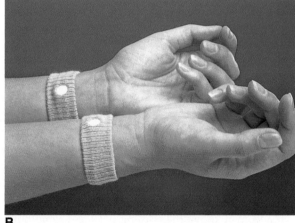

B

Fig. 9-19   A, Pericardium 6 (p6) acupressure point for nausea. **B,** Sea Bands used for stimulation of acupressure point p6. (**B,** Courtesy Sea-Band International, Newport, RI.)

NURSE ALERT *Although complementary and alternative medications (CAM) may benefit the woman during pregnancy, some practices should be avoided because they may cause miscarriage or preterm labor. It is important to ask the woman what therapies she may be using.*

Recognizing potential complications.   One of the most important responsibilities of care providers is to alert the pregnant woman to signs and symptoms that indicate a potential complication of pregnancy. The woman needs to know how and to whom to report such warning signs. Therefore the pregnant woman and her family can be reassured if they receive and use a printed form written at the appropriate literacy level, in their language and reflective of their culture, listing the signs and symptoms that warrant an investigation and the telephone numbers to call with questions or in an emergency.

The nurse must answer questions honestly as they arise during pregnancy. Pregnant women often have difficulty deciding when to report signs and symptoms. The mother is encouraged to refer to the printed list of potential complications and to listen to her body. If she senses that something is wrong, she should call her care provider. Several signs

and symptoms must be discussed more extensively. These include vaginal bleeding, alteration in fetal movements, symptoms of gestational hypertension, rupture of membranes, and preterm labor (see Signs of Potential Complications box on p. 250).

Recognizing preterm labor.   Teaching each expectant mother to recognize preterm labor is necessary for early diagnosis and treatment. Preterm labor occurs after the twentieth week but before the thirty-seventh week of pregnancy and consists of uterine contractions that, if untreated, cause the cervix to open earlier than normal and result in preterm birth.

Although the exact etiology of preterm labor is unknown, it is assumed to have multiple causes. An increased incidence of preterm birth is associated with sociodemographic factors such as poverty, low educational level, lack of social support, smoking, domestic violence, and stress (Freda, 2003; Freda & Patterson, 2003; Moos, 2004). Other risk factors include a previous preterm labor (McPheeters et al., 2005), current multifetal gestation, and some uterine and cervical variations (March of Dimes Birth Defects Foundation, 2005). The rate

PATIENT INSTRUCTIONS FOR SELF-CARE
How to Recognize Preterm Labor

Because the onset of preterm labor is subtle and often hard to recognize, it is important to know how to feel your abdomen for uterine contractions. You can feel for contractions in the following way. While lying down, place your fingertips on the top of your uterus. A contraction is the periodic tightening or hardening of your uterus. If your uterus is contracting, you will actually feel your abdomen get tight or hard and then feel it relax or soften when the contraction is over.

If you think you are having any of the other signs and symptoms of preterm labor, empty your bladder, drink three to four glasses of water for hydration, lie down tilted toward your side, and place a pillow at your back for support.

Check for contractions for 1 hour. To tell how often contractions are occurring, check the minutes that elapse from the beginning of one contraction to the beginning of the next.

It is *not normal* to have frequent uterine contractions (every 10 minutes or more often for 1 hour).

Contractions of labor are regular, frequent, and hard. They also may be felt as a tightening of the abdomen or a backache. This type of contraction causes the cervix to efface and dilate.

Call your doctor, nurse-midwife, clinic, or labor and birth unit, or go to the hospital if any of the following signs occur:
- You have uterine contractions every 10 minutes or more often for 1 hour or
- You have any of the other signs and symptoms for 1 hour or
- You have any bloody spotting or leaking of fluid from your vagina

It is often difficult to identify preterm labor. Accurate diagnosis requires assessment by the health care provider, usually in the hospital or clinic.

Post these instructions where they can be seen by everyone in the family.

---

is almost twice as high in the African-American population as in Caucasians. The pathology associated with preterm labor also is unclear, and more research is necessary to identify the pathophysiology of preterm labor and effective treatment strategies.

If a woman knows the warning signs and symptoms of preterm labor and seeks care early enough, prevention of preterm birth may be possible. Warning signs and symptoms of preterm labor are given in the Patient Instructions for Self-Care box. Fig. 9-20 shows the possible locations of symptoms in the body.

Sexual counseling

Sexual counseling of expectant couples includes countering misinformation, providing reassurance of normality, and suggesting alternative behaviors. The uniqueness of each couple is considered within a biopsychosocial framework

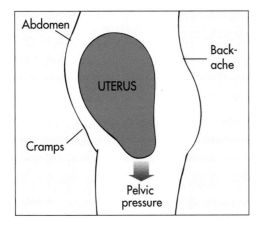

Fig. 9-20 Symptoms of preterm labor.

(see the Patient Instructions for Self-Care box on p. 271. Nurses can initiate discussion about sexual adaptations that must be made during pregnancy, but they themselves need a sound knowledge base about the physical, social, and emotional responses to sex during pregnancy. Not all maternity nurses are comfortable dealing with the sexual concerns of their patients; therefore those nurses who are aware of their personal strengths and limitations in dealing with sexual content are better prepared to make referrals if necessary (Westheimer & Lopater, 2005).

Many women merely need permission to be sexually active during pregnancy. Many other women, however, need to be given information about the physiologic changes that occur during pregnancy, have the myths that are associated with sex during pregnancy dispelled, and participate in open discussions of intercourse positions that decrease pressure on the gravid abdomen (Westheimer & Lopater, 2005). Such tasks are within the purview of the nurse and should be an integral component of the health care rendered.

Some couples need to be referred for sex therapy or family therapy. Couples with long-standing problems with sexual dysfunction that are intensified by pregnancy are candidates for sex therapy. Whenever a sexual problem is a symptom of a more serious relationship problem, the couple would benefit from family therapy.

Countering misinformation. Many myths and much of the misinformation related to sex and pregnancy are masked by seemingly unrelated issues. For example, a discussion about the baby's ability to hear and see in utero may be prompted by questions about the baby being an "unseen observer" of the couple's lovemaking. The counselor must be extremely sensitive to the questions behind such questions when counseling in this highly charged emotional area.

PATIENT INSTRUCTIONS FOR SELF-CARE
Sexuality in Pregnancy

- Be aware that maternal physiologic changes, such as breast enlargement, nausea, fatigue, abdominal changes, perineal enlargement, leukorrhea, pelvic vasocongestion, and orgasmic responses, may affect sexuality and sexual expression.
- Discuss responses to pregnancy with your partner.
- Keep in mind that cultural prescriptions ("dos") and proscriptions ("don'ts") may affect your responses.
- Although your libido may be depressed during the first trimester, it often increases during the second and third trimesters.
- Discuss and explore with your partner:
  - Alternative behaviors (e.g., mutual masturbation, foot massage, cuddling)

- Alternative positions (e.g., female superior, side-lying) for sexual intercourse
- Intercourse is safe as long as it is not uncomfortable. There is no correlation between intercourse and miscarriage, but observe the following precautions:
- Abstain from intercourse if you experience uterine cramping or vaginal bleeding; report event to your caregiver as soon as possible.
- Abstain from intercourse (or any activity that results in orgasm) if you have a history of cervical incompetence, until the problem is corrected.
- Continue to use "safer sex" behaviors. Women at risk for acquiring or conveying STIs are encouraged to use condoms during sexual intercourse throughout pregnancy.

STI, Sexually transmitted infection.

Suggesting alternative behaviors. Research has not demonstrated conclusively that coitus and orgasm are contraindicated at any time during pregnancy for the obstetrically and medically healthy woman (Cunningham et al., 2005). However, a history of more than one miscarriage; a threatened miscarriage in the first trimester; impending miscarriage in the second trimester; and PROM, bleeding, or abdominal pain during the third trimester warrant caution when it comes to coitus and orgasm.

Solitary and mutual masturbation and oral-genital intercourse may be used by couples as alternatives to penile-vaginal intercourse. Partners who enjoy cunnilingus (oral stimulation of the clitoris or vagina) may feel "turned off" by the normal increase in the amount and odor of vaginal discharge during pregnancy. Couples who practice cunnilingus should be cautioned against the blowing of air into the vagina, particularly during the last few weeks of pregnancy when the cervix may be slightly open. An air embolism can occur if air is forced between the uterine wall and the fetal membranes and enters the maternal vascular system through the placenta.

Showing the woman or couple pictures of possible variations of coital position often is helpful (Fig. 9-21). The

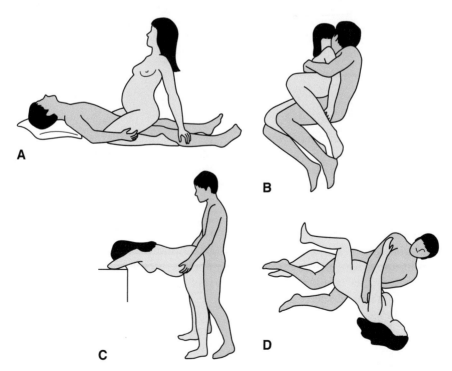

Fig. 9-21 Positions for sexual intercourse during pregnancy. **A,** Female superior. **B,** Side by side. **C,** Rear entry. **D,** Side-lying, facing each other.

PLAN OF CARE | *Discomforts of Pregnancy and Warning Signs*

FIRST TRIMESTER

NURSING DIAGNOSIS Anxiety related to deficient knowledge about schedule of prenatal visits throughout pregnancy as evidenced by woman's questions and concerns

Expected Outcome *Woman will verbalize correct appointment schedule for the duration of the pregnancy and feelings of being "in control."*

Nursing Interventions/*Rationales*

- Provide information regarding schedule of visits, tests, and other assessments and interventions that will be provided throughout the pregnancy *to empower patient to function in collaboration with the caregiver and diminish anxiety.*
- Allow woman time to describe level of anxiety *to establish basis for care.*
- Provide information to woman regarding prenatal classes and labor area tours *to decrease feelings of anxiety about the unknown.*

NURSING DIAGNOSIS Imbalanced nutrition: less than body requirements, related to nausea and vomiting as evidenced by woman's report and weight loss

Expected Outcome *Woman will gain 1 to 2.5 kg during the first trimester.*

Nursing Interventions/*Rationales*

- Verify prepregnant weight *to plan a realistic diet according to individual woman's nutritional needs.*
- Obtain diet history *to identify current meal patterns and foods that may be implicated in nausea.*
- Advise woman to consume small frequent meals and avoid having empty stomach *to avoid further nausea episodes.*
- Suggest that woman eat a simple carbohydrate such as dry crackers before arising in the morning *to avoid empty stomach and decrease incidence of nausea and vomiting.*
- Advise woman to call health care provider if vomiting is persistent and severe *to identify possible incidence of hyperemesis gravidarum.*

NURSING DIAGNOSIS Fatigue related to hormonal changes in the first trimester as evidenced by woman's complaints

Expected Outcome *Woman will report a decreased number of episodes of fatigue.*

Nursing Interventions/*Rationales*

- Rest as needed *to avoid increasing feeling of fatigue.*
- Eat a well-balanced diet *to meet increased metabolic demands and avoid anemia.*
- Discuss the use of support systems to help with household responsibilities *to decrease workload at home and decrease fatigue.*
- Reinforce to woman the transitory nature of first trimester fatigue *to provide emotional support.*
- Explore with the woman a variety of techniques to prioritize roles *to decrease family expectations.*

SECOND TRIMESTER

NURSING DIAGNOSIS Constipation related to progesterone influence on GI tract as evidenced by woman's report of altered patterns of elimination

Expected Outcome *Woman will report a return to normal bowel elimination pattern after implementation of interventions.*

Nursing Interventions/*Rationales*

- Provide information to woman regarding pregnancy-related causes: progesterone slowing gastrointestinal motility, growing uterus compressing intestines, and influence of iron supplementation *to provide basic information for self-care during pregnancy.*
- Assist woman to plan a diet that will promote regular bowel movements, such as increasing amount of oral fluid intake to at least six to eight glasses of water a day, increasing the amount of fiber in daily diet, and maintaining moderate exercise program *to promote self-care.*
- Reinforce for woman that she should not take any laxatives, stool softeners, or enemas without first consulting the health care provider *to prevent any injuries to woman or fetus.*

---

female-superior, side-by-side, rear-entry, and side-lying positions are possible alternative positions to the traditional male-superior position. The woman astride (superior position) allows her to control the angle and depth of penile penetration, as well as to protect her breasts and abdomen. The side-by-side position or any position that places less pressure on the pregnant abdomen and requires less energy may be preferred during the third trimester.

Multiparous women sometimes have significant breast tenderness in the first trimester. A coital position that avoids direct pressure on the woman's breasts and decreased breast fondling during love play can be recommended to such couples. The woman also should be reassured that this condition is normal and temporary.

Some women complain of lower abdominal cramping and backache after orgasm during the first and third trimesters. A back rub can often relieve some of the discomfort and provide a pleasant experience. A tonic uterine contraction, often lasting up to a minute, replaces the rhythmic contractions of orgasm during the third trimester. Changes in the FHR without fetal distress also have been reported.

The objective of "safer sex" is to provide prophylaxis against the acquisition and transmission of STIs (e.g., herpes simplex virus [HSV], HIV). Because these diseases may be transmitted to the woman and her fetus, the use of condoms is recommended throughout pregnancy if the woman is at risk for acquiring an STI.

Well-informed nurses who are comfortable with their own sexuality and the sexual counseling needs of expectant couples can offer information and advice in this valuable but often neglected area. They can establish an open environment in which couples can feel free to introduce their concerns about sexual adjustment and seek support and guidance.

PLAN OF CARE   *Discomforts of Pregnancy and Warning Signs—cont'd*

NURSING DIAGNOSIS Anxiety related to deficient knowledge about course of first pregnancy as evidenced by woman's questions regarding possible complications of second and third trimesters

Expected Outcomes *Woman will correctly list signs of potential complications that can occur during the second and third trimesters and exhibit no overt signs of stress.*

Nursing Interventions/*Rationales*

- Provide information concerning the potential complications or warning signs that can occur during the second and third trimesters, including possible causes of signs and the importance of calling the health care provider immediately *to ensure identification and treatment of problems in a timely manner.*
- Provide a written list of complications *to have a reference list for emergencies.*

THIRD TRIMESTER

NURSING DIAGNOSIS Fear related to deficient knowledge regarding onset of labor and the processes of labor related to inexperience as evidenced by woman's questions and statement of concerns

Expected Outcomes *Woman will verbalize basic understanding of signs of labor onset and when to call the health care provider, identify resources for childbirth education, and express increasing confidence in readiness to cope with labor.*

Nursing Interventions/*Rationales*

- Provide information regarding signs of labor onset, when to call the health care provider, and give written information regarding local childbirth education classes *to empower and promote self-care.*
- Promote ongoing effective communication with health care provider *to promote trust and decrease fear of unknown.*
- Provide the woman with decision-making opportunities *to promote effective coping.*

- Provide opportunity for woman to verbalize fears regarding childbirth *to assist in decreasing fear through discussion.*

NURSING DIAGNOSIS Disturbed sleep patterns related to discomforts or insomnia of third trimester as evidenced by woman's report of inadequate rest

Expected Outcomes *Woman will report an improvement of quality and quantity of rest and sleep.*

Nursing Interventions/*Rationales*

- Assess current sleep pattern and review need for increased requirement during pregnancy *to identify need for change in sleep patterns.*
- Suggest change of position to side-lying with pillows between legs or to semi-Fowler position *to increase support and decrease any problems with dyspnea or heartburn.*
- Reinforce the possibility of the use of various sleep aides such as relaxation techniques, reading, and decreased activity before bedtime *to decrease the possibility of anxiety or physical discomforts before bedtime.*

NURSING DIAGNOSIS Ineffective sexuality patterns related to changes in comfort level and fatigue

Expected Outcome *Woman will verbalize feelings regarding changes in sexual desire.*

Nursing Interventions/*Rationales*

- Assess couple's usual sexuality patterns *to determine how patterns have been altered by pregnancy.*
- Provide information regarding expected changes in sexuality patterns during pregnancy *to correct any misconceptions.*
- Allow the couple to express feelings in a nonjudgmental atmosphere *to promote trust.*
- Refer couple for counseling as appropriate *to assist the couple to cope with sexuality pattern changes.*
- Suggest alternative sexual positions *to decrease pressure on enlarging abdomen of woman and increase sexual comfort and satisfaction of couple.*

GI, Gastrointestinal.

Psychosocial support

Esteem, affection, trust, concern, consideration of cultural and religious responses, and listening are all components of the emotional support given to the pregnant woman and her family. The woman's satisfaction with her relationships—partner and familial—and their support, her feeling of competence, and her sense of being in control are important issues to be addressed in the third trimester. A discussion of fetal responses to stimuli, such as sound and light, as well as patterns of sleeping and waking, can be helpful. Other issues of concern that may arise for the pregnant woman and couple include fear of pain, loss of control, and possible birth of the infant before reaching the hospital; anxieties about parenthood; parental concerns about the safety of the mother and unborn child; parental concerns about siblings and their acceptance of the new baby; parental concerns about social and economic responsibilities; and parental concerns arising from conflicts in cultural, religious, or personal value systems. In addition, the father's or partner's commitment to the pregnancy and to the couple's relationship and concerns about sexuality and its expression are topics for discussion for many couples. Providing the prospective mother and father with an opportunity to discuss their concerns and validating the normality of their responses can meet their needs to varying degrees. Nurses also must recognize that men feel more vulnerable during their partner's pregnancy. Anticipatory guidance and health promotion strategies can help partners cope with their concerns. Health care providers can stimulate and encourage open dialogue between the expectant father and mother.

Evaluation

Evaluation of the effectiveness of care of the woman during pregnancy is based on the previously stated outcomes. More effort is needed in evaluating outcomes of nursing care during the prenatal period. A formal systematic follow-up on quality of care is not common but should be developed and incorporated in all settings (see Plan of Care on p. 272-273).

VARIATIONS IN PRENATAL CARE ■

The course of prenatal care described thus far may seem to suggest that the experiences of childbearing women are similar and that nursing interventions are uniformly consistent across all populations. Although typical patterns of response to pregnancy are easily recognized and many aspects of prenatal care indeed are consistent, pregnant women enter the health care system with individual concerns and needs. The nurse's ability to assess unique needs and to tailor interventions to the individual is the hallmark of expertise in providing care. Variations that influence prenatal care include culture, age, and number of fetuses.

Cultural Influences

Prenatal care as we know it is a phenomenon of Western medicine. In the U.S. biomedical model of care, women are encouraged to seek prenatal care as early as possible in their pregnancy by visiting a physician, and/or a nurse-midwife. Such visits are usually routine and follow a systematic sequence, with the initial visit followed by monthly, then semimonthly, and then weekly visits. Monitoring weight and BP; testing blood and urine; teaching specific information about diet, rest, and activity; and preparing for childbirth are common components of prenatal care. This model not only is unfamiliar but also seems strange to women of other cultures. Different models for providing prenatal care for women throughout the world are being explored (Chalmers, Mangiaterra, & Porter, 2001).

Many cultural variations are found in prenatal care. Even if the prenatal care described is familiar to a woman, some practices may conflict with the beliefs and practices of a subculture group to which she belongs. Because of these and other factors, such as lack of money, lack of transportation, and language barriers, women from diverse cultures do not participate in the prenatal care system, for instance by keeping prenatal appointments (Shaffer, 2002). Such behavior may be misinterpreted by nurses as uncaring, lazy, or ignorant.

A concern for modesty also is a deterrent to many women seeking prenatal care. For some women, exposing body parts, especially to a man, is considered a major violation of their modesty. For many women, invasive procedures, such as a vaginal examination, may be so threatening that they cannot be discussed even with their own husbands; therefore many women prefer a female health care provider. Too often, health care providers assume women lose this modesty during pregnancy and labor, but actually most women value and appreciate efforts to maintain their modesty.

For many cultural groups, a physician is deemed appropriate only in times of illness, and because pregnancy is considered a normal process and the woman is in a state of health,

the services of a physician are considered inappropriate. Even if what are considered problems with pregnancy by standards of Western medicine do develop, they may not be perceived as problems by members of other cultural groups.

Although pregnancy is considered normal by many, certain practices are expected of women of all cultures to ensure a good outcome. **Cultural prescriptions** tell women what to do, and **cultural proscriptions** establish taboos. The purposes of these practices are to prevent maternal illness resulting from a pregnancy-induced imbalanced state and to protect the vulnerable fetus. Prescriptions and proscriptions regulate the woman's emotional response, clothing, activity and rest, sexual activity, and dietary practices. Exploration of the woman's beliefs, perceptions of the meaning of childbearing, and health care practices may help health care providers foster her self-actualization, promote attainment of the maternal role, and positively influence her relationship with her spouse.

To provide culturally sensitive care, the nurse must be knowledgeable about practices and customs, although it is not possible to know all there is to know about every culture and subculture or the many lifestyles that exist. It is important to learn about the varied cultures in which specific nurses practice. When exploring cultural beliefs and practices related to childbearing, the nurse can support and nurture those beliefs that promote physical or emotional adaptation. However, if potentially harmful beliefs or activities are identified, the nurse should carefully provide education and propose modifications.

Emotional response

Virtually all cultures emphasize the importance of maintaining a socially harmonious and agreeable environment for a pregnant woman. An absence of stress is important in ensuring a successful outcome for the mother and baby. Harmony with other people must be fostered, and visits from extended family members may be required to demonstrate pleasant and noncontroversial relationships. If discord exists in a relationship, it is usually dealt with in culturally prescribed ways.

Besides proscriptions regarding food, other proscriptions involve forms of magic. For example, some Mexicans believe that pregnant women should not witness an eclipse of the moon because it may cause a cleft palate in the infant. They also believe that exposure to an earthquake may precipitate preterm birth, miscarriage, or even a breech presentation. In some cultures a pregnant woman must not ridicule someone with an affliction for fear her child might be born with the same handicap. A mother should not hate a person lest her child resemble that person, and dental work should not be done because it may cause a baby to have a "harelip." A widely held folk belief in some cultures is that the pregnant woman should refrain from raising her arms above her head, because such movement ties knots in the umbilical cord and may cause it to wrap around the baby's neck. Another belief is that placing a knife under the bed of a laboring woman will "cut" her pain.

Clothing

Although most cultural groups do not prescribe specific clothing to be worn during pregnancy, modesty is an expectation of many. Some Mexican women of the Southwest wear a cord beneath the breasts and knotted over the umbilicus. This cord, called a muñeco, is thought to prevent morning sickness and ensure a safe birth. Amulets, medals, and beads also may be worn to ward off evil spirits.

Physical activity and rest

Norms that regulate the physical activity of mothers during pregnancy vary tremendously. Many groups, including Native Americans and some Asian groups, encourage women to be active, to walk, and to engage in normal, although not strenuous, activities to ensure that the baby is healthy and not too large. Conversely, other groups such as Filipinos believe that any activity is dangerous, and others willingly take over the work of the pregnant woman. Some Filipinos believe that this inactivity protects the mother and child. The mother is encouraged simply to produce the succeeding generation. If health care providers do not know of this belief, they could misinterpret this behavior as laziness or noncompliance with the desired prenatal health care regimen. It is important for the nurse to find out the way each pregnant woman views activity and rest.

Sexual activity

In most cultures, sexual activity is not prohibited until the end of pregnancy. Some Latinos view sexual activity as necessary to keep the birth canal lubricated. Conversely, some Vietnamese may have definite proscriptions against sexual intercourse, requiring abstinence throughout the pregnancy because it is thought that sexual intercourse may harm the mother and fetus.

Diet

Nutritional information given by Western health care providers also may be a source of conflict for many cultural groups, but such a conflict commonly is not known by health care providers unless they understand the dietary beliefs and practices of the people for whom they are caring. For example, Muslims have strict regulations regarding preparation of food, and if meat cannot be prepared as prescribed, they may omit meats from their diets. Many cultures permit pregnant women to eat only warm foods.

Age Differences

The age of the childbearing couple may have a significant influence on their physical and psychosocial adaptation to pregnancy. Normal developmental processes that occur in both very young and older mothers are interrupted by pregnancy and require a different type of adaptation to pregnancy than that of the woman of typical childbearing age. Although the individuality of each pregnant woman is recognized, special needs of expectant mothers 15 years of age or younger or those 35 years of age or older are summarized.

Adolescents

Teenage pregnancy is a worldwide problem (Cherry, Dillon, & Rugh, 2001). About 1 million adolescent females in the United States, or four out of every 10 girls, become pregnant each year. Most of the pregnancies are unintended; 56% end in live birth; 29% ended in induced abortion; and 15% in miscarriage (Arias, MacDorman, Strobino, & Guyer, 2003). Adolescents are responsible for almost 500,000 births in the United States annually. Hispanic adolescents currently have the highest birth rate, although the rate for African-American adolescents also is high. Of girls who become pregnant, 21% are repeat pregnancies (Arias et al., 2003). Most of these young women are unmarried, and many are not ready for the emotional, psychosocial, and financial responsibilities of parenthood.

Despite these alarming statistics and the fact that the United States has the highest adolescent birth rate in the industrialized world, the birth rate for adolescents has steadily declined since 1991 (Arias et al., 2003). Concentrated national efforts have generated a host of adolescent pregnancy-prevention programs that have had varying degrees of success (Ford et al., 2002). Characteristics of programs that make a difference are those that have sustained commitment to adolescents over a long time, involve the parents and other adults in the community, promote abstinence and personal responsibility, and assist adolescents to develop a clear strategy for reaching future goals such as a college education or a career.

When adolescents do become pregnant and decide to give birth, they are much less likely than older women to receive adequate prenatal care, with many receiving no care at all (Ford et al., 2002). These young women also are more likely to smoke and less likely to gain adequate weight during pregnancy. As a result of these and other factors, babies born to adolescents are at greatly increased risk of LBW, of serious and long-term disability, and of dying during the first year of life.

Delayed entry into prenatal care may be the result of late recognition of pregnancy, denial of pregnancy, or confusion about the available services. Such a delay in care may leave an inadequate time before birth to attend to correctable problems. The very young pregnant adolescent is at higher risk for each of the confounding variables associated with poor pregnancy outcomes (e.g., socioeconomic factors) and for those conditions associated with a first pregnancy regardless of age (e.g., gestational hypertension). However, when prenatal care is initiated early and consistently, and confounding variables are controlled, very young pregnant adolescents are at no greater risk (nor are their infants) for an adverse outcome than are older pregnant women. The role of the nurse in reducing the risks and consequences of adolescent pregnancy is therefore twofold: first, to encourage early and continued prenatal care, and second, to refer the adolescent, if necessary, for appropriate social support services, which can help reverse the effects of a negative socioeconomic environment (Fig. 9-22) (see Plan of Care).

PLAN OF CARE *Pregnant Adolescent*

NURSING DIAGNOSIS Imbalanced nutrition: less than body requirements related to intake insufficient to meet metabolic needs of fetus and adolescent patient

Expected Outcomes *Patient will gain weight as prescribed by age, take prenatal vitamins and iron as prescribed, and maintain normal hematocrit and hemoglobin.*

Nursing Interventions/*Rationales*

- Assess current diet history and intake *to determine prescriptions for additions or changes in present dietary pattern.*
- Compare prepregnancy weight with current weight *to determine if pattern is consistent with appropriate fetal growth and development.*
- Provide information concerning food prescriptions for appropriate weight gain, considering preferences for "fast food" and peer influences *to correct any misconceptions and increase chances for compliance with diet.*
- Include patient's immediate family or support system during instruction *to ensure that person preparing family meals receives information.*

NURSING DIAGNOSIS Risk for injury, maternal or fetal, related to inadequate prenatal care and screening

Expected Outcomes *Patient will experience uncomplicated pregnancy and deliver a healthy fetus at term.*

Nursing Interventions/*Rationales*

- Provide information using therapeutic communication and confidentiality *to establish relationship and build trust.*
- Discuss importance of ongoing prenatal care and possible risks to adolescent patient and fetus *to reinforce that ongoing assessment is crucial to health and well-being of patient and fetus, even if patient feels well. The adolescent patient is at greater risk for certain complications that may be avoided or managed early if prenatal visits are maintained.*
- Discuss risks of alcohol, tobacco, and recreational drug use during pregnancy *to minimize risks to patient and fetus, because adolescent patient has a higher abuse rate than the rest of the pregnant population.*
- Assess for evidence of sexually transmitted infection (STI) and provide information regarding safer sexual practice *to minimize risk to patient and fetus, because adolescent is at greater risk for STIs.*
- Screen for preeclampsia on an ongoing basis *to minimize risk, because adolescent population is at greater risk for preeclampsia.*

NURSING DIAGNOSIS Social isolation related to body image changes of pregnant adolescent as evidenced by patient statements and concerns

Expected Outcomes *Patient will identify support systems and report decreased feelings of social isolation.*

Nursing Interventions/*Rationales*

- Establish a therapeutic relationship *to listen objectively and establish trust.*

- Discuss with patient changes in relationships that have occurred as a result of the pregnancy *to determine extent of isolation from family, peers, and father of the baby.*
- Provide referrals and resources appropriate for developmental stage of patient *to give information for patient support.*
- Provide information regarding parenting classes, breastfeeding classes, and childbirth-preparation classes *to give further information and group support, which lessens social isolation.*

NURSING DIAGNOSIS Interrupted family processes related to adolescent pregnancy

Expected Outcome *Patient will reestablish relationship with her mother and father of baby.*

Nursing Interventions/*Rationales*

- Encourage communication with mother *to clarify roles and relationships related to birth of infant.*
- Encourage communication with father of baby (if she desires continued contact) *to ascertain level of support to be expected of father of baby.*
- Refer to support group *to learn more effective ways of problem solving and reducing conflict within the family.*

NURSING DIAGNOSIS Disturbed body image related to situational crisis of pregnancy

Expected Outcome *Pregnant adolescent will verbalize positive comments regarding her body image during the pregnancy.*

Nursing Interventions/*Rationales*

- Assess pregnant adolescent's perception of self related to pregnancy *to provide basis for further interventions.*
- Give information regarding expected body changes occurring during pregnancy *to provide a realistic view of these temporary changes.*
- Provide opportunity to discuss personal feelings and concerns *to promote trust and support.*

NURSING DIAGNOSIS Risk for impaired parenting related to immaturity and lack of experience in new role of adolescent mother

Expected Outcome *Parents will demonstrate parenting roles with confidence.*

Nursing Interventions/*Rationales*

- Provide information on growth and development *to enhance knowledge so that adolescent mother can have basis for caring for her infant.*
- Refer to parenting classes *to enhance knowledge and obtain support for providing appropriate care to newborn and infant.*
- Initiate discussion of child care *to assist adolescent in problem solving for future needs.*
- Assess parenting abilities of adolescent mother and father *to provide baseline for education.*
- Provide information on parenting classes that are appropriate for parents' developmental stage to give opportunity *to share common feelings and concerns.*
- Assist parents to identify pertinent support systems *to give assistance with parenting as needed.*

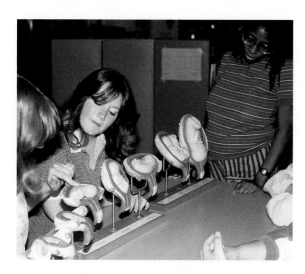

Fig. 9-22 Pregnant adolescents reviewing fetal development. (Courtesy Marjorie Pyle, RNC, Lifecircle, Costa Mesa, CA.)

Women older than 35 years

Two groups of older parents have emerged in the population of women having a child late in their childbearing years. One group consists of women who have many children or who have an additional child during the menopausal period. The other group consists of women who have deliberately delayed childbearing until their late thirties or early forties.

Multiparous women. Multiparous women may have never used contraceptives because of personal choice or lack of knowledge concerning contraceptives. They also may be women who have used contraceptives successfully during the childbearing years, but as menopause approaches, they may cease menstruating regularly or stop using contraceptives and consequently become pregnant. The older multiparous woman may feel that pregnancy separates her from her peer group and that her age is a hindrance to close associations with young mothers. Other parents welcome the unexpected infant as evidence of continuing maternal and paternal roles.

Primiparous women. The number of first-time pregnancies in women between the ages of 35 and 40 years has increased significantly over the past three decades (Tough et al., 2002). Seeing women in their late thirties or forties during their first pregnancy is no longer unusual for health care providers. Reasons for delaying pregnancy include a desire to obtain advanced education, career priorities, and use of better contraceptive measures. Women who are infertile do not delay pregnancy deliberately but may become pregnant at a later age as a result of fertility studies and therapies.

These women choose parenthood. They often are successfully established in a career and a lifestyle with a partner that includes time for self-attention, the establishment of a home with accumulated possessions, and freedom to travel. When asked the reason they chose pregnancy later in life, many reply, "Because time is running out."

The dilemma of choice includes the recognition that being a parent will have positive and negative consequences.

Couples should discuss the consequences of childbearing and childrearing before committing themselves to this lifelong venture. Partners in this group seem to share the preparation for parenthood, planning for a family-centered birth, and desire to be loving and competent parents; however, the reality of child care may prove difficult for such parents.

First-time mothers older than 35 years select the "right time" for pregnancy; this time is influenced by their awareness of the increasing possibility of infertility or of genetic defects in the infants of older women. Such women seek information about pregnancy from books, friends, and electronic resources. They actively try to prevent fetal disorders and are careful in searching for the best possible maternity care. They identify sources of stress in their lives. They have concerns about having enough energy and stamina to meet the demands of parenting and their new roles and relationships.

If older women become pregnant after treatment for infertility, they may suddenly have negative or ambivalent feelings about the pregnancy. They may experience a multifetal pregnancy that may create emotional and physical problems. Adjusting to parenting two or more infants requires adaptability and additional resources.

During pregnancy, parents explore the possibilities and responsibilities of changing identities and new roles. They must prepare a safe and nurturing environment during pregnancy and after birth. They must integrate the child into an established family system and negotiate new roles (parent roles, sibling roles, grandparent roles) for family members.

Adverse perinatal outcomes are more common in older primiparas than in younger women, even when they receive good prenatal care. Tough and colleagues (2002) reported that women aged 35 years and older are more likely than are younger primiparas to have LBW infants, premature birth, and multiple births. The occurrence of these complications is quite stressful for the new parents, and nursing interventions that provide information and psychosocial support are needed, as well as care for physical needs. In addition, in women aged 35 years or older there is an increased risk of maternal mortality. Pregnancy-related deaths result from hemorrhage, infection, embolisms, hypertensive disorders of pregnancy, cardiomyopathy, and strokes (Callaghan & Berg, 2003).

Multifetal pregnancy

When the pregnancy involves more than one fetus, **multifetal pregnancy,** both the mother and fetuses are at increased risk for adverse outcomes. The maternal blood volume is increased, resulting in an increased strain on the maternal cardiovascular system. Anemia often develops because of a greater demand for iron by the fetuses. Marked uterine distention and increased pressure on the adjacent viscera and pelvic vasculature and diastasis of the two rectus abdominis muscles (see Fig. 8-12) may occur. Placenta previa develops more commonly in multifetal pregnancies because of the large size or placement of the placentas (Clark, 2004).

Premature separation of the placenta may occur before the second and any subsequent fetuses are born.

Twin pregnancies often end in prematurity. Spontaneous rupture of membranes before term is common. Congenital malformations are twice as common in monozygotic twins as in singletons, although there is no increase in the incidence of congenital anomalies in dizygotic twins. In addition, two-vessel cords—that is, cords with a vein and a single umbilical artery instead of two—occur more often in twins than in singletons, but this abnormality is most common in monozygotic twins. The clinical diagnosis of multifetal pregnancy is accurate in about 90% of cases. The likelihood of a multifetal pregnancy is increased if any one or a combination of the following factors is noted during a careful assessment:

- History of dizygous twins in the female lineage
- Use of fertility drugs
- More rapid uterine growth for the number of weeks of gestation
- Hydramnios
- Palpation of more than the expected number of small or large parts
- Asynchronous fetal heart beats or more than one fetal electrocardiographic tracing
- Ultrasonographic evidence of more than one fetus

The diagnosis of multifetal pregnancy can come as a shock to many expectant parents, and they may need additional support and education to help them cope with the changes they face. The mother needs nutrition counseling so that she gains more weight than that needed for a singleton birth, counseling that maternal adaptations will probably be more uncomfortable, and information about the possibility of a preterm birth.

If the presence of more than three fetuses is diagnosed, the parents may receive counseling regarding selective reduction of the pregnancies to reduce the incidence of premature birth and improve the opportunities for the remaining fetuses to grow to term gestation (Malone & D'Alton, 2004). This situation poses an ethical dilemma for many couples, especially those who have worked hard to overcome problems with infertility and harbor strong values regarding right to life (Strong, 2003). Nurse-initiated discussion to identify what resources could help the couple (e.g., a minister, priest, or mental health counselor) can make the decision-making process somewhat less traumatic.

The prenatal care given women with multifetal pregnancies includes changes in the pattern of care and modifications in other aspects such as the amount of weight gained and the nutritional intake necessary. The prenatal visits of these women are scheduled at least every 2 weeks in the second trimester and weekly thereafter. In twin gestations the recommended weight gain is 16 to 20 kg. Iron and vitamin supplementation is desirable. As preeclampsia and eclampsia are increased in multifetal pregnancies, nurses aggressively work to prevent, identify, and treat these complications of pregnancy.

The considerable uterine distention involved can cause the backache commonly experienced by pregnant women to be even worse. Maternal support hose may be worn to control leg varicosities. If risk factors such as premature dilation of the cervix or bleeding are present, abstinence from orgasm and nipple stimulation during the last trimester is recommended to help avert preterm labor. Frequent ultrasound examinations, nonstress tests, and FHR monitoring will be performed. Some practitioners recommend bed rest beginning at 20 weeks in women carrying multiple fetuses to prevent preterm labor. Other practitioners question the value of prolonged bed rest. If bed rest is recommended, the mother assumes a lateral position to promote increased placental perfusion. If birth is delayed until after the thirty-sixth week, the risk of morbidity and mortality decreases for the neonates.

Multiple newborns will likely place a strain on finances, space, workload, and the woman's and family's coping capability. Lifestyle changes may be necessary. Parents will need assistance in making realistic plans for the care of the babies (e.g., whether to breastfeed and whether to raise them as "alike" or as separate persons). Parents should be referred to national organizations such as Parents of Twins and Triplets, Mothers of Twins, and the La Leche League for further support (see Resources at end of chapter).

CHILDBIRTH AND PERINATAL EDUCATION

The goal of childbirth and perinatal education is to assist individuals and their family members to make informed, safe decisions about pregnancy, birth, and early parenthood. It also is to assist them to comprehend the long-lasting potential that empowering birth experiences have in the lives of women and that early experiences have on the development of children and the family. The perinatal education program is an expansion of the earlier childbirth education movement that originally offered a set of classes in the third trimester of pregnancy to prepare parents for birth. Today perinatal education programs consist of a menu of class series and activities from preconception through the early months of parenting.

All health-promoting education should be provided in a context that emphasizes how well designed a healthy body is to adapt to the changes that accompany pregnancy. Without this context of health, routine care and testing for risks may contribute to a mindset of families that pregnancy is a pathologic as opposed to a healthy mind-body-spirit event.

Some of the decisions the childbearing family must consider are the decision to have a baby, followed by choices of a care provider and type of care (a midwifery model [natural oriented] versus a medical [intervention oriented] model); the place for birth (hospital, birthing center, home); and the type of infant feeding (breast or bottle) and care. If a woman has had a previous cesarean birth, she may

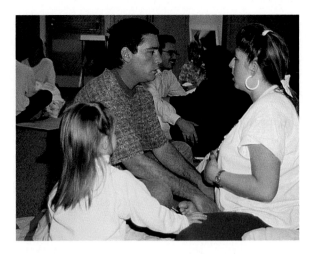

Fig. 9-23 Learning relaxation exercises with the whole family. (Courtesy Marjorie Pyle, RNC, Lifecircle, Costa Mesa, CA.)

consider having a vaginal birth. This section discusses these choices and the nurse's role in educating childbearing families to make informed decisions about them.

Previous pregnancy and childbirth experiences are important elements that influence current learning needs. The patient's (and support person's) age, cultural background, personal philosophy with regard to childbirth, socioeconomic status, spiritual beliefs, and learning styles all need to be assessed to develop the best plan to help the woman meet her needs.

Most childbirth education classes are attended by the pregnant woman and her partner, although a friend, teenage daughter, or parent may be the designated support person (Fig. 9-23). Classes may also be held for grandparents and siblings to prepare them for their attendance at birth and/or the arrival of the baby (see Fig. 9-4). Siblings often see a film about birth and learn ways they can help welcome the baby. They also learn to cope with changes that include a reduction in parental time and attention. Grandparents learn about current child care practices and how to help their adult children adapt to parenting in a supportive way.

Perinatal Care Choices

The Coalition to Improve Maternity Services (CIMS), a group of more than 50 nursing and maternity care–oriented organizations, produced a document to assist women in selecting their perinatal care. After some explanation of choices, women are encouraged to ask potential care providers the following questions:

- Who can be with me during labor and birth?
- What happens during a normal labor and birth in your setting?
- How do you allow for differences in culture and beliefs?
- Can I walk and move around during labor? What position do you suggest for birth?

- How do you make sure everything goes smoothly when my nurse, doctor, nurse-midwife, or agency work with one another?
- What things do you normally do to a woman in labor?
- How do you help mothers stay as comfortable as they can be? Besides drugs, how do you help mothers relieve the pain of labor?
- What if my baby is born early or has special problems?
- Do you circumcise babies?
- How do you help mothers who want to breastfeed?

The entire document can be obtained at www.motherfriendly.org. By using a related CIMS questionnaire provided by Hotelling (2004), hospitals and birthing centers can apply to CIMS to be designated "Mother-Friendly," and such ratings can be passed on to expectant parents.

Childbirth Education Programs

Childbirth, when one is prepared and well supported, presents to women a unique and powerful opportunity to find their core strength in a manner that forever changes their self-perception. Expectant parents and their families have different interests and information needs as the pregnancy progresses.

Early pregnancy ("early bird") classes provide fundamental information. Classes are developed around the following areas: (1) early fetal development, (2) physiologic and emotional changes of pregnancy, (3) human sexuality, and (4) the nutritional needs of the mother and fetus. Environmental and workplace hazards may be addressed. Exercises, nutrition, warning signs, drugs, and self-medication are topics of interest and concern.

Midpregnancy classes emphasize the woman's participation in self-care. Classes provide information on preparation for breastfeeding and formula feeding, infant care, basic hygiene, common complaints and simple safe remedies, infant health, parenting, and updating and refining the birth plans.

Late pregnancy classes emphasize labor and birth. Different methods of coping with labor and birth have been developed and are often the basis for various prenatal classes. These include Lamaze, Bradley, and Dick-Read. A hospital tour is usually included.

Throughout the series of classes there is discussion of support systems that people can use during pregnancy and after birth. Such support systems help parents function independently and effectively. During all the classes the open expression of feelings and concerns about any aspect of pregnancy, birth, and parenting is welcomed.

Fathers or partners often worry about their role during childbirth classes and labor and birth, as well as the safety of their partner and baby during the birth. Many fathers elect to participate actively during labor and the birth of their child. As noted earlier, however, some men, through personal or cultural conception of the father role, neither want nor intend to participate. It is important that the partners agree on each other's roles.

EVOLVE/CD: Case Study—Second Trimester

Pain management

Fear of pain in labor is a key issue for pregnant women and the reason many give for attending childbirth education classes. Numerous studies show that women who have received childbirth preparation later report no less pain but do report greater ability to cope with the pain during labor and birth and increased birth satisfaction than unprepared women. Therefore although pain management strategies are an essential component of childbirth education, pain eradication is not the primary source of birth satisfaction. Control in childbirth, meaning participation in decision making, has been repeatedly found to be the primary source of birth satisfaction.

Pain management strategies are an essential component of childbirth education. Couples need information about the advantages and disadvantages of pain medication and about other techniques for coping with labor. An emphasis on nonpharmacologic pain management strategies helps couples manage the labor and birth with dignity and increased comfort. Most instructors teach a flexible approach, which helps couples learn and master many techniques that can be used during labor. Couples are taught techniques such as massage, pressure on the palms or soles of the feet, hot compresses to the perineum, perineal massage, applications of heat or cold, breathing patterns, and focusing of attention on visual or other stimuli as ways to increase coping and decrease the distress from labor pain (see Chapter 12 for further discussion).

Current practices in childbirth education

A variety of approaches to childbirth education have evolved as childbirth educators attempt to meet learning needs. In addition to classes designed specifically for pregnant adolescents, their partners, and/or parents, classes exist for other groups with special learning needs. These include classes for first-time mothers over age 35, single women, adoptive parents, and parents of twins. Refresher classes for parents with children not only review coping techniques for labor and birth but also help couples prepare for sibling reactions and adjustments to a new baby. Cesarean birth classes are offered for couples who have this kind of birth scheduled because of breech position or other risk factors. Other classes focus on vaginal birth after cesarean (VBAC), because many women successfully give birth vaginally after previous cesarean birth.

Strategies for childbirth education

Because of the multicultural composition of the population in North America, there is great diversity in attitudes, expectations, and behaviors judged appropriate during pregnancy and early parenthood. No one approach can meet all needs. For example, classes for new immigrants are particularly effective when taught in a native language (e.g., Spanish, Tagalog, Cantonese). For classes to be meaningful, parent educators must understand the value systems in other cultures and their influence on issues such as nutrition, exercise, valuing of early prenatal care, maternal weight gain, and infant feeding practices. Parent educators must establish rapport, be understood, and build on cultural practices, reinforcing the positive and promoting change only if a practice, such as pica, is directly harmful.

OPTIONS FOR CARE PROVIDERS ■

Often the first decision the woman makes is who will be her primary health care provider for the pregnancy and birth. This decision is doubly important because it usually affects where the birth will take place. The nurse can provide information about the different types of health care providers and what kind of care to expect from each type.

Physicians

Physicians (obstetricians, family practice physicians) attend about 91% of births in the United States and Canada (Martin et al., 2003). They see low risk and high risk patients. Care often includes pharmacologic and medical management of problems as well as use of technologic procedures. Family practice physicians may need backup by obstetricians if a specialist is needed for a problem (e.g., a cesarean birth). Most physicians manage births in a hospital setting.

Nurse-Midwives

Nurse-midwives are registered nurses with advanced training in care of obstetric patients. They provide care for about 8% of the births in the United States and Canada (Martin et al., 2003). Nurse-midwives may practice with physicians or independently with a contracted health care provider agency for physician backup. They usually see low risk obstetric patients. Care is often noninterventionist, and the woman and her family are encouraged to be active participants in the care. Nurse-midwives must refer patients to physicians for complications. Most births are managed in hospital settings or alternative birth centers; a small number may be managed in a home setting.

Direct entry midwives

Direct entry midwives are trained in midwifery schools, or universities as a profession distinct from nursing. Increasing numbers of midwives in the United Kingdom and Ireland fall into this category.

Independent midwives

Independent midwives, who also may be called *lay midwives,* are nonprofessional caregivers. Their training varies greatly, from formal training to self-teaching. They manage about 1% of births in the United States and Canada. Patients who develop problems need to be seen by a physician. A majority (i.e., 61%) of births are managed in the home setting.

Doulas

A doula is professionally trained to provide labor support, including physical, emotional, and informational support to women and their partners during labor and birth. The

BOX 9-7

Questions to Ask When Choosing a Doula

To discover the specific training, experience, and services offered by anyone who provides labor support, potential patients, nursing supervisors, physicians, midwives, and others should ask the following questions of that person:

- What training have you had?
- Tell me about your experience with birth, personally and as a doula.
- What is your philosophy about childbirth and supporting women and their partners through labor?
- May we meet to discuss our birth plans and the role you will play in supporting me through childbirth?
- May we call you with questions or concerns before and after the birth?
- When do you try to join women in labor? Do you come to our home or meet us at the hospital?
- Do you meet with us after the birth to review the labor and answer questions?
- Do you work with one or more backup doulas for times when you are not available? May we meet them?
- What is your fee?

From Simkin, P., & Way, K. (1998). *DONA position paper: The doula's contributions to modern maternity care.* Seattle, WA: Doulas of North America.

doula does not become involved with clinical tasks (Doulas of North America [DONA], 1999a, 1999b, 1999c). A doula typically meets with the mother and her partner before labor to ascertain their expectations and desires for the birth experience. Working collaboratively with other health care providers and the woman's supportive individuals, the doula focuses efforts on assisting the woman to achieve her goals. Box 9-7 provides questions to ask when interviewing a prospective doula. See Resources at end of chapter for organizations that offer information or referral services.

Although the doula role originally developed as an assistant during labor, some women need assistance during the postpartum period. There are small but growing numbers of postnatal doulas, who provide assistance to the new mother as she develops competence with infant care, feeding, and other maternal tasks.

Birth Setting Choices

With careful thought, the concept of natural or family- or woman-centered maternity care can be implemented in any setting. The three primary options for birth settings today are the hospital, birth center, and home. Women consider several factors in choosing a setting for childbirth, including the preference of their health care provider, characteristics of the birthing unit, and preference of their third-party payer. Approximately 99% of all births in the United States take place in a hospital setting (Martin et al., 2003). However, the types of labor and birth services vary greatly, from the traditional labor and delivery rooms with separate postpartum and newborn units, to in-hospital birthing centers where all or almost all care takes place in a single unit.

Labor, delivery, recovery, postpartum (birthing) rooms

Labor, delivery, and recovery (LDR) and labor, delivery, recovery, and postpartum (LDRP) rooms offer families a comfortable, private space for childbirth (Fig. 9-24). Women are admitted to LDR units, labor and give birth,

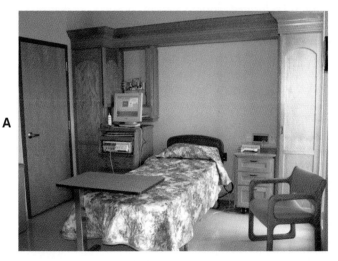
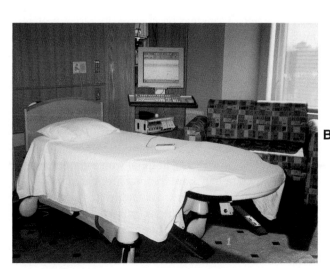

Fig. 9-24 **A,** Labor, delivery, and recovery (LDR) unit. **B,** Labor, delivery, recovery, and postpartum (LDRP) unit. Note sofa in background that converts to a bed. (**A,** Courtesy Julie Perry Nelson, Gilbert, AZ; **B,** Courtesy Dee Lowdermilk, Chapel Hill, NC.)

and spend the first 1 to 2 hours postpartum there for immediate recovery and to have time with their families to bond with their newborns. After this period of recovery, the mothers and newborns are transferred to a postpartum unit and nursery or mother-baby unit for the duration of their stay.

In LDRP units, total care is provided from admission for labor through postpartum discharge in the same room and usually by the same nursing staff. The woman and her family may stay in this unit for 6 to 48 hours after giving birth. The units are furnished to provide a homelike atmosphere, as LDR units are, but have accommodations for family members to stay overnight.

Both units are equipped with fetal monitors, emergency resuscitation equipment for both mother and newborn, and heated cribs or warming units for the newborn. Often this equipment is out of sight in cabinets or closets when it is not being used.

Birth centers

Free-standing birth centers are usually built in locations separate from the hospital but may be located nearby in case transfer of the woman or newborn is needed. These birth centers are intended to offer families a safe and cost-effective alternative to hospital or home birth. The centers are usually staffed by nurse-midwives or physicians who also have privileges at the local hospital. Only women at low risk for complications are included for care. Attendance at childbirth and parenting classes is required of all patients. The family is admitted to the birth center for labor and birth and will remain there until discharge, which often takes place within 6 hours of the birth.

Birth centers typically have homelike accommodations, including a double bed for the couple and a crib for the newborn (Fig. 9-25, *A*). Emergency equipment and drugs are stored discreetly within cupboards, out of view but easily accessible. Private bathroom facilities are incorporated into each birth unit. There may be an early labor lounge or a living room and small kitchen (Fig. 9-25, *B*).

Services provided by the free-standing birth centers include those necessary for safe management during the childbearing cycle. Patients must understand that some situations require transfer to a hospital, and they must agree to abide by those guidelines. Expectant families develop birth plans— that is, the practices and procedures they would like to either include or exclude from their childbirth experience.

Birth centers as well as a hospital with a comprehensive birthing program may have resources for parents such as a lending library that includes books and videotapes; reference files on related topics; recycled maternity clothes, baby clothes, and equipment; and supplies and reference materials for childbirth educators. The centers may also have referral files for community resources that offer services relating to childbirth and early parenting, including support groups (e.g., for single parents, for postbirth support, and for

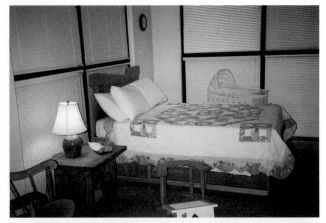

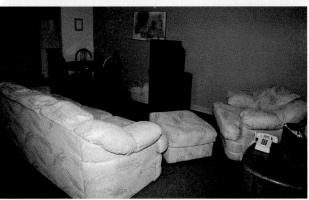

Fig. 9-25 Birth center. **A,** Note double bed, baby crib, and birthing stool. **B,** Lounge and kitchen. (**A,** Courtesy Dee Lowdermilk, Chapel Hill, NC. Photo location: The Women's Birth and Wellness Center). **B,** Courtesy Michael S. Clement, MD, Mesa, AZ. Photo location: Bethany Birth Center, Phoenix, AZ.)

parents of twins), genetic counseling, women's issues, and consumer action.

When birth occurs in a birth center or a home setting, it should be located close to a major hospital so that quick transfer to that institution is possible if necessary. Ambulance service and emergency procedures must be readily available. Fees vary with the services provided but typically are less than or equal to those charged by local hospitals. Some base fees on the ability of the family to pay (a reduced-fee sliding scale). Several third-party payers, as well as Medicaid and the Civilian Health and Medical Programs of the Uniformed Services (TRICARE/CHAMPUS), recognize and reimburse these centers.

Home birth

Home birth has always been popular in certain countries, such as Sweden and The Netherlands. In developing countries, hospitals or adequate lying-in facilities often are unavailable to most pregnant women, and home birth is a necessity. In North America, home births account for less than 1% of births (Martin et al., 2003).

National groups supporting home birth are the Home Oriented Maternity Experience (HOME) and the National Association of Parents for Safe Alternatives in Childbirth (NAPSAC). These groups work to foster more humane childbearing practices at all levels, integrating the alternatives for childbirth to meet the needs of the total population.

With a home birth the family is in control of the experience, and the birth may be more physiologically natural in familiar surroundings. The mother may be more relaxed than she would be in the hospital environment. The family can assist in and be a part of the birth, and the mother-father and partner-infant (and sibling-infant) contact is immediate and sustained. Home birth may be less expensive than a hospital confinement. Serious infection may be less likely (assuming strict aseptic principles are followed) because it is usual for people to be relatively immune to the bacteria in their own homes.

Although some physicians and nurses support home births that use good medical and emergency backup systems, many regard this practice as exposing the mother and the fetus to unnecessary danger. Therefore home births are not widely accepted by the North American medical community. This makes it difficult for a family to find a qualified health care provider willing to give prenatal care and to attend the birth. Backup emergency care by a physician in a hospital may be difficult to arrange in advance. If an emergency birth is necessary, no effective way exists to do this rapidly in the home setting.

Factors increasing the safety of birth at home. Most health care providers agree that if home birth is the woman's choice, certain criteria promote a safe home birth experience. The woman must be comfortable with her decision to have her baby at home. She should be in good health. Home birth is not indicated for women with a high risk pregnancy. A drive to the hospital (if needed) should take no more than 10 to 15 minutes. The woman should be attended by a well-trained physician or midwife with adequate medical supplies and resuscitation equipment, including oxygen.

Critical Thinking Exercise

Deciding about a Home Birth

Millie, 28 years old and gravida 1, para 0, is interested in having a home birth. She is currently 14 weeks pregnant, and her pregnancy is progressing normally. According to an ultrasound examination she has one fetus, which is of appropriate size for gestational age with no detectable anomalies. She asks a nurse in the obstetric clinic how to find a midwife who will attend a home birth.

1 Evidence—Is there sufficient evidence to draw conclusions about the safety of a home birth for Millie?
2 Assumptions—Describe the underlying assumptions for each of the following issues:
   a. Assessments that are necessary to identify whether it is feasible and safe for Millie to have a home birth
   b. Supports necessary for a home birth
   c. How to identify providers who are willing to attend a home birth
   d. Ethics of the nurse assisting Millie to find a midwife who will attend a home birth
3 What implications and priorities for nursing care can be drawn at this time?
4 Does the evidence objectively support your conclusion?
5 Are there alternative perspectives to your conclusion?

COMMUNITY ACTIVITY

Select an immigrant or other minority group in your community and identify childbirth-related beliefs and practices that are unique to that group. Are there stores in the area that sell items that meet the needs of that group? Does the community center have activities or classes that are directed toward that group? Are there childbirth education programs available that provide essential information while incorporating cultural patterns? As a nurse, what could you contribute to the community that would help meet the needs of that group?

Key Points

- The prenatal period is a preparatory one both physically, in terms of fetal growth and parental adaptations, and psychologically, in terms of anticipation of parenthood.
- Parent-child, sibling-child, and grandparent-child relationships are affected by pregnancy.
- Discomforts and changes of pregnancy can cause anxiety to the woman and her family and require sensitive attention and a plan for teaching self-care measures.
- Education about healthy ways of using the body (e.g., exercise, body mechanics) is essential given maternal anatomic and physiologic responses to pregnancy.
- Important components of the initial prenatal visit include detailed and carefully recorded findings from the interview, a comprehensive physical examination, and selected laboratory tests.
- Even in normal pregnancy the nurse must remain alert to hazards such as supine hypotension,

Continued

Key Points—cont'd

warning signs and symptoms, and signs of family maladaptations.

- BP is evaluated on the basis of absolute values and length of gestation and interpreted in light of modifying factors.
- Each pregnant woman needs to know how to recognize and report preterm labor.
- Childbirth education is a process designed to help parents make the transition from the role of expectant parents to the role and responsibilities of parents of a new baby.

- The likelihood of physical abuse increases during pregnancy.
- Nurses must be knowledgeable about practices and customs related to childbearing to provide culturally sensitive care.
- Cultural prescriptions and proscriptions influence responses to pregnancy and to the health care delivery system.

Answer Guidelines to Critical Thinking Exercise

Deciding about a Home Birth

1 Yes, there is sufficient evidence to draw conclusions about the safety of a home birth for Millie.
2 a. Millie needs to have a low risk pregnancy, have education about requirements for a home birth, have supports available, be able to secure the equipment necessary, and have made plans for hospital or emergency care as needed.
  b. Millie needs to have a partner or family or friends who will support her; there needs to be a backup plan for emergencies.
  c. Midwives are listed in telephone directories. Names of home birth midwives can be obtained from midwifery associations, boards of registered nursing, telephone directories, and by word of mouth.

  d. Women have the right to select their care provider. Part of the role of a nurse is appropriate referral; therefore referral to a home birth midwife is ethical.
3 Priorities for care include assuring that Millie has access to prenatal care, providing information about home birth and other options for care such as a birth center, and making appropriate referrals.
4 Yes, information about the importance of prenatal care and the safety of home birth is available and supports the conclusion.
5 The nurse might explore with Millie her reasons for seeking a home birth, her tolerance of pain and willingness to forego use of analgesic medications during labor, and her previous experiences with physicians, nurses, and midwives.

Resources

Association of Labor Assistants and Childbirth
  Educators (ALACE)
P.O. Box 382724
Cambridge, MA 02238
617-441-2500

Baby Center (source for expectant parents)
www.babycenter.com

Babies Online (source of articles on pregnancy and baby care)
www.babiesonline.com

Childbirth Graphics
P.O. Box 21207
Waco, TX 76702
800-229-3366
www.childbirthgraphics.com

Childbirth.org (source of links to other sites related to pregnancy
  and birth)
www.childbirth.org

Coalition to Improve Maternity Services (CIMS)
P.O. Box 246
Ponte Verde Beach, FL 32004
888-282-CIMS
www.motherfriendly.org

COPE (Coping with the Overall Pregnancy/Parenting Experience)
37 Clarendon St.
Boston, MA 02116
617-357-5588

Doulas of North America (DONA)
1100 23rd Ave., East
Seattle, WA 98112
206-324-5440
www.dona.org

Healthy Mothers, Healthy Babies Coalition
Washington, DC 20024
202-863-2458

International Childbirth Education Association (ICEA)
P.O. Box 20048
Minneapolis, MN 55420
800-624-4934
www.icea.org

La Leche League International
P.O. Box 4097
Schaumburg, IL 60168
800-525-3243
www.lalecheleague.org

Lamaze International
1200 19th St., NW, Suite 300
Washington, DC 20036
202-223-4579 (fax)
202-857-1100
800-368-4404
www.lamaze-childbirth.com

Lesbian Mother's Support Society
www.lesbian.org/lesbian-moms

March of Dimes Birth Defects Foundation
1275 Mamaroneck Ave.
White Plains, NY 10605
914-997-4537 (fax)
800-658-6674
www.marchofdimes.com

Midwife Alliance of North America (MANA)
309 Main St.
Concord, NH 03301
316-283-4543

National Center for Complementary and Alternative Medicine (NCCAM) Clearinghouse
P.O. Box 7923
Gaithersburg, MD 20898
www.nccam.nih.gov

National Organization of Fathers of Twins Clubs, Inc.
www.nofotc.org

National Organization of Mothers of Twins Clubs, Inc.
Albuquerque, NM 87192
505-275-0955
www.nomotc.org

National Organization on Adolescent Pregnancy, Parenting, and Prevention
2401 Pennsylvania Ave., Suite 350
Washington, DC 20037
202-293-8370

Parenthood After Thirty
451 Vermont
Berkeley, CA 94707
415-524-6635

Parents of Twins and Triplets on the Net
www.potatonet.org

Sex Information and Education Council of the United States (provides publications [e.g., *Sexual relations in pregnancy and postpartum*] and teaching aids)
130 W. 42nd St., Suite 350
New York, NY 10036
www.siecus.org

Stepping Up: Prevention Strategies for Pregnancy, Parenting and Infancy
www.steppingup.washington.edu

References

American College of Obstetricians and Gynecologists (ACOG). (2002). Exercise during pregnancy and the postpartum period. ACOG Committee Opinion #267. *Obstetrics & Gynecology, 99*(1), 171-173.

American College of Obstetricians and Gynecologists (ACOG). (2003). Immunization during pregnancy. ACOG Committee Opinion #282, *Obstetrics & Gynecology, 101*(1), 207-212.

American Dietetic Association. (2002). Position of the American Dietetic Association: Nutrition and lifestyle for a healthy pregnancy. *Journal of the American Dietetic Association, 102*(10), 1479-1490.

Andres, R. (2004). Effects of therapeutic, diagnostic, and environmental agents and exposure to social and illicit drugs. In R. Creasy, R. Resnik, & J. Iams, (Eds.). *Maternal-fetal medicine: Principles and practice* (5th ed.). Philadelphia: Saunders.

Arias, E., MacDorman, M., Strobino, D., Guyer, B. (2003). Annual summary of vital statistics-2002. *Pediatrics, 112*(6), 1215-1230

Artal, R., & Subak-Sharpe, G. (1998). *Pregnancy and exercise.* New York: Delacorte Press.

Association of Women's Health, Obstetric and Neonatal Nurses. (1999). *HIV testing and disclosure for pregnant women and newborns.* Policy Position Statement. Washington, DC: AWHONN.

Barish, R. (2004). In-flight radiation exposure during pregnancy. *Obstetrics & Gynecology, 103*(6), 1326-1330.

Beal, M. (1998). Women's use of complementary and alternative therapies in reproductive health. *Journal of Nurse-Midwifery, 43*(3), 224-233.

Benn, P., Egan, J., Fang, M., & Smith-Bindman, R. (2004) Changes in the utilization of prenatal diagnosis. *Obstetrics & Gynecology, 103*(6), 1255-1260.

Boggess, K., Lieff, S., Murtha, A., Moss, K., Beck, J., & Offenbacher, S. (2003). Maternal periodontal disease is associated with an increased risk for preeclampsia. *Obstetrics & Gynecology, 101*(2), 227-231.

Boyle, G., Banks, J., Petrizzi, M., & Larimore, W. (2003). Sharing maternity care. *Family Practice Management, 10*(3), 37-40.

Bricker, L., & Neilson, J. (2000). Routine Doppler ultrasound in pregnancy (Cochrane Review). In *The Cochrane Library,* Issue 3. Oxford: Update Software.

Brocklehurst, P. (2002). Interventions for reducing the risk of mother-to-child transmission of HIV infection (Cochrane Review). In *The Cochrane Library,* Issue 3. Oxford: Update Software.

Brocklehurst, P., & Volmink, J. (2002). Antiretrovirals for reducing the risk of mother-to-child transmission of HIV infection (Cochrane Review). In *The Cochrane Library,* Issue 3. Oxford: Update Software.

Callaghan, W., & Berg, C., (2003). Pregnancy related mortality among women aged 35 years and older, United States, 1991-1997. *Obstetrics & Gynecology, 102*, (5, Part 1,) 1015-1021.

Carl, D., Roux, G., & Matacale, R. (2000). Exploring dental hygiene and perinatal outcomes: Oral health implications for pregnancy and early childhood. *AWHONN Lifelines, 4*(1), 22-27.

Chalmers, B., Mangiaterra, V., & Porter, R. (2001). WHO principles of prenatal care: The essential antenatal, perinatal, and postpartum care course. *Birth, 28*(3), 202-207.

Chandler, D. (2002). Late entry into prenatal care in a rural setting. *Journal of Midwifery and Women's Health, 47*(1), 28-34.

Cherry, A., Dillon, M., & Rugh, D. (2001). *Teenage pregnancy: A global view.* Westport: Greenwood Press.

Clark, S. (2004). Placenta previa and abruption placentae, In R. Creasy, R. Resnik, & J. Iams (Eds.), *Maternal-fetal medicine: Principles and practice.* (5th ed.). Philadelphia: Saunders.

Corbett, R., Ryan, C., & Weinrich, S. (2003). Pica in pregnancy. *MCN, American Journal of Maternal Child Nursing, 28*(3), 183-191.

Cunningham, F, Leveno, K., Bloom, S., Hauth, J., Gilstrap, L., & Wenstrom, K. (2005). *Williams obstetrics* (22nd ed.). New York: McGraw Hill.

Doulas of North America (DONA). (1999a). *Do I need a doula?* Internet document available at http://www.dona.com (accessed September 22, 2005).

Doulas of North America (DONA). (1999b). *Doulas of North America position paper: The doula's contribution to modern maternity care.* Internet document available at http://www.dona.com (accessed September 22, 2005).

Doulas of North America (DONA). (1999c). *Mission statement.* Internet document available at http://www.dona.com (accessed September 22, 2005).

Fetrick, A., Christensen, M., & Mitchell, C. (2003). Does public health nurse home visitation make a difference in the health outcomes of pregnant clients and their offspring? *Public Health Nursing, 20*(3), 184-189.

Foley, E. (2002). Drug screening and criminal prosecution of pregnant women. *Journal of Obstetric, Gynecologic, and Neonatal Nursing, 33*(2), 133-137.

Ford, K. et al. (2002). Effects of a prenatal care intervention for adolescent mothers on birth weight, repeat pregnancy, and educational outcomes at one year postpartum. *Journal of Perinatal Education, 11*(1), 35-38.

Freda, M. (2003). Nursing's contribution to the literature on preterm labor and birth. *Journal of Obstetric, Gynecologic, and Neonatal Nursing, 32*(5), 659-667.

Freda, M., & Patterson, E. (2003). *Preterm labor and birth: Prevention and nursing management* (3rd ed.) (Nursing Module). New York: March of Dimes Birth Defects Foundation.

Fries, M., Bashford, M., & Nunes, M. (2005). Implementing prenatal screening for cystic fibrosis in routine obstetric practice. *American Journal of Obstetrics and Gynecology, 192*(2), 527-534.

Giannelli, M., Doyle, P., Roman, E., Pelerin, M., & Hermon, C. (2003). The effect of caffeine consumption and nausea on the risk of miscarriage. *Padiatric and Perinatal Epidemiology, 17*(4), 316-323.

Gilbert, E., & Harmon, J. (2003). *Manual of high risk pregnancy and delivery* (3rd ed.). St. Louis: Mosby.

Graves, J., Miller, E., & Sellers, A. (2002). Maternal serum triple analyte screening in pregnancy. *American Family Physician, 65*(5), 915-920.

Handler, A., Rosenberg, D., Raube, K., & Lyons, S. (2003). Prenatal care characteristics and African-American women's satisfaction with care in a managed care organization. *Women's Health Issues, 13*(3), 93-103.

Harris, L., & Paltrow, L. (2003). The status of pregnant women and fetuses in U.S. criminal law. *Journal of the American Medical Association, 289*(13), 1697-1699.

Himmelberger, S. (2002). Preventing group B strep in newborns. *AWHONN Lifelines, 6*(4), 339-342.

Hotelling, B. (2004). Is your perinatal practice mother-friendly? A strategy for improving maternity care. *Birth, 32*(2), 143-147.

Jared, J. et al. (1999). Perioperative periodontal disease and low birth weight: A critical link? *Access, 13*(3), 32, 34-37.

Jenkins, T. & Wapner, R. (2004). Prenatal diagnosis of congenital disorders. In R. Creasy, R. Resnik, & J. Iams (Eds.). *Maternal-fetal medicine: Principles and practice.* (5th ed.). Philadelphia: Saunders

Jepson, R., Mihaljevic, L., & Craig, J. (2005). Cranberries for preventing urinary tract infections (Cochrane Review). In *The Cochrane Library*, Issue 2. Oxford: Update Software.

Johnson, T., & Niebyl, J. (2002). Preconception and prenatal care: Part of the continuum. In S. Gabbe, J. Niebyl, & J. Simpson (Eds.), *Obstetrics: Normal and problem pregnancies* (4th ed.). New York: Churchill Livingstone.

Katz, V., Farmer, R., Tufariello, J., & Carpenter, M. (2001). Why we should eliminate the due date: A truth in jest. *Obstetrics & Gynecology, 98*(6), 1127-1129.

Kehringer, K. (2003). Informed consent: Hospitals must obtain informed consent prior to drug testing pregnant patients. *The Journal of Law, Medicine, & Ethics, 32*(3), 455-457.

Kiel, R., Nashelsky, J., Robbins, B., & Bondi, S. (2003). Does cranberry juice prevent or treat urinary tract infection? *The Journal of Family Practice, 52*(2), 154-155.

Kramer, M. (2001). Regular aerobic exercise during pregnancy (Cochrane Review). In *The Cochrane Library,* Issue 1. Oxford: Update Software.

Kroelinger, C., & Oths, K. (2000). Partner support and pregnancy wantedness. *Birth, 27*(2), 112-119.

Lawrence, R., & Lawrence, R. (2005). *Breastfeeding: A guide for the medical profession* (6th ed.). St. Louis: Mosby.

Lederman, R. (1996). *Psychosocial adaptation in pregnancy* (2nd ed.). New York: Springer.

Lewallen, L. (2004). Healthy behaviors and sources of health information among low-income pregnant women. *Public Health Nursing, 21*(3), 200-206.

Lumley J., Oliver S., & Waters, E. (1999). Interventions for promoting smoking cessation during pregnancy (Cochrane Review). In *The Cochrane Library,* Issue 2, 2004. Chichester, UK: John Wiley & Sons.

Malone, F., & D'Alton, M. (2004). Multiple gestation. Clinical characteristics and management. In R. Creasy, R. Resnik, & J. Iams (Eds.), *Maternal-fetal medicine: Principles and practice* (5th ed.). Philadelphia: Saunders.

March of Dimes Birth Defects Foundation. (2005). *PeriStats (2005): Born too soon and too small in the United States.* Internet document available at www.marchofdimes.com/peristats (accessed May 15, 2005).

Martin, J., Hamilton, B., Sutton, P., Ventura, S., Menacker, F., & Munson, M. (2003). Births: Final data for 2002. *National vital statistics reports 52*(10). Hyattsville, Maryland: National Center for Health Statistics.

Martin, J., Kochanek, K., Strobino, D., Guyer, B., & MacDorman, M. (2005). Annual summary of vital statistics—2003. *Pediatrics, 115*(3), 619-634.

Martin, S., Mackie, L., Kupper, L., Buescher, P., Moracco, K. (2001). Physical abuse of women before, during, and after pregnancy. *Journal of the American Medical Association, 285*(12), 1581-1584.

May, K. (1982). Three phases of father involvement in pregnancy. *Nursing Research, 31*(6), 337-342.

McFarlane, J., Parker, B., & Cross, B. (2001). *Abuse during pregnancy: A protocol for prevention and intervention* (2nd ed.) (Nursing Module). New York: March of Dimes Birth Defects Foundation.

McPheeters, M., Miller, W., Hartman, K., Savitz, D., Kaufamn, J., Garrett, J., & Thorp, J. (2005). The epidemiology of threatened preterm labor: A prospective cohort study. *American Journal of Obstetrics & Gynecology, 192*(4), 1325-1330.

Mercer, R. (1995). *Becoming a mother.* New York: Springer.

Moos, M. K. (2004). Understanding prematurity: Sorting fact from fiction. *AWHONN Lifelines, 8*(1), 32-37.

Morris, S., & Johnson, N. (2005). Exercise in pregnancy: A critical appraisal of the literature. *Journal of Reproductive Medicine, 50*(3), 181-188.

National High Blood Pressure Education Program. (2003). *Seventh report of the Joint National Committee on Prevention, Detection, Evaluation, and Treatment of High Blood Pressure,* Bethesda, MD: U.S. Department of Health and Human Services, National Institutes of Health, National Heart, Lung, & Blood Institute.

Pavill, B. (2002). Fathers and breastfeeding: Consider these ways to get dad involved. *AWHONN Lifelines, 6*(4), 324-331.

Peters, R., & Flack, J. (2004). Hypertensive disorders of pregnancy. *Journal of Obstetric, Gynecologic, and Neonatal Nursing, 33*(2), 209-220.

Raz, R., Chazan, B., & Dan, M. (2004). Cranberry juice and urinary tract infection. *Clinical Infectious Diseases, 38*(10), 1413-1419.

Rubin, R. (1975). Maternal tasks in pregnancy. *Maternal-Child Nursing Journal, 4*(3), 143-153.

Rubin, R. (1984). *Maternal identity and the maternal experience.* New York: Springer.

Sampselle, C. (2003). Behavior interventions in young and middle-aged women: Simple interventions to combat a complex problem. *American Journal of Nursing, 103*(suppl), 9-19.

Schirmer, G. (1998). *Herbal medicine.* Bedford, TX: MED2000, Inc.

Seidel, H., Ball, J., Dains, J., & Benedict, G. (2003). *Mosby's guide to physical examination* (5th ed.). St. Louis: Mosby.

Shaffer, C. (2002). Factors influencing the access to prenatal care by Hispanic pregnant women. *Journal of the American Academy of Nurse Practitioners, 14*(2), 93-98.

Simkin, P., & Way, K. (1998). *DONA position paper: The doula's contributions to modern maternity care.* Seattle, WA: Doulas of North America.

Smith, C., Crowther, C., Willson, K., Hotham, N., & McMillian, V. (2004). A randomized controlled trial of ginger to treat nausea and vomiting in pregnancy. *Obstetrics & Gynecology 103*(4), 639-645.

Strong, C. (2003). Too many twins, triplets, quadruplets, and so on: a call for new priorities. *Journal of Law, Medicine & Ethics (31),* 272-282.

Sword, W. (2003). Prenatal care use among women of low income: A matter of "taking care of self." *Qualitative Health Research, 13*(3): 319-332.

Tiran, D., & Mack, S. (2000). *Complementary therapies for pregnancy and childbirth* (2nd ed). Edinburgh: Baillière Tindall.

Todd, S., LaSala, K., & Neil-Urban, S. (2001). An integrated approach to prenatal smoking cessation interventions. *MCN American Journal of Maternal Child Nursing, 26*(4), 185-191.

Torstein, V., Bakketeig, L.S., Trygg, K.U., Lund-Larsen, K, & Jacobsen, G. (2003). High caffeine consumption in the third trimester of pregnancy: Gender-specific effects on fetal growth. *Paediatric and Perinatal Epidemiology, 17,* 324-331.

Tough, S., Newburn-Cook, C. Johnston, D., Svenson, L., Rose, S., & Belik, J. (2002). Delayed childbearing and its impact on population rate changes in lower birth weight, multiple birth, and preterm delivery. *Pediatrics, 109*(3), 399-403.

Villar, J., Carroli, G., Khan-Neelofur, D., Piaggio, G., & Gulmezoglu, M. (2001). Patterns of routine antenatal care for low-risk pregnancy (Cochrane Review). In *The Cochrane Library,* Issue 4. Oxford: Update Software.

Wagner, C., Katikaneni, L., Cox, T., & Ryan, R. (1998). The impact of prenatal drug exposure on the neonate. *Obstetrics and Gynecology Clinics of North America, 2*(1), 169-194.

Walker, L., Cooney, A., & Riggs, M. (1999). Psychosocial and demographic factors related to health behaviors in the 1st trimester. *Journal of Obstetric, Gynecologic, and Neonatal Nursing, 28*(6), 606-614.

Westheimer, R. & Lopater, S. (2005). *Human sexuality: A psychosocial perspective* (2nd ed.). Philadelphia: Lippincott Williams & Wilkins.

Yu, S., Park, C., & Schwalberg, R. (2002). Factors associated with smoking cessation among U.S. pregnant women. *Maternal and Child Health Journal, 6*(2), 89-97.

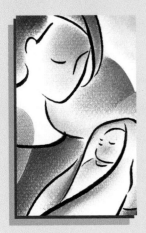

CHAPTER 10

Maternal and Fetal Nutrition

SHANNON E. PERRY

LEARNING OBJECTIVES

- *Explain recommended maternal weight gain during pregnancy.*
- *Compare the recommended level of intake of energy sources, protein, and key vitamins and minerals during pregnancy and lactation.*
- *Give examples of the food sources that provide the nutrients required for optimal maternal nutrition during pregnancy and lactation.*
- *Examine the role of nutrition supplements during pregnancy.*

- *List five nutritional risk factors during pregnancy.*
- *Compare the dietary needs of adolescent and mature pregnant women.*
- *Give examples of cultural food patterns and possible dietary problems for two ethnic groups or for two alternative eating patterns.*
- *Assess nutritional status during pregnancy.*

KEY TERMS AND DEFINITIONS

adequate intakes (AIs) Recommended nutrient intakes estimated to meet the needs of almost all healthy people in the population; provided for nutrients or age-group categories where the available information is not sufficient to warrant establishing recommended dietary allowances

anthropometric measurements Body measurements, such as height and weight

body mass index (BMI) Method of calculating appropriateness of weight for height (BMI = weight/height^2)

Dietary Reference Intakes (DRIs) Nutritional recommendations for the United States, consisting of the recommended dietary allowances, adequate intakes, and tolerable upper intake levels; the upper limit of intake associated with low risk in almost all members of a population

intrauterine growth restriction (IUGR) Fetal undergrowth from any cause

kcal Kilocalorie; unit of heat content or energy equal to 1000 small calories

lactose intolerance Inherited absence of the enzyme lactase

physiologic anemia Relative excess of plasma leading to a decrease in hemoglobin concentration and hematocrit; normal adaptation during pregnancy

pica Unusual oral craving during pregnancy (e.g., for laundry starch, dirt, red clay)

pyrosis A burning sensation in the epigastric and sternal region from stomach acid (heartburn)

Recommended Dietary Allowances (RDAs) Recommended nutrient intakes estimated to meet the needs of almost all (97% to 98%) of the healthy people in the population

ELECTRONIC RESOURCES

Additional information related to the content in Chapter 10 can be found on

the companion website at **evolve**
http://evolve.elsevier.com/Lowdermilk/Maternity/
- NCLEX Review Questions
- WebLinks

or on the interactive companion CD
- NCLEX Review Questions
- Critical Thinking Exercise—Nutrition Education
- Plan of Care—Nutrition during Pregnancy

*N*utrition is one of the many factors that influence the outcome of pregnancy (Fig. 10-1). However, maternal nutritional status is an especially significant factor, both because it is potentially alterable and because good nutrition before and during pregnancy is an important preventive measure for a variety of problems. These problems include birth of low-birth-weight (LBW) and preterm infants. It is essential that the importance of good nutrition be emphasized to all women of childbearing potential. Nutrition assessment, intervention, and evaluation must be an integral part of the nursing care provided to all pregnant women.

The Pregnancy Nutrition Surveillance System (PNSS) was developed to help health professionals identify and reduce pregnancy-related health risks (Centers for Disease Control and Prevention [CDC], 2004). The data collected from programs such as the Special Supplemental Nutrition Program for Women, Infants, and Children (WIC) and prenatal clinics funded by Maternal and Child Health Program Block Grants are submitted to the CDC. Annual data summaries allow states to monitor trends in prevalence of prenatal risk factors that predict low birth weight and infant mortality, as well as monitor infant feeding practices.

NUTRIENT NEEDS BEFORE CONCEPTION

The first trimester of pregnancy is a crucial one for embryonic and fetal organ development. A healthful diet before conception is the best way to ensure that adequate nutrients are available for the developing fetus. Folate or folic acid intake is of particular concern in the periconceptual period. Folate is the form in which this vitamin is found naturally in foods, and folic acid is the form used in fortification of grain products and other foods and in vitamin supplements. Neural tube defects, or failure in closure of the neural tube, are more common in infants of women with poor folic acid intake. It is estimated that the incidence of neural tube defects could be halved if all women had an adequate folic acid intake during the periconceptual period (Kilpatrick & Laros, 2004). All women capable of becoming pregnant are advised to consume 400 mcg of folic acid daily in fortified foods (e.g., ready-to-eat cereals and enriched grain products) or supplements in addition to a diet rich in folate-containing foods such as green leafy vegetables, whole grains, and fruits.

Both maternal and fetal risks in pregnancy are increased when the mother is significantly underweight or overweight when pregnancy begins. Ideally, all women would achieve a desirable body weight before conception.

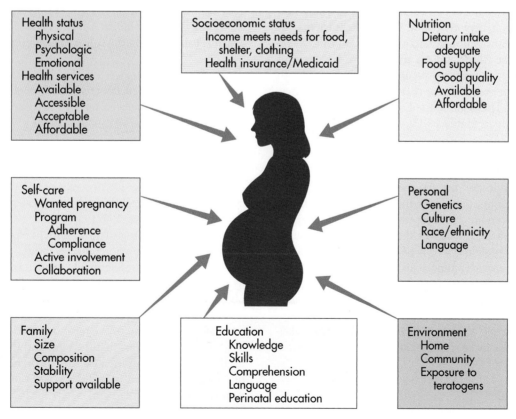

Fig. 10-1 Factors that affect the outcome of pregnancy.

NUTRIENT NEEDS DURING PREGNANCY

Nutrient needs are determined, at least in part, by the stage of gestation. The amount of fetal growth varies during the different stages of pregnancy. During the first trimester, the synthesis of fetal tissues places relatively few demands on maternal nutrition. Therefore during the first trimester, when the embryo or fetus is very small, the needs are only slightly increased over those before pregnancy. In contrast, the last trimester is a period of noticeable fetal growth when most of the fetal stores of energy sources and minerals are deposited. Basal metabolic rates (BMRs), when expressed as kilocalories (kcal) per minute, are approximately 20% higher in pregnant women than in nonpregnant women. This increase includes the energy cost for tissue synthesis.

The Food and Nutrition Board of the National Academy of Sciences publishes recommendations for the people of the United States, the Dietary Reference Intakes (DRIs). The DRIs consist of Recommended Dietary Allowances (RDAs) and Adequate Intakes (AIs), as well as Upper Limits (ULs), guidelines for avoiding excessive intakes of nutrients that may be toxic if consumed in excess. RDAs for some nutrients have been available for many years, and they have been revised periodically. RDAs are recommendations for daily nutritional intakes that meet the needs of almost all (97% to 98%) of the healthy members of the population. AIs are similar to the RDAs and are believed to cover the needs of virtually all healthy individuals in a group, except that they deal with nutrients for which there are not enough data to be certain of their requirements. The RDAs and AIs include a wide variety of nutrients and food components, and they are divided into age, sex, and life-stage categories (e.g., infancy, pregnancy, and lactation). They can be used as goals in planning the diets of individuals (Table 10-1).

Energy Needs

Energy (kilocalories or kcal) needs are met by carbohydrate, fat, and protein in the diet. No specific recommendations exist for the amount of carbohydrate and fat in the diet of the pregnant woman. However, intake of these nutrients should be adequate to support the recommended weight gain. Although protein can be used to supply energy, its primary role is to provide amino acids for the synthesis of new tissues (see the discussion on protein later in this chapter). The RDA during the second and third trimesters of pregnancy is 300 kcal greater than prepregnancy needs. Very underweight or active women or those with multifetal gestations will require more than 300 additional kcal to sustain the desired rate of weight gain.

Weight gain

The optimal weight gain during pregnancy is not known precisely. It is known, however, that the amount of weight gained by the mother during pregnancy has an important bearing on the course and outcome of pregnancy. Adequate weight gain does not necessarily indicate that the diet is nutritionally adequate, but it is associated with a reduced risk of giving birth to a small-for-gestational-age (SGA) or preterm infant.

The desirable weight gain during pregnancy varies among women. The primary factor to consider in making a weight gain recommendation is the appropriateness of the prepregnancy weight for the woman's height. Maternal and fetal risks in pregnancy are increased when the mother is either significantly underweight or overweight before pregnancy, and when weight gain during pregnancy is either too low or too high. Severely underweight women are more likely to have preterm labor and to give birth to LBW infants. Women with inadequate weight gain have an increased risk of giving birth to an infant with intrauterine growth restriction (IUGR). Greater-than-expected weight gain during pregnancy may occur for many reasons, including multiple gestation, edema, preeclampsia, and overeating. When obesity is present (either preexisting or developed during pregnancy), there is an increased likelihood of macrosomia and fetopelvic disproportion; operative birth; emergency cesarean birth; postpartum hemorrhage; wound, genital tract, or urinary tract infection; birth trauma; and late fetal death. Obese women are more likely than normal-weight women to have gestational hypertension and gestational diabetes; their risk of giving birth to a child with a major congenital defect is double that of normal-weight women.

A commonly used method of evaluating the appropriateness of weight for height is the body mass index (BMI), which is calculated by the following formula:

$$BMI = weight/height^2$$

where the weight is in kilograms and height is in meters. Therefore for a woman who weighed 51 kg before pregnancy and is 1.57 m tall:

$$BMI = 51/(1.57)^2, \text{ or } 20.7$$

Prepregnant BMI can be classified into the following categories: less than 19.8, underweight or low; 19.8 to 26, normal; 26 to 29, overweight or high; and greater than 29, obese (Institute of Medicine, 1992).

For women with single fetuses, current recommendations are that women with a normal BMI should gain 11.5 to 16 kg during pregnancy, underweight women should gain 12.5 to 18 kg, overweight women should gain 7 to 11.5 kg, and obese women should gain at least 7 kg (Institute of Medicine, 1992). Adolescents are encouraged to strive for weight gains at the upper end of the recommended range for their BMI because it appears that the fetus and the still-growing mother compete for nutrients. The risk of mechanical complications at birth is reduced if the weight gain of short adult women (shorter than 157 cm) is near the lower end of their recommended range. In twin gestations, gains of approximately 16 to 20 kg appear to be associated with the best outcomes (Malone & D'Alton, 2004).

CD: Critical Thinking Exercise—Nutrition Education

Pattern of weight gain

Weight gain should take place throughout pregnancy. The risk of giving birth to an SGA infant is greater when the weight gain early in pregnancy has been poor. The likelihood of preterm birth is greater when the gains during the last half of pregnancy have been inadequate. These risks exist even when the total gain for the pregnancy is in the recommended range.

The optimal rate of weight gain depends on the stage of pregnancy. During the first and second trimesters, growth takes place primarily in maternal tissue; during the third trimester, growth occurs primarily in fetal tissues. During the first trimester there is an average total weight gain of only 1 to 2.5 kg. Thereafter the recommended weight gain increases to approximately 0.4 kg/week for a woman of normal weight (Fig. 10-2). The recommended weekly weight gain for overweight women during the second and third trimesters is 0.3 kg, and for underweight women it is 0.5 kg. The recommended caloric intake corresponds to this pattern of gain. For the first trimester there is no increment; during the second and third trimesters an additional 300 kcal/day over the prepregnant intake is recommended. The amount of food providing 300 kcal is not great. It can be provided by one additional serving from any one of the following groups: milk, yogurt, or cheese (all skim milk products); fruits; vegetables; and bread, cereal, rice, or pasta.

The reasons for an inadequate weight gain (less than 1 kg/month for normal-weight women or less than 0.5 kg/month for obese women during the last two trimesters) or excessive weight gain (more than 3 kg/month) should be evaluated thoroughly. Possible reasons for deviations from the expected

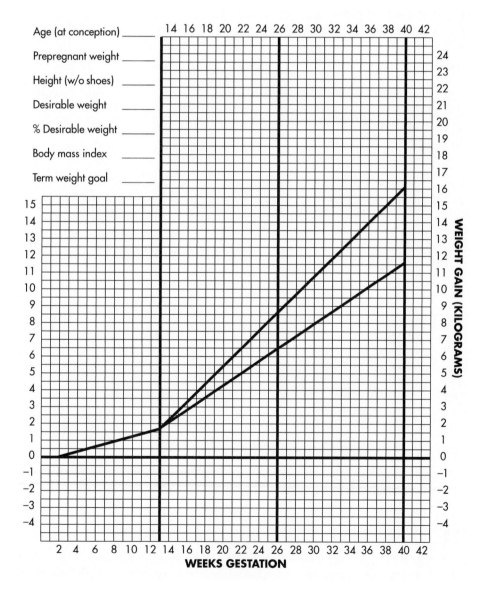

Fig. 10-2 Prenatal weight gain chart for plotting weight gain of normal-weight women. NOTE: Young adolescents, African-American women, and smokers should aim for the upper end of the recommended range; short women (<157 cm) should strive for gains at the lower end of the range.

TABLE 10-1

Recommendations for Daily Intakes of Selected Nutrients during Pregnancy and Lactation

NUTRIENT (UNIT)	RECOMMENDATION FOR NONPREGNANT WOMAN*	RECOMMENDATION FOR PREGNANCY*	RECOMMENDATION FOR LACTATION*	ROLE IN RELATION TO PREGNANCY AND LACTATION	FOOD SOURCES
Energy (kilocalories [kcal] or kilojoules [kJ]†)	Variable	First trimester, same as nonpregnant; second and third trimesters, nonpregnant + 300 kcal or 72 kJ	Nonpregnant + 500 kcal or 120 kJ	Growth of fetal and maternal tissues; milk production	Carbohydrate, fat, and protein
Protein (g)	50	60	65	Synthesis of the products of conception; growth of maternal tissue and expansion of blood volume; secretion of milk protein during lactation	Meats, eggs, cheese, yogurt, legumes (dry beans and peas, peanuts), nuts, grains
MINERALS					
Calcium (mg)	1300/1000	1300/1000	1300/1000	Fetal and infant skeleton and tooth formation; maintenance of maternal bone and tooth mineralization	Milk, cheese, yogurt, sardines or other fish eaten with bones left in, deep green leafy vegetables except spinach or Swiss chard, calcium-set tofu, baked beans, tortillas
Iron (mg)	15/18	30	10/9	Maternal hemoglobin formation, fetal liver iron storage	Liver, meats, whole grain or enriched breads and cereals, deep green leafy vegetables, legumes, dried fruits
Zinc (mg)	9/8	12/11	13/12	Component of numerous enzyme systems, possibly important in preventing congenital malformations	Liver, shellfish, meats, whole grains, milk
Iodine (mcg)	150	220	290	Increased maternal metabolic rate	Iodized salt, seafood, milk and milk products, commercial yeast breads, rolls, and donuts
Magnesium (mg)	360/310-320	400/350-360	360/310-320	Involved in energy and protein metabolism, tissue growth, muscle action	Nuts, legumes, cocoa, meats, whole grains

FAT-SOLUBLE VITAMINS

Vitamin				Function	Sources
A (mcg)	700	750/770	1200/1300	Essential for cell development, tooth bud formation, bone growth	Deep green leafy vegetables; dark yellow vegetables; and fruits, chili peppers, liver, fortified margarine and butter
D (mcg)	5	5	5	Involved in absorption of calcium and phosphorus, improves mineralization	Fortified milk and margarine, egg yolk, butter, liver, seafood
E (mg)	15	15	19	Antioxidant (protects cell membranes from damage), especially important for preventing breakdown of RBCs	Vegetable oils, green leafy vegetables, whole grains, liver, nuts and seeds, cheese, fish

WATER-SOLUBLE VITAMINS

Vitamin				Function	Sources
C (mg)	65/75	80/85	115/120	Tissue formation and integrity, formation of connective tissue, enhancement of iron absorption	Citrus fruits, strawberries, melons, broccoli, tomatoes, peppers, raw deep green leafy vegetables
Folate (mcg)	400	600	500	Prevention of neural tube defects, support for increased maternal RBC formation	Fortified ready-to-eat cereals and other grain products, green leafy vegetables, oranges, broccoli, asparagus, artichokes, liver
B$_6$ or pyridoxine (mg)	1.2/1.3	1.9	2.0	Involved in protein metabolism	Meat, liver, deep green vegetables, whole grains
B$_{12}$ (mcg)	2.4	2.6	2.8	Production of nucleic acids and proteins, especially important in formation of RBCs and neural functioning	Milk and milk products, egg, meat, liver, fortified soy milk

Recommendations are the Dietary Reference Intakes (RDA or AI, see text), where available.

Sources: Food and Nutrition Board, National Academy of Sciences, Institute of Medicine, 1997; *Dietary Reference Intakes for calcium, phosphorus, magnesium, vitamin D, and fluoride*, 1998; *Dietary Reference Intakes for thiamine, riboflavin, niacin, vitamin B$_6$, folate, vitamin B$_{12}$, pantothenic acid, biotin, and choline*, 2000; *Dietary Reference Intakes for vitamin A, vitamin K, arsenic, boron, chromium, copper, iodine, iron, manganese, molybdenum, nickel, silicon, vanadium, and zinc*, Washington, DC, National Academy Press. Where DRIs are not available, the values are taken from Food and Nutrition Board, National Academy of Sciences, National Research Council: *Recommended dietary allowances*, ed 10, Washington, DC, 1989, National Academy Press.

*When two values appear, separated by a diagonal slash, the first is for females younger than 19 years, and the second is for those 19 to 50 years of age.

†The international metric unit of energy measurement is the joule (J).

1 kcal = 4.184 kJ.

RBCs, red blood cells.

rate of weight gain, besides inadequate or excessive dietary intake, include measurement or recording errors, differences in weight of clothing, time of day, and accumulation of fluids. An exceptionally high gain is likely to be caused by an accumulation of fluids, and a gain of more than 3 kg in a month, especially after the twentieth week of gestation, often heralds the development of preeclampsia.

Hazards of restricting adequate weight gain

Figure-conscious women may find it difficult to make the transition from guarding against weight gain before pregnancy to valuing weight gain during pregnancy. In counseling these women the nurse can emphasize the positive effects of good nutrition as well as the adverse effects of maternal malnutrition (manifested by poor weight gain) on infant growth and development. This counseling includes information on the components of weight gain during pregnancy (Table 10-2) and the amount of this weight that will be lost at birth. Early in a woman's pregnancy, explaining ways to lose weight in the postpartum period helps relieve her concerns. Because lactation can help to reduce maternal energy stores gradually, this provides an opportunity to promote breastfeeding.

Pregnancy is not a time for a weight-reduction diet. Even overweight or obese pregnant women need to gain at least enough weight to equal the weight of the products of conception (fetus, placenta, and amniotic fluid). If they limit their caloric intake to prevent weight gain, they may also excessively limit their intake of important nutrients. Moreover, dietary restriction results in catabolism of fat stores, which in turn augments the production of ketones. The long-term effects of mild ketonemia during pregnancy are not known, but ketonuria has been found to be correlated with the occurrence of preterm labor. It should be stressed to obese women (and to all pregnant women) that the quality of the weight gain is important, with emphasis placed on the consumption of nutrient-dense foods and the avoidance of empty-calorie foods.

Weight gain is important, but pregnancy is not an excuse for uncontrolled dietary indulgence. Excessive weight gained

Critical Thinking Exercise

Nutrition and the Underweight Pregnant Adolescent

Carmen, of Hispanic heritage, is 15 years old and is 3 months pregnant. She comes to her initial appointment for diagnosis and care. She appears to be underweight for her height. To provide optimum care for her, you plan to calculate her prepregnancy BMI. When her pregnancy is confirmed, you are asked to compose a food plan with Carmen that meets the minimum daily requirements and allows for growth of the pregnancy. You know that it is important to include consideration of personal preferences and cultural factors in your plan. With Carmen, identify barriers to implementing the plan.

1 Evidence—Is there sufficient evidence to draw conclusions about an appropriate nutrition plan, taking into consideration personal preferences and cultural factors?
2 Assumptions—Describe underlying assumptions about each of the following issues:
   a. Dietary Reference Intakes for pregnancy and lactation
   b. Indicators of nutritional risk in pregnancy
   c. Daily food guide for pregnancy and lactation
   d. Sources of calcium for women who do not drink milk
3 What implications and priorities for nursing care can be drawn at this time?
4 Does the evidence objectively support your conclusion?
5 Are there alternative perspectives to your conclusion?

during pregnancy may be difficult to lose after pregnancy, thus contributing to chronic overweight or obesity, an etiologic factor in a host of chronic diseases including hypertension, diabetes mellitus, and arteriosclerotic heart disease. The woman who gains 18 kg or more during pregnancy is especially at risk.

Protein

Protein, with its essential constituent nitrogen, is the nutritional element basic to growth. Adequate protein intake is essential to meet increasing demands in pregnancy. These demands arise from the rapid growth of the fetus; the enlargement of the uterus and its supporting structures, mammary glands, and placenta; an increase in maternal circulating blood volume and subsequent demand for increased amounts of plasma protein to maintain colloidal osmotic pressure; and the formation of amniotic fluid.

Milk, meat, eggs, and cheese are complete-protein foods with a high biologic value. Legumes (dried beans and peas), whole grains, and nuts are also valuable sources of protein. In addition, these protein-rich foods are a source of other nutrients such as calcium, iron, and B vitamins; plant sources of protein often provide needed dietary fiber. The recommended daily food plan (Table 10-3) is a guide to the

TABLE 10-2

Tissues Contributing to Maternal Weight Gain at 40 Weeks of Gestation

TISSUE	KILOGRAMS	POUNDS
Fetus	3-3.9	7-8.5
Placenta	.9-1.1	2-2.5
Amniotic fluid	.9	2
Increase in uterine tissue	.9	2
Breast tissue	.5-1.8	1-4
Increased blood volume	1.8-2.3	4-5
Increased tissue fluid	1.4-2.3	3-5
Increased stores (fat)	1.8-2.7	4-6

TABLE 10-3

Daily Food Guide for Pregnancy and Lactation

FOOD GROUP	SERVING SIZE	SUGGESTED NUMBER OF SERVINGS		
		NONPREGNANT, NONLACTATING WOMAN	PREGNANT WOMAN	LACTATING WOMAN
GRAIN PRODUCTS Include whole-grain and enriched breads, cereals, pasta, and rice.	1 slice bread; ½ bun, bagel, or English muffin; 1 oz ready-to-eat cereal; ½ c cooked grains	6-11	6-11	6-11
VEGETABLES Eat dark green leafy and deep yellow often. Eat dried beans and peas often; count ½ c cooked dried beans or peas as a serving of vegetables or 1 oz from meat group.	1 c raw leafy greens; ½ c of others	3-5	3-5	3-5
FRUITS Include citrus fruits, strawberries, or melons frequently.	1 medium apple, orange, banana, peach, etc; ½ c small or diced fruit; ¾ c juice	2-4	2-4	2-4
MILK AND MILK PRODUCTS	1 c milk or yogurt; 1½ oz cheese	2-3	3 or more	4 or more
MEAT, POULTRY, FISH, DRY BEANS, NUTS, AND EGGS Eat peanut butter or nuts rarely to avoid excessive fat intake. Limit egg intake to reduce cholesterol intake; trim fat from meat, and remove skin from poultry.	½ c cooked dried beans, 1 egg, or 1½ T peanut butter is equivalent to 1 oz of meat	Up to 6 oz total	Up to 6 oz total	Up to 6 oz total

c, cup; *T,* tablespoon.

amounts of these foods that would supply the quantities of protein needed. The recommendations provide for only a modest increase in protein intake over the prepregnant levels in adult women. Protein intake in many people in the United States is relatively high, so many women may not need to increase their protein intake at all during pregnancy. Three servings of milk, yogurt, or cheese (four for adolescents) and 5 to 6 oz (140 to 168 g) (two servings) of meat, poultry, or fish supply the recommended protein for the pregnant woman. Additional protein is provided by vegetables and breads, cereals, rice, and pasta. Pregnant adolescents, women from impoverished backgrounds, and women adhering to unusual diets, such as a macrobiotic (highly restricted vegetarian) diet, are those most likely to have inadequate protein intake. The use of high-protein supplements is not recommended, because these have been associated with an increased incidence of preterm births.

Fluids

Essential during the exchange of nutrients and waste products across cell membranes, water is the main substance of cells, blood, lymph, amniotic fluid, and other vital body fluids. It also aids in maintaining body temperature. A good fluid intake promotes good bowel function, which is sometimes a problem during pregnancy. The recommended daily intake is about six to eight glasses (1500 to 2000 ml) of fluid. Water, milk, and juices are good fluid sources. Dehydration may increase the risk of cramping, contractions, and preterm labor.

Women who consume more than 300 mg of caffeine daily (equivalent to about 500 to 750 ml of coffee) may be at increased risk of miscarriage and of giving birth to infants with IUGR. The ill effects of caffeine have been proposed to result from vasoconstriction of the blood vessels supplying the uterus or from interference with cell division in the developing fetus. Consequently, caffeine-containing products such as caffeinated coffee, tea, soft drinks, and cocoa beverages should be avoided or consumed only in limited quantities.

Aspartame (NutraSweet, Equal), acesulfame potassium (Sunett), and sucralose (Splenda), artificial sweeteners commonly used in low- or no-calorie beverages and low-calorie food products, have not been found to have adverse effects on the normal mother or fetus. Aspartame, which contains phenylalanine, should be avoided by the woman with phenylketonuria (PKU) (Box 10-1).

BOX 10-1

Use of Artificial Sweeteners during Pregnancy

All of the following sweeteners are approved for use in all age groups, including pregnant women, in the United States:

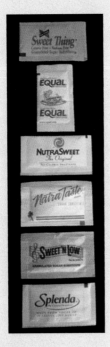

ACESULFAME K
- Brand names: Sunett, Sweet One
- Primary uses: baked goods, frozen desserts, candies, beverages
- Sweetness: 200 times sweeter than sugar
- Shelf life: long
- Suitability for cooking: good, does not break down when heated
- Health concerns: none known

ASPARTAME
- Brand names: Equal, NutraSweet, NatraTaste
- Primary uses: beverages, frozen desserts, dairy products, chewing gum, breakfast cereals, table-top sweetener
- Sweetness: 180 times sweeter than sugar
- Shelf life: relatively short (about 5 months in a soft drink)
- Suitability for cooking: breaks down and loses sweetness if cooked at high temperatures or for long periods
- Health concerns: contains phenylalanine, a consideration in the diets of people with phenylketonuria

NEOTAME
- Brand names: none (not currently available)
- Primary uses: approved in the United States but not currently marketed; proposed for use in beverages, frozen desserts, yogurt, chewing gum, toppings, fillings, fruit spreads, table-top sweetener
- Sweetness: 8000 times sweeter than sugar
- Shelf life: similar to aspartame (about 5 months in a soft drink)
- Suitability for cooking: good, but loses sweetness if cooked at high temperatures or for prolonged periods
- Health concerns: none known; contains phenylalanine but not in a form that can be metabolized

SACCHARIN
- Brand name: Sweet 'n Low
- Primary uses: fountain drinks, chewable vitamins and medications, table-top sweetener
- Sweetness: 300 times sweeter than sugar
- Shelf life: long
- Suitability for cooking: good, does not lose sweetness during cooking
- Health concerns: linked to bladder cancer in rats

SUCRALOSE
- Brand name: Splenda
- Primary uses: baked goods, beverages, frozen desserts, gelatins, table-top sweetener
- Sweetness: 600 times sweeter than sugar
- Shelf life: long
- Suitability for cooking: very good, does not break down during cooking (maltodextrin is added to give products better bulk and texture)
- Health concerns: none known

SUGAR ALCOHOLS (not technically artificial sweeteners; contain almost as many calories as sugar)
- Types: sorbitol, xylitol, lactitol, mannitol, and maltitol
- Primary uses: sugar-free candy, cookies, and chewing gum
- Sweetness: most are about 70% as sweet as sugar; xylitol equals sugar in sweetness
- Shelf life: long
- Suitability for cooking: good
- Advantages over sugar: do not promote tooth decay, more slowly metabolized so that they do not create a rapid peak in blood glucose
- Health concerns: diarrhea can occur with large intakes

Sugar is important for the volume and moisture of baked goods. Artificial sweeteners may produce a good-tasting product, but some sugar is necessary in many recipes to yield normal volume and texture.

Minerals and Vitamins

In general the nutrient needs of pregnant women, except perhaps for folate and iron, can be met through dietary sources. Counseling about the need for a varied diet rich in vitamins and minerals should be a part of every pregnant woman's early prenatal care and should be reinforced throughout pregnancy. Supplements of certain nutrients (listed in the following discussion) are recommended whenever the woman's diet is very poor or whenever significant nutritional risk factors are present. Nutritional risk factors in pregnancy are listed in Box 10-2.

Iron

Iron is needed both to allow transfer of adequate iron to the fetus and to permit expansion of the maternal red blood cell (RBC) mass. Beginning in the latter part of the first trimester, the blood volume of the mother increases steadily, peaking at about 1500 ml more than that in the nonpregnant state. In twin gestations, the increase is at least 500 ml greater than that in pregnancies with single fetuses. Plasma volume increases more than RBC mass, with the difference between plasma and RBCs being greatest during the second trimester. The relative excess of plasma causes a modest decrease in the hemoglobin concentration and hematocrit, termed *physiologic anemia of pregnancy*. This is a normal adaptation during pregnancy.

However, poor iron intake and absorption, which can result in iron deficiency anemia, is relatively common among women in the childbearing years. It affects nearly one fifth of the pregnant women in industrialized countries. The maternal mortality rate is increased among anemic women, who are poorly prepared to tolerate hemorrhage at the time of birth. In addition, anemic women may have a greater likelihood of cardiac failure during labor, postpartum infections, and poor wound healing. The fetus is also affected by maternal anemia. The risk of preterm birth is about threefold

greater in anemic women, and fetal iron stores may also be reduced by maternal anemia. Anemia is more common among adolescents and African-American women than among adult Caucasian women.

The Institute of Medicine (1992) recommended that all pregnant women receive a supplement of 30 mg of ferrous iron daily, starting by 12 weeks of gestation. (Iron supplements may be poorly tolerated during the nausea that is prevalent in the first trimester.) If maternal iron deficiency anemia is present (preferably diagnosed by measurement of serum ferritin, a storage form of iron), increased dosages (60 to 100 mg daily) are recommended. Certain foods taken with an iron supplement can promote or inhibit absorption of iron from the supplement. Even when a woman is taking an iron supplement, she should include good food sources of iron in her daily diet (see Table 10-1).

Calcium

There is no increase in the DRI of calcium during pregnancy and lactation, in comparison with the recommendation for the nonpregnant woman (see Table 10-1). The DRI (1000 mg daily for women age 19 and older and 1300 mg for those younger than age 19) appears to provide sufficient calcium for fetal bone and tooth development to proceed while maternal bone mass is maintained.

Milk and yogurt are especially rich sources of calcium, providing approximately 300 mg/cup (240 ml). Nevertheless, many women do not consume these foods or do not consume adequate amounts to provide the recommended intakes of calcium. One problem that can interfere with milk consumption is lactose intolerance, which is an inability to digest milk sugar (lactose) and is caused by the absence of the lactase enzyme in the small intestine. Lactose intolerance is relatively common in adults, particularly African-Americans, Asians, Native Americans, and Inuits. Milk consumption may cause abdominal cramping, bloating, and diarrhea in such people. Yogurt, sweet acidophilus milk, buttermilk, cheese, chocolate milk, and cocoa may be tolerated even when fresh fluid milk is not. Commercial products that contain lactase (e.g., Lactaid) are widely available. Many supermarkets stock lactase-treated milk. The lactase in these products hydrolyzes, or digests, the lactose in milk, making it possible for lactose-intolerant people to drink milk.

In some cultures, adults rarely drink milk. For example, Puerto Ricans and other Hispanic people may use milk only as an additive in coffee. Pregnant women from these cultures may need to consume nondairy sources of calcium. Vegetarian diets may also be deficient in calcium (Box 10-3). If calcium intake appears low and the woman does not change her dietary habits despite counseling, a daily supplement containing 600 mg of elemental calcium may be needed. Calcium supplements may also be recommended when a pregnant woman experiences leg cramps caused by an imbalance in the calcium/phosphorus ratio.

BOX 10-2

Indicators of Nutritional Risk in Pregnancy

- Adolescence
- Frequent pregnancies: three within 2 years
- Poor fetal outcome in a previous pregnancy
- Poverty
- Poor diet habits with resistance to change
- Use of tobacco, alcohol, or drugs
- Weight at conception under or over normal weight
- Problems with weight gain
- Any weight loss
- Weight gain of less than 1 kg/mo after the first trimester
- Weight gain of more than 1 kg/wk after the first trimester
- Multifetal pregnancy
- Low hemoglobin or hematocrit values (or both)

EVIDENCE-BASED PRACTICE
Calcium Supplementation for Preventing Preeclampsia

BACKGROUND

- Hypertensive disorders of pregnancy are associated with maternal and fetal death and morbidity. Hypertension leads to poor uterine perfusion, preterm birth, fetal distress, low birth weight, and perinatal fetal mortality. In the mother, preeclampsia can lead to edema; seizures; renal failure; the syndrome of hemolysis, elevated liver enzymes, and low platelets (HELLP); admission to intensive care; cesarean birth; and maternal death. *Gestational hypertension* is usually defined as new-onset diastolic blood pressure over 90 mm Hg, or a rise over baseline for systolic blood pressure of 30 mm Hg or for diastolic pressure of 15 mm Hg. Preeclampsia is diagnosed when gestational hypertension is accompanied by proteinuria of 2+, or 300 mg in 24 hours. Blood pressure climbs when the endothelial walls become inflamed from unknown causes. Low calcium intake may stimulate either parathyroid hormone or renin release, which increases cellular uptake of calcium, leading to vasospasm. Calcium supplementation reduces parathyroid hormone, thus reducing intravascular inflammation, and may be a treatment for gestational hypertension. Calcium may also relax the smooth muscles in the uterus, reducing the risk of preterm labor. Calcium is cost-effective, familiar, and available. No risk of renal stones has been noted.

OBJECTIVES

- The goal of the review was to determine whether calcium supplementation during pregnancy affected preeclampsia, and related adverse maternal and fetal outcomes. Of interest were comparisons of women at low risk for preeclampsia with high risk mothers (teens, women with history of preeclampsia or prepregnancy hypertension, increased sensitivity to angiotensin II) and comparisons of women with low dietary calcium baselines (under 900 mg/day) with women with adequate dietary calcium. The intervention was oral calcium, at least 1 g/day. The controls took a placebo. Maternal outcome measures included hypertension, proteinuria, placental abruption, cesarean birth, mother's length of stay, eclampsia, renal failure, HELLP, intensive care unit admission, and maternal death. Fetal or neonatal outcomes included preterm labor (before 37 weeks), low birth weight, small size for gestational age, admission to neonatal intensive care unit (NICU), length of stay longer than 7 days, perinatal death, long-term disability, and childhood hypertension (greater than 95th percentile).

METHODS
Search Strategy

- The reviewers searched the Cochrane database, MEDLINE, 30 journals and conferences, and a weekly current awareness service of 37 journals. Search keywords were *calcium, hypertension, pregnancy, blood pressure,* and combinations of these terms.
- Eleven randomized, placebo-controlled trials were selected, representing 6894 women from Argentina, the United States, Australia, Ecuador, and India. The trials were published from 1989 to 2001.

Statistical Analyses

- Similar data were pooled, and effect size (the difference between intervention and control groups in each trial) was calculated. The calculations comparing high risk and low risk women, and baseline low and adequate dietary calcium, were analyzed post hoc (after the main calculations).

FINDINGS

- Calcium supplementation was associated with significantly less high blood pressure than placebo. The difference was more marked in the group of women at high risk for gestational hypertension and in the group of women with low baseline dietary calcium. Preeclampsia was likewise significantly reduced with calcium in low risk women and markedly reduced in high risk women and women with low baseline dietary calcium, but the effect was not significant with women who had adequate baseline dietary calcium. The risk of preterm birth and low birth weight was significantly decreased among high risk women taking calcium. There was no difference in caesarean births, admission to NICU, or perinatal death. Data were inadequate to make determinations about maternal death or serious morbidity, placental abruptions, mother's length of stay, small-for-gestational-age babies, or childhood disabilities. One follow-up study of children at 7 years of age found fewer elevated blood pressures in the calcium group than placebo, suggesting a lingering benefit for the offspring. No side effects of calcium were recorded in these trials.

LIMITATIONS

- The doses and types of calcium differed, as did the definitions of high risk and the baseline dietary calcium intake, causing heterogeneity in the trials and limiting generalizability. Some randomization was not well described. In general, however, these were strong trials in that they were large, double-blinded, and placebo-controlled trials.

CONCLUSIONS

- Supplemental calcium is associated with less hypertension and less preeclampsia, as well as less preterm birth and low birth weight, especially in those women at high risk.

IMPLICATIONS FOR PRACTICE

- Health care providers should support calcium supplementation for women at high risk for gestational hypertension, as well as in communities with low baseline calcium intake.

IMPLICATIONS FOR FURTHER RESEARCH

- Research should focus on women at high risk for gestational hypertension and communities with low baseline dietary calcium, and on ideal dosages of calcium. The one study of long-term benefits for offspring was promising. Researchers should distinguish between small-for-gestational-age babies and preterm babies, because they are different conditions and have different prognoses.

Reference: Atallah, A., Hofmeyr, G., & Duley, L. (2003). Calcium supplementation during pregnancy for preventing hypertensive disorders and related problems (Cochrane Review). In *The Cochrane Library,* Issue 2, 2004. Chichester, UK: John Wiley & Sons.

Calcium Sources for Women Who Do Not Drink Milk

Each of the following provides approximately the same amount of calcium as 1 cup of milk.

FISH
3-oz can of sardines
4½-oz can of salmon (if bones are eaten)

BEANS AND LEGUMES
3 cups cooked dried beans
2½ cups refried beans
2 cups baked beans with molasses
1 cup tofu (calcium is added in processing)

GREENS
1 cup collards
1½ cups kale or turnip greens

BAKED PRODUCTS
3 pieces cornbread
3 English muffins
4 slices French toast
2 waffles (7 inches in diameter)

FRUITS
11 dried figs
1⅛ cups orange juice with calcium added

SAUCES
3 oz pesto sauce
5 oz cheese sauce

Sodium

During pregnancy the need for sodium increases slightly, primarily because the body water is expanding (e.g., the expanding blood volume). Sodium is essential for maintaining body water balance. In the past, dietary sodium was routinely restricted in an effort to control the peripheral edema that commonly occurs during pregnancy. It is now recognized that moderate peripheral edema is normal in pregnancy, occurring as a response to the fluid-retaining effects of elevated levels of estrogen. An excessive emphasis on sodium restriction may make it difficult for pregnant women to achieve an adequate diet. Grain, milk, and meat products, which are good sources of other nutrients needed during pregnancy, are significant sources of sodium. In addition, sodium restriction may stress the adrenal glands and the kidney as they attempt to retain adequate sodium. In general, sodium restriction is necessary only if the woman has a medical condition such as renal or liver failure or hypertension.

Excessive intake of sodium is discouraged during pregnancy just as it is in nonpregnant women, because it may contribute to abnormal fluid retention and edema. Table salt (sodium chloride) is the richest source of sodium. Most canned foods contain added salt unless the label specifically states otherwise. Large amounts of sodium are also found in many processed foods, including meats (e.g., smoked or cured meats, cold cuts, and corned beef), baked goods, mixes for casseroles or grain products, soups, and condiments. Products low in nutritive value and excessively high in sodium include pretzels, potato and other chips, pickles, catsup, prepared mustard, steak and Worcestershire sauces, some soft drinks, and bouillon. A moderate sodium intake can usually be achieved by salting food lightly in cooking; adding no additional salt at the table; and avoiding low-nutrient, high-sodium foods.

Zinc

Zinc is a constituent of numerous enzymes involved in major metabolic pathways. Zinc deficiency is associated with malformations of the central nervous system in infants. When large amounts of iron and folic acid are consumed, the absorption of zinc is inhibited and serum zinc levels are reduced as a result. Because iron and folic acid supplements are commonly prescribed during pregnancy, pregnant women should be encouraged to consume good sources of zinc daily (see Table 10-1). Women with anemia who receive high-dose iron supplements also need supplements of zinc and copper (King, 2000).

Fluoride

There is no evidence that prenatal fluoride supplementation reduces the child's likelihood of tooth decay during the preschool years (Fluoride Recommendations Work Group, 2001). No increase in fluoride intake over the nonpregnant DRI is currently recommended during pregnancy.

Fat-soluble vitamins

Fat-soluble vitamins—A, D, E, and K—are stored in the body tissues. With chronic overdoses these vitamins can reach toxic levels. Because of the high potential for toxicity, pregnant women are advised to take fat-soluble vitamin supplements only as prescribed. Vitamins A and D deserve special mention.

Adequate intake of vitamin A is needed so that sufficient amounts can be stored in the fetus. Dietary sources can readily supply sufficient amounts. Congenital malformations have occurred in infants of mothers who took excessive amounts of vitamin A during pregnancy, and therefore supplements are not recommended for pregnant women. Vitamin A analogs such as isotretinoin (Accutane), which are prescribed for the treatment of cystic acne, are a special concern. Isotretinoin use during early pregnancy has been associated with an increased incidence of heart malformations, facial abnormalities, cleft palate, hydrocephalus, and deafness and blindness in the infant, as well as an increased risk of miscarriage. Topical agents such as tretinoin (Retin-A) do not appear to enter the circulation in any substantial amounts, but their safety in pregnancy has not been confirmed.

Vitamin D plays an important role in absorption and metabolism of calcium. The main food sources of this vitamin are enriched or fortified foods such as milk and ready-to-eat cereals. Vitamin D is also produced in the skin by the action of ultraviolet light (in sunlight). Severe deficiency may lead to neonatal hypocalcemia and tetany, as well as hypoplasia of the tooth enamel. Women with lactose intolerance and those who do not include milk in their diet for any reason are at risk for vitamin D deficiency. Other risk factors are having dark skin; habitually using clothing that covers most of the skin (e.g., Arab women with extensive body covering); and living in northern latitudes where sunlight exposure is limited, especially during the winter. Use of recommended amounts of sunscreen with a sun protection factor (SPF) rating of 15 reduces skin vitamin D production by as much as 99% (Scanlon, 2001), reinforcing the need for regular intake of fortified foods or a supplement.

Water-soluble vitamins

Body stores of water-soluble vitamins are much smaller than those of fat-soluble vitamins. Water-soluble vitamins, in contrast to fat-soluble vitamins, are readily excreted in the urine. Therefore good sources of these vitamins must be consumed frequently. Toxicity with overdose is less likely than with fat-soluble vitamins.

Because of the increase in RBC production during pregnancy, as well as the nutritional requirements of the rapidly growing cells in the fetus and placenta, pregnant women should consume about 50% more folic acid than nonpregnant women, or about 0.6 mg (600 mcg) daily. In the United States all enriched grain products (this includes most white breads, flour, and pasta) must contain folic acid at a level of 1.4 mg/kg of flour. This level of fortification is designed to supply approximately 0.1 mg of folic acid daily in the average American diet and has significantly increased folic acid consumption in the population as a whole. All women of childbearing potential need careful counseling about including good sources of folic acid in their diet (Box 10-4; see Table 10-1). Supplemental folic acid is usually prescribed to ensure that intake is adequate. Women who have borne a child with a neural tube defect are advised to consume 4 mg of folic acid daily, and a supplement is required for them to achieve this level of intake.

Pyridoxine, or vitamin B_6, is involved in protein metabolism. Although levels of a pyridoxine-containing enzyme have been reported to be low in women with preeclampsia, there is no evidence that supplementation prevents or corrects the condition. No supplement is recommended routinely, but women with poor diets and those at nutritional risk (see Box 10-2) may need a supplement providing 2 mg/day.

Vitamin C, or ascorbic acid, plays an important role in tissue formation and enhances the absorption of iron. The vitamin C needs of most women are readily met by a diet that includes at least one daily serving of citrus fruit or juice or another good source of the vitamin (see Table 10-1), but women who smoke need more. For women at nutritional

---

BOX 10-4

Food Sources of Folate

FOODS PROVIDING 500 mcg OR MORE PER SERVING
- Liver: Chicken, turkey, goose (3½ oz)

FOODS PROVIDING 200 mcg OR MORE PER SERVING
- Liver: Lamb, beef, veal (3½ oz)

FOODS PROVIDING 100 mcg OR MORE PER SERVING
- Legumes, cooked (½ cup)
  - Peas: Black-eyed peas, chickpeas (garbanzos)
  - Beans: Black, kidney, pinto, red, navy
  - Lentils
- Vegetables (½ cup)
  - Asparagus
  - Spinach, cooked
- Papaya (1 medium)
- Breakfast cereal, ready-to-eat (½-1 cup)
- Wheat germ (½ cup)

FOODS PROVIDING 50 mcg OR MORE PER SERVING
- Vegetables (cup)
  - Broccoli
  - Beans: lima, baked, or pork and beans
  - Greens: collards or mustard, cooked
  - Spinach, raw
- Fruits (½ cup)
  - Avocado
  - Orange or orange juice
- Pasta, cooked (1 cup)
- Rice, cooked (1 cup)

FOODS PROVIDING 20 mcg OR MORE PER SERVING
- Bread (1 slice)
- Egg (1 large)
- Corn (½ cup)

---

risk, a supplement of 50 mg/day is recommended. However, if the mother takes excessive doses of this vitamin during pregnancy, a vitamin C deficiency may develop in the infant after birth.

Multivitamin and multimineral supplements during pregnancy

The consensus of the 1992 Institute of Medicine committee is that food can and should be the normal vehicle to meet the additional needs imposed by pregnancy, except for iron. Recall that a supplemental dose of 30 mg/day is recommended. In addition, the recommended folate intake may be difficult for some women to achieve. Some women habitually consume diets that are deficient in necessary nutrients and, for whatever reason, may be unable to change this intake. For these women, a multivitamin-multimineral supplement should be considered to ensure that they consume the RDA for most known vitamins and minerals. It is important that the pregnant woman understand that the use of a vitamin-mineral supplement does not lessen the need to consume a nutritious, well-balanced diet.

Other Nutritional Issues during Pregnancy

Pica and food cravings

Pica, the practice of consuming nonfood substances (e.g., clay, dirt, and laundry starch) or excessive amounts of foodstuffs low in nutritional value (e.g., cornstarch, ice, baking powder, and baking soda), is often influenced by the woman's cultural background (Fig. 10-3). In the United States it appears to be most common among African-American women, women from rural areas, and women with a family history of pica. Regular and heavy consumption of low-nutrient products may cause more nutritious foods to be displaced from the diet, and the items consumed may interfere with the absorption of nutrients, especially minerals. Women with pica have lower hemoglobin levels than those without pica. The possibility of pica must be considered when pregnant women are found to be anemic. The nurse should provide counseling about the health risks associated with pica.

The existence of pica, as well as details of the type and amounts of products ingested, is likely to be discovered only by the sensitive interviewer who has developed a relationship of trust with the woman. It has been proposed that pica and food cravings (e.g., the urge to consume ice cream, pickles, or pizza) during pregnancy are caused by an innate drive to consume nutrients missing from the diet. However, research has not supported this hypothesis.

Adolescent pregnancy needs

Many adolescent females have diets that provide less than the recommended intakes of key nutrients, including energy, calcium, and iron. Pregnant adolescents and their infants are at increased risk of complications during pregnancy and parturition. Growth of the pelvis is delayed in comparison with growth in stature, and this helps to explain why cephalopelvic disproportion and other mechanical problems associated with labor are common among young adolescents. Competition for nutrients between the growing adolescent and the fetus may also contribute to some of the poor outcomes apparent in teen pregnancies. Pregnant adolescents are encouraged to choose a weight gain goal at the upper end of the range for their BMI.

Efforts to improve the nutritional health of pregnant adolescents focus on improving the nutrition knowledge, meal planning, and food preparation and selection skills of young women; promoting access to prenatal care; developing nutrition interventions and educational programs that are effective with adolescents; and striving to understand the factors that create barriers to change in the adolescent population.

Preeclampsia

The cause of preeclampsia is not known. There has been speculation that the poor intake of several nutrients, including calcium, magnesium, vitamin B$_6$, and protein, might foster its development. There is no definite evidence that nutritional deficiencies are causes or that nutritional supplements can help prevent it. At present, a diet adequate in the recommended nutrients (see Table 10-1) appears to be the best means of reducing the risk of preeclampsia.

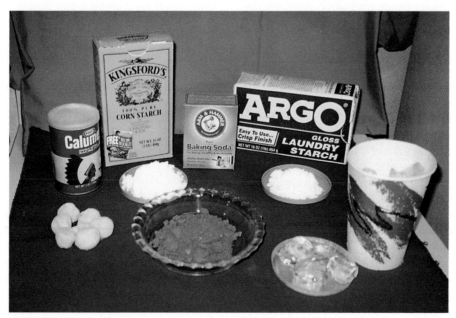

Fig. 10-3 Nonfood substances consumed in pica: (center) red clay from Georgia (left to right); Nzu from Eastern Nigeria, baking powder, corn starch, baking soda, laundry starch, and ice. Some individuals practice *poly-pica* (consuming more than one of these substances.) (Courtesy Shannon Perry, Phoenix, AZ.)

Exercise during pregnancy

Moderate exercise during pregnancy yields numerous benefits, including improving muscle tone, potentially shortening the course of labor, and promoting a sense of well-being. If no medical or obstetric problems contraindicate physical activity, pregnant women should perform 30 minutes of moderate physical exercise on most, if not all, days of the week (American College of Obstetricians and Gynecologists [ACOG], 2002). Two nutritional concepts are especially important for women who choose to exercise during pregnancy. First, a liberal amount of fluid should be consumed before, during, and after exercise because dehydration can trigger premature labor. Second, the calorie intake should be sufficient to meet the increased needs of pregnancy and the demands of exercise.

NUTRIENT NEEDS DURING LACTATION

Nutritional needs during lactation are similar in many ways to those during pregnancy (see Table 10-1). Needs for energy (calories), protein, calcium, iodine, zinc, the B vitamins (thiamine, riboflavin, niacin, pyridoxine, and vitamin B_{12}), and vitamin C remain greater than nonpregnant needs. The recommendations for some of these (e.g., vitamin C, zinc, and protein) are slightly to moderately higher than during pregnancy (see Table 10-1). This allowance covers the amount of the nutrients released in the milk, as well as the needs of the mother for tissue maintenance. In the case of iron and folic acid, the recommendation during lactation is lower than during pregnancy. Both of these nutrients are essential for RBC formation and therefore for maintaining the increase in the blood volume that occurs during pregnancy. With the decrease in maternal blood volume to nonpregnant levels after birth, maternal iron and folic acid needs also decrease. Many lactating women have a delay in the return of menses; this conserves blood cells and reduces iron and folic acid needs. It is especially important that the calcium intake be adequate; if it is not and the women does not respond to diet counseling, a supplement of 600 mg of calcium per day may be needed.

The recommended energy intake is an increase of 500 kcal more than the woman's nonpregnant intake. The Institute of Medicine (1992) recommends that lactating women consume at least 1800 kcal/day; it is difficult to obtain adequate nutrients for maintenance of lactation at levels below that. Because of the deposition of energy stores, the woman who has gained the optimal amount of weight during pregnancy is heavier after birth than at the beginning of pregnancy. As a result of the caloric demands of lactation, however, the lactating mother usually experiences a gradual but steady weight loss. Most women rapidly lose several pounds during the first month after birth whether or not they breastfeed. After the first month the average loss during lactation is 0.5 to 1 kg a month.

Fluid intake must be adequate to maintain milk production, but the mother's level of thirst is the best guide to the right amount. There is no need to consume more fluids than those needed to satisfy thirst.

Smoking, alcohol intake, and excessive caffeine intake should be avoided during lactation. Smoking may not only impair milk production but also may expose the infant to the risk of passive smoking. It is speculated that the infant's psychomotor development may be affected by maternal alcohol use, and alcoholic beverages (two drinks per day) may impair the milk ejection reflex. Caffeine intake may lead to a reduced iron concentration in milk and consequently contribute to the development of anemia in the infant. The caffeine concentration in milk is only approximately 1% of the mother's plasma level, but caffeine seems to accumulate in the infant. Breastfed infants of mothers who drink large amounts of coffee or caffeine-containing soft drinks may be unusually active and wakeful.

CARE MANAGEMENT

During pregnancy, nutrition plays a key role in achieving an optimum outcome for the mother and her unborn baby. Motivation to learn about nutrition is usually higher during pregnancy as parents strive to "do what's right for the baby." Optimum nutrition cannot eliminate all problems that may arise during pregnancy, but it does establish a good foundation for supporting the needs of the mother and her unborn baby.

Assessment and Nursing Diagnoses

Assessment is based on a diet history (a description of the woman's usual food and beverage intake and factors affecting her nutritional status, such as medications being taken and adequacy of income to allow her to purchase the necessary foods) obtained from an interview and review of the woman's health records, physical examination, and laboratory results. Ideally, a nutritional assessment is performed before conception so that any recommended changes in diet, lifestyle, and weight can be undertaken before the woman becomes pregnant.

Diet history

Obstetric and gynecologic effects on nutrition. Nutritional reserves may be depleted in the multiparous woman or one who has had frequent pregnancies (especially three pregnancies within 2 years). A history of preterm birth or the birth of an LBW or SGA infant may indicate inadequate dietary intake. Preeclampsia may also be a factor in poor maternal nutrition. Birth of a large-for-gestational-age (LGA) infant may indicate the existence of maternal diabetes mellitus. Previous contraceptive methods also may affect reproductive health. Increased menstrual blood loss often occurs during the first 3 to 6 months after placement of an intrauterine contraceptive device. Consequently the user may have low iron stores or even iron deficiency anemia. Oral contraceptive agents, on the other hand, are associated with decreased menstrual losses and increased iron stores. Oral contraceptives, however, may interfere with folic acid metabolism.

Medical history. Chronic maternal illnesses such as diabetes mellitus, renal disease, liver disease, cystic fibrosis or other malabsorptive disorders, seizure disorders and the use of anticonvulsant agents, hypertension, and PKU may affect a woman's nutritional status and dietary needs. In women with illnesses that have resulted in nutritional deficits or that require dietary treatment (e.g., diabetes mellitus, PKU), it is extremely important for nutritional care to be started and for the condition to be optimally controlled before conception. A registered dietitian can provide in-depth counseling for the woman who requires a therapeutic diet during pregnancy and lactation.

Usual maternal diet. The woman's usual food and beverage intake, adequacy of income and other resources to meet her nutritional needs, any dietary modifications, food allergies and intolerances, and all medications and nutrition supplements being taken, as well as pica and cultural dietary requirements, should be ascertained. In addition, the presence and severity of nutrition-related discomforts of pregnancy, such as morning sickness, constipation, and pyrosis (heartburn), should be determined. The nurse should be alert to any evidence of eating disorders such as anorexia nervosa, bulimia, or frequent and rigorous dieting before or during pregnancy.

The impact of food allergies and intolerances on nutritional status ranges from very important to almost none. Lactose intolerance is of special concern in pregnant and lactating women because no other food group equals milk and milk products in terms of calcium content. If a woman has lactose intolerance, the interviewer should explore her intake of other calcium sources (see Box 10-3).

The assessment must include an evaluation of the woman's financial status and her knowledge of sound dietary practices. The quality of the diet improves with increasing socioeconomic status and educational level. Poor women may not have access to adequate refrigeration and cooking facilities and may find it difficult to obtain adequate nutritious food. The pregnancy rates are high among homeless women, and many such women cannot or do not take advantage of services such as food stamps.

Box 10-5 provides a simple tool for obtaining diet history information. When potential problems are identified, they should be followed up with a careful interview.

Physical examination. Anthropometric (body) measurements provide short- and long-term information about a woman's nutritional status and are therefore essential to the assessment. At a minimum, the woman's height and weight must be determined at the time of her first prenatal visit, and her weight should be measured at each subsequent visit (see earlier discussion of BMI).

A careful physical examination can reveal objective signs of malnutrition (Table 10-4). It is important to note, however, that some of these signs are nonspecific and that the physiologic changes of pregnancy may complicate the interpretation of physical findings. For example, lower extremity edema often occurs in calorie and protein deficiency, but it may also be a normal finding in the third trimester of pregnancy. Interpretation of physical findings is made easier by a thorough health history and by laboratory testing, if indicated.

Laboratory testing. The only nutrition-related laboratory testing needed by most pregnant women is a hematocrit or hemoglobin measurement to screen for the presence of anemia. Because of the physiologic anemia of pregnancy, the reference values for hemoglobin and hematocrit must be adjusted during pregnancy. The lower limit of the normal range for hemoglobin during pregnancy is 11 g/dl in the first and third trimesters and 10.5 g/dl in the second trimester (compared with 12 g/dl in the nonpregnant state). The lower limit of the normal range for hematocrit is 33% during the first and third trimesters and 32% in the second trimester (compared with 36% in the nonpregnant state). Cutoff values for anemia are higher in women who smoke or who live at high altitudes, because the decreased oxygen-carrying capacity of their RBCs causes them to produce more RBCs than other women.

A woman's history or physical findings may indicate the need for additional testing, such as a complete blood cell count with a differential to identify megaloblastic or macrocytic anemia and measurement of levels of specific vitamins or minerals believed to be lacking in the diet.

The assessment gives a basis for making appropriate nursing diagnoses.

- *Imbalanced nutrition: less than body requirements related to*
  —inadequate information about nutritional needs and weight gain during pregnancy
  —misperceptions regarding normal body changes during pregnancy and inappropriate fear of becoming fat
  —inadequate income or skills in meal planning and preparation
- *Imbalanced nutrition: more than body requirements related to*
  —excessive intake of energy (calories) or decrease in activity during pregnancy
  —use of unnecessary dietary supplements
- *Constipation related to*
  —decrease in gastrointestinal motility because of elevated progesterone levels
  —compression of intestines by the enlarging uterus
  —oral iron supplementation

Expected Outcomes of Care

An individualized plan of care based on the nursing diagnoses should be developed in collaboration with the woman. For many women with uncomplicated pregnancies,

BOX 10-5

Food Intake Questionnaire

Which of the following did you eat or drink yesterday? If the way you ate yesterday wasn't the way you usually eat, choose a recent day that was typical for you.

FOOD OR DRINK	NUMBER OF SERVINGS	FOOD OR DRINK	NUMBER OF SERVINGS
Beer, wine, other alcoholic drinks	___	Orange or grapefruit juice	___
Tea	___	Fruit juice other than orange or grapefruit	___
Coffee	___		
Fruit drink	___	Soft drinks	___
Water	___	Milk	___
Cheese	___	Cereal with milk	___
Macaroni and cheese	___	Yogurt	___
Other foods with cheese (such as lasagna, enchiladas, cheeseburgers)	___	Pizza	___
		Melon (such as watermelon, cantaloupe, honeydew)	___
Orange or grapefruit	___		
Bananas	___	Berries (kind_____)	___
Peaches or apricots	___	Apples	___
Green salad	___	Other fruit	___
Spinach or greens	___	Broccoli	___
Green peas	___	Green beans	___
Sweet potatoes	___	Potatoes (other than fried)	___
Carrots	___	Corn	___
Meat	___	Other vegetables	___
Fish	___	Chicken or turkey	___
Peanut butter	___	Egg	___
Dried beans or peas	___	Nuts	___
Bacon or sausage	___	Hot dog	___
Bread	___	Cold cuts (e.g., bologna)	___
Rice	___	Roll/bagel	___
Spaghetti or other pasta	___	Noodles	___
Tortillas	___	Chips	___
French fries	___	Cake	___
Cookie	___	Donut or pastry	___
Pie	___		

Are you often bothered by any of the following? (Circle all that apply)

   Nausea   Vomiting   Heartburn   Constipation

Are you on a special diet? No ___ Yes ___ If yes, what kind? _____

Do you try to limit the amount or kind of food you eat to control your weight? No ___ Yes ___

Do you avoid any foods for health or religious reasons? No ___ Yes ___ If yes, what foods? _____

Do you take any prescribed drugs or medications? No___ Yes ___
   If yes, what are they? _____

Do you take any over-the-counter medications (such as aspirin, cold medicines, Tylenol)?
   No ___ Yes ___ If yes, what are they? _____

Do you take any herbal supplements?
   No ___ Yes ___ If yes, what are they? _____

Do you ever have trouble affording the food you need? No ___ Yes ___

Do you have any help getting the food you need? No ___ Yes ___ (Circle all that apply)
   Food stamps   WIC   School lunch or breakfast
   Food from a food pantry, soup kitchen, or food bank

the nurse can serve as the primary source of nutrition education during pregnancy. The registered dietitian, who has specialized training in diet evaluation and planning, nutritional needs during illness, and ethnic and cultural food patterns, as well as translating nutrient needs into food patterns, often serves as a consultant. Pregnant women with serious nutritional problems, those with intervening illnesses such as diabetes (either preexisting or gestational), and any others requiring in-depth dietary counseling should be referred to the dietitian. The nurse, dietitian, physician, and nurse-midwife collaborate in helping the woman achieve nutrition-related expected outcomes. Some

TABLE 10-4

Physical Assessment of Nutritional Status

SIGNS OF GOOD NUTRITION	SIGNS OF POOR NUTRITION
GENERAL APPEARANCE	
Alert, responsive, energetic, good endurance	Listless, apathetic, cachectic, easily fatigued, looks tired
MUSCLES	
Well developed, firm, good tone, some fat under skin	Flaccid, poor tone, undeveloped, tender, "wasted" appearance
NERVOUS CONTROL	
Good attention span, not irritable or restless, normal reflexes, psychologic stability	Inattentive, irritable, confused, burning and tingling of hands and feet, loss of position and vibratory sense, weakness and tenderness of muscles, decrease or loss of ankle and knee reflexes
GASTROINTESTINAL FUNCTION	
Good appetite and digestion, normal regular elimination, no palpable organs or masses	Anorexia, indigestion, constipation or diarrhea, liver or spleen enlargement
CARDIOVASCULAR FUNCTION	
Normal heart rate and rhythm, no murmurs, normal blood pressure for age	Rapid heart rate, enlarged heart, abnormal rhythm, elevated blood pressure
HAIR	
Shiny, lustrous, firm, not easily plucked, healthy scalp	Stringy, dull, brittle, dry, thin and sparse, depigmented, can be easily plucked
SKIN (GENERAL)	
Smooth, slightly moist, good color	Rough, dry, scaly, pale, pigmented, irritated, easily bruised, petechiae
FACE AND NECK	
Skin color uniform, smooth, pink, healthy appearance; no enlargement of thyroid gland; lips not chapped or swollen	Scaly, swollen, skin dark over cheeks and under eyes, lumpiness or flakiness of skin around nose and mouth; thyroid enlarged; lips swollen, angular lesions or fissures at corners of mouth
ORAL CAVITY	
Reddish pink mucous membranes and gums; no swelling or bleeding of gums; tongue healthy pink or deep reddish in appearance, not swollen or smooth, surface papillae present; teeth bright and clean, no cavities, no pain, no discoloration	Gums spongy, bleed easily, inflamed or receding; tongue swollen, scarlet and raw, magenta color, beefy, hyperemic and hypertrophic papillae, atrophic papillae; teeth with unfilled caries, absent teeth, worn surfaces, mottled
EYES	
Bright, clear, shiny, no sores at corners of eyelids, membranes moist and healthy pink color, no prominent blood vessels or mound of tissue (Bitot's spots) on sclera, no fatigue circles beneath	Eye membranes pale, redness of membrane, dryness, signs of infection, Bitot's spots, redness and fissuring of eyelid corners, dryness of eye membrane, dull appearance of cornea, soft cornea, blue sclerae
EXTREMITIES	
No tenderness, weakness, or swelling; nails firm and pink	Edema, tender calves, tingling, weakness; nails spoon-shaped, brittle
SKELETON	
No malformations	Bowlegs, knock-knees, chest deformity at diaphragm, beaded ribs, prominent scapulas

common nutrition-related outcomes are that the woman will take the following actions:

- Achieve an appropriate weight gain during pregnancy. An appropriate goal for weight gain takes into account such factors as prepregnancy weight, whether she is overweight or obese or underweight, and whether the pregnancy is single or multifetal.
- Consume adequate nutrients from the diet and supplements to meet estimated needs.
- Cope successfully with nutrition-related discomforts associated with pregnancy, such as morning sickness, pyrosis (heartburn), and constipation.
- Avoid or reduce potentially harmful practices such as smoking, alcohol consumption, and caffeine intake.
- Return to prepregnancy weight (or an appropriate weight for height) within 6 months of giving birth.

Plan of Care and Interventions

Nutritional care and teaching generally involve the following: (1) acquainting the woman with nutritional needs during pregnancy and, if necessary, the characteristics of an adequate diet; (2) helping her individualize her diet so that she achieves an adequate intake while conforming to her personal, cultural, financial, and health circumstances; (3) acquainting her with strategies for coping with the nutrition-related discomforts of pregnancy; (4) helping her use nutrition supplements appropriately; and (5) consulting with and making referrals to other professionals or services as indicated. Two programs that provide nutrition services are the food stamp program and WIC. These programs provide vouchers for selected foods to pregnant and lactating women, as well as infants and children at nutritional risk. WIC foods include items such as eggs, cheese, milk, juice, and fortified cereals—foods chosen because they provide iron, protein, vitamin C, and other vitamins.

Adequate dietary intake

Diet teaching can take place in a one-on-one interview or in a group setting. In either case, teaching should emphasize the importance of choosing a varied diet composed of readily available foods, rather than specialized diet supplements. Good nutrition practices (and avoidance of poor practices such as smoking and alcohol or drug use) are essential content for prenatal classes designed for women in early pregnancy (see Guidelines/Guías box).

MyPyramid (Fig. 10-4), an update of the Food Guide Pyramid, can be used as a guide for making daily food choices during pregnancy and lactation, just as it is during other stages of the life cycle. Five categories are specified: grains, vegetables, fruits, milk, and meats and beans. At least 3 oz of whole grain breads, cereals, rice, and pasta per day is recommended. Other daily recommendations are 2½ cups of vegetables, 2 cups of fruits, 3 cups of low-fat or fat-free milk or milk products, and 5½ oz of protein (meat and beans). Most of the fat in the diet should come from fish, nuts, and vegetable oils. The importance of consuming adequate amounts from the

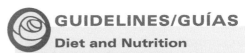

GUIDELINES/GUÍAS
Diet and Nutrition

- You need to gain weight.
- *Usted necesita aumentar de peso.*

- You need to control your weight gain.
- *Usted necesita controlar su aumento de peso.*

- Eat nutritious foods.
- *Coma alimentos nutritivos.*

- Eat foods high in protein, calcium, vitamins, and iron.
- *Coma alimentos altos en proteínas, calcio, vitaminas, y hierro.*

- Eat a lot of fruits and vegetables.
- *Coma muchas frutas y vegetales.*

- Drink four glasses of milk a day.
- *Tome cuatro vasos de leche diariamente.*

- Drink low-fat instead of whole milk.
- *Tome la leche baja en grasa en lugar de la leche entera.*

- Avoid salty foods like sausage, hot dogs, and french fries.
- *Evite alimentos muy salados como calchichas, perros calientes, y papitas fritas.*

- Avoid fried foods.
- *Evite las frituras.*

- Avoid caffeine.
- *Evite la cafeína.*

- There is caffeine in Coca-Cola, tea, and chocolate.
- *Hay cafeína en la Coca-Cola, el té, y el chocolate.*

- Take prenatal vitamins.
- *Tome vitaminas prenatales.*

milk, yogurt, and cheese group needs to be emphasized, especially for adolescents and women under age 25, who are still actively adding calcium to their skeletons. Staying within daily calorie needs and exercising a minimum of 30 minutes per day is important.

Pregnancy. The pregnant woman must understand what adequate weight gain during pregnancy means, recognize the reasons for its importance, and be able to evaluate her own gain in terms of the desirable pattern. Many women, particularly those who have worked hard to control their weight before pregnancy, may find it difficult to understand why the weight gain goal is so high when a newborn infant is so small. The nurse can explain that maternal weight gain consists of increments in the weight of many tissues, not just the growing fetus (see Table 10-2).

Dietary overindulgence, which may result in excessive fat stores that persist after giving birth, should be discouraged. Nevertheless, it is best not to focus unduly on weight gain because this could result in feelings of stress and guilt in the woman who does not follow the preferred pattern of gain. Teaching regarding weight gain during pregnancy is summarized in Box 10-6.

Postpartum. The need for a varied diet with portions of food from all food groups continues throughout lactation. As mentioned previously, the lactating woman should be

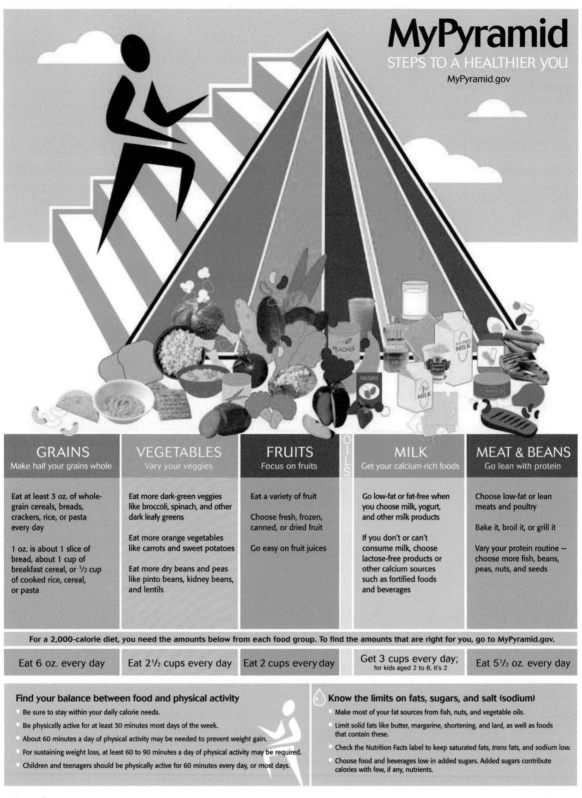

MyPyramid
STEPS TO A HEALTHIER YOU
MyPyramid.gov

GRAINS	VEGETABLES	FRUITS	OILS	MILK	MEAT & BEANS
Make half your grains whole	Vary your veggies	Focus on fruits		Get your calcium-rich foods	Go lean with protein
Eat at least 3 oz. of whole-grain cereals, breads, crackers, rice, or pasta every day 1 oz. is about 1 slice of bread, about 1 cup of breakfast cereal, or ½ cup of cooked rice, cereal, or pasta	Eat more dark-green veggies like broccoli, spinach, and other dark leafy greens Eat more orange vegetables like carrots and sweet potatoes Eat more dry beans and peas like pinto beans, kidney beans, and lentils	Eat a variety of fruit Choose fresh, frozen, canned, or dried fruit Go easy on fruit juices		Go low-fat or fat-free when you choose milk, yogurt, and other milk products If you don't or can't consume milk, choose lactose-free products or other calcium sources such as fortified foods and beverages	Choose low-fat or lean meats and poultry Bake it, broil it, or grill it Vary your protein routine — choose more fish, beans, peas, nuts, and seeds

For a 2,000-calorie diet, you need the amounts below from each food group. To find the amounts that are right for you, go to MyPyramid.gov.

Eat 6 oz. every day	Eat 2½ cups every day	Eat 2 cups every day		Get 3 cups every day; for kids aged 2 to 8, it's 2	Eat 5½ oz. every day

Find your balance between food and physical activity
- Be sure to stay within your daily calorie needs.
- Be physically active for at least 30 minutes most days of the week.
- About 60 minutes a day of physical activity may be needed to prevent weight gain.
- For sustaining weight loss, at least 60 to 90 minutes a day of physical activity may be required.
- Children and teenagers should be physically active for 60 minutes every day, or most days.

Know the limits on fats, sugars, and salt (sodium)
- Make most of your fat sources from fish, nuts, and vegetable oils.
- Limit solid fats like butter, margarine, shortening, and lard, as well as foods that contain these.
- Check the Nutrition Facts label to keep saturated fats, *trans* fats, and sodium low.
- Choose food and beverages low in added sugars. Added sugars contribute calories with few, if any, nutrients.

MyPyramid.gov
STEPS TO A HEALTHIER YOU

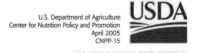
U.S. Department of Agriculture
Center for Nutrition Policy and Promotion
April 2005
CNPP-15

USDA is an equal opportunity provider and employer

Fig. 10-4 MyPyramid: a guide to daily food choices. (Modified from U.S. Department of Health and Human Services and U.S. Department of Agriculture. *Dietary Guidelines for Americans,* 2005, 6th ed. Washington, DC: U.S. Government Printing Office and U.S. Department of Agriculture Center for Nutrition Policy and Promotion, April 2005, CNPP-16).

Weight Gain during Pregnancy

- Progressive weight gain during pregnancy is essential to ensure normal fetal growth and development and the deposition of maternal stores that promote successful lactation.
- Recommended weight gain during pregnancy is determined largely by prepregnancy weight for height: normal-weight women, 11.5-16 kg; underweight women, 12.5-18 kg; overweight women, 7-11.5 kg.
- Weight gain should be achieved through a balanced diet of regular foods chosen from all the different food groups (see Table 10-3).
- The pattern of weight gain is important: approximately 0.4 kg/week during the second and third trimesters for normal-weight women; 0.5 kg/week for underweight women; and 0.3 kg/week for overweight women.

advised to consume at least 1800 kcal daily, and she should receive counseling if her diet appears to be inadequate in any nutrients. Special attention should be given to her zinc, vitamin B_6, and folic acid intake because the recommendations for these remain higher than for nonpregnant women (see Table 10-1). Sufficient calcium is needed to allow for both milk formation and for maintenance of maternal bone mass. It may be difficult for lactating women to consume enough of these nutrients without careful diet planning.

The woman who does not breastfeed loses weight gradually if she consumes a balanced diet that provides slightly less than her daily energy expenditure. Lactating and nonlactating women should know that fat is the most concentrated source of calories in the diet (9 kcal/g versus 4 kcal/g in carbohydrates and proteins). Therefore the first step in weight reduction (or preventing excessive weight gain) is to evaluate sources of fat in the diet and explore with the woman ways of reducing them. Even foods such as vegetables that are naturally low in fat can become high in fat when fried or sautéed, served with excessive amounts of salad dressing, consumed with high-fat dips or sauces, or seasoned with butter or bacon drippings. A reasonable weight loss goal for nonlactating women is 0.5 to 1 kg/week; a loss of 1 kg/month is recommended for most lactating women who need to lose weight. A woman who is lactating may be able to lose up to 2 kg/month without decreasing her milk supply.

Daily food guide and menu planning. The daily food plan (see Table 10-2 and Fig. 10-4) can be used as a guide for educating women about nutritional needs during pregnancy and lactation. This food plan is general enough to be used by women from a variety of cultures, including those following a vegetarian diet. One of the more helpful teaching strategies is to assist the woman to plan daily menus that follow the food plan and are affordable, have realistic preparation times, and are compatible with personal preferences and cultural practices. Information regarding cultural food patterns is provided later in this chapter.

Medical nutrition therapy. During pregnancy and lactation, the food plan for women with special medical nutrition therapy (therapeutic diets) may have to be modified. The registered dietitian can instruct these women about their diets and assist them in meal planning. However, the nurse should understand the basic principles of the diet and be able to reinforce the diet teaching.

The nurse should be especially aware of the dietary modifications necessary for women with diabetes mellitus (either gestational or preexisting). This is necessary because this disease is relatively common and because fetal deformity and death occur more often in pregnancies complicated by hyperglycemia or hypoglycemia (see discussion of diabetes in Chapter 22).

Counseling about iron supplementation

As mentioned earlier, the nutritional supplement most commonly needed during pregnancy is iron. However, a variety of dietary factors can affect the completeness of absorption of an iron supplement. The following points should be addressed in patient education:

- Bran, milk, egg yolks, coffee, tea, or oxalate-containing vegetables such as spinach and Swiss chard will inhibit iron absorption if consumed at the same time as iron.
- Iron absorption is promoted by a diet rich in vitamin C (e.g., citrus fruits and melons) or "heme iron" (found in red meats, fish, and poultry).
- Iron supplements are best absorbed on an empty stomach; to this end they can be taken between meals with beverages other than milk, tea, or coffee.
- Some women have gastrointestinal discomfort when they take the supplement on an empty stomach; therefore a good time for them to take the supplement is just before bedtime.
- Constipation is common with iron supplementation.
- Iron supplements should be kept away from any children in the household because their ingestion could result in acute iron poisoning and even death.

Coping with nutrition-related discomforts of pregnancy

The most common nutrition-related discomforts of pregnancy are nausea and vomiting (or "morning sickness"), constipation, and pyrosis.

Nausea and vomiting. Nausea and vomiting are most common during the first trimester. Usually, nausea and vomiting cause only mild to moderate problems nutritionally, although they may cause substantial discomfort. Antiemetic medications, vitamin B_6, and p6 acupressure may be effective in reducing the severity of nausea (Jewell & Young, 2004). The pregnant woman may find the following suggestions helpful in alleviating the problems:

- Eat dry, starchy foods such as dry toast, Melba toast, or crackers on awakening in the morning and at other times when nausea occurs.

- Avoid consuming excessive amounts of fluids early in the day or when nauseated (but compensate by drinking fluids at other times).
- Eat small amounts frequently (every 2 to 3 hours), and avoid large meals that distend the stomach.
- Avoid skipping meals and thereby becoming extremely hungry, which may worsen nausea. Have a snack such as cereal with milk, a small sandwich, or yogurt before bedtime.
- Avoid sudden movements. Get out of bed slowly.
- Decrease intake of fried and other fatty foods. Starches such as pastas, rice, and breads and low-fat, high-protein foods such as skinless broiled or baked poultry, cooked dry beans or peas, lean meats, and broiled or canned fish are good choices.
- Some women find that tart foods or drinks (e.g., lemonade) or salty foods (e.g., potato chips) are tolerated during periods of nausea.
- Fresh air may help relieve nausea. Keep the environment well ventilated (e.g., open a window), go for a walk outside, or decrease cooking odors by using an exhaust fan.
- During periods of nausea, eat foods served at cool temperatures and foods that give off little aroma.
- Try herbal teas such as those made with raspberry leaf or peppermint to decrease nausea.
- Ginger root may be effective in reducing nausea.
- Avoid brushing teeth immediately after eating.

Hyperemesis gravidarum (severe and persistent vomiting causing weight loss, dehydration, and electrolyte abnormalities) occurs in up to 1% of pregnant women. Intravenous fluid and electrolyte replacement is usually necessary for women who lose 5% of their body weight. Often this is followed by improved tolerance of oral intake; therapy then consists of frequent consumption of small amounts of low-fat foods. Enteral tube feeding using small-bore nasogastric tubes has been successful for some women. Because pulmonary aspiration of the feeding is a potential complication if vomiting occurs, antiemetic medications are sometimes used in conjunction with tube feedings. Tube feedings may be used to supplement oral intake, with the volume of the tube feeding gradually being decreased as oral intake improves. In some instances, total parenteral nutrition (balanced intravenous feedings of amino acids, carbohydrate, lipid, vitamins, and minerals) is used to nourish women with hyperemesis gravidarum when their nutritional status has been severely impaired.

Constipation. Improved bowel function generally results from increasing the intake of fiber (e.g., wheat bran and whole-wheat products, popcorn, and raw or lightly steamed vegetables) in the diet. Fiber helps retain water within the stool, creating a bulky stool that stimulates intestinal peristalsis. The recommendation for adults for fiber is 25 to 35 g/day. An increase of approximately 15% would be optimal. An adequate fluid intake (at least 50 ml/kg/day) helps hydrate the fiber and increase the bulk of the stool. Making a habit

of regular exercise that uses large muscle groups (walking, swimming, cycling) also helps stimulate bowel motility.

Pyrosis. Pyrosis, or heartburn, is usually caused by reflux of gastric contents into the esophagus. This condition can be minimized by eating small, frequent meals rather than two or three larger meals daily. Because fluids increase the distention of the stomach, they should not be consumed with foods. The woman needs to be sure to drink adequate amounts between meals. Avoiding spicy foods may help alleviate the problem. Lying down immediately after eating and wearing clothing that is tight across the abdomen can contribute to the problem of reflux.

Cultural influences

Consideration of a woman's cultural food preferences enhances communication and provides a greater opportunity for following the agreed-on pattern of intake. Women in most cultures are encouraged to eat a diet typical for them. The nurse needs to be aware of what constitutes a typical diet for each cultural or ethnic group. However, several variations may occur within one cultural group. Therefore a careful exploration of individual preferences is needed. Although some ethnic and cultural food beliefs may seem, at first glance, to conflict with the dietary instruction provided by physicians, nurses, and dietitians, it is often possible for the empathic health care provider to identify cultural beliefs that are congruent with the modern understanding of pregnancy and fetal development. Many cultural food practices have some merit or the culture would not have survived. Food cravings during pregnancy are considered normal by many cultures, but the kinds of cravings often are culturally specific. In most cultures women crave acceptable foods, such as chicken, fish, and greens among African-Americans. Cultural influences on food intake usually lessen if the woman and her family become more integrated into the dominant culture. Nutrition beliefs and the practices of selected cultural groups are summarized in Table 10-5.

Vegetarian diets. Vegetarian diets represent another cultural effect on nutritional status. Foods basic to almost all vegetarian diets are vegetables, fruits, legumes, nuts, seeds, and grains. However, there are many variations in vegetarian diets. Semivegetarians, who are not truly vegetarians, include fish, poultry, eggs, and dairy products in their diets but do not eat beef or pork. Such a diet can be completely adequate for pregnant women. Besides plant products, lacto-ovovegetarians also eat dairy products and eggs. Iron and zinc intake may not be adequate in these women, but such diets can be otherwise nutritionally sound. Strict vegetarians, or vegans, consume only plant products. Because vitamin B_{12} is found only in foods of animal origin, this diet is therefore deficient in vitamin B_{12}. As a result, strict vegetarians should take a supplement or regularly consume vitamin B_{12}–fortified foods (e.g., soy milk). Vitamin B_{12} deficiency can result in megaloblastic anemia, glossitis (inflamed red tongue), and neurologic deficits in the mother. Infants born to affected mothers are likely to have megaloblastic anemia and exhibit neurodevelopmental

TABLE 10-5

Characteristic Food Patterns of Selected Cultures

MILK GROUP	PROTEIN GROUP	FRUITS AND VEGETABLES	BREADS AND CEREALS	POSSIBLE DIETARY PROBLEMS
NATIVE AMERICAN (MANY TRIBAL VARIATIONS; MANY "AMERICANIZED")				
Fresh milk Evaporated milk for cooking Ice cream Cream pie	Pork, beef, lamb, rabbit Fowl, fish, eggs Legumes Sunflower seeds Nuts: walnuts, acorn, pine, peanut butter Game meat	Green peas, beans Beets, turnips Leafy green and other vegetables Grapes, bananas, peaches, other fresh fruits Roots	Refined bread Whole wheat Cornmeal Rice Dry cereals "Fry" bread Tortillas	Obesity, diabetes, alcoholism, nutritional deficiencies expressed in dental problems and iron deficiency anemia Inadequate amounts of all nutrients Excessive use of sugar
MIDDLE EASTERN* (ARMENIAN, GREEK, SYRIAN, TURKISH)				
Yogurt Little butter	Lamb Nuts Dried peas, beans, lentils Sesame seeds	Peppers, tomatoes, cabbage, grape leaves, cucumbers, squash Dried apricots, raisins, dates	Cracked wheat and dark bread	Fry many meats and vegetables Lack of fresh fruits Insufficient foods from milk group High consumption of sweetenings, lamb fat, and olive oil
AFRICAN-AMERICAN (PARTICULARLY SOUTHERN AND RURAL)				
Milk† Ice cream Cheese: longhorn, American	Pork: all cuts, plus organs, chitterlings Beef, lamb Chicken, giblets Eggs Nuts Legumes Fish, game	Leafy vegetables Green and yellow vegetables Potato: white, sweet Stewed fruit Bananas and other fresh fruit	Cornmeal and hominy grits Rice Biscuits, pancakes, white breads Puddings: bread, rice	Extensive use of frying, smothering in gravy, or simmering Fats: salt pork, bacon drippings, lard, and gravies High consumption of sweets Insufficient citrus Vegetables often boiled for long periods with pork fat and much salt Limited amounts from milk group†
CHINESE (CANTONESE MOST PREVALENT)				
Milk: water buffalo	Pork sausage‡ Eggs and pigeon eggs Fish Lamb, beef, goat Fowl: chicken, duck Nuts Legumes Soybean curd (tofu)	Many vegetables Radish leaves Bean, bamboo sprouts	Rice/rice flour products Cereals, noodles Wheat, corn, millet seed	Tendency of some immigrants to use large amounts of grease in cooking Limited use of milk and milk products Often low in protein, calories, or both Soy sauce (high sodium)

MSG, monosodium L-glutamate.
*Religious holidays may involve fasting, which is believed to increase the likelihood of preterm labor. Fasting requirement may be waived during pregnancy.
†Lactose intolerance relatively common in adults.
‡Lower in fat content than Western sausage.

TABLE 10-5

Characteristic Food Patterns of Selected Cultures—cont'd

MILK GROUP	PROTEIN GROUP	FRUITS AND VEGETABLES	BREADS AND CEREALS	POSSIBLE DIETARY PROBLEMS
FILIPINO (SPANISH-CHINESE INFLUENCE)				
Flavored milk Milk in coffee Cheese: gouda, cheddar	Pork, beef, goat, rabbit Chicken Fish Eggs, nuts, legumes	Many vegetables and fruits	Rice, cooked cereals Noodles: rice, wheat	Limited use of milk and milk products Tendency to prewash rice Tendency to have only small portions of protein foods
ITALIAN				
Cheese Some ice cream	Meat Eggs Dried beans	Leafy vegetables Potatoes Eggplant, tomatoes, peppers Fruits	Pasta White breads, some whole wheat Farina Cereals	Prefer expensive imported cheeses; reluctant to substitute less expensive domestic varieties Tendency to overcook vegetables Limited use of whole grains High consumption of sweets Extensive use of olive oil Insufficient servings from milk group
JAPANESE (ISEI, MORE JAPANESE INFLUENCE; NISEI, MORE WESTERNIZED)				
Increasing amounts being used by younger generations	Pork, beef, chicken Fish Eggs Legumes: soys, red, lima beans Tofu Nuts	Many vegetables and fruits Seaweed	Rice, rice cakes Wheat noodles Refined bread, noodles	Excessive sodium: pickles, salty crisp seaweed, MSG, and soy sauce Insufficient servings from milk group May use prewashed rice
HISPANIC, MEXICAN-AMERICAN				
Milk Cheese Flan, ice cream	Beef, pork, lamb, chicken, tripe, hot sausage, beef intestines Fish Eggs Nuts Dry beans: pinto, chickpeas (often eaten more than once daily)	Spinach, wild greens, tomatoes, chilies, corn, cactus leaves, cabbage, avocado, potatoes Pumpkin, zapote, peaches, guava, papaya, citrus	Rice, cornmeal Sweet bread, pastries Tortilla: corn, flour Vermicelli (fideo)	Limited meats primarily due to cost Limited use of milk and milk products Large amounts of lard Abundant use of sugar Tendency to boil vegetables for long periods

Continued

TABLE 10-5

Characteristic Food Patterns of Selected Cultures—cont'd

MILK GROUP	PROTEIN GROUP	FRUITS AND VEGETABLES	BREADS AND CEREALS	POSSIBLE DIETARY PROBLEMS
PUERTO RICAN				
Limited use of milk products Coffee with milk (café con leche)	Pork Poultry Eggs (Fridays) Dried codfish Beans (habichuelas)	Avocado, okra Eggplant Sweet yams Starchy vegetables and fruits (viandas)	Rice Cornmeal	Small amounts of pork and poultry Extensive use of fat, lard, salt pork, and olive oil Lack of milk products
SCANDINAVIAN (DANISH, FINNISH, NORWEGIAN, SWEDISH)				
Cream Butter Cheeses	Wild game Reindeer Fish (fresh or dried) Eggs	Berries Dried fruit Vegetables: cole slaw, roots	Whole wheat, rye, barley, sweets (cookies and sweet breads)	Insufficient fresh fruits and vegetables High consumption of sweets, pickled or salted meats, and fish
SOUTHEAST ASIAN (VIETNAMESE, CAMBODIAN)				
Generally not taken Coffee with condensed cow's milk Plain yogurt Ice cream (rare) Soybean milk	Fish (daily): fresh, dried, salted Poultry/eggs: duck, chicken Pork Beef (seldom) Dry beans Tofu	Seasonal variety: fresh or preserved Green, leafy vegetables Yams Corn	Rice: grains, flour, noodles French bread "Cellophane" (bean starch) noodles	Fresh milk products generally not consumed Poultry/eggs may be limited Meat considered "unclean" is avoided Preference for a diet high in salt and pepper, as well as rice and pork High intake of MSG and soy sauce
JEWISH: ORTHODOX*				
Milk† Cheese†	Meat (bloodless; Kosher prepared): beef, lamb, goat, deer, poultry (all types), no pork Fish with fins and scales only No crustaceans	Wide variety	Wide variety	High intake of sodium in meat products

delays. Iron, calcium, zinc, and vitamin B_6 intake may also be low in women on this diet, and some strict vegetarians have excessively low caloric intakes. The protein intake should be assessed especially carefully because plant proteins tend to be incomplete in that they lack one or more amino acids required for growth and maintenance of body tissues. The daily consumption of a variety of different plant proteins (grains, dried beans and peas, nuts, and seeds) helps provide all of the essential amino acids.

Evaluation

In evaluating the adequacy of nutritional intake during pregnancy, the woman's weight gain can be compared with standardized grids showing recommended patterns (see Fig. 10-2). These grids are based on mean data and do not always account for factors such as ethnic or racial variations. To evaluate the adequacy of the woman's diet, it can be compared with the plan in Table 10-2. It is essential that individual factors affecting nutritional needs and dietary intake be considered.

Physical examination and laboratory testing can be used to confirm that nutritional status is adequate (see the section on assessment). When weight gain is inadequate or when nutritional deficits are present, the nurse must reassess the woman and her understanding of her nutritional needs, reinforce teaching as needed, and continue to reevaluate her nutritional status regularly (see Plan of Care).

PLAN OF CARE *Nutrition during Pregnancy*

NURSING DIAGNOSIS Deficient knowledge related to nutritional requirements during pregnancy

Expected Outcome *The patient will delineate nutritional requirements and exhibit evidence of incorporating requirements into diet.*

Nursing Interventions/*Rationales*

- Review basic nutritional requirements for a healthy diet using recommended dietary guidelines and MyPyramid *to provide knowledge baseline for discussion.*
- Discuss increased nutrient needs (calories, protein, minerals, vitamins) that occur as a result of being pregnant *to increase knowledge needed for altered dietary requirements.*
- Discuss the relationship between weight gain and fetal growth *to reinforce interdependence of fetus and mother.*
- Calculate the appropriate total weight gain range during pregnancy using the woman's body mass index (BMI) as a guide and discuss recommended rates of weight gain during the various trimesters of pregnancy *to provide concrete measures of dietary success.*
- Review food preferences, cultural eating patterns or beliefs, and prepregnancy eating patterns *to enhance integration of new dietary needs.*
- Discuss how to fit nutritional needs into usual dietary patterns and how to alter any identified nutritional deficits or excesses *to increase chances of success with dietary alterations.*
- Discuss food aversions or cravings that may occur during pregnancy and strategies to deal with these if they are detrimental to fetus (e.g., pica) *to ensure well-being of fetus.*
- Have woman keep a food diary delineating eating habits, dietary alterations, aversions, and cravings *to track eating habits and potential problem areas.*

NURSING DIAGNOSIS Imbalanced nutrition: more than body requirements related to excessive intake or inadequate activity levels (or both)

Expected Outcome *The patient's weekly weight gain will be reduced to the appropriate rate using her BMI and recommended weight gain ranges as guidelines.*

Nursing Interventions/*Rationales*

- Review recent diet history (including food cravings) using a food diary, 24-hour recall, or food frequency approach *to ascertain food excesses contributing to excess weight gain.*
- Review normal activity and exercise routines *to determine level of energy expenditure;* discuss eating patterns and reasons that lead to increased food intake (e.g., cultural beliefs or myths, increased stress, boredom) *to identify habits that contribute to excess weight gain.*

- Review optimal weight gain guidelines and their rationale *to ensure that woman is knowledgeable about healthful weight gain rates.*
- Set target weight gains for the remaining weeks of the pregnancy *to establish goals.*
- Discuss with the woman what changes can be made in diet, activity, and lifestyle *to enhance chances of meeting weight gain goals and dietary needs.* Weight-reduction diets should be avoided, *because they may deprive the mother and fetus of needed nutrients and lead to ketonemia.*

NURSING DIAGNOSIS Imbalanced nutrition: less than body requirements related to inadequate intake of needed nutrients

Expected Outcome *The woman's weekly weight gain will be increased to the appropriate rate using her BMI and recommended weight gain ranges as guidelines.*

Nursing Interventions/*Rationales*

- Review recent diet history (including food aversions) using a food diary, 24-hour recall, or food frequency approach *to ascertain dietary inadequacies contributing to lack of sufficient weight gain.*
- Review normal activity and exercise routines *to determine level of energy expenditure;* discuss eating patterns and reasons that lead to decreased food intake (e.g., morning sickness, pica, fear of becoming fat, stress, boredom) *to identify habits that contribute to inadequate weight gain.*
- Review optimal weight gain guidelines and their rationale *to ensure that woman is knowledgeable about healthful weight gain rates.*
- Set target weight gains for the remaining weeks of the pregnancy *to establish goals.*
- Review increased nutrient needs (calories, protein, minerals, vitamins) that occur as a result of being pregnant *to ensure that woman is knowledgeable about altered dietary requirements.*
- Review relationship between weight gain and fetal growth *to reinforce that adequate weight gain is needed to promote fetal well-being.*
- Discuss with woman what changes can be made in diet, activity, and lifestyle *to enhance chances of meeting set weight gain goals and nutrient needs of mother and fetus.*
- If woman has fear of being fat, if symptoms of an eating disorder are evident, or if problems in adjusting to a changing body image surface, refer woman to the appropriate mental health professional for evaluation, because intensive treatment and follow-up may be required *to ensure fetal health.*

COMMUNITY ACTIVITY

Visit a prenatal clinic. Identify sources of nutrition education that are evident in the waiting room. Does the clinic employ a nutritionist or dietitian? Who provides nutrition counseling in the clinic? Are print materials available in multiple languages? Are interpreters available? Are there sources of free materials on nutrition that could be placed in the clinic? Are the nutrition education materials culturally relevant? Identify strengths and weaknesses of nutrition education in that setting. Develop a feasible plan for improving nutrition education in the clinic.

Key Points

- A woman's nutritional status before, during, and after pregnancy contributes significantly to her well-being and that of her infant.
- Many physiologic changes occurring during pregnancy influence the need for additional nutrients and the efficiency with which the body uses them.
- Both the total maternal weight gain and the pattern of weight gain are important determinants of the outcome of pregnancy.
- The appropriateness of the mother's prepregnancy weight for height (BMI) is a major determinant of her recommended weight gain during pregnancy.
- Nutritional risk factors include adolescent pregnancy, nicotine use, alcohol or drug use, bizarre or faddish food habits, a low weight for height, and frequent pregnancies.
- Iron supplementation is usually routinely recommended during pregnancy. Other supplements may be warranted when nutritional risk factors are present.
- The nurse and the woman are influenced by cultural and personal values and beliefs during nutrition counseling.
- Pregnancy complications that may be nutrition related include anemia, preeclampsia, gestational diabetes, and IUGR.
- Dietary adaptation can be an effective intervention for some of the common discomforts of pregnancy, including nausea and vomiting, constipation, and heartburn.

Answer Guidelines to Critical Thinking Exercise

Nutrition and the Underweight Pregnant Adolescent

1 Yes. A dietary assessment using a food intake questionnaire should be conducted and a physical assessment of nutritional status performed. Based on these data, the desired pattern of weight gain during pregnancy, and a knowledge of characteristic food patterns of Hispanic people, planning can begin.

2 a. A list of Dietary Reference Intakes for pregnancy and lactation can be shared with Carmen. Through discussion, you can determine whether Carmen is ingesting adequate amounts of these important elements and whether supplementation of vitamins and minerals is necessary.

   b. While reviewing indicators of nutritional risk in pregnancy with Carmen, problem areas can be identified, and recommendations for change provided as needed.

   c. The daily food guide for pregnancy and lactation can be shared with Carmen. It can provide a basis for planning appropriate menus to provide the necessary nutrients and provide more energy (calories) to increase her weight gain, taking into consideration the growth needs of an adolescent

   d. As someone of Hispanic heritage, Carmen may be lactose intolerant and may need sources of calcium other than milk. Through careful questioning, her lactose status can be determined and counseling can be provided about nonmilk sources of calcium.

3 As part of her prenatal care, Carmen (and all pregnant women) should receive nutrition counseling. Carmen is currently underweight. Carmen can be assisted to plan menus that allow a weight gain to support growth of the pregnancy and the fetus and provide nutrients to support her own growth.

4 Yes, there is ample evidence about DRIs in pregnancy and lactation. Nutrition counseling should be part of the plan of care for Carmen.

5 Often adolescents have inadequate intakes of appropriate nutritional elements. They may try to maintain a slender appearance. Women who are underweight are at risk for preterm birth as well as for having a fetus with IUGR. Carmen could be trying to hide her pregnancy by limiting her weight gain. Fast food choices as well as ethnic and cultural patterns of eating could be factors. Enlisting the support of her family would likely be helpful in planning appropriate meals.

Resources

American Botanical Council
P.O. Box 144345
Austin, TX 78714-4345
512-926-4900
www.herbalgram.org

American Diabetes Association
Diabetes Information Service Center
1660 Duke St.
Alexandria, VA 22314
800-342-2383
www.diabetes.org

American Dietetic Association
216 West Jackson Blvd., Suite 800
Chicago, IL 60606-6995
www.eatright.org

American Medical Association
Department of Foods and Nutrition
515 N. State St.
Chicago, IL 60610
www.ama-assn.org

Anorexia Nervosa and Related Eating Disorders, Inc.
www.anred.com

Body Mass Index Calculator
National Heart, Lung, and Blood Institute Information Center
P.O. Box 30105
Bethesda, MD 20824-0105
301-592-8573
www.nhlbisupport.com/bmi

Center for Food Safety and Applied Nutrition
Food and Drug Administration
200 C St., SW
Washington, DC 20250
202-720-2791
www.usda.gov/usda.htm

Food and Nutrition Board
Institute of Medicine
2101 Constitution Ave., NW
Washington, DC 20418
202-334-1732
www.iom.edu
email: fnb@nas.edu

MyPyramid:
www.mypyramid.gov

National Dairy Council
6300 N. River Rd.
Rosemont, IL 60018
www.nutritionexplorations.org

Nutritional content of foods:
www.nal.usda.gov/fnic/foodcomp

Office of Dietary Supplements
National Institutes of Health
31 Center Dr., Room 1829
Bethesda, MD 20892-2086
301-435-2920
www.ods.od.nih.gov

RDAs according to age and sex:
www.nal.usda.gov

Society for Nutrition Education
1001 Connecticut Ave., NW, Suite 529
Washington, DC 20036-5528
202-452-8534
www.sne.org
email: info@sne.org

Special Supplemental Nutrition Program for Women, Infants, and
    Children (WIC)
Food and Consumer Service
3101 Park Center Dr., Room 819
Alexandria, VA 22302
703-305-2286
www.usda.gov

U.S. Department of Agriculture
Food and Nutrition Information Center
14th and Independence Ave., SW
Washington, DC 20250
202-720-2791
www.usda.gov

References

American College of Obstetricians and Gynecologists (ACOG). (2002). Exercise during pregnancy and the postpartum period. ACOG Committee Opinion No. 267. *Obstetrics & Gynecology, 99*(1), 171-173.

Atallah, A., Hofmeyr, G., & Duley, L. (2003). Calcium supplementation during pregnancy for preventing hypertensive disorders and related problems (Cochrane Review). In *The Cochrane Library,* Issue 2, 2004. Chichester, UK: John Wiley & Sons.

Boushey, C., Edmonds, J., & Welshimer, K. (2001). Estimates of the effects of folic-acid fortification and folic-acid bioavailability for women. *Nutrition, 17*(10), 873-879.

Centers for Disease Control and Prevention (CDC). (2004). *PNSS pregnancy nutrition surveillance system.* Internet document available at www.ced.gov/nccdphp/dnpa/PNSS.htm (accessed August 22, 2004).

Fluoride Recommendations Work Group. (2001). Recommendations for using fluoride to prevent and control dental caries in the United States. *Morbidity and Mortality Weekly Report, 50*(RR-14), 1-42.

Food and Nutrition Board, Institute of Medicine. (1997). *Dietary reference intakes for calcium, phosphorus, magnesium, vitamin D, and fluoride.* Washington, DC: National Academy Press.

Food and Nutrition Board, Institute of Medicine. (1998). *Dietary reference intakes for thiamine, riboflavin, niacin, vitamin B_6, folate, vitamin B_{12}, pantothenic acid, biotin, and choline.* Washington, DC: National Academy Press.

Food and Nutrition Board, Institute of Medicine. (2000). *Dietary reference intakes for vitamin C, vitamin E, selenium, and carotenoids.* Washington, DC: National Academy Press.

Food and Nutrition Board, Institute of Medicine. (2001). *Dietary reference intakes for vitamin A, vitamin K, arsenic, boron, chromium, copper, iodine, iron, manganese, molybdenum, nickel, silicon, vanadium, and zinc.* Washington, DC: National Academy Press.

Food and Nutrition Board, National Academy of Science, National Research Council. (1989). *Recommended dietary allowances* (10th ed.). Washington, DC: National Academy Press.

Institute of Medicine. (1992). *Nutrition during pregnancy and lactation: An implementation guide.* Washington, DC: National Academy Press.

Jewell, D., & Young, G. (2004). Interventions for nausea and vomiting in early pregnancy (Cochrane Review). In *The Cochrane Library,* Issue 4, 2004. Chichester, UK: John Wiley & Sons.

Kilpatrick, S., & Laros, R. (2004). Maternal hematologic disorders. In R. Creasy, R. Resnik, & J. Iams (Eds.), *Maternal-fetal medicine: Principles and practice* (5th ed.). Philadelphia: Saunders.

King, J. (2000). Determinants of maternal zinc status during pregnancy. *American Journal of Clinical Nutrition, 71*(5 suppl), 1334S-1343S.

Malone, F., & D'Alton, M. (2004). Multiple gestation: Clinical characteristics and management. In R. Creasy, R. Resnik, & J. Iams (Eds.), *Maternal-fetal medicine: Principles and practice* (5th ed.). Philadelphia: Saunders.

Scanlon, K. (Ed.). (2001). *Final report of the vitamin D expert panel.* Atlanta, GA: Centers for Disease Control and Prevention.

CHAPTER 11

Labor and Birth Processes

DEITRA LEONARD LOWDERMILK

LEARNING OBJECTIVES

- *Explain the five factors that affect the labor process.*
- *Describe the anatomic structure of the bony pelvis.*
- *Recognize the normal measurements of the diameters of the pelvic inlet, cavity, and outlet.*
- *Explain the significance of the size and position of the fetal head during labor and birth.*
- *Summarize the cardinal movements of the mechanism of labor for a vertex presentation.*
- *Assess the maternal anatomic and physiologic adaptations to labor.*
- *Describe fetal adaptations to labor.*

KEY TERMS AND DEFINITIONS

asynclitism Oblique presentation of the fetal head at the superior strait of the pelvis; the pelvic planes and those of the fetal head are not parallel

attitude Relation of fetal parts to each other in the uterus (e.g., all parts flexed, or all parts flexed except neck is extended)

biparietal diameter Largest transverse diameter of the fetal head; measured between the parietal bones

bloody show Vaginal discharge that originates in the cervix and consists of blood and mucus; increases as cervix dilates during labor

dilation Stretching of the external os from an opening a few millimeters in size to an opening large enough to allow the passage of the fetus

effacement Thinning and shortening or obliteration of the cervix that occurs during late pregnancy or labor or both

engagement In obstetrics, the entrance of the fetal presenting part into the superior pelvic strait and the beginning of the descent through the pelvic canal

Ferguson reflex Reflex contractions (urge to push) of the uterus after stimulation of the cervix

fontanels Broad areas, or soft spots, consisting of a strong band of connective tissue contiguous with cranial bones and located at the junctions of the bones

lie Relationship existing between the long axis of the fetus and the long axis of the mother; in a longitudinal lie, the fetus is lying lengthwise or vertically, whereas in a transverse lie, the fetus is lying crosswise or horizontally in the uterus

lightening Sensation of decreased abdominal distention produced by uterine descent into the pelvic cavity as the fetal presenting part settles into the pelvis; usually occurs 2 weeks before the onset of labor in nulliparas

molding Overlapping of cranial bones or shaping of the fetal head to accommodate and conform to the bony and soft parts of the mother's birth canal during labor

position Relationship of a reference point on the presenting part of the fetus, such as the occiput, sacrum, chin, or scapula, to its location in the front, back, or sides of the maternal pelvis

presentation That part of the fetus that first enters the pelvis and lies over the inlet; may be head, face, breech, or shoulder

presenting part That part of the fetus that lies closest to the internal os of the cervix

station Relationship of the presenting fetal part to an imaginary line drawn between the ischial spines of the pelvis

suboccipitobregmatic diameter Smallest diameter of the fetal head; follows a line drawn from the middle of the anterior fontanel to the undersurface of the occipital bone

Valsalva maneuver Any forced expiratory effort against a closed airway, such as holding one's breath and tightening the abdominal muscles (e.g., pushing during the second stage of labor)

vertex Crown, or top, of the head

*D*uring late pregnancy the woman and fetus prepare for the labor process. The fetus has grown and developed in preparation for extrauterine life. The woman has undergone various physiologic adaptations during pregnancy that prepare her for birth and motherhood. Labor and birth represent the end of pregnancy, the beginning of extrauterine life for the newborn, and a change in the lives of the family. This chapter discusses the factors affecting labor, the process involved, the normal progression of events, and the adaptations made by both the woman and fetus.

FACTORS AFFECTING LABOR

At least five factors affect the process of labor and birth. These are easily remembered as the five *P*s: passenger (fetus and placenta), passageway (birth canal), powers (contractions), position of the mother, and psychologic response. The first four factors are presented here as the basis of understanding the physiologic process of labor. The fifth factor is discussed in Chapter 12. Other factors that may be a part of the woman's labor experience may be important as well. VandeVusse (1999) identified external forces including place of birth, preparation, type of provider (especially nurses), and procedures. Physiology (sensations) was identified as an internal force. These factors are discussed generally in Chapter 14 as they relate to nursing care during labor. Further research investigating essential forces of labor is recommended.

Passenger

The way the passenger, or fetus, moves through the birth canal is determined by several interacting factors: the size of the fetal head, fetal presentation, fetal lie, fetal attitude, and fetal position. Because the placenta also must pass through the birth canal, it can be considered a passenger along with the fetus; however, the placenta rarely impedes the process of labor in normal vaginal birth, except in cases of placenta previa.

Size of the fetal head

Because of its size and relative rigidity, the fetal head has a major effect on the birth process. The fetal skull is composed of two parietal bones, two temporal bones, the frontal bone, and the occipital bone (Fig. 11-1, *A*). These bones are united by membranous sutures: the sagittal, lambdoidal, coronal, and frontal (Fig. 11-1, *B*). Membrane-filled spaces

called fontanels are located where the sutures intersect. During labor, after rupture of membranes, palpation of fontanels and sutures during vaginal examination reveals fetal presentation, position, and attitude.

The two most important fontanels are the anterior and posterior ones (see Fig. 11-1, *B*). The larger of these, the anterior fontanel, is diamond shaped, is about 3 cm by 2 cm, and lies at the junction of the sagittal, coronal, and frontal sutures. It closes by 18 months after birth. The posterior fontanel lies at the junction of the sutures of the two parietal bones and the occipital bone, is triangular, and is about 1 cm by 2 cm. It closes 6 to 8 weeks after birth.

Sutures and fontanels make the skull flexible to accommodate the infant brain, which continues to grow for some time after birth. Because the bones are not firmly united, however, slight overlapping of the bones, or molding of the shape of the head, occurs during labor. This capacity of the bones to slide over one another also permits adaptation to the various diameters of the maternal pelvis. Molding can be extensive, but the heads of most newborns assume their normal shape within 3 days after birth.

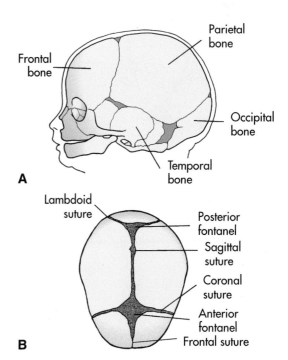

Fig. 11-1 Fetal head at term. **A,** Bones. **B,** Sutures and fontanels.

Although the size of the fetal shoulders may affect passage, their position can be altered relatively easily during labor, so one shoulder may occupy a lower level than the other. This creates a shoulder diameter that is smaller than the skull, facilitating passage through the birth canal. The circumference of the fetal hips is usually small enough not to create problems.

Fetal presentation

Presentation refers to the part of the fetus that enters the pelvic inlet first and leads through the birth canal during labor at term. The three main presentations are cephalic presentation (head first), occurring in 96% of births (Fig. 11-2); breech presentation (buttocks or feet first), occurring in 3% of births (Fig. 11-3, *A-C*); and shoulder presentation, seen in 1% of births (Fig. 11-3, *D*). The presenting part is that part of the fetal body first felt by the examining finger during a vaginal examination. In a cephalic presentation the presenting part is usually the occiput; in a breech presentation it is the sacrum; in the shoulder presentation it is the scapula.

When the presenting part is the occiput, the presentation is noted as vertex (see Fig. 11-2). Factors that determine the presenting part include fetal lie, fetal attitude, and extension or flexion of the fetal head.

Fetal lie

Lie is the relation of the long axis (spine) of the fetus to the long axis (spine) of the mother. The two primary lies are longitudinal, or vertical, in which the long axis of the fetus is parallel with the long axis of the mother (see Fig. 11-2); and transverse, horizontal, or oblique, in which the long axis of the fetus is at a right angle diagonal to the long axis of the mother (see Fig. 11-3, *D*). Longitudinal lies are either cephalic or breech presentations, depending on the fetal structure that first enters the mother's pelvis. Vaginal birth cannot occur when the fetus stays in a transverse lie. An oblique lie, one in which the long axis of the fetus is lying at an angle to the long axis of the mother, is less common and usually converts to a longitudinal or transverse lie during labor (Cunningham et al., 2005).

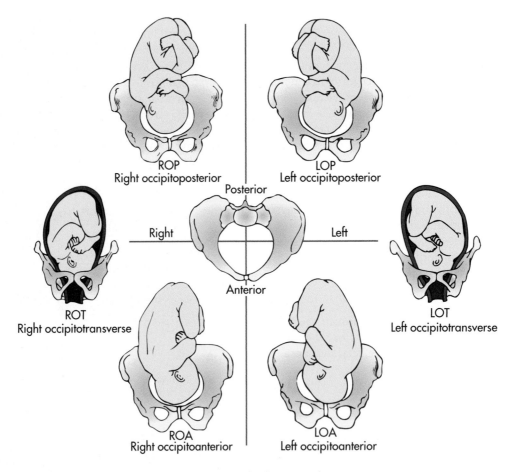

ROP
Right occipitoposterior

LOP
Left occipitoposterior

Posterior

Right ———— Left

Anterior

ROT
Right occipitotransverse

LOT
Left occipitotransverse

ROA
Right occipitoanterior

LOA
Left occipitoanterior

Lie: Longitudinal or vertical
Presentation: Vertex
Reference point: Occiput
Attitude: Complete flexion

Fig. 11-2 Examples of fetal vertex (occiput) presentations in relation to front, back, or side of maternal pelvis.

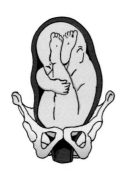

A Frank breech

Lie: Longitudinal or vertical
Presentation: Breech (incomplete)
Presenting part: Sacrum
Attitude: Flexion, except for legs at knees

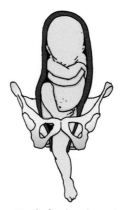

B Single footling breech

Lie: Longitudinal or vertical
Presentation: Breech (incomplete)
Presenting part: Sacrum
Attitude: Flexion, except for one leg extended at hip and knee

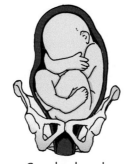

C Complete breech

Lie: Longitudinal or vertical
Presentation: Breech (sacrum and feet presenting)
Presenting part: Sacrum (with feet)
Attitude: General flexion

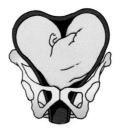

D Shoulder presentation

Lie: Transverse or horizontal
Presentation: Shoulder
Presenting part: Scapula
Attitude: Flexion

Fig. 11-3   Fetal presentations. **A-C,** Breech (sacral) presentation. **D,** Shoulder presentation.

Fetal attitude

Attitude is the relation of the fetal body parts to each other. The fetus assumes a characteristic posture (attitude) in utero partly because of the mode of fetal growth and partly because of the way the fetus conforms to the shape of the uterine cavity. Normally the back of the fetus is rounded so that the chin is flexed on the chest, the thighs are flexed on the abdomen, and the legs are flexed at the knees. The arms are crossed over the thorax, and the umbilical cord lies between the arms and the legs. This attitude is termed *general flexion* (see Fig. 11-2).

Deviations from the normal attitude may cause difficulties in childbirth. For example, in a cephalic presentation, the fetal head may be extended or flexed in a manner that presents a head diameter that exceeds the limits of the maternal pelvis, leading to prolonged labor, forceps- or vacuum-assisted birth, or cesarean birth.

Certain critical diameters of the fetal head are usually measured. The biparietal diameter, which is about 9.25 cm at term, is the largest transverse diameter and an important

indicator of fetal head size (Fig. 11-4, *B*). In a well-flexed cephalic presentation, the biparietal diameter will be the widest part of the head entering the pelvic inlet. Of the several anteroposterior diameters, the smallest and the most critical one is the suboccipitobregmatic diameter (about 9.5 cm at term). When the head is in complete flexion, this diameter allows the fetal head to pass through the true pelvis easily (Fig. 11-4, *A*; Fig. 11-5, *A*). As the head is more extended, the anteroposterior diameter widens, and the head may not be able to enter the true pelvis (see Fig. 11-5, *B, C*).

Fetal position

The presentation or presenting part indicates that portion of the fetus that overlies the pelvic inlet. Position is the relation of the presenting part (occiput, sacrum, mentum [chin], or sinciput [deflexed vertex]) to the four quadrants of the mother's pelvis (see Fig. 11-2). Position is denoted by a three-letter abbreviation. The first letter of the abbreviation denotes the location of the presenting part in the right (R) or left (L) side of the mother's pelvis. The middle letter stands

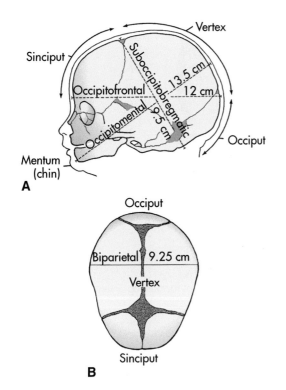

for the specific presenting part of the fetus (O for occiput, S for sacrum, M for mentum [chin], and Sc for scapula [shoulder]). The third letter stands for the location of the presenting part in relation to the anterior (A), posterior (P), or transverse (T) portion of the maternal pelvis. For example, ROA means that the occiput is the presenting part and is located in the right anterior quadrant of the maternal pelvis (see Fig. 11-2). LSP means that the sacrum is the presenting part and is located in the left posterior quadrant of the maternal pelvis (see Fig. 11-3).

Station is the relation of the presenting part of the fetus to an imaginary line drawn between the maternal ischial spines and is a measure of the degree of descent of the presenting part of the fetus through the birth canal. The placement of the presenting part is measured in centimeters above or below the ischial spines (Fig. 11-6). For example, when the lowermost portion of the presenting part is 1 cm above the spines, it is noted as being minus (−) 1. At the level of the spines, the station is said to be 0 (zero). When the presenting part is 1 cm below the spines, the station is said to be plus (+) 1. Birth is imminent when the presenting part is at +4 to +5 cm. The station of the presenting part should be determined when labor begins so that the rate of descent of the fetus during labor can be accurately determined.

Engagement is the term used to indicate that the largest transverse diameter of the presenting part (usually the biparietal diameter) has passed through the maternal pelvic

Fig. 11-4 Diameters of the fetal head at term. **A**, Cephalic presentations: occiput, vertex, and sinciput; and cephalic diameters: suboccipitobregmatic, occipitofrontal, and occipitomental. **B**, Biparietal diameter.

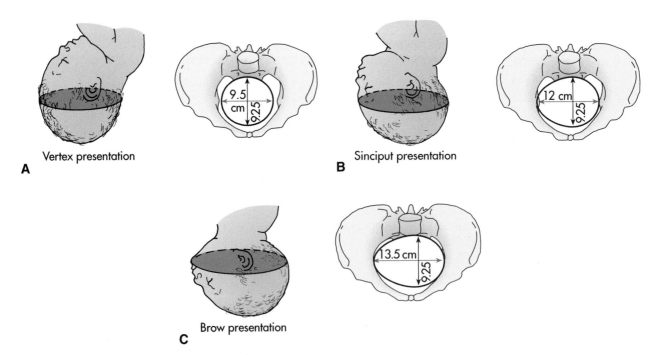

Fig. 11-5 Head entering pelvis. Biparietal diameter is indicated with shading (9.25 cm). **A**, Suboccipitobregmatic diameter: complete flexion of head on chest so that smallest diameter enters. **B**, Occipitofrontal diameter: moderate extension (military attitude) so that large diameter enters. **C**, Occipitomental diameter: marked extension (deflection), so that the largest diameter, which is too large to permit head to enter pelvis, is presenting.

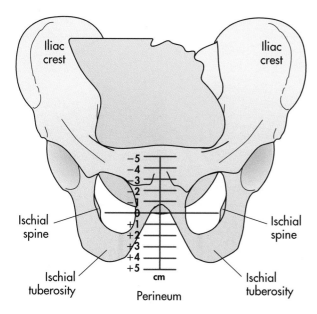

Fig. 11-6 Stations of presenting part, or degree of descent. The lowermost portion of the presenting part is at the level of the ischial spines, station 0.

brim or inlet into the true pelvis and usually corresponds to station 0. Engagement often occurs in the weeks just before labor begins in nulliparas and may occur before labor or during labor in multiparas. Engagement can be determined by abdominal or vaginal examination.

Passageway

The passageway, or birth canal, is composed of the mother's rigid bony pelvis and the soft tissues of the cervix, pelvic floor, vagina, and introitus (the external opening to the vagina). Although the soft tissues, particularly the muscular layers of the pelvic floor, contribute to vaginal birth of the fetus, the maternal pelvis plays a far greater role in the labor process because the fetus must successfully accommodate itself to this relatively rigid passageway. Therefore the size and shape of the pelvis must be determined before labor begins.

Bony pelvis

The anatomy of the bony pelvis is described in Chapter 4. The following discussion focuses on the importance of pelvic configurations as they relate to the labor process. (It may be helpful to refer to Fig. 4-4.)

The bony pelvis is formed by the fusion of the ilium, ischium, pubis, and sacral bones. The four pelvic joints are the symphysis pubis, the right and left sacroiliac joints, and the sacrococcygeal joint (Fig. 11-7, *A*). The bony pelvis is separated by the brim, or inlet, into two parts: the false pelvis and the true pelvis. The false pelvis is the part above the brim and plays no part in childbearing. The true pelvis, the part involved in birth, is divided into three planes: the inlet, or brim; the midpelvis, or cavity; and the outlet.

The pelvic inlet, which is the upper border of the true pelvis, is formed anteriorly by the upper margins of the

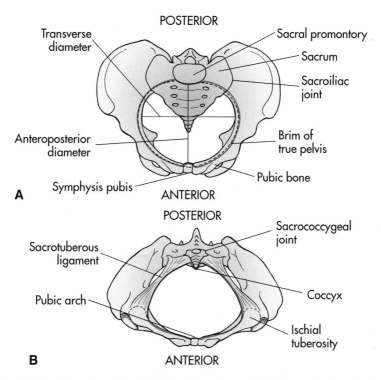

Fig. 11-7 Female pelvis. **A,** Pelvic brim above. **B,** Pelvic outlet from below.

pubic bone, laterally by the iliopectineal lines along the innominate bones, and posteriorly by the anterior, upper margin of the sacrum and the sacral promontory.

The pelvic cavity, or midpelvis, is a curved passage with a short anterior wall and a much longer concave posterior wall. It is bounded by the posterior aspect of the symphysis pubis, the ischium, a portion of the ilium, the sacrum, and the coccyx.

The pelvic outlet is the lower border of the true pelvis. Viewed from below, it is ovoid, somewhat diamond shaped, bounded by the pubic arch anteriorly, the ischial tuberosities laterally, and the tip of the coccyx posteriorly (Fig. 11-7, *B*). In the latter part of pregnancy, the coccyx is movable (unless it has been broken in a fall during skiing or skating, for example, and has fused to the sacrum during healing).

The pelvic canal varies in size and shape at various levels. The diameters at the plane of the pelvic inlet, midpelvis, and outlet, plus the axis of the birth canal (Fig. 11-8), determine whether vaginal birth is possible and the manner by which the fetus may pass down the birth canal.

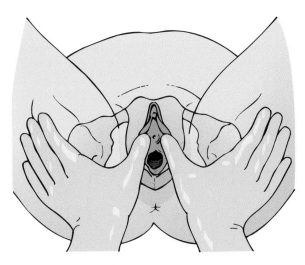

Fig. 11-9   Estimation of angle of subpubic arch. With both thumbs, examiner externally traces descending rami down to tuberosities. (From Barkauskas, V., Baumann, L., & Darling-Fisher, C. [2002]. *Health and physical assessment* [3rd ed.]. St. Louis: Mosby.)

The subpubic angle, which determines the type of pubic arch, together with the length of the pubic rami and the intertuberous diameter, is of great importance. Because the fetus must first pass beneath the pubic arch, a narrow subpubic angle will be less accommodating than a rounded wide arch. The method of measurement of the subpubic arch is shown in Fig. 11-9. A summary of obstetric measurements is given in Table 11-1.

The four basic types of pelves are classified as follows:
1. Gynecoid (the classic female type)
2. Android (resembling the male pelvis)
3. Anthropoid (resembling the pelvis of anthropoid apes)
4. Platypelloid (the flat pelvis)

The gynecoid pelvis is the most common, with major gynecoid pelvic features present in 50% of all women. Anthropoid and android features are less common, and platypelloid pelvic features are the least common. Mixed types of pelves are more common than are pure types (Cunningham et al., 2005). Examples of pelvic variations and their effects on mode of birth are given in Table 11-2.

Assessment of the bony pelvis can be performed during the first prenatal evaluation and need not be repeated if the pelvis is of adequate size and suitable shape. In the third trimester of pregnancy, the examination of the bony pelvis may be more thorough and the results more accurate because there is relaxation and increased mobility of the pelvic joints and ligaments owing to hormonal influences. Widening of the joint of the symphysis pubis and the resulting instability may cause pain in any or all of the pelvic joints.

Because the examiner does not have direct access to the bony structures and because the bones are covered with varying amounts of soft tissue, estimates of size and shape are approximate. Precise bony pelvis measurements can be determined by use of computed tomography, ultrasound, or

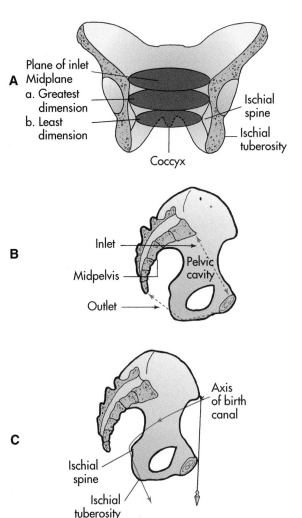

Fig. 11-8   Pelvic cavity. **A,** Inlet and midplane. Outlet now shown. **B,** Cavity of true pelvis. **C,** Note curve of sacrum and axis of birth canal.

TABLE 11-1

Obstetric Measurements

PLANE	DIAMETER	MEASUREMENTS
Inlet (superior strait)		
Conjugates		
Diagonal	12.5-13 cm	
Obstetric: measurement that determines whether presenting part can engage or enter superior strait	1.5-2 cm less than diagonal (radiographic)	
True (vera) (anteroposterior)	≥11 cm (12.5) (radiographic)	
		Length of diagonal conjugate (green line), obstetric conjugate (broken colored line), and true conjugate (black line)*
Midplane	10.5 cm	
Transverse diameter (interspinous diameter)		
The midplane of the pelvis normally is its largest plane and the one of greatest diameter		
		Measurement of interspinous diameter*
Outlet	≥8 cm	
Transverse diameter (intertuberous diameter) (biischial)		
The outlet presents the smallest plane of the pelvic canal		
		Use of Thom's pelvimeter to measure intertuberous diameter*

*From Seidel, H., Ball, J., Dains, J., & Benedict, G. (2003). *Mosby's guide to physical examination* (5th ed.). St. Louis: Mosby.

Comparison of Pelvic Types

	GYNECOID (50% OF WOMEN)	ANDROID (23% OF WOMEN)	ANTHROPOID (24% OF WOMEN)	PLATYPELLOID (3% OF WOMEN)
Brim	Slightly ovoid or transversely rounded	Heart shaped, angulated	Oval, wider anteroposteriorly	Flattened anteroposteriorly, wide transversely
	○ Round	♡ Heart	◯ Oval	⬭ Flat
Depth	Moderate	Deep	Deep	Shallow
Sidewalls	Straight	Convergent	Straight	Straight
Ischial spines	Blunt, somewhat widely separated	Prominent, narrow interspinous diameter	Prominent, often with narrow interspinous diameter	Blunted, widely separated
Sacrum	Deep, curved	Slightly curved, terminal portion often beaked	Slightly curved	Slightly curved
Subpubic arch	Wide	Narrow	Narrow	Wide
Usual mode of birth	Vaginal Spontaneous Occipitoanterior position	Cesarean Vaginal Difficult with forceps	Vaginal Forceps Spontaneous Occipitoposterior or occipitoanterior position	Vaginal Spontaneous

x-ray films. However, radiographic examination is rarely done during pregnancy because the x-rays may damage the developing fetus.

Soft tissues

The soft tissues of the passageway include the distensible lower uterine segment, cervix, pelvic floor muscles, vagina, and introitus. Before labor begins, the uterus is composed of the uterine body (corpus) and cervix (neck). After labor has begun, uterine contractions cause the uterine body to have a thick and muscular upper segment and a thin-walled, passive, muscular lower segment. A physiologic retraction ring separates the two segments (Fig. 11-10). The lower uterine segment gradually distends to accommodate the intrauterine contents as the wall of the upper segment thickens and its accommodating capacity is reduced. The contractions of the uterine body thus exert downward pressure on the fetus, pushing it against the cervix.

The cervix effaces (thins) and dilates (opens) sufficiently to allow the first fetal portion to descend into the vagina. As the fetus descends, the cervix is actually drawn upward and over this first portion.

The pelvic floor is a muscular layer that separates the pelvic cavity above from the perineal space below. This structure helps the fetus rotate anteriorly as it passes through the birth canal. As noted earlier, the soft tissues of the vagina develop throughout pregnancy until at term the vagina can dilate to accommodate the fetus and permit passage of the fetus to the external world.

Powers

Involuntary and voluntary powers combine to expel the fetus and the placenta from the uterus. Involuntary uterine contractions, called the *primary powers*, signal the beginning of labor. Once the cervix has dilated, voluntary bearing-down efforts by the woman, called the *secondary powers*, augment the force of the involuntary contractions.

Primary powers

The involuntary contractions originate at certain pacemaker points in the thickened muscle layers of the upper uterine segment. From the pacemaker points, contractions move downward over the uterus in waves, separated by short rest periods. Terms used to describe these involuntary contractions include *frequency* (the time from the beginning of one contraction to the beginning of the next), *duration* (length of contraction from the beginning to the end), and *intensity* (strength of contraction).

The primary powers are responsible for the effacement and dilation of the cervix and descent of the fetus. Effacement of the cervix means the shortening and thinning of the cervix during the first stage of labor. The cervix, normally 2 to 3 cm long and about 1 cm thick, is obliterated or "taken up" by a shortening of the uterine muscle bundles during the thinning of the lower uterine segment that occurs in advancing labor. Only a thin edge of the cervix can be palpated when effacement is complete. Effacement generally is advanced in first-time term pregnancy before more than slight dilation occurs. In subsequent pregnancies, effacement and

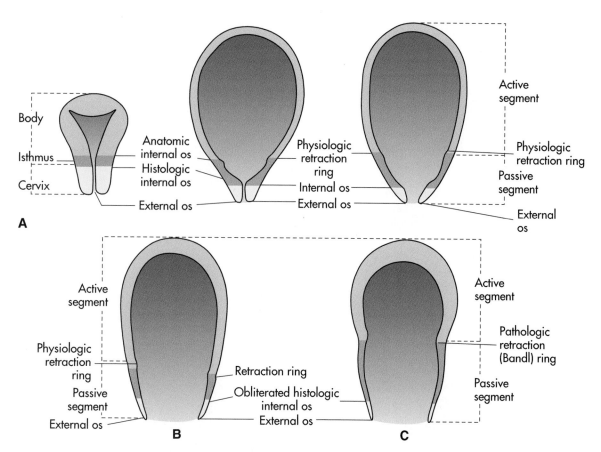

Fig. 11-10 **A,** Uterus in normal labor in early first stage, and **B,** in second stage. Passive segment is derived from lower uterine segment (isthmus) and cervix, and physiologic retraction ring is derived from anatomic internal os. **C,** Uterus in abnormal labor in second-stage dystocia. Pathologic retraction (Bandl) ring that forms under abnormal conditions develops from the physiologic ring.

dilation of the cervix tend to progress together. Degree of effacement is expressed in percentages from 0% to 100% (e.g., a cervix is 50% effaced) (Fig. 11-11, *A-C*).

Dilation of the cervix is the enlargement or widening of the cervical opening and the cervical canal that occurs once labor has begun. The diameter of the cervix increases from less than 1 cm to full dilation (approximately 10 cm) to allow birth of a term fetus. When the cervix is fully dilated (and completely retracted), it can no longer be palpated (Fig. 11-11, *D*). Full cervical dilation marks the end of the first stage of labor.

Dilation of the cervix occurs by the drawing upward of the musculofibrous components of the cervix, caused by strong uterine contractions. Pressure exerted by the amniotic fluid while the membranes are intact or by the force applied by the presenting part also can promote cervical dilation. Scarring of the cervix as a result of prior infection or surgery may slow cervical dilation.

In the first and second stages of labor, increased intrauterine pressure caused by contractions exerts pressure on the descending fetus and the cervix. When the presenting part of the fetus reaches the perineal floor, mechanical stretching of the cervix occurs. Stretch receptors

in the posterior vagina cause release of endogenous oxytocin that triggers the maternal urge to bear down, or the Ferguson reflex.

Uterine contractions are usually independent of external forces. For example, laboring women who are paraplegic will have normal but painless uterine contractions (Cunningham et al., 2005). However, uterine contractions may decrease temporarily in frequency and intensity if narcotic analgesic medication is given early in labor. Studies of effects of epidural analgesia have demonstrated prolonged length of labor for nulliparas both in the active phase of first stage labor and in the second stage (Alexander, Sharma, McIntire, & Leveno, 2002; Sharma & Leveno, 2003).

Secondary powers

As soon as the presenting part reaches the pelvic floor, the contractions change in character and become expulsive. The laboring woman experiences an involuntary urge to push. She uses secondary powers (bearing-down efforts) to aid in expulsion of the fetus as she contracts her diaphragm and abdominal muscles and pushes. These bearing-down efforts result in increased intraabdominal pressure that compresses

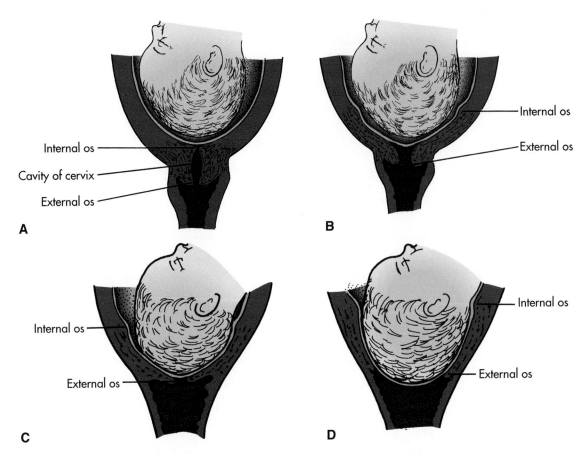

Internal os

Cavity of cervix

External os

A

Internal os

External os

B

Internal os

External os

C

Internal os

External os

D

Fig. 11-11 Cervical effacement and dilation. Note how cervix is drawn up around presenting part (internal os). Membranes are intact, and head is not well applied to cervix. **A,** Before labor. **B,** Early effacement. **C,** Complete effacement (100%). Head is well applied to cervix. **D,** Complete dilation (10 cm). Cranial bones overlap somewhat, and membranes are still intact.

the uterus on all sides and adds to the power of the expulsive forces.

The secondary powers have no effect on cervical dilation, but they are of considerable importance in the expulsion of the infant from the uterus and vagina after the cervix is fully dilated. Studies have shown that pushing in the second stage is more effective and the woman is less fatigued when she begins to push only after she has the urge to do so rather than beginning to push when she is fully dilated without an ✳ urge to do so (Roberts, 2002; 2003).

When and how a woman pushes in the second stage is a much-debated topic. Studies have investigated the effects of spontaneous bearing-down efforts, directed pushing, delayed pushing, Valsalva maneuver (closed glottis and ✳ prolonged bearing down), and open-glottis pushing (Hansen, Clark, & Foster, 2002; Mayberry et al., 2000; Minato, 2000/2001; Petrou, Coyle, & Fraser, 2000). Although no significant differences have been found in the duration of second-stage labor, adverse effects of certain types of pushing techniques have been reported. Fetal hypoxia and subsequent acidosis have been associated with prolonged breath holding and forceful pushing efforts (Roberts, 2002). Perineal tears have been associated with

directed pushing (Fraser et al., 2000). Continued study is needed to determine the effectiveness and appropriateness of strategies used by nurses to teach pushing techniques, the suitability and effectiveness of various pushing techniques related to nonreassuring fetal heart patterns, and the standards for length of duration of pushing in terms of maternal and fetal outcomes (Roberts, 2003).

Position of the Laboring Woman

Position affects the woman's anatomic and physiologic adaptations to labor. Frequent changes in position relieve fatigue, increase comfort, and improve circulation (Gupta & Nikodem, 2001). Therefore a laboring woman should be encouraged to find positions that are most comfortable for her (Fig. 11-12, *A*).

An upright position (walking, sitting, kneeling, or squatting) offers a number of advantages. Gravity can promote the descent of the fetus. Uterine contractions are generally stronger and more efficient in effacing and dilating the cervix, resulting in shorter labor (Gupta & Nikodem, 2001; Simkin & Ancheta, 2000).

An upright position also is beneficial to the mother's cardiac output, which normally increases during labor as

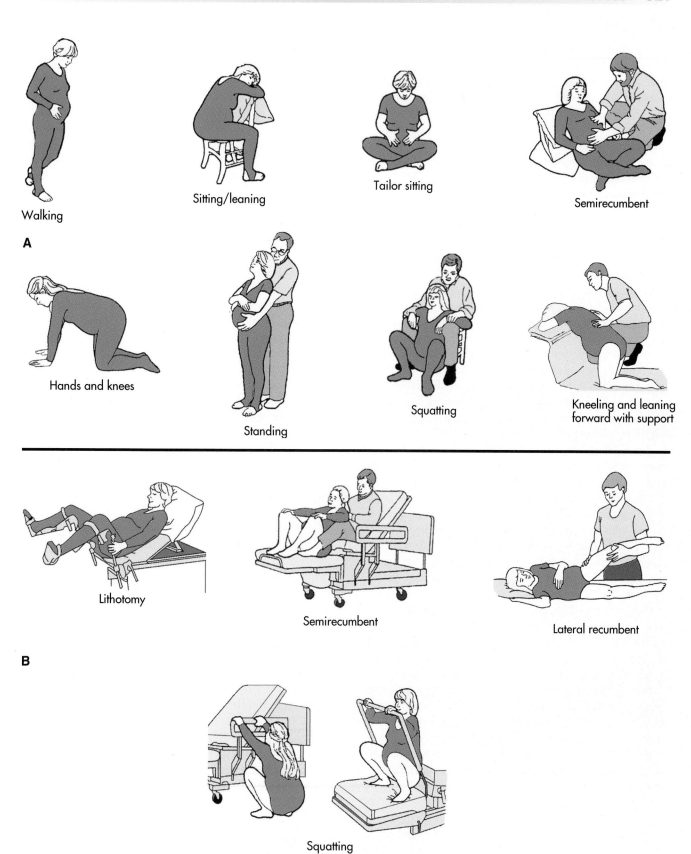

A

Walking

Sitting/leaning

Tailor sitting

Semirecumbent

Hands and knees

Standing

Squatting

Kneeling and leaning forward with support

B

Lithotomy

Semirecumbent

Lateral recumbent

Squatting

Fig. 11-12   Positions for labor and birth. **A,** Positions for labor. **B,** Positions for birth.

uterine contractions return blood to the vascular bed. The increased cardiac output improves blood flow to the utero-placental unit and the maternal kidneys. Cardiac output is compromised if the descending aorta and ascending vena cava are compressed during labor. Compression of these major vessels may result in supine hypotension that decreases placental perfusion. With the woman in an upright position, pressure on the maternal vessels is reduced, and compression is prevented. If the woman wishes to lie down, a lateral position is suggested (Blackburn, 2003).

The "all fours" position (hands and knees) may be used to relieve backache if the fetus is in an occipitoposterior position and may assist in anterior rotation of the fetus and in cases of shoulder dystocia (Hofmeyr & Kulier, 2000; Simkin & Ancheta, 2000).

Positioning for second-stage labor (Fig. 11-12, *B*) may be determined by the woman's preference, but it is constrained by the condition of the woman and fetus, the environment, and the health care provider's confidence in assisting with a birth in a specific position (Simkin & Ancheta, 2000). The predominant position in the United States in physician-attended births is the lithotomy position. Alternative positions and position changes that result in more births over an intact perineum are more commonly practiced by nurse-midwives (Shorten, Donsante, & Shorten, 2002).

A woman who pushes in a semirecumbent position needs adequate body support to push effectively because her weight will be on her sacrum, moving the coccyx forward and causing a reduction in the pelvic outlet. In a sitting or squatting position, abdominal muscles work in greater synchrony with uterine contractions during bearing-down efforts. Kneeling or squatting moves the uterus forward and aligns the fetus with the pelvic inlet and can facilitate the second stage of labor by increasing the pelvic outlet (Simkin & Ancheta, 2000).

The lateral position can be used by the woman to help rotate a fetus that is in a posterior position. It also can be used when there is a need for less force to be used during bearing down, such as when there is a need to control the speed of a precipitate birth (Simkin & Ancheta, 2000).

❋ No evidence exists that any of these positions suggested for second-stage labor increases the need for use of operative techniques (e.g., forceps- or vacuum-assisted birth, cesarean birth, episiotomy) or causes perineal trauma. No evidence has been found that use of any of these positions adversely affects the newborn (Mayberry et al., 2000).

PROCESS OF LABOR

The term *labor* refers to the process of moving the fetus, placenta, and membranes out of the uterus and through the birth canal. Various changes take place in the woman's reproductive system in the days and weeks before labor begins. Labor itself can be discussed in terms of the mechanisms involved in the process and the stages the woman moves through.

Signs Preceding Labor

In first-time pregnancies, the uterus sinks downward and forward about 2 weeks before term, when the fetus's presenting part (usually the fetal head) descends into the true pelvis. This settling is called **lightening,** or "dropping," and usually happens gradually. After lightening, women feel less congested and breathe more easily, but usually more bladder pressure results from this shift, and consequently a return of urinary frequency occurs. In a multiparous pregnancy, lightening may not take place until after uterine contractions are established and true labor is in progress.

The woman may complain of persistent low backache and sacroiliac distress as a result of relaxation of the pelvic joints. She may identify strong and frequent but irregular uterine (Braxton Hicks) contractions.

The vaginal mucus becomes more profuse in response to the extreme congestion of the vaginal mucous membranes. Brownish or blood-tinged cervical mucus may be passed **(bloody show).** The cervix becomes soft (ripens) and partially effaced and may begin to dilate. The membranes may rupture spontaneously.

Other phenomena are common in the days preceding labor: (1) loss of 0.5 to 1.5 kg in weight, caused by water loss resulting from electrolyte shifts that in turn are produced by changes in estrogen and progesterone levels; and (2) a surge of energy. Women speak of having a burst of energy that they often use to clean the house and put everything in order. Less commonly, some women have diarrhea, nausea, vomiting, and indigestion. Box 11-1 lists signs that may precede labor.

Onset of Labor

The onset of true labor cannot be ascribed to a single cause. Many factors, including changes in the maternal uterus, cervix, and pituitary gland, are involved. Hormones produced by the normal fetal hypothalamus, pituitary, and adrenal cortex probably contribute to the onset of labor. Progressive uterine distention, increasing intrauterine pressure, and aging of the placenta seem to be associated with increasing myometrial irritability. This is a result of increased concentrations of estrogen and prostaglandins, as well as decreasing progesterone levels. The mutually coordinated effects of these factors result in the occurrence of strong, regular, rhythmic

---

BOX 11-1

Signs Preceding Labor

- Lightening
- Return of urinary frequency
- Backache
- Stronger Braxton Hicks contractions
- Weight loss: 0.5-1.5 kg
- Surge of energy
- Increased vaginal discharge; bloody show
- Cervical ripening
- Possible rupture of membranes

uterine contractions. The outcome of these factors working together is normally the birth of the fetus and the expulsion of the placenta; however, how certain alterations trigger others and how proper checks and balances are maintained is not known.

Fetal fibronectin is a protein found in plasma and cervicovaginal secretions of pregnant women before the onset of labor. Assessment for the presence of fetal fibronectin is being used to predict the likelihood of preterm labor in women who are at increased risk for this complication. (Goldenberg et al., 2003). The value of detection of fetal fibronectin in management of women with preterm labor has yet to be determined, and therefore the test is not indicated for screening for preterm labor in low risk pregnant women (Bernhardt & Dorman, 2004).

Stages of Labor

Labor is considered "normal" when the woman is at or near term, no complications exist, a single fetus presents by vertex, and labor is completed within 18 hours. The course of normal labor, which is remarkably constant, consists of (1) regular progression of uterine contractions, (2) effacement and progressive dilation of the cervix, and (3) progress in descent of the presenting part. Four stages of labor are recognized. These stages are discussed in greater detail, along with nursing care for the laboring woman and family, in Chapter 14.

The first stage of labor is considered to last from the onset of regular uterine contractions to full dilation of the cervix. Commonly the onset of labor is difficult to establish because the woman may be admitted to the labor unit just before birth, and the beginning of labor may be only an estimate. The first stage is much longer than the second and third combined. Great variability is the rule, however, depending on the factors discussed previously in this chapter. Full dilation may occur in less than 1 hour in some multiparous pregnancies. In first-time pregnancy, complete dilation of the cervix can take up to 20 hours. Variations may reflect differences in the patient population (e.g., risk status, age) or in clinical management of the labor and birth (Albers, 1999).

The first stage of labor has been divided into three phases: a latent phase, an active phase, and a transition phase. During the latent phase, there is more progress in effacement of the cervix and little increase in descent. During the active phase and the transition phase, there is more rapid dilation of the cervix and increased rate of descent of the presenting part.

The second stage of labor lasts from the time the cervix is fully dilated to the birth of the fetus. The second stage takes an average of 20 minutes for a multiparous woman and 50 minutes for a nulliparous woman. Labor of up to 2 hours has been considered within the normal range for the second stage. Epidural analgesia will likely prolong the second stage (Zhang, Yancey, Klebanoff, Schwartz, & Schweitzer, 2001). Ethnicity may shorten the length of the

second stage of labor for African-American and Puerto Rican women (Diegmann, Andrews, & Niemczura, 2000).

Simkin and Ancheta (2000) described the latent and active phases of second-stage labor. The latent phase is a period that begins about the time of complete dilation of the uterus, when the contractions are weak or not noticeable and the woman is not feeling the urge to push, is resting, or is exerting only small bearing-down efforts with contractions. The active phase is a period when contractions resume, the woman is making strong bearing-down efforts, and the fetal station is advancing.

The third stage of labor lasts from the birth of the fetus until the placenta is delivered. The placenta normally separates with the third or fourth strong uterine contraction after the infant has been born. After it has separated, the placenta can be delivered with the next uterine contraction. The duration of the third stage may be as short as 3 to 5 minutes, although up to 1 hour is considered within normal limits. The risk of hemorrhage increases as the length of the third stage increases (Cunningham et al., 2005).

The fourth stage of labor arbitrarily lasts about 2 hours after delivery of the placenta. It is the period of immediate recovery, when homeostasis is reestablished. It is an important period of observation for complications, such as abnormal bleeding (see Chapter 25).

Mechanism of Labor

As already discussed, the female pelvis has varied contours and diameters at different levels, and the presenting part of the passenger is large in proportion to the passage. Therefore for vaginal birth to occur, the fetus must adapt to the

---

? Critical Thinking Exercise

Second Stage of Labor

During your clinical experience in the labor and birth unit, you are assigned to a woman having her first baby. Her cervix is fully dilated and effaced and the fetus is at station 0. She has an epidural and does not feel the urge to push, but her mother is telling her that she needs to push with each contraction, holding her breath as long as she can while she is pushing. What intervention would you suggest?

1 Evidence—Is there sufficient evidence to draw conclusions about what intervention is needed?
2 Assumptions—Describe underlying assumptions about the following issues:
   a. phases of second stage labor
   b. effects of epidurals on labor for nulliparas
   c. delayed versus directed pushing
   d. Valsalva maneuver (prolonged bearing down)
3 What implications and priorities for nursing care can be drawn at this time?
4 Does the evidence objectively support your conclusion?
5 Are there alternative perspectives to your conclusion?

EVIDENCE-BASED PRACTICE
Birthing Centers versus Hospital Births

BACKGROUND

- A frequent complaint of the hospital birthing experience is the focus on technology, what some have called the "cascade of interventions" that some women feel grows out of their control. One outcome of the consumer movement has been a demand for a more homelike birthing environment, with a focus on the natural process of birthing. In the 1970s and 1980s many women in the United States chose to give birth at home, attended by lay midwives or nurse-midwives. Hospitals responded to this with a mid-level solution: homelike birthing centers, staffed by professionals and in close proximity to specialty emergency services. Women at low risk for complications could be seen antenatally and could labor, give birth, and recover in the same environment, accompanied by family. Some birthing centers are owned and staffed by the institution; others are affiliated with a hospital but staffed independently. Birthing centers share a philosophy that many women can labor and deliver without medication and technology, if only they have the appropriate preparation and support. Birthing center staff feel that the pain cycle of fear-tension-pain can be broken by having the woman in a safe, supportive, familiar environment. Low risk obstetrics is lucrative for hospitals, and most have responded to the competition by offering attractive homelike birthing centers.

OBJECTIVES

- The reviewers planned to compare the maternal and fetal outcomes of birthing center to conventional hospital births. They hoped to compare hospital-based centers to free-standing centers. The intervention was labor and delivery at a birthing center, and the control was conventional hospital care. Outcome measures of interest were intrapartal medical interventions, complications, method of delivery, perinatal death, maternal satisfaction, neonatal health, and adjustment to parenting.

METHODS
Search Strategy

- The authors looked for randomized or quasi-randomized, controlled trials in Cochrane, MEDLINE, and Zetoc, a weekly awareness service of 37 relevant journals. Search keywords were not noted.
- The reviewers selected six trials, involving 8677 women, from the United Kingdom, Sweden, Canada, and Australia, published 1984 to 2000.

Statistical Analyses

- Similar data were pooled. Reviewers calculated relative risks for dichotomous (categoric) data, and weighted mean differences for continuous data. The reviewers accepted results outside the 95% confidence intervals as significant differences.

FINDINGS

- The birthing center group used less pain medication and less labor augmentation than the hospitalized group. The women were more mobile during labor. There were fewer fetal heart abnormalities and fewer operative deliveries (forceps, vacuum extraction, or cesarean birth). Episiotomy was less frequent, but perineal tears were more frequent. All of these differences were significant. There was no difference between groups in the number that had discontinued breastfeeding by 6 to 8 weeks postpartum. One trial noted significantly more sore nipples and mastitis in the birthing center group. There was a trend toward increased perinatal mortality rate in the birthing center group across three trials, but it did not reach the level of significance. No data were available on the type of caregivers or the continuity of care.

LIMITATIONS

- Substantial numbers of women (29% to 77%) in the birthing center groups transferred to the hospital during labor. Reasons included medical problems, no longer meeting the eligibility criteria for birthing center, and desire for epidural pain medication. This may introduce a selection bias.

CONCLUSIONS

- Women who give birth in a birthing center have fewer interventions than women who give birth in a hospital. Their outcomes are similar to the birth outcomes of women who give birth in a hospital.

IMPLICATIONS FOR PRACTICE

- The decreased use of pain medication and labor augmentation reflects their limited access in birthing centers. Electronic fetal monitors are not commonly used at birthing centers, so there would be fewer reports of fetal heart abnormalities, and women are freer to move around without monitors or intravenous lines. Many of the results mirror other evidence of the benefits of continuous support during labor and delivery (see "Evidence-Based Practice: Continuous Labor Support," Chapter 14). Hospitals would be wise to focus more on the benefits of continuous care for women in childbirth than on the décor of the environment.
- The trend toward increased perinatal mortality rate, although not significant, was consistent across three trials. The focus on normality may cause caregivers to miss subtle early warnings of problems or to delay action. All staff members need to be alert to trouble and able to expedite transfer to hospital care without delay.

IMPLICATIONS FOR FURTHER RESEARCH

- Solving the bias problem would be a significant step toward generalizable results. This includes randomization, dropouts, and addressing the inevitable transfers. Cost is a major driving force in policy and choice, yet it was not addressed in these trials. Further exploration of the perinatal mortality trend is warranted.

Reference: Hodnett, E., Downe, S., Edwards, N., Walsh, D. (2005). Home-like versus conventional institutional settings for birth (Cochrane Review). In *The Cochrane Library*, Issue 4, 2005. Chichester, UK: John Wiley & Sons.

birth canal during the descent. The turns and other adjustments necessary in the human birth process are termed the *mechanism of labor* (Fig. 11-13). The seven cardinal movements of the mechanism of labor that occur in a vertex presentation are engagement, descent, flexion, internal rotation, extension, external rotation (restitution), and finally birth by expulsion. Although these movements are discussed separately, in actuality a combination of movements occurs simultaneously. For example, engagement involves both descent and flexion.

Engagement

When the biparietal diameter of the head passes the pelvic inlet, the head is said to be engaged in the pelvic inlet (Fig. 11-13, *A*). In most nulliparous pregnancies, this occurs before the onset of active labor because the firmer abdominal muscles direct the presenting part into the pelvis. In multiparous pregnancies, in which the abdominal musculature is more relaxed, the head often remains freely movable above the pelvic brim until labor is established.

Asynclitism. The head usually engages in the pelvis in a synclitic position—one that is parallel to the anteroposterior plane of the pelvis. Frequently asynclitism occurs (the head is deflected anteriorly or posteriorly in the pelvis), which can facilitate descent because the head is being positioned to accommodate to the pelvic cavity (Fig. 11-14). Extreme asynclitism can cause cephalopelvic disproportion, even in a normal-size pelvis, because the head is positioned so that it cannot descend.

Descent

Descent refers to the progress of the presenting part through the pelvis. Descent depends on at least four forces: (1) pressure exerted by the amniotic fluid, (2) direct pressure exerted by the contracting fundus on the fetus, (3) force of the contraction of the maternal diaphragm and abdominal muscles in the second stage of labor, and (4) extension and straightening of the fetal body. The effects of these forces are modified by the size and shape of the maternal pelvic planes and the size of the fetal head and its capacity to mold.

The degree of descent is measured by the station of the presenting part (see Fig. 11-6). As mentioned, little descent occurs during the latent phase of the first stage of labor. Descent accelerates in the active phase when the cervix has dilated to 5 to 7 cm. It is especially apparent when the membranes have ruptured.

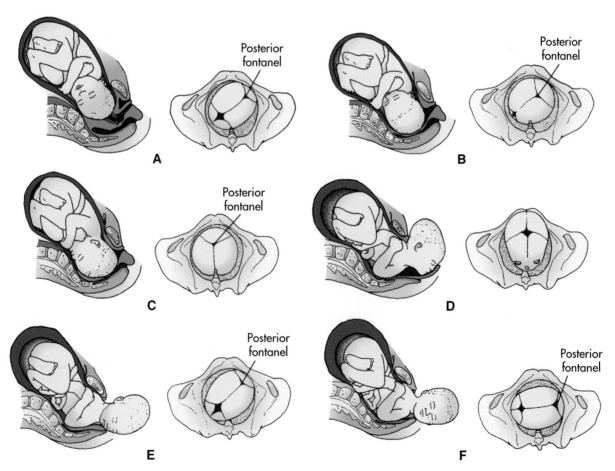

Fig. 11-13 Cardinal movements of the mechanism of labor. Left occipitoanterior (LOA) position. **A,** Engagement and descent. **B,** Flexion. **C,** Internal rotation to occipitoanterior position (OA). **D,** Extension. **E,** External rotation beginning (restitution). **F,** External rotation.

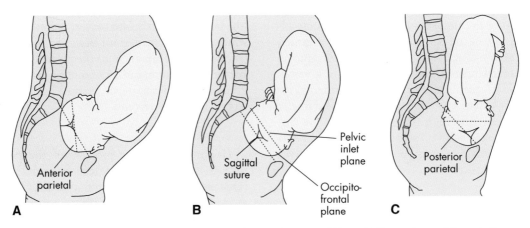

Fig. 11-14   Synclitism and asynclitism. **A,** Anterior asynclitism. **B,** Normal synclitism. **C,** Posterior asynclitism.

In a first-time pregnancy, descent is usually slow but steady; in subsequent pregnancies descent may be rapid. Progress in descent of the presenting part is determined by abdominal palpation (Leopold maneuvers) and vaginal examination until the presenting part can be seen at the introitus.

Flexion

As soon as the descending head meets resistance from the cervix, pelvic wall, or pelvic floor, it normally flexes, so that the chin is brought into closer contact with the fetal chest (see Fig. 11-13, *B*). Flexion permits the smaller suboccipitobregmatic diameter (9.5 cm) rather than the larger diameters to present to the outlet.

Internal rotation

The maternal pelvic inlet is widest in the transverse diameter; therefore the fetal head passes the inlet into the true pelvis in the occipitotransverse position. The outlet is widest in the anteroposterior diameter; for the fetus to exit, the head must rotate. Internal rotation begins at the level of the ischial spines but is not completed until the presenting part reaches the lower pelvis. As the occiput rotates anteriorly, the face rotates posteriorly. With each contraction, the fetal head is guided by the bony pelvis and the muscles of the pelvic floor. Eventually the occiput will be in the midline beneath the pubic arch. The head is almost always rotated by the time it reaches the pelvic floor (see Fig. 11-13, *C*). Both the levator ani muscles and the bony pelvis are important for achieving anterior rotation. A previous childbirth injury or regional anesthesia may compromise the function of the levator sling.

Extension

When the fetal head reaches the perineum for birth, it is deflected anteriorly by the perineum. The occiput passes under the lower border of the symphysis pubis first, and then the head emerges by extension: first the occiput, then the face, and finally the chin (see Fig. 11-13, *D*).

Restitution and external rotation

After the head is born, it rotates briefly to the position it occupied when it was engaged in the inlet. This movement is referred to as *restitution* (see Fig. 11-13, *E*). The 45-degree turn realigns the infant's head with her or his back and shoulders. The head can then be seen to rotate further. This external rotation occurs as the shoulders engage and descend in maneuvers similar to those of the head (see Fig. 11-13, *F*). As noted earlier, the anterior shoulder descends first. When it reaches the outlet, it rotates to the midline and is delivered from under the pubic arch. The posterior shoulder is guided over the perineum until it is free of the vaginal introitus.

Expulsion

After birth of the shoulders, the head and shoulders are lifted up toward the mother's pubic bone and the trunk of the baby is born by flexing it laterally in the direction of the symphysis pubis. When the baby has completely emerged, birth is complete, and the second stage of labor ends.

PHYSIOLOGIC ADAPTATION TO LABOR

In addition to the maternal and fetal anatomic adaptations that occur during birth, physiologic adaptations must occur. Accurate assessment of the laboring woman and fetus requires knowledge of these expected adaptations.

Fetal Adaptation

Several important physiologic adaptations occur in the fetus. These changes occur in fetal heart rate (FHR), fetal circulation, respiratory movements, and other behaviors.

Fetal heart rate

FHR monitoring provides reliable and predictive information about the condition of the fetus related to oxygenation. The average FHR at term is 140 beats/min. The normal range is 110 to 160 beats/min. Earlier in gestation the FHR is higher, with an average of approximately

160 beats/min at 20 weeks of gestation. The rate decreases progressively as the maturing fetus reaches term. However, temporary accelerations and slight early decelerations of the FHR can be expected in response to spontaneous fetal movement, vaginal examination, fundal pressure, uterine contractions, abdominal palpation, and fetal head compression. Stresses to the uterofetoplacental unit result in characteristic FHR patterns (see Chapter 13 for further discussion).

Fetal circulation

Fetal circulation can be affected by many factors, including maternal position, uterine contractions, blood pressure, and umbilical cord blood flow. Uterine contractions during labor tend to decrease circulation through the spiral arterioles and subsequent perfusion through the intervillous space. Most healthy fetuses are well able to compensate for this stress and exposure to increased pressure while moving passively through the birth canal during labor. Usually umbilical cord blood flow is undisturbed by uterine contractions or fetal position (Uçkar & Townsend, 1999).

Fetal respiration

Certain changes stimulate chemoreceptors in the aorta and carotid bodies to prepare the fetus for initiating respirations immediately after birth (Rosenberg, 2002; Uçkar & Townsend, 1999). These changes include the following:
- Fetal lung fluid is cleared from the air passages during labor and (vaginal) birth.
- Fetal oxygen pressure (PO_2) decreases.
- Arterial carbon dioxide pressure (PCO_2) increases.
- Arterial pH decreases.
- Bicarbonate level decreases.
- Fetal respiratory movements decrease during labor.

Maternal Adaptation

As the woman progresses through the stages of labor, various body system adaptations cause the woman to exhibit both objective and subjective symptoms (Box 11-2).

BOX 11-2

Maternal Physiologic Changes during Labor

- Cardiac output increases 10%-15% in first stage; 30%-50% in second stage.
- Heart rate increases slightly in first and second stages.
- Systolic blood pressure increases during uterine contractions in first stage; systolic and diastolic pressures increase during uterine contractions in second stage.
- White blood cell count increases.
- Respiratory rate increases.
- Temperature may be slightly elevated.
- Proteinuria may occur.
- Gastric motility and absorption of solid food is decreased; nausea and vomiting may occur during transition to second-stage labor.
- Blood glucose level decreases.

Cardiovascular changes

During each contraction, an average of 400 ml of blood is emptied from the uterus into the maternal vascular system. This increases cardiac output by about 12% to 31% in the first stage and by about 50% in the second stage. The heart rate increases slightly (Monga, 2004).

Changes in the woman's blood pressure also occur. Blood flow, which is reduced in the uterine artery by contractions, is redirected to peripheral vessels. As a result, peripheral resistance increases, and blood pressure increases (Monga, 2004). During the first stage of labor, uterine contractions cause systolic readings to increase by about 10 mm Hg; assessing blood pressure between contractions therefore provides more accurate readings. During the second stage, contractions may cause systolic pressures to increase by 30 mm Hg and diastolic readings to increase by 25 mm Hg, with both systolic and diastolic pressures remaining somewhat elevated even between contractions (Monga, 2004). Therefore the woman already at risk for hypertension is at increased risk for complications such as cerebral hemorrhage.

Supine hypotension (see Fig. 14-5) occurs when the ascending vena cava and descending aorta are compressed. The laboring woman is at greater risk for supine hypotension if the uterus is particularly large because of multifetal pregnancy, hydramnios, or obesity or if the woman is dehydrated or hypovolemic. In addition, anxiety and pain, as well as some medications, can cause hypotension.

The woman should be discouraged from using the Valsalva maneuver (holding one's breath and tightening abdominal muscles) for pushing during the second stage. This activity increases intrathoracic pressure, reduces venous return, and increases venous pressure. The cardiac output and blood pressure increase and the pulse slows temporarily. During the Valsalva maneuver, fetal hypoxia may occur. The process is reversed when the woman takes a breath.

The white blood cell (WBC) count can increase (Pagana & Pagana, 2003). Although the mechanism leading to this increase in WBCs is unknown, it may be secondary to physical or emotional stress or to tissue trauma. Labor is strenuous, and physical exercise alone can increase the WBC count.

Some peripheral vascular changes occur, perhaps in response to cervical dilation or to compression of maternal vessels by the fetus passing through the birth canal. Flushed cheeks, hot or cold feet, and eversion of hemorrhoids may result.

Respiratory changes

Increased physical activity with greater oxygen consumption is reflected in an increase in the respiratory rate. Hyperventilation may cause respiratory alkalosis (an increase in pH), hypoxia, and hypocapnia (decrease in carbon dioxide). In the unmedicated woman in the second stage, oxygen consumption almost doubles. Anxiety also increases oxygen consumption.

Renal changes

During labor, spontaneous voiding may be difficult for various reasons: tissue edema caused by pressure from the presenting part, discomfort, analgesia, and embarrassment. Proteinuria of +1 is a normal finding because it can occur in response to the breakdown of muscle tissue from the physical work of labor.

Integumentary changes

The integumentary system changes are evident, especially in the great distensibility (stretching) in the area of the vaginal introitus. The degree of distensibility varies with the individual. Despite this ability to stretch, even in the absence of episiotomy or lacerations, minute tears in the skin around the vaginal introitus do occur.

Musculoskeletal changes

The musculoskeletal system is stressed during labor. Diaphoresis, fatigue, proteinuria (+1), and possibly an increased temperature accompany the marked increase in muscle activity. Backache and joint ache (unrelated to fetal position) occur as a result of increased joint laxity at term. The labor process itself and the woman's pointing her toes can cause leg cramps.

Neurologic changes

Sensorial changes occur as the woman moves through phases of the first stage of labor and as she moves from one stage to the next. Initially she may be euphoric. Euphoria gives way to increased seriousness, then to amnesia between contractions during the second stage, and finally to elation or fatigue after giving birth. Endogenous endorphins (morphinelike chemicals produced naturally by the body) raise the pain threshold and produce sedation. In addition, physiologic anesthesia of perineal tissues, caused by pressure of the presenting part, decreases perception of pain.

Gastrointestinal changes

During labor, gastrointestinal motility and absorption of solid foods are decreased, and stomach-emptying time is slowed. Nausea and vomiting of undigested food eaten after onset of labor are common. Nausea and belching also occur as a reflex response to full cervical dilation. The woman may state that diarrhea accompanied the onset of labor, or the nurse may palpate the presence of hard or impacted stool in the rectum.

Endocrine changes

The onset of labor may be triggered by decreasing levels of progesterone and increasing levels of estrogen, prostaglandins, and oxytocin. Metabolism increases, and blood glucose levels may decrease with the work of labor.

Accurate assessment of the mother and fetus during labor and birth depends on knowledge of these expected adaptations so that appropriate interventions can be implemented.

COMMUNITY ACTIVITY

You have been asked by the staff at the community health center to prepare a childbirth class on the signs that precede labor for a group of Spanish-speaking nulliparas.
a. Identify essential content to be covered and describe how you would collect data about the group's knowledge and educational levels (e.g., through an interpreter).
b. Plan a 5- to 10-minute class, including audiovisuals. Discuss the plan with your faculty.
c. Give the class (through interpreter if needed), and ask the staff at the health center to evaluate it in terms of level of content and appropriate cultural content.

Key Points

- Labor and birth are affected by the five *Ps*: passenger, passageway, powers, position of the woman, and psychologic responses.
- Because of its size and relative rigidity, the fetal head is a major factor in determining the course of birth.
- The diameters at the plane of the pelvic inlet, midpelvis, and outlet, plus the axis of the birth canal, determine whether vaginal birth is possible and the manner in which the fetus passes down the birth canal.
- Involuntary uterine contractions act to expel the fetus and placenta during the first stage of labor; these are augmented by voluntary bearing-down efforts during the second stage.
- The first stage of labor lasts from the time dilation begins to the time when the cervix is fully dilated. The second stage of labor lasts from the time of full dilation to the birth of the infant. The third stage of labor lasts from the infant's birth to the expulsion of the placenta. The fourth stage is the first 2 hours after birth.
- The cardinal movements of the mechanism of labor are engagement, descent, flexion, internal rotation, extension, restitution and external rotation, and expulsion of the infant.
- Although the events precipitating the onset of labor are unknown, many factors, including changes in the maternal uterus, cervix, and pituitary gland, are thought to be involved.
- A healthy fetus with an adequate uterofetoplacental circulation will be able to compensate for the stress of uterine contractions.
- As the woman progresses through labor, various body systems adapt to the birth process.

Answer Guidelines to Critical Thinking Exercise

Second Stage of Labor

1 Yes, there is sufficient evidence to draw conclusions about what action should be implemented for this patient in second-stage labor.

2 a. There are variations in when a woman feels the initial urge to push. These are related to the fetal station and position of the presenting part. Second-stage labor has an early phase when the woman may not feel an urge to push; the uterine contractions may be weak. The active or last phase is when the woman feels a strong urge to push, usually when the fetal head has advanced to the pelvic floor and the Ferguson reflex is triggered. Passive descent and rotation of the fetal head (i.e., not encouraging the woman to push with contractions) in the early phase may prevent maternal and fetal complications. Pushing may also be more effective if the woman begins to push only after she has an urge to do so.

b. Nulliparas who have an epidural are more likely to have a longer second-stage labor than nulliparas who do not have an epidural, but research has not demonstrated harmful effects on the mother or fetus. With epidurals, the woman may not feel her contractions and may not feel an urge to push. A period of "laboring down" (not pushing with contractions) allows the fetus to descend and rotate and is one approach to managing patients with epidurals in second-stage labor.

c. Directed bearing down (pushing in a manner that the care provider thinks is effective or is based on the appearance of contractions on the electronic monitor) may trigger the Valsalva maneuver, which can cause an increase in maternal blood pressure and nonreassuring fetal heart rate patterns. The woman with an epidural may be directed to push too soon and may become tired before the contractions are strong again. Directed pushing also has been associated with perineal tears. Delayed or spontaneous pushing has been shown to have fewer effects on maternal blood pressure and

fetal status. Fewer interventions (e.g., episiotomies and forceps or vacuum assistance) are needed. Delayed pushing for women with epidurals (i.e., laboring down) allows fetal descent and rotation before pushing is initiated. Even though there is evidence to support this practice, it is not yet widely practiced in labor and birth units.

d. Use of prolonged strenuous pushing during contractions can affect maternal and fetal status. Maternal cardiac output may decrease, resulting in decreased blood flow to the uterus and decreased fetal oxygenation, resulting in fetal hypoxia and acidosis. This practice has been found to be harmful or ineffective and should be discouraged.

3 The nursing priority is to help the woman have a safe and effective second stage of labor with no maternal or fetal complications. Assessments for maternal and fetal effects of directed prolonged pushing need to be made. Explanations about the positive effects of delayed pushing are needed. The woman's mother needs to be included in the discussion about delayed pushing so that she becomes a better support for her daughter. When pushing is needed, demonstration of and encouragement for taking cleansing breaths as the contraction starts, pushing with the greatest force of the contraction, and taking breaths between bearing down efforts during the contraction are appropriate interventions. Continued nursing support, coaching, and encouragement for the patient and her mother during the second stage are needed.

4 Yes, there is evidence to support these conclusions about delayed second-stage pushing for nulliparous women with epidurals (Fraser, 2000; Hansen, Clark, & Foster, 2002; Mayberry, 2000.)

5 According to some researchers, there is no significant difference in the length of second-stage labor whether or not the woman delays pushing. If the patient wants to keep pushing, she should be encouraged to use the open-glottis method rather than the closed-glottis method.

Resources

Alexian Brothers Medical Center (information on stages of labor and other labor and birth topics)
Elk Grove, IL
847-437-5500
www.alexian.org/progserv/babies/babytoo.html

Baby Center (source for expectant parents)
www.babycenter.com/pregnancy

Childbirth Organization (source of links to other sites related to labor and birth
www.childbirth.org

Childbirth Graphics
P.O. Box 21207
Waco, TX 76702
800-229-3366
www.childbirthgraphics.com

References

Albers, L. (1999). The duration of labor in healthy women. *Journal of Perinatology, 19*(2), 114-119.

Alexander, J., Sharma, S., McIntire, D., & Leveno, K. (2002). Epidural analgesia lengthens the Friedman active phase of labor. *Obstetrics & Gynecology, 100*(1), 46-50.

Barkauskas, V., Baumann, L., & Darling-Fisher, C. (2002). *Health and physical assessment* (3rd ed.). St. Louis: Mosby.

Bernhardt, J., & Dorman, K. (2004). Pre-term birth risk assessment tools: Exploring fetal fibronectin and cervical length for validating risk. *AWHONN Lifelines, 8*(1), 38-44.

Blackburn, S. (2003). *Maternal, fetal, and neonatal physiology: A clinical perspective* (2nd ed.). St. Louis: Saunders.

Cunningham, F., Bloom, S., Gilstrap, L., Leveno, K., Hauth, J., & Wenstrom, K. (2005). *Williams obstetrics* (22nd ed.). New York: McGraw-Hill.

Diegmann, E., Andrews, C., & Niemczura, C. (2000). The length of the second stage of labor in uncomplicated, nulliparous African American and Puerto Rican women. *Journal of Midwifery & Women's Health, 45*(1), 67-71.

Fraser, W., Marcoux, S., Kraus, I., Douglas, J., Goulet, C., & Boulvain, M. (2000). Multicentered, randomized, controlled trial of delaying pushing for nulliparous women in the second stage of labor with continuous epidural analgesia. *American Journal of Obstetrics and Gynecology, 182*(5), 1165-1172.

Goldenberg, R., Iams, J., Mercer, B., Meis, P., Moawad, A., Das, A. et al. (2003). What have we learned about the predictors of preterm birth? *Seminars in Perinatology, 27*(3), 185-193.

Gupta, J., & Nikodem, V. (2001). Woman's position during second stage of labor (Cochrane Review). In *The Cochrane Library*, Issue 2. Oxford: Update Software.

Hansen, S., Clark, S., & Foster, J. (2002). Active pushing versus passive fetal descent in the second stage of labor: A randomized controlled trial. *Obstetrics & Gynecology, 99*(1), 29-34.

Hodnett, E. (2005). Home-like versus conventional institutional settings for birth (Cochrane Review). In *The Cochrane Library*, Issue 4, 2005. Chichester, UK: John Wiley & Sons.

Hofmeyr, G., & Kulier, R. (2000). Hands/knees posture in later pregnancy or labour for fetal malposition (lateral or posterior) (Cochrane Review). In *The Cochrane Library*, Issue 2. Oxford: Update Software.

Mayberry, L., Wood, S., Strange, L., Lee, L., Heisler, D., & Neilsen-Smith, K. (2000). *Second-stage labor management: Promotion of evidence-based practice and a collaborative approach to patient care.* Washington, DC: Association of Women's Health, Obstetric and Neonatal Nurses.

Minato, J. (2000/2001). Is it time to push? Examining rest in second-stage labor. *AWHONN Lifelines, 4*(6), 20-23.

Monga, M. (2004). Maternal cardiovascular and renal adaptations to pregnancy. In R. Creasy, R. Resnik, & J. Iams (Eds.), *Maternal-fetal medicine: Principles and practice* (5th ed.). Philadelphia: Saunders.

Pagana, K., & Pagana, T. (2003). *Mosby's diagnostic and laboratory test reference* (6th ed.). St. Louis: Mosby.

Petrou, S., Coyle, D., & Fraser, W. (2000). Cost-effectiveness of a delayed pushing policy for patients with epidural anesthesia: The PEOPLE (Pushing Early or Pushing Late with Epidural) Study Group. *American Journal of Obstetrics and Gynecology, 182*(5), 1158-1164.

Roberts, J. (2002). The "push" for evidence: Management of the second stage. *Journal of Midwifery & Women's Health, 47*(1), 2-15.

Roberts, J. (2003). A new understanding of the second stage of labor: Implications for nursing care. *Journal of Obstetric, Gynecologic, and Neonatal Nursing, 32*(6), 794-801.

Rosenberg, A. (2002). The neonate. In S. Gabbe, J. Niebyl, & J. Simpson (Eds.), *Obstetrics: Normal and problem pregnancies* (4th ed.). New York: Churchill Livingstone.

Seidel, H., Ball, J., Dains, J., & Benedict, G. (2003). *Mosby's guide to physical examination* (5th ed.). St. Louis: Mosby.

Sharma, S., & Leveno, K. (2003). Regional analgesia and progress of labor. *Clinical Obstetrics and Gynecology, 46*(3), 633-645.

Shorten, A., Donsante, J., & Shorten, B. (2002). Birth position, accoucheur, and perineal outcomes: Informing women about choices for vaginal birth. *Birth, 29*(1), 18-27.

Simkin, P., & Ancheta, R. (2000). *The labor progress handbook: Early interventions to prevent and treat dystocia.* Oxford: Blackwell Science Ltd.

Uçkar, E., & Townsend, N. (1999). Fetal adaptation. In L. Mandeville, & N. Troiano (Eds.), *AWHONN's high-risk and critical care intrapartum nursing* (2nd ed). Philadelphia: Lippincott.

VandeVusse, L. (1999). The essential forces of labor revisited: 13 *P*s reported in women's birth stories. *MCN American Journal of Maternal Child Nursing, 24*(4), 176-184.

Zhang, J., Yancey, M., Klebanoff, M., Schwartz, J., & Schweitzer, D. (2001). Does epidural analgesia prolong labor and increase risk of cesarean delivery? A natural experiment. *American Journal of Obstetrics and Gynecology, 185*(1), 128-134.

CHAPTER 12

Management of Discomfort

DEITRA LEONARD LOWDERMILK

LEARNING OBJECTIVES

- *Examine the various childbirth preparation methods.*
- *Describe breathing and relaxation techniques used for each stage of labor.*
- *Identify nonpharmacologic strategies to enhance relaxation and decrease discomfort during labor.*
- *Compare pharmacologic methods used to relieve discomfort in different stages of labor and for vaginal or cesarean births.*

- *Discuss the use of naloxone (Narcan).*
- *Apply the nursing process to the management of the discomfort of a woman in labor.*
- *Summarize the nursing responsibilities appropriate for a woman receiving analgesia or anesthesia during labor.*

KEY TERMS AND DEFINITIONS

analgesia Absence of pain without loss of consciousness

anesthesia Partial or complete absence of sensation with or without loss of consciousness

Bradley method Husband-coached childbirth preparation method using labor breathing techniques and environmental modification

counterpressure Pressure applied to the sacral area of the back during uterine contractions

Dick-Read method A prepared childbirth approach based on the premise that fear of pain produces muscular tension, producing pain and greater fear; includes teaching physiologic processes of labor, exercise to improve muscle tone, and techniques to assist in relaxation and prevent the fear-tension-pain mechanism

effleurage Gentle stroking used in massage, usually on the abdomen

epidural block Type of regional anesthesia produced by injection of a local anesthetic alone or in combination with a narcotic analgesic into the epidural (peridural) space

epidural blood patch A patch formed by a few milliliters of the mother's blood occluding a tear in the dura mater around the spinal cord that occurs during induction of spinal block; its purpose is to relieve headache associated with leakage of spinal fluid

gate-control theory of pain Pain theory used to explain the neurophysiologic mechanism underlying the perception of pain: the capacity of nerve pathways to transmit pain is reduced or completely blocked by using distraction techniques

Lamaze (psychoprophylaxis) method Childbirth preparation method developed in the 1950s by a French obstetrician, Fernand Lamaze, that gained popularity in the United States in the 1960s; requires practice at home and coaching during labor and birth; goals are to minimize fear and the perception of pain and to promote positive family relationships by using both mental and physical preparation, including breathing and relaxation techniques, effleurage, and focusing

local perinaeal infiltration anesthesia Process by which a substance such as a local anesthetic medication is deposited within the tissue to anesthetize a limited region of the body

neonatal narcosis Central nervous system depression in the newborn caused by an opioid (narcotic); may be signaled by respiratory depression, hypotonia, lethargy, and delay in temperature regulation

opioid (narcotic) agonist analgesics Medications that relieve pain by activating opioid receptors

opioid (narcotic) agonist-antagonist analgesics Medications that combine agonist activity (activates or stimulates a receptor to perform a function) and antagonist activity (blocks a receptor or medication designed to activate a receptor) to relieve pain without causing significant maternal or fetal or newborn respiratory depression

opioid (narcotic) antagonists Medications used to reverse the CNS depressant effects of an opioid, especially respiratory depression

pudendal nerve block Injection of a local anesthetic at the pudendal nerve root to produce numbness of the genital and perianal region

Continued

*P*ain is an unpleasant, complex, highly individualized phenomenon with both sensory and emotional components. Pregnant women commonly worry about the pain they will experience during labor and birth and how they will react to and deal with that pain. A variety of childbirth preparation methods can help the woman or couple cope with the discomfort of labor. The interventions selected depend on the situation and the preference of both the woman, her significant other, and her health care provider. The discomforts experienced during labor are discussed in this chapter, as are the nonpharmacologic and pharmacologic interventions to relieve the discomforts possible during the different stages of labor. This information provides the basis for understanding the nurse's role in the management of maternal discomfort during labor.

DISCOMFORT DURING LABOR AND BIRTH

Neurologic Origins

The pain and discomfort of labor have two origins, visceral and somatic (Lowe, 2002). During the first stage of labor, uterine contractions cause cervical dilation and effacement. Uterine ischemia (decreased blood flow and therefore local oxygen deficit) results from compression of the arteries supplying the myometrium during uterine contractions. Pain impulses during the first stage of labor are transmitted via the T11 to T12 spinal nerve segment and accessory lower thoracic and upper lumbar sympathetic nerves. These nerves originate in the uterine body and cervix.

The pain from cervical changes, distention of the lower uterine segment, and uterine ischemia that predominates during the first stage of labor is visceral pain. It is located over the lower portion of the abdomen. Referred pain occurs when the pain that originates in the uterus radiates to the abdominal wall, lumbosacral area of the back, iliac crests, and gluteal area and down the thighs. The woman usually has discomfort only during contractions and is free of pain between contractions, although some women have continuous contraction-related low back pain, even in the interval between contractions (Lowe, 2002).

During the second stage of labor the woman has somatic pain, which is often described as intense, sharp, burning, and well localized. Pain results from stretching and distention of perineal tissues and the pelvic floor to allow passage of the fetus, from distention and traction on the peritoneum and uterocervical supports during contractions, and from lacerations of soft tissue (e.g., cervix, vagina, perineum). Discomfort also can be produced by expulsive forces or by pressure exerted by the presenting part on the bladder, bowel, or other sensitive pelvic structures. Pain impulses during the second stage of labor are transmitted via the pudendal nerve through S2 to S4 spinal nerve segments and the parasympathetic system (Lowe, 2002).

Pain experienced during the third stage of labor and the afterpains of the early postpartum period are uterine, similar to the pain experienced early in the first stage of labor. Areas of discomfort during labor are shown in Fig. 12-1.

Factors Influencing Pain Response

A woman's pain during childbirth is unique to each woman and is influenced by a variety of physiologic, psychologic, and environmental factors.

Physiologic factors

A variety of physiologic factors can affect the intensity of pain experienced by women during childbirth. Women with a history of dysmenorrhea may experience increased pain during childbirth as a result of higher prostaglandin levels. Back pain associated with menstruation also may increase the

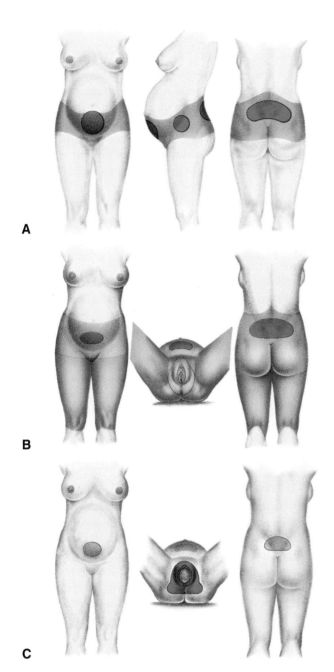

A

B

C

Fig. 12-1 Discomfort during labor. **A,** Distribution of labor pain during first stage. **B,** Distribution of labor pain during transition and early phase of second stage. **C,** Distribution of pain during late second stage and actual birth. (Gray areas indicate mild discomfort; light-colored areas indicate moderate discomfort; dark-colored areas indicate intense discomfort.)

likelihood of contraction-related low back pain. Upright positions, when assumed during labor, seem to result in decreased pain and an overall increase in comfort when compared with the supine position. Women also report that being able to move freely to find a position of comfort is an important factor in reducing pain and muscle tension and maintaining control during labor. Finally, the relation of fetal size to the dimensions of the maternal pelvis may influence pain intensity (Lowe, 2002; Simkin & O'Hara, 2002).

Endorphins are endogenous opioids secreted by the pituitary gland that act on the central and peripheral nervous systems to reduce pain. Beta-endorphin is the most potent of the endorphins. The physiologic role of endorphins is not completely understood. It is thought that endorphin levels increase during pregnancy and birth in humans. Higher endorphin levels may increase the ability of women in labor to tolerate acute pain and may reduce their irritability and anxiety. Levels of beta-endorphins are higher when a woman experiences a spontaneous, natural childbirth (Righard, 2001).

Culture

The obstetric population reflects the increasingly multicultural nature of U.S. society. As nurses care for women and families from a variety of cultural backgrounds, they must have knowledge and understanding of how culture mediates pain (Mattson, 2000). An understanding of the beliefs, values, and practices of various cultures helps the nurse provide appropriate culturally sensitive care (see Cultural Considerations box). It is important for the nurse to recognize that although a woman's behavior in response to pain may vary according to her cultural background, it may not accurately reflect the intensity of the pain she is experiencing. The nurse must assess the woman for the physiologic effects of pain and must listen to the words the woman uses to describe the sensory and affective qualities of her pain (Lowe, 2002).

Cultural Considerations

Some Cultural Beliefs about Pain

The following are examples of how women of different cultural backgrounds may react to pain. Because they are generalizations, the nurse must assess each woman experiencing pain related to childbirth.

Chinese women may not exhibit reactions to pain, although it is acceptable to exhibit pain during childbirth. They consider it impolite to accept something when it is first offered; therefore pain interventions must be offered more than once. Acupuncture may be used for pain relief.

Arab or Middle Eastern women may be vocal in response to labor pain. They may prefer medication for pain relief.

Japanese women may be stoic in response to labor pain, but they may request medication when pain becomes severe.

Southeast Asian women may endure severe pain before requesting relief.

Hispanic women may be stoic until late in labor, when they may become vocal and request pain relief.

Native American women may use medications or remedies made from indigenous plants. They are often stoic in response to labor pain.

African-American women may express pain openly. Use of medication for pain relief varies.

Anxiety

Anxiety is commonly associated with increased pain during labor. Mild anxiety is considered normal for a woman during labor and birth. However, excessive anxiety and fear cause more catecholamine secretion, which increases the stimuli to the brain from the pelvis because of decreased blood flow and increased muscle tension; this in turn magnifies pain (Lowe, 2002). Thus, as fear and anxiety heighten, muscle tension increases, the effectiveness of the uterine contractions decreases, the experience of discomfort increases, and a cycle of increased fear and anxiety begins. Ultimately this cycle will slow the progress of labor. The woman's "self-efficacy" or confidence in her ability to cope with pain will be diminished, potentially resulting in reduced effectiveness of pain relief measures being used.

Previous experience

For women who have had a difficult and painful previous birth experience, anxiety and fear from this past experience may lead to increased pain. Conversely, a woman who has experienced a labor and birth where pain coping skills were successful may experience increased anxiety when those previous coping skills are ineffective during a more difficult labor and birth.

Sensory pain for nulliparous women is often greater than that for multiparous women during early labor (dilation less than 5 cm) because their reproductive tract structures are less supple. During the transition phase of the first stage of labor and during the second stage of labor, multiparous women may experience greater sensory pain than nulliparous women because their more supple tissue increases the speed of fetal descent and thereby intensifies pain. The firmer tissue of nulliparous women results in a slower more gradual descent. Affective pain is usually greater for nulliparous women throughout the first stage of labor but decreases for both nulliparous and multiparous women during the second stage of labor (Lowe, 2002).

Women with a history of substance abuse experience as much pain during labor as other women. It is usually unnecessary to withhold pain medications. However, certain pain medications (e.g., opioid agonist-antagonists) can cause withdrawal symptoms in the woman with opioid addiction as well as in her newborn.

Pain is a personal response in each individual. As pain is experienced, people develop various coping mechanisms to deal with it. Emotional tension from anxiety and fear may increase pain and perception of pain during labor (see discussion of the Dick-Read method later in this chapter). Pain, or the possibility of pain, can induce fear in which anxiety borders on panic. Fatigue and sleep deprivation magnify pain. Parity may affect perception of labor pain because nulliparous women have longer labors and therefore greater fatigue, causing a vicious cycle of increased pain and a more likely use of pharmacologic support.

Childbirth preparation

Even pain stimuli that are particularly intense can, at times, be ignored. This is possible because certain nerve cell groupings within the spinal cord, brainstem, and cerebral cortex have the ability to modulate the pain impulse through a blocking mechanism. The gate-control theory of pain helps explain the way hypnosis and pain relief techniques taught in childbirth preparation classes work to relieve the pain of labor. According to this theory, pain sensations travel along sensory nerve pathways to the brain, but only a limited number of sensations, or messages, can travel through these nerve pathways at one time. Using distraction techniques such as massage or stroking, music, and imagery reduces or completely blocks the capacity of nerve pathways to transmit pain. These distractions are thought to work by closing down a hypothetic gate in the spinal cord, thus preventing pain signals from reaching the brain. Perception of pain is thereby diminished.

In addition, when the laboring woman engages in neuromuscular and motor activity, activity within the spinal cord itself further modifies the transmission of pain. Cognitive work involving concentration on breathing and relaxation requires selective and directed cortical activity that activates and closes the gating mechanism as well. The gate-control theory therefore underscores the need for a supportive birth setting that allows the laboring woman to relax and use various higher mental activities.

Comfort

Although the predominant medical approach to labor is that it is painful and the pain must be removed, an alternative view is that labor is a natural process and women can experience comfort and transcend the discomfort or pain. Having needs and desires met engenders a feeling of comfort. Comfort may be viewed as strengthening; this represents a paradigm shift in the interpretation of pain in labor (Koehn, 2000). The most helpful interventions in enhancing comfort are a caring nursing approach and a supportive presence.

Support

The pain occurring during childbirth and the management of this pain belong to the woman experiencing the pain; the nurse must engage in a cooperative effort to provide whatever external tools the woman requires to manage her pain experience. These tools include both nonpharmacologic and pharmacologic interventions. The presence of a person (e.g., doula, family member, friend) who provides physical, emotional, and psychologic support to the woman in labor is a beneficial form of care that significantly relieves pain, improves outcomes, decreases interventions (e.g., use of pharmacologic pain relief measures) and complication rates (e.g., cesarean births) associated with labor, and enhances overall maternal satisfaction (Hodnett, Gates, Hofmeyr, & Sakala, 2003; Righard, 2001; Simkin & O'Hara, 2002).

Environment

According to Lowe (2002), environment should be viewed in terms of the persons present (e.g., how they communicate, their philosophy of care, practice policies, and quality of support) and the physical space in which the labor occurs. The quality of the environment can influence a woman's ability to cope with the pain of labor. Women prefer to be cared for by familiar caregivers in a comfortable, homelike setting (Hodnett, 2002). An environment should be safe and private, allowing a woman to feel free to be herself as she tries out different comfort measures. Stimuli including light, noise, and temperature should be adjusted according to the woman's preferences. There should be space for movement, and equipment should be readily available for a variety of nonpharmacologic pain relief measures such as birth balls, comfortable chairs, tubs, and showers. The familiarity of the environment can be enhanced by bringing items from home such as pillows, objects for a focal point, music, and videos.

NONPHARMACOLOGIC MANAGEMENT OF DISCOMFORT

The alleviation of pain is important. Commonly, it is not the amount of pain the woman experiences, but whether she meets her goals for herself in coping with the pain that influences her perception of the birth experience as "good" or "bad." The observant nurse looks for clues to the woman's desired level of control in the management of pain and its relief.

The woman who chooses to deal with childbirth pain by using nonpharmacologic methods needs care and support from nurses and other care providers who are skilled in pain management. Many of the nonpharmacologic methods for relief of discomfort are taught in different types of prenatal preparation classes, or the woman or couple may have read various books and magazine articles on the subject in advance. Many of these methods require practice for best results (e.g., hypnosis, patterned breathing and controlled relaxation techniques, biofeedback), although the nurse may use some of them successfully without the woman or couple having prior knowledge (e.g., slow paced breathing, massage and touch, effleurage, counterpressure). Women should be encouraged to try a variety of methods and to seek alternatives, including pharmacologic methods, if the measure being used is no longer effective (Box 12-1).

Childbirth Preparation Methods

Historically, the major childbirth methods taught in the United States were the Dick-Read method, or natural childbirth method; the Lamaze method, or psychoprophylactic method; and the Bradley method, or husband-coached childbirth. In current practice the method of preparation has less emphasis; instead, emphasis is placed on getting expectant parents to attend childbirth preparation classes

---

BOX 12-1

Nonpharmacologic Strategies to Encourage Relaxation and Relieve Pain

CUTANEOUS STIMULATION STRATEGIES
- Counterpressure*
- Effleurage (light massage)*
- Therapeutic touch and massage*
- Walking*
- Rocking*
- Changing positions*
- Application of heat or cold*
- Transcutaneous electrical nerve stimulation
- Acupressure
- Water therapy (Showers, baths)
- Intradermal water block

SENSORY STIMULATION STRATEGIES
- Aromatherapy
- Breathing techniques*
- Music*
- Imagery*
- Use of focal points*

COGNITIVE STRATEGIES
- Childbirth education*
- Hypnosis
- Biofeedback

From Enkin, M. et al. (2001). Effective care in pregnancy and childbirth: A synopsis. *Birth,* 28(1), 41-51.
*Forms of care likely to be beneficial.

(U.S. Department of Health and Human Services [USDHHS], 2000).

How childbirth education influences a woman's response to pain is not completely understood. However, results of a number of studies suggest that not only is confidence greater after childbirth preparation but that this confidence increases the woman's ability to cope with labor and birth (Koehn, 2002).

Most proponents of prepared childbirth agree that the major causes of pain in labor are fear and tension. All childbirth methods attempt to reduce fear, tension, and pain by increasing the woman's knowledge of the labor and birth process, enhancing her self-confidence and sense of control, preparing a support person, and training the woman in physical conditioning and relaxation breathing. Women or couples should not expect a pain-free childbirth but rather a childbirth in which pain is controlled using a variety of methods including prepared childbirth techniques. No one approach can meet all needs.

Dick-Read method

To replace fear of the unknown with understanding and confidence, the **Dick-Read method** (Dick-Read, 1987) provides information on labor and birth, as well as nutrition, hygiene, and exercise. Classes include practice in three techniques: physical exercise to prepare the body for labor, conscious relaxation, and breathing patterns.

Conscious relaxation involves progressive relaxation of muscle groups in the entire body. With practice many women can relax on command, both during and between contractions. Some woman actually sleep between contractions.

Breathing patterns include deep abdominal respirations for most of labor, shallow breathing toward the end of the first stage, and, until recently, breath holding for the second stage of labor.

Teachers of the Dick-Read method also contend that the weight of the abdominal musculature of the contracting uterus increases pain. The woman is taught to force her abdominal muscles to rise as the uterus rises forward during a contraction, thus lifting the abdominal muscles off the contracting uterus.

Lamaze method

The Lamaze (psychoprophylaxis) method grew out of Pavlov's work on classical conditioning. According to Lamaze, pain is a conditioned response. Therefore women can also be conditioned not to experience pain in labor. The Lamaze method does this by conditioning women to respond to mock uterine contractions with controlled muscular relaxation and breathing patterns instead of crying out and losing control (Lamaze, 1972). Coping strategies also include concentrating on a focal point, such as a favorite picture or pattern, to keep nerve pathways occupied so that they cannot respond to painful stimuli.

The woman is taught to relax uninvolved muscle groups while she contracts a specific muscle group (Fig. 12-2). She applies this during labor by relaxing uninvolved muscles while her uterus contracts. The perception of maintaining control has also been found to be closely associated with satisfaction with the birth experience.

Lamaze teachers believe that chest breathing lifts the diaphragm off the contracting uterus, thus giving it more room to expand. The chest-breathing patterns are varied according to the intensity of the contractions and the progress of labor. Teachers also seek to eliminate fear by increasing the woman's understanding of her body functions and the neurophysiology of pain. Support in labor is provided by the woman's partner or other support person or by a specially trained labor attendant.

Bradley method

The Bradley method, also called *husband-coached childbirth,* was devised based on observations of animal behavior during birth. It emphasizes working in harmony with the body, using breath control and abdominal breathing, and promoting general body relaxation (Bradley, 1981).

The husband or partner takes an active role in assisting the woman to relax and use correct breathing techniques. This method also stresses environmental factors such as darkness, solitude, and quiet to make childbirth a more natural experience.

Specific Strategies
Focusing and relaxation

By reducing tension and stress, focusing and relaxation techniques allow a woman in labor to rest and to conserve energy for the task of giving birth. Attention-focusing and distraction techniques are forms of care likely to be beneficial in relieving labor pain (Enkin et al., 2000). Some women bring a favorite object such as a photograph or stuffed animal to the labor room and focus their attention on this object during contractions. Others choose to fix their attention on some object in the labor room. As the contraction begins, they focus on their chosen object and perform a breathing technique to reduce their perception of pain.

With imagery, the woman focuses her attention on a pleasant scene, a place where she feels relaxed, or an activity she enjoys. She can imagine walking through a restful garden or breathing in light, energy, and healing color and breathing out worries and tension. Choosing the subject for the imagery and practicing the technique during pregnancy will enhance effectiveness during labor (Koehn, 2000). These techniques, coupled with feedback relaxation, help the woman work with her contractions rather than against them. The support person monitors this process, telling the woman when to begin the breathing techniques (Fig. 12-3).

During childbirth preparation classes, the partner or coach can learn how to palpate a woman's body to detect tense and contracted muscles. The woman then learns how to relax the tense muscle in response to the gentle stroking of the muscle by the coach (see Fig. 12-2). In a common feedback mechanism, the woman and her coach say the word "relax" at the onset of each contraction and throughout it as needed. With practice the coach can effectively use support, feedback, and touch to facilitate the woman's relaxation and thereby reduce tension and stress and enhance the progress of labor (Humenick, Schrock, & Libresco, 2000). The nurse can assist the woman by providing a quiet environment and offering cues as needed.

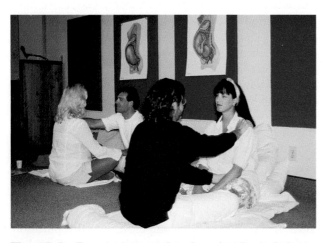

Fig. 12-2 Expectant parents learning relaxation techniques. (Courtesy Marjorie Pyle, RNC, Lifecircle, Costa Mesa, CA.)

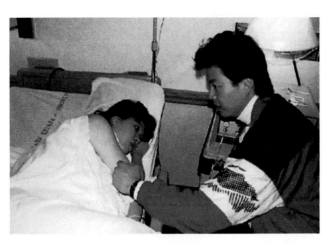

Fig. 12-3 Laboring woman using focusing and breathing techniques during a uterine contraction with coaching from her partner. (Courtesy Marjorie Pyle, RNC, Lifecircle, Costa Mesa, CA.)

Breathing techniques

Different approaches to childbirth preparation stress varying breathing techniques to provide distraction, thereby reducing the perception of pain and helping the woman maintain control throughout contractions. In the first stage of labor, such breathing techniques can promote relaxation of the abdominal muscles and thereby increase the size of the abdominal cavity. This lessens discomfort generated by friction between the uterus and abdominal wall during contractions. Because the muscles of the genital area also become more relaxed, they do not interfere with fetal descent. In the second stage, breathing is used to increase abdominal pressure and thereby assist in expelling the fetus. Breathing also can be used to relax the pudendal muscles to prevent precipitate expulsion of the fetal head.

For couples who have prepared for labor by practicing relaxing and breathing techniques, occasional reminders may be all that are necessary to help them along. For those who have had no preparation, instruction in simple breathing and relaxation can be given early in labor and often is surprisingly successful. Motivation is high, and readiness to learn is enhanced by the reality of labor.

Paced breathing. There are various breathing techniques for controlling pain during contractions (Box 12-2). The nurse needs to ascertain what, if any, techniques the laboring couple knows before giving them instruction. Simple patterns are more easily learned. Paced breathing is the technique most associated with prepared childbirth and includes slow-paced, modified-paced, and patterned-paced breathing techniques. Each labor is different, and nursing support includes assisting couples to adapt breathing techniques to their individual labor experience.

All patterns begin with a routine deep relaxing cleansing breath to "greet the contraction" and end with another deep breath exhaled to "gently blow the contraction away." In general, slow-paced breathing, at approximately half the woman's normal breathing rate, is initiated when the woman can no longer walk or talk through contractions. She should continue to use this technique for as long as it is effective in reducing the perception of pain and maintaining control. As contractions increase in frequency and intensity, the woman often needs to change to a more complex breathing technique, which is shallower and approximately twice her normal rate of breathing. This modified-paced pattern requires more concentration and therefore blocks more painful stimuli than the simpler slow-paced breathing pattern (Nichols, 2000; Perinatal Education Associates, 2003).

The most difficult time to maintain control during contractions comes when the cervix dilates from 8 cm to 10 cm. This phase is called the *transition phase* of the first stage of labor. Even for the woman who has prepared for labor, concentration on breathing techniques is difficult to maintain. The patterned-paced breathing technique is suggested for use during this phase. It may be the 4:1 pattern: breath, breath, breath, breath, blow (as though gently blowing out a candle).

BOX 12-2

Paced Breathing Techniques

CLEANSING BREATH

Relaxed breath in through nose and out mouth. Used at the beginning and end of each contraction.

SLOW-PACED BREATHING (APPROXIMATELY 6 TO 8 BREATHS PER MINUTE)

Not less than half normal breathing rate (number of breaths per minute divided by 2)
IN-2-3-4/OUT-2-3-4/IN-2-3-4/OUT-2-3-4. . .

MODIFIED-PACED BREATHING (APPROXIMATELY 32 TO 40 BREATHS PER MINUTE)

Not more than twice normal breathing rate (number of breaths per minute multiplied by 2)

IN-OUT/IN-OUT/IN-OUT/IN-OUT. . .

For more flexibility and variety the woman may combine the slow and modified breathing by using the slow breathing for beginnings and ends of contractions and modified breathing for more intense peaks. This technique conserves energy, lessens fatigue, and reduces risk for hyperventilation.

PATTERNED-PACED BREATHING (SAME RATE AS MODIFIED)

Enhances concentration
a. 3:1 Patterned breathing IN-OUT/IN-OUT/IN-OUT/IN-BLOW (repeat through contraction)
b. 4:1 Patterned breathing IN-OUT/IN-OUT/IN-OUT/IN-OUT/IN-BLOW (repeat through contraction)

Source: Nichols, F. (2000). Paced breathing techniques. In F. Nichols & S. Humenick (Eds.), *Childbirth education: Practice, research, and theory* (2nd ed.). Philadelphia: Saunders; Perinatal Education Associates. (2003). *Breathing through labor and birth.* Internet document available at http://www.birthsource.com/articlefile/Article39.html (accessed October 27, 2004).

This ratio may be increased to 6:1 or 8:1. An undesirable side effect of this type of breathing is hyperventilation. The woman and her support person must be aware of and watch for symptoms of the resultant respiratory alkalosis: light-headedness, dizziness, tingling of the fingers, or circumoral numbness. Respiratory alkalosis may be eliminated by having the woman breathe into a paper bag held tightly around the mouth and nose. This enables her to rebreathe carbon dioxide and replace the bicarbonate ion. The woman also can breathe into her cupped hands if no bag is available. Maintaining a breathing rate that is no more than twice the normal rate will lessen chances of hyperventilation. The partner can help the woman maintain her breathing rate with visual, tactile, or auditory cues (Nichols, 2000).

During second-stage pushing, the woman should find a breathing pattern that is relaxing and feels good for her and her baby. Any regular or rhythmic breathing during pushing should maintain a good oxygen flow to the fetus (Perinatal Education Associates, 2003).

Effleurage and counterpressure

Effleurage (light massage) and counterpressure have brought relief to many women during the first stage of labor. The gate-control theory may supply the reason for the effectiveness of these measures. Effleurage is light stroking, usually of the abdomen, in rhythm with breathing during contractions. It is used to distract the woman from contraction pain. Often the presence of monitor belts makes it difficult to perform effleurage on the abdomen; therefore a thigh or the chest may be used. As labor progresses, hyperesthesia may make effleurage uncomfortable and thus less effective.

Counterpressure is steady pressure applied by a support person to the sacral area with the fist or heel of the hand. This technique helps the woman cope with the sensations of internal pressure and pain in the lower back. It is especially helpful when back pain is caused by pressure of the occiput against spinal nerves when the fetal head is in a posterior position. Counterpressure lifts the occiput off these nerves, thereby providing pain relief. Although not an evidenced-based practice, pressure also may be applied bilaterally to the hips or knees to reduce low back pain (Simkin & Ancheta, 2000). The support person will need to be relieved occasionally because application of counterpressure is hard work.

Music

Music, taped or live, enhances relaxation during labor, thereby reducing stress, anxiety, and the perception of pain. It can be used to promote relaxation in early labor and to stimulate movement as labor progresses (Browning, 2000). Women should be taught about the effectiveness of using music during labor for relaxation and for reduction of the perception of pain. They should be encouraged to prepare their musical preferences in advance and bring a tape or compact disc player to the hospital or birthing center. Use of a headset or earphones may increase the effectiveness of the music because other sounds will be shut out. Live music provided at the bedside by a support person may also be very helpful in transmitting energy that decreases tension and elevates mood (Gentz, 2001). Changing the tempo of the music to coincide with the rate and rhythm of each breathing technique may facilitate proper pacing (Gentz, 2001).

Water therapy (hydrotherapy)

Bathing, showering, and jet hydrotherapy (whirlpool baths) with warm water (e.g., at or below body temperature) are nonpharmacologic measures that can be used to promote comfort and relaxation during labor (Fig. 12-4). Sitting in a tub of water up to the shoulders or lower for 1 to 2 hours has several immediate benefits. Buoyancy in the water results in general body relaxation and temporary relief from discomfort and pain (Nikodem, 2003). This reduces the woman's anxiety and enhances a feeling of well-being. Catecholamine production decreases. This triggers an increase in the levels of oxytocin (to stimulate uterine contractions) and endorphins (to reduce pain perception). In addition, the bubbles and gentle lapping of the water stimulate the nipples, also triggering an increase in oxytocin production; this has not been observed to cause uterine hyperstimulation. The cervix has often been observed to dilate 2 to 3 cm in 30 minutes of whirlpool therapy. Whirlpool baths in labor also have been found to have positive effects on analgesia requirements, instrumentation rates, condition of the perineum, and personal satisfaction with labor (Simkin & O'Hara, 2002). However, there is no clear evidence that these effects can be attributed solely to hydrotherapy (Benfield, 2002).

If the woman is having "back labor" as the result of an occiput posterior or transverse position, she is encouraged to assume the hands-and-knees or the side-lying position in the tub. Because these positions decrease pain and increase relaxation and production of oxytocin, the fetus can then rotate spontaneously to the occiput anterior position. Less effort is required when changing positions in water.

In some settings, jet hydrotherapy should be approved by the woman's primary health care provider. The woman's vital signs must be within normal limits, and she should be in the active phase of the first stage of labor (e.g., cervix at least 5 cm dilated). If she is in the latent phase, her contractions could slow (Mackey, 2001).

Fetal heart rate (FHR) monitoring is done by Doppler device, fetoscope, or wireless external monitor device (see Fig. 12-4, *C*). Placement of internal electrodes is contraindicated for jet hydrotherapy. The woman's membranes may be intact or ruptured. If they are ruptured, the fluid must be clear or only lightly stained with meconium (Mackey, 2001).

There is no limit to the time women can stay in the bath, and often women are encouraged to stay in it as long as desired. However, most women use jet hydrotherapy for 30 to 60 minutes at a time. During the bath, if the woman's temperature and the FHR increase, if the labor process becomes less effective (e.g., slows or becomes too intense), or if relief of pain is reduced, the woman can come out of the bath and

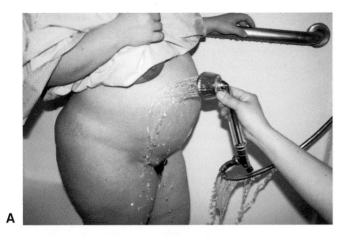

A

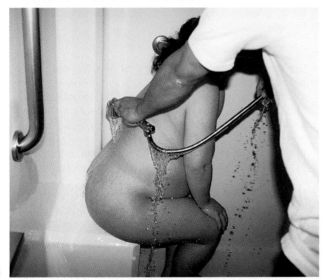

B

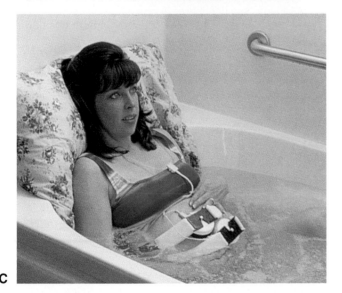

C

Fig. 12-4 Water therapy during labor. **A,** Use of shower during labor. **B,** Woman experiencing back labor relaxes as partner sprays warm water on her back. **C,** Laboring woman relaxes in Jacuzzi. Note that fetal monitoring can continue during time in the Jacuzzi. (**A** and **B** Courtesy Marjorie Pyle, RNC, Lifecircle, Costa Mesa, CA; **C** Courtesy Spacelabs Medical, Redmond, WA.)

Critical Thinking Exercise

Hydrotherapy

Yvonne is pregnant for the first time and is at term and in active labor. Her cervix is dilated 5 cm and her membranes are intact. She has declined pain medication but is somewhat uncomfortable during contractions. She thinks she would like to try the Jacuzzi tub to see if being in the water would make her feel more comfortable. However, she has concerns about the safety of being in the whirlpool bath during labor. She asks the nurse for information to help her decide what to do.

1. Evidence—Is there sufficient evidence to draw conclusions about what advice the nurse should give to Yvonne about hydrotherapy in labor?
2. Assumptions—What assumptions can be made about the following issues related to hydrotherapy:
   a. Degree of pain relief expected by the woman
   b. Effect on promotion of comfort
   c. Safety of hydrotherapy
3. What implications and priorities for nursing care can be drawn at this time?
4. Does the evidence objectively support your conclusion?
5. Are there alternative perspectives to your conclusion?

return at a later time. Repeated baths with occasional breaks may be more effective in relieving pain in long labors than extended amounts of time in the water. Fluids to maintain hydration and a cool face cloth for comfort are offered during the bath (Mackey, 2001; Simkin & O'Hara, 2002). The recommended temperature for the bath is between 36° and 38° C to avoid harmful effects (Florence & Palmer, 2003).

Transcutaneous electrical nerve stimulation

Transcutaneous electrical nerve stimulation (TENS) involves the placing of two pairs of flat electrodes on either side of the woman's thoracic and sacral spine (Fig. 12-5). These electrodes provide continuous low-intensity electrical impulses or stimuli from a battery-operated device. During a contraction the woman increases the stimulation from low to high intensity by turning control knobs on the device. High intensity should be maintained for at least 1 minute to facilitate release of endorphins. Women describe the resulting sensation as a tingling or buzzing and the pain relief as good or very good. TENS is most useful for lower back pain during the early first stage of labor. Using TENS poses no risk to the mother or fetus, and it is credited with reducing or eliminating the need for analgesia and with increasing the woman's perception of control over the experience. It may be effective because of the placebo effect; that is, confidence in the effectiveness of TENS may stimulate the release of endogenous opiates (endorphins) in the woman's body and thus alleviate the discomfort (Gentz, 2001). TENS is now considered a form of care with insufficient quality data �֍

BACKGROUND

- During labor, the buoyancy of water immersion may relieve pressure and tension, may decrease catecholamines and pain, may decrease maternal anxiety, may speed cervical dilation, and may increase uterine perfusion. The mother may benefit from decreased blood pressure and increased satisfaction. Water births may increase elasticity of the birth canal, resulting in fewer tears and episiotomies.
- Adverse maternal effects may include restricted mobility, risk for infection, and risk for water embolism. Reduced uterine tone may lead to decreased contraction effectiveness, postpartum bleeding, and need for manual removal of placenta.
- Adverse neonatal effects may include inhalation of water, possibly leading to hemodilution, or pneumonitis because of additives.

OBJECTIVES

- Research questions included evidence of benefits and risks of water immersion during pregnancy, early and late first-stage labor, and second-stage labor.
- The reviewers also questioned whether any difference in outcomes occurred in moving versus still water or if water additives, such as essential oils or salt, were present.
- Reviewers looked for the following outcomes in trials: maternal satisfaction, pain, use of analgesia and anesthesia, labor augmentation, maternal blood pressure and pulse, duration of labor and delivery, mode of delivery, perineal trauma, blood loss, postnatal infection, maternal self-esteem, postpartum depression, and breastfeeding. Fetal and infant outcomes were fetal heart rate patterns and neonatal Apgar score, cord pH, neonatal intensive care unit (NICU) admission, respiratory support, temperature at birth, infection, neurologic outcome (e.g., cerebral palsy, death, and cord injuries), and caregiver satisfaction and injuries.

METHODS
Search Strategy

- Search strategy involved searches in Cochrane Central Registry of Controlled trials, MEDLINE, hand searches in 30 journals, and a weekly alert service for 37 other journals. Keywords were not noted.
- Eight randomized, controlled trials were selected, for a total of 2939 women from Belgium, Australia, Sweden, South Africa, Canada, and the United States. The studies were published from 1993 to 2003. All studies used warm water immersion as their intervention, and standard institutional labor care for the controls.

Statistical Analyses

- Statistical analyses compared similar outcome measures. Interventions varied, such as water temperature (37° to 38° C) and the intermittent or continuous presence of a 1:1 caregiver.

FINDINGS

- During first-stage labor, women using water immersion demonstrated a statistically significant decrease in perception of pain and use of epidural, spinal, and cervical analgesia or anesthesia when compared with controls. Blood pressure was significantly lower for the water immersion group. No difference was noted between groups in labor or birth duration, operative or assisted birth, perineal trauma, tears, or episiotomies. Infants of mothers using water immersion during first-stage labor had no difference from the controls in number of low Apgar scores or NICU admissions. This was true even when the gestation was less than 34 weeks.
- During second-stage labor, one trial reported that women in the immersion group had greater satisfaction in coping with their pushing efforts than the controls.
- One study showed an increase in epidural use and labor augmentation if the water immersion was used early in labor, when compared with use during more advanced labor.

LIMITATIONS

- Small sample sizes limited all the studies. It is not possible to blind subjects or caregivers to the intervention. Comfort levels with the intervention differ across subjects and caregivers, which can bias pain perception, analgesia use, maternal satisfaction, self-esteem, and postpartum depression. Subjects did not always comply with the protocol to which they were randomized. One study found that 46% of its "immersion" group never got into the water. All studies reported some crossover between groups.
- Researchers used different definitions of labor, which can influence length and progression data. Trials varied on their tolerance of ruptured membranes; some required it and some excluded it, which can affect pain perception and analgesia use.
- Labor management varied across the trials, as did the presence of a 1:1 caregiver. There were differences in the pool shapes and differences in whether the water was still or moving, which may have affected comfort, position changes, and movement.

CONCLUSIONS

- Water immersion was associated with a significant decrease in the perception of pain and use of analgesia, and therefore may be of benefit for women in later first-stage labor. There were not enough data to recommend water immersion during second-stage labor.

IMPLICATIONS FOR PRACTICE

- Water immersion can be used to provide comfort in first-stage labor. Use of immersion must occur after labor is well established. Nurses can advocate for equipment in their birthing or labor and delivery units to enable them to offer this option. Having 1:1 caregivers to monitor safety and progress of labor is important.

IMPLICATIONS FOR FURTHER RESEARCH

- Standardized definitions, protocols, and outcome measures should be used in future research. Infection, a major concern, was not addressed. More well-designed trials evaluating water immersion during second-stage labor are needed.

Reference: Cluett, E., Nikoden, V., McCandlish, R., & Burns, E. (2004). Immersion in water in pregnancy, labour and birth (Cochrane Review). In *The Cochrane Library*, Issue 2, 2004. Chichester, UK: John Wiley & Sons.

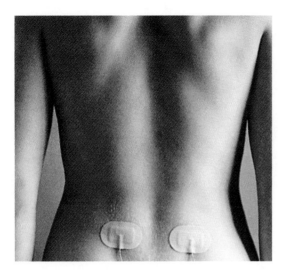

Fig. 12-5 Placement of transcutaneous electrical nerve stimulation (TENS) electrodes on back for relief of labor pain.

to recommend its use (Enkin et al., 2000). The nurse assists the woman in using TENS by explaining the device and its use, by carefully placing and securing the electrodes, and by closely evaluating its effectiveness.

Acupressure and acupuncture

Acupressure and acupuncture techniques can be used in pregnancy, in labor, and postpartum to relieve pain and other discomforts. Pressure, heat, or cold is applied to acupuncture points called *tsubos*. These points have an increased density of neuroreceptors and increased electrical conductivity. The effectiveness of acupressure has been attributed to the gate-control theory of pain and an increase in endorphin levels (Tiran & Mack, 2000). Acupressure is best applied over the skin without using lubricants. Pressure is usually applied with the heel of the hand, fist, or pads of the thumbs and fingers (Fig. 12-6). Tennis balls or other devices also may be used to apply pressure. Pressure is applied with

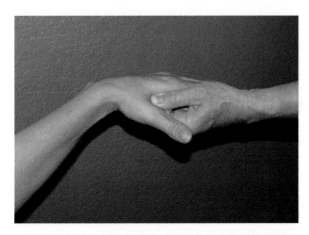

Fig. 12-6 Ho-Ku acupressure point (back of hand where thumb and index finger come together) used to enhance uterine contractions without increasing pain. (Courtesy Julie Perry Nelson, Gilbert, AZ.)

contractions initially and then continuously as labor progresses to the transition phase at the end of the first stage of labor (Koehn, 2000). Synchronized breathing by the caregiver and the woman is suggested for greater effectiveness. Acupressure points are found on the neck, shoulders, wrists, lower back including sacral points, hips, area below the kneecaps, ankles, nails on the small toes, and soles of the feet.

Acupuncture is the insertion of fine needles into specific areas of the body to restore the flow of qi (energy) and to decrease pain, which is thought to be obstructing the flow of energy. It should be done by a trained certified therapist. Current evidence implies that acupuncture may be beneficial for relief of labor pain; however, further study is indicated (Florence & Palmer, 2003).

Application of heat and cold

Warmed blankets, warm compresses, heated rice bags, a warm bath or shower, or a moist heating pad can enhance relaxation and reduce pain during labor. Heat relieves muscle ischemia and increases blood flow to the area of discomfort. Heat application is effective for back pain caused by a posterior presentation or general backache from fatigue ❋ (Simkin & O'Hara, 2002).

Cold application such as cool cloths or ice packs may be effective in increasing comfort when the woman feels warm 🔊 and may be applied to areas of pain. Cooling relieves pain by reducing the muscle temperature and relieving muscle spasms.

Heat and cold may be used alternately for a greater effect. Neither heat nor cold should be applied over ischemic or anesthetized areas because tissues can be damaged.

Touch and massage

Touch and massage have been an integral part of the traditional care process for women in labor. They are likely to ❋ be beneficial in relieving labor pain (Enkin et al., 2000).

Touch can be as simple as holding the woman's hand, stroking her body, and embracing her. When using touch to communicate caring, reassurance, and concern, it is important that the woman's preferences for touch (e.g., who can touch her, where they can touch her, and how they can touch her) and responses to touch be determined (Simkin & O'Hara, 2002). Touch also can involve very specialized techniques that require manipulation of the human energy field. Therapeutic touch (TT) uses the concept of energy fields within the body called *prana*. Prana are thought to be deficient in some people who are in pain. TT uses laying-on of hands by a specially trained person to redirect energy fields associated with pain (Scheiber & Selby, 2000). Research has demonstrated effectiveness of TT to enhance relaxation, reduce anxiety, and relieve pain (Marks, 2000); however, little is known about the use or effectiveness of TT for relieving labor pain.

Healing touch (HT) is another energy-based healing modality. Whereas TT emphasizes a single sequence of energy modulation, HT combines a variety of techniques from

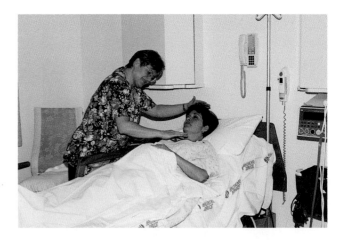

Fig. 12-7 Healing touch used for labor care. (Courtesy Wendy Wetzel, Flagstaff, AZ.)

a series of disciplines. This gives the practitioner an array of "tools" to use with patients. Practitioners are taught energetic diagnosis and treatment forms and the means of documenting the patient's response and progress. These techniques are said to align and balance the human energy field, thereby enhancing the body's ability to heal itself. HT has been used in labor management, but no studies have been published about its effectiveness (Hover-Kramer, Mentgen, & Scandrett-Hibdon, 2001) (Fig. 12-7).

Head, hand, back, and foot massage may be very effective in reducing tension and enhancing comfort. Hand and foot massage may be especially relaxing in advanced labor when hyperesthesia limits a woman's tolerance for touch on other parts of her body. The woman and her partner should be encouraged to experiment with different types of massage during pregnancy to determine what might feel best and be most relaxing during labor.

Hypnosis

Hypnosis, although not commonly used for pain management in the United States, is associated with shorter labors and less analgesia (Tiran & Mack, 2000). Hypnosis techniques used for labor and birth place an emphasis on enhancing relaxation and diminishing fear, anxiety, and perception of pain. The woman may be given direct suggestions about pain relief or indirect suggestions that she is experiencing diminished sensations (Ketterhagen, VandeVusse, & Berner, 2002). The woman receives posthypnotic suggestions, such as, "You will be able to push the baby out easily," to increase her confidence. To be successful, the woman must be educated regarding hypnosis and must practice the techniques during the prenatal period (Gentz, 2001).

Biofeedback

Biofeedback may provide another relaxation technique that can be used for labor. Biofeedback is based on the theory that if a person can recognize physical signals, certain internal physiologic events can be changed (i.e., whatever physical signs the woman has that are associated with her

pain). During the prenatal period, the woman must be educated to become aware of her body and its responses and how to relax for biofeedback to be effective. The woman must learn how to use thinking and mental processes (e.g., focusing) to control body responses and functions. Informational biofeedback helps couples develop awareness of their bodies and use strategies to change their responses to stress. If the woman responds to pain during a contraction with tightening of muscles, frowning, moaning, and breath holding, her partner uses verbal and touch feedback to help her relax. Formal biofeedback, which uses machines to detect skin temperature, blood flow, or muscle tension, also can prepare women to intensify their relaxation responses (DiFranco, 2000; Gentz, 2001; Snyder & Lindquist, 2000).

Aromatherapy

Aromatherapy uses oils distilled from plants, flowers, herbs, and trees to promote health and well-being and treat illnesses. The use of herbal teas and vapors is reported to have good effects in pregnancy and labor for some women (Tiran & Mack, 2000). Lavender, clary sage, and bergamot promote relaxation and can be used by adding a few drops to a warm bath, to warm water used for soaking compresses that can be applied to the body, to an aromatherapy lamp to vaporize a room, or to oil for a back massage (Tiran & Mack, 2000).

NURSE ALERT *Caution: Never apply the essential oils used for aromatherapy in full strength directly to the skin. Most oils should be diluted in a vegetable oil base before use. In addition, essential oils vary in terms of safe use during pregnancy (Gentz, 2001).*

Intradermal water block

An intradermal water block involves the injection of small amounts of sterile water (e.g., 0.05 to 0.1 ml) by using a fine needle (e.g., 25 gauge) into four locations on the lower back to relieve back pain. It may be effective in early labor and in an effort to delay the initiation of pharmacologic pain relief measures. Stinging will occur for about 20 to 30 seconds after injection, but back pain will be relieved for approximately 45 minutes to 2 hours. Effectiveness of this method may be related to the mechanisms of counterirritation (i.e., reducing localized pain in one area by irritating the skin in an area nearby), gate control, or an increase in the level of endogenous opioids (endorphins). When the effect wears off, the treatment can be repeated, or another method of pain relief can be used (Gentz, 2001; Simkin & O'Hara, 2002).

PHARMACOLOGIC MANAGEMENT OF DISCOMFORT

Pharmacologic measures for pain management should be implemented before pain becomes so severe that catecholamines increase and labor is prolonged. Pharmacologic and nonpharmacologic measures, when used together, increase the level of pain relief and create a more positive labor experience for the woman and her family. Nonpharmacologic measures can be used for relaxation and for pain relief, especially in early labor. Pharmacologic measures can be implemented as labor becomes more active and discomfort and pain intensify. Less pharmacologic intervention often is required because nonpharmacologic measures enhance relaxation and potentiate the analgesic's effect (Faucher & Brucker, 2000).

Sedatives

Sedatives relieve anxiety and induce sleep and may be given to a woman experiencing a prolonged latent phase of labor and when there is a need to decrease anxiety or promote sleep. They may also be given to augment analgesia and reduce nausea when an opioid is used. Barbiturates such as secobarbital sodium (Seconal) can cause undesirable side effects including respiratory and vasomotor depression affecting the woman and newborn. These effects are increased if a barbiturate is administered with another central nervous system (CNS) depressant such as an opioid analgesic. Because of these disadvantages, barbiturates are seldom used (Faucher & Brucker, 2000; Hawkins, Chestnut, & Gibbs, 2002).

Phenothiazines (e.g., promethazine [Phenergan], hydroxyzine [Vistaril]) do not relieve pain but decrease anxiety and apprehension, increase sedation, and may potentiate opioid analgesic effects (Florence & Palmer, 2003). Metoclopramide (Reglan) is an antiemetic that also can be used for this purpose.

Benzodiazepines (e.g., diazepam [Valium], lorazepam [Ativan]), when given with an opioid analgesic, seem to enhance pain relief and reduce nausea and vomiting, although the increased sedation experienced may be unacceptable to women in labor (Bricker & Lavender, 2002; Lehne, 2001).

Analgesia and Anesthesia

The use of analgesia and anesthesia was not generally accepted as part of obstetric management until Queen Victoria used chloroform during the birth of her son in 1853. Since then,

much study has gone into the development of pharmacologic measures for controlling discomfort during the birth period. The goal of researchers is to develop methods that will provide adequate pain relief to women without increasing maternal or fetal risk or affecting the progress of labor.

Nursing management of obstetric analgesia and anesthesia combines the nurse's expertise in maternity care with a knowledge and understanding of anatomy and physiology and of medications and their therapeutic effects, adverse reactions, and methods of administration.

Anesthesia encompasses analgesia, amnesia, relaxation, and reflex activity. Anesthesia abolishes pain perception by interrupting the nerve impulses to the brain. The loss of sensation may be partial or complete, sometimes with the loss of consciousness.

The term *analgesia* refers to the alleviation of the sensation of pain or the raising of the threshold for pain perception without loss of consciousness.

The type of analgesic or anesthetic chosen is determined in part by the stage of labor of the woman and by the method of birth planned (Box 12-3).

BOX 12-3

Pharmacologic Control of Discomfort by Stage of Labor and Method of Birth

FIRST STAGE
- Systemic analgesia
- Opioid agonist analgesics
- Opioid agonist-antagonist analgesics
- Epidural (block) analgesia
- Combined spinal-epidural (CSE) analgesia
- Paracervical block (rarely used)
- Nitrous oxide

SECOND STAGE
- Nerve block analgesia and anesthesia
- Local infiltration anesthesia
- Pudendal block
- Spinal (block) anesthesia
- Epidural (block) analgesia
- Combined spinal-epidural (CSE) analgesia
- Nitrous oxide

VAGINAL BIRTH
- Local infiltration anesthesia
- Pudendal block
- Epidural (block) analgesia and anesthesia
- Spinal (block) anesthesia
- Combined spinal-epidural (CSE) analgesia and anesthesia
- Nitrous oxide

CESAREAN BIRTH
- Spinal (block) anesthesia
- Epidural (block) anesthesia
- General anesthesia

Systemic analgesia

Systemic analgesia remains the major pharmacologic method for relieving the pain of labor when personnel trained in regional analgesia (e.g., epidural analgesia) are not available (Bricker & Lavender, 2002; Caton et al., 2002). It is a form of care with a trade-off between beneficial and adverse effects (Enkin et al., 2000). Systemic analgesics cross the maternal blood-brain barrier to provide central analgesic effects. They also cross through the placenta. Once transferred to the fetus, analgesics cross the fetal blood-brain barrier more readily than the maternal blood-brain barrier. The duration of action also will be longer because the systemic analgesics used during labor have a significantly longer half-life in the fetus and newborn. Effects on the fetus and newborn can be profound (e.g., respiratory depression, decreased alertness, delayed sucking), depending on the characteristics of the specific systemic analgesic used, the dosage given, and the route and timing of administration. IV administration is preferred to IM administration because the medication's onset of action is faster and more predictable; as a result, a higher level of pain relief usually occurs. IV patient-controlled analgesia (PCA) is now available for use during labor. With this method the woman self-administers small doses of an opioid analgesic by using a pump programmed for dose and frequency. Overall, a lower total amount of analgesic is used, and maternal satisfaction is high (Bricker & Lavender, 2002). Classifications of analgesic drugs used to relieve the pain of childbirth include opioid (narcotic) agonists and opioid (narcotic) agonist-antagonists.

Opioid agonist analgesics. Opioid (narcotic) agonist analgesics such as meperidine (Demerol) and fentanyl (Sublimaze) are effective for relieving severe, persistent, or recurrent pain. They have no amnesic effect but create a feeling of well-being or euphoria. These analgesics decrease gastric emptying and increase nausea and vomiting. Bladder and bowel elimination can be inhibited. Because heart rate (e.g., bradycardia, tachycardia), blood pressure (e.g., hypotension), and respiratory effort (e.g., depression) can be adversely affected, opioid analgesics should be used cautiously in women with respiratory and cardiovascular disorders. Safety precautions should be taken because sedation and dizziness can occur after administration, increasing the risk for injury. Research findings suggest that women who receive opioids for their labor pain have less effective pain

---

Medication Guide

Opioid Analgesics for Labor

MEPERIDINE (DEMEROL)

Action
Opioid agonist analgesic; stimulates mu and kappa opioid receptors to decrease transmission of pain impulses

Indication
Labor pain; postoperative pain after cesarean birth

Dosage and Route
25 mg IV; 50-75 mg IM or SC. May repeat in 1-3 hr; use of ataractic or antiemetic drugs may potentiate analgesic effect and decrease nausea and vomiting

Adverse Effects
Nausea and vomiting, sedation, confusion, drowsiness, tachycardia or bradycardia, hypotension, dry mouth, pruritus, urinary retention, respiratory depression (woman and newborn), decreased fetal heart rate (FHR) variability, decreased uterine activity if given in early labor

Nursing Considerations
Assess FHR and uterine activity; observe for respiratory depression; if birth occurs within 1-4 hr of dose, observe newborn for respiratory depression; have naloxone available as antidote; keep side rails up; continue use of nonpharmacologic pain relief measures

BUTORPHANOL TARTRATE (STADOL)

Action
Mixed agonist-antagonist analgesic; stimulates kappa opioid receptor and blocks mu opioid receptor

Indication
Labor pain; postoperative pain after cesarean birth

Dosage and Route
1 mg IV q3-4h; 2 mg IM q3-4h

Adverse Effects
Confusion, sedation, sweating; transient sinusoidal-like FHR rhythm; less respiratory depression than with meperidine, nausea, and vomiting

Nursing Considerations
See meperidine; may precipitate withdrawal symptoms in opioid-dependent women and their newborns

NALBUPHINE (NUBAIN)

Action
Mixed agonist-antagonist analgesic; stimulates kappa opioid receptor and blocks mu opioid receptor

Indication
Labor pain; postoperative pain after cesarean birth

Dosage and Route
10 mg IV; 10-20 mg IM q3-6h

Adverse Effects
See butorphanol

Nursing Considerations
See butorphanol

IM, Intramuscular; *IV,* intravenous; *SC,* subcutaneous.

Medication Guide

Fentanyl (Sublimaze) and Sufentanil (Sufenta)

Action

Opioid analgesics, rapid action with short duration (1-2 hr IM; ½-1 hr IV)

Indication

For epidural or intrathecal analgesia, alone or in combination with a local anesthetic

Dosage and Route

Fentanyl: IM 50 to 100 mcg, IV 25 to 50 mcg; epidural fentanyl: 1 to 2 mcg with 0.125% bupivacaine at rate of 8 to 10 ml/hr; sufentanil, 1 mcg with 0.125% bupivacaine at rate of 10 ml/hr; dosage regimens vary

Adverse Effects

Dizziness, drowsiness, allergic reactions, rash, pruritus, respiratory depression, nausea and vomiting, urinary retention

Nursing Considerations

Assess for respiratory depression; naloxone should be available as antidote

IM, Intramuscular; *IV,* intravenous.

relief and are less satisfied with their pain management method than women whose pain is managed by using epidural analgesia. Conversely, opioid use is associated with shorter labors, less oxytocin augmentation, and fewer instrumental vaginal births (e.g., forceps-assisted or vacuum-assisted birth) when compared with epidural analgesia (Bricker & Lavender, 2002; Caton et al., 2002; Leighton & Halpern, 2002).

Meperidine is historically the most commonly used opioid agonist analgesic for women in labor but it is no longer the preferred choice because other medications have fewer side effects (Florence & Palmer, 2003) (see Medication Guide).

Fentanyl (and sufentanil) is a potent, short-acting opioid agonist analgesic (see Medication Guide). Onset of the medication action after IV injection occurs within 2 minutes; the action peaks in 3 to 5 minutes; and the duration of action is about 30 to 60 minutes. Onset of the medication action occurs in 7 to 8 minutes after IM injection, reaches its peak effect in 20 to 30 minutes, and lasts for 1 to 2 hours. More frequent dosing is required with fentanyl because of its shorter duration of action. Additive CNS and respiratory depression occurs if fentanyl is given with alcohol, antihistamines, antidepressants, or sedative-hypnotics. Fentanyl is commonly used in combination with a local anesthetic agent for induction of spinal-epidural nerve block analgesia (Faucher & Brucker, 2000; Lehne, 2001) (see Medication Guide).

Opioid agonist-antagonist analgesics. An agonist is an agent that activates or stimulates a receptor to act; an antagonist is an agent that blocks a receptor or a medication designed to activate a receptor. Opioid (narcotic) agonist-antagonist analgesics such as butorphanol (Stadol) and nalbuphine (Nubain), in the doses used during labor, provide adequate analgesia without causing significant respiratory depression in the mother or neonate. They are less likely to cause nausea and vomiting when compared with meperidine, but sedation may be as great or greater. Both IM and IV routes of administration are used, with IV administration being more common. This classification of opioid analgesics is not suitable for women with an opioid dependence because the antagonist activity could precipitate withdrawal symptoms (abstinence syndrome) in both the mother and her newborn (Hawkins et al., 2002; Lehne, 2001) (see Medication Guide on p. 350 and Signs of Potential Complications boxes).

Opioid (narcotic) antagonists. Opioids such as meperidine and fentanyl can cause excessive CNS depression in the mother, the newborn, or both. Opioid antagonists such as naloxone (Narcan) can promptly reverse the CNS depressant effects, especially respiratory depression. In addition, the antagonist counters the effect of the stress-induced levels of endorphins. An opioid antagonist is especially valuable if labor is more rapid than expected and birth is anticipated when the opioid is at its peak effect. The antagonist may be given through the woman's IV line, or it can be administered intramuscularly (see Medication Guide). The woman should be told that the pain that was relieved with the use of the opioid analgesic will return with the administration of the opioid antagonist. Some authorities believe that unless maternal CNS depression is severe enough to affect her well-being and that of her fetus, the woman should not receive naloxone just before birth in an attempt to prevent neonatal CNS depression. Placental transfer of naloxone is unpredictable; the newborn may not require treatment with an opioid antagonist; and the sudden return of severe pain could have adverse physiologic and psychologic effects on the mother (Hawkins et al., 2002; Lehne, 2001).

signs of
POTENTIAL COMPLICATIONS

Maternal Opioid Abstinence Syndrome (Opioid/Narcotic Withdrawal)

Yawning, rhinorrhea (runny nose), sweating, lacrimation (tearing), mydriasis (dilation of pupils)
Anorexia
Irritability, restlessness, generalized anxiety
Tremor
Chills and hot flashes
Piloerection ("gooseflesh")
Violent sneezing
Weakness, fatigue, and drowsiness
Nausea and vomiting
Diarrhea, abdominal cramps
Bone and muscle pain, muscle spasm, kicking movements

Medication Guide

Naloxone (Narcan)

Action
Opioid antagonist

Indication
Reverses opioid-induced respiratory depression in woman or newborn; may be used to reverse pruritus from epidural opioids

Dosage and Route
Adult
Narcotic overdose: 0.4 to 2 mg IV, may repeat IV at 2- to 3-min intervals up to 10 mg; if IV route unavailable, IM or SC administration may be used
Postoperative narcotic depression: Initial dose 0.1 to 0.2 mg IV at 2- to 3-min intervals to desired degree of reversal; may repeat dose in 1 to 2 hours if needed

Newborn
Narcotic-induced depression: Initial dose is 0.01 mg/kg IV, IM, or SC; may be repeated at 2- to 3-min intervals until desired degree of reversal obtained

Adverse Effects
Maternal hypotension and hypertension, tachycardia, nausea and vomiting, sweating, and tremulousness

Nursing Considerations
Woman should delay breastfeeding until medication is out of system; do not give if woman is opioid dependent—may cause abrupt withdrawal; if given to woman for reversal of respiratory depression caused by opioid analgesic, pain will return suddenly

IM, Intramuscular; *IV,* intravenous; *SC,* subcutaneous.

NURSE ALERT *An opioid antagonist must be administered cautiously to an opioid-dependent woman because it may precipitate abstinence syndrome (withdrawal symptoms) in both the mother and her newborn (see Signs of Potential Complications box).*

An opioid antagonist can be given to the newborn as one part of the treatment for neonatal narcosis, which is a state of CNS depression in the newborn produced by an opioid. Prophylactic administration of naloxone is controversial. Affected infants may exhibit respiratory depression, hypotonia, lethargy, and a delay in temperature regulation. Risk for hypoxia, hypercarbia, and acidosis increases if neonatal narcosis is not treated promptly. Treatment involves ventilation, administration of oxygen, and gentle stimulation. Naloxone is administered, if still required, to reverse CNS depression. More than one dose of naloxone may be required because its half-life is shorter than the half-life of opioids. Alterations in neurologic and behavioral responses may be evident in the newborn for as long as 2 to 4 days after birth. Some depression of attention and social responsiveness can be evident for up to 6 weeks after birth. The significance of these neurobehavioral changes is unknown (Hawkins et al., 2002; Lehne, 2001).

Nerve block analgesia and anesthesia

A variety of local anesthetic agents are used in obstetrics to produce regional analgesia (some pain relief and motor block) and anesthesia (complete pain relief and motor block). Most of these agents are related chemically to cocaine and end with the suffix *-caine.* This helps to identify a local anesthetic.

The principal pharmacologic effect of local anesthetics is the temporary interruption of the conduction of nerve impulses, notably pain. Examples of common agents are bupivacaine, lidocaine, mepivacaine, ropivacaine, and chloroprocaine. The solution strength of the local anesthetic agent and the amount used will depend on the type of nerve block being performed (Florence & Palmer, 2003).

Rarely, people are sensitive (allergic) to one or more local anesthetics. Such a reaction may include respiratory depression, hypotension, and other serious adverse effects. Epinephrine, antihistamines, oxygen, and supportive measures should reverse these effects. Sensitivity may be identified by administering minute amounts of the drug to be used to test for an allergic reaction.

Local perineal infiltration anesthesia. Local perineal infiltration anesthesia may be used when an episiotomy is to be performed or when lacerations need to be sutured after the birth in a woman who does not have regional anesthesia. Rapid anesthesia is produced by injecting approximately 10 to 20 ml of 1% lidocaine or 2% chloroprocaine into the skin and then subcutaneously into the region to be anesthetized. Epinephrine often is added to the solution to localize and intensify the effect of the anesthesia in a region and to prevent excessive bleeding and systemic absorption by constricting local blood vessels (Lehne, 2001). Repeated injections will prolong the anesthesia as long as needed.

Pudendal nerve block. Pudendal nerve block is useful for the second stage of labor, episiotomy, and birth. Although it does not relieve the pain from uterine contractions, it does relieve pain in the lower vagina, vulva, and perineum (Fig. 12-8, *A*). A pudendal nerve block should be administered 10 to 20 minutes before perineal anesthesia is needed.

The pudendal nerve traverses the sacrosciatic notch just medial to the tip of the ischial spine on each side. Injection of an anesthetic solution at or near these points anesthetizes the pudendal nerves peripherally (Fig. 12-9). The transvaginal approach is generally used because it is less painful for the woman, has a higher rate of success in blocking pain, and tends to cause fewer fetal complications (Hawkins et al., 2002). Pudendal block does not change maternal hemodynamic or respiratory functions, vital signs, or the FHR. However, the bearing-down reflex is lessened or lost completely.

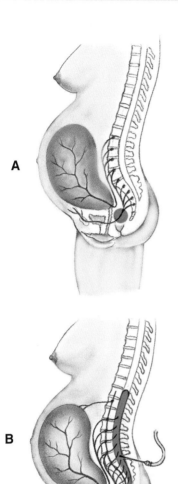

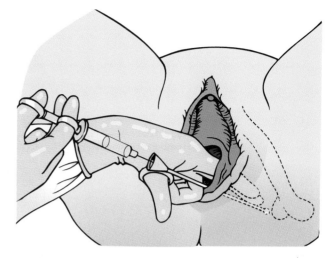

Fig. 12-9 Pudendal block. Use of needle guide (Iowa trumpet) and Luer-Lok syringe to inject medication.

Fig. 12-8 Pain pathways and sites of pharmacologic nerve blocks. **A,** Pudendal block: suitable during second and third stages of labor and for repair of episiotomy or lacerations. **B,** Epidural block: suitable for all stages of labor and for repair of episiotomy and lacerations.

Spinal anesthesia. In **spinal anesthesia (block)** an anesthetic solution containing a local anesthetic alone or in combination with fentanyl is injected through the third, fourth, or fifth lumbar interspace into the subarachnoid space (Fig. 12-10), where the anesthetic solution mixes with cerebrospinal fluid (CSF). This technique is commonly used for cesarean births. Low spinal anesthesia may be used for vaginal birth, but it is not suitable for labor. Spinal anesthesia used for cesarean birth provides anesthesia from the nipple (T6) to the feet. If it is used for vaginal birth, the anesthesia level is from the hips (T10) to the feet (Fig. 12-10, *C*).

For spinal anesthesia, the woman is sitting or lying on her side (e.g., modified Sims position) with back curved to widen the intervertebral space to facilitate insertion of a small-gauge spinal needle and injection of the anesthetic solution. The nurse supports the woman because she must remain still during the placement of the spinal needle. The insertion is made between contractions. After the anesthetic solution has been injected, the woman may be positioned upright to allow the heavier (hyperbaric) anesthetic solution to flow downward to obtain the lower level of anesthesia suitable for a vaginal birth. She may be positioned supine with head and shoulders slightly elevated and the uterus displaced with a wedge under one of her hips to obtain the higher level of anesthesia desired for cesarean birth. The anesthetic effect usually begins 1 to 2 minutes after the anesthetic solution is injected and lasts 1 to 3 hours, depending on the type of agent used (Hawkins et al., 2002) (Fig. 12-11).

Marked hypotension, impaired placental perfusion, and an ineffective breathing pattern may occur during spinal anesthesia. Before induction of the spinal anesthetic, the woman's fluid balance is assessed and IV fluid usually is administered to decrease the potential for hypotension caused by sympathetic blockade (vasodilation with pooling of blood in the lower extremities). After induction of the anesthetic, maternal blood pressure, pulse, and respirations and FHR and fetal heart pattern must be checked and documented every 5 to 10 minutes. If signs of serious maternal hypotension or fetal distress develop, emergency care must be given (see Emergency box).

Because the woman is unable to sense her contractions, she must be instructed when to bear down during a vaginal birth. If the birth occurs in a delivery room (rather than a labor-delivery-recovery room), the woman will need assistance in the transfer to a recovery bed after expulsion of the placenta.

Advantages of spinal anesthesia include ease of administration and absence of fetal hypoxia with maintenance of normotension. Maternal consciousness is maintained, excellent muscular relaxation is achieved, and blood loss is not excessive.

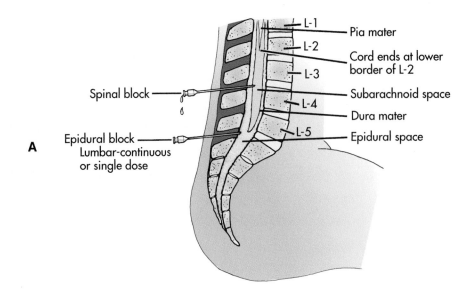

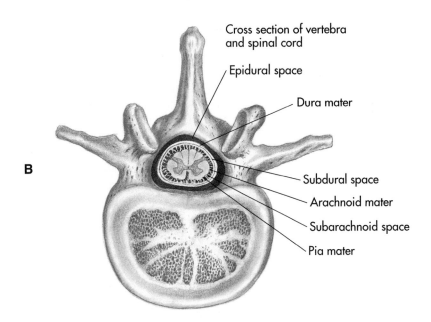

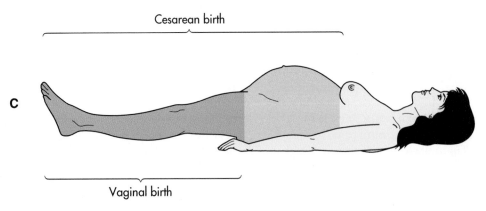

Fig. 12-10 **A,** Membranes and spaces of spinal cord and levels of sacral, lumbar, and thoracic nerves. **B,** Cross-section of vertebra and spinal cord. **C,** Level of anesthesia necessary for cesarean birth and for vaginal births.

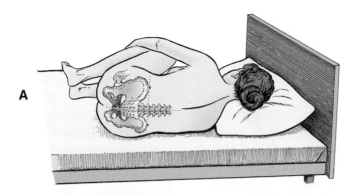

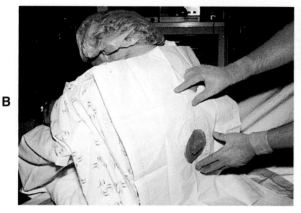

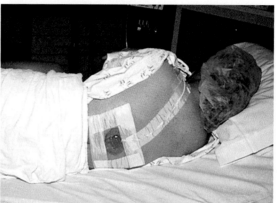

Fig. 12-11 Positioning for spinal and epidural blocks. **A,** Lateral position. **B,** Upright position. **C,** Catheter for epidural taped to woman's back with port segment located near shoulder. (**B** and **C,** Courtesy Michael S. Clement, MD, Mesa, AZ.)

EMERGENCY

Maternal Hypotension with Decreased Placental Perfusion

SIGNS AND SYMPTOMS

- Maternal hypotension (20% decrease from preblock baseline level or 100 mm Hg systolic)
- Fetal bradycardia
- Decreased beat-to-beat FHR variability

INTERVENTIONS

- Turn woman to lateral position or place pillow or wedge under hip (see Fig. 14-5) to deflect uterus.
- Maintain IV infusion at rate specified, or increase "as needed" administration per hospital protocol.
- Administer oxygen by face mask at 10-12 L/min or per protocol.
- Elevate the woman's legs.
- Notify the primary health care provider, anesthesiologist, and/or nurse anesthetist.
- Administer IV vasopressor (e.g., ephedrine 5-10 mg) per protocol if previous measures are ineffective.
- Remain with woman; continue to monitor maternal blood pressure and FHR every 5 minutes until her condition is stable or per primary health care provider's order.

FHR, Fetal heart rate; *IV,* intravenous.

Disadvantages of spinal anesthesia include medication reactions (e.g., allergy), hypotension, and an ineffective breathing pattern; cardiopulmonary resuscitation may be needed. When a spinal anesthetic is given, the need for operative birth (e.g., episiotomy, forceps-assisted birth, vacuum-assisted birth) tends to increase because voluntary expulsive efforts are reduced or eliminated. After birth the incidence of bladder and uterine atony, as well as postspinal headache, is higher.

Leakage of CSF from the site of puncture of the dura mater (membranous covering of the spinal cord) is thought to be the major causative factor in *postdural puncture headache (PDPH).* Presumably postural changes cause the diminished volume of CSF to exert traction on pain-sensitive CNS structures. Characteristically, assuming an upright position triggers or intensifies the headache, whereas assuming a supine position achieves relief in 30 minutes or less (Govenar, 2000). The resulting headache, auditory problems (e.g., tinnitus), and visual problems (e.g., blurred vision, photophobia) begin within 2 days of the puncture and may persist for days or weeks.

The likelihood of headache after dural puncture can be reduced, however, if the anesthesiologist uses a small-gauge spinal needle and avoids making multiple punctures of the meninges. Positioning the woman flat in bed (with only a

CD: Critical Thinking Exercise—Patient Receiving Epidural Block

small, flat pillow for her head) for at least 8 hours after spinal anesthesia also has been recommended to prevent headache, but no definitive evidence shows that this measure is effective. Positioning the woman on her abdomen, a difficult if not impossible position after a cesarean birth, is thought to decrease the loss of CSF through the puncture site. Hydration has been claimed to be of value in preventing and treating headache, but no compelling evidence supports its use (Cunningham et al., 2005). Initial treatment for a postdural puncture headache usually includes oral analgesics, bed rest in a quiet dimly lit or dark room, caffeine, and increased fluid intake (Govenar, 2000; Hawkins et al., 2002).

An autologous **epidural blood patch** is the most rapid, reliable, and beneficial relief measure for PDPH. The woman's blood (i.e., 10 to 20 ml) is injected slowly into the lumbar epidural space, creating a clot that patches the tear or hole in the dura mater around the spinal cord. It is considered if the headache does not resolve spontaneously or after use of more conservative, noninvasive techniques (Govenar, 2000) (Fig. 12-12).

After the blood patch procedure the woman should be observed for alteration of vital signs, pallor, clammy skin, and leakage of CSF. A bandage and cold pack are placed on the puncture site, and the woman rests in bed for approximately 1 hour. Discharge instructions include resting in bed for 24 to 48 hours, applying cold packs to the site as needed for comfort, avoiding analgesics that affect platelet aggregation (e.g., nonsteroidal antiinflammatory drugs [NSAIDs]) for 2 days, drinking plenty of fluids, and observing for signs of infection at the site and for neurologic symptoms such as pain, numbness and tingling in legs, and difficulty with walking or elimination. The woman should be cautioned to avoid lifting, straining at stool, coughing, tub bathing, or swimming for at least 2 days (Govenar, 2000; Hawkins et al., 2002).

Epidural anesthesia or analgesia (block). Relief from the pain of uterine contractions and birth (vaginal and cesarean) can be relieved by injecting a suitable local

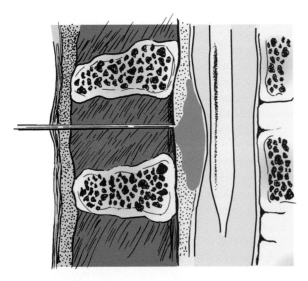

Fig. 12-12 Blood-patch therapy for spinal headache.

? Critical Thinking Exercise

Epidurals and Labor Progress

Dodie received combined spinal-epidural analgesia during the active phase of first stage labor. She is now in transition and is concerned about whether she will be able to push effectively in the second stage. She has heard that women who have epidurals have to push longer and sometimes even have to have a cesarean birth. How would you respond to these concerns?

1 Evidence—Is there sufficient evidence to draw conclusions about what advice the nurse should give to Dodie about epidurals and labor progress?
2 Assumptions—What assumptions can be made about the following issues related to epidurals:
   a. Effects on labor progress
   b. Effects on cesarean rates
   c. Effects on neonates
   d. Use of upright positions in second-stage labor in women with epidurals
3 What implications and priorities for nursing care can be drawn at this time?
4 Does the evidence objectively support your conclusion?
5 Are there alternative perspectives to your conclusion?

---

anesthetic agent (e.g., bupivacaine, ropivacaine), an opioid analgesic (e.g., fentanyl, sufentanil), or both into the epidural (peridural) space. Injection is made between the fourth and fifth lumbar vertebrae for a lumbar **epidural block** (see Figs. 12-8, *B*, and 12-10, *A*) and infrequently through the sacral hiatus for a caudal epidural block. Depending on the type and amount of medication(s) used, an anesthetic or analgesic effect will occur with varying degrees of motor impairment.

Lumbar epidural anesthesia and analgesia. Lumbar epidural anesthesia and analgesia is the most effective pharmacologic pain relief method for labor currently available. As a result, it is the most commonly used method for relieving pain during labor in the United States. More than half of the women giving birth each year choose epidural analgesia (Lieberman & O'Donoghue, 2002). For relieving the discomfort of labor and vaginal birth, a block from T10 to S5 is required. For cesarean birth, a block from at least T8 to S1 is essential. The diffusion of epidural anesthesia depends on the location of the catheter tip, the dose and volume of the anesthetic agent used, and the woman's position (e.g., horizontal or head-up position) (Cunningham et al., 2005).

For the induction of a lumbar epidural block, the woman is positioned as for a spinal block. She may sit with her back curved or she may assume a modified Sims position with her shoulders parallel, legs slightly flexed, and back arched (see Fig. 12-10).

After the epidural has been started, the woman is positioned preferably on her side so that the uterus does not compress the ascending vena cava and descending aorta, which can impair venous return, reduce cardiac output and blood pressure, and decrease placental perfusion. Her position should be alternated from side to side every hour. Upright positions and ambulation may be encouraged, depending on the degree of motor impairment. Oxygen should be available if hypotension occurs despite maintenance of hydration with IV fluid and displacement of the uterus to the side. Ephedrine (a vasopressor used to increase maternal blood pressure) and increased IV fluid infusion may be needed (see Emergency box). The FHR, fetal heart pattern, and progress in labor must be monitored carefully because the woman in labor may not be aware of changes in the strength of the uterine contractions or the descent of the presenting part.

Several methods can be used for an epidural block. An intermittent block is achieved by using repeated injections of anesthetic solution; it is the least common method. The most commonly used method is the continuous block, achieved by using a pump to infuse the anesthetic solution through an indwelling plastic catheter. Patient-controlled epidural analgesia (PCEA) is the newest method; it uses an indwelling catheter and a programmed pump that allows the woman to control the dosing. The advantages of an epidural block are numerous: the woman remains alert and able to participate, good relaxation is achieved, airway reflexes remain intact, only partial motor paralysis develops, gastric emptying is not delayed, and blood loss is not excessive. Fetal complications are rare but may occur in the event of rapid absorption of the medication or marked maternal hypotension. The dose, volume, and type of medication(s) used can be modified to allow the woman to push and to assume upright positions and even walk, to produce perineal anesthesia, and to permit forceps-assisted, vacuum-assisted, or cesarean birth if required (Cunningham et al., 2005).

The disadvantages of epidural block also are numerous. The woman's ability to move freely is limited, related to the use of an IV infusion and electronic monitoring, orthostatic hypotension and dizziness, sedation, and weakness of the legs. CNS effects such as excitation, bizarre behavior, tinnitus, disorientation, paresthesia, and convulsions can occur if a solution containing a local anesthetic agent is accidentally injected into a blood vessel. Respiratory arrest can occur if the relatively high dosage used with an epidural block is accidentally injected into the subarachnoid space. Women who receive an epidural have a higher rate of fever (i.e., intrapartum temperature of 38° C or higher), especially when labor lasts longer that 12 hours; the temperature elevation most likely is related to thermoregulatory changes, although infection cannot be ruled out. The elevation in temperature can result in fetal tachycardia and neonatal workup for sepsis, whether or not signs of infection are present. Hypotension as a result of sympathetic blockade can be an outcome of an epidural block (see Emergency Box). Urinary retention and stress incontinence can occur in the immediate postpartum period. This temporary difficulty in urinary elimination could be related not only to the effects of the epidural block but also to the increased duration of labor and need for instrumental

birth associated with the block (Lieberman & O'Donoghue, 2002). Pruritus (itching) is a side effect associated with the use of an opioid, especially fentanyl. A relation between epidural analgesia and longer second-stage labor, increased incidence of fetal malposition, use of oxytocin, and forceps-assisted or vacuum-assisted birth has been documented. Current research findings have been unable to demonstrate a significant increase in cesarean birth associated with epidural analgesia (Lieberman & O'Donoghue, 2002; Sharma & Leveno, 2003). Occasionally a PDPH can occur after accidental perforation of the dura mater during the administration of the epidural block. Because a larger needle is used for an epidural block, the risk for severe headache is high as a result of greater CSF loss (Hawkins et al., 2002). For some women, the epidural block is not effective, and a second form of analgesia is required to establish effective pain relief. When women progress rapidly in labor, pain relief may not be obtained before birth occurs.

Combined spinal-epidural analgesia. Using opioids such as fentanyl and sufentanil to potentiate the effects of local anesthetic agents has resulted in the reduction of the amount of the local anesthetic used, thereby reducing motor blockade. A combined spinal-epidural (CSE) technique is an increasingly popular approach that can be used to block pain transmission without compromising motor ability. There is a high concentration of opioid receptors along the pain pathway in the spinal cord, in the brainstem, and in the thalamus. Because these receptors are highly sensitive to opioids, a small quantity of an opioid-agonist analgesic produces marked pain relief lasting for several hours. The opioid is injected into the subarachnoid space for rapid activation of the opioid receptors. A catheter is left in place in the epidural space to extend the duration of the analgesia by using a lower dose of a local anesthetic agent (Hawkins et al., 2002). Although women can walk (hence the term "walking epidural"), they often choose not to do so because of sedation and fatigue, abnormal sensations perceived in their legs, weakness of the legs, and a feeling of insecurity. Often health care providers are reluctant to encourage or assist women to ambulate for fear of injury (Mayberry, Clemmens, & De, 2002). However, women can be assisted to change positions and use upright positions during labor and birth (Mayberry, Strange, Suplee, & Gennaro, 2003).

CSE analgesia may be associated with fetal bradycardia, necessitating close assessment of FHR and fetal heart pattern (Lieberman & O'Donoghue, 2002).

Epidural and intrathecal opioids. Opioids also can be used alone, eliminating the effect of a local anesthetic altogether. The use of epidural or intrathecal (spinal) opioids without the addition of a local anesthetic agent during labor has several advantages. Opioids administered in this manner do not cause maternal hypotension or affect vital signs. The woman feels contractions but not pain. Her ability to bear down during the second stage of labor is preserved because the pushing reflex is not lost, and her motor power remains intact.

Fentanyl, sufentanil, or preservative-free morphine may be used. Fentanyl and sufentanil produce short-acting analgesia (i.e., 1.5 to 3.5 hours), and morphine may provide pain relief for 4 to 7 hours. Morphine may be combined with fentanyl or sufentanil. For most women, intrathecal opioids do not provide adequate analgesia for second-stage labor pain, episiotomy, or birth (Cunningham et al., 2005). Pudendal nerve blocks or local perineal infiltration anesthesia may be necessary.

A more common indication for the administration of epidural or intrathecal analgesics is the relief of postoperative pain. For example, women who give birth by cesarean can receive fentanyl or morphine through a catheter. The catheter may then be removed, and the women are usually free of pain for 24 hours. Occasionally the catheter is left in place in the epidural space in case another dose is needed.

Women receiving epidurally administered morphine after the cesarean birth are up soon after surgery with surprising ease and are able to care for their newborns. The early ambulation and freedom from pain also facilitate bladder emptying, enhance peristalsis, and prevent clot formation in the lower extremities (e.g., thrombophlebitis). To those women who have had a previous cesarean birth and have had the usual postoperative pain, the effects of this approach seem miraculous. However, the mother may not understand why she may have pain after the opioid effect wears off.

Side effects of opioids administered by the epidural and intrathecal routes include nausea, vomiting, pruritus, urinary retention, and delayed respiratory depression. These side effects are more common when morphine is administered. Antiemetics, antipruritics, and opioid antagonists are used to relieve these symptoms. For example, naloxone (Narcan), promethazine (Phenergan), or metoclopramide (Reglan) may be administered. Hospital protocols should provide specific instructions for the treatment of these side effects. Use of epidural opioids is not without risks. Respiratory depression is a serious concern; for this reason the woman's respiratory rate should be assessed and documented every hour for 24 hours, or as designated by hospital protocol. Naloxone should be readily available for use if the respiratory rate decreases to less than 10 breaths per minute or if the oxygen saturation rate decreases to less than 89%. Administration of oxygen by face mask also may be initiated, and the anesthesiologist should be notified.

Contraindications to epidural blocks. Some contraindications to epidural analgesia include (Hawkins et al., 2002) the following:

- Active antepartum hemorrhage. Acute hypovolemia leads to increased sympathetic tone to maintain the blood pressure. Any anesthetic technique that blocks the sympathetic fibers can produce significant hypotension that can endanger the mother and baby.
- Anticoagulant therapy or bleeding disorder. If a woman is receiving anticoagulant therapy or has a bleeding disorder, injury to a blood vessel may cause the formation of a hematoma that may compress the

cauda equina or the spinal cord and lead to serious CNS complications.

- Infection at the injection site. Infection can be spread through the peridural or subarachnoid spaces if the needle traverses an infected area.
- Allergy to the anesthetic drug.
- Maternal refusal.
- Some types of maternal cardiac conditions.

Epidural block effects on neonate. Debate persists concerning the effects of epidural anesthesia and analgesia on the newborn's neurobehavioral responses. Findings from studies that examine associations between neurobehavioral outcome and epidural block are far from consistent. For example, studies comparing the neonatal neurobehavioral scores for infants born to mothers who did and mothers who did not receive epidural analgesia either have shown little or no difference in the scores or have shown that the infants of mothers who received epidural anesthesia did not score as well on neurobehavioral tests. In one research study, infants exposed to an epidural block tended to have less muscle tone but were better able to orient and habituate to sound when compared with infants whose mother received opioids during labor (Lieberman & O'Donoghue, 2002).

Nitrous oxide for analgesia

Nitrous oxide mixed with oxygen can be inhaled in a low concentration (50% or less) to reduce but not eliminate pain during the first and second stages of labor. At the lower doses used for analgesia, the woman remains awake, and the danger of aspiration is avoided because the laryngeal reflexes are unaffected. It can be used in combination with other non-pharmacologic and pharmacologic measures for pain relief.

A face mask or mouthpiece is used to self-administer the gas. The woman should place the mask over her mouth and nose or insert the mouthpiece 30 seconds before the onset of a contraction (if regular) or as soon as a contraction begins (if irregular). When she inhales, a valve opens, and the gas is released. She should continue to inhale the gas slowly and deeply until the contraction starts to subside. When inhalation stops, the valve closes. Onset of action is 50 seconds; therefore beginning the inhalation process 30 seconds before the onset of a contraction provides the best pain relief. During the interval between contractions, the woman should remove the device and breathe normally (Rosen, 2002).

Most women who use nitrous oxide obtain adequate pain relief and are satisfied with the method. The nurse should observe the woman for nausea and vomiting, drowsiness, dizziness, hazy memory, and loss of consciousness. Loss of consciousness is more likely to occur if opioids are used with the nitrous oxide. The use of nitrous oxide does not appear to depress uterine contractions or cause adverse reactions in the fetus and newborn (Rosen, 2002).

Nitrous oxide for pain relief during labor is more readily available in Canada and European countries than in the United States (Caton et al., 2002).

General anesthesia

General anesthesia rarely is used for uncomplicated vaginal birth and is infrequently used for cesarean birth. It may be necessary if there is a contraindication to a spinal or epidural block or if indications necessitate rapid birth (vaginal or cesarean) without sufficient time to perform a block. In addition, being awake and aware during major surgery may be unacceptable for some women having a cesarean birth.

If general anesthesia is being considered, the nurse gives the woman nothing by mouth and ensures that an IV infusion is in place. If time allows, the nurse premedicates the woman with a nonparticulate (clear) oral antacid (e.g., sodium citrate, Bicitra, Alka-Seltzer) to neutralize the acidic contents of the stomach. Aspiration of highly acidic gastric contents will damage lung tissue. Some anesthesiologists and physicians also order the administration of a histamine (H_2)-receptor blocker such as cimetidine (Tagamet) to decrease the production of gastric acid and metoclopramide (Reglan) to increase gastric emptying (Hawkins et al., 2002). Before the anesthesia is given, a wedge should be placed under one of the woman's hips to displace the uterus. Uterine displacement prevents aortocaval compression, which interferes with placental perfusion.

Thiopental, a short-acting barbiturate, or ketamine is administered intravenously to render the woman unconscious, and then succinylcholine, a muscle relaxer, is administered to facilitate passage of an endotracheal tube. Sometimes the nurse is asked to assist with applying cricoid pressure before intubation as the woman begins to lose consciousness. This maneuver blocks the esophagus and prevents aspiration should the woman vomit or regurgitate (Fig. 12-13). Pressure is released once the endotracheal tube is securely in place.

After the woman is intubated, nitrous oxide and oxygen in a 50:50 mixture are administered. A low concentration of a volatile halogenated agent (e.g., isoflurane) also may be administered to increase pain relief and to reduce maternal awareness and recall (Hawkins et al., 2002). In higher concentrations, isoflurane or methoxyflurane relaxes the uterus quickly and facilitates intrauterine manipulation, version, and extraction. However, at higher concentrations, these agents cross the placenta readily and can produce narcosis in the fetus and could reduce uterine tone after birth, increasing the risk for hemorrhage.

Priorities for recovery room care are to maintain an open airway and cardiopulmonary function and to prevent postpartum hemorrhage. Routine postpartum care is organized to facilitate parent-child attachment as soon as possible and to answer the mother's questions. When appropriate, the nurse assesses the mother's readiness to see the baby, as well as her response to the anesthesia and to the event that necessitated general anesthesia (e.g., emergency cesarean birth when vaginal birth was anticipated).

CARE MANAGEMENT ■

The choice of pain relief depends on a combination of factors, including the woman's special needs and wishes, the availability of the desired method(s), the knowledge and expertise in nonpharmacologic and pharmacologic methods of the health care providers involved in the woman's care, and the phase and stage of labor. The nurse is responsible for assessing maternal and fetal status, establishing mutual goals with the woman (and her family), formulating nursing diagnoses, planning and implementing nursing care, and evaluating the effects of care. It is essential for the nurse to document carefully all aspects of care management.

Assessment and Nursing Diagnoses

The assessment of the woman, her fetus, and her labor is a joint effort of the nurse and the primary health care providers, who consult with the woman regarding their findings and recommendations. The needs of each woman are different, and

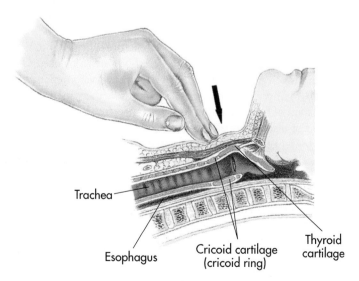

Fig. 12-13 Technique for applying pressure on cricoid cartilage to occlude esophagus to prevent pulmonary aspiration of gastric contents during induction of general anesthesia.

many factors must be considered before deciding whether nonpharmacologic methods, pharmacologic methods, or a combination of both will be used to manage labor pain. It is critical that the nurse take note of all pain characteristics including location, intensity, quality, frequency, duration, and effectiveness of relief measures. The nurse should never assume that because a woman is in labor, her pain must be uterine in origin. Because pain is a subjective phenomenon, the nurse must listen to the woman's description of her pain. One self-assessment tool that can be used is a visual analogue scale (VAS). The VAS allows the woman to indicate on a line how severe or intense she perceives her pain to be from "no pain" to "pain as bad as it could possibly be." The McGill Pain Questionnaire provides a more complete picture of the pain experience because the woman is able to describe the sensory and emotional or affective dimensions of her pain rather than just its intensity (Lowe, 2002). Self-assessment is recommended to ensure that pain management is based on the subjective nature of the woman's pain rather than just on the nurse's judgment. It is not unusual for a nurse to overestimate or underestimate the pain being experienced by the patient. Baker, Ferguson, Roach, and Dawson (2001) found that nurse-midwives consistently underestimated pain intensity that women described as severe. When there are major cultural differences between the health care provider and the patient, inaccurate interpretation of pain intensity often occurs (Lowe, 2002) (see Guidelines/Guías box).

History

The woman's prenatal record is read and relevant information identified. This includes the woman's parity, estimated date of birth, and complications and medications during pregnancy. If the woman has a history of allergies, this is noted, and a warning is displayed in a prominent place (Mahlmeister, 2003). A history of smoking and neurologic and spinal disorders also is noted.

Interview

Interview data consist of the time of the woman's last meal and the type of food and fluid consumed; the nature of any existing respiratory condition (e.g., cold, allergy); and unusual reactions (e.g., allergy) to medications, cleansing agents, latex, or tape. The woman is asked whether she attended childbirth preparation classes. The extent of her preparation and her preferences for management of discomfort including a birth plan are reviewed. Her knowledge of the options for the management of discomfort also is assessed. Information on the woman's perception of discomfort and her expressed need for medication is added to the database. Relevant events that have occurred since the woman's last contact with her primary health care provider also are reviewed (e.g., infections, diarrhea, a change in fetal movement patterns). If verbal and physical signs indicate the existence of substance abuse (e.g., opioids, alcohol), the nurse should ask the woman to identify the type of substance used, the last time it was taken, and the method of administration.

GUIDELINES/GUÍAS
Pain Management

- Do you want to get up and walk?
- ¿Desea levantarse y caminar?
- Do you want pain medication?
- ¿Quiere medicina para el dolor?
- I am going to give you the pain medicine in an injection.
- Le voy a dar la medicina para el dolor por inyección.
- I am going to give you the pain medicine through an IV.
- Le voy a dar la medicina para el dolor por el suero.
- This is a pain reliever called Demerol/Stadol/Nubain.
- Ésta es una medicina para aliviar el dolor que se llama Demerol/Stadol/Nubain.
- The effects of this medicine are relatively short.
- Los efectos de esta medicina son de corta duración.
- The epidural is a stronger method of pain relief.
- La anestesia epidural es un método más potente para aliviar el dolor.
- You should not be able to feel the contraction pain.
- No debe de sentir el dolor de las contracciones.

Physical examination

The character and status of the labor and fetal response are assessed during a physical examination. The nurse evaluates the woman's hydration status by assessing intake and output measurements, the moistness of the mucous membranes, skin turgor, and concentration of urine. Bladder distention is noted. Any evidence of skin infection near sites of possible needle insertion is recorded and reported. Signs of apprehension such as fist clenching and restlessness also are noted.

If the woman is in labor, the status of maternal vital signs, FHR and fetal heart pattern, uterine contractions, amniotic membranes and fluid, cervical effacement and dilation, and fetal descent is determined. The anticipated time until birth is estimated if possible. The length of labor and degree of fatigue are other important considerations. If pharmacologic methods are to be used, the type of analgesia or anesthesia chosen will vary depending on the status of the maternal-fetal unit, the progress of labor, and the method of birth planned (see Box 12-3).

Laboratory tests

The results of laboratory tests are reviewed to determine whether the woman is experiencing anemia (hemoglobin and hematocrit), a coagulopathy or bleeding disorder (prothrombin time and platelet count), or infection (white blood cell count and differential).

Signs of potential problems

Any medication can cause a minor or severe allergic reaction. As part of the assessment for such allergic reactions, the nurse should monitor the woman's vital signs, respiratory status, cardiovascular status, integument, and platelet and white blood cell count. The woman is observed for side effects of drug therapy, especially drowsiness. Minor reactions can consist of a rash, rhinitis, fever, asthma, or pruritus. Management of the less acute allergic response is not an emergency (Lehne, 2001).

Severe reactions may occur suddenly and lead to shock. The most dramatic form of anaphylaxis is sudden severe bronchospasm, vasospasm, severe hypotension, and death. Signs of anaphylaxis are largely caused by contraction of smooth muscles and may begin with irritability, extreme weakness, nausea, and vomiting. This may lead to dyspnea, cyanosis, convulsions, and cardiac arrest. An acute allergic reaction (anaphylaxis) must be diagnosed and treated immediately. Treatment usually consists of 1:1000 epinephrine injected subcutaneously or intramuscularly, followed by parenteral administration of antihistamines. Supportive care is given to alleviate the symptoms; the type of care is determined by the rapidly assessed cardiovascular and respiratory response of the woman to the primary interventions (Lehne, 2001). Cardiopulmonary resuscitation may be necessary.

NURSE ALERT *Complications may occur with epidural analgesia, including injection-related emergencies and compression problems. These complications can require immediate interventions. Nurses must be prepared to provide safe and effective care during the emergency situation. Clear procedures or protocols should be in place in labor and birth units delineating responsibilities and actions needed (Mahlmeister, 2003).*

The nurse also must be alert for changes in fetal well-being; nonreassuring changes in FHR and fetal heart pattern should be noted and reported to the primary health care provider.

The following nursing diagnoses are relevant in the management of discomfort during labor and birth:

- *Acute pain related to*
  - −processes of labor and birth
- *Risk for ineffective tissue perfusion related to*
  - −effects of analgesia or anesthesia
  - −maternal position
- *Hypothermia related to*
  - −effects of analgesia or anesthesia
- *Situational low self-esteem related to*
  - −negative perception of the woman's (or her family's) behavior
- *Fear related to deficient knowledge of*
  - −procedure for epidural analgesia
  - −expected sensation during spinal anesthesia
- *Risk for maternal injury related to*
  - −effects of analgesia and anesthesia on sensation and motor control

Expected Outcomes of Care

The expected outcomes of nursing care in the management of the discomfort of labor and birth include the following:

- The woman will promptly report the characteristics of her pain and discomfort.
- The woman will verbalize understanding of her needs and rights with regard to pain relief management that uses a variety of nonpharmacologic and pharmacologic methods reflecting her preferences.
- The woman will have adequate pain relief without adding maternal risk (e.g., through the use of appropriate nonpharmacologic methods and appropriate medication, including the appropriate dose, timing, and route of administration).
- The fetal status will remain reassuring, and the newborn will adjust to extrauterine life without problems related to management of maternal pain.

Plan of Care and Interventions

A plan of care is developed for each woman to address her particular clinical and nursing problems. The nurse collaborates with the primary health care provider and laboring woman in selecting those aspects of care relevant to the woman and her family.

Nonpharmacologic interventions

The nurse supports and assists the woman as she uses nonpharmacologic interventions for pain relief and relaxation. During labor, the nurse should ask the woman how she feels, to evaluate the effectiveness of the specific pain management techniques used. Appropriate interventions can then be planned or continued for effective care, such as trying other nonpharmacologic methods or combining nonpharmacologic methods with medications (see Plan of Care).

The woman's perception of her behavior during labor is of utmost importance. If she planned a nonmedicated birth but then needs and accepts medication, her self-esteem may falter. Verbal and nonverbal acceptance of her behavior is given as necessary by the nurse and reinforced by discussion and reassurance after birth. Providing explanations about the fetal response to maternal discomfort, the effects of maternal stress and fatigue on the progress of labor, and the medication itself is a supportive measure. The woman also may experience anxiety and stress related to anticipated or actual pain. Stress can cause increased maternal catecholamine production. Increased levels of catecholamines have been linked to dysfunctional labor and fetal and neonatal distress and illness. Nurses must be able to implement strategies aimed at reducing this stress (Hodnett, 2002; Lowe, 2002).

Informed consent

The primary health care provider and anesthesia care provider are responsible for informing women of the alternative methods of pharmacologic pain relief available in the hospital. A description of the various anesthetic techniques

---

PLAN OF CARE *Nonpharmacologic Management of Discomfort*

NURSING DIAGNOSIS Anxiety related to lack of confidence in ability to cope effectively with pain during labor

Expected Outcome *Woman will express decrease in anxiety and experience satisfaction with her labor and birth performance.*

Nursing Interventions/*Rationales*

- Assess whether woman and significant other have attended childbirth classes, her knowledge of labor process, and her current level of anxiety *to plan supportive strategies.*
- Encourage support person to remain with woman in labor *to provide support and increase probability of response to comfort measures.*
- Teach or review nonpharmacologic techniques available to decrease anxiety and pain during labor (e.g., focusing and feedback, breathing techniques, effleurage, and sacral pressure) *to enhance chances of success in using techniques.*
- Explore other techniques that the woman or significant other may have learned in childbirth classes (e.g., hypnosis, yoga, acupressure, biofeedback, therapeutic touch, aromatherapy, imaging, music) *to provide largest repertoire of coping strategies.*
- Explore use of hydrotherapy if ordered by physician and if woman meets use criteria (i.e., vital signs within normal limits [WNL], cervix 4 to 5 cm dilated, active phase of first stage labor) *to aid relaxation and stimulate production of natural oxytocin.*
- Explore use of transcutaneous electrical nerve stimulation per physician order *to provide an increased perception of control over pain and an increase in release of endogenous opiates.*
- Assist woman to change positions and to use pillows *to reduce stiffness, aid circulation, and promote comfort.*

- Assess bladder for distention and encourage voiding often *to avoid bladder distention and subsequent discomfort.*
- Encourage rest between contractions *to minimize fatigue.*
- Keep woman and significant other informed about progress *to allay anxiety.*
- Guide couple through the labor stages and phases, helping them use and modify comfort techniques that are appropriate to each phase *to ensure greatest effectiveness of techniques employed.*
- Support couple if pharmacologic measures are required to increase pain relief, explaining safety and effectiveness *to reduce anxiety and maintain self-esteem and sense of control over labor process.*

NURSING DIAGNOSIS Health-seeking behavior (labor) related to desire for a healthy outcome of labor and birth

Expected Outcome *Woman will participate in care planning for labor.*

Nursing Interventions/*Rationales*

- Discuss woman's birth plan and knowledge about the birth process *to collect data for plan of care.*
- Provide information about the labor process *to correct any misconceptions.*
- Inform woman about her labor status and fetus's well-being *to promote comfort and confidence.*
- Discuss rationales for all interventions *to incorporate woman into plan of care.*
- Incorporate nonpharmacologic interventions into plan of care *to increase woman's sense of control during labor.*
- Provide emotional support and ongoing positive feedback *to enhance positive coping mechanisms.*

---

and what they entail is essential to informed consent, even if the woman received information about analgesia and anesthesia earlier in her pregnancy. The discussion of pain management options ideally should take place in the third trimester so the woman has time to consider alternatives. Nurses play a part in the informed consent by clarifying and describing procedures or by acting as the woman's advocate and asking the primary health care provider for further explanations. The procedure and its advantages and disadvantages must be thoroughly explained.

LEGAL TIP Informed Consent for Anesthesia

The woman receives (in an understandable manner) the following:

- *Explanation of alternative methods of anesthesia and analgesia available*
- *Description of anesthetic and procedure for administration*
- *Description of the benefits, discomforts, risks, and consequences for the mother and the fetus*
- *Explanation of how complications can be treated*
- *Information that the anesthetic is not always effective*
- *Indication that the woman may withdraw consent at any time*

- *Opportunity to have any question answered*
- *Opportunity to have components of the consent explained in the woman's own words*

The consent form will

- *Be written or explained in the woman's primary language*
- *Have the woman's signature*
- *Have the date of consent*
- *Carry the signature of anesthetic care provider, certifying that the woman has received and appears to understand the explanation*

Timing of administration

It is often the nurse who notifies the primary health care provider that the woman is in need of pharmacologic measures to relieve her discomfort. Orders are often written for the administration of pain medication as needed by the woman and based on the nurse's clinical judgment. Generally, pharmacologic measures for pain relief are not implemented until labor has advanced to the active phase of the first stage of labor and the cervix is dilated approximately 4 to 5 cm to avoid suppressing the progress of labor (see Box 12-3). Conversely, nonpharmacologic measures can be used to relieve pain in early labor while relieving stress and enhancing progress.

Preparation for procedures

The methods of pain relief available to the woman are reviewed, and information is clarified as necessary. The procedure and what will be asked of the woman (e.g., to maintain flexed position during insertion of epidural needle) must be explained. The woman also can benefit from knowing the way that the medication is to be given, the interval before the medication takes effect, and the expected pain relief from the medication. Skin-preparation measures are described, and an explanation is given for the need to empty the bladder before the analgesic or anesthetic is administered and the reason for keeping the bladder empty. When an indwelling catheter is to be threaded into the epidural space, the woman should be told that she may have a momentary twinge down her leg, hip, or back, and that this feeling is not a sign of injury.

Administration of medication

Accurate monitoring of the progress of labor forms the basis for the nurse's judgment that a woman needs pharmacologic control of discomfort. Knowledge of the medications used during childbirth is essential. The most effective route of administration is selected for each woman; then the medication is prepared and administered correctly.

Intravenous route.   The preferred route of administration of medications such as meperidine, fentanyl, or nalbuphine is through IV tubing, administered into the port nearest the woman while the infusion of the IV solution is stopped. The medication is given slowly in small doses during a contraction. It may be given over the period of three to five consecutive contractions if needed to complete the dose. It is given during contractions to decrease fetal exposure to the medication because uterine blood vessels are constricted during contractions, and the medication stays within the maternal vascular system for several seconds before the uterine blood vessels reopen. When the medication is infused, the IV infusion is then restarted slowly to prevent a bolus of medication from being administered. With this method of injection, along with smaller but more frequent dosing, the amount of medication crossing the placenta to the fetus is reduced while the woman's degree of pain relief is maximized. The IV route is associated with the following advantages:

- The onset of pain relief is more predictable.
- Pain relief is obtained with small doses of the drug.
- The duration of effect is more predictable.

Intramuscular route.   IM injections of analgesics, although still used, are not the preferred route for administration for women in labor. Identified disadvantages of the IM route include the following:

- The onset of pain relief is delayed.
- Higher doses of medication are required.
- Medication from muscle tissue is released at an unpredictable rate and is available for transfer across the placenta to the fetus.

IM injections given in the upper arm (deltoid muscle) seem to result in more rapid absorption and higher blood levels of the medication (Bricker & Lavender, 2002). If regional anesthesia is planned later in labor, the autonomic blockade from the regional (e.g., epidural) anesthesia increases blood flow to the gluteal region and accelerates absorption of medication that may be sequestered there. The maternal plasma level of the medication necessary to bring pain relief usually is reached 45 minutes after IM injection, followed by a decline in plasma levels. The maternal medications levels (after IM injections) also are unequal because of uneven distribution (maternal uptake) and metabolism. The primary advantage of using the IM route is quick administration by the health care provider.

Spinal nerve blocks.   An IV infusion is usually established before the induction of spinal nerve blocks (e.g., epidural, subarachnoid). Anesthesia protocols often include the prophylactic administration of IV fluid before epidural and spinal anesthesia for blood volume expansion to prevent maternal hypotension. However, routine preloading with IV fluids before epidural analgesia is a form of care with a trade-off between beneficial and adverse effects (Enkin et al., 2000).

Lactated Ringer's and normal saline solutions are commonly used infusion solutions. Infusion solutions without dextrose are preferred, especially when the solution must be infused rapidly (e.g., to treat dehydration or to maintain blood pressure) because solutions containing dextrose rapidly increase maternal blood glucose levels. The fetus responds to high blood glucose levels by increasing insulin production; neonatal hypoglycemia may result. In addition, dextrose changes the osmotic pressure so that fluid is excreted from the kidneys more rapidly.

Because spinal nerve blocks can reduce bladder sensation, resulting in difficulty voiding, the woman should empty her bladder before the induction of the block and should be encouraged to void at least every 2 hours thereafter. The nurse should palpate for bladder distention and measure urinary output to ensure that the bladder is being completely emptied. A distended bladder can inhibit uterine contractions and fetal descent, resulting in a slowing of the progress of labor. The status of the maternal-fetal unit and the progress of labor must be established before the block is performed. The nurse or the woman's partner must assist the woman to assume and maintain the correct position for induction of epidural and spinal anesthesia (see Fig. 12-11).

Safety and general care

After a spinal nerve block is administered, the woman is protected from injury by raising the side rails and placing a call bell within easy reach when the nurse is not in attendance. Oxygen and suction should be readily available at the bedside. The nurse must make sure there is no prolonged pressure on an anesthetized part (e.g., lying on one side with weight on one leg, tight linen on feet). If stirrups are used for birth, the nurse should pad them, adjust both stirrups to the same level and angle, place both of the woman's legs into them simultaneously while avoiding putting pressure on the popliteal angle, and apply restraints (if used) without restricting circulation.

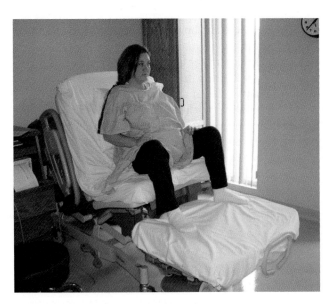

Fig. 12-14 Modified throne position for labor. (Courtesy Julie Perry Nelson, Gilbert, AZ.)

Depending on the level of motor blockade, the woman should be assisted to remain as mobile as possible. When in bed, her position should be alternated from side to side every hour to ensure adequate distribution of the anesthetic solution and to maintain circulation to the uterus and placenta. Assisting the woman to assume upright positions such as sitting (e.g., modified throne position in which the woman sits on the bed with the bottom part lowered to place her feet below her body) (Fig. 12-14), tug-of-war position (woman tugs on towel or sheet that is tied to the bar on the bed or held by the nurse), and squatting by using the head of the bed for support will facilitate fetal descent and enhance bearing-down efforts (Gilder, Mayberry, Gennaro, & Clemmons, 2002). Upright positions are very important in the prevention of operative births (e.g., forceps-assisted or vacuum-assisted birth) and should be encouraged when the woman has a low-dose epidural or CSE (Mayberry et al., 2003). To prevent injury, the nurse must assess the level of motor of function (e.g., woman takes three unassisted steps with accompaniment, woman stands and closes eyes while nurse notes degree of unsteadiness, woman is able to flex legs or rise from a supine position), level of sensation in legs (e.g., degree of numbness), and level of sedation before the woman is assisted out of bed and periodically thereafter (Mayberry, Clemmens, & De, 2002). The woman should sit on the side of the bed before standing to determine if orthostatic hypotension occurs. If she is not dizzy or light-headed, then she can stand at the side of the bed and even walk.

Health care providers should recognize that the second stage of labor is often prolonged in women who use epidural analgesia for pain management. Research evidence indicates that as long as the well-being of the maternal-fetal unit is established, a period of "laboring down" to allow the fetus to descend and rotate with uterine contractions and the use of open-glottis pushing techniques when the fetus has reached a 1+ station and is rotating to an anterior position are the best approaches to use for the management of second-stage labor (Mayberry, Clemmens, & De, 2002). Use of upright positions for second stage labor can be encouraged, including squatting and sitting upright (Mayberry, Clemmens, & De, 2003) (see Chapter 14 for a full discussion of second stage labor management).

The nurse monitors and records the woman's response to nonpharmacologic pain relief methods and to medication(s). This includes the degree of pain relief, the level of apprehension, the return of sensations and perception of pain, and allergic or adverse reactions (e.g., hypotension, respiratory depression, hypothermia, fever, pruritus, nausea, and vomiting). The nurse continues to monitor maternal vital signs, blood pressure, the strength and frequency of uterine contractions, changes in the cervix and station of the presenting part, the presence and quality of the bearing-down reflex, bladder filling, and state of hydration. Determining the fetal response after administration of analgesia or anesthesia is vital. The woman is asked if she (or the family) has any questions. The nurse also assesses the woman's and her family's understanding of the need for ensuring her safety (e.g., keeping side rails up, calling for assistance as needed).

The time that elapses between the administration of an opioid and the baby's birth is documented. Medications given to the newborn to reverse opioid effects are recorded. After birth the woman who has had spinal, epidural, or general anesthesia is assessed for return of sensory and motor function in addition to the usual postpartum assessments. Both the nurse and the anesthesia provider are responsible for documenting assessments and care in relation to the epidural (Mahlmeister, 2003).

Evaluation
Evaluation of the effectiveness of care of the woman needing management of discomfort during labor and birth is based on the previously stated outcomes.

COMMUNITY ACTIVITY

1 Attend a childbirth education class session on pain management during labor and birth. Answer the following questions, and perform the following evaluations:
   a. What nonpharmacologic methods were discussed?
   b. What pharmacologic methods were discussed?
   c. Was the information presented in a nonbiased manner?
   d. Was the information evidence based?
   e. Evaluate the session in terms of the goals stated for the class.

f. Evaluate how well the participants could demonstrate nonpharmacologic methods (e.g., breathing techniques).

g. Was the information culturally appropriate for all participants; How so or why not?

h. How could the class have been improved?

2 Identify sources in your area for childbirth education classes. Your analysis should address the following points:

a. Ways in which pregnant women can find out about classes in the area (e.g., how and where advertised)

b. Convenience of location; times of classes

c. Costs

d. Choices of classes offered (e.g., number of sessions, topics, target audiences, languages)

e. Suggestions for improving any of the above

Key Points

- The expected outcome of preparation for childbirth and parenting is "education for choice."

- Nonpharmacologic pain and stress management strategies are valuable for managing labor discomfort alone or in combination with pharmacologic methods.

- The gate-control theory of pain and the stress response are the bases for many of the nonpharmacologic methods of pain relief.

- The type of analgesic or anesthetic to be used is determined in part by the stage of labor and the method of birth.

- Sedatives may be appropriate for women in prolonged early labor when there is a need to decrease anxiety or to promote sleep or therapeutic rest.

- Naloxone (Narcan) is an opioid antagonist that can reverse opioid effects, especially respiratory depression.

- Pharmacologic control of discomfort during labor requires collaboration among the health care providers and the laboring woman.

- The nurse must understand medications, their expected effects, their potential adverse reactions, and their methods of administration.

- Maintenance of maternal fluid balance is essential during spinal and epidural nerve blocks.

- Maternal analgesia or anesthesia potentially affects neonatal neurobehavioral response.

- The use of opioid agonist-antagonist analgesics in women with preexisting opioid dependence may cause symptoms of abstinence syndrome (opioid withdrawal).

- General anesthesia is rarely used for vaginal birth but may be used for cesarean birth or whenever rapid anesthesia is needed in an emergency.

Answer Guidelines to Critical Thinking Exercise

Hydrotherapy

1 Yes, there is sufficient evidence to draw conclusions about what advice to give to Yvonne about hydrotherapy.

2 a. Most women desire pain relief in labor. Satisfaction with their experience of labor is related to how well their expectations met reality, not necessarily how much pain they experienced. Nurses need to support the laboring woman to make informed choices that meet the woman's expectations but also ensure the safety of the woman and infant.

b. Studies on the effect of hydrotherapy on labor pain (Benfield, 2002; Nikodem, 2003; Simkin & O'Hara, 2002) suggest that immersion has a number of physiologic effects that can affect the perception of pain in labor. Women may relax in the warmth and buoyancy of the water; vasodilation is promoted; and catecholamine production is reduced. Increased relaxation and decreased pain have been noted in study participants.

c. Potential harmful effects of hydrotherapy include hyperthermia, hypothermia, and infection (especially if membranes are ruptured). Water temperature in the range of 36° to 38° C has been suggested to avoid potentially adverse effects. Increased risk of infection in low risk women with or without ruptured membranes or their infants has not been established.

3 The priority is to provide information to Yvonne about the potential benefits and risks of hydrotherapy, then to support her

if she chooses to use the Jacuzzi. Implications for care would be to check the temperature of the water to make sure it stays within the recommended range, to perform maternal and fetal assessments as per protocol or health care provider's orders, to assess pain level during the bath, and to help Yvonne get into and out of the tub safely.

4 Subjective responses of women in studies suggest there is evidence to support use of hydrotherapy. However, there are few randomized controlled trials available to evaluate the effects of hydrotherapy on labor pain or to identify or confirm adverse effects. Florence and Palmer (2003) suggest that hydrotherapy can be used as a primary measure or an additional measure for managing labor pain.

5 There are many nonpharmacologic methods of pain relief that are beneficial (e.g., massage, music, aromatherapy, and warm showers). One or more of these can be encouraged if Yvonne decides not to use the Jacuzzi.

Epidurals and Labor Progress

1 Yes, there is sufficient evidence to draw conclusions about what advice to give Dodie concerning epidurals and labor progress and the incidence of cesarean births.

2 a. Studies have demonstrated that both first and second stages of labor are lengthened with epidural analgesia, and oxytocin use and assisted vaginal births are increased (Sharma & Leveno,

2003). Combined spinal-epidural analgesia provides effective labor pain relief with little effect on uterine contractions or maternal pushing efforts (Florence and Palmer, 2003).

   b. Studies on effects of epidurals on cesarean birth rates are difficult to interpret because many have flawed design problems; however, Sharma and Leveno (2003) conclude that cesarean rates are not increased.

   c. Sharma and Leveno report that most studies conclude that there are few if any fetal or neonatal effects and none that were clinically significant. Harmful FHR patterns have not been related to epidural analgesia, although fetal bradycardia has been reported when combined spinal-epidural analgesia is used. Apgar scores and umbilical cord blood gas levels have shown no adverse effects on the neonate.

   d. Mayberry and others (2003) studied the use of upright positions during second-stage labor in women who had been given low-dose epidural analgesia. In this descriptive study, the women were able to assume upright positions when provided with physical and emotional support. Upright positions and frequent position changes are recommended by AWHONN in the guidelines for second stage labor management; however, no specific suggestions were made for women who had epidurals because of a lack of research.

3 The priority is to assure Dodie that she will have support and encouragement during the second stage and that interventions will be implemented to promote a successful vaginal birth. Implications for care include position changes and continued fetal and maternal assessments to evaluate progress and to identify potential problems. Dodie may be encouraged to "labor down" until the fetus has moved down in the birth canal and pushing can be more effective.

4 The evidence does not strongly support the conclusion that use of upright positions prevents longer labors, but it is more objective in supporting giving Dodie assurance about having a successful vaginal birth.

5 Dodie may decide that she would like to let the analgesia wear off somewhat so that she can better feel the contraction and push more effectively.

Resources

Academy for Guided Imagery, Inc.
30765 Pacific Coast Hwy., Suite 369
Malibu, CA 90265
800-726-2070
www.academyforguidedimagery.com

American Academy of Husband-Coached Childbirth
   (Bradley Method of Natural Childbirth)
P.O. Box 5224
Sherman Oaks, CA 91413
800-422-4784
www.bradleybirth.com

Birthworks, Inc.
P.O. Box 2045
Medford, NJ 08055
888-862-4784
www.birthworks.org

Childbirth and Postpartum Professional Association (CAPPA)
P.O. Box 491448
Lawrenceville, GA 30043
888-692-2772
www.mycappa.net

Cutting Edge Press (source for information and equipment
   regarding childbirth support measures by Polly Perez)
www.childbirth.org/CEP.html

Healing Touch International, Inc.
12477 W. Cedar Dr., Suite 202
Lakewood, CO 80228
303-989-7982
www.healingtouch.net

HypnoBirthing Institute
P.O. Box 810
Epsom, NH 03234
877-798-3286
www.hypnobirthing.com

Lamaze International
2025 M St., Suite 800
Washington, DC 20036-3309
800-368-4404
www.lamaze.org

Maternity Center Association
281 Park Ave., South, 5th Floor
New York, NY 10010
212-777-5000
www.maternitywise.org

Perinatal Education Associates, Inc.
98 E. Franklin St., Suite B
Centersville, OH 45459
1-866-882-4784
www.birthsource.com

Read Natural Childbirth Foundation
P.O. Box 150956
San Rafael, CA 94915
415-456-8462

Touch Research Institutes
University of Miami School of Medicine
P.O. Box 016820
Miami, FL 33101
305-243-6781
www.miami.edu/touch-research/home.html

References

Baker, A., Ferguson, S., Roach, G., & Dawson, D. (2001). Perceptions of labour pain by mothers and their attending midwives. *Journal of Advanced Nursing, 35*(2), 171-179.

Benfield, R. (2002). Hydrotherapy in labor. *Image: Journal of Nursing Scholarship, 34*(4), 347-352.

Bradley, R. (1981). *Husband-coached childbirth* (3rd ed.). New York: HarperCollins.

Bricker, L., & Lavender, T. (2002). Parenteral opioids for labor pain relief: A systematic review. *American Journal of Obstetrics and Gynecology, 186*(5), S94-S109.

Browning, C. (2000). Using music during childbirth. *Birth, 27*(4), 272-276.

Caton, D., Corry, M., Frigoletto, F., Hopkins, D., Lieberman, E., Mayberry L., et al. (2002). The nature and management of labor pain: Executive summary. *American Journal of Obstetrics and Gynecology, 186*(5), S1-S15.

Cluett, E., Nikoden, V., McCandlish, R., & Burns, E. (2004). Immersion in water in pregnancy, labour and birth (Cochrane Review). In *The Cochrane Library*, Issue 2, 2004. Chichester, UK: John Wiley & Sons.

Cunningham, F., Leveno, K., Bloom, S., Hauth, J., Gilstrap, L., & Wenstrom, K. (2005). *Williams obstetrics* (22nd ed.). New York: McGraw-Hill.

Dick-Read, G. (1987). *Childbirth without fear* (5th ed.). New York: Harper-Collins.

DiFranco, J. (2000). Biofeedback. In F. Nichols & S. Humenick (Eds.), *Childbirth education: Practice, research, and theory* (2nd ed.). Philadelphia: Saunders.

Enkin, M., Keirse, M., Neilson, J., Crowther, C., Dudley, L., Hodnett, E., & Hofmeyr, G. (2000). *A guide to effective care in pregnancy and childbirth* (3rd ed.). Oxford, NY: Oxford University Press.

Enkin, M., Keirse, M., Neilson, J., Crowther, C., Duley, L., Hodnett, E., & Hofmeyr, G. (2001). Effective care in pregnancy and childbirth: A synopsis. *Birth, 28*(1), 41-51.

Faucher, M., & Brucker, M. (2000). Intrapartum pain: Pharmacologic management. *Journal of Obstetric, Gynecologic, and Neonatal Nursing, 29*(2), 169-180.

Florence, D., & Palmer, D. (2003). Therapeutic choices for the discomforts of labor. *Journal of Perinatal and Neonatal Nursing, 17*(4), 238-249.

Gentz, B. (2001). Alternative therapies for the management of pain in labor and delivery. *Clinical Obstetrics and Gynecology, 44*(4), 704-732.

Gilder, K., Mayberry, L., Gennaro, S., & Clemmons, D. (2002). Maternal positions in labor with epidural analgesia: Results from a multisite survey. *AWHONN Lifelines, 6*(1), 40-45.

Govenar, J. (2000). Handling headache after dural puncture. *RN, 63*(12), 26-31.

Hawkins, J., Chestnut, D., & Gibbs, C. (2002). Obstetric anesthesia. In S. Gabbe, J. Niebyl, & J. Simpson (Eds.), *Obstetrics: Normal and problem pregnancies* (4th ed.). (pp. 431-472). Philadelphia: Churchill Livingstone.

Hodnett, E. (2002). Pain and women's satisfaction with the experience of childbirth: A systematic review. *American Journal of Obstetrics and Gynecology, 186*(5), S160-S172.

Hodnett, E., Gates, S., Hofmeyr, G., Sakala, C. (2003). Continuous support for women during childbirth (Cochrane Review). In *The Cochrane Library*, Issue 3. Oxford: Update Software.

Hover-Kramer, D., Mentgen, J., & Scandrett-Hibdon, S. (2001). *Healing touch: A resource for health care professionals*. Albany, NY: Delmar.

Humenick, S., Schrock, P., & Libresco, M. (2000). Relaxation. In F. Nichols & S. Humenick (Eds.), *Childbirth education: Practice, research, and theory* (2nd ed.). Philadelphia: Saunders.

Ketterhagen, D., VandeVusse, L., & Berner, M. (2002). Self-hypnosis: Alternative anesthesia for childbirth. *MCN American Journal of Maternal Child Nursing, 27*(6), 335-340.

Koehn, M. (2000). Alternative and complementary therapies for labor and birth: An application of Kolcaba's theory of holistic comfort. *Holistic Nursing Practice, 15*(1), 66-77.

Koehn, M. (2002). Childbirth education outcomes: An integrated review. *Journal of Perinatal Education, 11*(3), 10-19.

Lamaze, F. (1972). *Painless childbirth*. New York: Pocket Books.

Lehne, R. (2001). *Pharmacology for nursing care* (4th ed.). Philadelphia: Saunders.

Leighton, B., & Halpern, S. (2002). The effects of epidural analgesia on labor, maternal, and neonatal outcomes: A systematic review. *American Journal of Obstetrics and Gynecology, 186*(5), S69-S77.

Lieberman, E., & O'Donoghue, C. (2002). Unintended effects of epidural anesthesia during labor: A systematic review. *American Journal of Obstetrics and Gynecology, 186*(5), S31-S68.

Lowe, N. (2002). The nature of labor pain. *American Journal of Obstetrics and Gynecology, 186*(5), S16-S24.

Mackey, M. (2001). Use of water in labor and birth. *Clinical Obstetrics and Gynecology, 44*(4), 733-749.

Mahlmeister, L. (2003). Nursing responsibilities in preventing, preparing for, and managing epidural emergencies. *Journal of Perinatal and Neonatal Nursing, 17*(1), 19-32.

Marks, G. (2000). Alternative therapies. In F. Nichols & S. Humenick (Eds.), *Childbirth education: Practice, research, and theory* (2nd ed.). Philadelphia: Saunders.

Mattson, S. (2000). Striving for cultural competence: Providing care for the changing face of the U.S. *AWHONN Lifelines, 4*(3), 48-52.

Mayberry, L., Clemmens, D., & De, A. (2002). Epidural analgesia side effects, co-interventions, and care of women during childbirth: A systematic review. *American Journal of Obstetrics and Gynecology, 186*(5), S81-S93.

Mayberry, L., Strange, L., Suplee, P., & Gennaro, S. (2003). Use of upright positioning with epidural analgesia: Findings from an observational study. *MCN American Journal of Maternal Child Nursing, 28*(3), 152-159.

Nichols, F. (2000) Paced breathing techniques. In F. Nichols & S. Humenick (Eds.), *Childbirth education: Practice, research, and theory* (2nd ed.). Philadelphia: Saunders.

Nikodem, V. (2003). Immersion in water in pregnancy, labour, and birth (Cochrane Review). In *The Cochrane Library*, Issue 2. Oxford: Update Software.

Perinatal Education Associates. (2003). *Breathing through labor and birth*. Internet document available at http://www.birthsource.com (accessed October 27, 2004).

Righard, L. (2001). Making childbirth a normal process. *Birth, 28*(1), 1-4.

Rosen, M. (2002). Nitrous oxide for relief of labor pain: A systematic review. *American Journal of Obstetrics and Gynecology, 186*(5), S110-S126.

Scheiber, B., & Selby, C. (Eds.). (2000). *Therapeutic touch*. New York: Prometheus Books.

Sharma, S., & Leveno, K. (2003). Regional analgesia and progress of labor. *Clinical Obstetrics and Gynecology, 46*(3), 633-645.

Simkin, P., & Ancheta, R. (2000). *The labor progress handbook: Early interventions to prevent and treat dystocia*. Malden, MA: Blackwell Science.

Simkin, P., & O'Hara, M. (2002). Nonpharmacologic relief of pain during labor: Systematic reviews of five methods. *American Journal of Obstetrics and Gynecology, 186*(5), S131-S159.

Snyder, M., & Lindquist, R. (Eds.). (2000). *Complementary/alternative therapies in nursing* (4th ed.). New York: Springer.

Tiran, D., & Mack, S. (2000). *Complementary therapies for pregnancy and childbirth* (2nd ed.). Edinburgh: Baillière-Tindall.

U.S. Department of Health and Human Services (USDHHS). (2000). *Healthy People 2010* (conference edition, Vol. II). Washington, DC: USDHHS.

CHAPTER 13

Fetal Assessment during Labor

DEITRA LEONARD LOWDERMILK

LEARNING OBJECTIVES

- *Identify typical signs of nonreassuring fetal heart rate (FHR) patterns.*
- *Compare FHR monitoring done by intermittent auscultation (IA) with external and internal electronic methods.*
- *Explain the baseline FHR and evaluate periodic changes.*
- *Describe nursing measures that can be used to maintain FHR patterns within normal limits.*
- *Differentiate among the nursing interventions used for managing specific FHR patterns, including tachycardia and bradycardia; increased and decreased variability; and late and variable decelerations.*
- *Review the documentation of the monitoring process necessary during labor.*

KEY TERMS AND DEFINITIONS

acceleration Increase in fetal heart rate (FHR); usually interpreted as a reassuring sign

amnioinfusion Infusion of normal saline warmed to body temperature through an intrauterine catheter into the uterine cavity in an attempt to increase the fluid around the umbilical cord and prevent compression during uterine contractions

baseline fetal heart rate Average FHR during a 10-minute period that excludes periodic and episodic changes and periods of marked variability

bradycardia Baseline FHR below 110 beats per minute (beats/min)

deceleration Slowing of FHR attributed to a parasympathetic response and described in relation to uterine contractions. Types of decelerations include:

  early deceleration A visually apparent gradual decrease of FHR before the peak of a contraction and return to baseline as the contraction ends; caused by fetal head compression

  late deceleration A visually apparent gradual decrease of FHR with the lowest point of the deceleration occurring after the peak of the contraction and returning to baseline after the contraction ends; caused by uteroplacental insufficiency

  variable deceleration A visually abrupt decrease in FHR below the baseline occurring any time during the uterine contracting phase and caused by compression of the umbilical cord.

electronic fetal monitoring (EFM) Electronic surveillance of FHR by external and internal methods

episodic changes Changes from baseline patterns in the FHR that are not associated with uterine contractions

hypoxemia Reduction in arterial Po_2 resulting in metabolic acidosis by forcing anaerobic glycolysis, pulmonary vasoconstriction, and direct cellular damage

hypoxia Insufficient availability of oxygen to meet the metabolic needs of body tissue

intermittent auscultation Listening to fetal heart sounds at periodic intervals using nonelectronic or ultrasound devices placed on the maternal abdomen

nonreassuring FHR patterns FHR patterns that indicate the fetus is not well oxygenated and requires intervention

periodic changes Changes from baseline of the fetal heart rate that occur with uterine contractions

tachycardia Baseline FHR above 160 beats/min

tocolysis Inhibition of uterine contractions through administration of medications; used as an adjunct to other interventions in the management of fetal compromise related to increased uterine activity

uteroplacental insufficiency Decline in placental function (exchange of gases, nutrients, and wastes) leading to fetal hypoxia and acidosis; evidenced by late FHR decelerations in response to uterine contractions

Valsalva maneuver Any forced expiratory effort against a closed airway, such as holding one's breath and tightening the abdominal muscles (e.g., pushing during the second stage of labor)

variability Normal irregularity of fetal cardiac rhythm or fluctuations from the baseline FHR of two cycles or more

he ability to assess the fetus by auscultation of the fetal heart was initially described more than 300 years ago. With the advent of the fetoscope and stethoscope after the turn of the twentieth century, the listener could hear clearly enough to count the fetal heart rate (FHR). When electronic FHR monitoring made its debut for clinical use in the early 1970s, it was anticipated that its use would effect a decrease in cerebral palsy and be more sensitive than stethoscopic auscultation in predicting and preventing fetal compromise (Simpson & Knox, 2000). Although neither of these possibilities has been realized, electronic fetal monitoring (EFM) is a useful tool for visualizing FHR patterns on a monitor screen or printed tracing.

Pregnant women should be informed about the equipment and procedures used and the risks, benefits, and limitations of intermittent auscultation (IA) and EFM. This chapter discusses the basis for fetal monitoring, the types of monitoring, and nursing assessment and management of nonreassuring fetal status.

BASIS FOR MONITORING

Understanding fetal and uteroplacental circulation is important in understanding FHR and uterine activity (UA) monitoring (see Chapter 7).

Fetal Response

Because labor is a period of physiologic stress for the fetus, frequent monitoring of fetal status is part of the nursing care during labor. The fetal oxygen supply must be maintained during labor to prevent fetal compromise and to promote newborn health after birth. The fetal oxygen supply can decrease in a number of ways:

1. Reduction of blood flow through the maternal vessels as a result of maternal hypertension (chronic hypertension or gestational hypertension); hypotension (caused by supine maternal position, hemorrhage, or epidural analgesia or anesthesia); or hypovolemia (caused by hemorrhage)
2. Reduction of the oxygen content in the maternal blood as a result of hemorrhage or severe anemia
3. Alterations in fetal circulation, occurring with compression of the umbilical cord (transient, during uterine contractions [UCs]; or prolonged, resulting from

cord prolapse); placental separation or complete abruption; or head compression (head compression causes increased intracranial pressure and vagal nerve stimulation with an accompanying decrease in the FHR)
4. Reduction in blood flow to the intervillous space in the placenta secondary to uterine hypertonus (generally caused by excessive exogenous oxytocin) or secondary to deterioration of the placental vasculature associated with maternal disorders such as hypertension or diabetes mellitus

Fetal well-being during labor can be measured by the response of the FHR to UCs. In general, reassuring FHR patterns are characterized by the following:

• A baseline FHR in the normal range of 110 to 160 beats per minute (beats/min) with no periodic changes and a moderate baseline variability (see later discussion p. 374)
• Accelerations with fetal movement

Uterine Activity

A normal UA pattern in labor is characterized by the following:

• Contractions occurring every 2 to 5 minutes and lasting less than 90 seconds
• Contractions moderate to strong in intensity, as detected by palpation, or intensity is less than 80 mm Hg, as measured by an intrauterine pressure catheter (IUPC)
• Thirty seconds or more elapsing between the end of one contraction and the beginning of the next contraction
• Between contractions, uterine relaxation should be detected by palpation or by an average intrauterine pressure of 20 mm Hg or less (Tucker, 2004).

Fetal Compromise

The goals of intrapartum FHR monitoring are to identify and differentiate the reassuring patterns from the nonreassuring patterns, which can be indicative of fetal compromise. Nursing care focuses on interventions promoting adequate fetal oxygenation and interventions for nonreassuring patterns if they occur.

Nonreassuring FHR patterns are those associated with fetal hypoxemia, which is a deficiency of oxygen in the arterial blood. If uncorrected, hypoxemia can deteriorate to severe fetal hypoxia, which is an inadequate supply of oxygen at the cellular level. Nonreassuring FHR patterns include the following:

- Progressive increase or decrease in baseline rate
- Tachycardia of 160 beats/min or more
- Progressive decrease in baseline variability
- Severe variable decelerations (FHR less than 60 beats/min lasting longer than 30 to 60 seconds, with rising baseline, decreasing variability, or slow return to baseline)
- Late decelerations of any magnitude, especially those that are repetitive and uncorrectable
- Absent or undetected FHR variability
- Prolonged deceleration (greater than 60 to 90 seconds)
- Severe bradycardia (less than 70 beats/min)

MONITORING TECHNIQUES

The ideal method of fetal assessment during labor continues to be debated. Results from research studies indicate that both IA of the FHR and electronic FHR monitoring are associated with similar fetal outcomes in low risk intrapartum patients (Feinstein, Sprague, & Trepanier, 2000; Thacker, Stroup, & Chang, 2001). Although IA is a high-touch, low-technology method of assessing fetal status during labor that places fewer restrictions on maternal activity, more than 80% of laboring women in the United States are monitored electronically for at least part of their labor (Albers, 2001). The lack of evidence on the efficacy of EFM should be a factor to consider in decision making about which method of fetal assessment is offered to low risk laboring women (Wood, 2003).

Intermittent Auscultation

Intermittent auscultation uses listening to fetal heart sounds at periodic intervals to assess the FHR. IA of the fetal heart can be performed with a Leff scope, a DeLee-Hillis fetoscope, or a Doppler ultrasound device. If a Leff scope is used, the domed side should be opened to the connective tubing to the earpieces. The domed side is then applied to the maternal abdomen. The fetoscope is applied to the listener's forehead because bone conduction amplifies the fetal heart sounds for counting. The ultrasound device transmits ultrahigh-frequency sound waves reflecting movement of the fetal heart and converts these sounds into an electronic signal that can be counted (Fig. 13-1).

One procedure for performing auscultation is as follows:
1. Perform Leopold maneuvers (see p. 412) by palpating the maternal abdomen to identify fetal presentation and position.
2. Place the listening device over the area of maximal intensity (see Fig. 14-6 on p. 413) and clarity of the fetal heart sounds to obtain the clearest and loudest sound, which is easiest to count. Apply ultrasound gel to Doppler ultrasound device if used.

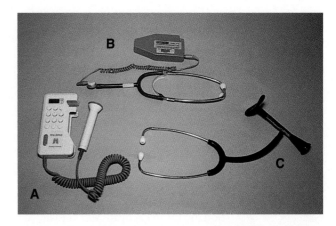

Fig. 13-1 **A,** Ultrasound fetoscope. **B,** Ultrasound stethoscope. **C,** DeLee-Hillis fetoscope. (Courtesy Michael S. Clement, MD, Mesa, AZ.)

3. Palpate the abdomen for the absence of UA to be able to count the FHR between contractions.
4. Count the maternal radial pulse while listening to the FHR to differentiate it from the fetal rate.
5. Count the FHR for 30 to 60 seconds between contractions to identify the baseline rate. This rate can be assessed only during the absence of UA.
6. Auscultate the FHR during a contraction and for 30 seconds after the end of the contraction to identify any increases or decreases in FHR in response to the contraction.

By using IA the nurse can assess the baseline FHR, rhythm, and increases and decreases from baseline (Feinstein, 2000). The method and frequency of fetal surveillance during labor will vary depending on maternal-fetal risk factors and the preference of the facility. In the absence of risk factors, one recommended practice is to auscultate the FHR as follows (American Academy of Pediatrics [AAP] & American College of Obstetricians and Gynecologists [ACOG], 2002; Association of Women's Health, Obstetric and Neonatal Nurses, [AWHONN], 2003):
- *First stage*
  Active phase: every 30 minutes
- *Second stage*
  Every 15 minutes

If risk factors are present, the FHR is auscultated as follows:
- *First stage*
  Active phase: every 15 minutes
- *Second stage*
  Every 5 minutes

There is no recommended practice for assessing the FHR in the latent phase of first-stage labor; however, AWHONN (2003) suggests that the FHR be assessed as frequently as maternal vital signs. The FHR also is assessed before and after ambulation, rupture of membranes, and administration of medications and anesthesia, and more frequently when nonreassuring FHR patterns are heard (AWHONN, 2003; Tucker, 2004).

NURSE ALERT *When the FHR is auscultated and documented, it is inappropriate to use the descriptive terms associated with EFM (e.g., moderate variability, variable deceleration) because most of the terms are visual descriptions of the patterns produced on the monitor tracing. Terms that are numerically defined, however, such as bradycardia and tachycardia, can be used.*

Every effort should be made to use the method of fetal assessment the woman desires, if possible. However, auscultation of the FHR in accordance with the frequency guidelines just given may be difficult in today's busy labor and birth units. When used as the primary method of fetal assessment, auscultation requires a 1:1 nurse-to-patient staffing ratio. If acuity and census change so that auscultation standards are no longer met, the nurse must inform the physician or nurse-midwife that continuous EFM will be used until staffing can be arranged to meet the standards.

The woman can become anxious if the examiner cannot readily count the fetal heartbeats. It often takes time for the inexperienced listener to locate the heartbeat and find the area of maximal intensity. To allay the mother's concerns, she can be told that the nurse is "finding the spot where the sounds are loudest." If it takes considerable time to locate the fetal heartbeats, the examiner can reassure the mother by offering her an opportunity to listen to them, too. If the examiner cannot locate the fetal heartbeat, assistance should be requested. In some cases ultrasound can be used to help locate the fetal heartbeat. Seeing the FHR on the ultrasound screen will be reassuring to the mother if there was initial difficulty in locating the best area for auscultation.

When using IA, UA is assessed by palpation. The examiner should keep his or her hand placed over the fundus before, during, and after contractions. The contraction intensity is usually described as mild, moderate, or strong. The contraction duration is measured in seconds, from the beginning to the end of the contraction. The frequency of contractions is measured in minutes, from the beginning of one contraction to the beginning of the next contraction. The examiner should keep his or her hand on the fundus after the contraction is over to evaluate uterine resting tone or relaxation between contractions. Resting tone between contractions is usually described as soft or relaxed (Goodwin, 2000).

Accurate and complete documentation of fetal status and UA is especially important when IA and palpation are being used because no paper tracing record of these assessments is provided as with continuous EFM. Labor flow records or computer charting systems that prompt notations of all assessments are useful for ensuring such comprehensive documentation.

Electronic Fetal Monitoring

The purpose of electronic FHR monitoring is the ongoing assessment of fetal oxygenation. FHR tracings are analyzed for characteristic patterns that signify specific hypoxic and nonhypoxic events (King & Parer, 2000; Parer & King, 2000).

The two modes of electronic fetal monitoring include the external mode, which uses external transducers placed on the maternal abdomen to assess FHR and UA, and the internal mode, which uses a spiral electrode applied to the fetal presenting part to assess the FHR and an IUPC to assess UA and pressure. The differences between the external and internal modes of EFM are summarized in Table 13-1.

External monitoring

Separate transducers are used to monitor the FHR and UCs (Fig. 13-2). The ultrasound transducer works by reflecting high-frequency sound waves off a moving interface: in this case, the fetal heart and valves; therefore short-term variability and beat-to-beat changes in the FHR cannot be assessed accurately by this method. It is sometimes difficult to reproduce a continuous and precise record of the FHR because of artifacts introduced by fetal and maternal movement. The FHR is printed on specially formatted monitor paper. The standard paper speed is 3 cm/min. Once the area of maximal intensity of the FHR has been located, conductive gel is applied to the surface of the ultrasound transducer, and the transducer is then positioned over this area.

The tocotransducer (tocodynamometer) measures UA transabdominally. The device is placed over the fundus above the umbilicus. UCs or fetal movements depress a pressure-sensitive surface on the side next to the abdomen. The tocotransducer can measure and record the frequency, regularity, and approximate duration of UCs but not their intensity. This method is especially valuable for measuring UA during the first stage of labor in women with intact membranes or for antepartum testing. Because the tocotransducer of most electronic fetal monitors is designed for assessing UA in the term pregnancy, it may not be sensitive enough to detect preterm

CD: Critical Thinking Exercise—Fetal Monitoring

TABLE 13-1

TABLE 13-1

External and Internal Modes of Monitoring

EXTERNAL MODE	INTERNAL MODE
FETAL HEART RATE	
Ultrasound transducer: High-frequency sound waves reflect mechanical action of the fetal heart. Noninvasive. Does not require rupture of membranes or cervical dilation. Used during both the antepartum and intrapartum periods.	*Spiral electrode:* This electrode converts the fetal electrocardiogram (ECG) as obtained from the presenting part to the fetal heart rate (FHR) via a cardiotachometer. This method can be used only when membranes are ruptured and the cervix is sufficiently dilated during the intrapartum period. Electrode penetrates into fetal presenting part by 1.5 mm and must be attached securely to ensure a good signal.
UTERINE ACTIVITY	
Tocotransducer: This instrument monitors frequency and duration of contractions by means of a pressure-sensing device applied to the maternal abdomen. Used during both the antepartum and the intrapartum periods.	*Intrauterine pressure catheter (IUPC):* This instrument monitors the frequency, duration, and intensity of contractions. The two types of IUPCs are a fluid-filled system and a solid catheter. Both measure intrauterine pressure at the catheter tip and convert the pressure into millimeters of mercury on the uterine activity panel of the strip chart. Both can be used only when membranes are ruptured and the cervix is sufficiently dilated during the intrapartum period.

Modified from Tucker, S. (2004). *Pocket guide to fetal monitoring and assessment* (5th ed.). St. Louis: Mosby.

UA. When monitoring the woman in preterm labor, remember that the fundus may be located below the level of the umbilicus. The nurse may need to rely on the woman to indicate when UA is occurring and to use palpation as an additional way of assessing contraction frequency.

The external transducer is easily applied by the nurse, but it must be repositioned as the woman or fetus changes position (see Fig. 13-2, *B*). The woman is asked to assume a semi-sitting or a lateral position. The equipment is removed periodically to wash the applicator sites and to give back rubs. Use of an external transducer confines the woman to bed. Portable telemetry monitors allow observation of the FHR and UC patterns by means of centrally located electronic display stations. These portable units permit the

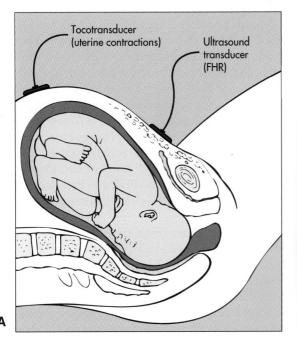

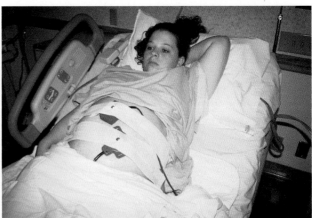

Fig. 13-2   **A,** External noninvasive fetal monitoring with tocotransducer and ultrasound transducer. **B,** Ultrasound transducer is placed below umbilicus, over the area where fetal heart rate is best heard, and tocotransducer is placed on uterine fundus. (**B,** Courtesy Marjorie Pyle, RNC, Lifecircle, Costa Mesa, CA.)

woman to walk around during electronic monitoring. Other monitoring equipment can be used when the woman is submerged in water (see Fig. 12-4, *C*).

Internal monitoring

The technique of continuous internal monitoring allows an accurate appraisal of fetal well-being during labor (Fig. 13-3). For this type of monitoring, the membranes must be ruptured, the cervix sufficiently dilated (2-3 cm), and the presenting part low enough to allow placement of the electrode. A small spiral electrode attached to the presenting part shows a continuous FHR on the fetal monitor strip.

Internal monitoring of the FHR may be implemented without internal monitoring of UA. For UA to be monitored, a solid or fluid-filled IUPC is introduced into the uterine cavity. A solid catheter has a pressure-sensitive tip that measures changes in intrauterine pressure. A catheter filled with sterile water also can be used. As the catheter is compressed during a contraction, pressure is placed on the pressure transducer or strain gauge; this pressure is then converted into a pressure reading in millimeters of mercury. The average pressure during a contraction ranges from 50 to 85 mm Hg. The IUPC can measure the frequency, duration, and intensity of UCs.

The FHR and UA are displayed on the monitor paper, with the FHR in the upper section and UA in the lower section. Fig. 13-4 contrasts the internal and external modes of electronic monitoring. Note that each small square represents 10 seconds; each larger box of six squares equals 1 minute (when paper is moving through the monitor at 3 cm/min).

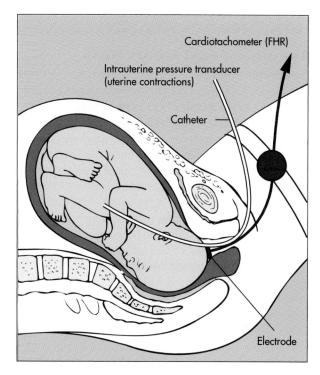

Fig. 13-3 Diagrammatic representation of internal invasive fetal monitoring with intrauterine pressure catheter and spiral electrode in place (membranes ruptured and cervix dilated).

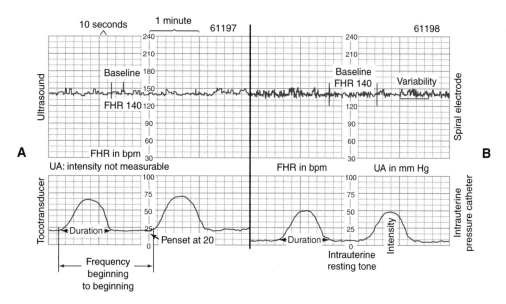

Fig. 13-4 Display of fetal heart rate and uterine activity on monitor paper. **A,** External mode with ultrasound and tocotransducer as signal source. **B,** Internal mode with spiral electrode and intrauterine catheter as signal source. Frequency of contractions is measured from the beginning of one contraction to the beginning of the next. (From Tucker, S. [2004]. *Pocket guide to fetal monitoring and assessment* [5th ed.]. St. Louis: Mosby.)

FETEL HEART RATE PATTERNS ▣

Baseline Fetal Heart Rate

The intrinsic rhythmicity of the fetal heart, the central nervous system (CNS), and the fetal autonomic nervous system control the FHR. An increase in sympathetic response results in acceleration of the FHR, whereas an augmentation in parasympathetic response produces a slowing of the FHR. Usually a balanced increase of sympathetic and parasympathetic response occurs during contractions, with no observable change in the baseline FHR.

Baseline fetal heart rate is the average rate during a 10-minute segment that excludes periodic or episodic changes, periods of marked variability, and segments of the baseline that differ by more than 25 beats/min (National Institute of Child Health and Human Development [NICHD], 1997). The normal range at term is 110 to 160 beats/min.

Variability of the FHR can be described as irregular fluctuations in the baseline FHR of two cycles per minute or greater (NICHD, 1997). It is a characteristic of baseline FHR and does not include accelerations or decelerations of the FHR. Variability has been described as short term (beat to beat) or long term (rhythmic waves or cycles from baseline). The current definition for research does not distinguish between short-term and long-term variability because in actual practice they are viewed together (NICHD, 1997); however, this definition does identify four ranges of variability as seen in Fig. 13-5. These are based on visualization of the amplitude of the FHR in the peak-to-trough segment in beats per minute and include the following:

- Absent or undetected variability
- Minimal variability (greater than undetected but not more than 5 beats/min)
- Moderate variability (6 to 25 beats/min)
- Marked variability (greater than 25 beats/min)

In many facilities, short-term and long-term variability continue to be used to describe the FHR fluctuations. Short-term variability is commonly described as either absent or present while long-term variability may be described using the above categories (Tucker, 2004).

Absence of or undetected variability is considered nonreassuring. Diminished variability can result from fetal hypoxemia and acidosis, as well as from certain drugs that depress the CNS, including analgesics, narcotics (meperidine [Demerol]), barbiturates (secobarbital [Seconal] and pentobarbital [Nembutal]), tranquilizers (diazepam [Valium]), ataractics (promethazine [Phenergan]), and general anesthetics. In addition, a temporary decrease in variability can occur when the fetus is in a sleep state. These sleep states do not usually last longer than 30 minutes. Table 13-2 contrasts key differences between increased and decreased variability.

A sinusoidal pattern—a regular smooth, undulating wave-like pattern—is not included in the current research definition of FHR variability. This uncommon pattern occurs when fetal hypoxia results from Rh isoimmunization or fetal anemia (Fig. 13-6).

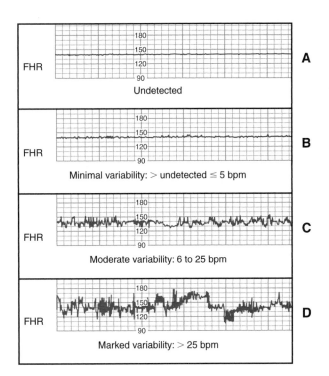

Fig. 13-5 Fetal heart rate variability. **A,** Absent or undetected. **B,** Minimal. **C,** Moderate. **D,** Marked. (Modified from Tucker, S. [2004]. *Pocket guide to fetal monitoring and assessment* [5th ed.]. St. Louis: Mosby.)

Tachycardia is a baseline FHR greater than 160 beats/min for a duration of 10 minutes or longer. It can be considered an early sign of fetal hypoxemia, especially when associated with late decelerations and minimal or absent variability. Fetal tachycardia can result from maternal or fetal infection, such as prolonged rupture of membranes with amnionitis; from maternal hyperthyroidism or fetal anemia; or in response to drugs such as atropine, hydroxyzine (Vistaril), terbutaline, or illicit drugs such as cocaine or methamphetamines.

Bradycardia is a baseline FHR less than 110 beats/min for a duration of 10 minutes or longer. (Bradycardia should be distinguished from prolonged deceleration patterns, which are periodic changes described later in this chapter.)

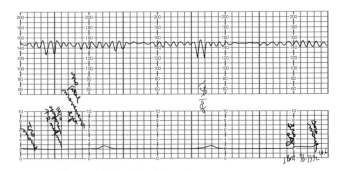

Fig. 13-6 Sinusoidal fetal heart rate. Note the rhythmic undulating pattern. (From: Tucker, S. [2004]. *Pocket guide to fetal monitoring and assessment* [5th ed.]. St. Louis: Mosby.)

TABLE 13-2

Increased and Decreased Variability

INCREASED VARIABILITY	DECREASED VARIABILITY
CAUSE	
Early mild hypoxemia	Hypoxia or acidosis
Fetal stimulation by the following:	CNS depressants
Uterine palpation	Analgesics or narcotics
Uterine contractions	Meperidine (Demerol)
Fetal activity	Alphaprodine (Nisentil)
Maternal activity	Morphine
Drugs:	Pentazocine (Talwin)
Illicit drugs (e.g., cocaine and methamphetamines)	Barbiturates
Sympathomyometic (e.g., terbutaline and asthma	Secobarbital (Seconal)
drugs)	Pentobarbital (Nembutal)
	Amobarbital (Amytal)
	Tranquilizers
	Diazepam (Valium)
	Ataractics
	Promethazine (Phenergan)
	Propiomazine (Largon)
	Hydroxyzine (Vistaril)
	Promazine (Sparine)
	Parasympatholytics
	Atropine
	General anesthetics
	Prematurity: <24 wk
	Fetal sleep cycles
	Congenital abnormalities
	Fetal cardiac dysrhythmias
CLINICAL SIGNIFICANCE	
Significance of marked variability not known; increased variability from a previous average variability is earliest FHR sign of mild hypoxemia	Benign when associated with periodic fetal sleep states, which last 20 to 30 min; if caused by drugs, variability usually increases as drugs are excreted
	Decreased variability is not reassuring and is considered a sign of fetal stress *unless* it has an identifiable temporary (e.g., fetal sleep) or correctable cause
	Decreased variability associated with uncorrectable late decelerations indicates presence of fetal acidosis and can result in low Apgar scores
NURSING INTERVENTION	
Priority depends on cause: Observe FHR tracing carefully for any nonreassuring patterns, including decreasing variability and late decelerations; if using external mode of monitoring, consider using internal mode (spiral electrode) for a more accurate tracing. Intervention usually not required unless nonreassuring FHR pattern develops	Dependent on cause; intervention not warranted if associated with fetal sleep states or temporarily associated with CNS depressants; consider performing external stimulation or scalp stimulation during a vaginal examination to elicit an acceleration of FHR or return to moderate variability; consider application of spiral electrode; assist health care provider with fetal oxygen saturation monitoring if ordered; prepare for birth if so indicated by the primary health care provider

From Tucker, S. (2004). *Pocket guide to fetal monitoring and assessment* (5th ed.). St. Louis: Mosby.
CNS, Central nervous system; *FHR,* fetal heart rate.

It can be considered a later sign of fetal hypoxia and is known to occur before fetal death. Bradycardia can result from placental transfer of drugs such as anesthetics, prolonged compression of the umbilical cord, maternal hypothermia, and maternal hypotension. Maternal supine hypotension syndrome, caused by the weight and pressure of the gravid uterus on the inferior vena cava, decreases the return of blood flow to the maternal heart, which then reduces maternal cardiac output and blood pressure. These responses in the mother subsequently result in a decrease in the FHR and fetal bradycardia. Table 13-3 contrasts tachycardia with bradycardia.

Tachycardia and Bradycardia

TACHYCARDIA	BRADYCARDIA
DEFINITION FHR >160 beats/min lasting >10 min	FHR <110 beats/min lasting >10 min
CAUSE Early fetal hypoxemia Maternal fever Parasympatholytic drugs (atropine, hydroxyzine) β-Sympathomimetic drugs (ritodrine, isoxsuprine) Intraamniotic infection Maternal hyperthyroidism Fetal anemia Fetal heart failure Fetal cardiac dysrhythmias Illicit drugs (cocaine, methamphetamines)	Late fetal hypoxemia or hypoxia β-Adrenergic blocking drugs (propranolol; anesthetics for epidural, spinal, caudal, and pudendal blocks) Maternal hypotension Prolonged umbilical cord compression Fetal congenital heart block Maternal hypothermia Prolonged maternal hypoglycemia
CLINICAL SIGNIFICANCE Persistent tachycardia in absence of periodic changes does not appear serious in terms of neonatal outcome (especially true if tachycardia is associated with maternal fever); tachycardia is a nonreassuring sign when associated with late decelerations, severe variable decelerations, or absence of variability	Bradycardia with moderate variability and absence of periodic changes is not a sign of fetal compromise if FHR remains >80 beats/min; bradycardia caused by hypoxia is a nonreassuring sign when associated with loss of variability and late decelerations
NURSING INTERVENTION Priority dependent on cause: —reduce maternal fever with antipyretics as ordered, hydration, and cooling measures —oxygen at 8-10 L/min by face mask may be of some value —carry out health care provider's orders based on alleviating cause (e.g., assist with fetal pulse oximetry if performed to collect more data about cause)	Priority dependent on cause and based on stage of labor, fetal position and station, and fetal status —intervention not warranted in fetus with heart block diagnosed by ECG —scalp stimulation may be performed to determine whether the fetus has the ability to compensate physiologically for stress (FHR will accelerate) —all interventions to improve fetal oxygenation (i.e., lateral maternal positioning, hydration, correction of maternal hypotension, maternal oxygenation and discontinuing oxytocin) may be implemented —carry out health care provider's orders based on alleviating cause

From Tucker, S. (2004). *Pocket guide to fetal monitoring and assessment* (5th ed.). St. Louis: Mosby.
ECG, Electrocardiography; *FHR,* fetal heart rate.

Changes in Fetal Heart Rate

Changes in FHR from the baseline are categorized as periodic or episodic. Periodic changes are those that occur with UCs. Episodic changes are those that are not associated with UCs. These patterns include accelerations and decelerations (NICHD, 1997).

Accelerations

Acceleration of the FHR is defined as a visually apparent abrupt increase in FHR above the baseline rate. The increase is 15 beats/min or greater and lasts 15 seconds or more, with the return to baseline less than 2 minutes from the beginning of the acceleration. In preterm gestations the definition of an acceleration is a peak of 10 beats/min or more above baseline for at least 10 seconds. Acceleration of the FHR for more than 10 minutes is considered a change in baseline rate.

Accelerations can be periodic or episodic. Periodic accelerations are caused by dominance of the sympathetic nervous response and are usually encountered with breech presentations. Pressure of the contraction applied to the fetal buttocks results in accelerations, whereas pressure applied to the head results in decelerations. Accelerations may occur, however, during the second stage of labor in cephalic presentations. Episodic accelerations (Fig. 13-7, *B*) of the FHR occur during fetal movement and are indications of fetal well-being.

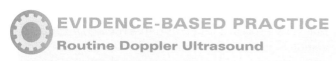

EVIDENCE-BASED PRACTICE
Routine Doppler Ultrasound

BACKGROUND

- Prenatal diagnosticians have used a noninvasive technique called *Doppler ultrasound* since 1977 to visualize the movement of blood in a vessel by detecting the change of frequency of reflected sound. With Doppler ultrasound the movement of blood in the umbilical artery and the uteroplacental circulation gives information about the quality of perfusion to the fetus. This can screen women with high risk pregnancies for conditions leading to intrauterine growth restriction and gestational hypertension perfusion disorders. There is evidence that Doppler ultrasound is a better indicator of fetal well-being than the biophysical profile or electronic fetal monitoring.

- Use of screening tests in pregnancy should be preceded by questions about the proven clinical effectiveness of testing: sensitivity (ability to detect a problem), specificity (ability to rule out the problem for truly normal subjects), risks of the testing procedure, and what treatments are reasonably available for those with abnormal results. Testing can produce anxiety, inappropriate intervention, and iatrogenic (caused by the caregiver) morbidity and mortality. Questions have been raised in the past about the safety of repeated fetal ultrasound examination in general. Although the procedure is of unquestionable value in high risk pregnancies, these questions regarding the routine use of Doppler ultrasound in low risk pregnancies should be answered, and the answers should be backed up by supportive evidence from randomized, controlled trials.

OBJECTIVES

- The authors of the review sought to assess the safety and efficacy of Doppler ultrasound in low risk pregnancies. The intervention was the use of Doppler ultrasound on women with low risk pregnancies. Maternal outcomes included fetal monitoring, kick counts, biophysical profile, ultrasound, operative delivery, and psychologic effects. Perinatal outcomes included birth weight, gestational age at birth, preterm birth, respiratory status, Apgar score, admission to special care nursery, morbidity, neural development at 2 years, and perinatal death.

METHODS
Search Strategy

- The authors searched the Cochrane database. Search keywords were not noted.
- Five trials, including 14,338 women, were selected from France, the United Kingdom, and Australia, dated 1992 to 1997.

Statistical Analyses

- Statistical analyses included pooling similar data for metaanalysis and analyzing differences between the Doppler group and controls for each outcome studied. The reviewers accepted results outside the 95% confidence interval as significant.

FINDINGS

- No differences between the two groups were found in antenatal admissions or obstetric interventions. One trial found increased perinatal mortality rate in the Doppler group, but when these data were added to the pooled data, the overall difference was not significant. One trial found that the Doppler group was more likely to have repeat tests. No trials evaluated the ability of second-trimester Doppler ultrasound to predict preeclampsia, intrauterine growth restriction, or adverse pregnancy outcome. No data were found on acute neonatal problems, long-term neurologic development, or maternal psychologic factors. One trial found that there was an increase in birth weight below the 10th percentile in women who had intensive repeated fetal ultrasound and Doppler ultrasound examinations, when compared with women who had only selected Doppler tests.

LIMITATIONS

- Interventions varied among trials: some evaluated umbilical artery Doppler alone; others evaluated both umbilical artery and uteroplacental blood flow. One trial compared patients who underwent repeated ultrasound examination plus Doppler with patients who underwent Doppler ultrasound examination only if indicated. Some studies did not allow controls to receive the intervention, and some did allow it. Parameters of measurement differed for the Doppler ultrasound examination. One trial had differing protocols for high risk and low risk women. The homogeneity of the protocols limits generalizability. Many women dropped out of some studies. No trials included management protocols for abnormal results.

CONCLUSIONS

- There is no supporting evidence that routine use of Doppler ultrasound in low risk pregnancy is beneficial to mother or baby. The study showing the intrauterine growth restriction (birth weight less than 10th percentile) suggests that repeated ultrasound examinations may be harmful to the fetus. Doppler ultrasound remains a valuable tool when indicated for high risk pregnancies.

IMPLICATIONS FOR PRACTICE

- Nurses can question the practice of routine Doppler ultrasound in low risk pregnancy. They can educate patients about the risks and benefits of these routines. As patients become more knowledgeable, they can discuss with their primary health care provider the indications for the test.

IMPLICATIONS FOR FURTHER RESEARCH

- Large trials are needed to determine Doppler ultrasound's ability to predict preeclampsia, intrauterine growth restriction, and other adverse outcomes in low risk pregnancies. Outcomes should include maternal psychologic effects, neonatal morbidity, and long-term neurologic development of the baby. Of particular interest is resolving the issue of the safety of ultrasound.

Reference: Bricker, L., & Neilson, J. (2000). Routine Doppler ultrasound in pregnancy (Cochrane Review). In *The Cochrane Library*, Issue 2, 2004. Chichester, UK: John Wiley & Sons.

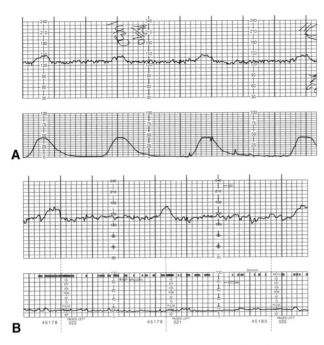

Fig. 13-7 **A,** Acceleration of fetal heart rate (FHR) with uterine contractions. **B,** Acceleration of FHR movement. (From Tucker, S. [2004]. *Pocket guide to fetal monitoring and assessment* [5th ed.]. St. Louis: Mosby.)

Decelerations

A deceleration (caused by dominance of parasympathetic response) may be benign or nonreassuring. Three types of decelerations are encountered during labor: *early, late,* and *variable.* FHR decelerations are described by their visual relation to the onset and end of a contraction and by their shape.

Early decelerations. Early deceleration of the FHR is a visually apparent gradual decrease and return to baseline FHR in response to fetal head compression. It is a normal and benign finding (NICHD, 1997). The deceleration generally starts before the peak of the UC and returns to the baseline at the same time as the UC returns to its baseline. Early decelerations may also occur during UCs, during vaginal examinations, as a result of fundal pressure, and during placement of the internal mode of fetal monitoring. When present, they usually occur during the first stage of labor when the cervix is dilated 4 to 7 cm. Early decelerations sometimes are seen during the second stage when the woman is pushing.

Because early decelerations are considered to be benign, interventions are not necessary. It is valuable to identify early decelerations so that they can be distinguished from late or variable decelerations, which can be nonreassuring and for which interventions are appropriate. The different characteristics of accelerations of the FHR and early decelerations are contrasted in Table 13-4.

Late decelerations. Late deceleration of the FHR is a visually apparent gradual decrease in and return to base-

line FHR associated with UCs (NICHD, 1997). The deceleration begins after the contraction has started, and the lowest point of the deceleration occurs after the peak of the contraction. The deceleration usually does not return to baseline until after the contraction is over (Fig. 13-8, *B*).

Uteroplacental insufficiency causes late decelerations. Persistent and repetitive late decelerations usually indicate the presence of fetal hypoxemia stemming from insufficient placental perfusion. They can be associated with fetal hypoxemia progressing to hypoxia and acidemia progressing to acidosis. They should be considered an ominous sign when they are uncorrectable, especially if they are associated with decreased variability and tachycardia. Late decelerations caused by the maternal supine hypotension syndrome are usually correctable when the woman turns on her side to displace the weight of the gravid uterus off the vena cava. Such lateral positioning allows better return of maternal blood flow to the heart, which in turn increases cardiac output and blood pressure.

Late decelerations caused by uteroplacental insufficiency can result from uterine hyperstimulation with oxytocin, gestational hypertension, postdate or postterm pregnancy, amnionitis, small-for-gestational-age (SGA) fetus, maternal diabetes, placenta previa, abruptio placentae, conduction anesthetics (producing maternal hypotension), maternal cardiac disease, and maternal anemia. The clinical significance and nursing interventions are described in Table 13-5.

Variable decelerations. Variable deceleration is defined as a visual abrupt decrease in FHR below the baseline. The decrease is 15 beats/min or more, lasts at least 15 seconds, and returns to baseline in less than 2 minutes from the time of onset (NICHD, 1997). Variable decelerations occur any time during the uterine contracting phase and are caused by compression of the umbilical cord. Table 13-5 contrasts late deceleration with variable deceleration.

The pattern of variable decelerations differs from those of early and late decelerations, which closely approximate the shape of the corresponding UC. Instead, variable decelerations often have a U or V shape, characterized by a rapid descent to and ascent from the nadir (or depth) of the deceleration (Fig. 13-8, *C*). Some variable decelerations are preceded and followed by brief accelerations of the FHR, known as "shouldering," which is an appropriate compensatory response to compression of the umbilical cord.

Variable decelerations may be related to partial, brief compression of the cord. If encountered in the first stage of labor, they usually can be resolved by changing the mother's position, such as from one side to the other. Oxygen administration by face mask to the mother is sometimes helpful. Variable decelerations are most commonly found during the second stage of labor as a result of umbilical cord compression during fetal descent (Freeman, Garite, & Nageotte, 2003). If repetitive variable decelerations occur during the second stage, it is important to discourage the woman from pushing with every contraction

Text continued on p. 382.

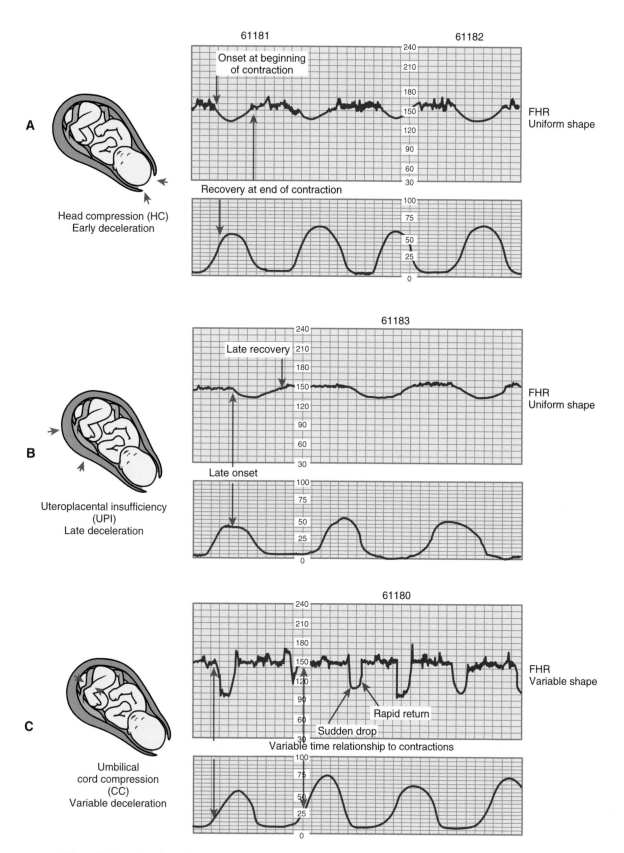

Fig. 13-8 Deceleration patterns. **A,** Early decelerations caused by head compression. **B,** Late decelerations caused by uteroplacental insufficiency. **C,** Variable decelerations caused by cord compression. (From Tucker, S. [2004]. *Pocket guide to fetal monitoring and assessment* [5th ed.]. St. Louis: Mosby.)

Accelerations and Early Decelerations

	ACCELERATION	EARLY DECELERATION
Description	Transitory increase of fetal heart rate (FHR) above baseline (see Fig. 13-7)	Transitory decrease of FHR below baseline concurrent with uterine contractions (see Fig. 13-8, *A*)
Shape	May resemble shape of uterine contraction or be spikelike	Uniform shape; mirror image of uterine contraction
Onset	Onset to peak (30 sec; often precedes or occurs simultaneously with uterine contraction)	Early in contraction phase before peak of contraction
Recovery	Less than 2 min from onset	By end of contraction as uterine pressure returns to its resting tone
Amplitude	Usually 15 beats/min above baseline	Usually proportional to amplitude of contraction; rarely decelerates below 100 beats/min
Baseline	Usually associated with average baseline variability	Usually associated with average baseline variability
Occurrence	Variable; may be repetitive with each contraction	Repetitious (occurs with each contraction); usually occurs between 4- and 7-cm dilation and in second stage of labor
Cause	Spontaneous fetal movement Vaginal examination Reaction to external sounds Electrode application, scalp stimulation Breech presentation, occiput posterior position Uterine contractions Fundal pressure Abdominal palpation	Head compression resulting from the following: —Uterine contractions —Vaginal examination —Fundal pressure —Placement of internal mode of monitoring
Clinical significance	Acceleration with fetal movement signifies fetal well-being, representing fetal alertness or arousal states	Reassuring pattern not associated with fetal hypoxemia, acidemia, or low Apgar scores
Nursing intervention	None required	None required

From Tucker, S. (2004). *Pocket guide to fetal monitoring and assessment* (5th ed.). St. Louis: Mosby.

Late Decelerations and Variable Decelerations

	LATE DECELERATION	VARIABLE DECELERATION
Description	Transitory gradual decrease in fetal heart rate (FHR) below baseline rate in contracting phase (see Fig. 13-8, *B*)	Abrupt decrease in FHR that is variable in duration, intensity, and timing related to onset of contractions (see Fig. 13-8, *C*)
Shape	Uniform; mirror image of uterine contraction; may be deep or shallow	Variable; characterized by sudden decrease in FHR in V, U, or W shape
Onset	Late in contraction phase; after peak of contraction; nadir of deceleration occurs after peak of contraction	Onset of deceleration to the beginning of nadir, <30 sec; decrease in FHR baseline is ≥15 beats/min, lasting ≥15 sec; variable times in contracting phase; often preceded by transitory acceleration
Recovery	Well after end of contraction	Return to baseline is rapid and <2 min from onset, sometimes with transitory acceleration or acceleration immediately before and after deceleration (shouldering or "overshoot"); slow return to baseline with severe variable decelerations

TABLE 13-5

Late Decelerations and Variable Decelerations—cont'd

	LATE DECELERATION	VARIABLE DECELERATION
Deceleration	Usually proportional to amplitude of contraction; rarely decelerates to <100 beats/min; however, shallow late decelerations have the same significance	*Mild:* decelerates to any level, <30 sec with abrupt return to baseline *Moderate:* decelerates to <70 beats/min for 30 to 60 sec or <70 to 80 bpm for 60 sec *Severe:* decelerates to <70 beats/min for >60 sec, with slow return to baseline
Baseline	Often associated with loss of variability and increasing baseline rate	Mild variables usually associated with average baseline variability; moderate and severe variables often associated with decreasing variability and increasing baseline rate
Occurrence	Occurs with each contraction; may be observed at any time during labor	Variable; commonly observed late in labor with fetal descent and pushing
Cause	Uteroplacental insufficiency caused by the following: —Uterine hyperactivity or hypertonicity —Maternal supine hypotension —Epidural or spinal anesthesia —Placenta previa —Abruptio placentae —Hypertensive disorders —Postmaturity —Intrauterine growth restriction —Diabetes mellitus —Intraamniotic infection	Umbilical cord compression caused by the following: —Maternal position with cord between fetus and maternal pelvis —Cord around fetal neck, arm, leg, or other body part —Short cord —Knot in cord —Prolapsed cord
Clinical significance	Nonreassuring pattern associated with fetal hypoxemia, acidemia, and low Apgar scores; considered ominous if persistent and uncorrected, especially when associated with fetal tachycardia and loss of variability	Variable decelerations occur in ~50% of all labors and usually are transient and correctable *Reassuring* variable decelerations last <45 sec and abruptly return to the FHR baseline; normal baseline rate continues; variability does not decrease *Nonreassuring* variable decelerations decrease to ≤70 beats/min for ≥60 sec and have a prolonged return to baseline; baseline rate increases, variability is absent Nonreassuring variable decelerations are associated with fetal acidemia, hypoxemia, and low Apgar scores; severe variable decelerations with average baseline variability just before birth are usually well tolerated
Nursing interventions	The usual priority is: —Change maternal position (lateral) —Correct maternal hypotension by elevating legs —Increase rate of maintenance IV solution. —Palpate uterus to assess for hyperstimulation —Discontinue oxytocin if infusing —Administer oxygen at 8-10 L/min with tight face mask —Consider internal monitoring for a more accurate fetal and uterine assessment —Fetal scalp or acoustic stimulation —Assist with fetal oxygen saturation monitoring if ordered —Assist with birth (cesarean or vaginal assisted) if pattern cannot be corrected	The usual priority is: —Change maternal position (side to side, knee chest) —if decelerations are severe, proceed with following measures: a. Discontinue oxytocin if infusing b. Administer oxygen at 8-10 L/min with tight face mask c. Assist with vaginal or speculum examination to assess for cord prolapse d. Assist with amnioinfusion if ordered e. Assist with fetal oxygen saturation monitoring if ordered f. Assist with birth (vaginal assisted or cesarean) if pattern cannot be corrected

From Tucker, S. (2004). *Pocket guide to fetal monitoring and assessment* (5th ed.). St. Louis: Mosby.
IV, Intravenous.

so that the fetus has time to recover. Variable decelerations are associated with neonatal depression only when cord compression is severe or prolonged (i.e., tight nuchal cord, short cord, knot in cord, prolapsed cord). Further descriptions of the types of variable decelerations, the clinical significance, and nursing interventions are given in Table 13-5.

Prolonged decelerations. A prolonged deceleration is a visually apparent decrease in FHR below the baseline 15 beats/min or more and lasting more than 2 minutes but less than 10 minutes. A deceleration lasting more than 10 minutes is considered a baseline change (NICHD, 1997). Generally the benign causes are pelvic examination, application of a spiral electrode, rapid fetal descent, and sustained maternal Valsalva maneuver. Other, less benign, causes are progressive severe variable decelerations, sudden umbilical cord prolapse, hypotension produced by spinal or epidural analgesia or anesthesia, paracervical anesthesia, tetanic contraction, and maternal hypoxia, which may occur during a seizure. When the deceleration lasts longer than 1 to 2 minutes, a loss of variability with rebound tachycardia usually occurs. Occasionally a period of late decelerations follows. Prolonged decelerations usually are isolated events that end spontaneously. However, when a prolonged deceleration is seen late in the course of severe variable decelerations or during a prolonged series of late decelerations, the prolonged deceleration may occur just before fetal death.

NURSE ALERT *Nurses should notify the physician or nurse-midwife immediately and initiate appropriate treatment for nonreassuring patterns when they see a prolonged deceleration.*

CARE MANAGEMENT

The care given to women being monitored by EFM or auscultation is the same as that given to the woman having a low risk labor. Care of the woman being monitored by internal methods may vary. FHR pattern recognition and intervention may require a nurse to have additional education and clinical experience.

Assessment and Nursing Diagnoses

The assessment of the woman includes the maternal temperature, pulse, respiratory rate, blood pressure, position, comfort, voiding pattern, status of membranes, UC pattern, cervical effacement and dilation, and emotional status. The fetal assessment includes the fetal presentation, fetal position, FHR, and identification of both reassuring and nonreassuring FHR patterns. A checklist may be used by the nurse to assess the FHR (Box 13-1). All of the assessment information must be documented in the woman's medical record.

BOX 13-1

Checklist for Fetal Heart Rate and Uterine Activity Assessment (Revised)

Patient's name _____ Date/time _____

1. What is the baseline fetal heart rate (FHR)?
   _____ Beats/min
   Check one of the following as observed on the monitor strip:
   _____ Average baseline FHR (110 to 160 beats/min)
   _____ Tachycardia (>160 beats/min)
   _____ Bradycardia (<110 beats/min)
2. What is the baseline variability?
   _____ Absence of variability
   _____ Minimal variability (barely detectable up to 5 beats/min)
   _____ Moderate variability (6 to 25 beats/min)
   _____ Marked variability (>25 beats/min)
3. Are there any periodic or episodic changes in FHR?
   _____ Accelerations with fetal movement
   _____ Repetitive accelerations with each contraction
   _____ Early decelerations (head compression)
   _____ Late decelerations (uteroplacental insufficiency)
   _____ Variable decelerations (cord compression)
        _____ Reassuring (<30 to 45 seconds, abrupt return to baseline, normal baseline, moderate variability)
        _____ Nonreassuring(>60 seconds, slow return to baseline, increasing baseline rate, absence of variability)
   _____ Prolonged deceleration (>2 minutes to 10 minutes)
4. What is the uterine activity/contraction pattern?
   _____ Frequency (beginning to beginning of UC)
   _____ Duration (beginning to end of UC)
   Abdominal palpation method
   _____ Strength (mild, moderate, strong)
   _____ Resting time (from end of one contraction to beginning of next one)
   Internal monitoring (IUPC)
   _____ Intensity (mm Hg pressure)
   _____ Resting tone (mm Hg pressure)
   COMMENTS: _____

   PANEL NUMBER: _____
   WHAT CAN BE OR SHOULD HAVE BEEN DONE?:
   _____
   _____
   _____

Modified from Tucker, S. (2004). *Pocket guide to fetal monitoring and assessment* (5th ed.). St. Louis: Mosby.

Evaluation of the EFM equipment also must be done to ensure that the equipment is working properly and to allow an accurate assessment of the woman and fetus. A checklist for fetal monitoring equipment can be used to evaluate the equipment functions (Box 13-2).

BOX 13-2

Checklist for Fetal Monitoring Equipment

PREPARATION OF MONITOR

1. Is the paper inserted correctly?
2. Are transducer cables plugged into the appropriate outlet of the monitor?
3. Is paper speed set to 3 cm/min?

ULTRASOUND TRANSDUCER

1. Has ultrasound transmission gel been applied to the transducer?
2. Was the fetal heart rate (FHR) tested and noted on the monitor paper?
3. Does a signal light flash or an audible beep occur with each heart beat?
4. Is the belt secure and snug but comfortable for the laboring woman?

TOCOTRANSDUCER

1. Is the tocotransducer firmly positioned at the site of the least maternal tissue?
2. Has it been applied without gel or paste?
3. Was the uterine activity (UA) reference knob pressed between contractions to adjust the UA baseline to print at the 20 mm Hg line?
4. Is the belt secure and snug but comfortable for the laboring woman?

SPIRAL ELECTRODE

1. Is the connector attached firmly to the leg plate?
2. Is the spiral electrode attached to the presenting part of the fetus?
3. Is the inner surface of the leg plate covered with electrode gel (if necessary)?
4. Is the leg plate properly secured to the woman's thigh?

INTERNAL CATHETER/STRAIN GAUGE

1. Is the length line on the catheter visible at the introitus?
2. Is it noted on the monitor paper that a UA test or calibration was done?
3. Has the monitor been set to zero according to manufacturer's directions?
4. Is the IUPC properly secured to the woman's thigh?

Modified from Tucker, S. (2004). *Pocket guide to fetal monitoring and assessment* (5th ed.). St. Louis: Mosby.

Nursing diagnoses for the woman who is being monitored electronically for fetal status are based on assessment findings. Possible diagnoses include the following:

- *Decreased maternal cardiac output related to*
  - −supine hypotension secondary to maternal position
- *Anxiety related to*
  - −lack of knowledge concerning fetal monitoring during labor
  - −restriction of mobility or movement during EFM
- *Impaired fetal gas exchange related to*
  - −umbilical cord compression
  - −placental insufficiency

- *Acute pain related to*
  - −use of belts to position transducers
  - −maternal position
  - −vaginal examinations associated with application of maternal or fetal internal monitoring equipment or fetal blood sampling
- *Risk for fetal injury related to*
  - −unrecognized hypoxemia, hypoxia, or anoxia
  - −infection secondary to internal monitoring or scalp blood sampling

Expected Outcomes of Care

The primary goals of nursing care are to have a healthy fetal and maternal outcome. The interventions implemented to achieve these outcomes are determined by knowledge of fetal status and by standards for care. The planning process includes accommodating the wishes of the woman and family, answering questions, and explaining nursing interventions.

Expected outcomes for the pregnant woman and family and the fetus include the following:

- The pregnant woman and family will verbalize their understanding of the need for monitoring.
- The pregnant woman and family will recognize and avoid situations that compromise maternal and fetal circulation.
- The fetus will not have any hypoxemic, hypoxic, or anoxic episodes.
- Should fetal compromise occur, it will be identified promptly, and appropriate nursing interventions such as intrauterine resuscitation will be initiated and the physician or nurse-midwife notified.

Plan of Care and Interventions

It is the responsibility of the nurse providing care to women in labor to assess FHR patterns, implement independent nursing interventions, document observations and actions according to the established standard of care, and report nonreassuring patterns to the primary care provider (e.g., physician, certified nurse-midwife). See Box 13-3 for a sample protocol for FHR monitoring by IA and EFM during labor.

Although the use of EFM can be reassuring to many parents, it can be a source of anxiety to some. Therefore the nurse must be particularly sensitive to and respond appropriately to the emotional, informational, and comfort needs of the woman in labor and those of her family (Fig. 13-9 and Box 13-4).

Electronic fetal monitoring pattern recognition

Nurses must evaluate many factors to determine whether an FHR pattern is reassuring or nonreassuring. A complete description of FHR tracings includes both qualitative and quantitative descriptions of baseline rate and variability, presence of accelerations, periodic or episodic decelerations, and changes in the FHR pattern over time (NICHD, 1997). Nurses evaluate these factors based on other obstetric

BOX 13-3

Protocol for Fetal Heart Rate Monitoring

MATERNAL AND FETAL ASSESSMENTS

- Obtain a 20-min strip of electronic fetal monitoring (EFM) for all patients admitted to labor unit.

Low Risk Patient

- Auscultate or assess tracing every 30 min in active phase of first stage of labor.
- Auscultate or assess tracing every 15 min in second stage.

High Risk Patient

- Auscultate or assess tracing every 15 min in active phase and every 5 min in second stage.

Auscultation: All Patients

- Count baseline fetal heart rate (FHR) between contractions.
- Assess FHR during the contraction and for 30 sec after the contraction.
- Note increases or decreases of FHR.
- Assess FHR before ambulation.
- Interpret FHR data, nursing interventions, and patient responses.
- Notify primary health care provider.

EFM: All Patients

- Assess and interpret baseline FHR, variability of FHR, and presence or absence of decelerations and accelerations.

Assessments for All Patients

- Assess uterine activity for frequency and duration, the intensity of contractions, and uterine resting tone.
- Assess FHR immediately after rupture of membranes, vaginal examinations, and any invasive procedure.

MATERNAL CARE

- Assist woman to a comfortable position other than supine.
- Change maternal position at least every 2 hr.

EXTERNAL MONITORING
Ultrasound Transducer
Function

- Monitors FHR with high-frequency sound waves.

Nursing Care

- Tap transducer before use to ensure sound transmission.
- Apply ultrasound transmission gel to transducer, clean abdomen and transducer, and reapply gel every 2h and as needed.
- Massage reddened skin areas gently and reposition belt or adhesive device every 2h and as needed.
- Auscultate FHR with stethoscope or fetoscope if in doubt as to validity of tracing.
- Position and reposition transducer prn to ensure receipt of clear, interpretable FHR data.

Tocotransducer
Function

- Monitors uterine activity via a pressure-sensing device placed on the maternal abdomen.

Nursing Care

- Position and reposition every 2h and as needed on the fundus, where there is the least maternal tissue.
- Keep abdominal strap snug but comfortable for the laboring woman.
- Adjust knob between contractions to print between 10 and 20 mm Hg on the monitor strip paper.
- Palpate fundus every 30 to 60 min to assess strength of contraction; only frequency and duration of contractions can be assessed with tocotransducer.
- Do not determine woman's need for analgesia based on uterine activity displayed on monitor strip.
- Gently massage reddened areas under transducer and belt hourly and as needed.

INTERNAL MONITORING
Spiral Electrode
Function

- Obtains fetal electrocardiogram (ECG) from presenting part and converts it into FHR.

Nursing Care

- Ensure that the connector to the scalp electrode is appropriately attached to leg plate.
- Reapply electrode paste to leg plate if needed.
- Observe FHR tracing on monitor strip for variability.

complications, progress in labor, and analgesia or anesthesia. They also must consider the estimated time interval until birth. Interventions are therefore based on clinical judgment of a complex, integrated process (Haggerty & Nuttall, 2000).

LEGAL TIP **Fetal Monitoring Standards**

Nurses who care for women during childbirth are legally responsible for correctly interpreting FHR patterns, initiating appropriate nursing interventions based on those patterns, and documenting the outcomes of those interventions. Perinatal nurses are responsible for the timely notification of the physician or nurse-midwife in the event of nonreassuring FHR patterns. Perinatal nurses also are responsible for initiating the institutional chain of command should differences in opinion arise among health care providers concerning the interpretation of the FHR pattern and the intervention required.

Nursing management of nonreassuring patterns. The term *intrauterine resuscitation* is sometimes used to refer to those interventions initiated when a nonreassuring FHR pattern is noted; they are directed primarily toward improving uterine and intervillous space blood flow and secondarily toward increasing maternal oxygenation and cardiac output (Parilla, 2002). The following preventive interventions are described in this chapter: avoiding the supine position and encouraging maternal position changes; encouraging

Protocol for Fetal Heart Rate Monitoring—cont'd

- Turn electrode counterclockwise to remove; never pull straight out from presenting part.
- Administer perineal care after the woman voids during labor and prn.

Intrauterine Catheter
Function
- Catheter (solid or fluid filled) that monitors intraamniotic pressure internally.

Nursing Care
- Ensure that the length line on catheter is visible at introitus.
- For closed-system catheters, set baseline rate between uterine contractions when uterus is relaxed.
- Flush open-system catheter with sterile water before insertion and prn.
- For open-system catheters, turn stopcock off to woman, then with pressure valve of strain gauge released, flush strain gauge, remove syringe, and set stylus to 0 lines of chart paper; test further according to manufacturer's instructions every 3-4h and as needed.
- Check proper functioning by tapping catheter, asking woman to cough, or applying fundal pressure; observe appropriate inflection on strip chart.
- Keep catheter or cable secured to woman's leg to prevent dislodgment.

REPORTABLE CONDITIONS
- Presence of nonreassuring patterns:
  - Severe variable decelerations
  - Late decelerations
  - Absence of variability
  - Prolonged deceleration
  - Severe bradycardia
- Worsening of any pattern
- Presence of identifiable fetal dysrhythmias
- Difficulty in obtaining adequate FHR tracing or inadequate audible FHR

EMERGENCY MEASURES
- Implement the following measures immediately in the event of nonreassuring patterns. The priority will depend

on the type of nonreassuring FHR pattern is present (refer to Tables 13-2, 13-3, and 13-5):
- Reposition patient in lateral position to increase uteroplacental perfusion or relieve cord compression.
- Administer oxygen at 8-10 L/min or per hospital protocol by face mask.
- Discontinue oxytocin if infusing.
- Correct maternal hypovolemia by increasing intravenous (IV) rate per protocol or as ordered.
- Assess for bleeding or other cause of pattern change, such as maternal hypotension.
- Notify primary health care provider.
- Assist with other methods of assessment such as fetal oxygen saturation monitoring or interventions such as amnioinfusion.
- Anticipate emergency preparation for surgical intervention if nonreassuring pattern continues despite interventions.

DOCUMENTATION*
Patient Record: Auscultation
- FHR baseline, rate and rhythm, increases or decreases

Patient Record: EFM
- Method of monitoring, change in method, and adjustments to equipment
- FHR range, variability, presence of decelerations or accelerations
- Uterine activity as determined by palpation or by external or internal monitoring
- Interpretation of FHR data, nursing interventions, and patient responses
- Notification of primary health care provider

Monitor Strip
- Patient identification data
- Assessments, procedures, and interventions (medications, etc.)
- Notification of primary health care provider
- Significant occurrences (sterile vaginal examination, rupture of membranes, etc.)
- Adjustments of the monitor equipment

*If computer charting system is used, follow institutional policies and system guidelines and protocols.

spontaneous short bursts of pushing in response to involuntary bearing-down urges; and encouraging pushing with mouth open and glottis open with vocalizing. Previously it was thought that the left lateral maternal position preferentially promoted maternal cardiac output, thereby enhancing blood flow to the fetus. However, it is now known that either the right or left lateral maternal position effectively enhances uteroplacental blood flow. The key issue is to avoid positioning the laboring woman on her back to reduce the risk of supine hypotension, which leads to decreased placental perfusion.

Compression of the umbilical cord vessels results in variable decelerations. Amnioinfusion is an intervention that can help relieve such pressure on a nonprolapsed umbilical cord. If maternal hypotension caused by acute hemorrhage (hypovolemia) occurs, the rapid infusion of blood volume expanders may be ordered. Until the infusion is established, the nurse can elevate the woman's legs. Blood pooled in the legs, especially as a result of sympathetic blockade (e.g., epidural anesthesia), will then drain quickly into the central venous circulation, and this will augment the effective intravascular volume (Parilla, 2002).

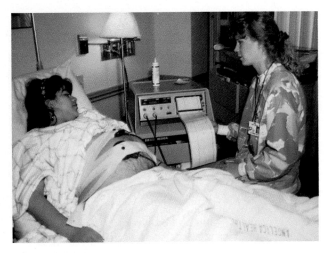

Fig. 13-9 Nurse explains electronic fetal monitoring as ultrasound transducer monitors the fetal heart rate. (Courtesy Marjorie Pyle, RNC, Lifecircle, Costa Mesa, CA.)

Oxytocin always should be infused via a piggyback connection near the indwelling needle. If FHR patterns change for any reason, oxytocin stimulation of the uterine muscle must be discontinued. This consists of turning off the intravenous (IV) line from the piggyback (containing oxytocin) and opening the primary infusion line.

Nurses must assign priorities to interventions to maximize the efficacy of the intrauterine resuscitation. The *first priority* is to open the maternal and fetal vascular systems, the *second priority* is to increase blood volume, and the *third priority* is to optimize oxygenation of the circulating blood volume. For example, to relieve an acute FHR deceleration, the nurse can do the following:

- Assist the woman to the side-lying position if she is not already in a lateral position.
- Increase the maternal blood volume by increasing the rate of the primary IV infusion or by raising the woman's legs.
- Provide oxygen by face mask.

Some interventions are specific to the FHR pattern. Nursing interventions appropriate for the management of tachycardia and bradycardia are given in Table 13-2, and those appropriate for the management of increased or decreased variability are given in Table 13-3. No specific nursing interventions are required for the management of FHR acceleration or early deceleration (see Table 13-4). However, late and some types of variable FHR decelerations require aggressive intervention (see Table 13-5). The primary health care provider decides whether medical intervention should be instituted, what intervention is indicated, or whether immediate vaginal or cesarean birth should be performed.

Other methods of assessment and intervention

Other methods of assessment and intervention are designed to be used in conjunction with EFM in an effort to identify and intervene in the presence of a nonreassuring

---

BOX 13-4

Patient and Family Teaching When Electronic Fetal Monitor Is Used

The following guidelines relate to patient teaching and the functioning of the monitor.
- Explain the purpose of monitoring.
- Explain each procedure.
- Provide rationale for maternal position other than supine.
- Explain that fetal status can be continuously assessed by electronic fetal monitoring (EFM), even during contractions.
- Explain that the lower tracing on the monitor strip paper shows uterine activity; the upper tracing shows the fetal heart rate (FHR).
- Reassure woman and partner that prepared childbirth techniques can be implemented without difficulty.
- Explain that, during external monitoring, effleurage can be performed on sides of abdomen or upper portion of thighs.
- Explain that breathing patterns based on the time and intensity of contractions can be enhanced by the observation of uterine activity on the monitor strip paper, which shows the onset of contractions.
- Note peak of contraction; knowing that contraction will not get stronger and is half over is usually helpful.
- Note diminishing intensity.
- Coordinate with appropriate breathing and relaxation techniques.
- Reassure woman and partner that the use of internal monitoring does not restrict movement, although she is confined to bed.*
- Explain that use of external monitoring usually requires the woman's cooperation during positioning and movement.
- Reassure woman and partner that use of monitoring does not imply fetal jeopardy.
- Reassure her that the equipment is removed periodically to permit the applicator sites to be washed and other care to be given.

*Portable telemetry monitors allow the FHR and uterine contraction patterns to be observed on centrally located display stations. These portable units permit ambulation during electronic monitoring.

FHR. These methods include FHR response to stimulation, fetal oxygen saturation monitoring, fetal blood sampling, amnioinfusion, and tocolysis. Umbilical cord acid-base determination is an assessment technique that is a useful adjunct to the Apgar score in assessing the immediate condition of the newborn.

Fetal heart rate response to stimulation. Stimulation of the fetus is done to elicit an acceleration of the FHR of 15 beats/min for at least 15 seconds (Tucker, 2004). The two methods of fetal stimulation currently in practice are scalp stimulation (using digital pressure during a vaginal examination) and vibroacoustic stimulation (using an artificial larynx or fetal acoustic stimulation device over the fetal head for 1 to 2 seconds). An FHR acceleration usually indicates fetal well-being. If the fetus does not have an acceleration, however, it does not necessarily indicate fetal compromise, but further evaluation of fetal well-being is needed.

Fetal oxygen saturation monitoring. Continuous monitoring of fetal oxygen saturation ($FSpO_2$) or fetal pulse oximetry (FPO) is a method of fetal assessment that was approved for clinical use by the Food and Drug Administration in May 2000 (Porter, 2000). FPO works in a way similar to the pulse oximetry used in children and adults. A specially designed sensor is inserted next to the fetal cheek or temple area to assess oxygen saturation. The sensor is then connected to a monitor, and the data are displayed on the UA panel of the fetal monitor tracing. The normal range of oxygen saturation in the adult is 95% to 100%. The normal range for the healthy fetus is 30% to 70% (Simpson & Porter, 2001), with the cutoff value for the critical threshold of $FSpO_2$ at 30% (Garite et al., 2000).

FPO may be used if certain criteria are met, including a single fetus with at least 36 weeks of gestation in a vertex presentation with a nonreassuring FHR pattern. The membranes should be ruptured, the cervix dilated at least 2 cm, and the fetal station at least a −2 or less (Garite et al., 2000). The value of $FSpO_2$ monitoring is that in the event of nonreassuring FHR patterns, it could support the decision about whether labor should continue or whether to intervene with an expeditious assisted vaginal or cesarean birth of the fetus (Simpson, 2003).

When the use of FPO becomes more widely practiced, the labor nurse's role will expand to include this type of monitoring in practice (Porter, 2000). Simpson and Porter (2001) suggested that nurses will be involved in identifying potential candidates for monitoring, inserting the sensor (according to state nurse practice acts and institutional policies), interpreting data, documenting findings, and communicating with the primary health care provider.

Fetal scalp blood sampling. Sampling of the fetal scalp blood was designed to assess the fetal pH, PO_2, and PCO_2. The procedure is performed by obtaining a sample of fetal scalp blood through the dilated cervix after the membranes have ruptured. The scalp is swabbed with a disinfecting solution before making the puncture, and the sample is then collected. However, the blood gas values vary so rapidly with transient circulatory changes that fetal blood sampling is seldom performed in the United States (Gilstrap, 2004). When used, it is usually in tertiary centers with the capability for repetitive sampling and rapid report of results. The circulatory changes that cause the variability and thus undermine the utility of this procedure are maternal acidosis or alkalosis, caput succedaneum, the stage of labor, and the time relation of scalp sampling to UCs.

Amnioinfusion. Amnioinfusion is used during labor either to supplement the amount of amniotic fluid to reduce the severity of variable decelerations caused by cord compression or to dilute meconium-stained amniotic fluid with saline or lactated Ringer's solution (Hofmeyr, 2002;

Parer & Nageotte, 2004). The procedure to supplement amniotic fluid is indicated for patients with oligohydramnios, secondary to uteroplacental insufficiency, premature rupture of membranes, or postmaturity, who are at risk for variable decelerations because of umbilical cord compression.

Oligohydramnios is an abnormally small amount of amniotic fluid or the absence of amniotic fluid. Without the buffer of amniotic fluid, the umbilical cord can easily become compressed during contractions or fetal movement, diminishing the flow of blood between the fetus and placenta, as evidenced by variable decelerations. Amnioinfusion replaces the "cushion" for the cord and relieves both the frequency and intensity of variable decelerations.

Amnioinfusion also is indicated in the presence of moderate to thick meconium to dilute and flush out the meconium with the intent of avoiding meconium-aspiration syndrome in the neonate (Hofmeyr, 2002).

Risks of amnioinfusion are overdistention of the uterine cavity and increased uterine tone. Techniques of amnioinfusion treatment vary, but usually fluid is administered through an IUPC. The woman's membranes must be ruptured for the IUPC placement. The fluid is administered by attaching plastic (IV) tubing to a liter of normal saline or lactated Ringer's solution through a port in the IUPC. Double-lumen IUPCs are preferred because the IUP can be monitored without stopping the procedure. The fluid is usually warmed with a blood warmer before administration for the preterm or SGA fetus (Torgersen, 2004). The flow rate can be by bolus or continuous flow or by a combination of these two methods.

Intensity and frequency of UCs should be continually assessed during the procedure. The recorded uterine resting tone during amnioinfusion will appear higher than normal because of resistance to outflow and turbulence at the end of the catheter. The true resting tone can be checked by discontinuing the amnioinfusion when using a single-lumen IUPC (Tucker, 2004).

Tocolytic therapy. Tocolysis (relaxation of the uterus) can be achieved through the administration of drugs that inhibit UCs. This therapy can be used as an adjunct to other interventions in the management of fetal stress when the fetus is exhibiting nonreassuring patterns associated with increased UA. Tocolysis improves blood flow through the placenta by inhibiting UCs. Tocolysis may be considered by the primary health care provider and implemented when other interventions to reduce UA, such as maternal position change and discontinuance of an oxytocin infusion, have no effect on diminishing the UCs. A tocolytic drug such as magnesium sulfate or terbutaline can be administered intravenously to decrease UA (Tucker, 2004). If the FHR pattern improves, the woman may be allowed to continue labor; if there is no improvement, immediate cesarean birth may be needed.

Umbilical cord acid-base determination. In assessing the immediate condition of the newborn after birth, a sample of cord blood is a useful adjunct to the Apgar

Types of Acidosis

BLOOD GASES*	RESPIRATORY	METABOLIC	MIXED
pH	↓ (<7.1)	↓ (<7.1)	↓ (<7.1)
Pco_2 (mm Hg)	↑ (>60)	Normal (<60)	↑ (>60)
Hco_3^- (mEq/L)	Normal (16-24)	↓ (<16)	↓ (<16)
Base	Normal (<12)	↑ (>12)	↑ (>12)

Sources: Gilstrap, L. (2004). Fetal acid-base balance. In R. Creasy, R. Resnik, & J. Iams (Eds.). *Maternal-fetal medicine: Principles and practice* (5th ed.). Philadelphia: Saunders; Pagana, K., & Pagana, T. (2002). *Mosby's manual of diagnostic and laboratory tests* (2nd ed.). St Louis: Mosby; Tucker, S. (2004). *Pocket guide to fetal monitoring and assessment* (5th ed.). St. Louis: Mosby.
*Arterial values.

score. The procedure is generally done by withdrawing blood from the umbilical artery and having the blood tested for pH, Pco_2, and Po_2. Umbilical cord gas measurements reflect the acid-base status of the newborn at birth, a measurement not reflected in the Apgar score (Gilstrap, 2004). If acidosis is present (e.g., pH 7.10 to 7.18) the type of acidosis is determined (respiratory, metabolic, or mixed) by analyzing the blood gas values (Table 13-6).

Patient and family teaching

Part of the nurse's role includes acting as a partner with the woman to achieve a high-quality birthing experience. In addition to teaching and supporting the woman and her family with understanding of the laboring and birth process, breathing techniques, use of equipment, and pain management techniques, the nurse can assist with two factors that have an effect on fetal status: pushing and positioning. The nurse should provide information and support to the woman with regard to these two factors.

Maternal positioning. Maternal supine hypotensive syndrome is caused by the weight and pressure of the gravid uterus on the inferior vena cava when the woman is in a supine position. This decreases venous return to the woman's heart and cardiac output and subsequently reduces her blood pressure. The low maternal blood pressure decreases intervillous space blood flow during UCs and results in fetal hypoxia. This is reflected on the fetal monitor as a nonreassuring FHR pattern, usually late decelerations. The nurse should solicit the woman's cooperation in avoiding the supine position. The woman should be encouraged to maintain a side-lying position or semi-Fowler's position with a lateral tilt to the uterus.

Discouraging the Valsalva maneuver. The Valsalva maneuver can be described as the process of making a forceful bearing-down attempt while holding one's breath with a closed glottis and tightening the abdominal muscles. This process stimulates the parasympathetic division of the autonomic nervous system, producing a vagal response, and results in the decrease of the maternal heart rate and blood pressure. Prolonged pushing in this manner can decrease placental blood flow, alter maternal and fetal oxygenation, decrease the fetal pH and Po_2, increase the fetal Pco_2, and increase the likelihood of fetal hypoxemia, as reflected in FHR pattern changes.

During the second stage of labor, when the woman needs to push, an alternative to breath holding with a closed glottis is to perform the open-mouth and open-glottis breathing-pushing technique. The nurse should instruct the woman to keep her mouth and glottis open and to let air escape from the lungs during the pushing process. This may result in an audible grunting sound and will prevent the Valsalva maneuver. Some providers of care prefer the laboring-down process or delayed pushing, which is to refrain from pushing in the early second stage of labor. The natural forces of labor contractions are used to move the fetus down the birth canal, and then focused pushing is used for a short period to expel the fetus from the birth canal.

Documentation

Clear and complete documentation on the woman's monitor strip is started before the initiation of monitoring and consists of identifying information plus other relevant data. This documentation is continued and updated according to institutional protocol as monitoring progresses. In some institutions, observations noted and interventions implemented are recorded on the monitor strip to produce a comprehensive document that chronicles the course of labor and the care rendered. In other institutions this documentation is confined to the labor flow record or computer chart. Advocates of documenting on both the medical record and the EFM strip cite as advantages of this approach the ease of writing directly on the strip while at the bedside or inputting the data on a computer-based documentation system and the improved accuracy in documenting critical events and the interventions implemented. Others believe that charting on the EFM strip constitutes duplicate documentation of the same information noted in the medical record, and thus it is unnecessary additional paperwork for the nurse.

One way of documenting that frequent maternal-fetal assessments have been done at the bedside is either to initial the EFM strip or to depress the "mark" button during these assessments. Data-entry devices are now available with some EFM systems; assessments are keyed in and subsequently printed on the strip. A disadvantage of documenting on both the EFM strip and the medical record is that frequently the times noted for events and interventions on the EFM strip do not correlate with what is later documented in the medical record. These inaccuracies can lead those involved in the retrospective review process carried out during litigation to infer that documentation errors have occurred. Therefore if institutional policy mandates documentation on both the monitor strip and the medical record, it is critically important for the nurse to make sure the times and notations of events and interventions recorded in each place agree. No one method of documentation is right; rather, the nurse must be aware of and follow individual institutional policies, as well as participate in formulating such policies (McCartney, 2002). Many of the aspects of care and events that can be documented on the patient's medical record or the monitor strip are listed in Box 13-5.

Evaluation

Evaluation is a continuous process. The nurse can assume that care was effective when the outcomes for care have been achieved (see Plan of Care).

PLAN OF CARE *Electronic Fetal Monitoring during Labor*

NURSING DIAGNOSIS Maternal anxiety related to lack of knowledge about use of electronic monitor

Expected Outcomes *The patient will exhibit increased understanding about fetal monitoring and signs of reduced anxiety (i.e., absence of physical indicators, absence of perceived threat, and absence of feelings of dread).*

Nursing Interventions/*Rationales*

- Explain and demonstrate to woman and labor support partner how the electronic monitor (internal or external) works in assessing FHR and in detecting and assessing quality of uterine contractions *to remove fear of unknown and ensure that woman can move with the monitor.*
- When making adjustment to the monitor, explain to the couple what is being done and why, *to promote understanding and allay anxiety.*
- Explain that although a side-lying position or semi-Fowler's position provides for optimal monitoring, position changes decrease discomfort; therefore encourage frequent changes in position (other than supine) and explain any monitoring adjustments that are being made as a result *to reduce discomfort and allay anxiety.*

NURSING DIAGNOSIS Risk for fetal injury related to inaccurate placement of transducers or electrodes, misinterpretation of results, or failure to use other assessment techniques to monitor fetal well-being

Expected Outcomes *Fetal well-being is adequately assessed, and any fetal compromise is identified immediately.*

Nursing Interventions/*Rationales*

- Carefully follow guidelines and checklist for application and initiation of monitoring *to ensure proper placement of monitoring devices and production of accurate output from monitoring devices.*
- Check placement throughout monitoring process *to ensure that devices remain correctly placed.*
- Regularly assess and record results of electronic EFM (FHR and variability, decelerations, accelerations, uterine activity, contractions, uterine resting tone) *to provide consistent and timely evaluation of fetal well-being and progress of labor.*
- Auscultate FHR and palpate contractions on a regular basis *to provide a cross-check on the EFM output and ensure fetal well-being.*

NURSING DIAGNOSIS Risk for maternal injury related to incorrect placement of external or internal monitors or misinterpretation of contraction pattern

Expected Outcome *Maternal well-being is assessed continuously, and any alterations are identified promptly.*

Nursing Interventions/*Rationales*

- Palpate uterine contractions *to correlate data with electronic monitoring results.*
- Periodically recheck placement *to verify that all monitoring devices are accurately placed.*
- Assess uterine activity, contraction pattern, and baseline *to provide ongoing evaluation and basis for further interventions.*
- Use correct aseptic technique for insertion of internal monitors *to prevent infection.*
- Monitor maternal temperature, as well as color, odor, and amount of amniotic fluid, *to determine indicators of infection.*

NURSING DIAGNOSIS Risk for impaired physical mobility related to restriction of movement with monitoring devices

Expected Outcome *Woman will be able to change positions and ambulate at intervals.*

Nursing Interventions/*Rationales*

- Discontinue continuous EFM at intervals *to change position and increase mobility.*
- Encourage woman to change position and reposition monitor as needed *to decrease complications of immobility.*
- Place external monitor manually at intervals *to collect data while woman is out of bed.*

EFM, Electronic fetal monitoring; *FHR,* fetal heart rate.

CD: Plan of Care—*Electronic fetal monitoring during labor*

BOX 13-5

Documentation

OBSERVATIONS

Maternal
- Vital signs: BP, TPR
- Oxygen saturation if monitored
- Uterine activity: frequency, duration, intensity, resting tone
- Behavior: anxiety, irritability, fear of losing control
- Breathing pattern
- Position; activity (ambulating, BRP, use of birthing ball, etc.)
- Rupture of membranes; time, color, amount, odor
- Voidings; nausea, vomiting
- Urge to push; bearing down; pushing

Fetal
- FHR, variability, periodic or episodic changes
- Fetal movement
- Oxygen saturation if monitored
- Presentation, position, station

ADJUSTMENTS
- Relocation of transducers
- Replacement of electrode

- Replacement of IUPC
- Adjustment or flushing of IUPC
- Testing of monitor
- Monitor paper changes; time lapse
- Interruption or removal of monitoring equipment

INTERVENTIONS
- Maternal position change
- Administration of oxygen
- Parenteral fluids; changes in flow rate
- Amnioinfusion
- Fetal scalp stimulation
- Medication administration
- Oxytocin
- Analgesics
- Anesthetics
- Tocolytics
- Primary health care provider notification, reason, and response
- Birth data

BP, Blood pressure; *BRP,* bath room privileges; *FHR,* fetal heart rate; *IUPC,* intrauterine pressure catheter; *TPR,* Temperature, Pulse, and Respirations.

COMMUNITY ACTIVITY

You have been asked to give a class on fetal assessment during labor to couples attending childbirth classes at the local clinic. The class is a mix of low and high risk patients. The objective of the class is to provide them with information for making an informed decision about the choice between intermittent auscultation and electronic fetal monitoring.

1 Prepare the class using an ethical decision model such as described in the Wood article in your reference list.
2 Summarize the topics you will include and identify the evidence on which these topics are based.
3 Suggest questions that the women can ask their health care providers about fetal monitoring choices.

Key Points

- Fetal well-being during labor is gauged by the response of the FHR to UCs.
- FHR characteristics include the baseline FHR and periodic changes in the FHR.
- The monitoring of fetal well-being includes FHR assessment, watching for meconium-stained amniotic fluid, and assessment of maternal vital signs and UA.
- It is the responsibility of the nurse to assess FHR patterns, implement independent nursing interventions, and report nonreassuring patterns to the physician or nurse-midwife.
- AWHONN and ACOG have established and published health care provider standards and guidelines for fetal heart monitoring.
- The emotional, informational, and comfort needs of the woman and her family must be addressed when the mother and her fetus are being monitored.
- Documentation is initiated and updated according to institutional protocol.

Answer Guidelines to Critical Thinking Exercise

Fetal Monitoring

1 There is not enough evidence that says there are significant differences in infant outcomes between infants of low risk mothers who had EFM and infants of those who had IA of the FHR. There is some evidence that there is an increase in operative births when EFM is used (Albers, 2001; Thacker, Stroup, & Chang, 2001).

2 a. IA is as effective in low risk and high risk women as continuous monitoring. The monitoring guidelines are different. In low risk women in active labor IA is done every

30 min; in second stage—every 15 min. For high risk women, every 15 min in active labor and every 5 min in second stage.

b. There are no significant differences in infant outcomes when the above monitoring guidelines have been used.

c. A 1:1 nurse:patient ratio is needed for IA; EFM is routinely used in most health care facilities because of budget and staff limitations.

3 The priority for the nurse is to respond to Keri's concern about a safe outcome. Keri needs to be assured that her baby will be assessed and interventions will be implemented if nonreassuring signs occur. Then the nurse can provide information about fetal monitoring methods. If IA is a choice (hospital policy, health care provider approval), Keri should be given information about its effectiveness in low risk women and about its advantages and limitations. Keri also needs to know the difference between external and internal EFM and why each may be used in labor situations and the advantages and limitations. Keri's support persons should be included in the discussion. The doctor or nurse-midwife is informed of Keri's request and what information she has received from the nurse. A decision for using EFM or IA is then made between Keri and her primary health care provider.

4 Yes, there is objective evidence to support this response to Keri.

5 Keri may not be interested in learning about IA as a method, or it may not be available. Then the nurse should provide information about EFM and its advantages and limitations so that Keri does not have a false sense of security about the birth outcome just because her baby is being monitored with EFM.

Resources

American College of Nurse-Midwives
818 Connecticut Ave., NW, Suite 900
Washington, DC 20006
202-728-9860
www.midwife.org

American College of Obstetricians and Gynecologists (ACOG)
409 12th St., SW
Washington, DC 20024
800-762-2264
www.acog.com

Association of Women's Health, Obstetric and Neonatal Nurses (AWHONN)
2000 L St., NW, Suite 740
Washington, DC 20036
800-673-8499 (United States)
800-245-0231 (Canada)
www.awhonn.org

National Association of Parents and Professionals for Safe Alternatives in Childbirth (NAPSAC)
P.O. Box 267
Marble Hill, MO 63764
314-238-2010
www.napsac.org

National Institute of Child Health and Human Development (NICHD)
National Institutes of Health
9000 Rockville Pike
Bldg. 31, Room 2A32
Bethesda, MD 20892
301-496-4000
www.nih.gov

References

Albers, L. (2001). Monitoring the fetus in labor: Evidence to support the methods. *Journal of Midwifery & Women's Health, 46*(6), 366-373.

American Academy of Pediatrics (AAP) & American College of Obstetricians and Gynecologists (ACOG). (2002). *Guidelines for perinatal care* (5th ed.). Washington, DC: AAP & AGOG.

Association of Women's Health, Obstetric and Neonatal Nurses. (2003). *Fetal heart monitoring principles and practice* (3rd ed.). Dubuque, IA: Kendall/Hunt.

Bricker, L., & Neilson, J. (2000). Routine Doppler ultrasound in pregnancy (Cochrane Review). In *The Cochrane Library*, Issue 2, 2004. Chichester, UK: John Wiley & Sons.

Feinstein, N. (2000). Fetal heart rate auscultation: Current and future practice. *Journal of Obstetric, Gynecologic, and Neonatal Nursing, 29*(3), 306-315.

Feinstein, N., Sprague, A., & Trepanier, M. (2000). *Fetal heart rate auscultation*. Washington, DC: Association of Women's Health, Obstetric and Neonatal Nurses (AWHONN).

Freeman, R., Garite, T., & Nageotte, M. (2003). *Fetal heart rate monitoring* (3rd ed.). Philadelphia: Lippincott Williams & Wilkins.

Garite, T., Dilday, G., McNamara, H., Nageotte, M., Boehm, F., Dellinger, E., Knuppel, R. et al. (2000). A multicenter controlled trial of fetal pulse oximetry in the intrapartum management of nonreassuring fetal heart rate patterns. *American Journal of Obstetrics and Gynecology, 183*(5), 1049-1058.

Gilstrap, L. (2004). Fetal acid-base balance. In R. Creasy, R. Resnik, & J. Iams (Eds.), *Maternal-fetal medicine: Principles and practice* (5th ed.). Philadelphia: Saunders.

Goodwin, L. (2000). Intermittent auscultation of the fetal heart rate: A review of general principles. *Journal of Perinatal and Neonatal Nursing, 14*(3), 53-61.

Haggerty, L., & Nuttall, R. (2000). Experienced obstetric nurses' decision-making in fetal risk situations. *Journal of Obstetric, Gynecologic, and Neonatal Nursing, 29*(5), 480-490.

Hofmeyr, G. (2002). Amnioinfusion for meconium-stained liquor in labour (Cochrane Review). In *The Cochrane Library*, Issue 2, 2004, Oxford: Update Software.

King, T., & Parer, J. (2000). The physiology of fetal heart rate patterns and perinatal asphyxia. *Journal of Perinatal and Neonatal Nursing, 14*(3), 19-39.

McCartney, P. (2002). Electronic fetal monitoring and the legal medical record. *MCN American Journal of Maternal Child Nursing, 27*(4), 249.

National Institute of Child Health and Human Development (NICHD) Research Planning Workshop. (1997). Electronic fetal heart rate monitoring: Research guidelines for interpretation. *American Journal of Obstetrics and Gynecology, 177*(6), 1385-1390.

Pagana, K., & Pagana, T. (2002). *Mosby's manual of diagnostic and laboratory tests* (2nd ed.). St. Louis: Mosby.

Parer, J., & King, T. (2000). Fetal heart rate monitoring: Is it salvageable? *American Journal of Obstetrics and Gynecology, 182*(4), 982-987.

Parer, J., & Nageotte, M. (2004). Intrapartum fetal surveillance. In R. Creasy, R. Resnik, & J. Iams (Eds.), *Maternal-fetal medicine: Principles and practice* (5th ed.). Philadelphia: Saunders.

Parilla, B. (2002). Estimation of fetal well-being. In A. Fanaroff & R. Martin (Eds.), *Neonatal-perinatal medicine: Diseases of the fetus and infant* (7th ed.). St. Louis: Mosby.

Porter, M. (2000). Fetal pulse oximetry: An adjunct to electronic fetal heart rate monitoring. *Journal of Obstetric, Gynecologic, and Neonatal Nursing, 29*(5), 537-548.

Simpson, K. (2003). Fetal pulse oximetry update. *AWHONN Lifelines, 7*(5), 411-412.

Simpson, K., & Knox, G. (2000). Risk management and electronic fetal monitoring: Decreasing risk of adverse outcomes and liability exposure. *Journal of Perinatal and Neonatal Nursing, 14*(3), 40-52.

Simpson, K., & Porter, M. (2001). Fetal oxygen saturation monitoring: Using this new technology for fetal assessment during labor. *AWHONN Lifelines, 5*(2), 26-33.

Thacker, S., Stroup, D., & Chang, M. (2001). Continuous electronic heart rate monitoring for fetal assessment during labor (Cochrane Review). In *The Cochrane Library,* Issue 2, 2001. Oxford: Update Software.

Torgersen, K. (2004). Intrapartum fetal assessment. In S. Mattson and J. Smith (Eds.). *Core curriculum for maternal-newborn nursing* (3rd ed). St. Louis: Elsevier.

Tucker, S. (2004). *Pocket guide to fetal monitoring and assessment* (5th ed.). St. Louis: Mosby.

Wood, S. (2003). Should women be given a choice about fetal assessment in labor? *MCN American Journal of Maternal Child Nursing, 28*(5), 292-298.

CHAPTER 14

Nursing Care during Labor and Birth

DEITRA LEONARD LOWDERMILK

LEARNING OBJECTIVES

- Review the factors included in the initial assessment of the woman in labor.
- Describe the ongoing assessment of maternal progress during the first, second, and third stages of labor.
- Recognize the physical and psychosocial findings indicative of maternal progress during labor.
- Describe fetal assessment during labor.
- Identify signs of developing complications during labor and birth.
- Identify nursing interventions for each stage of labor and birth.

- Examine the influence of cultural and religious beliefs and practices on the process of labor and birth.
- Evaluate research findings on the importance of support (family, doula, nurse) in facilitating maternal progress during labor and birth.
- Describe the role and responsibilities of the nurse during an emergency childbirth.
- Identify the effect of perineal trauma on the woman.
- Discuss ways the nurse can increase the use of evidence-based practices in caring for a woman during labor and birth.

KEY TERMS AND DEFINITIONS

active phase Phase in the first stage of labor when the cervix dilates from 4 to 7 cm

amniotomy Artificial rupture of the fetal membranes (AROM), using a plastic Amnihook or surgical clamp

bloody or pink show Blood-tinged mucoid vaginal discharge that originates in the cervix and indicates passage of the mucous plug (operculum) as the cervix ripens before labor and dilates during labor; it increases as labor progresses

crowning Phase in the descent of the fetus when the top of the head can be seen at the vaginal orifice as the widest part of the head (biparietal diameter) distends the vulva just before birth

doula Experienced female assistant hired to give the woman support during labor and birth

episiotomy Surgical incision of the perineum at the end of the second stage of labor to facilitate birth and to avoid laceration of the perineum

fern test The appearance of a fernlike pattern found on microscopic examination of certain fluids such as amniotic fluid

first stage of labor Stage of labor from the onset of regular uterine contractions to full effacement and dilation of the cervix

latent phase Phase in the first stage of labor when the cervix dilates from 0 to 3 cm

Leopold maneuvers Four maneuvers for diagnosing the fetal position by external palpation of the mother's abdomen

lithotomy position Position in which the woman lies on her back with her knees flexed and with

abducted thighs drawn up toward her chest; stirrups attached to an examination table can be used to facilitate assuming and maintaining this position

nitrazine test Evaluation of body fluids using a test strip to determine the fluid's pH; urine will exhibit an acidic result, and amniotic fluid will exhibit an alkaline result

nuchal cord Encircling of fetal neck by one or more loops of umbilical cord

Ritgen maneuver Technique used to control the birth of the head; upward pressure from the coccygeal region to extend the head during the actual birth

rupture of membranes (ROM) Integrity of the amniotic membranes is broken either spontaneously or artificially (amniotomy)

second stage of labor Stage of labor from full dilation of the cervix to the birth of the baby

spontaneous rupture of membranes (SROM, SRM) Rupture of membranes by natural means, most often during labor

third stage of labor Stage of labor from the birth of the baby to the separation and expulsion of the placenta

transition phase Phase in the first stage of labor when the cervix dilates from 8 to 10 cm

uterine contractions Primary powers of labor that act involuntarily to dilate and efface the cervix, expel the fetus, facilitate separation of the placenta, and prevent hemorrhage

For most women, labor begins with the first uterine contraction, continues with hours of hard work during cervical dilation and birth, and ends as the woman and her significant others begin the attachment process with the newborn. Nursing care management focuses on assessment and support of the woman and her significant others throughout labor and birth, with the goal of ensuring the best possible outcome for all involved.

FIRST STAGE OF LABOR

CARE MANAGEMENT

The first stage of labor begins with the onset of regular uterine contractions and ends with full cervical effacement and dilation. Care begins when the woman reports one or more of the following:

- Onset of progressive, regular uterine contractions that increase in frequency, strength, and duration
- Blood-tinged mucoid vaginal discharge (bloody or pink show) indicating that the mucous plug (operculum) has passed
- Fluid discharge from the vagina (spontaneous rupture of membranes [SROM; SRM])

The first stage of labor consists of the following three phases: the latent phase (up to 3 cm of dilation), the active phase (4 to 7 cm of dilation), and the transition phase (8 to 10 cm of dilation). Most nulliparous women seek admission to the hospital in the latent phase because they have not experienced labor before and are unsure of the "right" time to come in. Multiparous women usually do not come to the hospital until they are in the active phase.

The nursing process is used as a framework for managing the care of women and their significant others during all stages of labor. Involving the laboring woman as a partner in the formulation of an individualized plan of care helps preserve the woman's sense of control, facilitates her participation in her own childbirth experience, and enhances her self-esteem and level of satisfaction.

Women often have lingering impressions of their childbirth experiences. Caregivers who are respectful, supportive, available, protective, encouraging, kind, patient, professional, calm, and comforting help these women to remember their childbirth experiences in positive terms. Frustrations women feel regarding their childbirth experiences stem from pain, lack of control, lack of knowledge, or the negative behaviors of some caregivers (Hanson, VandeVusse, & Harrod, 2001; Tumblin & Simkin, 2001).

Assessment and Nursing Diagnoses

Assessment begins at the first contact with the woman, whether by telephone or in person. Many women call the hospital or birthing center first to receive validation that it is all right for them to come in for evaluation or admission. The manner in which the nurse communicates with the woman during this first contact can set the tone for a positive birth experience. A caring attitude by the nurse encourages the woman to verbalize questions and concerns. If possible, the nurse should have the woman's prenatal record in hand when speaking to her or admitting her for evaluation of labor. Copies of records are often filed on the perinatal unit at some time during the woman's third trimester.

Certain factors are assessed initially to determine whether the woman is in true or false labor and whether she should come for further assessment or admission (see Teaching Guidelines box).

The pregnant woman may call the primary health care provider or come to the hospital while in false labor or early in the latent phase of the first stage of labor. She may feel discouraged on learning that the contractions that feel so strong and regular to her are not true contractions because they are not causing cervical dilation or are still not strong or frequent enough for admission.

If the woman lives near the hospital, she may be asked to stay home or return home to allow labor to progress (i.e., until the uterine contractions are more frequent and intense). The ideal setting for the low risk woman at this time is the familiar environment of her home. The nurse can use a telephone interview (Box 14-1) to assess the woman's status and to give instructions regarding the optimal time for admission and to reinforce teaching regarding the signs that require immediate notification of the primary health care provider. Measures the woman and her significant others can

TEACHING GUIDELINES
How to Distinguish True Labor from False Labor

TRUE LABOR
- Contractions
  - Occur regularly, becoming stronger, lasting longer, and occurring closer together
  - Become more intense with walking
  - Usually felt in lower back, radiating to lower portion of abdomen
  - Continue despite use of comfort measures
- Cervix (by vaginal examination)
  - Shows progressive change (softening, effacement, and dilation signaled by the appearance of bloody show)
  - Moves to an increasingly anterior position
- Fetus
  - Presenting part usually becomes engaged in the pelvis, which results in increased ease of breathing; at the same time, the presenting part presses downward and compresses the bladder, resulting in urinary frequency

FALSE LABOR
- Contractions
  - Occur irregularly or become regular only temporarily
  - Often stop with walking or position change
  - Can be felt in the back or abdomen above the navel
  - Often can be stopped through the use of comfort measures
- Cervix (by vaginal examination)
  - May be soft, but there is no significant change in effacement or dilation or evidence of bloody show
  - Is often in a posterior position
- Fetus
  - Presenting part is usually not engaged in the pelvis

use to enhance the progress of labor, reduce anxiety, and maintain comfort are described.

A warm shower can be relaxing for the woman in early labor. Soothing back, foot, and hand massage or a warm drink of preferred liquids such as tea or milk can help the woman to rest and even to sleep, especially if false or early labor is occurring at night. Diversional activities such as walking outdoors or in the house, reading, watching television, doing needlework, or talking with friends can reduce the perception of early discomfort, help the time pass, and reduce anxiety.

The woman who lives at a considerable distance from the hospital may be admitted in early labor. The same measures used by the woman at home should be offered to the hospitalized woman in early labor.

Admission to labor unit

When the woman arrives at the perinatal unit, assessment is the top priority (Fig. 14-1). The nurse first performs a screening assessment by using the techniques of interview and physical assessment and reviews the laboratory and diagnostic test findings to determine the health status of the

BOX 14-1

Telephone Interview with Woman in Latent Phase of Labor

The perinatal nurse performs the following steps of the nursing process.

ASSESSMENT
- Gathers data regarding the woman's status, including signs and symptoms indicative of true or false labor (uses prenatal chart if available)
- Discusses instructions given by the woman's primary health care provider regarding when to come for admission

PLANNING AND IMPLEMENTATION
- Decides whether the woman will come for labor assessment and admission or be encouraged to stay at home until contractions increase in duration, frequency, and intensity
- Assures the woman that she is welcome to call the perinatal unit at any time to discuss her labor status
- Answers questions the woman and her family may have regarding labor or provides instruction as needed (e.g., which entrance of the hospital to use)

- Suggests a variety of positions she can assume to maximally enhance uteroplacental and renal blood flow (e.g., side-lying position) and enhance the progress of labor (e.g., upright positions and ambulation)
- Suggests diversional activities, such as walking, reading, watching television, talking to friends
- Suggests measures to maintain comfort, such as a warm shower, back or foot massage
- Discusses the oral intake of foods and fluids appropriate for early labor (light foods or fluids or clear liquids depending on the preference of her primary health care provider)
- Instructs the woman to come in immediately if membranes rupture, bleeding occurs, or fetal movements change

EVALUATION
- Evaluates whether instructions and information have been understood by the woman by asking her to verbalize her understanding

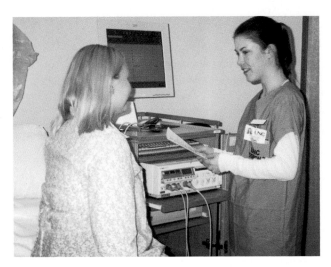

Fig. 14-1 Woman being assessed for admission to the labor and birth unit. (Courtesy Dee Lowdermilk, Chapel Hill, NC.)

woman and her fetus and the progress of her labor. The primary health care provider is notified, and if the woman is admitted, a detailed systems assessment is done.

LEGAL TIP Obstetric Triage and EMTALA

The Emergency Medical Treatment and Active Labor Act (EMTALA) is a federal regulation enacted to ensure that a woman gets emergency treatment or active labor care whenever such treatment is sought. Nurses working in labor and birth units must be familiar with their responsibilities according to the EMTALA regulations, which include providing services to pregnant women when they experience an urgent pregnancy problem. A pregnant woman presenting in an obstetric triage is considered to be in "true" labor until a qualified health care provider certifies that she is not. Agencies need to have specific policies and procedures in place so that compliance with the EMTALA regulations is achieved while safe and efficient care is provided (Caliendo, Millbauer, Moore, & Kitchen, 2004).

When the woman is admitted, she usually is moved from an observation area to the labor room; the labor, delivery, and recovery (LDR) room; or the labor, delivery, recovery, and postpartum (LDRP) room. Because first impressions are important, the woman and her partner are welcomed by name and introduced to the staff members who will be involved in the woman's care. Women often express concern regarding the number of persons intruding on their labor experience, especially if the role of the person and purpose for his or her presence are not clearly identified (Hanson, Vande-Vusse, & Harrod, 2001).

If the woman wishes, her partner is included in the assessment and admission process. Significant others not participating in this process may be directed to the appropriate waiting area, if that is the policy of the unit. Family-centered care is the trend in maternity today. This approach views labor as wellness and the woman and her support persons as active participants in the process of labor and birth. LDR or

LDRP rooms are essential components of family-centered care, and the woman is encouraged to have anyone she wishes present for her support. After birth the mother, baby, and support persons are permitted to stay together to celebrate the arrival of a new family member (Zwelling & Phillips, 2001).

The woman is asked to undress and put on her own gown or a hospital gown. An admissions band is placed on the woman's wrist. Her personal belongings are put away safely or given to family members, according to agency policy. Often women who participate in expectant parents classes bring a birth bag or Lamaze bag with them. The woman and her partner are oriented regarding the layout and operation of the unit and room, including the use of the call light and telephone system, and how to adjust lighting in the room and the different bed positions.

The nurse assures the woman that she is in competent, caring hands and that she and her partner can ask questions related to her care and her status and those of her fetus at any time during labor. The woman's anxiety can be minimized by explaining terms commonly used during labor. The woman's interest, response, and prior experience guide the depth and breadth of these explanations.

Admission data. Admission forms such as the one in Fig. 14-2 can provide guidelines for the acquisition of important assessment information when a woman in labor is being evaluated or admitted. Additional sources of data include the prenatal record, the initial interview, physical examination to determine baseline physiologic parameters, laboratory and diagnostic test results, expressed psychosocial and cultural factors, and the clinical evaluation of labor status.

Prenatal data. The nurse reviews the prenatal record to identify the woman's individual needs and risks. If the woman has not had any prenatal care or her prenatal record is unavailable, certain baseline information must be obtained. If the woman is having discomfort, the nurse should ask questions between contractions when the woman can concentrate more fully on her answers. At times the partner or support person(s) may need to be secondary sources of essential information.

It is important to know the woman's age so that the plan of care can be tailored to the needs of her age group. For example, a 14-year-old girl and a 40-year-old woman have different but specific needs, and their ages place them at risk for different problems. Height and weight relations are important to determine because a weight gain greater than that recommended may place the woman at a higher risk for cephalopelvic disproportion and cesarean birth. This is especially true for women who are petite and have gained 16 kg or more. Other factors to consider are the woman's general health status, current medical conditions or allergies, respiratory status, and previous surgical procedures.

Her obstetric and pregnancy history are carefully noted. These include gravidity, parity, and problems such as history of vaginal bleeding, gestational hypertension, anemia, gestational diabetes, infections (e.g., bacterial or sexually transmitted), and immunodeficiency.

Obstetric Admitting Record Page 1 of 2

Basic Admission Data Date __ / __ / __ Time _____
☐ Ambulatory ☐ Direct admit ☐ Stretcher
☐ Wheelchair ☐ Transfer from_____

| G | T | Pt | A | L | L M P | / / | E D D | / / | Age |

E D D By fetal assessment / /

Race/Ethnicity_____
Occupation_____ Education_____
Marital status S M Sep D W Religion_____
MD/CNM_____ Tel no | Support person/Relationship Tel no

Reasons for Admission
☐ **Onset of labor**
☐ Induction of labor
☐ Spontaneous abortion
☐ Cesarean section
  ☐ Primary ☐ Repeat
  (reason for primary_____)
☐ VBAC
☐ Tubal ligation
☐ Vaginal bleeding
☐ PROM
☐ Preterm labor
Detail reasons for admission_____

Observation evaluation
☐ Fetal status
  ☐ Ultrasound
  ☐ Amniocentesis
  ☐ NST
  ☐ CST
☐ Medical complications
_____
☐ Obstetric complications
_____

Patient Triage Data
Contractions ☐ **None** ☐ Palpation ☐ Tocotransducer
  Frequency_____ Duration_____ Intensity_____
  Began on __ / __ / __ Time_____
Membranes ☐ **Intact** ☐ Bulging
  ☐ Ruptured (Date __ / __ / __ Time_____)
Fluid ☐ Clear ☐ Bloody ☐ Foul smelling
  ☐ Meconium stained ☐ No foul odor
Vaginal bleeding ☐ **None** ☐ Normal show
  ☐ Bleeding (describe_____)

Cervical Exam
  Station_____ Effacement_____ Dilatation_____ cms
  Presentation
  ☐ Vertex ☐ Transverse lie
  ☐ Face/Brow ☐ Compound
  ☐ Breech (type_____) ☐ Unknown
Medication allergy/Sensitivity ☐ **None**
  ☐ Identify_____
Other allergy/Sensitivity ☐ **None**
  ☐ Identify_____

Patient Care Data

Personal Effects	Disposition		
Item	With patient	With support person	Other (describe)

Illness (≤ 14 days prior to admission) ☐ **None**
  ☐ Type/Treatment_____
Recent Exposure to Communicable Disease ☐ **None**
  ☐ Type/Date_____ __ / __ / __
Last Oral Intake
  Fluids __ / __ / __ Time_____
  Solids __ / __ / __ Time_____
Medications ☐ **None**
  Type/Dose Last taken With patient Disposition
      No Yes
      ☐ ☐

Alcohol/Drug use ☐ No ☐ Yes
  Substances Amt/Day Last used
  _____ _____ __ / __ / __ Time_____
  _____ _____ __ / __ / __ Time_____

Plans for Birth and Hospital Stay
Support person present in L&D ☐ No ☐ Yes_____
Other family members in L&D ☐ No ☐ Yes_____
Anesthesia ☐ **None**
  ☐ Local ☐ Epidural ☐ Spinal ☐ General
Delivery site
  ☐ DR ☐ Birthing room ☐ LDR ☐ LDRP ☐ OR
Personal requests_____
Adoption ☐ No
  ☐ Yes Contact with infant ☐ No ☐ Yes
      Adoption contact_____
Feeding preference ☐ Breast ☐ Bottle
Room preference ☐ Private ☐ Semi-Private
  ☐ Rooming-In
☐ Tubal ligation Authorization signed ☐ Yes ☐ No
☐ Circumcision Authorization signed ☐ Yes ☐ No

Psychosocial Data
Communication Deficit ☐ **None**
  ☐ Identify_____

Other children ☐ No ☐ Yes Age/Sex_____
_____ , _____ , _____

Partner involved ☐ Yes ☐ No

Admitting signature_____ Time_____

Fig. 14-2 Obstetric admitting record. (Permission to use and/or reproduce this copyrighted material has been granted by the owner, MNRS-Briggs Corporation, Des Moines, IA.)

Continued

Obstetric Admitting Record	Page 2 of 2	

Psychosocial Data (Cont'd.)

Basic needs met   Yes   No   If no, explain

- Housing ☐ ☐ _____
- Clothing ☐ ☐ _____
- Food ☐ ☐ _____
- Transportation ☐ ☐ _____

Free from apparent physical/emotional abuse ☐Yes ☐No
If no, explain_____

Life Stress   No   Yes   If no, explain
- Living ☐ ☐ _____
- Working ☐ ☐ _____
- Serious illness ☐ ☐ _____

Self Care Needs ☐None ☐Needs help with_____

Emotional status   ☐Happy   ☐Ambivalent
   ☐Anxious   ☐Depressed   ☐Angry

Discharge Planning Data

Discharge planning initiated ☐**Yes** ☐No
Discharge needs identified_____

Social service referral ☐No ☐Yes ___ / ___ / ___
Planned length of stay_____days

Significant Prenatal Data

Prenatal Records Available on Admission
☐**Yes** ☐No
Source of prenatal data_____
First prenatal visit___ / ___ / ___
Attended prenatal classes ☐**Yes** ☐No
Infant care provider:

Lab Findings
☐**None**

Blood type & Rh _____
Rubella titer _____
Serology _____
HbSAg _____

Fetal Assessment Tests
☐**None**

Date	Test	Result
/		
/		
/		
/		

Maternal Problems Identified ☐**None**

	Active	Resolved
1._____	☐	☐
2._____	☐	☐
3._____	☐	☐

Fetal Problems Identified ☐**None**

	Active	Resolved
1._____	☐	☐
2._____	☐	☐
3._____	☐	☐

Physical Assessment

Detail all abnormal findings

Height		Wt pregrav/grav	
Temp	Pulse	Resp	BP

System	Normal	Abnormal
HEENT	☐	☐
Neurologic	☐	☐
Skin	☐	☐
Breasts	☐	☐
Extremities	☐	☐
Cardiovascular	☐	☐
Respiratory	☐	☐
Abdomen	☐	☐
Gastrointestinal	☐	☐
Urinary	☐	☐
Genitalia	☐	☐

Specimens obtained (check all that apply)

Urine test	Time	Results	Blood test	Time	Results
☐Urinalysis			☐Hgb		
☐C + S			☐Hct		
☐Glucose			☐VDRL/RPR		
☐Albumin			☐Type/Screen		
☐Ketones			☐		
☐pH			☐		
☐Blood			☐		

Fetal Evaluation Data

Fundal height_____cms FHR_____
Estimated ☐Fetoscope
fetal weight_____ ☐Doppler
Weeks gestation (est) ☐Fetal monitor
By dates_____wks ☐Other
By ultrasound_____wks
   Date___ / ___ / ___

Multiple gestation ☐**No** ☐Yes

Infant	Presentation	Position
1. _____	_____	_____
2. _____	_____	_____
3. _____	_____	_____

Initial Problems Identified ☐**None**
1. _____
2. _____
3. _____

Physician/CNM_____
Notified by_____
   Date___ / ___ / ___Time_____

_____
Admitting signature

_____
Examiner signature
   Date___ / ___ / ___Time_____

Fig. 14-2, cont'd

If this is not the woman's first labor and birth experience, it is important to note the characteristics of her previous experiences. This information includes the duration of previous labors, the type of anesthesia used, the kind of birth (e.g., spontaneous vaginal, forceps-assisted, vacuum-assisted, or cesarean birth) and the condition of the newborn. The woman's perception of her previous labor and birth experiences should be explored because it may influence her attitude toward her current experience. Women can retain long-term memories of their childbirth experiences. The memory of labor and birth events including her behavior and that of health care providers (e.g., physician, nurse-midwife, nurses, doula, partner) can affect a woman's postpartum emotional adjustment, self-esteem, and ability to parent effectively (Hanson, VandeVusse, & Harrod, 2001).

It is important to confirm the expected date of birth (EDB). Other data in the prenatal record include patterns of maternal weight gain, physiologic measurements such as maternal vital signs (blood pressure, temperature, pulse, respirations); fundal height; baseline fetal heart rate (FHR); and laboratory and diagnostic test results. Laboratory tests include the woman's blood type and Rh factor; a complete or partial blood cell count (CBC, hemoglobin, and hematocrit); the 50-g blood glucose test; determination of the rubella titer; serologic tests (Venereal Disease Research Laboratories [VDRL] or rapid plasma reagin [RPR] test) for syphilis; hepatitis B surface antigen (HBsAg); culture for group B streptococci; and urinalysis. Additional tests may include a tuberculosis screen with purified protein derivative (PPD); screening for the human immunodeficiency virus (HIV); and a screen for sickle cell trait or other genetic disorders (e.g., maternal serum alpha-fetoprotein). Diagnostic tests include amniocentesis, nonstress test (NST), contraction stress test (CST), biophysical profile (BPP), and ultrasound examination.

Interview. The woman's primary complaint or reason for coming to the hospital is determined in the interview. Her primary complaint may be that her bag of waters (BOW, amniotic membranes) ruptured, with or without contractions. The woman may have come in for an obstetric check, which is a period of observation reserved for women who are unsure about the onset of their labor. This allows time on the unit for the diagnosis of labor without official admission and minimizes or avoids cost to the patient when used by the hospital and approved by the woman's health insurance plan.

Even the experienced mother may have difficulty determining the onset of labor. The woman is asked to recall the events of the previous days and to describe the following:

- Time and onset of contractions and progress in terms of frequency and duration
- Location and character of discomfort from contractions (e.g., back pain, suprapubic discomfort)
- Persistence of contractions despite changes in maternal position and activity (e.g., walking or lying down)

- Presence and character of vaginal discharge or show
- The status of amniotic membranes, such as a gush or seepage of fluid (rupture of membranes [ROM])

If there has been a discharge that may be amniotic fluid, she is asked the date and time the fluid was first noted and the fluid's characteristics (e.g., amount, color, unusual odor). In many instances, a sterile speculum examination and a nitrazine (pH) or fern test can confirm that the membranes are ruptured (see Procedure box).

These descriptions help the nurse assess the degree of progress in the process of labor. Bloody or pink show is distinguished from bleeding by the fact that it is pink and feels sticky because of its mucoid nature. It is scant to begin with and increases with effacement and dilation of the cervix. A woman may report a scant brownish to bloody discharge that may be attributed to cervical trauma resulting from vaginal examination or coitus within the last 48 hours.

In case general anesthesia may be required in an emergency, it is important to assess the woman's respiratory status. The nurse determines this by asking the woman if she has a "cold" or related symptoms (e.g., "stuffy nose," sore throat, or cough). The status of allergies is rechecked, including allergies to medications used in obstetrics, such as lidocaine (Xylocaine). Some allergic responses cause swelling of the mucous membranes of the respiratory tract, which could interfere with breathing and the administration of inhalation anesthesia.

Because vomiting and subsequent aspiration into the respiratory tract can complicate an otherwise normal labor, the nurse records the time and type of the woman's last solid and liquid intake.

Any information not found in the prenatal record is obtained during the admission assessment. Pertinent data include the birth plan (Box 14-2), the choice of infant feeding method, the type of pain management, and the name of the pediatric health care provider. A patient profile is obtained that identifies the woman's preparation for childbirth, the support person or family members desired during childbirth and their availability, and ethnic or cultural expectations and needs. The woman's use of alcohol, drugs, and tobacco before or during pregnancy should be determined. Screening of the neonate for substances abused by the mother may be required. After birth the nurse would assess the neonate for signs indicating maternal substance use during pregnancy (e.g., abstinence syndrome, characteristic size and appearance).

The nurse reviews the birth plan; if no written plan has been prepared, the nurse helps the woman formulate a birth plan by describing options available and finds out the woman's wishes and preferences. The nurse prepares the woman for the possibility that changes may be needed in her plan as labor progresses and assures her that information will be provided so that she can make informed decisions. The nurse uses the information in the birth plan to individualize the care given the woman during labor.

Procedure

Tests for Rupture of Membranes

NITRAZINE TEST FOR pH

- Explain procedure to woman or couple.

Procedure

- Wash hands.
- Use nitrazine test paper, a dye-impregnated test paper for determining pH (differentiates amniotic fluid, which is slightly alkaline, from urine and purulent material [pus], which are acidic).
- Wearing a sterile glove lubricated with water, place a piece of test paper at the cervical os.

OR

- Use a sterile, cotton-tipped applicator to dip deep into vagina to pick up fluid; touch applicator to test paper. (Procedure may be done during speculum examination.)

Read Results

- Membranes probably intact: identifies vaginal and most body fluids that are acidic:

Yellow	pH 5.0
Olive-yellow	pH 5.5
Olive-green	pH 6.0

- Membranes probably ruptured: identifies amniotic fluid that is alkaline:

Blue-green	pH 6.5
Blue-gray	pH 7.0
Deep blue	pH 7.5

- Realize that false test results are possible because of presence of bloody show, insufficient amniotic fluid, or semen.
- Provide pericare as needed.
- Remove gloves and wash hands.

Document Results

- Results are positive or negative.

TEST FOR FERNING OR FERN PATTERN

- Explain procedure to woman or couple.
- Wash hands, apply sterile gloves, obtain specimen of fluid (usually during sterile speculum examination).
- Spread a drop of fluid from vagina on a clean glass slide with a sterile, cotton-tipped applicator.
- Allow fluid to dry.
- Examine slide under microscope: observe for appearance of ferning (a frondlike crystalline pattern) (do not confuse with cervical mucus test, when high levels of estrogen cause the ferning).
- Observe for absence of ferning (alerts staff to possibility that amount of specimen was inadequate or that specimen was urine, vaginal discharge, or blood).
- Provide pericare as needed.
- Remove gloves and wash hands.

Document Results

- Results are positive or negative.

BOX 14-2

The Birth Plan

The birth plan should include the woman's or couple's preferences related to the following:

- Presence of birth companions such as the partner, older children, parents, friends, and doula, and the role each will play
- Presence of other persons such as students, male attendants, interpreters
- Clothing to be worn
- Environmental modifications such as lighting, music, privacy, focal point, items from home such as pillows
- Labor activities such as preferred positions for labor and for birth, ambulation, birth balls, showers and whirlpool baths, oral food and fluid intake
- List of comfort and relaxation measures
- Labor and birth medical interventions such as pharmacologic pain relief measures, intravenous therapy, electronic monitoring, induction or augmentation measures, episiotomy
- Care and handling of the newborn immediately after birth such as cutting of the cord, eye care, breastfeeding
- Cultural and religious requirements related to the care of the mother, newborn, and placenta

The childbirth.org website (http://www.childbirth.org) provides couples with an interactive birth plan along with examples of birth plans.

The nurse should discuss with the woman and her partner their plans for preserving childbirth memories by using photography and videotaping and provide information about the agency's policies regarding these practices and under what circumstances they are allowed. Protection of privacy and safety and infection control are major concerns for the parents-to-be and the agency. If a birth video is made, consideration should be given to the woman's reaction to viewing the video after birth. She may need help in interpreting the events, behaviors, and reactions she sees depicted in the video, because her impression of her childbirth experience, including her behavior, can have a profound effect on her future labor and birth experiences. Women may have an idealized view of what their birth video will depict, based on childbirth videos viewed during an expectant childbirth class (Hanson, VandeVusse, & Harrod, 2001).

Psychosocial factors. The woman's general appearance and behavior (and those of her partner) provide valuable clues to the type of supportive care she will need. However, the nurse should keep in mind that general appearance and behavior may vary, depending on the stage and phase of labor (Table 14-1).

Women with a history of sexual abuse. Memories of sexual abuse can be triggered during labor by intrusive procedures such as vaginal examinations; loss of control; being confined to bed and "restrained" by monitors, intravenous (IV) lines, and epidurals; being watched by students;

TABLE 14-1

Woman's Responses and Support Person's Actions during First Stage of Labor

WOMAN'S RESPONSES	NURSE OR SUPPORT PERSON'S ACTIONS*
DILATION OF CERVIX 0-3 CM (LATENT) (contractions 30-45 sec long, 5-30 min apart, mild to moderate)	
Mood: alert, happy, excited, mild anxiety	Provides encouragement, feedback for relaxation, companionship
Settles into labor room; selects focal point	Assists woman to cope with contractions
Rests or sleeps, if possible	Encourages use of focusing techniques
Uses breathing techniques	Helps to concentrate on breathing techniques
Uses effleurage, focusing, and relaxation techniques	Uses comfort measures
	Assists woman into comfortable position
	Informs woman of progress; explains procedures and routines
	Gives praise
	Offer fluids, food, ice chips as ordered
DILATION OF CERVIX 4-7 CM (ACTIVE) (contractions 40-70 sec long, 3-5 min apart, moderate to strong)	
Mood: seriously labor oriented, concentration and energy needed for contractions, alert, more demanding	Acts as buffer; limits assessment techniques to between contractions
	Assists woman to cope with contractions
Continues relaxation, focusing techniques	Encourages woman as needed to help her maintain breathing techniques
Uses breathing techniques	Uses comfort measures
	Assists with frequent position changes, emphasizing side-lying and upright positions
	Encourages voluntary relaxation of muscles of back, buttocks, thighs, and perineum; performs effleurage
	Applies counterpressure to sacrococcygeal area
	Encourages and praises
	Keeps woman aware of progress
	Offers analgesics as ordered
	Checks bladder; encourages her to void
	Gives oral care; offers fluids, food, ice chips as ordered
DILATION OF CERVIX 8-10 CM (TRANSITION) (contractions 45-90 sec long, 2-3 min apart, strong)	
Mood: irritable, intense concentration, symptoms of transition (e.g., nausea, vomiting)	Stays with woman; provides constant support
	Assists woman to cope with contractions
Continues relaxation, needs greater concentration to do this	Reminds, reassures, and encourages woman to reestablish breathing pattern and concentration as needed
Uses breathing techniques	Alerts woman to begin breathing pattern before contraction becomes too intense
Uses pattern-paced breathing (i.e., 4:1 breathing pattern) if using psychoprophylactic techniques	Prompts panting respirations if woman begins to push prematurely
	Uses comfort measures
Uses panting to overcome urge to push if appropriate	Accepts woman's inability to comply with instructions
	Accepts irritable response to helping, such as counterpressure
	Supports woman who has nausea and vomiting; gives oral care as needed; gives reassurance regarding signs of end of first stage
	Uses relaxation techniques (effleurage and voluntary relaxation)
	Keeps woman aware of progress

*Provided by nurses and support persons in collaboration with the nurse.

and having intense sensations in the uterus and genital area, especially at the time when she must push the baby out. Women who are abuse survivors may fight the labor process by reacting in panic or anger toward care providers, may take control of everyone and everything related to their childbirth, may surrender by being submissive and dependent, or may retreat by mentally dissociating themselves from the sensations of labor and birth (Hobbins, 2004).

The nurse can help these women to associate the sensations they are experiencing with the process of childbirth and not with their past abuse. The woman's sense of control should be maintained by explaining all procedures and why they are needed, validating her needs and paying close attention to her requests, proceeding at the woman's pace by waiting for her to give permission to touch her, accepting her often extreme reactions to labor, and protecting her privacy by limiting the amount of exposure of her body and the number of persons involved in her care. It is recommended that all laboring women be cared for in this manner, because it is not unusual for a woman to choose not to reveal a history of sexual abuse. These care measures can help a woman to perceive her childbirth experience in positive terms and to parent her new baby effectively (Hobbins, 2004).

Stress in labor.   The way in which women and their support person or family members approach labor is related to the manner in which they have been socialized to the childbearing process. Their reactions reflect their life experiences regarding childbirth—physical, social, cultural, and religious. Feelings a woman has about her pregnancy and fears regarding childbirth should be discussed. This is especially important if the woman is a primigravida who has not attended childbirth classes or is a multiparous woman who has had a previous negative childbirth experience. Major fears and concerns relate to the process and effects of childbirth, maternal and fetal well-being, and the attitude and actions of the health care staff. Unresolved fears increase a woman's stress and can inhibit the process of labor as a result of the inhibiting effects of catecholamines associated with the stress response on uterine contractions (Melender, 2002).

Women in labor usually have a variety of concerns that they will voice if asked but rarely volunteer. It is important to ask the woman what she expects or to suggest that the woman ask her primary health care provider about an issue. The following are common concerns of women in labor: Will my baby be all right? Will I be able to stand labor? Will my labor be long? How will I act? Will I need medication? Will it work for me? Will my partner or someone be there to support me? Do I have to have an IV?

The nurse's responsibility to the woman in labor with regard to these concerns is to answer her questions or find the answers, to provide support for her and her support person or family, to take care of her in partnership with those persons the woman wants as her support team, and to serve as their advocate. Women feel empowered when they are given information they can understand and that shows support for their efforts. This feeling of empowerment gives women the sense that they have the freedom to participate fully in their labor and birth and fosters a positive perception of the experience. In contrast, a woman's level of anxiety and fear may increase when she does not understand what is being said. The woman who is unfamiliar with expressions such as "bloody show," "the membranes ruptured," "scalp electrode," and "baby's lying on the cord" could panic. Many such expressions sound violent and could conjure up thoughts of injury or pain.

The nurse communicates to the woman that she is not expected to act in any particular way and that the process will end in the birth of her baby, which is the only expectation she should have. Women need to trust in their own innate ability to give birth, and nurses need to support and protect the woman's efforts to achieve this outcome (Lothian, 2001).

The father, coach, or significant other(s) also experiences stress during labor. The nurse can assist and support these individuals by identifying their needs and expectations and by helping make sure these are met. The nurse can ascertain what role the support person intends to fulfill and whether he or she is prepared for that role by making observations and asking her/himself such questions as, "Has the couple attended childbirth classes?" "What role does this person expect to play?" "Does he or she do all the talking?" "Is he or she nervous, anxious, aggressive, or hostile?" "Does he or she look hungry, tired, worried, or confused?" "Does he or she watch television, sleep, or stay out of the room instead of paying attention to the woman?" "Where does he or she sit?" "Does he or she touch the woman; what is the character of the touch?" The nurse should be sensitive to the needs of support persons and provide teaching and support as appropriate.

Cultural factors.   It is important to note the woman's ethnic or cultural and religious background to anticipate nursing interventions that should be added to or eliminated from the individualized plan of care (Fig. 14-3). The woman should be encouraged to request specific caregiving behaviors and practices that are important to her. If a special request contradicts usual practices in that setting, the woman or the nurse can ask the woman's primary health care provider to write an order to accommodate the special request. For example, in many cultures, it is unacceptable to have a male caregiver examine a pregnant woman. In

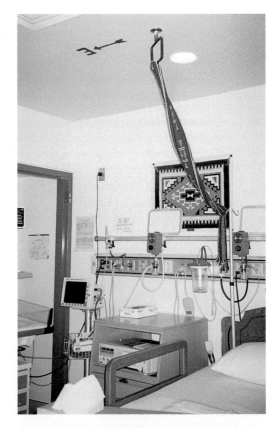

Fig. 14-3   Birthing room specific to a Native American population. Note the arrow pointing east, the rug on the wall, and the cord hanging from the ceiling. (Courtesy Patricia Hess, San Francisco, CA; Chinle Comprehensive Health Care Center, Chinle, AZ.)

Cultural Considerations

Birth Practices in Different Cultures

SOUTH KOREA
Stoic response to labor pain; fathers usually not present.

JAPAN
Natural childbirth methods practiced; may labor silently; may eat during labor; father may be present.

CHINA
Stoic response to pain; fathers usually not present; side-lying position preferred for labor and birth, because this position is thought to reduce infant trauma.

INDIA
Natural childbirth methods preferred; father is usually not present; female relatives usually present.

IRAN
Fathers not present; female support and female care-givers preferred.

MEXICO
May be stoic about discomfort until second stage, then may request pain relief; fathers and female relatives may be present.

LAOS
May use squatting position for birth; fathers may or may not be present; female attendants preferred.

From D'Avanzo, C., & Geissler, E. (2003). *Pocket guide to cultural assessment.* (3rd ed.). St. Louis: Mosby.

some cultures it is traditional to take the placenta home; in others the woman is given only certain nourishments during labor. Some women believe that cutting the body, as with an episiotomy, allows the spirit to leave the body and that rupturing the membranes prolongs, not shortens, labor. It is important that the rationale for required care measures be carefully explained (Mattson, 2000) (see Cultural Considerations box).

Within cultures, women may have the "right" way to behave in labor instilled in them and may react to the pain experienced in that way. These behaviors can range from total silence to moaning or screaming, but they are not in and of themselves a gauge of the degree of pain. A woman who moans with contractions may not be in as much physical pain as a woman who is silent but winces during contractions (Table 14-2). Some women feel it is shameful to scream or cry out in pain if a man is present. If the woman's support person is her mother, she may perceive the need to "behave" more strongly than if her support person is the father of the baby. She will perceive herself as failing or succeeding on the basis of her ability to adhere to these "standards" of behavior. Conversely, a woman's behavior in response to pain may influence the support received from significant others. In some cultures, women who lose control and cry out in pain may be scolded, whereas in other cultures, support persons will become more helpful (D'Avanzo & Geissler, 2003).

The choice of birth companion is influenced by the woman's cultural and religious background and by trends in the society in which she lives. For example, in Western societies, the father is viewed as the ideal birth companion. For European-American couples, attending childbirth classes together has become a traditional, expected activity. In some other cultures the father's presence during labor and birth is inappropriate—for example Mexican, Filipino, Chinese, Islamic, and Ethiopian (D'Avanzo & Geissler, 2003). However, among the Laotian (Hmong), the father plays an important role in the birth. If couples from these cultures immigrate to the United States or Canada, their roles may change. The nurse will need to talk to the woman and her support persons to determine the roles they wish to assume.

The non–English-speaking woman in labor. A woman's level of anxiety in labor increases when she does not understand what is happening to her or what is being said. Some misunderstanding may occur with English-speaking women and cause some stress, but the effect of misunderstanding on non–English-speaking women is much more dramatic. These women often feel a complete loss of control over their situation if no health care provider is present who speaks their language. They can panic and withdraw or become physically abusive when someone tries to do something they perceive might harm them or their babies. Sometimes a support person is able to serve as an interpreter. However, this must be done with caution because the interpreter may not be able to convey exactly what the nurse or others are saying or what the woman is saying, which can increase the woman's stress level even more.

Ideally, a bilingual nurse will care for the woman. Alternatively, an employee or volunteer interpreter may be contacted for assistance (see Box 2-1). Ideally, the interpreter is from the woman's culture. For some women a female interpreter may be more acceptable. If no one in the hospital is able to interpret, a service can be called so that interpretation can take place over the telephone. Another alternative is for the labor and birth unit staff to prepare a set of cards with graphic illustrations that depict common situations. These cards can be used to communicate with non–English-speaking women. Even when the nurse has limited ability to communicate verbally with the woman, in most instances the nurse's efforts to communicate are meaningful and appreciated by the woman. Speaking slowly and avoiding complex words and medical terms can help a woman and her partner to understand (Mattson, 2000) (see Guidelines/Guías box).

Physical examination

The initial physical examination includes a general systems assessment; performance of Leopold maneuvers to determine fetal presentation and position and the point of maximal intensity (PMI) for auscultating the FHR; assessment of fetal status; assessment of uterine contractions; and vaginal examination to assess the status of cervical effacement and dilation, fetal descent, and amniotic membranes

TABLE 14-2

Sociocultural Basis of Pain Experience

WOMAN IN LABOR	NURSE
PERCEPTION OF MEANING	
Origin: Cultural concept of and personal experience with pain; for example:	Origin: Cultural concept of and personal experience with pain; in addition, nurse becomes accustomed to working with certain "expected" pain trajectories. For example, in obstetrics, pain is expected to increase as labor progresses, be intermittent, and have an end point; relief can be derived from medications once labor is well established and fetus or newborn can cope with amount and elimination of medications; relief can also come from woman's knowledge, attitude, and support from family or friends.
Pain in childbirth is inevitable, something to be endured.	
Pain in childbirth can be avoided completely.	
Pain in childbirth is punishment for sin.	
Pain in childbirth can be controlled.	
COPING MECHANISMS	
Woman may exhibit the following behaviors:	Nurse may respond by:
Be traditionally vocal or nonvocal; crying out or groaning, or both, may be part of her ritual response to pain	Using physical factors effectively (e.g., using tone of voice, closeness in space, and touch as media for conveying message of interest and caring)
Use counterstimulation to minimize pain (e.g., rubbing, applying heat, or applying counterpressure)	Using avoidance, belittling, or other distracting actions as protective device for self
Use relaxation, distraction, or autosuggestion as pain-countering techniques	Offering comfort measures and other nonpharmacologic methods of pain relief
Resist any use of "needles" as modes of administering pain relief agents	Using pharmacologic resources at hand judiciously
	Assuming accountability for control and management of pain
EXPECTATIONS OF OTHERS	
Nurse may be seen as someone who will accept woman's statement of pain and act as her advocate.	Only certain verbal or nonverbal responses to pain may be accepted as appropriate responses.
Medical personnel may be expected to relieve woman of all pain sensations.	Couple that is prepared for childbirth may be expected to refuse medication and to wish to "do everything on their own."
Nurse may be expected to be interested, gentle, kind, and accepting of behavior exhibited.	Woman's definition of pain may not be accepted; that is, woman may wish to experience and participate in controlling pain or may not be able to accept any pain as reasonable.

GUIDELINES/GUÍAS

Labor Assessment

- What time did the contractions begin?
- *¿A qué hora le empezaron las contracciones?*

- How far apart are the contractions?
- *¿Con qué frecuencia tiene las contracciones?*

- Have the membranes ruptured? When?
- *¿Se le rompió la fuente? ¿Cuándo?*

- Have you had bleeding?
- *¿Ha tenido hemorragia?*

- What color was the fluid? Red? Pink?
- *¿Qué color tenía el líquido? ¿Rojo? ¿Rosado?*

- How much? A cupful? A tablespoon? A teaspoon?
- *¿Cuánto? ¿Una taza? ¿Una cucharada? ¿Una cucharadita?*

- When was the last time you ate or drank anything?
- *¿Cuándo fue la última vez que comió o tomó algo?*

- Have you had any problems with this pregnancy?
- *¿Ha tenido algún problema con este embarazo?*

- Are you taking any medications?
- *¿Toma algún medicamento?*

- Are you allergic to penicillin or other medicines?
- *¿Es alérgica a la penicilina u otras medicinas?*

- Please sign this consent form.
- *Por favor, firme este formulario de autorización.*

and fluid. The findings of the admission physical examination serve as a baseline for assessing the woman's progress from that point.

It is important to obtain as many related pieces of information as possible before planning and implementing care. Women often focus on the nature of their contractions as the clearest indicator of how far advanced their labor is. However, the findings from the vaginal examination are more valid indicators of the phase of labor, especially for nulliparous women.

The information yielded by a complete and accurate assessment during the initial examination serves as the basis for determining whether the woman should be admitted and what her ongoing care should be. Expected maternal progress and minimal assessment guidelines during the first stage of labor are presented in Table 14-3 and the Care Path for the low risk woman in the first stage of labor.

Standard Precautions should guide all assessment and care measures (Box 14-3). The assessment findings are explained to the woman whenever possible. Throughout labor, accurate documentation, following agency policy, is done as soon as possible after a procedure has been performed (Fig. 14-4).

General systems assessment. A brief systems assessment is performed. This includes an assessment of the heart, lungs, and skin; an examination to determine the presence and extent of edema of the legs, face, hands, and sacrum; and testing of deep tendon reflexes and for clonus.

Vital signs. Vital signs (temperature, pulse, respirations, and blood pressure) are assessed on admission, and the initial values are used as the baseline for comparison with subsequent values. If the blood pressure is elevated, it should be reassessed 30 minutes later, between contractions, using a correct-size blood pressure cuff to obtain a reading after the woman has relaxed. To prevent supine hypotension and fetal distress, the woman should be encouraged to lie on her side and not supine (Fig. 14-5). Her temperature is monitored so that signs of infection or a fluid deficit (e.g., dehydration associated with inadequate intake of fluids) can be identified.

Text continued on p. 412.

TABLE 14-3

Expected Maternal Progress in First Stage of Labor

CRITERION	LATENT (0-3 cm)	ACTIVE (4-7 cm)	TRANSITION (8-10 cm)
	PHASES MARKED BY CERVICAL DILATION*		
Duration†	About 6-8 hr	About 3-6 hr	About 20-40 min
Contractions			
Strength	Mild to moderate	Moderate to strong	Strong to very strong
Rhythm	Irregular	More regular	Regular
Frequency	5-30 min apart	3-5 min apart	2-3 min apart
Duration	30-45 sec	40-70 sec	45-90 sec
Descent			
Station of	Nulliparous: 0	Varies: +1 to +2 cm	Varies: +2 to +3 cm
presenting part	Multiparous: −2 cm to 0	Varies: +1 to +2 cm	Varies: +2 to +3 cm
Show			
Color	Brownish discharge, mucous plug, or pale pink mucus	Pink to bloody mucus	Bloody mucus
Amount	Scant	Scant to moderate	Copious
Behavior and appearance‡	Excited; thoughts center on self, labor, and baby; may be talkative or silent, calm or tense; some apprehension; pain controlled fairly well; alert, follows directions readily; open to instructions	Becomes more serious, doubtful of control of pain, more apprehensive; desires companionship and encouragement; attention more inwardly directed; fatigue evidenced; malar (cheeks) flush; has some difficulty following directions	Pain described as severe; backache common; frustration, fear of loss of control, and irritability may be voiced; vague in communications; amnesia between contractions; writhing with contractions; nausea and vomiting, especially if hyperventilating; hyperesthesia; circumoral pallor, perspiration of forehead and upper lips; shaking tremor of thighs; feeling of need to defecate, pressure on anus

*In the nullipara, effacement is often complete before dilation begins; in the multipara, it occurs simultaneously with dilation.
†Duration of each phase is influenced by such factors as parity, maternal emotions, position, level of activity, and fetal size, presentation and position. For example, the labor of a nullipara tends to last longer, on average, than the labor of a multipara. Women who ambulate and assume upright positions or change positions frequently during labor tend to experience a shorter first stage. Descent is often prolonged in breech presentations and occiput posterior positions.
‡Women who have epidural analgesia for pain relief may not demonstrate some of these behaviors.

CARE PATH · *Low Risk Woman in First Stage of Labor*

CARE MANAGEMENT	CERVICAL DILATION		
	0-3 cm (LATENT)	4-7 cm (ACTIVE)	8-10 cm (TRANSITION)
I. ASSESSMENT MEASURES*	**Frequency**	**Frequency**	**Frequency**
Blood pressure, pulse, respirations	Every 30-60 min	Every 30 min	Every 15-30 min
Temperature†	Every 4 hr	Every 4 hr	Every 4 hr
Uterine activity	Every 30-60 min	Every 15-30 min	Every 10-15 min
Fetal heart rate (FHR)	Every 30-60 min	Every 15-30 min	Every 15-30 min
Vaginal show	Every 30-60 min	Every 30 min	Every 15 min
Behavior, appearance, mood, energy level of woman; condition of partner	Every 30 min	Every 15 min	Every 5 min
Vaginal examination‡	As needed to identify progress	As needed to identify progress	As needed to identify progress
II. PHYSICAL CARE MEASURES§	Stay at home for as long as possible Relaxation measures; rest and sleep if at night Activity—ambulation; emphasize upright positions Diversional activities Nourishment—light foods and full liquids Encourage to void every 2 hr Perform basic hygiene measures	Coach breathing techniques Encourage effleurage Assist in using relaxation techniques between contractions Encourage ambulation, upright positions Assist with position changes Use comfort measures desired by woman: massage, hot or cold packs, touch, etc. Initiate hydrotherapy (shower, bath, Jacuzzi) Provide nourishment as desired Encourage voiding every 2 hr Assist with hygiene, perineal care Provide pharmacologic pain relief as requested by the woman and ordered by the primary health care provider indicated Provide relief for partner	Coach breathing techniques Reduce touch if increased sensitivity is noted Help to relax between contractions Assist with position changes Use comfort measures according to acceptance level Continue hydrotherapy if effective Provide clear liquids: sips, ice chips Encourage voiding every 2 hr Provide hygiene measures, emphasizing mouth and perineal care Provide pharmacologic pain relief as requested by the woman and ordered by the primary health care provider Prepare for birth
III. EMOTIONAL SUPPORT	Review birth plan Review process of labor—what to expect, pain management techniques available Redemonstrate breathing techniques Keep informed: progress, procedures	Provide feedback about performance Reduce distractions during contractions Role model comfort measures Reassure, encourage, praise Take charge, talk through contraction until control regained Continue to keep informed	Provide continuous support Reduce distractions Role model care measures to assist partner Continue reassurance, praise, and encouragement Keep informed Take charge as needed

*Full assessment using interview, physical examination, and laboratory testing is performed on admission. Subsequently, frequency of assessment is determined by the risk status of the maternal-fetal unit. More frequent assessment is required in high risk situations. Frequency of assessment and method of documentation are also determined by agency policy, which is usually based on the recommended care standards of medical and nursing organizations.

†If membranes have ruptured, the temperature should be assessed every 1 to 2 hr; assess orally or tympanically between contractions.

‡Perform vaginal examination at admission and thereafter only when signs indicate that progress has occurred (e.g., significant increase in frequency, duration, and intensity of contractions; rupture of membranes; perineal pressure); strict aseptic technique should be used. In the presence of vaginal bleeding, the primary health care provider performs the examination under a double setup in a delivery room, or an ultrasonography is performed to determine placental location.

§Physical care measures are performed by the nurse working together with the woman's partner and significant others. The woman is capable of greater independence in the latent phase but needs more assistance during the active and transition phases.

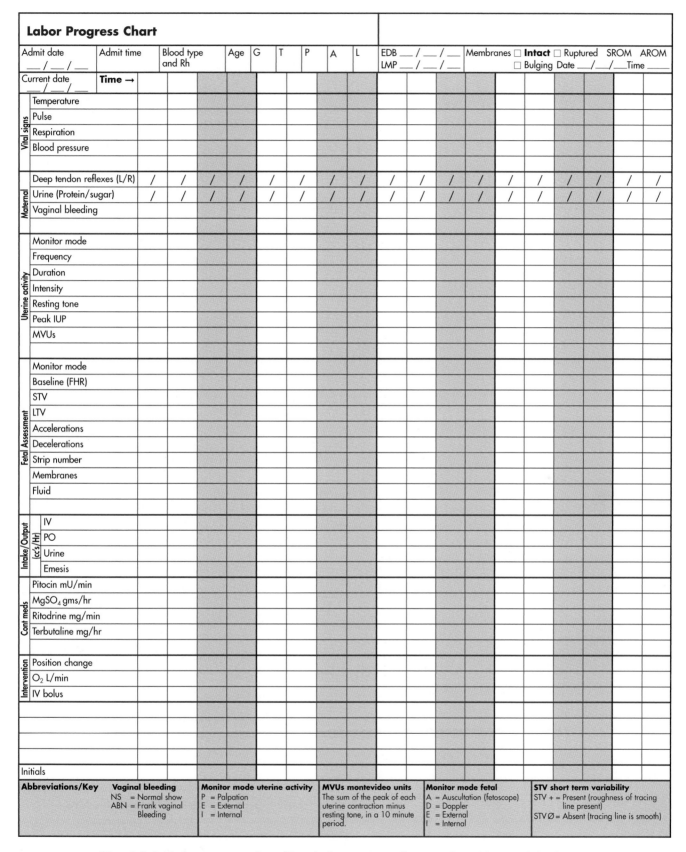

Fig. 14-4 Labor progress chart. (Permission to use and/or reproduce this copyrighted material has been granted by the owner, MNRS-Briggs Corporation, Des Moines, IA.)

Continued

Labor Progress Chart

Medication Allergy/Sensitivity ☐ None

(Identify)_____

Chart_____ of_____

/	/	/	/	/	/	/	/	/	/	/	/	/	/	/	/	/	/	/	/
/	/	/	/	/	/	/	/	/	/	/	/	/	/	/	/	/	/	/	/

LVT (long term variability)
0-2   BPM = Absent
3-5   BPM = Minimal
6-25 BPM = Average
>25 BPM = Marked

Accelerations
+ = 15 BPM ↑ × 15 sec
0 = Absent

Decelerations
N = None
E = Early
V = Variable
L = Late
P = Prolonged

Membranes
I = Intact
B = Bulging
R = Ruptured

Fluid
C = Clear
M = Meconium stained
B = Bloody
F = Foul smelling
NF = Not foul smelling

Fig. 14-4, cont'd

Labor Progress Chart

Time →			
Mark X • 10			
-4 9			
-3 **D** 8			
-2 **i** 7			
S -1 **l** 6			
t 0 **a** 5			
a +1 **t** 4			
i +2 **i** 3			
o +3 **o** 2			
n **n**			
Effacement % and/or position			
Examined by:			

IV Record

Start date	Time	Solution	Amount (cc's)	Medication/Dose added	Initials	Infused date	Time	Amount infused

Teaching

Topic	Date time	Comments
Oriented		
Labor review		
Support person		
Pre-Op		
Safety		

Interval Medications

Date time	Medication/Dose	Route	Site	Initials		Initials	Signature

Progress Notes

Date	Time	

Fig. 14-4, cont'd

Continued

Labor Progress Chart

Progress Notes (Cont'd.)

Date	Time	

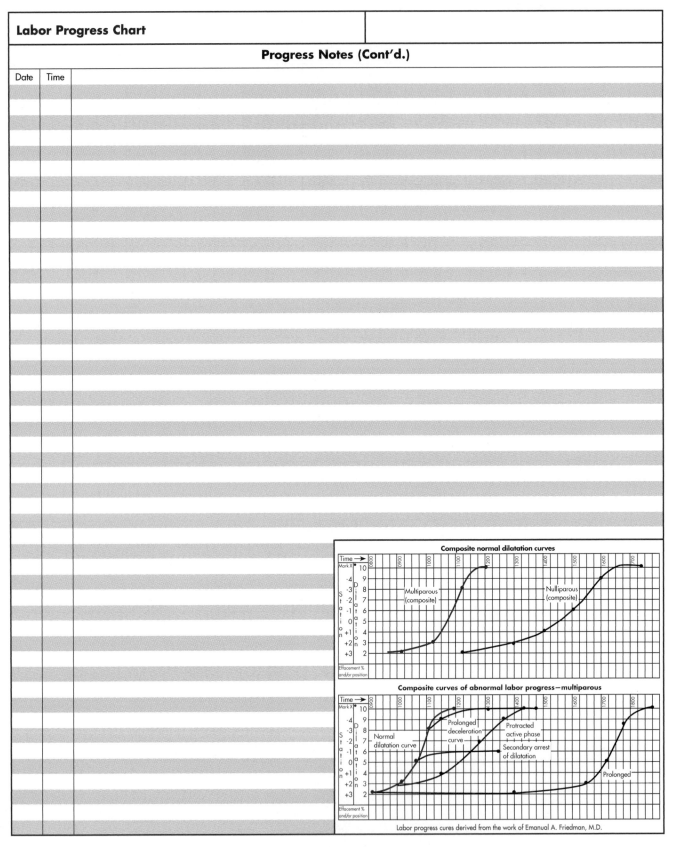

Fig. 14-4, cont'd

BOX 14-3

Standard Precautions during Childbirth

Birth is a time when nurses and other health care providers are exposed to a great deal of maternal and newborn blood and body fluids. Observation of Standard Precautions is necessary to prevent the transmission of infection. Perinatal infections most often are transmitted through contact with body fluids. The Standard Precautions applicable to childbirth include the following:

- Wash hands before and after putting on gloves and performing procedures.
- Wear gloves (clean or sterile, as appropriate) when performing procedures that require contact with the woman's genitalia and body fluids, including bloody show (e.g., during vaginal examination, amniotomy, hygienic care of the perineum, insertion of an internal scalp electrode and intrauterine pressure monitor, and catheterization).
- Wear a mask that has a shield or protective eyewear, and a cover gown when assisting with the birth. Cap and shoe covers are worn for cesarean birth but are optional for vaginal birth in a birthing room. Gowns worn by the primary health care provider who is attending the birth should have a waterproof front and sleeves and should be sterile.
- Drape the woman with sterile towels and sheets as appropriate. Explain to the woman what can and cannot be touched.
- Help the woman's partner put on appropriate coverings for the type of birth, such as cap, mask, gown, and shoe covers. Show the partner where to stand and what can and cannot be touched.
- Wear gloves and gown when handling the newborn immediately after birth.
- Use an appropriate method to suction the newborn's airway, such as a bulb syringe, mechanical wall suction, or De Lee oral suction device, that prevents the newborn's mucus from getting into the user's mouth or airway.

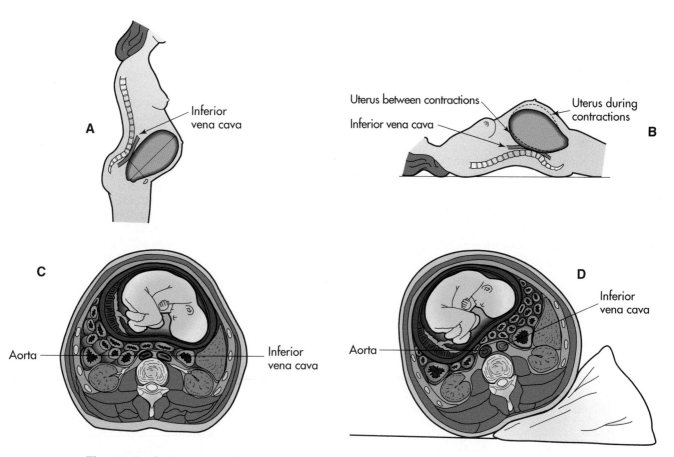

Fig. 14-5 Supine hypotension. Note relation of pregnant uterus to ascending vena cava in standing position (**A**), and in the supine position (**B**). **C,** Compression of aorta and inferior vena cava with woman in supine position. **D,** Compression of these vessels is relieved by placement of a wedge pillow under the woman's right side.

Leopold maneuvers (abdominal palpation).

Leopold maneuvers are performed with the woman briefly lying on her back (see Procedure box). These maneuvers help identify the (1) number of fetuses; (2) presenting part, fetal lie, and fetal attitude; (3) degree of the presenting part's descent into the pelvis; and (4) expected location of the point of maximal intensity (PMI) of the fetal heart tones (FHTs) on the woman's abdomen.

Assessment of FHTs and fetal heart rate pattern.

It is important for the nurse to understand the relation between the location of the PMI of the FHTs and fetal presentation, lie, and position. A high risk for childbirth complications may be revealed by variations in these findings. The PMI of the FHTs is the location on the maternal abdomen at which FHTs are the loudest (see Procedure Box). It is usually directly over the fetal back. The PMI also is an aid in determining the fetal presentation and position (Fig. 14-6). In a vertex presentation, FHTs are usually heard below the mother's umbilicus in either the right or left lower quadrant of the abdomen; in a breech presentation, FHTs are usually heard above the mother's umbilicus (Fig. 14-6, *A*). As the fetus descends and rotates internally, the FHTs are heard lower and closer to the midline of the maternal abdomen. The PMI of the fetus in the right occipitoanterior (ROA) position moves to the midline just over the symphysis pubis). Just before birth, the fetal position is occipitoanterior (OA), and the fetal back is directly above the symphysis pubis. Assessments recommended for determining fetal status in the low risk woman during each stage of labor are summarized in the Care Paths on p. 406 and p. 433. The FHR and pattern must be assessed (1) immediately after ROM, because this is the most common time for the umbilical cord to prolapse; (2) after any change in the contraction pattern or maternal status; and (3) before and after the woman receives medication or a procedure is performed (Tucker, 2004).

Assessment of uterine contractions.

A general characteristic of effective labor is regular uterine activity

---

Procedure

Leopold Maneuvers

LEOPOLD MANEUVERS

- Wash hands.
- Ask woman to empty bladder.
- Position woman supine with one pillow under her head and with her knees slightly flexed.
- Place small rolled towel under woman's right or left hip to displace uterus off major blood vessels (prevents supine hypotensive syndrome; see Fig. 14-5, *D*).
- *If right-handed, stand on woman's right, facing her:*
  1. Identify fetal part that occupies the fundus. The head feels round, firm, freely movable, and palpable by ballottement; the breech feels less regular and softer. This maneuver identifies fetal lie (longitudinal or transverse) and presentation (cephalic or breech) (Fig. A).
  2. Using palmar surface of one hand, locate and palpate the smooth convex contour of the fetal back and the irregularities that identify the small parts (feet, hands, elbows). This maneuver helps identify fetal presentation (Fig. B).
  3. With right hand, determine which fetal part is presenting over the inlet to the true pelvis. Gently grasp the lower pole of the uterus between the thumb and fingers, pressing in slightly (Fig. C). If the head is presenting and not engaged, determine the attitude of the head (flexed or extended).
  4. Turn to face the woman's feet. Using both hands, outline the fetal head (Fig. D) with the palmar surface of the fingertips. When the presenting part has descended deeply, only a small portion of it may be outlined. Palpation of the cephalic prominence helps identify the attitude of the head. If the cephalic prominence is found on the same side as the small parts, this means that the head must be flexed and the vertex is presenting (see Fig. D). If the cephalic prominence is on the same side as the back, this indicates that the presenting head is extended and the face is presenting.

- Document fetal presentation, position, and lie and whether presenting part is flexed or extended, engaged, or free floating. Use agency's protocol for documentation (e.g., "Vtx, LOA, floating").

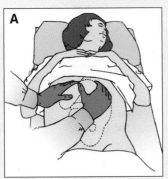
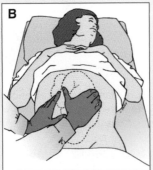
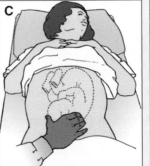
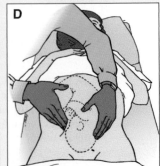

Procedure

Determination of Points of Maximal Intensity of Fetal Heart Tones

Wash hands.

Perform Leopold maneuvers.

Auscultate fetal heart tones (FHTs) based on fetal presentation identified with Leopold maneuvers. The PMI is the location at which the FHTs are the loudest, usually over the fetal back (see Fig. 14-6).

Chart PMI of FHTs using a two-line figure to indicate the four quadrants of the maternal abdomen, as follows: right upper quadrant (RUQ), left upper quadrant (LUQ), left lower quadrant (LLQ), and right lower quadrant (RLQ):

RUQ	LUQ
RLQ	LLQ

The umbilicus is the reference point for the quadrants (point at which the lines cross). The PMI for the fetus in vertex presentation, in general flexion with the back on the mother's right side, commonly is found in the mother's right lower quadrant and is recorded with an "X" or with the FHT, as follows:

X	or 140

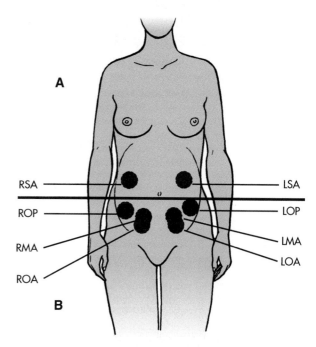

Fig. 14-6 Areas of maximal intensity of fetal heart tones (FHTs) for differing positions: *RSA*, right sacrum anterior; *ROP*, right occipitoposterior; *RMA*, right mentum anterior; *ROA*, right occipitoanterior; *LSA*, left sacrum anterior; *LOP*, left occipitoposterior; *LMA*, left mentum anterior; *LOA*, left occipitoanterior. **A**, Presentation is usually breech if FHTs are heard above umbilicus. **B**, Presentation is usually vertex if FHTs are heard below umbilicus.

(i.e., contractions becoming more frequent and increased duration), but uterine activity is not directly related to labor progress. Uterine contractions are the primary powers that act involuntarily to expel the fetus and the placenta from the uterus. Several methods are used to evaluate uterine contractions, including the woman's subjective description, palpation and timing of contractions by a health care provider, and electronic monitoring.

Each contraction exhibits a wavelike pattern. It begins with a slow increment (the "building up" of a contraction from its onset), gradually reaches an acme (intrauterine pressure less than 80 mm Hg), and then diminishes rapidly (decrement, the "letting down" of the contraction). An interval of rest (intrauterine pressure less than 20 mm Hg with a duration of at least 30 seconds) ends when the next contraction begins (Tucker, 2004). The outward appearance of the woman's abdomen during and between contractions and the pattern of a typical uterine contraction are shown in Fig. 14-7.

A uterine contraction is described in terms of the following characteristics:

- *Frequency*–How often uterine contractions occur; the time that elapses from the beginning of one contraction to the beginning of the next contraction
- *Intensity*–The strength of a contraction at its peak
- *Duration*–The time that elapses between the onset and the end of a contraction

- *Resting tone*–The tension in the uterine muscle between contractions; relaxation of the uterus

Uterine contractions are assessed by palpation or by an external or internal electronic monitor. Frequency and duration can be measured by all three methods of uterine activity monitoring. The accuracy of determining intensity varies by the method used. Palpation is more subjective and is a less precise way of determining the intensity of uterine contractions. The following terms are used to describe what is felt on palpation:

- *Mild*–Slightly tense fundus that is easy to indent with fingertips (feels like touching finger to tip of nose)
- *Moderate*–Firm fundus that is difficult to indent with fingertips (feels like touching finger to chin)
- *Strong*–Rigid, boardlike fundus that is almost impossible to indent with fingertips (feels like touching finger to forehead)

Women in labor tend to describe the pain of contractions in terms of the sensations they are experiencing in the lower abdomen or back, which may be unrelated to the firmness of the uterine fundus. Therefore their assessment of the strength of their contractions can be less valid than that of the health care provider, although the amount of discomfort reported is valid.

External electronic monitoring provides information about the relative strength of the uterine contractions. Internal electronic monitoring with an intrauterine pressure

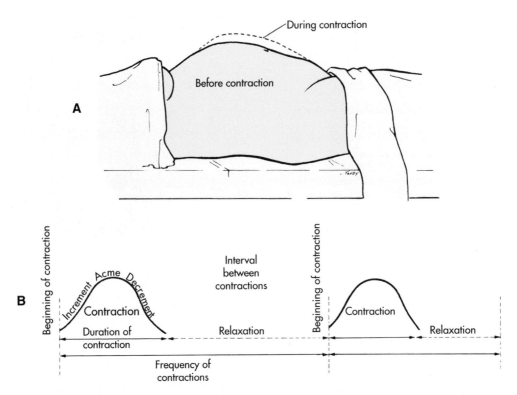

Fig. 14-7 Assessment of uterine contractions. **A,** Abdominal contour before and during uterine contraction. **B,** Wavelike pattern of contractile activity.

catheter is the most accurate way of assessing the intensity of uterine contractions.

On admission, a 20- to 30-minute baseline monitoring of uterine contractions and the FHR and pattern commonly is done. The minimal assessment times during the various phases of labor are given in the Care Paths on pp. 406 and 433, and the findings expected as labor progresses are summarized in Tables 14-3 and 14-7.

The nurse's responsibility in the monitoring of uterine contractions is to ascertain whether they are powerful and frequent enough to accomplish the work of expelling the fetus and the placenta.

NURSE ALERT *If the characteristics of contractions are found to be abnormal, either exceeding or falling below what is considered acceptable in terms of the standard characteristics, the nurse should report this to the primary health care provider.*

Cervical effacement, dilation, fetal descent. Uterine activity must be considered in the context of its effect on cervical effacement and dilation and on the degree of descent of the presenting part (see Chapter 11). The effect on the fetus also must be considered. The progress of labor can be effectively verified through the use of graphic charts (partograms) on which cervical dilation and station (descent) are plotted. This type of graphic charting assists in early identification of deviations from expected labor patterns. Fig. 14-8 provides examples of partograms. Hospitals and birthing centers may develop their own graphs for recording assess-

ments. Such graphs may include not only data on dilation and descent but also data on maternal vital signs, FHR, and uterine activity.

NURSE ALERT *It is important for the nurse to recognize that active labor can actually last longer than the expected labor patterns. This finding should not be a cause for concern unless the maternal-fetal unit exhibits signs of distress (e.g., nonreassuring FHR patterns, maternal fever) (Cesario, 2004).*

Vaginal examination. The vaginal examination reveals whether the woman is in true labor and enables the examiner to determine whether the membranes have ruptured (Fig. 14-9). Because this examination is often stressful and uncomfortable for the woman, it should be performed only when indicated by the status of the woman and her fetus. For example, a vaginal examination should be performed on admission, when significant change has occurred in uterine activity, on maternal perception of perineal pressure or the urge to bear down, when membranes rupture, or when variable decelerations of the FHR are noted. A full explanation of the examination and support of the woman are important factors in reducing the stress and discomfort associated with the examination. Chapter 5 describes a typical vaginal examination.

Laboratory and diagnostic tests

Analysis of urine specimen. A clean-catch urine specimen may be obtained to gather further data about the pregnant woman's health. It is a convenient and

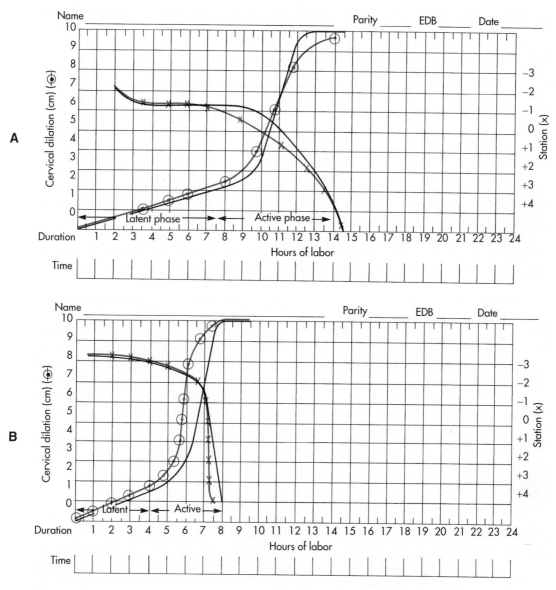

Fig. 14-8   Partograms for assessment of patterns of cervical dilation and descent. Individual woman's labor patterns *(colored)* are superimposed on prepared labor graph *(black)* for comparison. **A,** Labor of a nulliparous woman. **B,** Labor of a multiparous woman. The rate of cervical dilation is plotted with the circled plot points. A line drawn through these symbols depicts the slope of the curve. Station is plotted with Xs. A line drawn through the Xs reveals the pattern of descent.

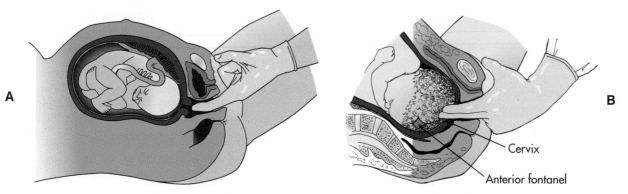

Fig. 14-9   Vaginal examination. **A,** Undilated, uneffaced cervix; membranes intact. **B,** Palpation of sagittal suture line. Cervix effaced and partially dilated.

simple procedure that can provide information about her hydration status (e.g., specific gravity, color, amount), nutritional status (e.g., ketones), infection status (e.g., leukocytes), and the status of possible complications such as preeclampsia, shown by finding protein in the urine. The results can be obtained quickly and help the nurse determine appropriate interventions to implement.

Blood tests. The blood tests performed vary with the hospital protocol and the woman's health status. An example of a minimal assessment is a hematocrit determination, in which the specimen is centrifuged in the perinatal unit. Blood can be obtained by a finger stick or from the hub of a catheter used to start an IV line. More comprehensive blood assessments such as white blood cell count, red blood cell count, the hemoglobin level, hematocrit, and platelet values are included in a CBC. A CBC may be ordered for women with a history of infection, anemia, gestational hypertension, or other disorders.

If the woman's blood type has not been verified, blood is drawn for the purpose of determining the type and Rh factor. If blood typing has already been done, the primary health care provider may choose not to repeat the test. If obvious signs of immunocompromise or substance abuse are present, other blood tests may be ordered.

Assessment of amniotic membranes and fluid. Labor is initiated at term by SROM in approximately 25% of pregnant women. A lag period, rarely exceeding 24 hours, may precede the onset of labor. Membranes (the BOW) also can rupture spontaneously any time during labor, but most commonly in the transition phase of the first stage of labor.

NURSE ALERT *The umbilical cord may prolapse when the membranes rupture. The FHR and pattern should be monitored closely for several minutes immediately after ROM to ascertain fetal well-being, and the findings should be documented.*

The tests used to assess amniotic fluid are discussed in the Procedure box on p. 400, and the characteristics of the fluid are described in Table 14-4. Artificial rupture of membranes (AROM, ARM), or amniotomy, may be done to augment or induce labor or to facilitate placement of internal monitors when fetal status indicates the need for some form of direct assessment (e.g., insertion of a fetal scalp electrode or an intrauterine pressure catheter).

Infection. When membranes rupture, microorganisms from the vagina can then ascend into the amniotic sac, causing chorioamnionitis and placentitis to develop. For this reason, maternal temperature and vaginal discharge are assessed frequently (every 1 to 2 hours) so that an infection developing after ROM can be identified early. Even when membranes are intact, however, microorganisms may ascend and cause PROM. There is controversy regarding whether prophylactic antibiotic therapy can protect against infection (chorioamnionitis), which involves

TABLE 14-4

Assessment of Amniotic Fluid Characteristics

CHARACTERISTIC OF FLUID	NORMAL FINDING	DEVIATION FROM NORMAL FINDING	CAUSE OF DEVIATION FROM NORMAL
Color	Pale, straw colored; may contain white flecks of vernix caseosa, lanugo, scalp hair	Greenish brown color Yellow-stained fluid Port wine colored	Hypoxic episode in fetus results in meconium passage into fluid May be normal finding in breech presentations related to pressure exerted on fetal abdominal wall during descent Fetal hypoxia ≥36 hr before ROM; fetal hemolytic disease; intrauterine infection Bleeding associated with premature separation of the placenta (abruptio placentae)
Viscosity and odor	Watery; no strong odor	Thick, cloudy, foul smelling	Intrauterine infection Large amount of meconium can make fluid thick
Amount (normally varies with gestational age)	400 ml (20 wk gestation) 1000 ml (36 to 38 wk gestation)	≥2000 ml (32 to 36 wk gestation) ≤500 ml (32 to 36 wk gestation)	Hydramnios; associated with congenital anomalies of the fetus when fetus cannot drink or fluid is trapped in the body (e.g., fetal gastrointestinal obstruction or atresias); increased risk with maternal pregestational or gestational diabetes mellitus Oligohydramnios; associated with incomplete or absent kidney; obstruction of urethra; fetus cannot secrete or excrete urine

ROM, Rupture of membranes.

signs of
POTENTIAL COMPLICATIONS

Labor

- Intrauterine pressure of ≥80 mm Hg (determined by intrauterine pressure catheter monitoring) or resting tone of ≥20 mm Hg
- Contractions consistently lasting ≥90 sec
- Contractions consistently occurring ≤2 min apart
- Relaxation between contractions lasting <30 sec
- Fetal bradycardia, tachycardia, decreased variability not associated with fetal sleep cycle or temporary effects of CNS depressant drugs given to the woman, or late or severe variable deceleration
- Irregular fetal heart rate; suspected fetal dysrhythmias
- Appearance of meconium-stained or bloody fluid from the vagina
- Arrest in progress of cervical dilation or effacement, descent of the fetus, or both
- Maternal temperature of ≥38° C
- Foul-smelling vaginal discharge
- Continuous bright- or dark-red vaginal bleeding

both the maternal and fetal sides of the membrane. Use of prophylactic antibiotics for prelabor ROM at term or
✳ preterm is a form of care of unknown effectiveness (Enkin et al., 2000).

The nurse's responsibility is to report findings promptly to the primary health care provider and to document findings in the labor record and on the monitor strip. If abnormal findings are noted, continuous electronic monitoring usually is implemented and maintained for the duration of labor. The presence of meconium-stained amniotic fluid alerts the nurse to the need to observe fetal status more closely. After birth, the newborn may be at risk for an alteration in respiratory status if meconium is aspirated into the lungs with the first breath.

Signs of potential problems

Assessment findings serve as a baseline for evaluating the woman's subsequent progress during labor. Although some problems of labor are anticipated, others may appear unexpectedly during the clinical course of labor (see Signs of Potential Complications box).

Nursing diagnoses

Nursing diagnoses determine the types of nursing actions needed to implement a plan of care. When establishing nursing diagnoses, the nurse should analyze the significance of findings ascertained during the assessment.

Nursing diagnoses appropriate for the first stage of labor include:

- *Anxiety related to*
  - negative experience with previous childbirth
  - cultural differences

- *Impaired urinary elimination related to*
  - reduced intake of oral fluids
  - diminished sensation of bladder fullness associated with epidural anesthesia or analgesia
- *Impaired fetal gas exchange related to*
  - maternal hypotension or hypertension
  - maternal position
  - compression of the umbilical cord
- *Situational low self-esteem (maternal) related to*
  - inability to meet self-expectations regarding performance during childbirth
  - loss of control during labor

Nursing diagnoses that represent potential areas for concern during the second stage of labor include the following:

- *Risk for injury to mother and fetus related to*
  - persistent use of Valsalva maneuver
- *Situational low self-esteem related to*
  - deficient knowledge of normal, beneficial effects of vocalization during bearing-down efforts
  - inability to carry out plan for birth without medication
- *Ineffective coping related to*
  - coaching that contradicts woman's physiologic urge to push
- *Anxiety related to*
  - inability to control defecation with bearing-down efforts
  - deficient knowledge regarding perineal sensations associated with the urge to bear down

Examples of nursing diagnoses relevant to the third stage of labor include the following:

- *Risk for deficient fluid volume related to*
  - blood loss occurring after placental separation and expulsion
  - inadequate contraction of the uterus
- *Anxiety related to*
  - lack of knowledge regarding separation and expulsion of the placenta
  - occurrence of perineal trauma and the need for repair
- *Fatigue related to*
  - energy expenditure associated with childbirth and the bearing-down efforts of the second stage

Expected Outcomes of Care

It is important for the nurse and woman to set and assign priorities to expected outcomes that focus on the woman, the fetus, and the woman's significant others. Appropriate nursing and patient actions are then determined so that these expected outcomes can be met. Planning with the woman is essential to ensure the achievement of expected outcomes and to maintain her sense of control over her own childbirth experience. Expected outcomes for the woman in the first stage of labor are that the woman will accomplish the following:

- Continue normal progression of labor while the FHR and pattern remain within the expected range and without signs of distress
- Maintain adequate hydration status through oral or IV intake
- Actively participate in the labor process
- Verbalize discomfort and indicate the need for measures that help reduce discomfort and promote relaxation
- Accept comfort and support measures from significant others and health care providers as needed
- Sustain no injury to herself or the fetus during labor and birth
- Initiate, along with the partner and family, the processes of bonding and attachment with the newborn
- Express satisfaction with her performance during labor and birth

Plan of Care and Interventions
Standards of care

Standards of care guide the nurse in preparing for and implementing procedures with the expectant mother (Box 14-4). Protocols for care based on standards include the following tasks:

- Check the primary health care provider's orders.
- Review the primary health care provider's orders for completeness and correctness (e.g., the dose and route of the analgesic to be administered).

BOX 14-4

Care Plan Using Protocols and Nursing Standards

CARE PLAN FOR LABOR   MARY JAMES
                                                UNIT NO. 4587024

Date Initiated: _____   Time: _____   RN: _____

OUTCOME STANDARDS
1 Patient will demonstrate normal labor progress while the fetus tolerates the labor process without demonstrating nonreassuring signs. Date met: _____
2 Patient will participate in decisions about her care. Date met: _____
3 Patient and her partner will verbalize knowledge of labor process and their expectations for the birth experience. Date met: _____

INITIATED Date/RN	PROBLEM	NURSING INTERVENTIONS	DISCONTINUED Date/RN
	Impaired maternal-fetal gas exchange	Implement fetal monitoring per protocol or orders from health care provider	
	Risk related to labor progress: • Impaired urinary elimination • Impaired tissue integrity related to birth	Provide nursing care per hospital procedure manual Implement labor care per protocol or care path Notify primary health care provider of problems (see Signs of Potential Complications box) Provide care for vaginal birth per hospital procedure manual Provide immediate care for newborn per hospital procedure manual Implement care for fourth stage of labor per protocol or care path	
	Anxiety related to maternal-fetal status	Encourage woman and her partner to express their concerns Keep couple informed of labor progress Involve woman in decision making regarding her care	
	Deficient knowledge about labor and procedures Acute pain related to process of labor	Explain procedures in terms woman can understand Promote use of relaxation techniques Provide comfort measures Offer pain medications as ordered Evaluate response to pain relief measures	
	Other problems		

- Check labels on IV solutions, drugs, and other materials used for nursing care.
- Check the expiration date on any packs of supplies used for procedures.
- Ensure that information on the woman's identification band is accurate (e.g., the band is the appropriate color for allergies).
- Use an empathic approach when giving care (see Guidelines/Guías box):
  —Use words the woman can understand when explaining procedures; repeat as necessary.
  —Respect the woman's individual needs and behaviors.
  —Establish rapport with the woman and her significant others.
  —Be kind, caring, and competent when performing necessary procedures.

GUIDELINES/GUÍAS

Care during Labor

- Lie down, please.
- *Acuéstese, por favor.*

- I am going to take your vital signs.
- *Voy a verificar sus signos vitales.*

- I am going to listen to the baby's heartbeat.
- *Voy a escuchar el latido del corazón del bebé.*

- This is a fetal monitor.
- *Este es un monitor fetal.*

- I need to examine you.
- *Necesito examinarle.*

- Do you need to use the bathroom?
- *¿Necesita usar el baño?*

- Would you like some pain medication?
- *¿Quisiera medicina para calmar el dolor?*

- Roll over on your side, please.
- *Póngase sobre un costado, por favor.*

- Relax.
- *Afloje los músculos.*

- Breathe deeply.
- *Respire profundamente.*

- Push.
- *Puje.*

- Do not push.
- *No puje.*

- Grab your knees and push.
- *Agárrese las rodillas y puje.*

- You are doing fine.
- *Bien. Muy bien.*

- Congratulations!
- *¡Felicidades!*

- You have a beautiful boy.
- *Usted tiene un niño precioso.*

- You have a beautiful girl.
- *Usted tiene una niña preciosa.*

—Be aware that pain and discomfort are as the woman describes them.
—Carry out appropriate comfort measures such as mouth care and back care
—Include the support persons in the care as desired by the woman and the support persons
—Recognize that a woman's current childbirth experience and the actions of nurses and other health care providers can have a positive or negative effect on the woman's future childbirth experiences.
- Use Standard Precautions, including precautions for invasive procedures (see Box 14-3).
- Document care according to hospital guidelines, and communicate information to the primary health care provider when indicated.

Physical nursing care during labor

The physical nursing care rendered to the woman in labor is an essential component of her care. The current emphasis on evidence-based practice supports the management of care by using this approach to enhance the safety, effectiveness, and acceptability of the physical care measures chosen to support the woman during labor and birth (Enkin et al., 2000). The various physical needs, the requisite nursing actions, and the rationale for care are presented in Table 14-5, the Plan of Care on p. 421, and the Care Path on p. 406.

General hygiene. Women in labor should be offered the use of showers or warm water baths, if they are available, to enhance the feeling of well-being and to minimize the discomfort of contractions (Benfield, 2002; Cluett, Nikodem, McCandlish, & Burns, 2004). Women also should be encouraged to wash their hands after voiding and to perform self-hygiene measures. Linen should be changed if it becomes wet or stained with blood, and linen savers (Chux) should be used and changed as needed.

Nutrient and fluid intake

Oral intake. Traditionally the laboring woman has been offered only clear liquids or ice chips or given nothing by mouth during the active phase of labor to minimize the risk of anesthesia complications and their sequelae should general anesthesia be required in an emergency. These sequelae include the aspiration of gastric contents and resultant compromise in oxygen perfusion, which may endanger the lives of the mother and fetus. This practice is being challenged today because regional anesthesia is used more often than general anesthesia, even for emergency cesarean births. Women are awake during regional anesthesia and are able to participate in their own care and protect their airway.

An adequate intake of fluids and calories is required to meet the energy demands and fluid losses associated with childbirth. The progress of labor slows, and ketosis develops if these demands are not met and fat is metabolized. Reduced energy for bearing-down efforts (pushing) increases the risk for a forceps- or vacuum-assisted birth. This is most

Text continued on p. 422.

TABLE 14-5

Physical Nursing Care during Labor

NEED	NURSING ACTIONS	RATIONALE
GENERAL HYGIENE		
Showers or bed baths, Jacuzzi bath	Assess for progress in labor	Determines appropriateness of the activity
	Supervise showers closely if woman is in true labor	Prevents injury from fall; labor may be accelerated
	Suggest allowing warm water to flow over back	Aids relaxation; increases comfort
Perineum	Cleanse frequently, especially after rupture of membranes and when show increases	Enhances comfort and reduces risk of infection
Oral hygiene	Offer toothbrush or mouthwash or wash the teeth with an ice-cold wet washcloth as needed	Refreshes mouth; helps counteract dry, thirsty feeling
Hair	Brush, braid per woman's wishes	Improves morale; increases comfort
Handwashing	Offer washcloths before and after voiding and as needed	Maintains cleanliness; prevents infection
Face	Offer cool washcloth	Provides relief from diaphoresis; cools and refreshes
Gowns and linens	Change as needed; fluff pillows	Improves comfort; enhances relaxation
NUTRIENT AND FLUID INTAKE		
Oral	Offer fluids and solid foods, following orders of primary health care provider and desires of laboring woman	Provides hydration and calories; enhances positive emotional experience and maternal control
Intravenous (IV)	Establish and maintain IV line as ordered	Maintains hydration; provides venous access for medications
ELIMINATION		
Voiding	Encourage voiding at least every 2 hr	A full bladder may impede descent of presenting part; overdistention may cause bladder atony and injury, as well as postpartum voiding difficulty
Ambulatory woman	Allow ambulation to bathroom according to orders of primary health care provider, if:	
	The presenting part is engaged	Reinforces normal process of urination
	The membranes are not ruptured	Precautionary measure to protect against prolapse of umbilical cord
	The woman is not medicated	Precautionary measure to protect against injury
Woman on bed rest	Offer bedpan	Prevents complications of bladder distention and ambulation
	Allow tap water to run; pour warm water over the vulva; give positive suggestion	Encourages voiding
	Provide privacy	Shows respect for woman
	Put up side rails on bed	Prevents injury from fall
	Place call bell within reach	Reinforces safe care
	Offer washcloth for hands	Maintains cleanliness; prevents infection
	Wash vulvar area	Maintains cleanliness; enhances comfort; prevents infection
Catheterization	Catheterize according to orders of primary health care provider or hospital protocol if measures to facilitate voiding are ineffective	Prevents complications of bladder distention
	Insert catheter between contractions	Minimizes discomfort
	Avoid force if obstacle to insertion is noted	"Obstacle" may be caused by compression of urethra by presenting part
Bowel elimination— sensation of rectal pressure	Perform vaginal examination	Prevents misinterpretation of rectal pressure from the presenting part as the need to defecate
		Determine degree of descent of presenting part
	Help the woman ambulate to bathroom or offer bedpan if rectal pressure is not from presenting part	Reinforce normal process of bowel elimination and safe care
	Cleanse perineum immediately after passage of stool	Reduces risk of infection and sense of embarrassment

PLAN OF CARE *Labor and Birth*

NURSING DIAGNOSIS Anxiety related to labor and the birthing process
Expected Outcome *Woman exhibits decreased signs of anxiety.*

Nursing Interventions/*Rationales*

- Orient woman and significant others to labor and birth unit and explain admission protocol *to allay initial feelings of anxiety.*
- Assess woman's knowledge, experience, and expectations of labor; note any signs or expressions of anxiety, nervousness, or fear *to establish a baseline for intervention.*
- Discuss the expected progression of labor and describe what to expect during the process *to allay anxiety associated with the unknown.*
- Actively involve woman in care decisions during labor, interpret sights and sounds of environment (monitor sights and sounds, unit activities), and share information on progression of labor (vital signs, fetal heart rate [FHR], dilation, effacement) *to increase her sense of control and allay fears.*

NURSING DIAGNOSIS Acute pain related to increasing frequency and intensity of contractions
Expected Outcome *Woman exhibits signs of ability to cope with discomfort.*

Nursing Interventions/*Rationales*

- Assess woman's level of pain and strategies that she has used to cope with pain *to establish a baseline for intervention.*
- Encourage significant other to remain as support person during labor process *to assist with support and comfort measures, because measures are often more effective when delivered by a familiar person.*
- Instruct woman and support person in use of specific techniques such as conscious relaxation, focused breathing, effleurage, massage, and application of sacral pressure *to increase relaxation, decrease intensity of contractions, and promote use of controlled thought and direction of energy.*
- Provide comfort measures such as frequent mouth care *to prevent dry mouth;* application of damp cloth to forehead, and changing of damp gown or bed covers *to relieve discomfort associated with diaphoresis.*
- Help woman change position *to reduce stiffness.*
- Explain what analgesics and anesthesia are available for use during labor and birth *to provide knowledge to help woman make decisions about pain control.*

NURSING DIAGNOSIS Risk for impaired urinary elimination related to sensory impairment secondary to labor
Expected Outcome *Bladder does not show signs of distention.*

Nursing Interventions/*Rationales*

- Palpate the bladder superior to the symphysis on a frequent basis (at least every 2 hours) *to detect a full bladder that occurs from increased fluid intake and inability to feel urge to void.*
- Encourage frequent voiding (at least every 2 hours) and catheterize if necessary *to avoid bladder distention because*

it impedes progress of fetus down birth canal and may result in trauma to the bladder.
- Assist to bathroom or commode to void if appropriate, provide privacy, and use techniques to stimulate voiding such as running water *to facilitate bladder emptying with an upright position (natural) and relaxation.*

NURSING DIAGNOSIS Risk for ineffective individual coping related to birthing process
Expected Outcome *Woman actively participates in the birth process with no evidence of injury to her or her fetus.*

Nursing Interventions/*Rationales*

- Constantly monitor events of second-stage labor and birth, including physiologic responses of woman and fetus and emotional responses of woman and partner, *to ensure maternal, partner, and fetal well-being.*
- Provide ongoing feedback to woman and partner *to allay anxiety and enhance participation.*
- Continue to provide comfort measures and minimize distractions *to decrease discomfort and aid in focus on the birth process.*
- Encourage woman to experiment with various positions *to assist downward movement of fetus.*
- Ensure that woman takes deep cleansing breaths before and after each contraction *to enhance gas exchange and oxygen transport to the fetus.*
- Encourage woman to push spontaneously when urge to bear down is perceived during a contraction *to aid descent and rotation of fetus.*
- Encourage woman to exhale, holding breath for short periods while bearing down, *to avoid holding breath and triggering a Valsalva maneuver and increasing intrathoracic and cardiovascular pressure and decreasing perfusion of placental oxygen, placing the fetus at risk.*
- Have woman take deep breaths and relax between contractions *to reduce fatigue and increase effectiveness of pushing efforts.*
- Have mother pant as fetal head crowns *to control birth of head.*
- Explain to woman and labor partner what is expected in the third stage of labor *to enlist cooperation.*
- Have woman maintain her position *to facilitate delivery of the placenta.*

NURSING DIAGNOSIS Fatigue related to energy expenditure during labor and birth
Expected Outcome *Woman's energy levels are restored.*

Nursing Interventions/*Rationales*

- Educate woman and partner about need for rest and help them plan strategies (e.g., restricting visitors, increasing role of support systems performing functions associated with daily routines) that allow specific times for rest and sleep *to ensure that woman can restore depleted energy levels in preparation for caring for a new infant.*
- Monitor woman's fatigue level and the amount of rest received *to ensure restoration of energy.*

CD: Plan of Care—Labor and Birth

Continued

PLAN OF CARE *Labor and Birth—cont'd*

NURSING DIAGNOSIS **Risk for deficient fluid volume related to decreased fluid intake and increased fluid loss during labor and birth**
Expected outcomes *Fluid balance is maintained, and there are no signs of dehydration.*

Nursing Interventions/Rationales
- Monitor fluid loss (i.e., blood, urine, perspiration) and vital signs; inspect skin turgor and mucous membranes for dryness *to evaluate hydration status.*

- Administer parenteral fluid per physician or nurse-midwife orders *to maintain hydration.*
- Monitor the fundus for firmness after placental separation to *ensure adequate contraction and prevent further blood loss.*
- Offer oral fluids following orders of physician or nurse-midwife and desire of laboring woman *to provide hydration.*

---

likely to occur in women who begin to labor early in the morning after a night without caloric intake. When women are permitted to consume fluids and food freely, they typically regulate their own oral intake, eating light foods (e.g., eggs, yogurt, ice cream, dry toast and jelly, fruit) and drinking fluids during early labor and tapering off to the intake of clear fluids and sips of water or ice chips as labor intensifies and the second stage approaches. Common practice is to allow clear liquids (e.g., water, tea, apple juice, clear sodas, gelatin, broth) during early labor, tapering off to ice chips and sips of water as labor progresses and becomes more active. Food and fluid consumed orally during labor can meet a laboring woman's hydration and energy demands more effectively and safely than fluid administered intravenously. In addition, the woman's sense of control

and level of comfort are enhanced (Scheepers et al., 2001). The CNM Data Group (1999) found that a woman's culture may influence what she will eat and drink during labor. In addition, women who used nonpharmacologic pain relief measures and labored in nonhospital settings were more likely to eat and drink during labor.

Withholding food and fluids in labor is a form of care unlikely to be beneficial, and offering oral fluids is demonstrably useful and should be encouraged (Enkin et al., 2000; Hofmeyr, 2005). Nurses should follow the orders of the woman's primary health care provider when offering the woman food or fluids during labor. As advocates, however, nurses can facilitate change by informing others of the current research findings that support the safety and effectiveness of the oral intake of food and fluid during labor and by initiating such research themselves.

Intravenous intake. Fluids are administered intravenously to the laboring woman to maintain hydration, especially when a labor is long and the woman is unable to ingest a sufficient amount of fluid orally or if she is receiving epidural or intrathecal anesthesia. However, routine use of IV fluids during labor is a form of care that is unlikely to be beneficial and may be harmful (Enkin et al., 2000). In most cases, an electrolyte solution without glucose is adequate and does not introduce excess glucose into the bloodstream. The latter is important because an excessive maternal glucose level results in fetal hyperglycemia and fetal hyperinsulinism. After birth, the neonate's high levels of insulin will then deplete his or her glucose stores, and hypoglycemia will result. Infusions containing glucose can also reduce sodium levels in both the woman and the fetus, leading to transient neonatal tachypnea. If maternal ketosis occurs, the primary health care provider may order an IV solution containing a small amount of dextrose to provide the glucose needed to assist in fatty acid metabolism.

Critical Thinking Exercise

Oral Intake in Labor

Margot is at 41 weeks of gestation in her first pregnancy. Her labor is being induced with IV oxytocin. She arrived at the labor unit at 7 AM, and it is now 2 PM. Her cervix is dilated 2 cm and effaced 40%. Her membranes are intact. She has a maintenance IV of 5% dextrose in lactated Ringer's solution (D5LR) at 100 ml/hr. She has been eating ice chips all morning but is now asking for something to drink as she has not eaten since 7 PM last night, and she feels hungry. How would you respond to her request?

1. Evidence—Is there sufficient evidence to draw conclusions about how the nurse should respond to her request?
2. Assumptions—Describe underlying assumptions about the following issues:
   a. Oral intake in labor
   b. Fasting in labor as a stressor
   c. Cultural influences on oral intake in labor
3. What implications and priorities for nursing care can be drawn at this time?
4. Does the evidence objectively support your conclusion?
5. Are there alternative perspectives to your conclusion?

NURSE ALERT *Nurses should carefully monitor the intake and output of laboring women receiving IV fluids because they also face an increased danger of hypervolemia as a result of the fluid retention that occurs during pregnancy.*

Elimination

Voiding. Voiding every 2 hours should be encouraged. A distended bladder may impede descent of the presenting part, inhibit uterine contractions, and lead to decreased bladder tone or atony after birth. Women who receive epidural analgesia or anesthesia are especially at risk for the retention of urine, and the need to void should be assessed more frequently in them.

The woman should be assisted to the bathroom to void, unless the primary health care provider has ordered bed rest; the woman is receiving epidural analgesia or anesthesia; internal monitoring is being used; or, in the nurse's judgment, ambulation would compromise the status of the laboring woman, her fetus, or both. External monitoring can usually be interrupted for the woman to go to the bathroom.

Catheterization. If the woman is unable to void and her bladder is distended, she may need to be catheterized. Most hospitals have protocols that rely on the nurse's judgment concerning the need for catheterization. Before performing the catheterization, the nurse should clean the vulva and perineum because vaginal show and amniotic fluid may be present. If there appears to be an obstacle that prevents advancement of the catheter, this is most likely the presenting part. If the catheter cannot be advanced, the nurse should stop the procedure and notify the primary health care provider of the difficulty.

Bowel elimination. Most women do not have bowel movements during labor because of decreased intestinal motility. Stool that has formed in the large intestine often is moved downward toward the anorectal area by the pressure exerted by the fetal presenting part as it descends. This stool is often expelled during second-stage pushing and birth. However, the passage of stool with bearing-down efforts increases the risk of infection and may embarrass the woman, thereby reducing the effectiveness of these efforts. To prevent these problems, the nurse should immediately cleanse the perineal area to remove any stool, while reassuring the woman that the passage of stool at this time is a normal and expected event, because the same muscles used to expel the baby also expel stool. Routine use of an enema to empty the rectum is considered to be harmful or ineffective and should be ✳ eliminated (Enkin et al., 2000).

When the presenting part is deep in the pelvis, even in the absence of stool in the anorectal area, the woman may feel rectal pressure and think she needs to defecate. If the woman expresses the urge to defecate, the nurse should perform a vaginal examination to assess cervical dilation and station. When a multiparous woman experiences the urge to defecate, this often means birth will follow quickly.

Ambulation and positioning. Freedom of maternal movement and choice of position throughout labor are forms of care likely to be beneficial for the laboring ✳ woman and should be encouraged (Enkin et al., 2000).

The potential advantages of ambulation include enhanced uterine activity, distraction from labor's discomforts, enhanced maternal control, and an opportunity for close interaction with the woman's partner and care provider as they help her to walk. Ambulation is associated with a reduced rate of operative birth (i.e., cesarean birth, use of forceps, and vacuum extraction) and less frequent use of opioid analgesics (Albers et al., 1997).

Walking, sitting, or standing during labor is more comfortable than lying down and facilitates the progress of labor (Simkin & Ancheta, 2000). Ambulation should be encouraged if membranes are intact, if the fetal presenting part is engaged after ROM, and if the woman has not received medication for pain (Fig. 14-10). Ambulation may be contraindicated, however, because of maternal or fetal status. The woman also may find it comfortable to stand and lean forward on her partner, doula, or nurse for support at times during labor (Fig. 14-11, *A*).

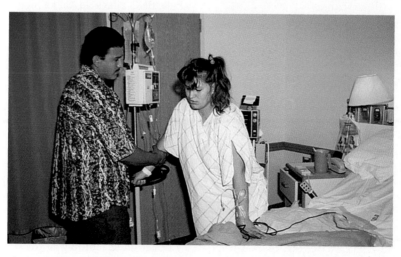

Fig. 14-10 Woman preparing to walk with partner. (Courtesy Marjorie Pyle, RNC, Lifecircle, Costa Mesa, CA.)

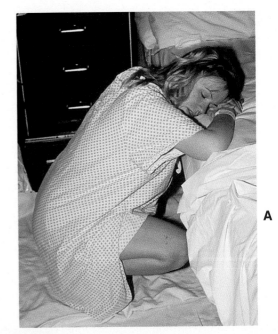

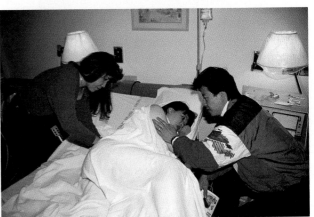

Fig. 14-12 Maternal positions for labor. **A,** Squatting. **B,** Lateral position. Support person is applying sacral pressure while partner provides encouragement. (Courtesy Marjorie Pyle, RNC, Lifecircle, Costa Mesa, CA.)

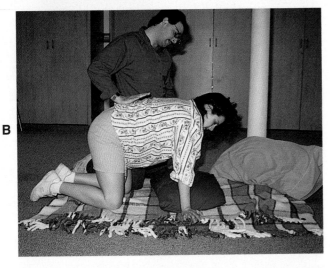

Fig. 14-11 **A,** Woman standing and leaning forward with support. **B,** Woman in hands-and-knees position. (Courtesy Marjorie Pyle, RNC, Lifecircle, Costa Mesa, CA.)

When the woman lies in bed, she will usually change her position spontaneously as labor progresses. If she does not change position every 30 to 60 minutes, she should be assisted to do so. The side-lying (lateral) position is preferred because it promotes optimal uteroplacental and renal blood flow and increases fetal oxygen saturation (Fig. 14-12, *B*). If the woman wants to lie supine, the nurse may place a pillow under one hip as a wedge to prevent the uterus from compressing the aorta and vena cava (see Fig. 14-5). Sitting is not contraindicated unless it adversely affects fetal status, which can be determined by checking the FHR and pattern. If the fetus is in the occiput posterior position, it may be

helpful to encourage the woman to squat during contractions, because this position increases pelvic diameter, allowing the head to rotate to a more anterior position (Fig. 14-12, *A*). A hands-and-knees position during contractions also is recommended to facilitate the rotation of the fetal occiput from a posterior to an anterior position, as gravity pulls the fetal back forward (Fig. 14-11, *B*).

Much research continues to be directed toward acquiring a better understanding of the physiologic and psychologic effects of maternal position in labor. The variety of positions that are recommended for the laboring woman are described in Box 14-5.

BOX 14-5

Some Maternal Positions during Labor and Birth*

SEMIRECUMBENT POSITION

With woman sitting with her upper body elevated to at least a 30-degree angle, place wedge or small pillow under hip to prevent vena caval compression and reduce likelihood of supine hypotension (see Fig. 14-5).

- The greater the angle of elevation, the more gravity or pressure is exerted that promotes fetal descent, the progress of contractions, and the widening of pelvic dimensions.
- Position is convenient for rendering care measures and for external fetal monitoring.

LATERAL POSITION (SEE FIG. 14-12, *B*)

Have woman alternate between left and right side-lying positions, and provide abdominal and back support as needed for comfort.

- Removes pressure from the vena cava and back, enhances uteroplacental perfusion, and relieves backache
- Makes it easier to perform back massage or counterpressure.
- Associated with less frequent, but more intense, contractions.
- Obtaining good external fetal monitor tracings may be more difficult.
- May be used as a birthing position.
- Takes pressure off perineum, allowing it to stretch gradually.
- Reduces risk for perineal trauma.

UPRIGHT POSITION

The gravity effect enhances the contraction cycle and fetal descent: the weight of the fetus places increasing pressure on the cervix; the cervix is pulled upward, facilitating effacement and dilation; impulses from the cervix to the pituitary gland increase, causing more oxytocin to be secreted; and contractions are intensified, thereby applying more forceful downward pressure on the fetus, but they are less painful.

- Fetus is aligned with pelvis, and pelvic diameters are widened slightly.
- Effective upright positions include the following:
  —Ambulation (see Fig. 14-10).
  —Standing and leaning forward with support provided by coach (see Fig. 14-11, *A*), end of bed, back of chair, or birth ball (see Fig. 14-13); relieves backache and facilitates application of counterpressure or back massage
  —Sitting up in bed, chair, or birthing chair, on toilet, or on bedside commode
  —Squatting (see Figs. 14-12, *A* and 14-17, *E*)

HANDS-AND-KNEES POSITION—IDEAL POSITION FOR POSTERIOR POSITIONS OF THE PRESENTING PART (SEE FIG. 14-11, *B*)

Assume an "all-fours" position in bed or on a covered floor; allows for pelvic rocking.

- Relieves backache characteristic of "back labor."
- Facilitates internal rotation of the fetus by increasing mobility of the coccyx, increasing the pelvic diameters, and using gravity to turn the fetal back and rotate the head.

*Assess the effect of each position on the laboring woman's comfort and anxiety level, progress of labor, and FHR pattern. Alternate positions every 30 to 60 min, allowing woman to take control of her position changes.

A birth ball (gymnastic ball, also used in physical therapy) can be used to support a woman's body as she assumes a variety of labor and birth positions (Fig. 14-13). The woman can sit on the ball while leaning over the bed, or she can lean over the ball to support her upper body and reduce stress on her arms and hands when she assumes a hands-and-knees position. The birth ball can encourage pelvic mobility and pelvic and perineal relaxation when the woman sits on the firm yet pliable ball and rocks in rhythmic movements. Warm compresses applied to the perineum and lower back can maximize this relaxation and comfort effect. The birth ball should be large enough so that when the woman sits, her knees are bent at a 90-degree angle and her feet are flat on the floor and approximately 2 feet apart.

Supportive care during labor and birth. Support during labor and birth involves emotional support, physical care and comfort measures, and provision of advice and information (Davies & Hodnett, 2002; Miltner, 2000). Effective support provided to women during labor can

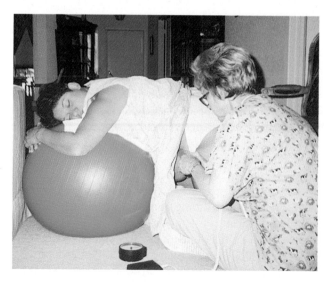

Fig 14-13 Woman laboring using birth ball. (Courtesy Polly Perez, Cutting Edge Press, Johnson, VT.)

result in shorter labors; reduced rates of complications and surgical or obstetric interventions (e.g., cesarean births, labor augmentations and inductions, episiotomies, forceps- and vacuum-assisted births); and enhanced self-esteem and satisfaction (Hodnett, 2001; Miltner, 2000). Physical, emotional, and psychologic support of the woman during labor and birth is a beneficial form of care demonstrated by clear research evidence (Enkin et al., 2000; MacKinnon, McIntyre, & Quance, 2005).

Labor rooms should be airy, clean, and homelike. The laboring woman should feel safe in this environment and free to be herself and to use the comfort and relaxation measures she prefers. To enhance relaxation, bright overhead lights should be turned off when not needed, and noise and intrusions should be kept to a minimum. The temperature is controlled to ensure the laboring woman's comfort. The room should be large enough to accommodate a comfortable chair for the woman's partner, the monitoring equipment, and hospital personnel. Couples may be encouraged to bring their own pillows to make the hospital surroundings more homelike and to facilitate position changes. Environmental modifications should reflect the preferences of the woman, including the number of visitors and availability of a telephone, television, and music. Nurses should ensure that each woman labors in an optimal birth environment (Hanson, VandeVusse, & Harrod, 2001).

Labor support by the nurse. The nurse can alleviate a woman's anxiety by explaining unfamiliar terms, providing information and explanations without her having to ask, and preparing her for sensations she will experience and procedures that will follow. By encouraging the woman or couple to ask questions and by providing honest, understandable answers, the nurse can play an important role in helping the woman achieve a satisfying birth experience (Hodnett, Gates, Hofmeyr, & Sakala, 2003; Hodnett et al., 2002; Miltner, 2002; Sauls, 2002).

Supportive nursing care for a woman in labor includes the following (Simkin, 2002):

- Helping the woman maintain control and participate to the extent she wishes in the birth of her infant
- Meeting the woman's expected outcomes for her labor
- Acting as the woman's advocate, supporting her decisions and respecting her choices as appropriate and relating her wishes as needed to other health care providers
- Helping the woman conserve her energy
- Helping control the woman's discomfort
- Acknowledging the woman's efforts, as well as those of her partner, during labor and providing positive reinforcement
- Protecting the woman's privacy and modesty

Couples who have attended childbirth education programs that teach the psychoprophylactic approach will know something about the labor process, coaching techniques, and comfort measures. The nurse should play a supportive role and keep such a couple informed of the progress. A review of methods learned in class may be needed.

Even when expectant parents have not attended childbirth classes, the nurse can teach them simple breathing and relaxation techniques during the early phase of labor. In this case, the nurse may provide more of the coaching and supportive care.

Comfort measures vary with the situation (Fig. 14-14). The nurse can draw on the couple's repertoire of comfort measures learned during the pregnancy. Such measures include maintaining a comfortable, supportive atmosphere in the labor and birth area; using touch therapeutically (e.g., heat or cold applied to the lower back in the event of back labor, a cool cloth applied to the forehead); providing non-pharmacologic measures to relieve discomfort (e.g., massage hydrotherapy, administering analgesics when necessary); and, most important of all, just being there (MacKinnon, McIntyre, & Quance, 2005; Simkin, 2002) (see Table 14-1; see also the Care Paths on pp. 406 and 433). See Chapter 12 for a full discussion of both pharmacologic and non-pharmacologic comfort measures.

Most women in labor respond positively to touch but permission should be obtained before any of these touching measures are used. They appreciate gentle handling by staff members. Back rubs and counterpressure may be offered, especially if the woman is experiencing back labor. A support person may be taught to exert counterpressure against the woman's sacrum over the occiput of the head of a fetus in a posterior position (see Fig. 14-12, *B*). The back pain is caused by the occiput pressing on spinal nerves, and counterpressure lifts the occiput off these nerves, thereby providing some relief from pain. The partner will need to be relieved after a while, however, because exerting counterpressure is hard work. Hand and foot massage also can be soothing and relaxing (Simkin, 2002). The woman's perception of the soothing qualities of touch changes as labor progresses. Many women become more sensitive to touch

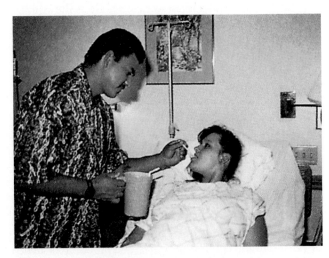

Fig. 14-14 Partner providing comfort measures. (Courtesy Marjorie Pyle, RNC, Lifecircle, Costa Mesa, CA.)

EVIDENCE-BASED PRACTICE
Continuous Labor Support

BACKGROUND

- Until the middle of the twentieth century, laboring women of all cultures had the support of other women to encourage and guide them through birth. Hospital births and the "cascade of medical interventions" have sparked calls for a return to a more humanized culture of birth, with the continuous presence of an emotionally supportive, reassuring person during labor. Labor support may enhance labor physiology and maternal confidence, mitigating the harsh environment of institutional routines, lack of privacy, and high rates of intervention. It may decrease stress and enhance passage of the fetus. Labor support has frequently been associated with decreased use of pain medication including epidural anesthesia, which may slow labor and lead to further interventions.
- In North America a trained birth assistant called a *doula* may fill this labor support role. Family members who have given birth themselves may also serve in this role. Observers have questioned the use of hospital staff in this role, as they are technologically oriented and may have conflicting demands on their time and loyalties.

OBJECTIVES

- The reviewers desired to assess the effects of continuous labor support on mothers and babies, when compared with standard institutional care.
- Outcome measures would ideally include:
  - Labor Events: amniotomy, augmented labor, electronic fetal monitoring, epidural analgesia, other pain medication, severe pain, and length of labor
  - Birth Events: cesarean birth, operative vaginal birth (forceps or vacuum), episiotomy, and perineal trauma
  - Newborn Events: 5-minute Apgar score, low cord pH, admission to special care nursery, and prolonged newborn hospital stay
  - Maternal Outcomes: anxiety during labor, dissatisfaction, difficulty coping, low coping, postpartum depression, low self-esteem, difficulty mothering, breastfeeding problems, pain, dyspareunia, problems with partner, and urinary and/or fecal incontinence

METHODS

Search Strategy

- The reviewers searched Cochrane, MEDLINE, 30 journals, and a weekly awareness service of 37 journals. Keywords were *labor, support, caregiver, doula, labor assistant, birth assistant, childbirth support,* and *labor companion.*
- Fifteen randomized, controlled trials involving 12,791 women provided high-quality data from hospitals in Australia, Belgium, Botswana, Canada, Finland, France, Greece, Guatemala, Mexico, South Africa, and the United States. All provided continuous presence during active labor as the intervention, and standard care for that institution as the control.

Statistical Analysis

- Statistical analyses included pooling of similar data. The reviewers analyzed certain variables, such as epidural analgesia, electronic fetal monitoring, employee or non-employee support person, and time of support onset. They analyzed how these variables may have influenced specific outcomes, such as pain medication, operative birth or normal spontaneous vaginal delivery (NSVD), low 5-minute Apgar scores, dissatisfaction, and postpartum depression.

FINDINGS

- The continuous support groups showed significant decreases in use of any pain medication and regional analgesia, decreased cesarean or operative birth, and maternal dissatisfaction. Reviewers found no difference between groups in augmented labor, low Apgar scores, special care nursery admissions, severe pain, perineal trauma, poor fetal outcomes, incontinence, or postpartum depression.
- When influences were compared with outcomes, the greatest benefits (decreased analgesia use, increased normal spontaneous vaginal births) were derived in settings where the support person was someone of the woman's own choosing and not staff. Benefit from support was dose related: the earlier the onset of support, the greater the effect.

LIMITATIONS

- This review had few limitations owing to the large numbers and similarities of interventions and outcome measures. There were differences in policies about other family members present, continuous electronic fetal monitoring, and epidural availability. The qualifications of the support people varied, although they were all women. Onset of support varied. Blinding of group randomization was not feasible. Attrition and dropouts were not always noted.

CONCLUSIONS

- All laboring women need continuous support. The greatest benefit may be early support from a trained or experienced nonstaff support person. The use of nurses or nurse-midwives for support may not decrease the cesarean birth rate, because of their interventionist training. Support may provide great benefits to a laboring woman in a resource-poor environment.

IMPLICATIONS FOR PRACTICE

- Childbirth educators can include in their classes the suggestion that a support person be selected to accompany the couple to labor. Nurses in the birthing setting can encourage laboring women to have continuous support and provide support to that person. Laboring women need to be given the choice of their support person.

IMPLICATIONS FOR FURTHER RESEARCH

- Further research is needed for maternal and infant health outcomes and for longer-term outcomes of postpartum depression and prolonged pain. Further information about costs, and comparisons of outcomes when support is provided by a trained doula or an experienced female family member or husband, would also be enlightening.

Reference: Hodnett, E., Gates, S., Hofmeyr, G., & Sakala, C. (2003). Continuous support for women during childbirth. *The Cochrane Database of Systematic Reviews*, Issue 3, 2003, Art. CD003766.

(hyperesthesia) as labor progresses. This is a typical response during the transition phase (see Table 14-3). They may tell their coach to leave them alone or not to touch them. The partner who is unprepared for this normal response may feel rejected and may react by withdrawing active support. The nurse can reassure him or her that this response is a positive indication that the first stage is ending and the second stage is approaching. Women with increased sensitivity to touch may have a positive response when touched on surfaces of the body where hair does not grow, such as the forehead, the palms of the hands, and the soles of the feet.

Labor support by the father or partner. Although another woman or a man other than the father may be the woman's partner, the father of the baby is usually the support person during labor. He often is able to provide the comfort measures and touch that the laboring woman needs. When the woman becomes focused on her pain, sometimes the partner can persuade her to try nonpharmacologic variations of comfort measures. In addition, he usually is able to interpret the woman's needs and desires for staff members.

Throughout the past 30 years, childbirth preparation education has been widely available. The father's ideal role was thought to be that of labor coach, and he was expected actively to help the woman cope with labor. However, this expectation may be unrealistic, because some men have concerns about their labor-coaching abilities. Men can assume one of at least three different roles during labor and birth: coach, teammate, or witness (Chapman, 1992). As a coach the father actively assists the woman during and after contractions. Men who are coaches express a strong need to be in control of themselves and of the labor experience. Women also express a great desire for the father to be physically involved in labor. The father who acts as the teammate assists the woman during labor and birth by responding to requests for physical or emotional support, or both. Teammates usually adopt the follower or helper role and look to the woman or nurse to tell them what to do. Women express a strong desire to have the father present and willing to help in any way. The father who acts as a witness acts as a companion, giving emotional and moral support. He watches the woman labor and give birth, but he often sleeps, watches television, or leaves the room for long periods. Witnesses believe that there is little they can do to help the woman physically and look to the nurses and health care providers to be in charge of the experience. Women do not expect more of this type of father than to just be present.

The feelings of a first-time father change as labor progresses. Although he is often calm at the onset of labor, feelings of fear and helplessness begin to dominate as labor becomes more active and the father realizes that labor is more work than he anticipated. The first-time father may feel excluded as birth preparations begin during the transition phase. Once the second stage begins and birth nears, the father's focus changes from the woman to the baby who is about to be born. The father will be exposed to many sights

---

BOX 14-6

Guidelines for Supporting the Father/Significant Other

- Orient to the labor room and the unit; explain location of the cafeteria, toilet, waiting room, and nursery; give information about visiting hours; introduce personnel by name, and describe their functions.
- Inform him of sights and smells he can expect to encounter; encourage him to leave the room if necessary.
- Respect his or the couple's decision about the degree of his involvement. Offer them freedom to make decisions.
- Tell him when his presence has been helpful, and continue to reinforce this throughout labor.
- Offer to teach him comfort measures.
- Inform him frequently of the progress of the labor and the woman's needs. Keep him informed about procedures to be performed.
- Prepare him for changes in the woman's behavior and physical appearance.
- Remind him to eat; offer him snacks and fluids if possible.
- Relieve him of the job of support person as necessary. Offer him blankets if he is to sleep in a chair by the bedside.
- Acknowledge the stress experienced by each partner during labor and birth and identify normal responses.
- Attempt to modify or eliminate unsettling stimuli, such as extra noise and extra light.

---

and smells he may never before have experienced. It is therefore important to tell him what to expect and to make him comfortable about leaving the room to regain his composure should something occur that surprises him. Before he leaves the room, provision should be made for someone else to support the woman during his absence. Staff members should tell the father that his presence is helpful and encourage him to be involved in the care of the woman to the extent to which he is comfortable. Ways in which the nurse can support the father-partner are detailed in Box 14-6. A well-informed father can make an important contribution to the health and well-being of the mother and child, their family interrelationship, and his self-esteem.

Labor support by doulas. Continuity of care has been cited by women as a critical component of a satisfying childbirth experience. This need can be met by a specially trained, experienced female labor attendant called a **doula.** The doula provides a continuous, one-on-one caring presence throughout the labor and birth of the woman she is attending. This is a beneficial form of care (Enkin et al., 2000). The primary role of the doula is to focus on the laboring woman and provide physical and emotional support by using soft, reassuring words; touching, stroking, and hugging; administering comfort measures to reduce pain and enhance relaxation; and walking with the woman, helping her to change positions, and coaching her bearing-down efforts. Doulas provide information and explain procedures and events. They advocate for the woman's right to participate actively in the management of her labor (Kayne, Greulich, & Albers, 2001; Trainor, 2002).

The doula also supports the woman's partner, who often feels unqualified to be the sole labor support. The doula can encourage and praise the partner's efforts, create a partnership as caregivers, and provide respite care. Doulas also facilitate communication between the laboring woman and her partner, as well as between the couple and the health care team (Tumblin & Simkin, 2001).

Continuous care provided by doulas significantly reduces the cesarean birth rate; duration of labor; use of oxytocin, analgesics, and forceps; and requests for epidural anesthesia. Laboring women also reported a higher level of satisfaction with their childbirth experience and greater success with breastfeeding (Klaus, Kennell, & Klaus, 1993; Trainor, 2002).

The role of the nurse and the doula are complementary. They should work together as a team, with the doula providing supportive nonmedical care measures and with the nurse focusing on monitoring the status of the maternal-fetal unit; implementing clinical care protocols, including pharmacologic interventions; and documenting assessment findings, actions, and responses.

Labor support by the grandparents. When grandparents act as labor coaches, it is especially important to support and treat them with respect. They may have a way to deal with pain relief based on their experience. They should be encouraged to help as long as their actions do not compromise the status of the mother or the fetus. One example of an acceptable practice would be giving the woman herbal teas during labor. The nurse acts as a role model for parents by treating grandparents with dignity and respect, by acknowledging the value of the grandparents' contributions to parental support, and by recognizing the difficulty parents have in witnessing their child's discomfort or crisis, regardless of the age of the child. If they have never witnessed a birth, the nurse may need to provide explanations of what is happening. Many of the activities used to support fathers also are appropriate for grandparents.

Siblings during labor and birth. The preparation of siblings for acceptance of the new child helps promote the attachment process. Such preparation and participation during pregnancy and labor may help the older children accept this change. The older child or children who know themselves to be important to the family become active participants. Rehearsal for the event before labor is essential.

The age and developmental level of children influence their responses; therefore preparation for the children to be present during labor is adjusted to meet each child's needs. The child younger than 2 years shows little interest in pregnancy and labor; for the older child, such preparation may reduce fears and misconceptions. Parents need to be prepared for labor and birth themselves and feel comfortable about the process and the presence of their children. Most parents have a "feel" for their children's maturational level

and their physical and emotional ability to observe and cope with the events of the labor and birth process. Preparation can include a description of the anticipated sights, events (e.g., ROM, monitors, IV infusions), smells, and sounds; a labor and birth demonstration; a tour of the birthing unit; and an opportunity to be around a real newborn. Children must learn that their mother will be working hard during labor and birth. She will not be able to talk to them during contractions. She may groan, scream, grunt, and pant at times as well as say things she would not say otherwise (e.g., "I can't take this anymore," "Take this baby out of me," or "This pain is killing me"). They can be told that labor is uncomfortable, but that their mother's body is made for the job. Storybooks about the birth process can be read to or by children to prepare them for the event. Films are available for preparing preschool and school-age children to participate in the labor and birth experience. Most agencies require that a specific person be designated to watch over the children who are participating in their mother's childbirth experience, to provide them with support, explanations, diversions, and comfort as needed. Health care providers involved in attending women during birth must be comfortable with the presence of children and the unpredictability of their questions, comments, and behaviors.

Emergency interventions. Emergency conditions that require immediate nursing intervention can arise with startling speed. Interventions for a nonreassuring FHR, inadequate uterine relaxation, vaginal bleeding, infection, and prolapse of the cord are detailed in the Emergency box.

Evaluation

Evaluation of progress and outcomes is a continuous activity during the first stage of labor. The nurse must carefully evaluate each interaction with the mother-to-be and her family and critically appraise how well the expected outcomes of care are being met.

SECOND STAGE OF LABOR

The **second stage of labor** is the stage in which the infant is born. This stage begins with full cervical dilation (10 cm) and complete effacement (100%) and ends with the baby's birth. The force exerted by uterine contractions, gravity, and maternal bearing-down efforts facilitates achievement of the expected outcome of a spontaneous, uncomplicated vaginal birth.

The second stage is composed of three phases: the latent, descent, and transition phases. These phases are characterized by maternal verbal and nonverbal behaviors, uterine activity, the urge to bear down, and fetal descent.

The latent phase is a period of rest and relative calm (i.e., "laboring down"). During this early phase, the fetus continues to descend passively through the birth canal and rotate to an anterior position as a result of ongoing uterine contractions. The woman is quiet and often relaxes with her eyes closed between contractions. The urge to bear down is not

EVOLVE/CD: Case Study—Second and Third Stages of Labor

Interventions for Emergencies

SIGNS
NONREASSURING FETAL HEART RATE PATTERN

- Fetal bradycardia (FHR <110 beats/min for >10 min)†
- Fetal tachycardia (FHR >160 beats/min for >10 min in term pregnancy)§
- Irregular FHR, abnormal sinus rhythm shown by internal monitor
- Persistent decrease in baseline FHR variability without an identified cause
- Late, severe variable, and prolonged deceleration patterns (>2 minutes to <10 minutes)
- Absence of FHTs

INADEQUATE UTERINE RELAXATION

- Intrauterine pressure >80 mm Hg (shown by intrauterine pressure catheter monitoring)
- Contractions consistently lasting >90 sec
- Contraction interval <2 min

VAGINAL BLEEDING

- Vaginal bleeding (bright red, dark red, or in an amount in excess of that expected during normal cervical dilation)
- Continuous vaginal bleeding with FHR changes
- Pain; may or may not be present

INFECTION

- Foul-smelling amniotic fluid
- Maternal temperature >38° C in presence of adequate hydration (straw-colored urine)
- Fetal tachycardia >160 beats/min for >10 min

PROLAPSE OF CORD

- Fetal bradycardia with variable deceleration during uterine contraction
- Woman reports feeling the cord after membranes rupture
- Cord lies alongside or below the presenting part of the fetus; can be seen or felt in or protruding from the vagina
- Major predisposing factors:
  - Rupture of membranes with a gush
  - Loose fit of presenting part in lower uterine segment
  - Presenting part not yet engaged
  - Breech presentation

INTERVENTIONS*
PRIORITIES ARE BASED ON WHAT SIGN IS PRESENT

Notify primary health care provider.‡
Change maternal position.
Discontinue oxytocin (Pitocin) infusion, if hyperstimulation is occurring.
Start an IV line if one is not in place.
Increase IV fluid rate, if fluid being infused, per protocol order.
Administer oxygen at 8 to 10 L/min by snug face mask.
Check maternal temperature for elevation.
Assist with amnioinfusion if ordered.
Stimulate fetal scalp or use sound stimulation.

Notify primary health care provider‡.
Discontinue oxytocin infusion, if being infused.
Change woman to side-lying position.
Start an IV line if one is not in place.
Increase IV fluid rate, if fluid is being infused.
Administer oxygen at 8 to 10 L/min by snug face mask.
Palpate and evaluate contractions.
Give tocolytics (terbutaline), as ordered.

Notify primary health care provider‡.
Assist with ultrasound examination if performed.
Start an IV line if one is not in place.
Anticipate emergency (stat) cesarean birth.
Do NOT perform a vaginal examination.

Notify primary health care provider‡.
Institute cooling measures for laboring woman.
Start an IV line if one is not in place.
Assist with or perform collection of catheterized urine specimen and amniotic fluid sample and send to the laboratory for urinalysis and cultures.

Call for assistance. Do not leave woman alone.
Have someone notify the primary health care provider immediately.
Glove the examining hand quickly and insert two fingers into the vagina to the cervix; with one finger on either side of the cord or both fingers to one side, exert upward pressure against the presenting part to relieve compression of the cord.
Place a rolled towel under the woman's hip.
Place woman in extreme Trendelenburg or modified Sims position or knee-chest position.
Wrap the cord loosely in a sterile towel saturated with warm sterile normal saline if the cord is protruding from the vagina.
Administer oxygen at 8 to 10 L/min by face mask until birth is accomplished.
Start IV fluids or increase existing drip rate.
Continue to monitor FHR by internal fetal scalp electrode, if possible.
Do not attempt to replace cord into cervix.
Prepare for immediate birth (vaginal or cesarean).

FHR, Fetal heart rate; *IV,* intravenous.
*Because emergency situations are often frightening events, it is important for the nurse to explain to the woman and her support person what is happening and how it is being managed.
†Practice is to intervene within 2 to 30 min of FHR <110 beats/min.
‡In most emergency situations, nurses take immediate action, following a protocol and standards of nursing practice. Another person can notify the primary health care provider, or this can be done by the nurse as soon as possible.
§Nonreassuring sign when associated with late decelerations or absence of variability, especially of >180 beats/min.

well established and may not be experienced at all or only during the acme of a contraction. Allowing a woman to rest during this phase, and waiting until the urge to push intensifies, has been found to reduce maternal fatigue, conserve energy for bearing-down efforts, and provide optimal maternal and fetal outcomes (Minato, 2000). Coaching a woman to push before her body signals readiness can result in a prolonged period of active pushing with limited to no progress. The woman may become dependent on her coach or nurses to tell her when and how to push (Roberts, 2002). However, women who have epidural analgesia may not feel the urge to bear down and will need coaching.

The descent phase or the phase of active pushing is characterized by strong urges to bear down as the reflex called the *Ferguson reflex* is activated when the presenting part presses on the stretch receptors of the pelvic floor. At this point, the fetal station is usually 1+, and the position is anterior. This stimulation causes the release of oxytocin from the posterior pituitary gland, which provokes stronger expulsive uterine contractions. The woman becomes more focused on bearing-down efforts, which become rhythmic. She changes positions frequently to find a more comfortable pushing position. The woman often announces the onset of contractions and becomes more vocal as she bears down. The urge to bear down intensifies as descent progresses.

In the transition phase, the presenting part is on the perineum, and bearing-down efforts are most effective for promoting birth. The woman may be more verbal about the pain she is experiencing; she may scream or swear and may act out of control (Roberts, 2002).

The nurse encourages the woman to "listen" to her body as she progresses through the phases of the second stage of labor. When a woman listens to her body to tell her when to bear down, she is using an internal locus of control and often feels more satisfied with her efforts to give birth to her baby. Her sense of self-esteem and accomplishment is enhanced, and her efforts become more effective. The woman's trust in her own body and her ability to give birth to her baby should be fostered (Mayberry et al., 2000).

If a woman is confined to bed, especially in a recumbent position, the rhythmic urge to bear down is delayed because gravity is not being used to press the presenting part against the pelvic floor. Being moved to another room and placed on a delivery table in the lithotomy position, as has been the custom in North America, also has an inhibiting effect on the urge to bear down. Today, Western societies have adopted the birthing practice of most non-Western societies in which labor and birth occur in the same room and women use various positions for bearing down, such as the side-lying position, kneeling, squatting, sitting, or standing.

The duration of the second stage of labor is influenced by several factors, such as the effectiveness of the primary and secondary powers of labor; the type and amount of analgesia or anesthesia used; the physical and emotional condition, position, activity level, parity, and pelvic adequacy of the laboring woman; the size, presentation, and position of the fetus; and the nature and source of support the woman receives.

For many multiparous women, birth occurs within minutes of complete dilation, perhaps only one push later. Nulliparous women usually push for 1 to 2 hours before giving birth. If the woman has been given epidural analgesia, pushing can last longer than 2 hours. Epidural analgesia blocks or reduces the urge to bear down and limits the woman's ability to attain an upright position to push. By adjusting doses to the lowest effective level, allowing the epidural to wear off at full dilation or after 1 hour of pushing, or using mixtures containing an opioid-agonist analgesic and a local anesthetic, the woman is able more fully to perceive the urge to bear down, to move more freely, and to attain an upright position with assistance as a result of increased strength and sensation in her legs. This approach can enhance the ability to bear down effectively and result in an uncomplicated vaginal birth (Mayberry et al., 2000). However, women also will have an increase in distress and the severity of pain. This results in an increase in sympathetic activity and the release of catecholamines. Catecholamines inhibit uterine contractions, potentially prolonging the second stage of labor. Allowing these women a "laboring down" period for fetal descent and rotation may result in a more positive outcome (Roberts, 2002).

Commonly, a second stage of more than 2 hours may be considered prolonged in women without regional analgesia and is reported to the primary health care provider. By using assessment findings such as the FHR and pattern, the descent of the presenting part, the quality of the uterine contractions, and the status of the woman, premature intervention with episiotomy or forceps- or vacuum- assisted birth can be avoided. If the status of the maternal-fetal unit is reassuring and progress is continuing, interventions to end the second stage of labor are unwarranted. Less emphasis should be placed on a definite time limit for the second stage. The duration of active pushing has been found to be more relevant to the newborn's condition at birth than the duration of the second stage of labor itself (Cesario, 2004; Minato, 2000; Roberts, 2002).

CARE MANAGEMENT

The only certain objective sign that the second stage of labor has begun is the inability to feel the cervix during vaginal examination, indicating that the cervix is fully dilated and effaced. The precise moment that this occurs is not easily determined because it depends on when a vaginal examination is performed to validate full dilation and effacement. This makes timing of the actual duration of the second stage difficult (Roberts, 2002). Other signs that suggest the onset of the second stage include the following:

- Sudden appearance of sweat on upper lip
- An episode of vomiting
- Increased bloody show
- Shaking of extremities

- Increased restlessness; verbalization (e.g., "I can't go on")
- Involuntary bearing-down efforts

These signs commonly appear at the time the cervix reaches full dilation; however, women with an epidural block may not exhibit such signs. Other indicators for each phase of the second stage are given in Table 14-6.

Women can begin to experience an irresistible urge to bear down before full dilation. For some women, this occurs as early as 5 cm of dilation. This is most often related to the station of the presenting part below the level of the ischial spines of the maternal pelvis. This occurrence creates a conflict between the woman, whose body is telling her to push, and her health care providers, who believe that pushing the fetal presenting part against an incompletely dilated cervix will result in cervical edema and lacerations, as well as a slowing down of labor progress. The premature urge to bear down must be evaluated as a phase of labor progress possibly indicating the onset of the second stage of labor. The timing of when a woman pushes in relation to whether or not her cervix is fully dilated should be based on research evidence rather than on tradition or routine practice. It may be safe and effective for a woman to push with the urge to bear down at the acme of a contraction if her cervix is soft, retracting, and 8 cm or more dilated and if the fetus is at 1+ station and rotating to an anterior position (Roberts, 2002).

Assessment is continuous during the second stage of labor. Professional standards and agency policy determine the specific type and timing of assessments, as well as the way in which findings are documented. The Care Path for the second and third stages of labor indicates typical assessments and the recommended frequency for their performance. Signs and symptoms of impending birth (see Table 14-6) may appear unexpectedly, requiring immediate action by the nurse (Box 14-7).

The nurse continues to monitor maternal-fetal status and events of the second stage and provide comfort measures for the mother, such as helping her change position; providing mouth care; maintaining clean, dry bedding; and keeping

Text continued on p. 435.

TABLE 14-6

Expected Maternal Progress in Second Stage of Labor

CRITERION	LATENT PHASE (AVERAGE DURATION, 10-30 MIN)	DESCENT PHASE (AVERAGE DURATION VARIES)*	TRANSITION PHASE (AVERAGE DURATION 5-15 MIN)
Contractions Magnitude (intensity) Frequency Duration	Period of physiologic lull for all criteria; period of peace and rest; "laboring down"	Significant increase 2-2.5 min 90 sec	Overwhelmingly strong Expulsive 1-2 min 90 sec
Descent, station	0 to +2	Increases and Ferguson reflex† activated, +2 to +4	Rapid, +4 to birth Fetal head visible in introitus
Show: color and amount		Significant increase in dark red bloody show	Bloody show accompanies birth of head
Spontaneous bearing-down efforts	Slight to absent, except during acme of strongest contractions	Increased urge to bear down	Greatly increased
Vocalization	Quiet; concern over progress	Grunting sounds or expiratory vocalization; announces contractions	Grunting sounds and expiratory vocalizations continue; may scream or swear
Maternal behavior	Experiences sense of relief that transition to second stage is finished Feels fatigued and sleepy Feels a sense of accomplishment and optimism, because the "worst is over" Feels in control	Senses increased urge to push Alters respiratory pattern: has short 4- to 5-sec breath holds with regular breaths in between, 5 to 7 times per contraction Makes grunting sounds or expiratory vocalizations Frequent repositioning	Describes extreme pain Expresses feelings of powerlessness Shows decreased ability to listen or concentrate on anything but giving birth Describes *ring of fire* (burning sensation of acute pain as vagina stretches and fetal head crowns) Often shows excitement immediately after birth of head

Source: Roberts, J. (2002). The "push" for evidence: Management of the second stage. *Journal of Midwifery & Women's Health, 47*(1), 2-15; Simkin, P., & Ancheta, R. (2000). *The labor progress handbook*. Malden, MA: Blackwell Science.
*Duration of descent phase can vary depending on maternal parity, effectiveness of bearing-down effort, and presence of spinal anesthesia or epidural analgesia.
†Pressure of presenting part on stretch receptors of pelvic floor stimulates release of oxytocin from posterior pituitary, resulting in more intense uterine contractions.

CARE PATH *Low Risk Woman in Second and Third Stages of Labor*

CARE MANAGEMENT	SECOND STAGE OF LABOR	THIRD STAGE OF LABOR
I. ASSESSMENT MEASURES*	**Frequency**	**Frequency**
Blood pressure, pulse, respirations	Every 5-30 min	Every 15 min
Uterine activity	Assess every contraction	Assess for signs of placental separation
Bearing-down effort	Assess each effort	
Fetal heart rate (FHR)	Every 5-15 min	Assist with determination of Apgar score at 1 and 5 min
Vaginal show	Every 15 min	Assess bleeding until placental expulsion
Signs of fetal descent: urge to bear down, perineal bulging, crowning	Every 10-15 min	
Behavior, appearance, mood, energy level of woman; condition of partner	Every 10-15 min	Assess response to completion of childbirth process, reaction to newborn
II. PHYSICAL CARE MEASURES†	**Latent phase:** Assist to rest in position of comfort Encourage relaxation to conserve energy Promote urge to push; if delayed: ambulation, shower, pelvic rock, position changes **Descent phase:** Assist to bear down effectively Help to use recommended positions that facilitate descent Encourage correct breathing during bearing-down efforts Help to relax between contractions Provide comfort measures as needed Cleanse perineum immediately if fecal material is expelled **Transition phase:** Assist to pant during contraction to avoid rapid birth of head Coach to gently bear down between contractions	Assist to bear down to facilitate delivery of separated placenta Administer oxytocic as ordered Provide pain relief as needed Provide hygiene and comfort measures as needed
III. EMOTIONAL SUPPORT	Keep informed of progress of fetal descent Provide feedback for bearing-down efforts Explain purpose if medications given Role model comfort measures Provide continuous nursing presence Create a quiet, calm environment Reassure, encourage, praise Take charge as needed, until woman regains confidence in ability to birth her baby Offer mirror to watch birth	Keep informed about progress of placental separation Explain purpose if medications given Describe status of perineal tissue and inform if repair is needed Introduce parents to their baby Assess and care for newborn within view of parents; delay eye prophylaxis to facilitate eye contact Provide private time for family to bond with their new baby and help them to create memories Encourage breastfeeding if desired

*Frequency of assessment is determined by the risk status of the maternal-fetal unit. More frequent assessment is required in high risk situations. Frequency of assessment and method of documentation are also determined by agency policy, which is usually based on the recommended care standards of medical and nursing organizations.

†Physical care measures are performed by the nurse working together with the woman's partner and significant others.

BOX 14-7

Guidelines for Assistance at the Emergency Birth of a Fetus in the Vertex Presentation

1. The woman usually assumes the position most comfortable for her. A lateral position is often recommended.

2. Reassure the woman that birth is usually uncomplicated and easy in these situations. Use eye-to-eye contact and a calm, relaxed manner. If there is someone else available, such as the partner, that person could help support the woman in the position, assist with coaching, and compliment her on her efforts.

3. Wash your hands and put on gloves, if available.

4. Place under woman's buttocks whatever clean material is available.

5. Avoid touching the vaginal area to decrease the possibility of infection.

6. As the head begins to crown, you should do the following:
   a. Tear the amniotic membrane if it is still intact.
   b. Instruct the woman to pant or pant-blow, thus minimizing the urge to push.
   c. Place the flat side of your hand on the exposed fetal head and apply *gentle* pressure toward the vagina to prevent the head from "popping out." The mother may participate by placing her hand under yours on the emerging head. NOTE: Rapid delivery of the fetal head must be prevented because a rapid change of pressure within the molded fetal skull follows, which may result in dural or subdural tears and may cause vaginal or perineal lacerations.

7. After the birth of the head, check for the umbilical cord. If the cord is around the baby's neck, try to slip it over the baby's head or pull it *gently* to get some slack so that you can slip it over the shoulders.

8. Support the fetal head as external rotation occurs. Then, with one hand on each side of the baby's head, exert *gentle* pressure downward so that the anterior shoulder emerges under the symphysis pubis and acts as a fulcrum; then, as *gentle* pressure is exerted in the opposite direction, the posterior shoulder, which has passed over the sacrum and coccyx, emerges.

9. Be alert! Hold the baby securely because the rest of the body may emerge quickly. The baby will be slippery!

10. Cradle the baby's head and back in one hand and the buttocks in the other. Keep the head down to drain away the mucus. Use a bulb syringe, if one is available, to remove mucus from the baby's mouth.

11. Dry the baby quickly to prevent rapid heat loss. Keep the baby at the same level as the mother's uterus until the end of the cord stops pulsating. NOTE: It is important to keep the baby at the same level as the mother's uterus to prevent the baby's blood from flowing to or from the placenta and the resultant hypovolemia or hypervolemia. Also, do not "milk" the cord.

12. Place the baby on the mother's abdomen, cover the baby (remember to keep the head warm, too) with the mother's clothing, and have her cuddle the baby. Compliment her (them) on a job well done, and on the baby, if appropriate.

13. Wait for the placenta to separate; *do not* tug on the cord. NOTE: Injudicious traction may tear the cord, separate the placenta, or invert the uterus. Signs of placental separation include a slight gush of dark blood from the introitus, lengthening of the cord, and change in the uterine contour from a discoid to globular shape.

14. Instruct the mother to push to deliver the separated placenta. Gently ease out the placental membranes using an up-and-down motion until the membranes are removed. If birth occurs outside a hospital setting, to minimize complications, do not cut the cord without proper clamps and a sterile cutting tool. Inspect the placenta for intactness. Place the baby on the placenta and wrap the two together for additional warmth.

15. Check the firmness of the uterus. Gently massage the fundus and demonstrate to the mother how she can massage her own fundus properly.

16. If supplies are available, clean the mother's perineal area and apply a peripad.

17. In addition to gentle massage of the fundus, the following measures can be taken to prevent or minimize hemorrhage:
    a. Put the baby to the mother's breast as soon as possible. Sucking or nuzzling and licking the nipple stimulates the release of oxytocin from the posterior pituitary. NOTE: If the baby does not or cannot nurse, manually stimulate the mother's nipples.
    b. Do not allow the mother's bladder to become distended. Assess the bladder for fullness and encourage her to void if fullness is found.
    c. Expel any clots from the mother's uterus.

18. Comfort or reassure the mother and her family or friends. Keep the mother and the baby warm. Give her fluids if available and tolerated.

19. If this is a multifetal birth, identify the infants in order of birth (using letters *A, B,* etc.).

20. Make notations regarding the following aspects of the birth:
    a. Fetal presentation and position
    b. Presence of cord around neck (nuchal cord) or other parts and number of times cord encircled part
    c. Color, character, and amount of amniotic fluid, if rupture of membranes occurs immediately before birth
    d. Time of birth
    e. Estimated time of determination of Apgar score (e.g., 1 and 5 min after birth), resuscitation efforts implemented, and ultimate condition of baby
    f. Sex of baby
    g. Time of placental expulsion, as well as the appearance and completeness of the placenta
    h. Maternal condition: affect, amount of bleeding, and status of uterine tonicity
    i. Any unusual occurrences during the birth (e.g., maternal or paternal response, verbalizations, or gestures in response to birth of baby)

TABLE 14-7

Woman's Responses and Support Person's Actions during Second Stage of Labor

WOMAN'S RESPONSES*	NURSE OR SUPPORT PERSON'S ACTIONS†
LATENT PHASE	
Experiences a short period of peace and rest	Encourages woman to "listen" to her body Continues support measures allowing woman to rest Suggests an upright position to encourage progression of descent if descent phase does not begin after 20 min
DESCENT PHASE	
Senses increased urgency to bear down as Ferguson reflex is activated Notes increase in intensity of uterine contractions; alters respiratory pattern: short 4- to 5-sec breath holds, five to seven times per contraction Makes grunting sounds or expiratory vocalizations	Encourages respiratory pattern of short breath holds and open-glottis pushing Stresses normality and benefits of grunting sounds and expiratory vocalizations Encourages bearing-down efforts with urge to push Encourages or suggests maternal movement and position changes (upright, if descent is not occurring) Encourages woman to "listen" to her body regarding movement and position change if descent is occurring Discourages long breath holds (no longer than 5 to 7 sec) If birth is to occur in a delivery room, transfers woman to delivery room early to avoid rushing, or, if permitted, offers her option of walking to delivery room Places woman in lateral recumbent position to slow descent if descent is too fast
TRANSITIONAL PHASE	
Behaves in manner similar to behavior during transition in first stage (8-10 cm) Experiences a sense of severe pain and powerlessness Shows decreased ability to listen Concentrates on birth of baby until head is born Experiences contractions as overwhelming in intensity Reports feeling ring of fire as head crowns Maintains respiratory pattern of three to five 7-sec breath holds per contraction, followed by forced expiration Eases head out with short expirations Responds with excitement and relief after head is born	Encourages slow, gentle pushing Explains that "blowing away the contraction" facilitates a slower birth of the head Provides mirror to help woman see or touch the emerging fetal head (best to extend over two to three contractions) to help her understand the perineal sensations Coaches woman to relax mouth, throat, and neck to promote relaxation of pelvic floor Applies warm compress to perineum to promote relaxation

*Woman's responses will be altered if epidural analgesia is being administered.
†Provided by nurses and support persons in collaboration with the nurse.

extraneous noise, conversation, and other distractions (e.g., laughing, talking of attending personnel in or outside the labor area) to a minimum. The woman is encouraged to indicate other support measures she would like (Table 14-7; also see Care Path for Low Risk Woman in Second and Third Stages of Labor on p. 433, and Plan of Care for Labor and Birth on p. 421).

In the hospital, birth may occur in an LDR, LDRP, or delivery room. If the mother is to be transferred to the delivery room for birth, the nurse accomplishes the transfer early enough to avoid rushing the woman. The birth area also is readied for the birth.

Maternal position

There is no single position for childbirth. Labor is a dynamic, interactive process involving the woman's uterus, pelvis, and voluntary muscles. In addition, angles between

the baby and the woman's pelvis constantly change as the infant turns and flexes down the birth canal. The woman may want to assume various positions for childbirth, and she should be encouraged and assisted in attaining and maintaining her position(s) of choice. Sitting and side-lying are the two most common positions assumed by women for their bearing-down efforts and birth.

Birth attendants play a major role in influencing a woman's choice of positions for birth, with nurse-midwives tending to advocate the nonlithotomy positions for the second stage of labor. Upright positions facilitate birth and fetal descent and reduce the duration of the second stage of labor and the need for episiotomy, forceps, or vacuum extractor in the following ways (Gupta & Hofmeyr, 2003):

- Straighten the longitudinal axis of the birth canal
- Use gravity to direct the fetal head toward the pelvic inlet, thereby facilitating descent

- Enlarge pelvic dimensions and restrict the encroachment of the sacrum and coccyx into the pelvic outlet
- Increase uteroplacental circulation, resulting in more intense, efficient uterine contractions
- Enhance the woman's ability to bear down effectively, thereby minimizing maternal exhaustion

The upright positions may, however, slightly increase the risk for second-degree lacerations and a blood loss greater than 500 ml. Further investigation is needed to determine the exact mechanism for these outcomes (Shorten, Donsante, & Shorten, 2002).

Squatting is highly effective in facilitating the descent and birth of the fetus. It is considered to be one of the best positions for the second stage of labor (Mayberry et al., 2000; Roberts, 2002). Women should assume a modified, supported squat until the fetal head is engaged, at which time a deep squat can be used. A firm surface is required for this position, and the woman will need side support (see Fig. 14-12, *A*). In a birthing bed a squat bar is available that she can use to help support herself (see Fig. 14-17, *E*). A birth ball also can be used to help a woman maintain the squatting position. The fetus will be aligned with the birth canal, and pelvic and perineal relaxation will be facilitated as she sits on the ball or holds it in front of her for support as she squats.

When a woman uses the standing position for bearing down, her weight is borne on both femoral heads, allowing the pressure in the acetabulum to cause the transverse diameter of the pelvic outlet to increase by up to 1 cm. This can be helpful if descent of the head is delayed because the occiput has not rotated from the lateral (transverse diameter of pelvis) to the anterior position. Birthing chairs or rocking chairs may be used to provide women with a good physiologic position to enhance bearing-down efforts during childbirth, although some women feel restricted by a chair. The upright position also provides a potential psychologic advantage in that it allows the mother to see the birth as it occurs and to maintain eye contact with the attendant. Most birthing chairs are designed so that if an emergency occurs, the chair can be adjusted to the horizontal or the Trendelenburg position.

Oversized beanbag chairs and large floor pillows may be used for both labor and birth. They can mold around and support the mother in whatever position she selects. These chairs are of particular value for mothers who wish to be actively involved in the birth process. Birthing stools can be used to support the woman in an upright position similar to squatting. Women may want to sit on the toilet or commode during pushing because they are concerned about stool incontinence during this stage. These women must be closely monitored, however, and removed from the toilet before birth becomes imminent. Because sitting on chairs, stools, toilets, or commodes can increase perineal edema and blood loss, it is important to assist the woman to change her position frequently.

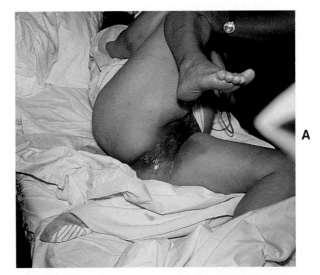

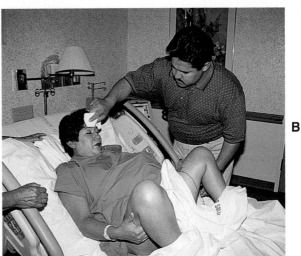

Fig. 14-15 **A,** Pushing, side-lying position. Perineal bulging can be seen. **B,** Pushing, semi-sitting position. (**A,** Courtesy Michael S. Clement, MD, Mesa, AZ. **B,** Courtesy Marjorie Pyle, RNC, Lifecircle, Costa Mesa, CA.)

The side-lying position, with the upper part of the woman's leg held by the nurse or coach or placed on a pillow, is an effective position for the second stage of labor (Fig. 14-15, *A*). Women using the lateral position have more control over their bearing-down efforts. In addition, a slower, more controlled descent of the fetus results in a reduced risk of perineal trauma (Gupta & Hofmeyr, 2003). Some women prefer a semi-sitting (semi-recumbent) position. To maintain good uteroplacental circulation and to enhance the woman's bearing-down efforts in this position, the woman's back and shoulders should be elevated to at least a 30-degree angle, and a wedge should be placed under one hip (Fig. 14-15, *B*). The episiotomy rate for nulliparas has been found to be highest in this position (Shorten, Donsante, & Shorten, 2002).

The hands-and-knees position, along with pelvic rocking and abdominal stroking, is an effective position for birth

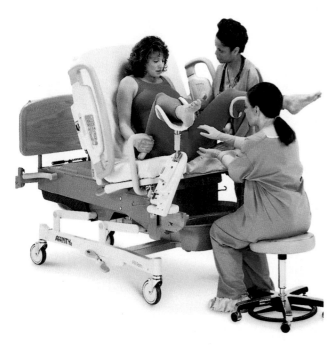

Fig. 14-16 Birthing bed. (Courtesy Hill-Rom, Batesville, IN.)

because it enhances placental perfusion, helps rotate the fetus from a posterior to an anterior position, and may facilitate the birth of the shoulders, especially if the fetus is large. Perineal trauma also may be reduced (Simkin & Ancheta, 2000) (see Fig. 14-11, *B*).

The birthing bed is commonly used today and can be set for different positions according to the woman's needs (Figs. 14-16 and 14-17). The woman can squat, kneel, sit, recline, or lie on her side, choosing the position most comfortable for her without having to climb into bed for the birth. At the same time, there is excellent exposure for examinations, electrode placement, and birth. The bed also can be positioned for the administration of anesthesia and is ideal to help women receiving an epidural to assume different positions to facilitate birth. The bed can be used to transport the woman to the operating room if a cesarean birth is necessary. Squat bars, over-the-bed tables, birth balls, and pillows can be used for support.

Bearing-down efforts

As the fetal head reaches the pelvic floor, most women experience the urge to bear down. Reflexively the woman will begin to exert downward pressure by contracting her abdominal muscles while relaxing her pelvic floor. This bearing down is an involuntary response to the Ferguson reflex. A strong expiratory grunt or groan (vocalization) often accompanies pushing when the woman exhales as she pushes.

When coaching women to push, the nurse should encourage them to push as they feel like pushing (instinctive, spontaneous pushing) rather than to give a prolonged push on command (Hansen, Clark, & Foster, 2002; Roberts, 2003).

Women will usually begin to push naturally as the contraction increases in intensity and the Ferguson reflex strengthens. The nurse should monitor the woman's breathing so that the woman does not hold her breath for more than 5 to 7 seconds at a time and should remind her to ventilate her lungs fully by taking deep cleansing breaths before and after each contraction. Bearing down while exhaling (open-glottis pushing) and taking breaths between bearing-down efforts help maintain adequate oxygen levels for the mother and fetus and result in approximately five pushes during a contraction, with each push lasting about 5 seconds (Mayberry et al., 2000). Women who use spontaneous pushing are less likely to have second- or third-degree lacerations or episiotomies (Roberts, 2002).

Prolonged breath-holding, or sustained, directed bearing down, which is still a common practice, may trigger the Valsalva maneuver, which occurs when the woman closes the glottis (closed-glottis pushing), thereby increasing intrathoracic and cardiovascular pressure, reducing cardiac output, and inhibiting perfusion of the uterus and the placenta. In addition, breath-holding for more than 5 to 7 seconds causes the perfusion of oxygen across the placenta to be diminished, resulting in fetal hypoxia. This approach to bearing down is harmful or ineffective and should be discouraged (Enkin et al., 2000).

A woman may reach the second stage of labor and then experience a lack of readiness to complete the process and give birth to her child. By recognizing that a woman may experience a need to hold back the birth of her baby, the nurse can then address the woman's concerns and effectively coach the woman during this stage of labor.

To ensure the slow birth of the fetal head, the woman is encouraged to control the urge to bear down by coaching her to take panting breaths or to exhale slowly through pursed lips as the baby's head crowns. At this point, the woman needs simple, clear directions from one person.

Amnesia between contractions often is pronounced in the second stage, and the woman may have to be roused to get her to cooperate in the bearing-down process. Parents who have attended childbirth education classes may have devised a set of verbal cues for the laboring woman to follow. It is helpful for them to have these cues printed on a card that can be attached to the head of the bed so that the nurse can better substitute as coach if the partner has to leave.

Fetal heart rate and pattern

As noted previously, the FHR must be checked. If the baseline rate begins to slow, if there is a loss of variability, or if deceleration patterns develop (e.g., late, variable), prompt treatment must be initiated. The woman can be turned on her side to reduce the pressure of the uterus against the ascending vena cava and descending aorta (see Fig. 14-5), and oxygen can be administered by mask at 8 to 10 L/min (Tucker, 2004). This is often all that is necessary to restore a reassuring pattern. If the FHR and pattern do

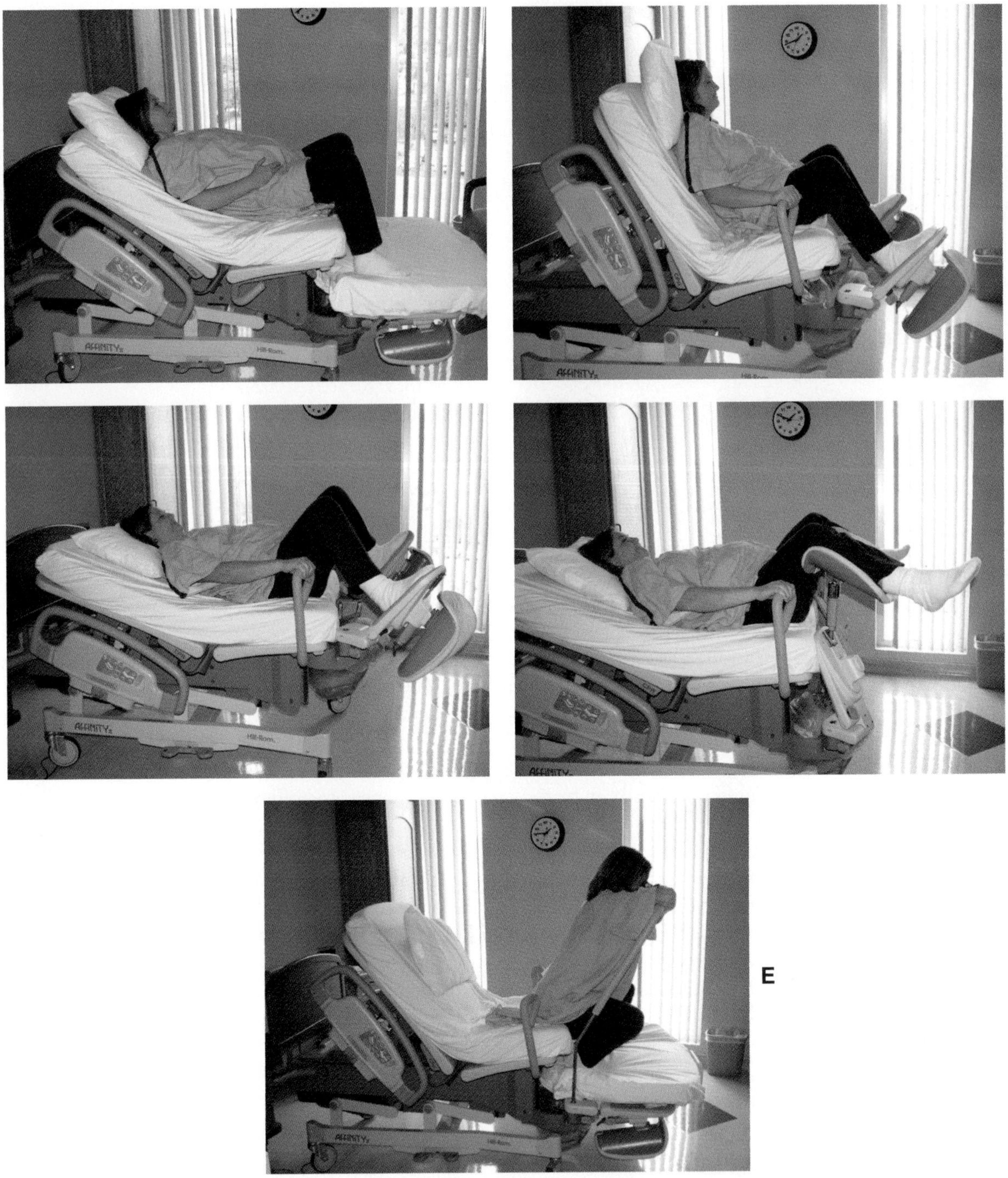

Fig. 14-17 The versatility of today's birthing bed makes it practical in a variety of settings. NOTE: OB table used for lithotomy position. **A,** Labor bed. **B,** Birth chair. **C,** Birth bed. **D,** OB table. **E,** Squatting or birth bar. (Courtesy Julie Perry Nelson, Gilbert, AZ.)

not become reassuring immediately, the primary health care provider should be notified quickly because medical intervention to hasten the birth may be indicated.

Support of the father or partner

During the second stage, the woman needs continuous support and coaching (see Table 14-7). Because the coaching process can be physically and emotionally tiring for support persons, the nurse offers them nourishment and fluids and encourages them to take short breaks. If birth occurs in an LDR or LDRP room, the partner may be allowed to wear street clothes or be required to wear a clean scrub outfit, cap, and mask (for the birth). The support person who attends the birth in a delivery room is instructed to put on a cover gown or scrub clothes, mask, hat, and shoe covers, as required by agency policy. The nurse also specifies support measures that can be used for the laboring woman and points out areas of the room in which the partner can move freely.

Partners are encouraged to be present at the birth of their infants if this is in keeping with their cultural and personal expectations and beliefs. In this way the psychologic closeness of the family unit is maintained, and the partner can continue to provide the supportive care given during labor. The woman and her partner need to have an equal opportunity to initiate the attachment process with the baby.

LEGAL TIP Documentation

Documentation of all observations (e.g., maternal vital signs, FHR and pattern, progress of labor) and nursing interventions, including patient response, should be done concurrent with care. The course of labor and the maternal-fetal response may change without warning. It is important that all documentation be accurate, complete, timely, and according to agency policy.

Supplies, instruments, and equipment

To prepare for birth in any setting, the birthing area is usually set up during the transition phase for nulliparous women and during the active phase for multiparous women.

The birthing bed or table is prepared, and instruments are arranged on the instrument table (Fig. 14-18). Standard procedures are followed for gloving, identifying and opening sterile packages, adding sterile supplies to the instrument table, unwrapping sterile instruments, and handing them to the primary health care provider. The crib or radiant warmer and equipment are readied for the support and stabilization of the infant (Fig. 14-19).

The items used for birth may vary among different facilities; therefore each facility's procedure manual should be consulted to determine the protocols specific to that facility.

The nurse estimates the time until the birth will occur and notifies the primary health care provider if he or she is not in the patient's room. Even the most experienced nurse can miscalculate the time left before birth occurs; therefore every nurse who attends a woman in labor must be prepared to assist with an emergency birth if the primary health care provider is not present (Box 14-8).

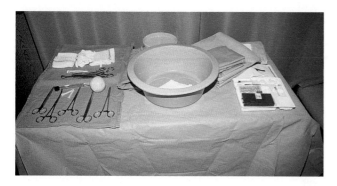

Fig. 14-18 Instrument table. (Courtesy Marjorie Pyle, RNC, Lifecircle, Costa Mesa, CA.)

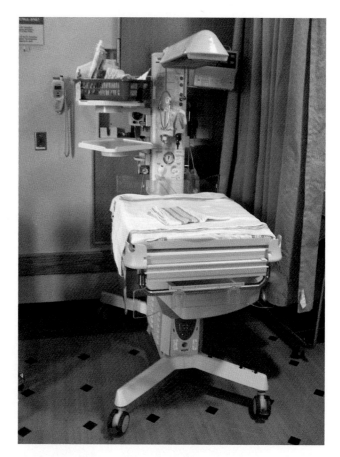

Fig. 14-19 Radiant warmer for newborn. (Courtesy Dee Lowdermilk, Chapel Hill, NC.)

Birth in a delivery room or birthing room

The woman will need assistance if she must move from the labor bed to the delivery table (Fig. 14-20). The various positions assumed for birth in a delivery room are the Sims or lateral position in which the attendant supports the upper part of the woman's leg, the dorsal position (supine position with one hip elevated), and the lithotomy position.

The lithotomy position has been the position most commonly used for birth in Western cultures, although this practice is slowly changing. The lithotomy position makes it more convenient for the primary health care provider to deal with complications that arise (see Fig. 14-17, *D*). To place the woman in this position, her buttocks are brought to the edge of the table and her legs are placed in stirrups. Care must be taken to pad the stirrups, to raise and place both legs simultaneously, and to adjust the shanks of the stirrups so that the calves of the legs are supported. There should be no pressure on the popliteal space. If the stirrups are not the same height, ligaments in the woman's back can be strained as she bears down, leading to considerable discomfort in the postpartum period. The lower portion of the table may be dropped down and rolled back under the table.

It should be noted that the routine use of a supine or lithotomy position for labor and birth has been identified

Video—Childbirth (vaginal and cesarean)

Text continued on p. 442.

BOX 14-8

Normal Vaginal Childbirth

FIRST STAGE

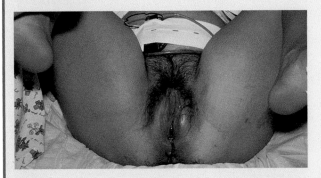

Anteroposterior slit. Vertex visible during contraction.

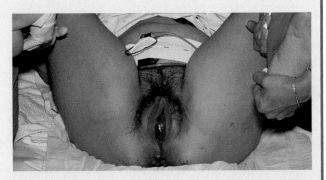

Oval opening. Vertex presenting. NOTE: Nurse *(on left)* is wearing gloves, but support person *(on right)* is not.

SECOND STAGE

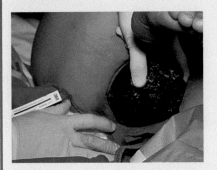

Crowning.

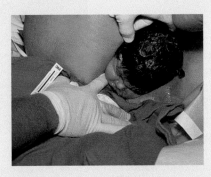

Nurse-midwife using Ritgen maneuver as head is born by extension.

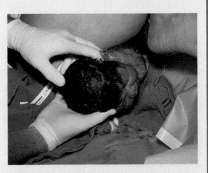

After nurse-midwife checks for nuchal cord, she supports head during external rotation and restitution.

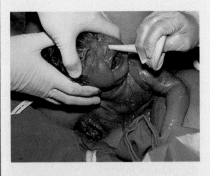

Use of bulb syringe to suction mucus.

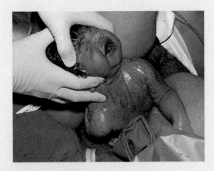

Birth of posterior shoulder.

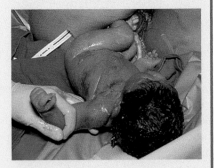

Birth of newborn by slow expulsion.

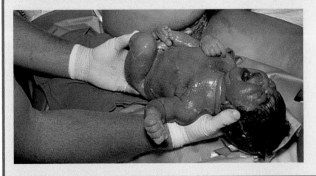

Second stage complete. Note that newborn is not completely pink yet.

Courtesy Michael S. Clement, MD, Mesa, AZ.

BOX 14-8

Normal Vaginal Childbirth—cont'd

THIRD STAGE

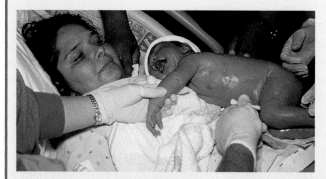

Newborn placed on mother's abdomen while cord is clamped and cut.

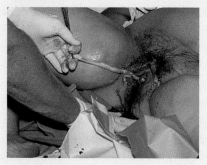

Note increased bleeding as placenta separates.

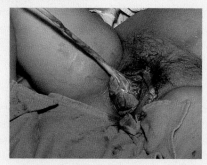

Expulsion of placenta.

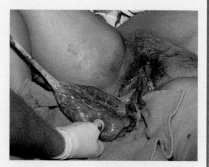

Expulsion is complete, marking the end of the third stage.

THE NEWBORN

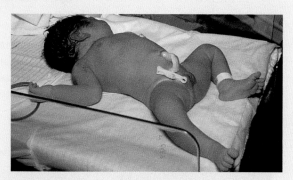

Newborn awaiting assessment. Note that color is almost completely pink.

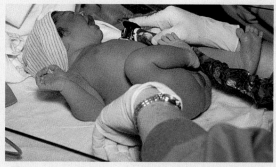

Newborn assessment under radiant warmer.

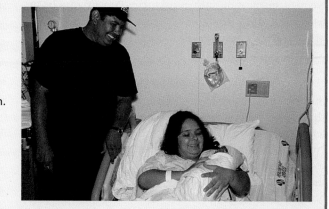

Parents admiring their newborn.

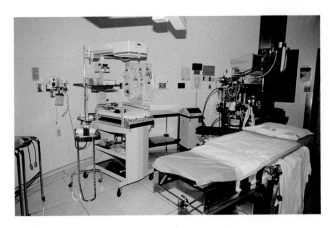

Fig. 14-20 Delivery room. (Courtesy Michael S. Clement, MD, Mesa, AZ.)

✳ as a clearly harmful or ineffective practice and should be discouraged (Enkin et al., 2000).

The maternal position for birth in a birthing room varies from a lithotomy position, with the woman's feet in stirrups, to one in which her feet rest on footrests while she holds onto a squat bar, to a side-lying position with the woman's upper leg supported by the coach, nurse, or squat bar. The foot of the bed can be removed so that the primary health care provider attending the birth can gain better perineal access for performing an episiotomy, delivering a large baby, using forceps or vacuum extractor, or getting access to the emerging head to facilitate suctioning. Otherwise the foot of the bed is left in place and lowered slightly to form a ledge that allows access for birth and that also serves as a place to lay the newborn (see Fig. 14-16).

Once the woman is positioned for birth either in a delivery room or birthing room, the vulva and perineum may be cleansed. Hospital protocols and the preferences of primary health care providers for cleansing may vary.

The labor nurse continues to coach and encourage the woman. The nurse auscultates the FHR or evaluates the monitor tracing every 5 to 15 minutes, depending on whether the woman is at low or high risk for problems or per protocol of the birthing facility, or continuously monitors the FHR with electronic monitoring. The primary health care provider is kept informed of the FHR and pattern (Tucker, 2004). An oxytocic medication such as oxytocin (Pitocin) may be prepared so that it is ready to be administered after expulsion of the placenta. Standard Precautions should always be followed as care is administered during the process of labor and birth (see Box 14-3).

In the delivery room the primary health care provider puts on a cap, a mask that has a shield or protective eyewear, and shoe covers. Hands are scrubbed, a sterile gown (with waterproof front and sleeves) is donned, and gloves are put on. Nurses attending the birth also may need to wear caps, protective eyewear, masks, gowns, and gloves. The woman may then be draped with sterile drapes. In the birthing room, Standard Precautions are observed, but the amount and types of protective coverings worn by those in attendance may vary.

Nursing contact with the parents is maintained by touching, verbal comforting, explaining the reasons for care, and sharing in the parents' joy at the birth of their child.

Water birth

There is evidence that immersion in water during first stage labor can reduce the amount of pain and anxiety in labor and does not appear to affect neonatal outcomes (Benfield, 2002; Cluett et al., 2004). However, the effects of immersion during birth and in the third stage have not been determined by randomized controlled trials that have a large enough sample to make a determination about maternal and neonatal outcomes.

If a woman wishes to have a water birth (Fig. 14-21) in the United States, the newborn will usually be removed from the water immediately after birth (Waterbirth International, 2005). The infant can be placed in the mother's arms until the cord is cut. The woman usually is assisted from the tub to the bed to deliver the placenta.

Mechanism of birth: vertex presentation

The three phases of the spontaneous birth of a fetus in a vertex presentation are (1) birth of the head, (2) birth of the shoulders, and (3) birth of the body and extremities (see Chapter 11).

With voluntary bearing-down efforts, the head appears at the introitus (Fig. 14-22). Crowning occurs when the widest part of the head (the biparietal diameter) distends the vulva just before birth. The birth attendant may apply mineral oil to the perineum and stretch it as the head is crowning. Immediately before birth, the perineal musculature becomes greatly distended. If an episiotomy (incision into the perineum to enlarge vaginal outlet) is necessary, it is done at this time to minimize soft tissue damage. Local anesthetic is administered before the episiotomy.

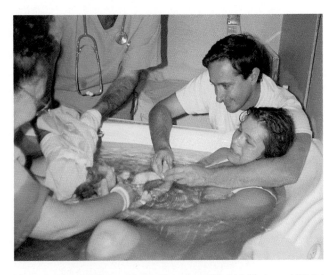

Fig. 14-21 Water birth. (Courtesy Global Maternal/Child Health Association, Inc., Wilsonville, OR.)

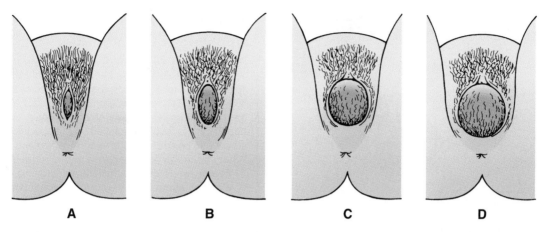

Fig. 14-22 Beginning birth with vertex presenting. **A,** Anteroposterior slit. **B,** Oval opening. **C,** Circular shape. **D,** Crowning.

The physician or nurse midwife may use a hands-on approach to control the birth of the head, believing that guarding the perineum results in a gradual birth that will prevent fetal intracranial injury, protect maternal tissues, and reduce postpartum perineal pain. This approach involves (1) applying pressure against the rectum, drawing it downward to aid in flexing the head as the back of the neck catches under the symphysis pubis; (2) then applying upward pressure from the coccygeal region (modified Ritgen maneuver) (Fig. 14-23) to extend the head during the actual birth, thereby protecting the musculature of the perineum; and (3) assisting the mother with voluntary control of the bearing-down efforts by coaching her to pant while letting uterine forces expel the fetus.

Some health care providers use a hands-poised (hands-off) approach when attending a birth. In this approach, hands are prepared to place light pressure on the fetal head to prevent rapid expulsion. Hands are not placed on the perineum or used to assist with birth of the shoulders and body.

The umbilical cord often encircles the neck (nuchal cord) but rarely so tightly as to cause hypoxia. After the head is born, gentle palpation is used to feel for the cord. If present, the cord should be slipped gently over the head (Fig. 14-24). If the loop is tight or if there is a second loop, the cord is clamped twice, cut between the clamps, and unwound from around the neck before the birth is allowed to continue. Mucus, blood, or meconium in the nasal or oral passages may prevent the newborn from breathing. To eliminate this problem, moist gauze sponges are used to wipe the nose and mouth. A bulb syringe is first inserted into the mouth and oropharynx to aspirate contents, and then the nares are cleared in the same fashion while the head is supported.

Prevention of meconium aspiration. If meconium has been present in the amniotic fluid during labor, preparations are made for wall suction, or in some cases a De Lee suction apparatus is placed on the sterile field for use. Fluids are withdrawn from the infant's mouth and nose before the first breath is taken to prevent meconium aspiration. Use of the De Lee device with oral suction to withdraw fluid

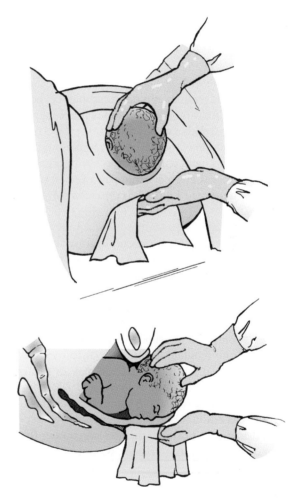

Fig. 14-23 Birth of head with modified Ritgen maneuver. Note control to prevent too rapid birth of head.

from the infant should be avoided unless the suction device is designed so that it can keep mucus from entering the user's airway.

The time of birth is the precise time when the entire body is out of the mother. In case of multiple births, each birth

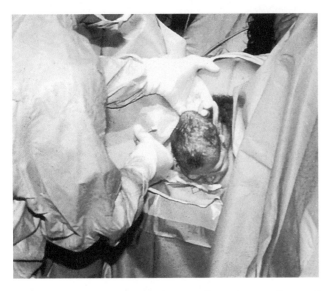

Fig. 14-24 Loosening nuchal cord (umbilical cord around neck). (Courtesy Marjorie Pyle, RNC, Lifecircle, Costa Mesa, CA.)

would be noted in the same way. Time of birth must be recorded on the record.

If the newborn's condition is not compromised, he or she may be placed on the mother's abdomen immediately after birth and covered with a warm, dry blanket. The cord may be clamped at this time, and the primary health care provider may ask if the woman's partner would like to cut the cord. If so, the partner is given a sterile pair of scissors and instructed to cut the cord 1 inch (2.5 cm) above the clamp (see Fig. 1-2).

Use of fundal pressure. Fundal pressure is the application of gentle, steady pressure against the fundus of the uterus to facilitate the vaginal birth. Historically it has been used when the administration of analgesia and anesthesia decreased the woman's ability to push during the birth, in cases of shoulder dystocia, and when second-stage fetal bradycardia or other nonreassuring FHR patterns were present. Use of fundal pressure by nurses is not advised because there is no standard technique available for this maneuver, and no current legal, professional, or regulatory standards exist for its use (Simpson & Knox, 2001). In cases of shoulder dystocia, fundal pressure is not recommended: the all-fours position (Gaskin maneuver), suprapubic pressure, and maternal position changes are among the recommended interventions (Baxley & Gobbo, 2004) (see Chapter 24).

Immediate assessments and care of the newborn

The care given immediately after the birth focuses on assessing and stabilizing the newborn. The nurse's primary responsibility at this time is the infant, because the primary health care provider is involved with the delivery of the placenta and the care of the mother. The nurse must watch the infant for any signs of distress and initiate appropriate interventions should any appear.

 Critical Thinking Exercise

Applying Fundal Pressure

Myra is a gravida 1, para 0 who has been in labor for 18 hours; her cervix has been completely effaced and 10 cm dilated for 2½ hours; the station has been at +1 for 45 minutes. She has been pushing for 2 hours and is exhausted. To assist in descent of the fetus, the primary health care provider has asked you to apply fundal pressure while he stretches the vaginal orifice and perineum. What should be your response to this request?

1 Evidence—Is there sufficient evidence to draw conclusions about what your proper action should be?
2 Assumptions—What assumptions can be made about the following issues?
   a. Benefits of fundal pressure
   b. Risks of fundal pressure
   c. Contraindications to fundal pressure
   d. Alternative approaches to the use of fundal pressure
3 What implications and priorities for nursing care can be drawn at this time?
4 Does the evidence objectively support your conclusion?
5 Are there alternative perspectives to your conclusion?

A brief assessment of the newborn can be performed while the mother is holding the infant. This includes checking the infant's airway and Apgar score. Maintaining a patent airway, supporting respiratory effort, and preventing cold stress by drying the newborn and covering the newborn with a warmed blanket or placing him or her under a radiant warmer are the major priorities in terms of the newborn's immediate care. Further examination, identification procedures, and care can be postponed until later in the third stage of labor or early in the fourth stage.

Perineal trauma related to childbirth

Lacerations. Most acute injuries and lacerations of the perineum, vagina, uterus, and their support tissues occur during childbirth. Some injuries to the supporting tissues, whether they were acute or nonacute and whether they were repaired or not, may lead to genitourinary and sexual problems later in life (e.g., pelvic relaxation, uterine prolapse, cystocele, rectocele, dyspareunia, urinary and bowel dysfunction).

Some damage occurs during every birth to the soft tissues of the birth canal and adjacent structures. The tendency to sustain lacerations varies with each woman; that is, the soft tissue in some women may be less distensible. Damage usually is more pronounced in nulliparous women because the tissues are firmer and more resistant than are those in multiparous women. Heredity also may be a factor. For example, the tissue of light-skinned women, especially those with reddish hair, is not so readily distensible as that of darker-skinned women, and healing may be less efficient. The perineal skin and vaginal mucosa may appear intact, but numerous small lacerations in underlying muscle and its fascia may be obscured. Damage to pelvic supports usually is readily apparent and is repaired after birth.

Immediate repair promotes healing, limits residual damage, and decreases the possibility of infection. Immediately after birth, the cervix, vagina, and perineum are inspected for damage. In addition, during the early postpartum period, the nurse and primary health care provider continue to inspect the perineum carefully and evaluate lochia and symptoms to identify any previously missed damage.

Perineal lacerations. Perineal lacerations usually occur as the fetal head is being born. The extent of the laceration is defined in terms of its depth:

1. *First degree:* Laceration that extends through the skin and structures superficial to muscles
2. *Second degree:* Laceration that extends through muscles of the perineal body
3. *Third degree:* Laceration that continues through the anal sphincter muscle
4. *Fourth degree:* Laceration that also involves the anterior rectal wall

Perineal injury often is accompanied by small lacerations on the medial surfaces of the labia minora below the pubic rami and to the sides of the urethra (periurethral) and clitoris. Lacerations in this highly vascular area often result in profuse bleeding. Special attention must be paid to third- and fourth-degree lacerations so that the woman retains fecal continence. Measures are taken to promote soft stools (e.g., roughage, fluid, activity, and stool softeners) to increase the woman's comfort and foster healing. Antimicrobial therapy may be instituted in some cases. Enemas and suppositories are contraindicated for these women.

Simple perineal injuries usually heal without permanent disability, regardless of whether they were repaired. However it is easier to repair a new perineal injury to prevent sequelae than it is to correct long-term damage.

Vaginal and urethral lacerations. Vaginal lacerations often occur in conjunction with perineal lacerations. Vaginal lacerations tend to extend up the lateral walls (sulci) and, if deep enough, involve the levator ani. Additional injury may occur high in the vaginal vault near the level of the ischial spines. Vaginal vault lacerations may be circular and may result from use of forceps to rotate the fetal head, rapid fetal descent, or precipitate birth.

Cervical injuries. Cervical injuries occur when the cervix retracts over the advancing fetal head. These cervical lacerations occur at the lateral angles of the external os; most are shallow, and bleeding is minimal. More extensive lacerations may extend to the vaginal vault or beyond it into the lower uterine segment; serious bleeding may occur. Extensive lacerations may follow hasty attempts to enlarge the cervical opening artificially or to deliver the fetus before full cervical dilation is achieved. Injuries to the cervix can have adverse effects on future pregnancies and childbirths.

Episiotomy. An episiotomy is an incision made in the perineum to enlarge the vaginal outlet. It is performed more commonly in the United States and Canada than in Europe. The side-lying position for birth, used routinely in Europe, causes less tension on the perineum, making possible a gradual stretching of the perineum with fewer indications for episiotomies.

Clear evidence exists that routine performance of an episiotomy for birth is a form of care that is likely to be harmful or ineffective (Enkin et al., 2000; Hofmeyr, 2005). Routine performance of episiotomies has declined in the United States since the 1990s, most likely related to the clear evidence regarding the harmful effects of episiotomy in terms of increased postpartum pain, blood loss, risk for infection, and occurrence of third- and fourth-degree lacerations (Weeks & Kozak, 2001). The practice in many settings now is to support the perineum manually during birth and allow the perineum to tear rather than perform an episiotomy. Tears are often smaller than an episiotomy, are repaired easily or not at all, and heal quickly. The pain and discomfort resulting from episiotomies can interfere with mother-infant interaction, breastfeeding, reestablishment of sexual relationship with partner, and even emotional recovery after birth.

The type of episiotomy is designated by the site and direction of the incision (Fig. 14-25). Midline (median) episiotomy is most commonly used in the United States. It is effective, easily repaired, and generally the least painful. However, midline episiotomies also are associated with a higher incidence of third- and fourth-degree lacerations. Sphincter tone is usually restored after primary healing and a good repair.

Mediolateral episiotomy is used in operative births when the need for posterior extension is likely. Although a fourth-degree laceration may be prevented, a third-degree laceration may occur. The blood loss also is greater and the repair more difficult and painful than with midline episiotomies. It is also more painful in the postpartum period, and the pain lasts longer.

Risk factors associated with perineal trauma (e.g., episiotomy, lacerations) include nulliparity, maternal position,

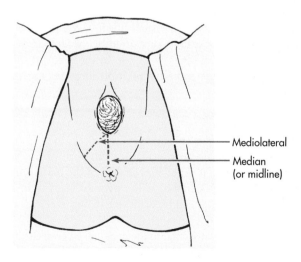

Mediolateral

Median (or midline)

Fig. 14-25 Types of episiotomies.

pelvic inadequacy (e.g., narrow subpubic arch with a constricted outlet), fetal malpresentation and position (e.g., breech, occiput posterior position), large (macrosomic) infants, use of instruments to facilitate birth, prolonged second stage of labor, fetal distress, and rapid labor in which there is insufficient time for the perineum to stretch. The rate of episiotomies also is higher when obstetricians rather than nurse midwives attend births. (Shorten, Donsante, & Shorten, 2002).

Alternative measures for perineal management, such as warm compresses, manual support, and massage (e.g., prenatal and intrapartum), have been shown to reduce, to varying degrees, the incidence of episiotomies, but further research is recommended. Use of Kegel exercises in the prenatal and postpartum periods improves and restores the tone and strength of the perineal muscles. Health practices, including good nutrition and appropriate hygienic measures, help maintain the integrity and suppleness of the perineal tissue. Nurses acting as advocates can encourage women to use alternative birthing positions that reduce pressure on the perineum (e.g., lateral position) and to use spontaneous bearing-down efforts. In addition, nurses can educate other health care providers about measures to preserve perineal integrity and to be more flexible in defining the maximal limit for the duration of the second stage of labor as long as the maternal-fetal unit is stable.

Emergency childbirth

Even under the best of circumstances, there probably will come a time when the perinatal nurse will be required to assist with the birth of an infant without medical assistance. Because it is neither possible nor desirable to prevent impending birth, the perinatal nurse must be able to function independently and be skilled in the safe birth of a vertex fetus (see Box 14-7).

A lateral Sims position may be the position of choice for birth when (1) the birth is progressing rapidly and there is insufficient time for slow distention of the perineum; (2) the fetal head seems too large to pass through the introitus without laceration, and episiotomy is not possible; or (3) the apparent size of the fetus is consistent with possible shoulder dystocia. In the lateral Sims position, less stress is placed on the perineum, and better visualization of the perineum is possible as the upper leg is supported by the woman's partner or the nurse (see Fig. 14-15, *A*). In the event of shoulder dystocia, the lateral Sims position increases the space needed for birth.

THIRD STAGE OF LABOR

The **third stage of labor** lasts from the birth of the baby until the placenta is expelled. The goal in the management of the third stage of labor is the prompt separation and expulsion of the placenta, achieved in the easiest, safest manner.

The placenta is attached to the decidual layer of the basal plate's thin endometrium by numerous fibrous anchor villi—much in the same way as a postage stamp is attached to a sheet of postage stamps. After the birth of the fetus, strong uterine contractions cause the placental site to shrink markedly. This causes the anchor villi to break and the placenta to separate from its attachments. Normally the first few strong contractions that occur 5 to 7 minutes after the baby's birth cause the placenta to be sheared away from the basal plate. A placenta cannot detach itself from a flaccid (relaxed) uterus because the placental site is not reduced in size.

Placental Separation and Expulsion

Placental separation is indicated by the following signs (Fig. 14-26):

- A firmly contracting fundus
- A change in the uterus from a discoid to a globular ovoid shape as the placenta moves into the lower uterine segment
- A sudden gush of dark blood from the introitus
- Apparent lengthening of the umbilical cord as the placenta descends to the introitus
- The finding of vaginal fullness (the placenta) on vaginal or rectal examination or of fetal membranes at the introitus

Depending on the preferences of the primary health care provider, an expectant or active approach may be used to manage the third stage of labor. Expectant management (watchful waiting) involves the natural, spontaneous separation and expulsion of the placenta by efforts of the mother with clamping and cutting of the cord after pulsation ceases. It may involve the use of gravity or nipple stimulation to facilitate separation and expulsion, but no oxytocic (uterotonic) medications are given. A quiet, relaxed environment that supports close skin-to-skin contact between mother and newborn also promotes the release of endogenous oxytocin.

Active management facilitates placenta separation and expulsion with administration of one or more oxytocic (uterotonic) medications after the birth of the anterior shoulder of the fetus, clamping and cutting of the umbilical cord immediately, and delivery of the placenta by application of controlled cord traction when signs of separation are noted. Research findings support the superiority of active management in terms of less blood loss and reduced risk of hemorrhage and other complications of the third stage of labor (Brucker, 2001; Prendiville, Elbourne, & McDonald, 2000). Active management of the third stage of labor is a beneficial form of care (Enkin et al., 2000).

To assist in the delivery of the placenta, the woman is instructed to push when signs of separation have occurred. If possible, the placenta should be expelled by maternal effort during a uterine contraction. Alternate compression and elevation of the fundus, plus minimal, controlled traction on the umbilical cord, may be used to facilitate delivery of the placenta and amniotic membranes. Oxytocics

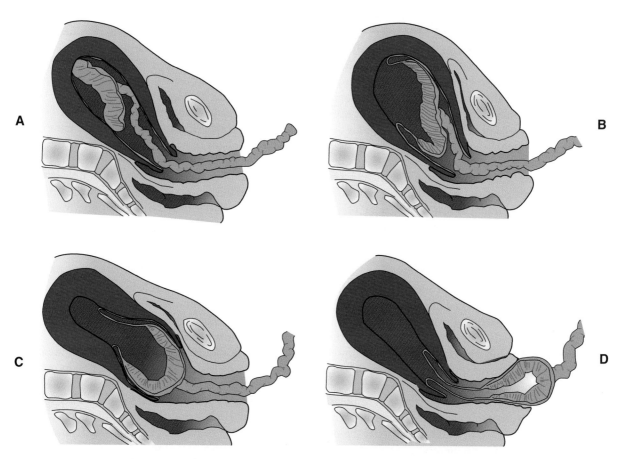

Fig. 14-26 Third stage of labor. **A,** Placenta begins to separate in central portion, accompanied by retroplacental bleeding. Uterus changes from discoid to globular shape. **B,** Placenta completes separation and enters lower uterine segment. Uterus is globular shape. **C,** Placenta enters vagina, cord is seen to lengthen, and there may be an increase in bleeding. **D,** Expulsion (delivery) of placenta and completion of third stage.

may be administered after the placenta is removed because they stimulate the uterus to contract, thereby helping to prevent hemorrhage.

Whether the placenta first appears by its shiny fetal surface (Schultze mechanism) or turns to show its dark roughened maternal surface first (Duncan mechanism) is of no clinical importance.

After the placenta and the amniotic membranes emerge, the primary health care provider examines them for intactness to ensure that no portion remains in the uterine cavity (i.e., no fragments of the placenta or membranes are retained) (Fig. 14-27).

Some women and their families may have culturally based beliefs regarding the care of the placenta and the manner of its disposal after birth, viewing the care and disposal of the placenta as a way of protecting the newborn from bad luck and illness. Requests by the woman to take the placenta home and dispose of it according to her customs may be at odds with health care agency policies, especially those related

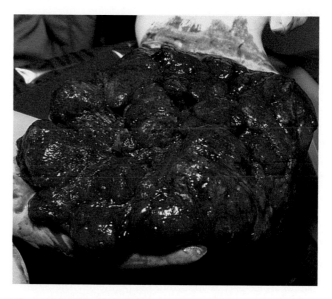

Fig. 14-27 Examination of the placenta. (Courtesy Michael S. Clement, MD, Mesa, AZ.)

to infection control and the disposal of biologic wastes. Many cultures follow specific rules regarding the disposal of the placenta in terms of method (burning, drying, burying, eating), site for disposal (in or near the home), and timing of disposal (immediately after birth, time of day, astrologic signs). Disposal rituals may vary according to the gender of the child and the length of time before another child is desired. If eaten, the placenta can be a means of restoring a woman's well-being after birth or ensuring high-quality breast milk. Health care providers can provide culturally sensitive health care by encouraging women and their families to express their wishes regarding the care and disposal of the placenta and by establishing a policy to fulfill these requests (D'Avanzo & Geissler, 2003; Lemon, 2002; Molina, 2001).

Maternal Physical Status

Physiologic changes after birth are profound. The cardiac output increases rapidly as maternal circulation to the placenta ceases and the pooled blood from the lower extremities is mobilized. The pulse rate slows in response to the change in cardiac output and tends to remain slightly slower than the prepregnancy rate for approximately 1 week.

Soon after the birth, the woman's blood pressure usually returns to prepregnancy levels. Several factors contribute to an elevated blood pressure at this time: the excitement of the second stage, certain medications, and the time of day (blood pressure is highest during the late afternoon). Analgesics and anesthetics may cause hypotension to develop in the hour after birth.

The major risk for women during the third stage of labor is postpartum hemorrhage. When the primary health care provider completes the delivery of the placenta, the nurse observes the mother for signs of excessive blood loss, including alteration in vital signs, pallor, light-headedness, restlessness, decreased urinary output, and alteration in level of consciousness and orientation.

Because of the rapid cardiovascular changes taking place (e.g., the increased intracranial pressure during pushing and the rapid increase in cardiac output), the risk of rupture of a preexisting cerebral aneurysm and the risk of formation of pulmonary emboli are greater than usual during this period. Another dangerous, unpredictable problem that may occur is the formation of an amniotic fluid embolism (see Chapter 24).

Women with a history of cardiac disorders are at increased risk for cardiac decompensation and pulmonary edema as a result of the circulatory changes associated with the birth of the fetus and expulsion of the placenta. The nurse should carefully assess the woman's respiratory pattern and effort, especially in the early postpartum period.

When the third stage is complete and any lacerations are repaired or an episiotomy is sutured, the vulvar area is gently cleansed with warm water or normal saline, and a perineal pad or an ice pack is applied to the perineum. The birthing bed or table is repositioned, and the woman's legs are lowered simultaneously from the stirrups if she gave birth in a lithotomy position. Drapes are removed, and dry linen is placed under the woman's buttocks; she is provided with a clean gown and a blanket, which is warmed, if needed. She is assisted into her bed if she is to be transferred from the birthing area to the recovery area; assistance also is necessary to move the woman from the birthing table onto a bed if the woman has had anesthesia and does not have full use of her lower extremities. The side rails are raised during the transfer. She may be given the baby to hold during the transfer or the father or partner may carry the baby or transport the baby in a crib, either to the nursery or to the recovery area. If the woman labors, gives birth, and recovers in the same bed and room, she is refreshed following the protocol already described. Maternal and neonatal assessments for the fourth stage of labor are instituted. Box 14-8 summarizes normal vaginal childbirth.

Care of the Family

Most parents enjoy being able to handle, hold, explore, and examine the baby immediately after birth. Both parents can assist with the thorough drying of the infant. The infant may be wrapped in a receiving blanket and placed on the woman's abdomen. If skin-to-skin contact is desired, the unwrapped infant may be placed on the woman's abdomen and then covered with a warm blanket.

Holding the newborn next to her skin helps the mother maintain the baby's body heat and provides skin-to-skin contact; care must be taken to keep the head warm. Stockinette caps are sometimes used to cover the newborn's head.

Many women wish to begin breastfeeding their newborns at this time to take advantage of the infant's alert state *(first period of reactivity)* and to stimulate the production of oxytocin that promotes contraction of the uterus. Others prefer to wait until the newborn, parents, and older siblings are together in the recovery area. In some cultures (e.g., Vietnamese and Hispanic), breastfeeding is not acceptable to some women until the milk comes in.

The woman usually feels some discomfort while the primary health care provider carries out the postbirth vaginal examination. The nurse can assist the woman to use breathing and relaxation or distraction techniques to assist her in dealing with the discomfort. During this time, the nurse assesses the newborn's physical condition; the baby can be weighed and measured, given eye prophylaxis and a vitamin K injection, given an identification bracelet, wrapped in warm blankets, and then given to the partner or back to the mother to hold when she is ready.

Family-newborn relationships

The woman's reaction to the sight of her newborn may range from excited outbursts of laughing, talking, and even crying to apparent apathy. A polite smile and nod may be her only acknowledgment of the comments of nurses and the primary health care provider. Occasionally the reaction is one of anger or indifference; the woman turns away from the baby, concentrates on her own pain, and sometimes makes hostile comments. These varied reactions can arise from pleasure, exhaustion, or deep disappointment. When

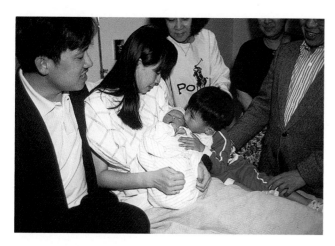

Fig. 14-28 Big brother becomes acquainted with new baby sister. (Courtesy Marjorie Pyle, RNC, Lifecircle, Costa Mesa, CA.)

evaluating parent-newborn interactions after birth, the nurse also should consider the cultural characteristics of the woman and her family and the expected behaviors of that culture. In some cultures, the birth of a male child is preferred, and women may grieve when a female child is born (D'Avanzo & Geissler, 2003).

Whatever the reaction and its cause may be, the woman needs continuing acceptance and support from all staff. Notation regarding the parents' reaction to the newborn can be made in the recovery record. Nurses can assess this reaction by asking themselves such questions as, "How do the parents look?" "What do they say?" "What do they do?" Further assessment of the parent-newborn relationship can be conducted as care is given during the period of recovery. This is especially important if warning signs (e.g., passive or hostile reactions to the newborn, disappointment with sex or appearance of the newborn, absence of eye contact, or limited interaction of parents with each other) were noted immediately after birth. The nurse may find it helpful to discuss any warning signs that may have been noted with the woman's primary health care provider.

Siblings, who may have appeared only remotely interested in the final phases of the second stage, tend to experience renewed interest and excitement when the newborn appears. They can be encouraged to hold the baby (Fig. 14-28).

Parents usually respond to praise of their newborn. Many need to be reassured that the dusky appearance of their baby's extremities immediately after birth is normal until circulation is well established. If appropriate, the nurse should explain the reason for the molding of the newborn's head. Information about hospital routine can be communicated. It is important, however, for nurses to recognize that the cultural background of the parents may influence their expectations regarding the care and handling of their newborn immediately after birth. For example, some traditional Southeast Asians believe that the head should not be touched because it is the most sacred part of a person's body. They also believe that praise of the baby is dangerous because jealous spirits may then cause the baby harm or take it away (D'Avanzo & Geissler, 2003). Hospital staff members, by their interest and concern, can provide the environment for making this a satisfying experience for parents, family, and significant others.

Determining a woman's satisfaction with and impressions of her childbirth experience is a critical component in the provision of high-quality maternal-newborn health care that meets the individual needs of women and families using these services.

COMMUNITY ACTIVITY

Conduct a survey in your area (e.g., county, health district) to determine what resources are available for childbirth preparation. These may include doula services, siblings at birth classes, grandparent classes, childbirth classes for new parents, review classes for parents who have children, support groups, and classes to introduce pets to new babies. Evaluate how well these resources and services are advertised and promoted and their accessibility (time and place) and affordability. Evaluate whether or not these services and resources consider differences in birth practices among the various ethnic groups that live in the area you surveyed.

Key Points

- The onset of labor may be difficult to determine for both nulliparous and multiparous women.

- The familiar environment of her home is most often the ideal place for a woman during the latent phase of the first stage of labor.

- The nurse assumes much of the responsibility for assessing the progress of labor and for keeping the primary health care provider informed about progress in labor and deviations from expected findings.

- The FHR and pattern reveal the fetal response to the stress of the labor process.

- Meconium-stained amniotic fluid is not always indicative of fetal distress associated with hypoxia.

- Assessment of the laboring woman's urinary output and bladder is critical to ensure her progress and to prevent injury to the bladder.

- Regardless of the actual labor and birth experience, the woman's or couple's perception of the birth experience is most likely to be positive when events

Continued

Key Points—cont'd

and performances are consistent with expectations, especially in terms of maintaining control and adequacy of pain relief.

- The woman's level of anxiety may increase when she does not understand what is being said to her about her labor because of the medical terminology used or because of a language barrier.

- Coaching, emotional support, and comfort measures assist the woman to use her energy constructively in relaxing and working with the contractions.

- The progress of labor is enhanced when a woman changes her position frequently during the first stage of labor.

- Doulas provide a continuous supportive presence during labor that can have a positive effect on the process of childbirth and its outcome.

- The cultural beliefs and practices of a woman and her significant others, including her partner, can have a profound influence on their approach to labor and birth.

- The nurse who is aware of particular sociocultural aspects of helping and coping acts as an advocate or protective agent for the woman or couple during labor.

- The quality of the nurse-patient relationship is a factor in the woman's ability to cope with the stressors of the labor process.

- Women with a history of sexual abuse often experience profound stress and anxiety during childbirth.

- Inability to palpate the cervix during vaginal examination indicates that complete effacement and full dilation have occurred and is the only certain, objective sign that the second stage has begun.

- Women may have an urge to bear down at various times during labor; for some it may be before the cervix is fully dilated, and for others it may not occur until the active phase of the second stage of labor.

- When allowed to respond to the rhythmic nature of the second stage of labor, the woman normally changes body positions, bears down spontaneously, and vocalizes (open-glottis pushing) when she perceives the urge to push (Ferguson reflex).

- Women should bear down several times during a contraction using the open-glottis pushing method; sustained closed-glottis pushing should be avoided because oxygen transport to the fetus will be inhibited.

- Nurses can use the role of advocate to prevent routine use of episiotomy and to reduce the incidence of lacerations by empowering women to take an active role in the birth and educating health care providers about approaches to managing childbirth that reduce the incidence of perineal trauma.

- Objective signs indicate that the placenta has separated and is ready to be expelled; excessive traction (pulling) on the umbilical cord, before the placenta has separated, can result in maternal injury.

- Siblings present for labor and birth need preparation and support for the event.

- Most parents and families enjoy being able to handle, hold, explore, and examine the baby immediately after the birth.

- Nurses should observe the progress in the development of parent-child relationships and be alert for warning signs that may appear during the immediate postpartum period.

- After an emergency childbirth out of the hospital, stimulation of the mother's nipple manually or by the infant's suckling stimulates the release of oxytocin from the maternal posterior pituitary gland; oxytocin stimulates the uterus to contract and thereby prevents hemorrhage.

Answer Guidelines to Critical Thinking Exercises

Oral Intake in Labor

1 Yes, there is evidence to support the nurse's response concerning Margot's request for something to eat and drink while in early labor.

2 a. Labor requires energy, and there is a loss of fluids during childbirth. Adequate intake of calories and fluids is needed to meet these needs and losses. If the needs are not met, labor progress can slow down and the woman can develop ketosis. She may also be at risk for not having enough energy to push during second stage, thus increasing her risk for a forceps- or vacuum-assisted birth.

b. Fasting in labor has been identified by many women as a stressor. Fasting has been described as a source of frustration related to feeling a sense of loss of control over being able to make a decision about eating or drinking in labor.

c. A woman's culture may influence whether she will want to eat or drink during labor. For example, in some cultures, a woman will drink only warm drinks as she believes that this practice will facilitate birth and the delivery of the placenta (CNM Data Group, 1999; D'Avanzo & Geissler, 2003).

3 One priority for the nurse would be to do a check for ketones in the urine at each void. Another priority is to assess the woman's energy level at frequent intervals. Oral fluids should be provided if ordered. If there is no order, the nurse should contact the doctor or nurse-midwife, provide information about Margot's labor status and her request for some type of nourishment, and advocate that the request be granted.

4 The evidence would seem to objectively support this action. Withholding fluids and food in labor is a form of care that is unlikely to be beneficial, and offering oral fluids should be en-

couraged (Enkin et al., 2000; Hofmeyr, 2005). Clear liquids are commonly given in early labor and can meet the woman's hydration needs and energy demands. The woman may also feel more comfortable and more in control (Scheepers et al., 2001). However, an exploratory study with Australian midwives concluded that there was not enough conclusive research evidence to support any stance on oral intake in labor (Parsons, 2004).

5 The nurse must follow the orders of the primary health care provider with regard to oral intake during labor. If the woman is allowed only ice chips, then the nurse must monitor energy and hydration levels closely and provide support and encouragement as well as comfort measures. The nurse can also advocate for policy changes by encouraging other health care providers to review research findings that support the safety and effectiveness of oral intake of flood and fluids during labor.

Applying Fundal Pressure

1 The use of fundal pressure in labor is controversial; clinical disagreements between physicians and nurses can arise when the use of fundal pressure is requested. Nurses may feel pressured to use this technique even when they feel it is not in the best interest of the mother and the fetus. There is no published evidence that fundal pressure is safe or effective. Very little about fundal pressure appears in the literature; often, when it is used, it is not documented in the medical record. To avert clinical disagreements, a plan for how such a request will be handled should be formulated.

2 a. Sometimes when AROM is indicated, pressure is used to guide the head of the fetus into the pelvis against the cervix to reduce the risk of prolapse of the cord. When the FHR is nonreassuring or difficult to trace electronically and a fetal scalp electrode (FSE) is to be placed but the fetal station is high, gentle fundal pressure may move the fetal head down and make it easier to apply the FSE. When the fetal head is crowning, maternal efforts are not enough for birth to occur, and the FHR is nonreassuring (indicating the need for an expeditious birth), fundal pressure may be the quickest way to effect birth.

b. Fetus and newborn: brachial plexus injury, fractures of the humerus and clavicle, spinal cord injury, subgaleal hemorrhage, and fetal death. Mother: perineal injuries (third- and fourth-degree lacerations), abdominal bruising, fractured ribs, liver rupture, uterine rupture, uterine inversion, possible amniotic fluid embolism. Nurse: back, arm, wrist, and hand injuries have been reported.

c. Fundal pressure should be avoided in the case of shoulder dystocia. If fundal pressure is applied, the anterior shoulder is likely to be further impacted, the birth delayed, and the risk of fetal injury increased. Suprapubic pressure is more commonly used to relieve shoulder dystocia.

d. Provider needs to be patient; pain relief measures should aim for epidural analgesia, not anesthesia; pushing may be delayed to allow passive descent to prevent maternal fatigue; directed coaching may be applied in pushing efforts.

3 The fetus needs to be assessed. If the FHR and fetal heart pattern are reassuring, there is no need to rush to birth and the mother can have a period of rest. Directed coaching in pushing can be provided.

4 There is little evidence in the literature about the risks and benefits of fundal pressure. The literature that exists mainly describes medicolegal problems when fundal pressure to relieve shoulder dystocia was used and it resulted in injury to the fetus or newborn. There is very limited information about the use of fundal pressure to shorten second-stage labor in low risk women.

5 The optimal solution to such requests is to develop an interdisciplinary plan to manage risk before the occasion for the request for application of fundal pressure arises. Each department must develop its own approach. The attorney and professional liability insurance carrier of the agency should be involved in the discussion. If nurses are to apply fundal pressure, they must be trained in the proper application. The use of fundal pressure should be documented.

Reference: Simpson, K., & Knox, G. (2001). Fundal pressure during the second stage of labor: Clinical perspectives and risk management issues. *MCN American Journal of Maternal Child Nursing, 26*(2), 64-71.

Resources

American College of Nurse Midwives
8403 Colesville Rd. Suite 1550
Silver Springs, MD 20910
240-485-1800
www.midwife.org

Association of Labor Assistants and Childbirth Educators (ALACE)
P.O. Box 390436
Cambridge, MA 02139
617-441-2500
www.alace.org

Childbirth Graphics
P.O. Box 21207
Waco, TX 76702-1207
800-299-3366
www.childbirthgraphics.com

Childbirth Organization
www.childbirth.org

Coalition for Improving Maternity Services (CIMS)
P.O. Box 2346
PonteVedra Beach, FL 32004
888-282-CIMS
www.motherfriendly.org

Doulas of North America (DONA)
P.O. Box 626
Jasper, IN 47547
888-788-DONA
www.dona.com

Gentlebirth
www.gentlebirth.org

Global Maternal/Child Health Association and Waterbirth International
P.O. Box 1400
Wilsonville, OR 97070
503-673-0026

International Childbirth Education Association, Inc. (ICEA)
P.O. Box 20048
Minneapolis, MN 55420
952-854-8660
www.icea.org

Midwives Alliance of North America (MANA)
375 Rockbridge Rd.
Suite 172-213
Lilburn, GA 30047
888-923-6262
www.mana.org

National Association of Childbearing Centers (NACC)
3123 Gottschall Rd.
Perkiomenville, PA 18074
215-234-8068
www.birthcenters.org

National Association of Parents and Professionals for Safe
  Alternatives in Childbirth (NAPSAC)
Rte 4, Box 646
Marble Hill, MO 63764
573-238-2010
www.napsac.org

Online Birth Center (OBC)
www.moonlily.com/obc

Waterbirth International
www.waterbirth.org

References

Albers, L. et al. (1997). The relationship of ambulation in labor to operative delivery. *Journal of Nurse Midwifery, 42*(1), 4-8.

Baxley, E., & Gobbo, R. (2004). Shoulder dystocia. *American Family Physician, 69*(7), 1707-1714.

Benfield, R. (2002). Hydrotherapy in labor. *Journal of Nursing Scholarship, 34*(4), 347-352.

Brucker, M. (2001). Management of the third stage of labor: An evidence-based approach. *Journal of Midwifery & Women's Health, 46*(6), 381-392.

Caliendo, C., Millbauer, L., Moore B., & Kitchen, E. (2004). Obstetric triage and EMTALA: Practice strategies for labor and delivery nursing units. *AWHONN Lifelines, 8*(5), 442-448.

Cesario, S. (2004). Reevaluation of the Friedman labor cure: A pilot study. *Journal of Obstetric, Gynecologic, and Neonatal Nursing, 33*(6), 713-722.

Chapman, L. (1992). Expectant father's roles during labor and birth. *Journal of Obstetric, Gynecologic, and Neonatal Nursing, 21*(2), 114-120.

Cluett, E., Nikodem, V., McCandlish, R., & Burns, E. (2004). Immersion in water in pregnancy, labour, and birth. *The Cochrane Database of Systematic Reviews.* Issue 3, Art. CD000111.

CNM Data Group. (1999). Oral intake in labor: Trends in midwifery practice. The CMN Data Group, 1996. *Journal of Nurse Midwifery, 44*(2), 135-138.

D'Avanzo, C., & Geissler, E. (2003). *Pocket guide to cultural assessment* (3rd ed.). St. Louis: Mosby.

Davies, B., & Hodnett, E. (2002). Labor support: Nurses' self-efficacy and views about factors influencing implementation. *Journal of Obstetric, Gynecologic, and Neonatal Nursing, 31*(1), 48-56.

Enkin, M. et al. (2000). *A guide to effective care in pregnancy and childbirth* (3rd ed.). Oxford, NY: Oxford University Press.

Gupta, J., & Hofmeyr, G. (2003). Position for women during second stage of labour for women with epidural anaesthesia. *The Cochrane Database of Systematic Reviews,* Issue 3, Art. CD002006.

Hansen, S., Clark, S., & Foster, J. (2002). Active pushing versus passive fetal descent in the second stage of labor: A randomized study. *Obstetrics and Gynecology, 99*(1), 29-34.

Hanson, L., VandeVusse, L., & Harrod, K. (2001). The theater of birth: Scenes from women's scripts. *Journal of Perinatal and Neonatal Nursing, 15*(2), 18-35.

Hobbins, D. (2004). Survivors of childhood sexual abuse: Implications for perinatal nursing. *Journal of Obstetric, Gynecologic, and Neonatal Nursing, 33*(4), 485-497.

Hodnett, E. (2001). Caregiver support for women during childbirth. *The Cochrane Database of Systematic Reviews,* Issue 1, Art. CD000199.

Hodnett, E., Gates, S., Hofmeyr, G., & Sakala, C. (2003). Continuous support for women during childbirth. *The Cochrane Database of Sysematic Reviews,* Issue 3, 2003, Art. CD003766.

Hodnett, E., Lowe, N., Hannah, M., Willan, A., Stevens, B., & Weston, J. (2002). Effectiveness of nurses as providers of birth support in North American hospitals. *Journal of the American Medical Association, 288*(11), 1373-1381.

Hofmeyr, G. (2005). Evidence-based intrapartum care. *Best Practices Research in Clinical Obstetrics and Gynaecology, 19*(1), 103-115.

Kayne, M., Greulich, M., & Albers, L. (2001). Doulas: An alternative yet complementary addition to care during childbirth. *Clinical Obstetrics and Gynecology, 44*(4), 692-703.

Klaus, M., Kennell, J., & Klaus, P. (1993). *Mothering the mother.* Redwood City, CA: Addison-Wesley.

Lemon, B. (2002). Exploring Latino rituals in birthing. *AWHONN Lifelines, 6*(5), 443-445.

Lothian, J. (2001). Back to the future: Trusting birth. *Journal of Perinatal and Neonatal Nursing, 15*(3), 13-22.

MacKinnon, K., McIntyre, M., & Quance, M. (2005). The meaning of the nurse's presence during childbirth. *Journal of Obstetric, Gynecologic, and Neonatal Nursing, 34*(1), 28-36.

Mattson, S. (2000). Working toward cultural competence: Making first steps through cultural assessment. *AWHONN Lifelines, 4*(4), 41-43.

Mayberry, L. et al. (2000). *Second stage labor management: Promotion of evidence-based practice and a collaborative approach to patient care.* Washington, DC: Association of Women's Health, Obstetric and Neonatal Nurses.

Melender, H. (2002). Experiences of fears associated with pregnancy and childbirth: A study of 329 pregnant women. *Birth, 29*(2), 101-111.

Miltner, R. (2000). Identifying labor support actions of intrapartum nurses. *Journal of Obstetric, Gynecologic, and Neonatal Nursing, 29*(5), 491-499.

Miltner, R. (2002). More than support: Nursing interventions provided to women in labor. *Journal of Obstetric, Gynecologic, and Neonatal Nursing, 31*(6), 753-761.

Minato, J. (2000). Is it time to push? Examining rest in second-stage labor. *AWHONN Lifelines, 4*(6), 20-23.

Molina, J. (2001). Traditional Native American practices in obstetrics. *Clinical Obstetrics and Gynecology, 44*(4), 661-670.

Parsons, M. (2004). A midwifery practice dichotomy on oral intake in labour. *Midwifery, 20*(1), 72-81.

Prendiville, W., Elbourne, D., & McDonald, S. (2000). Active versus expectant management in the third stage of labour. *The Cochrane Database of Systematic Reviews, Issue* 3, Art. CD000007.

Roberts, J. (2002). The "push" for evidence: Management of the second stage. *Journal of Midwifery & Women's Health, 47*(1), 2-15.

Roberts, J. (2003). A new understanding of the second stage of labor: Implications for care. *Journal of Obstetric, Gynecologic, and Neonatal Nursing, 32*(6), 794-801.

Sauls, D. (2002). Effects of labor support on mothers, babies, and birth outcomes. *Journal of Obstetric, Gynecologic, and Neonatal Nursing, 31*(6), 733-741.

Scheepers, H., Thans, H., deJong, P., Essed, G., LeCessie, S., & Kanhai, A. (2001). Eating and drinking in labor: The influence of caregiver advice on women's behavior. *Birth, 28*(2), 119-123.

Shorten, A., Donsante, J., & Shorten, B. (2002). Birth position, accoucheur, and perineal outcomes: Informing women about choices for vaginal birth. *Birth, 29*(1), 18-27.

Simkin, P. (2002). Supportive care during labor: A guide for busy nurses. *Journal of Obstetric, Gynecologic, and Neonatal Nursing, 31*(6), 721-732.

Simkin, P., & Ancheta, R. (2000). *The labor progress handbook.* Malden, MA: Blackwell Science.

Simpson, K., & Knox, G. (2001). Fundal pressure during the second stage of labor: Clinical perspectives and risk management issues. *MCN American Journal of Maternal Child Nursing, 26*(2), 64-71.

Trainor, C. (2002). Valuing labor support: A doula's perspective. *AWHONN Lifelines, 6*(5), 387-389.

Tucker, S. (2004). *Pocket guide to fetal monitoring and assessment* (5th ed.). St. Louis: Mosby.

Tumblin, A., & Simkin, P. (2001). Pregnant women's perception of their nurse's role during labor and delivery. *Birth, 28*(1), 52-56.

Waterbirth International. (2005). *Frequently Asked Questions. How long is the baby in the water?* Internet document available at http://waterbirth.org (accessed April 17, 2005).

Weeks, J., & Kozak, L. (2001). Trends in the use of episiotomy in the United States: 1980-1998. *Birth, 28*(3), 152-160.

Zwelling, E., & Phillips, C. (2001). Family-centered maternity care in the new millennium: Is it real or is it imagined? *Journal of Perinatal and Neonatal Nursing, 15*(3), 1-12.

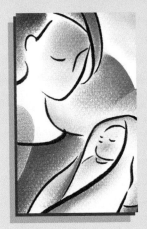

CHAPTER 15

Maternal Physiologic Changes

KELLY CRUM

LEARNING OBJECTIVES

- Describe the anatomic and physiologic changes that occur during the postpartum period.
- Identify characteristics of uterine involution and lochial flow and describe ways to measure them.

- List expected values for vital signs, deviations from normal findings, and probable causes of the deviations.

KEY TERMS AND DEFINITIONS

afterbirth pains (afterpains) Painful uterine cramps that occur intermittently for approximately 2 or 3 days after birth and that result from contractile efforts of the uterus to return to its normal involuted condition

autolysis The self-destruction of excess hypertrophied tissue

diastasis recti abdominis Separation of the two rectus muscles along the median line of the abdominal wall

involution Reduction in size of the uterus after birth, and its return to its nonpregnant condition

lochia Vaginal discharge during the puerperium consisting of blood, tissue, and mucus

lochia alba Thin, yellowish to white, vaginal discharge that follows lochia serosa on approxi-

mately the tenth day after birth and that may last from 2 to 6 weeks postpartum

lochia rubra Red, distinctly blood-tinged vaginal flow that follows birth and lasts 2 to 4 days

lochia serosa Serous, pinkish brown, watery vaginal discharge that follows lochia rubra until approximately the tenth day after birth

pelvic relaxation Lengthening and weakening of the fascial supports of pelvic structures

puerperium Period after the third stage of labor and lasting until involution of the uterus takes place, usually approximately 3 to 6 weeks; fourth trimester of pregnancy

subinvolution Failure of the uterus to reduce to its normal size and condition after pregnancy

ELECTRONIC RESOURCES

Additional information related to the content in Chapter 15 can be found on

the companion website at **evolve**
http://evolve.elsevier.com/Lowdermilk/Maternity/
- NCLEX Review Questions
- WebLinks

or on the interactive companion CD
- NCLEX Review Questions

The postpartum period is the interval between the birth of the newborn and the return of the maternal reproductive organs to their normal nonpregnant state. This period is sometimes referred to as the puerperium, or fourth trimester of pregnancy. Although the puerperium has traditionally been considered as lasting 6 weeks, this time frame varies among women. The distinct physiologic changes that occur during the reversal of the processes of pregnancy are normal. To provide care during the recovery period that is beneficial to the mother, her infant, and her family, the nurse must synthesize knowledge of maternal anatomy and physiology of the recovery period, the newborn's physical and behavioral characteristics, infant care activities, and family response to the birth of the infant. This chapter focuses on anatomic and physiologic changes that occur in the mother during the postpartum period.

REPRODUCTIVE SYSTEM AND ASSOCIATED STRUCTURES

Uterus

Involution process

The return of the uterus to a nonpregnant state after birth is known as involution. This process begins immediately after expulsion of the placenta with contraction of the uterine smooth muscle.

At the end of the third stage of labor the uterus is in the midline, approximately 2 cm below the level of the umbilicus, with the fundus resting on the sacral promontory. At this time the uterus weighs approximately 1000 g.

Within 12 hours the fundus may rise to approximately 1 cm above the umbilicus (Fig. 15-1). By 24 hours postpartum the uterus is about the same size it was at 20 weeks of gestation (Resnik, 2004). Involution progresses rapidly during the next few days. The fundus descends about 1 to 2 cm every 24 hours. By the sixth postpartum day the fundus is normally located halfway between the umbilicus and the symphysis pubis. The uterus should not be palpable abdominally after 2 weeks (Resnik, 2004).

The uterus, which at full term weighs approximately 11 times its prepregnancy weight, involutes to approximately 500 g by 1 week after birth and to 350 g by 2 weeks after birth. At 6 weeks it weighs 50 to 60 g (see Fig. 15-1).

Increased estrogen and progesterone levels are responsible for stimulating the massive growth of the uterus during pregnancy. Prenatal uterine growth results from both hyperplasia, an increase in the number of muscle cells, and from hypertrophy, an enlargement of the existing cells. Postpartally, the decrease in these hormones causes autolysis, the self-destruction of excess hypertrophied tissue. The additional cells laid down during pregnancy remain and account for the slight increase in uterine size after each pregnancy.

Subinvolution is the failure of the uterus to return to a nonpregnant state. The most common causes of subinvolution are retained placental fragments and infection.

Contractions

Postpartum hemostasis is achieved primarily by compression of intramyometrial blood vessels as the uterine muscle contracts rather than by platelet aggregation and clot formation. The hormone oxytocin, released from the pituitary gland, strengthens and coordinates these uterine contractions, which compress blood vessels and promote hemostasis. During the first 1 to 2 postpartum hours, uterine contractions may decrease in intensity and become uncoordinated. Because it is vital that the uterus remain firm and well contracted, exogenous oxytocin (Pitocin) is usually administered intravenously or intramuscularly immediately after expulsion of the placenta. Mothers who plan to breastfeed may also be encouraged to put the baby to breast immediately after birth because suckling stimulates oxytocin release from the posterior pituitary gland.

Afterpains

In first-time mothers, uterine tone is good, the fundus generally remains firm, and the mother does not perceive uterine cramping. Periodic relaxation and vigorous contraction are more common in subsequent pregnancies and may cause uncomfortable cramping called afterbirth pains (afterpains), which persist throughout the early puerperium. Afterpains are more noticeable after births in which the uterus was overdistended (e.g., large baby, multifetal gestation, polyhydramnios). Breastfeeding and exogenous oxytocic medication usually intensify these afterpains because both stimulate uterine contractions.

Placental site

Immediately after the placenta and membranes are expelled, vascular constriction and thromboses reduce the placental site to an irregular nodular and elevated area. Upward growth of the endometrium causes sloughing of necrotic tissue and prevents the scar formation that is characteristic of normal wound healing. This unique healing process enables the endometrium to resume its usual cycle of changes and to permit implantation and placentation in future pregnancies. Endometrial regeneration is completed by postpartum day 16, except at the placental site (Resnik, 2004). Regeneration at the placental site usually is not complete until 6 weeks after birth.

Lochia

Postchildbirth uterine discharge, commonly called lochia, initially is bright red (lochia rubra) and may contain small clots. For the first 2 hours after birth the amount of uterine discharge should be approximately that of a heavy menstrual period. After that time the lochial flow should steadily decrease.

Lochia rubra consists mainly of blood and decidual and trophoblastic debris. The flow pales, becoming pink or brown (lochia serosa) after 3 to 4 days. Lochia serosa consists of old blood, serum, leukocytes, and tissue debris. The median duration for lochia serosa discharge is 22 to 27 days (Bowes &

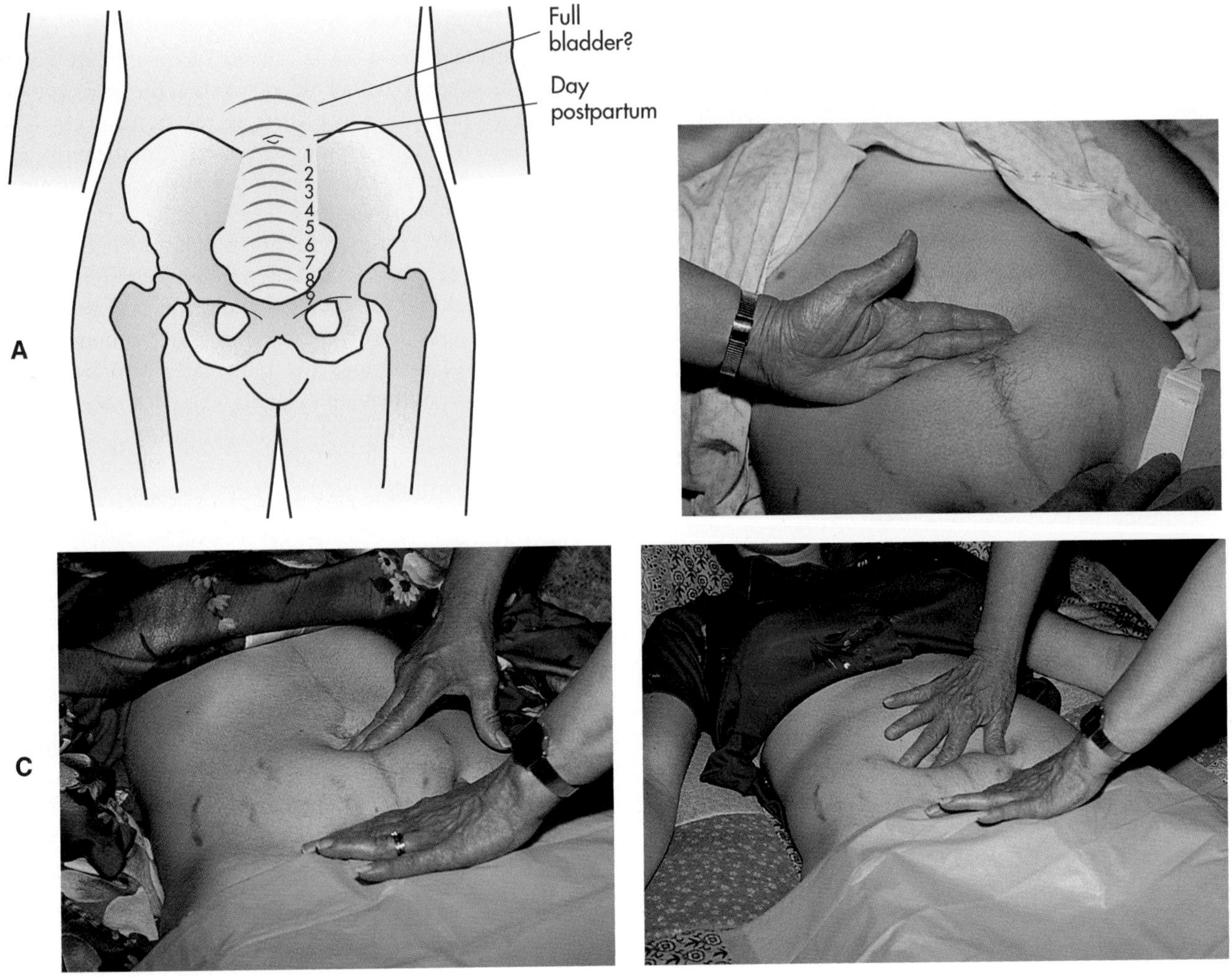

Fig. 15-1 Assessment of involution of uterus after childbirth. **A,** Normal progress, days 1 through 9. **B,** Size and position of uterus 2 hours after childbirth. **C,** Two days after childbirth. **D,** Four days after childbirth. (**B, C, D,** Courtesy Marjorie Pyle, RNC, Lifecircle, Costa Mesa, CA.)

Katz, 2002). In most women, about 10 days after childbirth the drainage becomes yellow to white (lochia alba). Lochia alba consists of leukocytes, decidua, epithelial cells, mucus, serum, and bacteria. Lochia alba usually continues for 10 to 14 days but may normally last longer (Simpson & Creehan, 2001).

If the woman receives an oxytocic medication, the flow of lochia is often scant until the effects of the medication wear off. The amount of lochia is typically smaller after cesarean births. Flow of lochia usually increases with ambulation and breastfeeding. Lochia tends to pool in the vagina when the woman is lying in bed; upon standing, the woman may experience a gush of blood. This gush should not be confused with hemorrhage.

Persistence of lochia rubra early in the postpartum period suggests continued bleeding as a result of retained fragments of the placenta or membranes. Recurrence of bleeding approximately 7 to 14 days after birth is from the healing placental site. About 10% to 15% of women will still be experiencing normal lochia serosa discharge at the 6-week

postpartum examination (Bowes & Katz, 2002). In the majority of women, however, a continued flow of lochia serosa or lochia alba by 3 to 4 weeks after birth may indicate endometritis, particularly if fever, pain, or abdominal tenderness is associated with the discharge. Lochia should smell like normal menstrual flow; an offensive odor usually indicates infection.

Not all postpartal vaginal bleeding is lochia; vaginal bleeding after birth may be a result of unrepaired vaginal or cervical lacerations. Table 15-1 distinguishes between lochial and nonlochial bleeding.

Cervix

The cervix is soft immediately after birth. Within 2 to 3 days postpartum it has shortened, become firm, and regained its form (Resnik, 2004). The cervix up to the lower uterine segment remains edematous, thin, and fragile for several days after birth. The ectocervix (portion of the cervix that protrudes into the vagina) appears bruised and has some small lacerations—optimal conditions for the development of

TABLE 15-1

Lochial and Nonlochial Bleeding

LOCHIAL BLEEDING	NONLOCHIAL BLEEDING
Lochia usually trickles from the vaginal opening. The steady flow is greater as the uterus contracts. A gush of lochia may result as the uterus is massaged. If it is dark in color, it has been pooled in the relaxed vagina, and the amount soon lessens to a trickle of bright red lochia (in the early puerperium).	If the bloody discharge spurts from the vagina, there may be cervical or vaginal tears in addition to the normal lochia. If the amount of bleeding continues to be excessive and bright red, a tear may be the source.

infection. The cervical os, which dilated to 10 cm during labor, closes gradually. Two fingers may still be introduced into the cervical os for the first 4 to 6 days postpartum; however, only the smallest curette can be introduced by the end of 2 weeks. The external cervical os never regains its prepregnant appearance; it is no longer shaped like a circle but appears as a jagged slit that is often described as a "fish mouth" (see Fig. 8-1 on p. 213). Lactation delays the production of cervical and other estrogen-influenced mucus and mucosal characteristics.

Vagina and Perineum

Postpartum estrogen deprivation is responsible for the thinness of the vaginal mucosa and the absence of rugae. The greatly distended, smooth-walled vagina gradually returns to its prepregnancy size by 6 to 10 weeks after childbirth (Resnik, 2004). Rugae reappear within 3 weeks, but they are never as prominent as they are in the nulliparous woman. Most rugae are permanently flattened. The mucosa remains atrophic in the lactating woman, at least until menstruation resumes. Thickening of the vaginal mucosa occurs with the return of ovarian function. Estrogen deficiency is also responsible for a decreased amount of vaginal lubrication. Localized dryness and coital discomfort (dyspareunia) may persist until ovarian function returns and menstruation resumes. The use of a water-soluble lubricant during sexual intercourse is usually recommended.

Initially, the introitus is erythematous and edematous, especially in the area of the episiotomy or laceration repair. It is usually barely distinguishable from that of a nulliparous woman if lacerations and an episiotomy have been carefully repaired, hematomas are prevented or treated early, and the woman observes good hygiene during the first 2 weeks after birth.

Most episiotomies are visible only if the woman is lying on her side with her upper buttock raised or if she is placed in the lithotomy position. A good light source is essential for visualization of some episiotomies. Healing of an episiotomy is the same as any surgical incision. Signs of infection (pain, redness, warmth, swelling, or discharge) or loss of approximation (separation of the edges of the incision) may occur. Healing should occur within 2 to 3 weeks.

Hemorrhoids (anal varicosities) are commonly seen (see Fig. 8-9 on p. 218). Internal hemorrhoids may evert while the woman is pushing during birth. Women often experience associated symptoms such as itching, discomfort, and bright red bleeding with defecation. Hemorrhoids usually decrease in size within 6 weeks of childbirth.

Pelvic muscular support

The supporting structure of the uterus and vagina may be injured during childbirth and may contribute to later gynecologic problems. Supportive tissues of the pelvic floor that are torn or stretched during childbirth may require up to 6 months to regain tone. Kegel exercises, which help to strengthen perineal muscles and encourage healing, are recommended after childbirth (see Teaching Guidelines, Chapter 4). Later in life, women can experience pelvic relaxation, the lengthening and weakening of the fascial supports of pelvic structures. These structures include the uterus, upper posterior vaginal wall, urethra, bladder, and rectum. Although pelvic relaxation can occur in any woman, it is usually a direct but delayed complication of childbirth (see Chapter 25).

ENDOCRINE SYSTEM ■

Placental Hormones

Significant hormonal changes occur during the postpartal period. Expulsion of the placenta results in dramatic decreases of the hormones produced by that organ. Decreases in human chorionic somatomammotropin, estrogens, cortisol, and the placental enzyme insulinase reverse the diabetogenic effects of pregnancy, resulting in significantly lower blood sugar levels in the immediate puerperium. Mothers with type 1 diabetes will be likely to require much less insulin for several days after birth. Because these normal hormonal changes make the puerperium a transitional period for carbohydrate metabolism, it is more difficult to interpret glucose tolerance tests during this time.

Estrogen and progesterone levels drop markedly after expulsion of the placenta and reach their lowest levels 1 week postpartum. Decreased estrogen levels are associated with breast engorgement and with the diuresis of excess extracellular fluid accumulated during pregnancy. In nonlactating women, estrogen levels begin to rise by 2 weeks after birth and by postpartum day 17 are higher than in women who breastfeed (Bowes & Katz, 2002).

β-Human chorionic gonadotropin (β-hCG) disappears from maternal circulation in 14 days (Resnik, 2004).

Pituitary Hormones and Ovarian Function

Lactating and nonlactating women differ considerably in the time when the first ovulation occurs and when menstruation resumes. The persistence of elevated serum prolactin levels in breastfeeding women appears to be responsible for suppressing ovulation. Because levels of follicle-stimulating hormone (FSH) have been shown to be identical in lactating and nonlactating women, it is thought that ovulation is suppressed in lactating women because the ovary does not respond to FSH stimulation when increased prolactin levels are present (Resnik, 2004).

Prolactin levels in blood rise progressively throughout pregnancy. In women who breastfeed, prolactin levels remain elevated into the sixth week after birth (Lawrence & Lawrence, 2004). Serum prolactin levels are influenced by the frequency of breastfeeding, the duration of each feeding, and the degree to which supplementary feedings are used. Individual differences in the strength of an infant's sucking stimulus probably also affect prolactin levels. In nonlactating women, prolactin levels decline after birth and reach the prepregnant range by the third postpartum week (Bowes & Katz, 2002).

Ovulation occurs as early as 27 days after birth in nonlactating women, with a mean time of about 70 to 75 days (Bowes & Katz, 2002). Approximately 70% of nonbreastfeeding women resume menstruating by 3 months after birth (Lawrence & Lawrence, 2004). In women who breastfeed, the mean length of time to initial ovulation is 6 months (Bowes & Katz, 2002). In lactating women, both resumption of ovulation and return of menses are determined in large part by breastfeeding patterns (Resnik, 2004). Many women ovulate before their first postpartum menstrual period occurs; therefore there is need to discuss contraceptive options early in the puerperium (Lawrence & Lawrence, 2004).

The first menstrual flow after childbirth is usually heavier than normal. Within three to four cycles the amount of menstrual flow returns to the woman's prepregnancy volume.

ABDOMEN

When the woman stands up during the first days after birth, her abdomen protrudes and gives her a still-pregnant appearance. During the first 2 weeks after birth the abdominal wall is relaxed. It takes approximately 6 weeks for the abdominal wall to return almost to its nonpregnancy state. The skin regains most of its previous elasticity, but some striae may persist. The return of muscle tone depends on previous tone, proper exercise, and the amount of adipose tissue. Occasionally, with or without overdistention because of a large fetus or multiple fetuses, the abdominal wall muscles separate, a condition termed *diastasis recti abdominis* (see Fig. 8-12). Persistence of this defect may be disturbing to the woman, but surgical correction rarely is necessary. With time, the defect becomes less apparent.

URINARY SYSTEM

The hormonal changes of pregnancy (i.e., high steroid levels) contribute to an increase in renal function; diminishing steroid levels after childbirth may partly explain the reduced renal function that occurs during the puerperium. Kidney function returns to normal within 1 month after birth. From 2 to 8 weeks are required for the pregnancy-induced hypotonia and dilation of the ureters and renal pelves to return to the nonpregnant state (Cunningham et al., 2005). In a small percentage of women, dilation of the urinary tract may persist for 3 months, which increases the chance of developing a urinary tract infection.

Urine Components

The renal glycosuria induced by pregnancy disappears, but lactosuria may occur in lactating women. The blood urea nitrogen increases during the puerperium as autolysis of the involuting uterus occurs. This breakdown of excess protein in the uterine muscle cells also results in a mild (+1) proteinuria for 1 to 2 days after childbirth in 40% to 50% of women (Simpson & Creehan, 2001). Ketonuria may occur in women with an uncomplicated birth or after a prolonged labor with dehydration.

Postpartal Diuresis

Within 12 hours of birth, women begin to lose excess tissue fluid accumulated during pregnancy. Profuse diaphoresis often occurs, especially at night, for the first 2 or 3 days after childbirth. Postpartal diuresis, caused by decreased estrogen levels, removal of increased venous pressure in the lower extremities, and loss of the remaining pregnancy-induced increase in blood volume, also aids the body in ridding itself of excess fluid. Fluid loss through perspiration and increased urinary output accounts for a weight loss of approximately 2.25 kg during the puerperium.

Urethra and Bladder

Birth-induced trauma, increased bladder capacity following childbirth, and the effects of conduction anesthesia combine to cause a decreased urge to void. In addition, pelvic soreness caused by the forces of labor, vaginal lacerations, or an episiotomy reduces or alters the voiding reflex. Decreased voiding combined with postpartal diuresis may result in bladder distention. Immediately after birth, excessive bleeding can occur if the bladder becomes distended because it pushes the uterus up and to the side and prevents the uterus from contracting firmly. Later in the puerperium overdistention can make the bladder more susceptible to infection and impede the resumption of normal voiding (Cunningham et al., 2005). With adequate emptying of the bladder, bladder tone is usually restored 5 to 7 days after childbirth.

EVIDENCE-BASED PRACTICE
Timing of Fluids and Food after Cesarean Birth

BACKGROUND

- Health care is full of assumptions and traditions that do not necessarily stem from evidence. It has long been customary to withhold fluids and food after major abdominal surgery until bowel function returns, evidenced by bowel sounds and passing of flatus and stool. The concern is the occurrence of paralytic ileus, a loss of peristalsis, characterized by abdominal tenderness and distention, nausea and vomiting, and lack of bowel sounds. Some health care providers have a policy of limiting food and fluids to women after cesarean birth, even if no handling of the bowel has occurred. Depending on the institution, fluids and food can be withheld up to 24 hours, followed by a transition day from clear to full liquids, and solids by the third day. This is in addition to the time that the woman has already been without food and fluids while in labor.

- Critics of this policy find this starvation unnecessary because simple cesarean birth is not associated with bowel manipulation. Indeed, there is some evidence that bowel function continues even after major manipulation, but with altered bowel sounds. Paralytic ileus is thought to be multifactorial, caused by neural and hormonal factors involving the sympathetic and parasympathetic nervous systems, use of narcotics, and type of anesthesia. Some researchers have found that fluids are well tolerated after cesarean birth and should be provided unless the operation involved extensive bowel manipulation or sepsis. Some institutions even offer fluids within 90 minutes after birth, and, if well tolerated, a regular diet soon thereafter.

OBJECTIVES

- Reviewers sought to clarify these different treatment alternatives and question the basis for delaying fluids and foods after cesarean birth. They sought to review trials that compared early and delayed reintroduction of fluids and food after cesarean birth. Outcome measures included occurrence of nausea, vomiting, crampy abdominal pain, bloating, and abdominal distention; presence of bowel action on the third postoperative day; delayed return to bowel sounds and action; ketosis; blood sugar values; duration of intravenous fluids; breastfeeding success; women's satisfaction; fatigue; need for analgesia; ambulation; and time spent in the hospital.

METHODS
Search Strategy

- The reviewers searched the Cochrane Database, MEDLINE, and the journals summarized by Zetoc, the British Library Electronic Table of Contents. Search words were *oral feed, oral fluid, oral hydration, oral intake, eat, drink, food, cesar, Caesar,* and *caesarean section.* Reviewers included six

randomized, controlled trials, published from 1993 to 2001. Information about total number of women and number of women per trial was not noted. Countries of origin also were not included in the review.

Statistical Analyses

- Statistical analyses of outcomes with early reintroduction of oral fluids and solids (usually within 6 to 8 hours postoperatively) were compared with delayed administration of fluids and solids, as defined by the trial authors. The authors accepted differences between groups that exceeded the 95% confidence interval as significant.

FINDINGS

- Early administration of oral fluids was associated with decreased time to first solids, decreased time to bowel sounds, and decreased length of hospitalization in the subgroup that had regional analgesia. Early fluids also led to a trend toward decreased abdominal distention, but this was not significant.

- There were no significant differences between early and delayed fluid administration in the following outcomes: nausea, vomiting, time to bowel action, time to passing flatus, paralytic ileus, and number of doses of analgesia taken postoperatively. No adverse outcomes were found with early postcesarean intake of fluids and food.

LIMITATIONS

- Protocols for times for offering fluids varied. Some trials may have offered clear liquids, some slush, and some fluid and food. Timing of intake varied. Because neither the number of the study participants nor the total number of studies reviewed was reported, it is not possible to assess whether small sample size led to bias.

- No data were available on intravenous hydration, biochemical changes, patient satisfaction, hunger, fatigue, and breastfeeding.

CONCLUSIONS

- There is no evidence from randomized trials to justify a policy of delaying fluids or food after uncomplicated cesarean birth.

IMPLICATIONS FOR PRACTICE

- Nurses in settings where food and fluid are withheld after cesarean birth should work to change the practice.

IMPLICATIONS FOR FURTHER RESEARCH

- The reviewers call for larger, well-designed trials. Further information is needed regarding the intake of fluids and food after complicated cesarean birth. It is unknown whether there are any differences in postoperative gastrointestinal recovery between planned and unplanned cesarean births.

Reference: Mangesi, L., & Hofmeyr, G. (2002). Early compared with delayed oral fluids and food after caesarean section (Cochrane Review). In *The Cochrane Library,* Issue 1, 2005. Chichester, UK: John Wiley & Sons.

GASTROINTESTINAL SYSTEM

Appetite

The mother usually is hungry shortly after the birth and can tolerate a light diet. Most new mothers are very hungry after full recovery from analgesia, anesthesia, and fatigue. Requests for double portions of food and frequent snacks are not uncommon.

Bowel Evacuation

A spontaneous bowel evacuation may not occur for 2 to 3 days after childbirth. This delay can be explained by decreased muscle tone in the intestines during labor and the immediate puerperium, prelabor diarrhea, lack of food, or dehydration. The mother often anticipates discomfort during the bowel movement because of perineal tenderness as a result of episiotomy, lacerations, or hemorrhoids and resists the urge to defecate. Regular bowel habits should be reestablished when bowel tone returns.

Operative vaginal birth (forceps or vacuum use) and anal sphincter lacerations are associated with an increased risk of postpartum anal incontinence. If it occurs, anal incontinence is often temporary and may resolve within 6 months (Bowes & Katz, 2002). Women should be taught during pregnancy about episiotomy and its possible sequelae. Pelvic floor (Kegel) exercises should be encouraged.

BREASTS

Promptly after birth, there is a decrease in the concentrations of hormones (i.e., estrogen, progesterone, hCG, prolactin, cortisol, and insulin) that stimulated breast development during pregnancy. The time it takes for these hormones to return to prepregnancy levels is determined in part by whether the mother breastfeeds her infant.

Breastfeeding Mothers

During the first 24 hours after birth, there is little, if any, change in the breast tissue. Colostrum, a clear yellow fluid, may be expressed from the breasts. The breasts gradually become fuller and heavier as the colostrum transitions to milk by about 72 to 96 hours after birth; this is often referred to as the "milk coming in." The breasts may feel warm, firm, and somewhat tender. Bluish-white milk with a skim-milk appearance (true milk) can be expressed from the nipples. As milk glands and milk ducts fill with milk, breast tissue may feel somewhat nodular or lumpy. Unlike the lumps associated with fibrocystic breast disease or cancer (which may be consistently palpated in the same location), the nodularity associated with milk production tends to shift in position. Some women experience engorgement, but with frequent breastfeeding and proper care, this is a temporary condition that typically lasts only 24 to 48 hours (See Chapter 20).

The nipples are examined for erectility and signs of irritation such as cracks, blisters, or reddening. Sore, damaged nipples are most often the result of incorrect latch (see Chapter 20).

Nonbreastfeeding Mothers

The breasts generally feel nodular in contrast to the granular feel of breasts in nonpregnant women. The nodularity is bilateral and diffuse. Prolactin levels drop rapidly. Colostrum is present for the first few days after childbirth. Palpation of the breast on the second or third day, as milk production begins, may reveal tissue tenderness in some women. On the third or fourth postpartum day, engorgement may occur. The breasts are distended (swollen), firm, tender, and warm to the touch (because of vasocongestion). Breast distention is caused primarily by the temporary congestion of veins and lymphatics rather than by an accumulation of milk. Milk is present but should not be expressed. Axillary breast tissue (the tail of Spence) and any accessory breast or nipple tissue along the milk line may be involved. Engorgement resolves spontaneously, and discomfort decreases usually within 24 to 36 hours. A breast binder or tight bra, ice packs, fresh cabbage leaves, or mild analgesics may be used to relieve discomfort. Nipple stimulation is avoided. If suckling is never begun (or is discontinued), lactation ceases within a few days to a week.

CARDIOVASCULAR SYSTEM

Blood Volume

Changes in blood volume after birth depend on several factors, such as blood loss during childbirth and the amount of extravascular water (physiologic edema) mobilized and excreted. Blood loss results in an immediate but limited decrease in total blood volume. Thereafter, most of the blood volume increase during pregnancy (1000 to 1500 ml) is eliminated within the first 2 weeks after birth (Simpson & Creehan, 2001).

Pregnancy-induced hypervolemia (an increase in blood volume of at least 35% more than prepregnancy values near term) allows most women to tolerate considerable blood loss during childbirth (Bowes & Katz, 2002). Many women lose approximately 500 ml of blood during vaginal birth of a single fetus and approximately twice this much during cesarean birth (Resnik, 2004).

Readjustments in the maternal vasculature after childbirth are dramatic and rapid. The woman's response to blood loss during the early puerperium differs from that in a nonpregnant woman. Three postpartal physiologic changes protect the woman by increasing the circulating blood volume: (1) elimination of uteroplacental circulation reduces the size of the maternal vascular bed by 10% to 15%, (2) loss of placental endocrine function removes the stimulus for vasodilation, and (3) mobilization of extravascular water stored during pregnancy occurs. Therefore hypovolemic shock usually does not occur in women who experience a normal blood loss.

Cardiac Output

Pulse rate, stroke volume, and cardiac output increase throughout pregnancy. Cardiac output remains increased for at least the first 48 hours postpartum because of an increase in stroke volume. This increased stroke volume is caused by the return of blood to the maternal systemic venous circulation, a result of rapid decrease in uterine blood flow and mobilization of extravascular fluid (Resnik, 2004). Cardiac output generally returns to normal by 6 weeks postpartum, but the rate of return appears to be variable (Resnik, 2004). Recent data suggest that stroke volume, cardiac output, and systemic vascular resistance remain elevated over nonpregnant values at least 12 weeks after delivery (Resnik, 2004).

Vital Signs

Few alterations in vital signs are seen under normal circumstances. Heart rate and blood pressure return to nonpregnant levels within a few days (Resnik, 2004) (Table 15-2). Respiratory function returns to nonpregnant levels by 6 to 8 weeks after birth. After the uterus is emptied, the diaphragm descends, the normal cardiac axis is restored, and the point of maximal impulse (PMI) and the electrocardiogram (ECG) are normalized.

TABLE 15-2

Vital Signs after Childbirth

NORMAL FINDINGS	DEVIATIONS FROM NORMAL FINDINGS AND PROBABLE CAUSES
TEMPERATURE	
Temperature during first 24 hours may rise to 38° C as a result of dehydrating effects of labor. After 24 hours the woman should be afebrile.	A diagnosis of puerperal sepsis is suggested if a rise in maternal temperature to 38° C is noted after the first 24 hours after childbirth and recurs or persists for 2 days. Other possibilities are mastitis, endometritis, urinary tract infection, and other systemic infections.
PULSE	
Pulse returns to nonpregnant levels within a few days postpartum, although the rate of return varies among individual women.	A rapid pulse rate or one that is increasing may indicate hypovolemia as a result of hemorrhage.
RESPIRATIONS	
Respirations should decrease to within the woman's normal prepregnancy range by 6 to 8 weeks after birth.	Hypoventilation may follow an unusually high subarachnoid (spinal) block or epidural narcotic after a cesarean birth.
BLOOD PRESSURE	
Blood pressure is altered *slightly* if at all. Orthostatic hypotension, as indicated by feelings of faintness or dizziness immediately after standing up, can develop in the first 48 hours as a result of the splanchnic engorgement that may occur after birth.	A low or decreasing blood pressure may reflect hypovolemia secondary to hemorrhage. However, it is a late sign, and other symptoms of hemorrhage usually alert the staff. An increased reading may result from excessive use of vasopressor or oxytocic medications. Because gestational hypertension can persist into or occur first in the postpartum period, routine evaluation of blood pressure is needed. If a woman complains of headache, hypertension must be ruled out as a cause before analgesics are administered.

Blood Components
Hematocrit and hemoglobin

During the first 72 hours after childbirth, there is a greater reduction of plasma volume than in the number of blood cells. This results in a rise in hematocrit and hemoglobin levels by the seventh day after the birth. There is no increased red blood cell (RBC) destruction during the puerperium, but any excess will disappear gradually in accordance with the life span of the RBC. The exact time at which RBC volume returns to prepregnancy values is not known, but it is within normal limits when measured 8 weeks after childbirth (Bowes & Katz, 2002).

White blood cell count

Normal leukocytosis of pregnancy averages approximately 12,000/mm^3. During the first 10 to 12 days after childbirth, values between 20,000 and 25,000/mm^3 are common. Neutrophils are the most numerous white blood cells. Leukocytosis coupled with the normal increase in erythrocyte sedimentation rate may obscure the diagnosis of acute infection at this time.

Coagulation factors

Clotting factors and fibrinogen are normally increased during pregnancy and remain elevated in the immediate puerperium. When combined with vessel damage and immobility, this hypercoagulable state causes an increased risk of thromboembolism, especially after a cesarean birth. Fibrinolytic activity also increases during the first few days after childbirth (Bowes & Katz, 2002). Factors I, II, VIII, IX, and X decrease within a few days to nonpregnant levels. Fibrin split products, probably released from the placental site, can also be found in maternal blood.

Varicosities

Varicosities (varices) of the legs and around the anus (hemorrhoids) are common during pregnancy. Varices, even the less common vulvar varices, regress (empty) rapidly immediately after childbirth. Surgical repair of varicosities is not considered during pregnancy. Total or nearly total regression of varicosities is expected after childbirth.

NEUROLOGIC SYSTEM ■

Neurologic changes during the puerperium are those that result from a reversal of maternal adaptations to pregnancy and those resulting from trauma during labor and childbirth.

Pregnancy-induced neurologic discomforts disappear after birth. Elimination of physiologic edema through the diuresis that follows childbirth relieves carpal tunnel syndrome by easing compression of the median nerve. The periodic numbness and tingling of fingers that afflicts 5%

 Critical Thinking Exercise

Complications of Immobility after Cesarean Birth

Your patient assignment today on the Mother-Baby Unit includes a patient who gave birth yesterday by cesarean. This patient has not yet gotten out of bed. She also refuses to turn herself in bed or perform deep breathing exercises because "both those things make me hurt." Based on your knowledge of postpartum physiology, you are concerned that she is at risk to develop a thromboembolism.

1 Evidence—Is there sufficient evidence to draw conclusions about risk factors for the development of a thromboembolism during the postpartum period in women who give birth by cesarean?

2 Assumptions—What assumptions can be made about the following issues:
   a. Differences in activity level between women who give birth vaginally and by cesarean during the immediate postpartum period
   b. The relationship between postoperative pain and the woman's activity level
   c. Cultural variations in reactions to pain and expression of pain
   d. Influence of supportive care by the nurse

3 What implications and priorities for nursing care can be drawn at this time?

4 Does the evidence objectively support your conclusion?

5 Are there alternative perspectives to your conclusion?

of pregnant women usually disappears after the birth unless lifting and carrying the baby aggravates the condition. Headache requires careful assessment. Postpartum headaches may be caused by various conditions, including postpartum-onset preeclampsia, stress, and leakage of cerebrospinal fluid into the extradural space during placement of the needle for epidural or spinal anesthesia. Depending on the cause and effectiveness of the treatment, the duration of the headaches can vary from 1 to 3 days to several weeks.

MUSCULOSKELETAL SYSTEM ■

Adaptations of the mother's musculoskeletal system that occur during pregnancy are reversed in the puerperium. These adaptations include the relaxation and subsequent hypermobility of the joints and the change in the mother's center of gravity in response to the enlarging uterus. The joints are completely stabilized by 6 to 8 weeks after birth. Although all other joints return to their normal prepregnancy state, those in the parous woman's feet do not. The new mother may notice a permanent increase in her shoe size.

INTEGUMENTARY SYSTEM

Chloasma of pregnancy (mask of pregnancy) usually disappears at the end of pregnancy. Hyperpigmentation of the areolae and linea nigra may not regress completely after childbirth. Some women will have permanent darker pigmentation of those areas. Striae gravidarum (stretch marks) on the breasts, abdomen, and thighs may fade but usually do not disappear.

Vascular abnormalities such as spider angiomas (nevi), palmar erythema, and epulis generally regress in response to the rapid decline in estrogens after the end of pregnancy. For some woman, spider nevi persist indefinitely.

Hair growth slows during the postpartum period. Some women actually experience hair loss, because the amount of hair lost is temporarily more than the amount regrown. The abundance of fine hair seen during pregnancy usually disappears after giving birth; however, any coarse or bristly hair that appears during pregnancy usually remains. Nails return to their prepregnancy consistency and strength.

Profuse diaphoresis that occurs in the immediate postpartum period is the most noticeable change in the integumentary system.

IMMUNE SYSTEM

No significant changes in the maternal immune system occur during the postpartum period. The mother's need for a rubella vaccination or for prevention of Rh isoimmunization is determined.

COMMUNITY ACTIVITY

Interview an office nurse or a nurse who acts in the role of a childbirth educator regarding what she or he teaches expectant parents and patients about postpartum physiologic changes. Does the nurse consider in-depth discussion of physiology to be necessary? Does the nurse have patient education materials related to postpartum physiology in languages other than English? Does the nurse discuss risk factors that the patient may have that would predispose her to postpartum complications? What actions are taken once it has been determined that the patient is at risk for developing postpartum complications?

Key Points

- The uterus involutes rapidly after birth and returns to the true pelvis within 2 weeks.
- The rapid drop in estrogen and progesterone levels after expulsion of the placenta is responsible for triggering many of the anatomic and physiologic changes in the puerperium.
- The return of ovulation and menses is determined in part by whether a woman breastfeeds her baby.
- Assessment of lochia and fundal height is essential to monitor the progress of normal involution and to identify potential problems.

- Few alterations in vital signs are seen after birth under normal circumstances.
- Activation of blood clotting factors, immobility, and sepsis predispose the woman to thromboembolism.
- Marked diuresis, decreased bladder sensitivity, and overdistention of the bladder can lead to problems with urinary elimination.
- Pregnancy-induced hypervolemia and postpartum physiologic changes allow the woman to tolerate considerable blood loss at birth.

Answer Guidelines to Critical Thinking Exercises

Concerns of a Breastfeeding Mother

1 Yes, there is sufficient evidence to draw conclusions about normal physiologic breast changes in lactating women and the reliability of breastfeeding as a contraceptive method. During lactation the breast may feel nodular or "lumpy" as a result of filled milk glands and milk ducts. The lumps often shift in position from day to day. At about six weeks after birth the breasts of a breastfeeding woman change in size to about what they were during or before pregnancy. Many women worry about their milk supply at this time because the change in breast tissue may coincide with an infant growth spurt. Although lumps may also be palpable in women with fibrocystic breast disease or breast cancer, the position of those lumps remains constant over time. Although most lactating women will not resume ovulation for several months after giving birth, breastfeeding cannot be considered a reliable contraceptive method. The return of ovulation is determined in large part by individual breastfeeding patterns and is influenced by such factors as the frequency and duration of breastfeeding sessions, the degree to which supplemental feeding is used, and the strength of each infant's sucking stimulus.

2 a. Breasts of lactating and nonlactating women will not feel the same when palpated.

b. Men and women may vary with regard to their interest in resuming sexual relations. Some couples resume sexual activity by 3 to 4 weeks after birth. By 6 weeks postpartum, episiotomy and/or lacerations should be healed well enough for sexual intercourse, although dyspareunia and vaginal dryness may be experienced. The woman may wish to delay intercourse because of fear of pain or because of fatigue resulting from the demands of caring for a newborn. The woman's partner may strongly desire to resume sexual activity and therefore may pressure her to participate even if she does not feel ready. Various positions may reduce pressure on tender tissues; the partner can insert a lubricated finger in the vagina to test for tender spots.

   c. The woman's preference regarding a contraceptive method should be honored if at all possible. Regardless of safety and effectiveness, women are not likely to consistently use a contraceptive method that they do not like. Some hormonal methods of contraception, such as those containing estrogen, should not be used while nursing because they adversely affect milk production. Although not as effective at pregnancy prevention as some other contraceptive options, foam and condoms may be acceptable choices because they provide some lubrication and thus may help to increase the woman's satisfaction with intercourse. The lactational amenorrhea method of birth control may be an option for Karen and her husband. They should receive information about a variety of contraceptive options so that they might make an informed decision.

3 Priority for nursing care at this time is to educate Karen about the normal breast changes associated with lactation and contraceptive options for the nursing woman. Karen should also be encouraged to discuss her contraceptive options with her health care provider before resuming sexual activity.

4 There is ample information available concerning breast changes during lactation and contraceptive options for the nursing mother.

5 Some women, whether breastfeeding or bottle-feeding, do not desire contraceptive use for a variety of reasons. Although some of these women may practice abstinence, many will resume unprotected sexual activity. Sterilization or vasectomy can be considered if their family is complete. Most medical professionals recommend waiting at least several months after giving birth before becoming pregnant again. This gives the woman's body time to replenish nutrient stores that were depleted during pregnancy.

Complications of Immobility after Cesarean Birth

1 Yes, there is sufficient evidence to draw conclusions about risk factors for developing a thromboembolism during the postpartum period, especially in postcesarean patients. The vessel damage that normally occurs during surgery and postoperative immobility are two contributing factors. Another contributing factor is the woman's hypercoagulable state. Clotting factors and fibrinogen are normally increased during pregnancy and remain elevated during the immediate postpartum period. Especially when blood pools in the lower extremities, clots are likely to form.

2 a. Women who give birth by cesarean are less likely than those who give birth vaginally to be active during the first day or so postpartum. Pain is an obvious reason for decreased activity. Other contributing factors to immobility include the presence of an indwelling urinary catheter and an intravenous line. Both of these are present in most postcesarean patients for at least 24 hours after surgery.

   b. Like other postoperative patients, postcesarean patients are less likely to be active when they are in pain. It is important to stay "on top of" a patient's pain by providing medication as soon as she begins to hurt rather than waiting until her pain is severe. Newer analgesic techniques, such as the use of epidural morphine, provide excellent postsurgical pain relief while minimizing the common complications, such as respiratory depression and constipation, experienced by patients receiving opioid medications. Patient controlled analgesia (PCA) can also be very effective in providing pain control.

   c. The physiology of pain response is the same for all. However, there are cultural variations in response to, and expression of, pain. Some cultures view verbal expression of pain negatively; others provide more support for the person who expresses pain. The culturally sensitive nurse will take into consideration the woman's culture when assessing and treating pain.

   d. A supportive nurse who provides explanations and rationale for suggested interventions (such as the importance of ambulation) and provides nonpharmacologic and pharmacologic pain relief measures will likely be able to influence her patients to ambulate as necessary. Taking time and providing encouragement are supportive interventions that will be appreciated.

3 The priorities for nursing care at this time are to educate this patient about the potential serious consequences of immobility and to encourage her to move as much as possible. Interventions to encourage activity would include providing assistance with changing positions (lying to sitting, sitting to standing, standing to walking) and ambulating, as well as administering analgesic medications before activity, to minimize pain. The patient might also be taught range-of-motion exercises for her legs and feet to be done in bed. This would improve lower extremity circulation and thus make thromboembolism formation less likely. She could also be assisted to sit on the side of the bed and dangle her legs.

4 There is a significant amount of information available concerning decreased activity because of pain in postsurgical patients and the risk of thromboembolism in postpartum women, especially when immobility is present.

5 A patient experiencing pain is not eager to move or do anything else that might cause the pain to increase. The postcesarean woman may be hesitant to move about in bed or to ambulate due to fear of disrupting or damaging the surgical incision site. She may fear that the wound will break open with activity. The nurse can offer simple explanations regarding the safety of ambulation in relation to the surgical incision, and can reassure the patient that she/he will be there to assist whenever the patient is ready to get out of bed.

Resources

American College of Nurse-Midwives
8403 Colesville Rd., Suite 1550
Silver Spring, MD 20910
240-485-1800
www.midwife.org

American College of Obstetricians and Gynecologists
409 12th St., SW
Washington, DC 20090-6920
202-638-5577
www.acog.com

Association of Women's Health, Obstetric and Neonatal Nurses
  (AWHONN)
2000 L St., NW, Suite 740
Washington, DC 20036
800-673-8499 (United States)
800-245-0231 (Canada)
www.awhonn.org

Coping with the Overall Pregnancy/Parenting Experience (COPE)
37 Clarendon St.
Boston, MA 02116
617-357-5588

Maternity Center Association, Inc.
281 Park Ave., South, 5th Floor
New York, NY 10010
212-777-5000
www.maternitywise.org

References

Bowes, W., & Katz, V. (2002). Postpartum care. In S. Gabbe, J. Niebyl, & J. Simpson (Eds.), *Obstetrics: Normal and problem pregnancies* (4th ed.). New York: Churchill Livingstone.

Cunningham, F., Leveno, K., Bloom, S., Hauth, J., Gilstrap, L., & Wenstrom, K. (2005). *Williams obstetrics* (22nd ed.). New York: McGraw-Hill.

Lawrence, R., & Lawrence, R. (2004). The breast and the physiology of lactation. In R. Creasy, R. Resnik, & J. Iams (Eds.), *Maternal-fetal medicine: Principles and practice* (5th ed.). Philadelphia: Saunders.

Mangesi, L., & Hofmeyr, G. (2002). Early compared with delayed oral fluids and food after caesarean section (Cochrane Review). In *The Cochrane Library*, Issue 1, 2005. Chichester, UK: John Wiley & Sons.

Resnik, R. (2004). The puerperium. In R. Creasy, R. Resnik, & J. Iams (Eds.), *Maternal-fetal medicine: Principles and practice* (5th ed.). Philadelphia: Saunders.

Simpson, K., & Creehan, P. (2001). AWHONN's *Perinatal nursing* (2nd ed.). Philadelphia: Lippincott.

CHAPTER 16

Nursing Care during the Fourth Trimester

KELLY CRUM

LEARNING OBJECTIVES

- Identify the priorities of maternal care given during the fourth stage of labor.
- Identify common selection criteria for safe early postpartum discharge.
- Summarize nursing interventions to prevent infection and excessive bleeding, to promote normal bladder and bowel patterns, and to care for the breasts of women who are breastfeeding or bottle-feeding.
- Explain the influence of cultural expectations on postpartum adjustment.
- Identify psychosocial needs of the woman in the early postpartum period.
- Discuss discharge teaching and postpartum home care.

KEY TERMS AND DEFINITIONS

couplet care One nurse, educated in both mother and infant care, functions as the primary nurse for both mother and infant (also known as *mother-baby care* or *single-room maternity care*)
engorgement Swelling of the breast tissue brought about by an increase in blood and lymph supplied to the breast, occurring as early milk (colostrum) transitions to mature milk, at about 72 to 96 hours after birth
fourth stage of labor The first 1 or 2 hours after birth
Homans sign Early sign of phlebothrombosis of the deep veins of the calf in which there are complaints of pain when the leg is in extension and the foot is dorsiflexed

thrombus Blood clot obstructing a blood vessel that remains at the place it was formed
uterine atony Relaxation of uterine muscle; leads to postpartum hemorrhage
warm line A help line, or consultation service, for families to access; most often for support of newborn care and postpartum care after hospital discharge

ELECTRONIC RESOURCES

Additional information related to the content in Chapter 16 can be found on

the companion website at **evolve**
http://evolve.elsevier.com/Lowdermilk/Maternity/
- NCLEX Review Questions
- Case Study—Fourth Trimester
- WebLinks

or on the interactive companion CD
- NCLEX Review Questions
- Case Study—Fourth Trimester
- Critical Thinking Exercise—Priority Nursing Care: Postpartum Unit
- Plan of Care—Postpartum Care-Vaginal Birth

The goal of nursing care in the immediate postpartum period is to assist women and their partners during their initial transition to parenting. The approach to the care of women after birth has changed from one modeled on sick care to one that is wellness oriented. Consequently, in the United States most women remain hospitalized no more than 1 or 2 days after vaginal birth, and some for as few as 6 hours. Because there is so much important information to be shared with these women in a very short time, it is vital that their care be thoughtfully planned and provided. Care is focused on the woman's physiologic recovery, her psychologic well-being, and her ability to care for herself and her new baby and includes other family members.

FOURTH STAGE OF LABOR

The first 1 to 2 hours after birth, sometimes called the fourth stage of labor, is a crucial time for mother and newborn. Both are not only recovering from the physical process of birth but are also becoming acquainted with each other and additional family members. During this time, maternal organs undergo their initial readjustment to the nonpregnant state and the functions of body systems begin to stabilize. Meanwhile, the newborn continues the transition from intrauterine to extrauterine existence.

The fourth stage of labor is an excellent time to begin breastfeeding because the infant is in an alert state and ready to nurse. Breastfeeding at this time also aids in the contraction of the uterus and the prevention of maternal hemorrhage. In most centers the mother remains in the labor and birth area during this recovery time. In an institution in which labor, delivery, and recovery (LDR) rooms are used, the woman stays in the same room in which she gave birth. In traditional settings, women are taken from the delivery room to a separate recovery area for observation. Arrangements for care of the newborn vary during the fourth stage of labor. In many settings, the baby remains at the mother's bedside, and the labor or birth nurse cares for both of them. In other institutions the baby is taken to the nursery for several hours of observation after an initial bonding period with the parents (Fig. 16-1).

Physical Assessment

If the recovery nurse has not previously cared for the new mother, her assessment begins with an oral report from the nurse who attended the woman during labor and birth and a review of the prenatal, labor, and birth records. Of primary importance are conditions that could predispose the mother to hemorrhage, such as precipitous labor, large baby, grand multiparity (i.e., having given birth to six or more viable infants), or induced labor. For healthy women, hemorrhage is probably the most dangerous potential complication during the fourth stage of labor.

During the first hour in the recovery room, physical assessments of the mother are frequent. All factors except

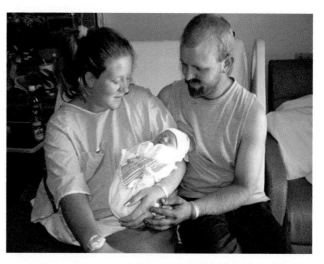

Fig. 16-1 Mother and father get acquainted with the newborn. (Courtesy Shannon Perry, Phoenix, AZ.)

temperature are assessed every 15 minutes for 1 hour. Temperature is assessed at the beginning and end of the recovery period. After the fourth 15-minute assessment, if all parameters have stabilized within the normal range, the process is usually repeated once in the second hour. Box 16-1 and Fig. 16-2 describe the physical assessment of the mother during the fourth stage of labor. Fig. 16-3 shows an easy-to-use flow sheet that combines the essential immediate postpartum and anesthesia recovery assessments.

During the fourth stage of labor, intense tremors that resemble shivering from a chill are commonly seen; they are not related to infection. Several theories have been offered to explain these tremors or shivering, such as their being the result of a sudden release of pressure on pelvic nerves after birth, a response to a fetus-to-mother transfusion that occurred during placental separation, a reaction to maternal adrenaline production during labor and birth, or a reaction to epidural anesthesia. Warm blankets and reassurance that the chills or tremors are common, are self-limiting, and last only a short time are useful interventions.

The nutritional status of the woman is assessed. Restriction of food and fluid intake and the loss of fluids (blood, perspiration, or emesis) during labor cause many women to express a strong desire to eat or drink soon after birth. In the absence of complications, a woman who has given birth vaginally; has recovered from the effects of the anesthetic; and has stable vital signs, a firm uterus, and small to moderate lochial flow may have fluids and a regular diet as desired (American Academy of Pediatrics [AAP] & American College of Obstetricians and Gynecologists [ACOG], 2002).

Postanesthesia Recovery

The woman who has given birth by cesarean or has received regional anesthesia for a vaginal birth requires special attention during the recovery period. Obstetric recovery areas are held to the same standard of care that would be expected

BOX 16-1

Assessment during Fourth Stage of Labor

- Before beginning the assessment, wash hands thoroughly, assemble necessary equipment, and explain the procedure to the patient.

BLOOD PRESSURE

- Measure blood pressure per assessment schedule.

PULSE

- Assess rate and regularity.

TEMPERATURE

- Determine temperature.

FUNDUS

- Put on clean examination gloves.
- Position woman with knees flexed and head flat.
- Just below umbilicus, cup hand and press firmly into abdomen. At the same time, stabilize the uterus at the symphysis with the opposite hand.
- If fundus is firm (and bladder is empty), with uterus in midline, measure its position relative to woman's umbilicus. Lay fingers flat on abdomen under umbilicus; measure how many fingerbreadths (fb) or centimeters (cm) fit between umbilicus and top of fundus. If the fundus is above the umbilicus, this is recorded as plus fb or cm; if below, as minus fb or cm.
- If fundus is not firm, massage it gently to contract and expel any clots before measuring distance from umbilicus.
- Place hands appropriately; massage gently only until firm.
- Expel clots while keeping hands placed as in Fig. 16-2. With upper hand, firmly apply pressure downward toward vagina; observe perineum for amount and size of expelled clots.

BLADDER

- Assess distention by noting location and firmness of uterine fundus and by observing and palpating bladder. Distended bladder is seen as a suprapubic rounded bulge that is dull to percussion and fluctuates like a water-filled balloon. When the bladder is distended, the uterus is usually boggy in consistency, well above the umbilicus, and to the woman's right side.
- Assist woman to void spontaneously. Measure amount of urine voided.
- Catheterize as necessary.
- Reassess after voiding or catheterization to make sure the bladder is not palpable and the fundus is firm and in the midline.

LOCHIA

- Observe lochia on perineal pads and on linen under the mother's buttocks. Determine amount and color, note size and number of clots; note odor.
- Observe perineum for source of bleeding (e.g., episiotomy, lacerations).

PERINEUM

- Ask or assist woman to turn on her side and flex upper leg on hip.
- Lift upper buttock.
- Observe perineum in good lighting.
- Assess episiotomy site or laceration repair for intactness, hematoma, edema, bruising, redness, and drainage.
- Assess for presence of hemorrhoids.

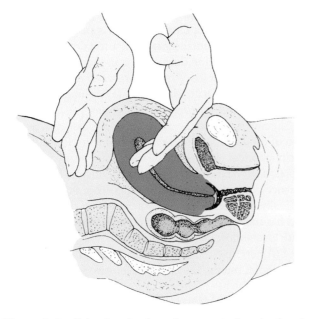

Fig. 16-2 Palpating fundus of uterus during the fourth stage of labor. Note that upper hand is cupped over fundus; lower hand dips in above symphysis pubis and supports uterus while it is massaged gently.

of any other postanesthesia recovery (PAR) room (AAP & ACOG, 2002). A PAR score is determined for each patient on arrival and updated as part of every 15-minute assessment. Components of the PAR score include activity, respirations, blood pressure, level of consciousness, and color.

NURSE ALERT *Regardless of her obstetric status, no woman should be discharged from the recovery area until she has completely recovered from the effects of anesthesia.*

If the woman received general anesthesia, she should be awake and alert and oriented to time, place, and person. Her respiratory rate should be within normal limits, and her oxygen saturation levels at least 95%, as measured by a pulse oximeter. If the woman received epidural or spinal anesthesia, she should be able to raise her legs, extended at the knees, off the bed or to flex her knees, place her feet flat on the bed, and raise her buttocks well off the bed. The numb or tingling, prickly sensation should be entirely gone from her legs. Often, it takes several hours for these anesthetic effects to disappear.

DIAGNOSIS:_____

PHYSICIAN:_____

ANESTHESIA:_____

ANESTHETIST:_____

ARMBANDS:_____mother _____infant

CLOTHING:_____c̄ family _____c̄ patient

ALLERGIES:_____

PAR SCORE: ADM:_____ DC:_____

ACTIVITY					
RESPIRATION					
BLOOD PRESSURE					
CONSCIOUS LEVEL					
COLOR					
TOTAL					

Activity

Able to move 4 extremities voluntarily or on command	2
Able to move 2 extremities voluntarily or on command	1
Able to move 0 extremities voluntarily or on command	0

Respiration

Able to deep breathe and cough freely	2
Dyspnea or limited breathing	1
Apneic	0

Blood Pressure

BP ± mm Hg of preanesthetic level	2
BP ± 25-50 mm HG of preanesthetic level	1
BP ± Greater than 50 mm HG of preanesthetic level	0

Conscious Level

Fully aware	2
Arousable on calling	1
Not responding	0

Color

Pink	2
Pale, dusky, blotchy, jaundiced, other	1
Cyanotic	0

Pain Scales
Wong Baker = WB
Numeric = N
Simple Descriptive = SD

Pain Characteristics
Location
Duration
Aggravating/Alleviating fx
Nature - dull, gnawing, hot, achy, sharp, burning, throbbing, shooting, stabbing

Observation Codes

A - Anxious	D - Depressed	H - Relaxed
B - Agitated,	E - Crying	V - VS Change
Restless	R - Restless	W - Withdrawn
C - Confused	G - Grimace	O - Other

Results Code
0 - No pain present
1 - Improved but still in pain
2 - No improvement

Pain Management Intervention
P - Pharmacological
NP - Non pharmacological

VITAL SIGNS:	TIME								
	BP								
	PULSE								
	RESP / O₂ Sat								
	TEMP								
FUNDUS FB-FINGERBREADTH B-BOGGY FM-FIRM MD-MIDLINE	FUNDUS								
LOCHIA CL-CLOTS MOD-MODERATE SM-SMALL LG-LARGE	LOCHIA								
BLADDER D-DISTENDED F-FOLEY ND-NON-DISTENDED	BLADDER								
EPISIOTOMY/INCISION NL-NORMAL D-DRY ABNL-ABNORMAL I-INTACT	EPIS / INC								
CLEAR CL WHEEZING W DIMINISHED D	BREATH SOUNDS								
q 1° q Shift	DTR / PROTEIN								
O₂ liters/min									
JP drain cc/hr									
INTAKE									
OUTPUT									
Pain Scale									
Observation Code									
Pain Management Intervention									
Results Code									
INITIALS									

DISCHARGE NOTE

Report Called To:_____

ANESTHESIA D/C:_____

EPIDURAL CATHETER: IN   OUT   NA

PCA

PCA Medication, Concentration and Volume
_____

Loading Dose _____

Continuous Rate _____ 4 hour limit _____

Lockout Interval _____

RN _____ RN _____

____ / ____ / _____ ____:____ am / pm

Meds / IV / Rate	Time / Initial
	/
	/
	/
	/
	/

INTAKE TOTAL
Shift 7A 3P 11P
_____

OUTPUT TOTAL
Shift 7A 3P 11P
_____

IV _____cc LTC
@ D/C

Signatures/Initials
_____
_____

Homans Sign   Pos ☐   Neg ☐

BONDING
☐ appropriate
☐ inappropriate
☐ NA (explain)
_____

Social Services
Notified
____ / ____ / ____
____:____ am/pm

TEACHING
☐ fundal massage
☐ TC & DB
☐ breastfeeding
☐ assistance on
    1st ambulation
☐ Pain Scale
☐ PCA pump

THE MED

Regional Medical Center at Memphis

MATERNITY RECOVERY ROOM RECORD

FORM NO. 68622 (10/01)   White (Chart)   Yellow (Pharmacy)

Fig. 16-3 An example of a maternity recovery room record. (Courtesy The Regional Medical Center at Memphis [The Med], Memphis, TN.)

Date of Birth: _____

Hour of Birth: _____

The uncomplicated vaginal birth patient's admission and discharge are based on a 24-hr length of stay after birth based on individual needs.

Time: _____

	RECOVERY	ADM. TO PP UNIT–8 HR	9-16 HR	17-24 HR/DISCHARGE
PRIMARY PHYSIOLOGIC FOCUS	Woman will have normal vital signs and moderate lochia as documented on flow sheet. Pain/discomfort will be controlled.	Woman will have normal vital signs and moderate lochia rubra. Pain/discomfort will be controlled.	Woman will have normal vital signs and minimal lochia rubra. Pain/discomfort will be controlled.	Woman will have normal vital signs and minimal lochia rubra. Pain/discomfort will be controlled.
	NA MET VARIANCE	**NA MET VARIANCE**	**NA MET VARIANCE**	**NA MET VARIANCE**
	Vital signs every 15 min ×1 hr, then every 4 hr. Assess pain and provide intervention as needed. Assess perineum/episiotomy. Assess lochia.	Vital signs every 4 hr. Assess pain and provide intervention as needed. Assess perineum/episiotomy. Assess lochia.	Vital signs every shift. Assess pain and provide intervention as needed. Assess perineum/episiotomy. Assess lochia.	Vital signs every shift. Assess pain and provide intervention as needed. Assess perineum/episiotomy. Assess lochia.
IVs/LABWORK/MEDICATIONS	**RECOVERY** Woman will have appropriate lab work done and medication given by time of transfer to Mother/Baby Unit.	**ADM. TO PP UNIT–8 HR** Woman will begin to verbalize understanding of hepatitis status and medication requirements.	**9-16 HR** Woman will have appropriate lab work done by 16 hr PP.	**17-24 HR/DISCHARGE** Woman will have appropriate lab work done and appropriate medications initiated.
	NA MET VARIANCE	**NA MET VARIANCE**	**NA MET VARIANCE**	**NA MET VARIANCE**
	CBC, if not done before birth. Urine drug screen if ordered. U/A-dipstick, if ordered. (Send to lab, if abnormal.)	Review hepatitis B status. Medication regimen initiated.	CBC. Review rubella status. Review Hgb and Hct.	Iron tablet. Prenatal vitamin. Rubella vaccine, if appropriate. Rh immune globulin, if indicated. Stool softener/laxative if needed.
NUTRITION/ELIMINATION	**RECOVERY** Woman will be up to bathroom before transfer.	**ADM. TO PP UNIT–8 HR** Woman will resume normal nutritional status and bladder function.	**9-16 HR** Woman will resume normal nutritional status and bladder function.	**17-24 HR/DISCHARGE** Woman will have normal bladder function.
	NA MET VARIANCE	**NA MET VARIANCE**	**NA MET VARIANCE**	**NA MET VARIANCE**
	Assess bladder fullness. Assist to bathroom. Assess for tolerance of oral intake.	Encourage ambulation. Encourage oral fluids. Assist to bathroom as needed. Assess bladder function. Encourage oral intake.	Encourage ambulation. Encourage oral fluids. Assist to bathroom as needed. Assess bladder function. Encourage oral intake.	Encourage ambulation. Encourage oral fluids. Assist to bathroom as needed. Stool softener/laxative prn.
PSYCHOSOCIAL	**RECOVERY** Woman and family will begin attachment behaviors with newborn.	**ADM. TO PP UNIT–8 HR** Woman and family will demonstrate appropriate attachment behaviors.	**9-16 HR** Family will verbalize comfort with new infant.	**17-24 HR/DISCHARGE** Family will verbalize comfort with new infant.
	NA MET VARIANCE	**NA MET VARIANCE**	**NA MET VARIANCE**	**NA MET VARIANCE**
	Encourage mother and family members to hold and touch infant. Provide skin-to-skin contact of mother and infant. Provide mother the opportunity to breastfeed, if applicable.	Offer flexible rooming-in with infant. Allow verbalization of woman's feelings. Assess discharge needs and need for social service consult.	Reinforce interventions.	Reinforce interventions. Completion of birth certificate. Arrange for home visit.

Date of Birth: _____

Hour of Birth: _____

The uncomplicated vaginal birth client's admission and discharge are based on a 24-hr length of stay after birth based on individual needs.

Time: _____

	RECOVERY	ADM. TO PP UNIT–8 HR	9-16 HR	17-24 HR/DISCHARGE
SELF-CARE ACTIVITY	Woman will begin self-care activities as tolerated.	Woman will be up to bathroom or shower with assistance.	Woman will be up to bathroom or shower independently.	Woman will be up to bathroom or shower independently.
	NA MET VARIANCE	NA MET VARIANCE	NA MET VARIANCE	NA MET VARIANCE
	Instruct woman in pericare and pad changes, and use of ice pack.	Reinforce proper pericare. Encourage woman to shower.	Reinforce proper pericare. Instruct in use of sitz bath.	Reinforce proper pericare. Instruct in use of sitz bath.
	RECOVERY	**ADM. TO PP UNIT–8 HR**	**9-16 HR**	**17-24 HR/DISCHARGE**
	Woman will begin to verbalize and/or demonstrate self-care and infant-care activities.	Woman will begin to verbalize and/or demonstrate infant- and self-care activities.	Woman and family will demonstrate appropriate infant-care activities.	Woman and family will demonstrate appropriate infant-care activities.
	NA MET VARIANCE	NA MET VARIANCE	NA MET VARIANCE	NA MET VARIANCE
TEACHING/ DISCHARGE PLANNING	Date:			
	Initials:			
	Teaching to include: • Breastfeeding latch-on and positioning, if applicable. • Appropriate handwashing techniques. • Cough and deep breathing exercises. • Pain-relief techniques or medication.	Teaching to include: • Breastfeeding or formula initial feeding information. • Breast care. • Perineal care. • Proper nutrition. • Safety issues.	Teaching to include: • Attendance at mother/baby-care class. • Breast care or formula information. • Newborn videos. • Lactation consult prn. • Appropriate handwashing techniques.	Teaching to include: • Reinforcement of teaching from mother/baby-care class. • Plans for self/infant follow-up. • Review IHSP.* • Review Baby Net program. • Telephone number for follow-up questions. • Home-going meds and purposes.
	1.	1.	1.	1.
	2.	2.	2.	2.
	3.	3.	3.	3.
	4.	4.	4.	4.

Variance Documentation: _____

_____

_____

_____

_____

*IHSP denotes a test done to determine whether follow-up is needed in the Infant Hearing Screening Program (IHSP).

Transfer from the Recovery Area

After the initial recovery period has been completed, the woman may be transferred to a postpartum room in the same or another nursing unit. In facilities with labor, delivery, recovery, and postpartum (LDRP) rooms, the nurse who provides care during the recovery period usually continues caring for the woman. Women who have received general or regional anesthesia must be cleared for transfer from the recovery area by a member of the anesthesia care team.

In preparing the transfer report the recovery nurse uses information from the records of admission, birth, and recovery. Information that must be communicated to the postpartum nurse includes identity of the health care provider; gravidity and parity; age; anesthetic used; any medications given; duration of labor and time of rupture of membranes; whether labor was induced or augmented; type of birth and repair; blood type and Rh status; group B streptococci status; status of rubella immunity; syphilis and hepatitis B serology test results (if positive); intravenous infusion of any fluids; physiologic status since birth; description of fundus, lochia, bladder, and perineum; gender and weight of infant; time of birth; chosen method of feeding; any abnormalities noted; and assessment of initial parent-infant interaction.

Most of this information is also documented for the nursing staff in the newborn nursery. In addition, specific information should be provided regarding the name of the pediatric care provider, the infant's Apgar scores, weight, voiding, stooling, and whether fed since birth. Nursing interventions that have been completed (e.g., eye prophylaxis, vitamin K injection) must also be recorded.

Women who give birth in birthing centers may go home within a few hours, after the woman's and infant's conditions are stable.

DISCHARGE—BEFORE 24 HOURS AND AFTER 48 HOURS

Early postpartum discharge, shortened hospital stay, and *1-day maternity stay* are all terms for the decreasing length of hospital stays of mothers and their babies after a low risk birth. The trend of shortened hospital stays is based largely on efforts to reduce health care costs coupled with consumer demands to have fewer medical interventions and more family-focused experiences (Meara, Kotagal, Atherton, & Lieu, 2004).

Laws Relating to Discharge

Health care providers have expressed concern with shortened stays because some medical problems do not show up in the first 24 hours after birth and new mothers have not had sufficient time to learn how to care for their newborns and identify newborn health problems such as jaundice and dehydration related to breastfeeding difficulties (Meara et al., 2004).

The concern for the potential increase in adverse maternal-infant outcomes from hospital early discharge practices led the American College of Obstetricians and Gynecologists (ACOG), the American Academy of Pediatrics (AAP), and other professional health care organizations to promote the enactment of federal and state maternity length-of-stay bills to ensure adequate care for both the mother and the newborn. The passage of the Newborns' and Mothers' Health Protection Act of 1996 provided minimum federal standards for health plan coverage for mothers and their newborns (AAP, 2004). Under the Newborns' and Mothers' Health Protection Act, all health plans are required to allow the new mother and newborn to remain in the hospital for a minimum of 48 hours after a normal vaginal birth and for 96 hours after a cesarean birth unless the attending provider, in consultation with the mother, decides on early discharge.

Criteria for Discharge

Early discharge with postpartum home care can be a safe and satisfying option for women and their families when it is comprehensive and based on individual needs (AAP, 2004). Hospital stays must be long enough to identify problems and to ensure that the woman is sufficiently recovered and is prepared to care for herself and the baby at home.

It is essential that nurses consider the medical needs of the woman and her baby and provide care that is coordinated to meet those needs in order to provide timely physiologic interventions and treatment to prevent morbidity and hospital readmission. With predetermined criteria for identifying low risk in the mothers and newborns (Box 16-2), the length of hospitalization can be based on medical need for care in an acute care setting or in consideration of the ongoing care needed in the home environment (AAP, 2004). Early follow-up visits are key to reducing readmissions of newborns (Meara et al., 2004).

Care paths provide the nurse with an organized approach toward meeting essential maternal-newborn care and teaching goals within a limited time frame (see Care Path on p. 471). Care paths can be developed for vaginal or cesarean births. Other methods such as postpartum order sets and maternal-newborn teaching checklists (Fig. 16-4) can be used to accomplish patient care and educational outcomes.

Hospital-based maternity nurses continue to play invaluable roles as caregivers, teachers, and patient and family advocates in developing and implementing effective home care strategies. The nurse participates in the determination of whether the mother and newborn meet the criteria for early discharge.

LEGAL TIP Early Discharge

Whether or not the woman and her family have chosen early discharge, the nurse and the primary health care provider are held responsible if the woman is discharged before her condition has stabilized within normal limits. If complications occur, the medical and nursing staff could be sued for abandonment.

BOX 16-2

Criteria for Early Discharge

MOTHER

- Uncomplicated pregnancy, labor, vaginal birth, and post-partum course
- No evidence of premature rupture of membranes
- Blood pressure, temperature stable and within normal limits
- Ambulating unassisted
- Voiding adequate amounts without difficulty
- Hemoglobin >10 g
- No significant vaginal bleeding; perineum intact or no more than second-degree episiotomy or laceration repair; uterus is firm
- Received instructions on postpartum self-care

INFANT

- Term infant (38 to 42 weeks) with weight appropriate for gestational age
- Normal findings on physical assessment
- Temperature, respirations, and heart rate within normal limits and stable for the 12 hours preceding discharge
- At least two successful feedings completed (normal sucking and swallowing)
- Urination and stooling have occurred at least once

- No evidence of significant jaundice in the first 24 hours after the birth
- No excessive bleeding at the circumcision site for at least 2 hours
- Screening tests performed according to state regulations; tests to be repeated at follow-up visit if done before the infant is 24 hours old
- Initial hepatitis B vaccine given or scheduled for first follow-up visit
- Laboratory data reviewed: maternal syphilis and hepatitis B status; infant or cord blood type and Coombs test results if indicated

GENERAL

- No social, family, or environmental risk factors identified
- Family or support person available to assist mother and infant at home
- Follow-up scheduled within 1 week if discharged before 48 hours after the birth
- Documentation of skill of mother in feeding (breastfeeding or bottle-feeding), cord care, skin care, perineal care, infant safety (use of car seat, sleeping positions), and recognizing signs of illness and common infant problems

EVOLVE/CD: Case Study—Fourth Trimester

Source: American Academy of Pediatrics (AAP). Committee on Fetus and Newborn. (2004). Hospital stay for healthy term infants. *Pediatrics, 113*(5), 1434-1436.

CARE MANAGEMENT— PHYSICAL NEEDS ■

Assessment and Nursing Diagnoses

A complete physical assessment, including measurement of vital signs, is performed on admission to the postpartum unit. If the woman's vital signs are within normal limits, they are usually assessed every 4 to 8 hours for the remainder of her hospitalization. Other components of the initial assessment include the mother's emotional status, energy level, degree of physical discomfort, hunger, and thirst. Intake and output assessments should always be included if an intravenous infusion or a urinary catheter is in place. If the woman gave birth by cesarean, her incisional dressing should also be assessed. To some degree, her knowledge level concerning self-care and infant care can also be determined at this time.

Ongoing physical assessment

The new mother should be evaluated thoroughly during each shift throughout hospitalization (Guidelines/Guías box). Physical assessments include evaluation of the breasts, uterine fundus, lochia, perineum, bladder and bowel function, vital signs, and legs. If a woman has an intravenous line in place, her fluid and hematologic status should be evaluated before it is removed. Signs of potential problems that

may be identified during the assessment process are listed in the Signs of Potential Complications box.

Routine laboratory tests

Several laboratory tests may be performed in the immediate postpartum period. Hemoglobin and hematocrit values are often evaluated on the first postpartum day to assess blood loss during childbirth, especially after cesarean birth. In some hospitals a clean-catch or catheterized urine specimen may be obtained and sent for routine urinalysis or culture and sensitivity, especially if an indwelling urinary catheter was inserted during the intrapartum period. In addition, if the woman's rubella and Rh status are unknown, tests to determine her status and need for possible treatment should be performed at this time.

Nursing diagnoses

Although all women experience similar physiologic changes during the postpartum period, certain factors act to make each woman's experience unique. From a physiologic standpoint the length and difficulty of the labor, type of birth (i.e., vaginal or cesarean), presence of episiotomy or lacerations, parity, and whether the mother plans to breastfeed or bottle-feed are factors to be considered with each woman. After analyzing the data obtained during the assessment process, the nurse establishes nursing diagnoses that will provide a guide for planning care. Examples of nursing diagnoses

Abbott Northwestern Hospital
A HealthSpan™ Organization
SELF/FAMILY LEARNING CHECKLIST

| Patient Name, Medical Record #, Date of Birth |

I learn best by: ☐ Group classes ☐ Individual instruction ☐ Video instruction ☐ Reading it myself

Please indicate your desired learning needs by placing a check in one of the columns next to each topic.

KEY 1 = Most important to learn before I go home
2 = I already know

(Please DATE when learning need is met.)

CARING FOR YOURSELF	1	2	DATE	CARING FOR BABY	1	2	DATE
Episiotomy and perineal care				Diapering			
Vaginal discharge				Baby bath, skin and cord care			
Hemorrhoids/Constipation				Circumcised/uncircumcised care			
Breast care				Burping			
Nutrition				Bowel movements/wet diapers			
Activity				Sleeping habits			
Post partal exercises				Newborn behavior			
Return of menstruation				Jaundice			
Family planning				Signs of illness			
Blood clots				Car seat safety			
Post partum emotions				General infant safety/poison control			
Post partum warning signs				Signs/symptoms of dehydration			
				Bulb syringe			
Cesarean Birth							
Incisional care				**BREAST FEEDING**			
				Sore nipples			
				Positioning			
				Frequency of feedings			
AFTER DISCHARGE				Expressing/storing milk			
When to call health care provider				Engorgement			
				Feeding water			
				Nursing while working			
OTHER				Weaning			
Working mothers							
Day care				**BOTTLE FEEDING**			
Sibling adjustment				Types of formula			
Single parent support				Preparing formula			
Time out for parents				Frequency of feedings			
Infant safety and security							
Infant as a Person Class							
New Parent Connection							

MEDICATIONS AT HOME

MEDICATIONS	STRENGTH	DOSAGE	FREQUENCY	PURPOSE/SPECIAL INSTRUCTIONS
			times per day	
			times per day	
			times per day	

RESOURCES REFERRALS
☐ Physician Discharge Instructions _____
☐ Home Care Agency _____
☐ Other Referrals _____

VALUABLES: ☐ Returned ☐ None   **MEDICATIONS:** ☐ Returned ☐ None   ☐ Room checked for belongings
Patient verbalized understanding of discharge information received.

PATIENT OR SUPPORT PERSON _____   NURSE'S SIGNATURE _____   DATE _____

SELF/FAMILY LEARNING CHECKLIST

Fig. 16-4 Self/family learning checklist. (Copyright Abbott Northwestern Hospital of Allina Health System, Minneapolis and St. Paul, MN.)

commonly established for the postpartum patient include the following:

- *Risk for deficient fluid volume (hemorrhage) related to*
  - —uterine atony after childbirth
- *Risk for constipation related to*
  - —postchildbirth discomfort
  - —childbirth trauma to tissues
  - —decreased intake of solid food and/or fluids
- *Acute pain related to*
  - —uterine involution
  - —trauma to perineum, episiotomy
  - —hemorrhoids
  - —engorged breasts
- *Disturbed sleep patterns related to*
  - —discomforts of postpartum period
  - —long labor process
  - —infant care and hospital routine
- *Ineffective breastfeeding related to*
  - —maternal discomfort
  - —infant positioning

Expected Outcomes of Care

The nursing plan of care includes both the postpartum woman and her infant, even if the nursery nurse retains primary responsibility for the infant. In many hospitals, **couplet care** (also called *mother-baby care* or *single-room maternity care*) is practiced. Nurses in these settings have been educated in both mother and infant care and function as primary nurses for both mother and infant, even if the infant is kept in the nursery. This approach is a variation of

GUIDELINES/GUÍAS

Postpartum Physical Assessment

- Are you planning to breastfeed or bottle-feed?
- *¿Piensa darle pecho o biberón al bebé?*

- Lie down, please.
- *Acuéstese, por favor.*

- I am going to take your vital signs.
- *Le voy a tomar sus signos vitales.*

- I need to take your blood pressure
- *Necesito tomarle la presión sanguínea.*

- Do you need to use the bathroom?
- *¿Necesita usar el baño?*

- I need to examine you.
- *Necesito examinarle.*

- Please spread your knees and legs apart.
- *Por favor, abra las rodillas y las piernas.*

- Roll over on your side, please.
- *Póngase sobre un costado, por favor.*

- Would you like some pain medication?
- *¿Desea medicina para calmar el dolor?*

- Would you like to take a sitz bath?
- *¿Desea tomar un baño de asiento?*

signs of POTENTIAL COMPLICATIONS

Physiologic Problems

TEMPERATURE
- More than 38° C after the first 24 hr

PULSE
- Tachycardia or marked bradycardia

BLOOD PRESSURE
- Hypotension or hypertension

ENERGY LEVEL
- Lethargy, extreme fatigue

UTERUS
- Deviated from the midline, boggy consistency, remains above the umbilicus after 24 hr

LOCHIA
- Heavy, foul odor, bright red bleeding that is not lochia

PERINEUM
- Pronounced edema, not intact, signs of infection, marked discomfort

LEGS
- Homans sign positive; painful, reddened area; warmth on posterior aspect of calf

BREASTS
- Redness, heat, pain, cracked and fissured nipples, inverted nipples, palpable mass

APPETITE
- Lack of appetite, nausea or vomiting

ELIMINATION
- Urine: inability to void, urgency, frequency, dysuria; bowel: constipation, diarrhea, epigastric pain

REST
- Inability to rest or sleep

NEUROLOGIC
- Headache, blurred vision

rooming-in, in which the mother and infant room together and mother and nurse share the care of the infant. The organization of the mother's care must take the newborn into consideration. The day actually revolves around the baby's feeding and care times.

Expected outcomes for the postpartum period are based on the nursing diagnoses identified for the individual patient. Examples of common expected outcomes for physiologic needs are that the woman will do the following:

- Demonstrate normal involution and lochial characteristics
- Remain comfortable and injury free
- Demonstrate normal bladder and bowel patterns

- Demonstrate knowledge of breast care, whether breast-feeding or bottle-feeding
- Integrate the newborn into the family

Plan of Care and Interventions

Once the nursing diagnoses are formulated, the nurse plans with the woman what nursing measures are appropriate and which are to be given priority. The nursing plan of care includes periodic assessments to detect deviations from normal physical changes, measures to relieve discomfort or pain, safety measures to prevent injury or infection, and teaching and counseling measures designed to promote the woman's feelings of competence in self-care and baby care. Family members are included in the teaching. The nurse evaluates continuously and is ready to change the plan if indicated. Almost all hospitals use standardized care plans or care paths as a basis for planning. The nurse's adaptation of the standardized plan to specific medical and nursing diagnoses results in individualized patient care (Plan of Care).

Nurses assume many roles while implementing the nursing care plan. They provide direct physical care, teach mother-baby care, and provide anticipatory guidance and counseling. Perhaps most important of all, they nurture the woman by providing encouragement and support as she begins to assume the many tasks of motherhood. Nurses who take the time to "mother the mother" do much to increase feelings of self-confidence in new mothers.

The first step in providing individualized care is to confirm the woman's identity by checking her wristband. At the same time the infant's identification number is matched with the corresponding band on the mother's wrist and, in some instances, the father's wrist. The nurse determines how the mother wishes to be addressed and then notes her preference in her record and in her nursing care plan.

The woman and her family are oriented to their surroundings. Familiarity with the unit, routines, resources, and personnel reduces one potential source of anxiety—the unknown. The mother is reassured through knowing whom and how she can call for assistance and what she can expect in the way of supplies and services. If the woman's usual daily routine before admission differs from the facility's routine, the nurse works with the woman to develop a mutually acceptable routine.

Infant abduction from hospitals in the United States has increased over the past few years. As a result, many units now have special limited entry systems in place. The mother should be taught to check the identity of any person who comes to remove the baby from her room. Hospital personnel usually wear picture identification badges. On some units, all staff members wear matching scrubs or special badges. Other units use closed-circuit television, computer monitoring systems, or fingerprint identification pads. As a rule, the baby is never carried in a staff member's arms between the mother's room and the nursery but is always wheeled in a bassinet, which also contains baby care supplies.

Patients and nurses must work together to ensure the safety of newborns in the hospital environment.

Prevention of infection

One important means of preventing infection is maintenance of a clean environment. Bed linens should be changed as needed. Disposable pads and draw sheets may need to be changed frequently. By not walking barefoot, women avoid contaminating the linens when they return to bed. Personnel must be conscientious about their handwashing techniques to prevent cross-infection. Standard Precautions must be practiced. Staff members with colds, coughs, or skin infections (e.g., a cold sore on the lips [herpes simplex virus type 1]) must follow hospital protocol when in contact with postpartum patients. In many hospitals, staff members with open herpetic lesions, strep throat, conjunctivitis, upper respiratory infections, or diarrhea are encouraged to avoid contact with mothers and infants by staying home until the condition is no longer contagious.

Proper care of the episiotomy site and any perineal lacerations prevents infection in the genitourinary area and aids the healing process. Educating the woman to wipe from front to back (urethra to anus) after voiding or defecating is a simple first step. In many hospitals a squeeze bottle filled with warm water or an antiseptic solution is used after each voiding to cleanse the perineal area. Heat lamps and sitz baths, once commonly used to promote healing, are now much less frequently used for this purpose (Box 16-3). The woman should change her perineal pad from front to back each time she voids or defecates and wash her hands thoroughly before and after doing so.

Prevention of excessive bleeding

The most common cause of excessive bleeding after birth is **uterine atony,** failure of the uterine muscle to contract firmly. The two most important interventions for preventing excessive bleeding are maintaining good uterine tone and preventing bladder distention. If uterine atony occurs, the relaxed uterus distends with blood and clots, blood vessels in the placental site are not clamped off, and excessive bleeding results.

Excessive blood loss after childbirth may also be caused by vaginal or vulvar hematomas, unrepaired lacerations of the vagina or cervix, and retained placental fragments.

NURSE ALERT *A perineal pad saturated in 15 minutes or less and pooling of blood under the buttocks are indications of excessive blood loss, requiring immediate assessment, intervention, and notification of the physician or nurse-midwife.*

Accurate visual estimation of blood loss is an important nursing responsibility. Blood loss is usually described subjectively as scant, light, moderate, or heavy (profuse). Fig. 16-5 shows examples of perineal pad saturation corresponding to each of these descriptions.

Although postpartal blood loss may be estimated by observing the amount of staining on a perineal pad, it is

PLAN OF CARE *Postpartum Care—Vaginal Birth*

NURSING DIAGNOSIS Risk for deficient fluid volume related to uterine atony and hemorrhage

Expected Outcome *Fundus is firm, lochia is moderate, and there is no evidence of hemorrhage.*

Nursing Interventions/*Rationales*

- Monitor lochia (color, amount, consistency), and count and weigh sanitary pads if lochia is heavy *to evaluate amount of bleeding.*
- Monitor and palpate fundus for location and tone *to determine status of uterus and dictate further interventions because atonic uterus is most common cause of postpartum hemorrhage.*
- Monitor intake and output, assess for bladder fullness, and encourage voiding *because a full bladder interferes with involution of the uterus.*
- Monitor vital signs (increased pulse and respirations, decreased blood pressure) and skin temperature and color *to detect signs of hemorrhage or shock.*
- Monitor postpartum hematology studies *to assess effects of blood loss.*
- If fundus is boggy, apply gentle massage and assess tone response *to promote uterine contractions and increase uterine tone.* (Do not overstimulate because doing so can cause fundal relaxation.)
- Express uterine clots *to promote uterine contraction.*
- Explain to the woman the process of involution and teach her to assess and massage the fundus and to report any persistent bogginess *to involve her in self-care and increase sense of self-control.*
- Administer oxytocic agents per physician or nurse-midwife order and evaluate effectiveness *to promote continuing uterine contraction.*
- Administer fluids, blood, blood products, or plasma expanders as ordered *to replace lost fluid and lost blood volume.*

NURSING DIAGNOSIS Acute pain related to postpartum physiologic changes (hemorrhoids, episiotomy, breast engorgement, cracked and sore nipples)

Expected Outcome *Woman exhibits signs of decreased discomfort.*

Nursing Interventions/*Rationales*

- Assess location, type, and quality of pain *to direct intervention.*
- Explain to the woman the source and reasons for the pain, its expected duration, and treatments *to decrease anxiety and increase sense of control.*
- Administer prescribed pain medications *to provide pain relief.*
- If pain is perineal (episiotomy, hemorrhoids), apply ice packs in the first 24 hours *to reduce edema and vulvar irritation and reduce discomfort;* encourage sitz baths using cool water for first 24 hours *to reduce edema* and warm water thereafter *to promote circulation;* apply witch hazel compresses *to reduce edema;* teach woman to use prescribed perineal creams, sprays, or ointments *to depress response of peripheral nerves;* teach woman to tighten buttocks before sitting and to sit on flat, hard surfaces *to compress buttocks and reduce pressure on the perineum.* (Avoid donuts and soft pillows as they separate the buttocks and decrease venous blood flow, increasing pain.)
- If pain is from breasts and woman is breastfeeding, encourage use of a well-fitted, supportive bra *to increase comfort;* ascertain that infant has latched on correctly *to prevent sore nipples.*

- If breasts are engorged, have woman apply ice packs to breasts 15 minutes on, 45 minutes off, apply cabbage leaves in same manner *to relieve discomfort.* Use warm compresses or take a warm shower before breastfeeding *to stimulate milk flow and relieve stasis.* Hand express milk or pump milk *to relieve discomfort if infant is unable to latch on and feed.*
- If nipples are sore, have woman rub breast milk into nipples after feeding and air-dry nipples; apply purified lanolin or other breast creams as prescribed; and wear breast shields in her bra *to minimize nipple irritation.* Assist woman to correct latch problem *to prevent further nipple soreness.*
- If pain is from breast and woman is not breastfeeding, encourage use of a well-fitted, supportive bra or breast binder and application of ice packs and/or cabbage leaves *to suppress milk production and decrease discomfort.*

NURSING DIAGNOSIS Disturbed sleep patterns related to excitement, discomfort, and environmental interruptions

Expected Outcome *Woman sleeps for uninterrupted periods of time and feels rested after waking.*

Nursing Interventions/*Rationales*

- Establish woman's routine sleep patterns and compare with current sleep patterns, exploring things that interfere with sleep, *to determine scope of problem and direct interventions.*
- Individualize nursing routines to fit woman's natural body rhythms (i.e., wake-sleep cycles), provide a sleep-promoting environment (i.e., darkness, quiet, adequate ventilation, appropriate room temperature), prepare for sleep using woman's usual routines (i.e., back rub, soothing music, warm milk), teach use of guided imagery and relaxation techniques *to promote optimum conditions for sleep.*
- Avoid things or routines (i.e., caffeine, foods that induce heartburn, fluids, strenuous mental or physical activity) *that may interfere with sleep.*
- Administer sedation or pain medication as prescribed *to enhance quality of sleep.*
- Advise woman or partner to limit visitors and activities *to avoid further taxation and fatigue.*
- Teach woman to use infant nap time as a time for her also *to nap and replenish energy and decrease fatigue.*

NURSING DIAGNOSIS Risk for impaired urinary elimination related to perineal trauma and effects of anesthesia

Expected Outcome *Woman will void within 6 to 8 hours after birth and will empty bladder completely.*

Nursing Interventions/*Rationales*

- Assess position and character of uterine fundus and bladder *to determine if any further interventions are indicated because of displacement of the fundus or distention of the bladder.*
- Measure intake and output *to assess for evidence of dehydration and subsequent anticipated decrease in urine output.*
- Encourage voiding by walking woman to bathroom, running water over perineum, running water in sink, providing privacy *to encourage voiding.*
- Encourage oral intake *to replace fluids lost during childbirth and prevent dehydration.*
- Catheterize as necessary by indwelling or straight method *to ensure bladder emptying and allow uterine involution.*

BOX 16-3

Interventions for Episiotomy, Lacerations, and Hemorrhoids

Explain both procedure and rationale before implementation.

CLEANSING
- Wash hands before and after cleansing perineum and changing pads.
- Wash perineum with mild soap and warm water at least once daily.
- Cleanse from symphysis pubis to anal area.
- Apply peripad from front to back, protecting inner surface of pad from contamination.
- Wrap soiled pad and place in covered waste container.
- Change pad with each void or defecation or at least four times per day.
- Assess amount and character of lochia with each pad change.

ICE PACK
- Apply a covered ice pack to perineum from front to back.
  - During first 2 hours to decrease edema formation and increase comfort
  - After the first 2 hours following the birth to provide anesthetic effect

SQUEEZE BOTTLE
- Demonstrate for and assist woman; explain rationale.
- Fill bottle with tap water warmed to approximately 38° C (comfortably warm on the wrist).
- Instruct woman to position nozzle between her legs so that squirts of water reach perineum as she sits on toilet seat. Explain that it will take the whole bottle of water to cleanse perineum.
- Remind her to blot dry with toilet paper or clean wipes.
- Remind her to avoid contamination from anal area.
- Apply clean pad.

SITZ BATH
Built-in Type
- Prepare bath by thoroughly scrubbing with cleaning agent and rinsing.
- Pad with towel before filling.

- Fill one half to one third with water of correct temperature (38° to 40.6° C). Some women prefer cool sitz baths. Ice is added to water to lower the temperature to the level comfortable for the woman.
- Encourage woman to use at least twice a day for 20 minutes.
- Place call light within easy reach.
- Teach woman to enter bath by tightening gluteal muscles and keeping them tightened and then relaxing them after she is in the bath.
- Place dry towels within reach.
- Ensure privacy.
- Check woman in 15 minutes; assess pulse as needed.

Disposable Type
- Clamp tubing and fill bag with warm water.
- Raise toilet seat, place bath in bowl with overflow opening directed toward back of toilet.
- Place container above toilet bowl.
- Attach tube into groove at front of bath.
- Loosen tube clamp to regulate rate of flow: fill bath to about one half full; continue as above for built-in sitz bath.

DRY HEAT
- Inspect lamp for defects.
- Cover lamp with towels.
- Position lamp 50 cm from perineum; use three times a day for 20-minute periods.
- Teach regarding use of 40-W bulb at home.
- Provide draping over woman.
- If same lamp is being used by several women, clean it carefully between uses.

TOPICAL APPLICATIONS
- Apply anesthetic cream or spray after cleansing perineal area: use sparingly three to four times per day.
- Offer witch hazel pads (Tucks) after voiding or defecating; woman pats perineum dry from front to back, then applies witch hazel pads.

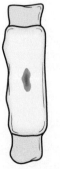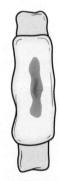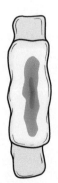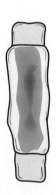

Fig. 16-5 Blood loss after birth is assessed by the extent of perineal pad saturation as (from left to right) scant (<2.5 cm), light (<10 cm), moderate (>10 cm), or heavy (one pad saturated within 2 hours).

difficult to judge the amount of lochial flow based only on observation of perineal pads. More objective estimates of blood loss include measuring serial hemoglobin or hematocrit values; weighing blood clots and items saturated with blood (1 ml equals 1 g); and establishing how many milliliters it takes to saturate perineal pads being used (Simpson & Creehan, 2001).

Any estimation of lochial flow is inaccurate and incomplete without consideration of the time factor. The woman who saturates a perineal pad in 1 hour or less is bleeding much more heavily than the woman who saturates one perineal pad in 8 hours.

Luegenbiehl (1997) found that nurses in general tend to overestimate, rather than underestimate, blood loss. Different brands of perineal pads vary in their saturation volume and soaking appearance. For example, blood placed on some brands tends to soak down into the pad, whereas on other brands it tends to spread outward. Nurses should determine saturation volume and soaking appearance for the brands used in their institution so that they may improve accuracy of blood loss estimation.

NURSE ALERT *The nurse always checks under the mother's buttocks as well as on the perineal pad. Blood may flow between the buttocks onto the linens under the mother, although the amount on the perineal pad is slight; thus excessive bleeding may go undetected.*

Blood pressure is not a reliable indicator of impending shock from early hemorrhage. More sensitive means of identifying shock are provided by respirations, pulse, skin condition, urinary output, and level of consciousness (Benedetti, 2002). The frequent physical assessments performed during the fourth stage of labor are designed to provide prompt identification of excessive bleeding (Emergency box).

EMERGENCY

Hypovolemic Shock

SIGNS AND SYMPTOMS

- Persistent significant bleeding—perineal pad soaked within 15 minutes; may not be accompanied by a change in vital signs or maternal color or behavior.
- Woman states she feels weak, light-headed, "funny," or "sick to my stomach" or that she "sees stars."
- Woman begins to act anxious or exhibits air hunger.
- Woman's skin turns ashen or grayish.
- Skin feels cool and clammy.
- Pulse rate increases.
- Blood pressure declines.

INTERVENTIONS

- Notify primary health care provider.
- If uterus is atonic, massage gently and expel clots to cause uterus to contract; compress uterus manually, as needed, using two hands. Add oxytocic agent to intravenous drip, as ordered.
- Give oxygen by face mask or nasal prongs at 8 to 10 L/min.
- Tilt the woman onto her side or elevate the right hip; elevate her legs to at least a 30-degree angle.
- Provide additional or maintain existing intravenous infusion of lactated Ringer's solution or normal saline solution to restore circulatory volume.
- Administer blood or blood products, as ordered.
- Monitor vital signs.
- Insert an indwelling urinary catheter to monitor perfusion of kidneys.
- Administer emergency drugs, as ordered.
- Prepare for possible surgery or other emergency treatments or procedures.
- Chart incident, medical and nursing interventions instituted, and results of treatments.

Maintenance of uterine tone

A major intervention to restore good tone is stimulation by gently massaging the uterine fundus until firm (see Fig. 16-2). Fundal massage may cause a temporary increase in the amount of vaginal bleeding seen as pooled blood leaves the uterus. Clots may also be expelled. The uterus may remain boggy even after massage and expulsion of clots.

Fundal massage can be a very uncomfortable procedure. Understanding the causes and dangers of uterine atony and the purpose of fundal massage can help the woman to be more cooperative. Teaching the patient to massage her own fundus enables her to maintain some control and decreases her anxiety.

Additional interventions likely to be used are administration of intravenous fluids and oxytocic medications (drugs that stimulate contraction of the uterine smooth muscle). (See Table 25-1 for information about common oxytocic medications.)

Prevention of bladder distention. A full bladder causes the uterus to be displaced above the umbilicus and well to one side of midline in the abdomen. It also prevents the uterus from contracting normally. Nursing interventions focus on helping the woman to empty her bladder spontaneously as soon as possible. The first priority is to assist the woman to the bathroom or onto a bedpan if she is unable to ambulate. Having the woman listen to running water, placing her hands in warm water, or pouring water from a squeeze bottle over her perineum may stimulate voiding. Other techniques include assisting the woman into the shower or sitz bath and encouraging her to void, or placing oil of peppermint in a bedpan under the woman (the vapors may relax the urinary meatus and trigger spontaneous voiding). Administering analgesics, if ordered, may be indicated because some women may fear voiding because of anticipated pain. If these measures are unsuccessful, a sterile catheter may be inserted to drain the urine.

Promotion of comfort, rest, ambulation, and exercise

Comfort. Most women experience some degree of discomfort during the postpartum period. Common causes of discomfort include afterbirth pains (afterpains), episiotomy or perineal lacerations, hemorrhoids, and breast engorgement. The woman's description of the type and severity of her pain is the best guide in choosing an appropriate intervention. To confirm the location and extent of discomfort, the nurse inspects and palpates areas of pain as appropriate for redness, swelling, discharge, and heat and observes for body tension, guarded movements, and facial tension. Blood pressure, pulse, and respirations may be elevated in response to acute pain. Diaphoresis may accompany severe pain. A lack of objective signs does not necessarily mean there is no pain, because there may also be a cultural component to the expression of pain. Nursing interventions are intended to eliminate the pain sensation entirely or reduce it to a tolerable level that allows the woman to care for herself and her baby. Nurses may use both nonpharmacologic and pharmacologic interventions to promote comfort. Pain relief is enhanced by using more than one method or route.

Nonpharmacologic interventions. Warmth, distraction, imagery, therapeutic touch, relaxation, and interaction with the infant may decrease the discomfort associated with afterbirth pain. Simple interventions that can decrease the discomfort associated with an episiotomy or perineal lacerations include encouraging the woman to lie on her side whenever possible and to use a pillow when sitting. Other interventions include application of an ice pack; topical application (if ordered); dry heat; cleansing with a squeeze bottle; and a cleansing shower, tub bath, or sitz bath. Many of these interventions are also effective for hemorrhoids, especially ice packs, sitz baths, and topical applications (such as witch hazel pads). Box 16-3 gives more specific information about these interventions.

The discomfort associated with engorged breasts may be lessened by applying ice, heat, or cabbage leaves to the breasts and wearing a well-fitted support bra. Decisions about specific interventions for engorgement are based on whether the woman chooses breastfeeding or bottle-feeding (see Chapter 20).

Pharmacologic interventions. Most health care providers routinely order a variety of analgesics to be administered as needed, including both narcotic and nonnarcotic (nonsteroidal antiinflammatory) medications, with their dosage and time frequency ranges. Topical application of antiseptic or anesthetic ointment or spray is a common pharmacologic intervention for perineal pain. Patient-controlled analgesia pumps and epidural analgesia are technologies commonly used to provide pain relief after cesarean birth.

> **NURSE ALERT** *The nurse should carefully monitor all women receiving opioids because respiratory depression and decreased intestinal motility are side effects.*

Many women want to participate in decisions about analgesia. Severe pain, however, may interfere with active participation in choosing pain relief measures. If an analgesic is to be given, the nurse must make a clinical judgment of the type, dosage, and frequency from the medications ordered. The woman is informed of the prescribed analgesic and its common side effects; this teaching is documented.

Breastfeeding mothers often have concerns about the effects of an analgesic on the infant. Although nearly all drugs present in maternal circulation are also found in breast milk, many analgesics commonly used during the postpartum period are considered relatively safe for breastfeeding mothers. Often, the timing of medications can be adjusted to minimize infant exposure. A mother may be given pain medication immediately after breastfeeding so that the interval between medication administration and the next nursing period is as long as possible. The decision to administer medications of any type to a breastfeeding mother must always be made by carefully weighing the woman's need against actual or potential risks to the infant.

If acceptable pain relief has not been obtained in 1 hour and there has been no change in the initial assessment, the nurse may need to contact the primary care provider for additional pain relief orders or further directions. Unrelieved pain results in fatigue, anxiety, and a worsening perception of the pain. It might also indicate the presence of a previously unidentified or untreated problem.

Rest. The excitement and exhilaration experienced after the birth of the infant may make rest difficult. The new mother, who is often anxious about her ability to care for her infant or is uncomfortable, may also have difficulty sleeping. The demands of the infant, the hospital environment and routines, and the presence of frequent visitors contribute to alterations in her sleep pattern.

Fatigue. Fatigue is common in the postpartum period (Troy, 2003) and involves both physiologic components, associated with long labors, cesarean birth, anemia, and breastfeeding, and psychologic components, related to depression and anxiety. Infant behavior may also contribute to fatigue, particularly for mothers of more difficult infants.

Interventions must be planned to meet the woman's individual needs for sleep and rest. Back rubs, other comfort measures, and medication for sleep for the first few nights may be necessary. The side-lying position for breastfeeding minimizes fatigue in nursing mothers (Troy, 2003). Support and encouragement of mothering behaviors help reduce anxiety. Hospital and nursing routines may be adjusted to meet individual needs. In addition, the nurse can help the family limit visitors and provide a comfortable chair or bed for the partner.

Ambulation. Early ambulation is successful in reducing the incidence of thromboembolism and in promoting the woman's more rapid recovery of strength. Free movement is encouraged once anesthesia wears off unless an analgesic has been administered. After the initial recovery period is over, the mother is encouraged to ambulate frequently.

> **NURSE ALERT** *Having a hospital staff or family member present the first time the woman gets out of bed after birth is wise because she may feel weak, dizzy, faint, or light-headed.*

The rapid decrease in intraabdominal pressure after birth results in a dilation of blood vessels supplying the intestines (splanchnic engorgement) and causes blood to pool in the viscera. This condition contributes to the development of orthostatic hypotension when the woman who has recently given birth sits or stands up, first ambulates, or takes a warm shower or sitz bath. The nurse also needs to consider the baseline blood pressure; amount of blood loss; and type, amount, and timing of analgesic or anesthetic medications administered when assisting a woman to ambulate.

Prevention of clot formation is important. Women who must remain in bed after giving birth are at increased risk for the development of a thrombus. They may have antiembolic stockings (TED hose) and/or a Sequential Compression

EVIDENCE-BASED PRACTICE
Promoting Breastfeeding

BACKGROUND

- Well-documented benefits of breastfeeding include significantly reduced mortality in preterm infants; reduced morbidity from gastrointestinal, respiratory, urinary tract, and middle ear infections; and less atopic illness. In developing countries the protective effect against infant and child mortality lasts into the second year of life. Breastfed infants demonstrate significantly higher cognitive abilities and have significantly lower blood pressure through the midteen years.

- Women also experience associated health benefits with breastfeeding. A World Health Organization (WHO) review recommends exclusive breastfeeding for 6 months, with introduction of solids and continued breastfeeding thereafter. Yet breastfeeding initiation remains discouragingly low in some areas. In developed countries, the typical breastfeeding mother is advantaged, and mothers who are teenagers with low income and less education are the least likely to initiate or continue breastfeeding. Developing countries, on the other hand, are more likely to see breastfeeding in the lower socioeconomic classes than in the educated, advantaged class. Hospitals may be discouraging breastfeeding by dispensing commercial discharge packs with free formula samples, a practice that the UNICEF-WHO Baby Friendly Initiative hopes to make illegal in as many countries as possible, as a standard of good practice. Many interventions, including the "Ten Steps to Successful Breastfeeding" developed by UNICEF-WHO, have been developed to encourage women to initiate and sustain breastfeeding.

OBJECTIVES

- The reviewers hoped to describe the forms of support for breastfeeding women, the timing, and the settings. They wished to evaluate the effectiveness of the interventions, especially with low-income populations, to determine whether the postnatal intervention is strengthened by an antenatal component, to distinguish the different care providers and training, and to explore whether the background breastfeeding rates of a country influence the success of a breastfeeding intervention. The control group received standard care.

METHODS
Search Strategy

- Search strategy includes searching Cochrane, MEDLINE, EMBASE, Zetoc, Midwives Information and Resource Service and asking experts. Search keywords were not noted.
- The authors found 20 eligible randomized or quasi-randomized, controlled trials involving 23,712 women from Brazil, the United States, Nigeria, Canada, Iran, Bangladesh, the United Kingdom, Belarus, Mexico, and Sweden, dated 1979 to 2000.

Statistical Analyses

- Similar data were pooled in a meta-analysis. Reviewers calculated relative risks for dichotomous (categorical) data, and weighted mean differences for continuous data. The authors accepted differences outside the 95% confidence interval as significant.

FINDINGS

- Overall, there were significant beneficial effects on any breastfeeding outcomes in groups that received extra breastfeeding support, and breastfeeding duration was significantly longer. Treatment effect was greater in areas with a greater background breastfeeding rate in the population. The supported groups were significantly more likely to breastfeed exclusively than the women in control groups. Professional support staff were more effective at preventing the cessation of breastfeeding, up to 9 months. Lay support staff were effective at reducing the cessation of breastfeeding in women who were exclusively breastfeeding, compared with controls. Face-to-face contact was more effective than phone calls. Of the training courses for support personnel, the UNICEF-WHO training courses had the most beneficial effect on exclusive and prolonged breastfeeding. Exclusive breastfeeding was especially beneficial to infants with diarrhea. Breastfeeding women expressed greater satisfaction than controls.

- In a related review of commercial discharge packs, nine trials of 3720 women found a decrease in exclusive breastfeeding duration when the women were given formula samples by the hospital.

LIMITATIONS

- The outcomes are measured in myriad ways, such as breastfeeding duration from 2 weeks to 1 year, in a variety of increments. The interventions are not described and therefore not reproducible in many studies. Follow-up was varied. The strengths of the study were the power of the numbers and the consistency of the findings.

CONCLUSIONS

- Increased support for breastfeeding does increase the initiation, duration of exclusive breastfeeding, and duration of any breastfeeding, with beneficial results for infants. The UNICEF-WHO training courses are effective for personnel. Face-to-face contact is most effective. There is no evidence that antenatal breastfeeding support improves outcomes. Exclusive breastfeeding is very effective in managing infant diarrhea. Finally, a background culture of breastfeeding seems to act synergistically with support to encourage breastfeeding.

IMPLICATIONS FOR PRACTICE

- Nurses can ensure that all mothers receive support for breastfeeding. They can advocate for a hospital discharge pack with breastfeeding-related items, such as breast pads and pump, and breastfeeding information. They can strive to have their hospital meet the criteria for Baby Friendly status.

IMPLICATIONS FOR FURTHER RESEARCH

- Further research is needed to assess the effectiveness of support personnel and training in a variety of settings, especially in areas of low incidence of breastfeeding. Cost-effectiveness is an important outcome. Implementation of the Baby Friendly Initiative needs ongoing monitoring. Qualitative research is needed to identify elements of effective support strategies.

References: Donnelly, A. et al. (2001). Commercial hospital discharge packs for breastfeeding women (Cochrane Review). In *The Cochrane Library*, Issue 2, 2004. Chichester, UK: John Wiley & Sons; Indoria, S., & Wade, A. (2001). Support for breastfeeding women (Cochrane Review). In *The Cochrane Library*, Issue 2, 2004. Chichester, UK: John Wiley & Sons; Sikorski, J. et al. (2001). Support for breastfeeding women (Cochrane Review). In *The Cochrane Library*, Issue 2, 2004. Chichester, UK: John Wiley & Sons.

Device (SCD boots) ordered prophylactically. If a woman remains in bed longer than 8 hours (e.g., for postpartum magnesium sulfate therapy for preeclampsia), exercise to promote circulation in the legs is indicated, using the following routine:

- Alternate flexion and extension of feet.
- Rotate ankle in circular motion.
- Alternate flexion and extension of legs.
- Press back of knee to bed surface; relax.

If the woman is susceptible to thromboembolism, she is encouraged to walk about actively for true ambulation and is discouraged from sitting immobile in a chair. Women with varicosities are advised to wear support hose. If a thrombus is suspected, as evidenced by complaint of pain in calf muscles or warmth, redness, or tenderness in the suspected leg (positive Homans sign), the primary health care provider should be notified immediately; meanwhile the woman should be confined to bed, with the affected limb elevated on pillows.

Exercise. Most women who have just given birth are extremely interested in regaining their nonpregnant figures. Postpartum exercise can begin soon after birth, although the woman should be encouraged to start with simple exercises and gradually progress to more strenuous ones. Fig. 16-6 illustrates a number of exercises appropriate for the new mother. Abdominal exercises are postponed until approximately 4 weeks after cesarean birth.

Kegel exercises to strengthen pelvic muscle tone are extremely important, particularly after vaginal birth. Kegel exercises help women regain the muscle tone that is often lost as pelvic tissues are stretched and torn during pregnancy and birth. Women who maintain muscle strength may benefit years later by maintaining urinary continence.

It is essential that women learn to perform Kegel exercises correctly (see Patient Teaching in Chapter 4, p. 93). Approximately one fourth of all women who learn Kegel exercises do them incorrectly and may increase their risk of incontinence (Sampselle et al., 2000). This may occur when women inadvertently bear down on the pelvic floor muscles, thrusting the perineum outward. The woman's technique can be assessed during the pelvic examination at her checkup by inserting two fingers intravaginally and checking whether the pelvic floor muscles correctly contract and relax.

Promotion of nutrition

During the hospital stay, most women display a good appetite and eat well; nutritious snacks are usually welcomed. Women may request that family members bring to the hospital favorite or culturally appropriate foods (Fig. 16-7 on p. 484). Cultural dietary preferences must be respected. This interest in food presents an ideal opportunity for nutritional counseling on dietary needs after pregnancy, such as for breastfeeding, preventing constipation and anemia, promoting weight loss, and promoting healing and well-being (see Chapter 10). Prenatal vitamins and iron supplements are often continued until 6 weeks postpartum or until the ordered supply has been used.

Promotion of normal bladder and bowel patterns

Bladder function. After giving birth the mother should void spontaneously within 6 to 8 hours. The first several voidings should be measured to document adequate emptying of the bladder. A volume of at least 150 ml is expected for each voiding. Some women experience difficulty in emptying the bladder, possibly a result of diminished bladder tone, edema from trauma, or fear of discomfort. Nursing interventions for inability to void and bladder distention are discussed on p. 479.

Bowel function. Interventions to promote normal bowel elimination include educating the woman about measures to avoid constipation, such as ensuring adequate roughage and fluid intake and promoting exercise. Alerting the woman to side effects of medications such as narcotic analgesics (e.g., decreased gastrointestinal tract motility) may encourage her to implement measures to reduce the risk of constipation. Stool softeners or laxatives may be necessary during the early postpartum period. With early discharge a new mother may be home before having a bowel movement. Some mothers experience gas pains. Antigas medications may be ordered. Ambulation or rocking in a rocking chair may stimulate passage of flatus and relief of discomfort.

Breastfeeding promotion and lactation suppression

Breastfeeding promotion. The first 1 to 2 hours after childbirth is an excellent time to encourage the mother to breastfeed. The infant is typically in an alert state and will suckle if put to the breast. Breastfeeding aids in the contraction of the uterus and prevention of maternal hemorrhage. This is an opportune time to instruct the mother in breastfeeding and to assess the physical appearance of the breasts and nipples. (See Chapter 20 for further information on assisting the breastfeeding woman.)

Lactation suppression. Suppression of lactation is necessary when the woman has decided not to breastfeed or in the case of neonatal death. Wearing a well-fitted support bra or breast binder continuously for at least the first 72 hours after giving birth is important. Women should avoid breast stimulation, including running warm water over the breasts, newborn suckling, or pumping of the breasts. A few nonbreastfeeding mothers experience severe breast engorgement (swelling of breast tissue caused by increased blood and lymph supply to the breasts as the body produces milk, occurring at about 72 to 96 hours after birth). If breast engorgement occurs, it can usually be managed satisfactorily with nonpharmacologic interventions.

Ice packs to the breasts are helpful in decreasing the discomfort associated with engorgement. The woman should use a 15-minutes-on–45-minutes-off schedule (to prevent the rebound swelling that can occur if ice is used continuously), or she can place fresh cabbage leaves inside her bra. Cabbage leaves have been used to treat swelling in other cultures for years (Ayers, 2000; Mass, 2004). The exact mechanism of ac-

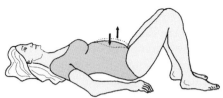

Abdominal Breathing. Lie on back with knees bent. Inhale deeply through nose. Keep ribs stationary and allow abdomen to expand upward. Exhale slowly but forcefully while contracting the abdominal muscles; hold for 3 to 5 seconds while exhaling. Relax.

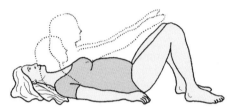

Reach for the Knees. Lie on back with knees bent. While inhaling, deeply lower chin onto chest. While exhaling, raise head and shoulders slowly and smoothly and reach for knees with arms outstretched. The body should only rise as far as the back will naturally bend while waist remains on floor or bed (about 6 to 8 inches). Slowly and smoothly lower head and shoulders back to starting position. Relax.

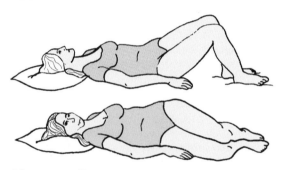

Double Knee Roll. Lie on back with knees bent. Keeping shoulders flat and feet stationary, slowly and smoothly roll knees over to the left to touch floor or bed. Maintaining a smooth motion, roll knees back over to the right until they touch floor or bed. Return to starting position and relax.

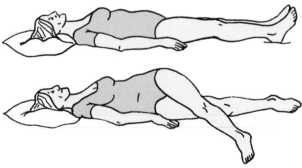

Leg Roll. Lie on back with legs straight. Keeping shoulders flat and legs straight, slowly and smoothly lift left leg and roll it over to touch the right side of floor or bed and return to starting position. Repeat, rolling right leg over to touch left side of floor or bed. Relax.

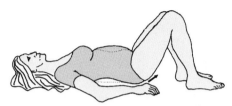

Combined Abdominal Breathing and Supine Pelvic Tilt (Pelvic Rock). Lie on back with knees bent. While inhaling deeply, roll pelvis back by flattening lower back on floor or bed. Exhale slowly but forcefully while contracting abdominal muscles and tightening buttocks. Hold for 3 to 5 seconds while exhaling. Relax.

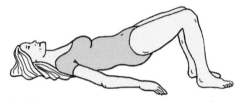

Buttocks Lift. Lie on back with arms at sides, knees bent, and feet flat. Slowly raise buttocks and arch back. Return slowly to starting position.

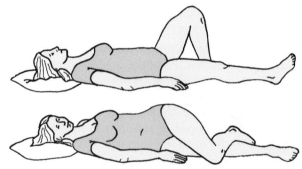

Single Knee Roll. Lie on back with right leg straight and left leg bent at the knee. Keeping shoulders flat, slowly and smoothly roll left knee over to the right to touch floor or bed and then back to starting position. Reverse position of legs. Roll right knee over to the left to touch floor or bed and return to starting position. Relax.

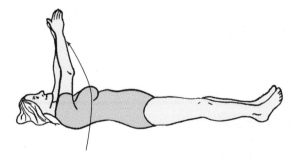

Arm Raises. Lie on back with arms extended at 90-degree angle from body. Raise arms so they are perpendicular and hands touch. Lower slowly.

Fig. 16-6   Postpartum exercise should begin as soon as possible. The woman should start with simple exercises and gradually progress to more strenuous ones.

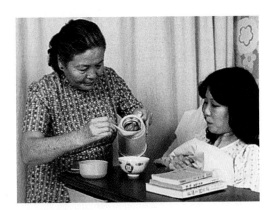

Fig. 16-7 Special foods are considered essential for recovery in the Asian culture. (Courtesy Concept Media, Irvine, CA.)

tion is not known, but it is thought that naturally occurring plant estrogens or salicylates may be responsible for the effects. The leaves are replaced each time they wilt. A mild analgesic may also be necessary to help the mother through this uncomfortable time. Medications that were once prescribed for lactation suppression (e.g., estrogen, estrogen and testosterone, bromocriptine) are no longer used.

Health promotion for future pregnancies and children

Rubella vaccination. For women who have not had rubella (10% to 20% of all women) or women who are serologically not immune (titer of 1:8 or enzyme immunoassay level less than 0.8), a subcutaneous injection of rubella vaccine is recommended in the postpartum period to prevent the possibility of contracting rubella in future pregnancies. Seroconversion occurs in approximately 90% of women vaccinated after birth. The live attenuated rubella virus is not communicable in breast milk; therefore breastfeeding mothers can be vaccinated. However, because the virus is shed in urine and other body fluids, the vaccine should not be given if the mother or other household members are immunocompromised. Rubella vaccine is made from duck eggs, so women who have allergies to these eggs may develop a hypersensitivity reaction to the vaccine, for which they will need adrenaline. A transient arthralgia or rash is common in vaccinated women but is benign. Because the vaccine may be teratogenic, women who receive the vaccine must be informed about this fact.

LEGAL TIP Rubella Vaccination

Informed consent for rubella vaccination in the postpartum period includes information about possible side effects and the risk of teratogenic effects. Women must understand that they must practice contraception to avoid pregnancy for 1 month after being vaccinated (ACOG, 2002).

Prevention of Rh isoimmunization. Injection of Rh immune globulin (a solution of gamma globulin that contains Rh antibodies) within 72 hours after birth prevents sensitization in the Rh-negative woman who has had a fetomaternal transfusion of Rh-positive fetal red blood cells (RBCs) (Medication Guide). Rh immune globulin promotes lysis of fetal Rh-positive blood cells before the mother forms her own antibodies against them.

Medication Guide

Rh Immune Globulin, RhoGAM, Gamulin Rh, HypRho-D, Rhophylac

ACTION

Suppression of immune response in nonsensitized women with Rh-negative blood who receive Rh-positive blood cells because of fetomaternal hemorrhage, transfusion, or accident

INDICATIONS

Routine antepartum prevention at 20 to 30 weeks gestation in women with Rh-negative blood; suppress antibody formation after birth, miscarriage or pregnancy termination, abdominal trauma, ectopic pregnancy, amniocentesis, version, or chorionic villi sampling

DOSAGE AND ROUTE

Standard dose 1 vial (300 mcg) intramuscularly (IM) in deltoid or gluteal muscle; microdose 1 vial (50 mcg) IM in deltoid muscle; Rhophylac can be given IM or IV (available in prefilled syringes)

ADVERSE EFFECTS

Myalgia, lethargy, localized tenderness and stiffness at injection site, mild and transient fever, malaise, headache, rarely nausea, vomiting, hypotension, tachycardia, possible allergic response

NURSING CONSIDERATIONS

- Give standard dose to mother at 28 weeks pf gestation as prophylaxis, or after an incident or exposure risk that occurs after 28 weeks of gestation (e.g., amniocentesis, second trimester miscarriage or abortion, after external version attempt) and within 72 hours after birth if baby is Rh positive.
- Give microdose for first trimester miscarriage or abortion, ectopic pregnancy, chorionic villus sampling.
- Verify that the woman is Rh negative and has not been sensitized, that Coombs' test is negative, and that baby is Rh positive. Provide explanation to the woman about procedure, including the purpose, possible side effects, and effect on future pregnancies. Have the woman sign a consent form if required by agency. Verify correct dosage and confirm lot number and woman's identity before giving injection (verify with another RN or use other procedure per agency policy); document administration per agency policy. Observe patient for at least 20 minutes after administration for allergic response.
- The medication is made from human plasma (a consideration if woman is a Jehovah's Witness). The risk of transmitting infectious agents, including viruses, cannot be completely eliminated.

NURSE ALERT *After birth, Rh immune globulin is administered to all Rh-negative, antibody (Coombs')-negative women who give birth to Rh-positive infants. Rh immune globulin is administered to the mother intramuscularly or intravenously. It should never be given to an infant.*

The administration of 300 microgram (1 vial) of Rh immune globulin is usually sufficient to prevent maternal sensitization. If a large fetomaternal transfusion is suspected, however, the dosage needed should be determined by performing a Kleihauer-Betke test, which detects the amount of fetal blood in the maternal circulation. If more than 15 ml of fetal blood is present in maternal circulation, the dosage of Rh immune globulin must be increased.

A 1:1000 dilution of Rh immune globulin is crossmatched to the mother's RBCs to ensure compatibility. Because Rh immune globulin is usually considered a blood product, precautions similar to those used for transfusing blood are necessary when it is given. The identification number on the patient's hospital wristband should correspond to the identification number found on the laboratory slip. The nurse must also check to see that the lot number on the laboratory slip corresponds to the lot number on the vial. Finally, the expiration date on the vial should be checked to ensure a usable product.

Rh immune globulin suppresses the immune response. Therefore the woman who receives both Rh immune globulin and rubella vaccine must be tested at 3 months to see if she has developed rubella immunity. If not, the woman will need another dose of rubella vaccine.

There is some disagreement about whether Rh immune globulin should be considered a blood product. Health care providers need to discuss the most current information about this issue with women whose religious beliefs conflict with having blood products administered to them.

Evaluation

The nurse can be reasonably assured that care was effective when the expected outcomes of care for physical needs have been achieved.

CARE MANAGEMENT—PSYCHOSOCIAL NEEDS

Meeting the psychosocial needs of new mothers involves assessing the parents' reactions to the birth experience, feelings about themselves, and interactions with the new baby and other family members (Fig. 16-8). Specific interventions are then planned to increase the parents' knowledge and self-confidence as they assume the care and responsibility of the new baby and integrate this new member into their existing family structure in a way that meets their cultural expectations (see Chapter 17).

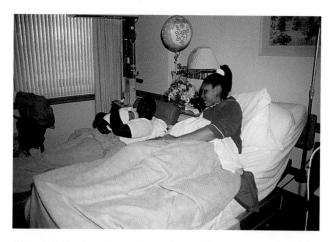

Fig. 16-8 Bonding and attachment begun early after birth are fostered in the postpartum period. (Courtesy Marjorie Pyle, RNC, Lifecircle, Costa Mesa, CA.)

Assessment and Nursing Diagnoses
Impact of the birth experience

Many women indicate a need to examine the birth process itself and look at their own intrapartal behavior in retrospect. Their partners may express similar desires. If their birth experience was different from their birth plan (e.g., induction, epidural anesthesia, cesarean birth), both partners may need to mourn the loss of their expectations before they can adjust to the reality of their actual birth experience. Inviting them to review the events and describe how they feel helps the nurse assess how well they understand what happened and how well they have been able to put their childbirth experience into perspective.

Maternal self-image

An important assessment concerns the woman's self-concept, body image, and sexuality. How this new mother feels about herself and her body during the puerperium may affect her behavior and adaptation to parenting. The woman's self-concept and body image may also affect her sexuality. Overweight women may experience symptoms of depression and anxiety up to 14 months postpartum (Carter, Baker, & Brownell, 2000).

Feelings related to sexual adjustment after childbirth are often a cause of concern for new parents. Women who have recently given birth may be reluctant to resume sexual intercourse for fear of pain or may worry that coitus could damage healing perineal tissue. Because many new parents are anxious for information but reluctant to bring up the subject, postpartum nurses should matter-of-factly include the topic of postpartum sexuality during their routine physical assessment. While examining the episiotomy site, for example, the nurse can say, "I know you're sore right now, but it probably won't be long until you (or you and your partner) are ready to make love again. Have you thought about what that might be like? Would you like to ask me questions?" This approach assures the woman and her partner that resuming sexual activity is a

Critical Thinking Exercise

Return to Nonpregnant Appearance

Deidra is 10 days postpartum. Before pregnancy, her weight was appropriate for her height. However, during pregnancy, she gained 46 pounds. She gave birth vaginally to an 8-pound, 6-ounce boy and is breastfeeding the baby. Deidra is concerned about regaining her figure after childbirth and voices concerns that she will never regain the figure she once had.

1 Evidence—Is there sufficient evidence to draw conclusions about counseling women with regard to regaining their nonpregnant appearance?

2 Assumptions—What assumptions can be made about the following issues:
   a. Appropriate diet for the postpartum mother who wants to improve her appearance
   b. The relationship between breastfeeding and postpartum weight loss
   c. Exercises for the postpartum woman who wants to improve her appearance
   d. The relationship between perceived body image and self-esteem in postpartum women

3 What implications and priorities for nursing care can be drawn at this time?

4 Does the evidence objectively support your conclusion?

5 Are there alternative perspectives to your conclusion?

legitimate concern for new parents and indicates the nurse's willingness to answer questions and share information.

Adaptation to parenthood and parent-infant interactions

The psychosocial assessment also includes evaluating adaptation to parenthood, as evidenced by mother's and father's reactions to and interactions with the new baby. Clues indicating successful adaptation begin to appear early in the postbirth period as parents react positively to the newborn infant and continue the process of establishing a relationship with their infant.

Parents are adapting well to their new roles when they exhibit a realistic perception and acceptance of their newborn's needs and his or her limited abilities, immature social responses, and helplessness. Examples of positive parent-infant interactions include taking pleasure in the infant and in the tasks done for and with her or him, understanding the infant's emotional states and providing comfort, and reading the infant's cues for new experiences and sensing the infant's fatigue level (see Chapter 17).

Should these indicators be missing, the nurse needs to investigate further what is hindering the normal adaptation process. There are several questions that the nurse can ask, such as "Do you feel sad often?" or "Are there concerns that you have about being a good parent?" that will help to determine if the woman is experiencing the normal "baby blues" or if there is another more serious underlying process taking place (i.e., postpartum depression) (Jesse & Graham, 2005). See Chapter 25 for further discussion of postpartum depression.

Family structure and functioning

A woman's adjustment to her role as mother is affected greatly by her relationships with her partner, her mother and other relatives, and any other children. Nurses can help ease the new mother's return home by identifying possible conflicts among family members and helping the woman plan strategies for dealing with these problems before discharge. Such a conflict could arise when couples have very different ideas about parenting. Dealing with the stresses of sibling rivalry and unsolicited grandparent advice can also affect the woman's psychological well-being. Only by asking about other nuclear and extended family members can the nurse discover potential problems in such relationships and help plan workable solutions for them.

Impact of cultural diversity

The final component of a complete psychosocial assessment is the woman's cultural beliefs and values. Much of a woman's behavior during the postpartum period is strongly influenced by her cultural background. Nurses are likely to come into contact with women from many different countries and cultures. All cultures have developed safe and satisfying methods of caring for new mothers and babies. Only by understanding and respecting the values and beliefs of each woman can the nurse design a plan of care to meet her individual needs.

Sometimes the psychosocial assessment indicates serious actual or potential problems that must be addressed. The Signs of Potential Complications box lists several psychosocial needs that, at a minimum, warrant ongoing evaluation

 Critical Thinking Exercise

Cultural Influences during the Postpartum Period

Terri, who is Asian, gave birth to her first child yesterday. This morning she refuses to eat her breakfast or take a shower, stating that to do either would cause an imbalance in her system. Although her chart indicates that she intends to breastfeed, she requests formula for her baby.

1 Evidence—Is there sufficient evidence to draw conclusions about the cultural beliefs of Asians as they relate to the postpartum period and breastfeeding?

2 Assumptions—What assumptions can be made about the following issues?
   a. Culturally appropriate diet, activity, and hygiene for the postpartum Asian woman
   b. Providing appropriate care for the newborn, including breastfeeding, in the Asian culture
   c. Role of other family members and friends in providing care to the postpartum woman and newborn
   d. Difficulty in establishing lactation if breastfeeding is not begun immediately

3 What implications and priorities for nursing care can be drawn at this time?

4 Does the evidence objectively support your conclusion?

5 Are there alternative perspectives to your conclusion?

signs of
POTENTIAL COMPLICATIONS

Psychosocial Needs

- Unable or unwilling to discuss labor and birth experience
- Refers to self as ugly and useless
- Excessively preoccupied with self (body image)
- Markedly depressed
- Lacks a support system
- Partner or other family members react negatively to the baby
- Refuses to interact with or care for baby. For example, does not name baby, does not want to hold or feed baby, is upset by vomiting and wet or dirty diapers. (Cultural appropriateness of actions needs to be considered.)
- Expresses disappointment over baby's sex
- Sees baby as messy or unattractive
- Baby reminds mother of family member or friend she does not like
- Has difficulty sleeping
- Experiences loss of appetite

following hospital discharge. Patients exhibiting these needs should be referred to appropriate community resources for assessment and management.

After analyzing the data obtained during the assessment process, the nurse establishes nursing diagnoses to provide a guide for planning care. Nursing diagnoses related to psychosocial issues that are frequently established for the postpartum patient include the following:

- *Interrupted family processes related to*
  - −unexpected birth of twins
- *Impaired verbal communication related to*
  - −patient's hearing impairment
  - −nurse's language not the same as patient's
- *Impaired parenting related to*
  - −long, difficult labor
  - −unmet expectations of labor and birth
- *Anxiety related to*
  - −newness of parenting role, sibling rivalry, or response of grandparent
- *Risk for situational low self-esteem related to*
  - −body image changes

Expected Outcomes of Care

Expected psychosocial outcomes during the postpartum period are based on the nursing diagnoses identified for the individual woman and her family. Examples of common expected outcomes include that the woman (family) will do the following:

- Identify measures that promote a healthy personal adjustment in the postpartum period
- Maintain healthy family functioning based on cultural norms and personal expectations

Plan of Care and Interventions

The nurse functions in the roles of teacher, encourager, and supporter rather than doer while implementing the psychosocial plan of care for a postpartum woman. Implementation of the psychosocial care plan involves carrying out specific activities to achieve the expected outcome of care planned for each individual woman. Topics that should be included in the psychosocial plan of care include promotion of parenting skills and family member adjustment to the newborn infant (see Chapter 17).

Cultural issues must also be considered when planning care. There are many traditional health beliefs and practices among the different cultures within the U.S. population. Traditional health practices that are used to maintain health or to avoid illnesses deal with the whole person (i.e., body, mind, and spirit) and tend to be culturally based.

Women from various cultures may view health as a balance between opposing forces (e.g., cold versus hot), being in harmony with nature, or just "feeling good." Traditional practices may include the observance of certain dietary restrictions, clothing, or taboos for balancing the body; participation in certain activities such as sports and art for maintaining mental health; and use of silence, prayer, or meditation for developing spiritually. Practices (e.g., using religious objects or eating garlic) are used to protect oneself from illness and may involve avoiding people who are believed to create hexes or spells or who have an "evil eye." Restoration of health may involve taking folk medicines (e.g., herbs, animal substances) or using a traditional healer.

Childbirth occurs within this sociocultural context. Rest, seclusion, dietary restraints, and ceremonies honoring the mother are all common traditional practices that are followed for the promotion of the health and well-being of the mother and baby.

There are several common traditional health practices used and beliefs held by women and their families during the postpartum period. In Asia, for example, pregnancy is considered to be a "hot" state, and childbirth results in a sudden loss of this state (Kim-Godwin, 2003). Therefore balance must be restored by facilitating the return of the hot state, which is present physically or symbolically in hot food, hot water, and warm air.

Another common belief is that the mother and baby remain in a weak and vulnerable state for a period of several weeks after birth. During this time the mother may remain in a passive role, taking no baths or showers, and may stay in bed to prevent cold air from entering her body.

Women who have immigrated to the United States or other Western nations without their extended families may not have much help at home, making it difficult for them to observe these activity restrictions (Davis, 2001). The Cultural Considerations box lists some common cultural beliefs about the postpartum period and family planning.

It is important that nurses consider all cultural aspects when planning care and not use their own cultural beliefs as the framework for that care. Although the beliefs and

Cultural Considerations

Postpartum Period and Family Planning

POSTPARTUM CARE

- *Chinese, Mexican, Korean, and Southeast Asian women* may wish to eat only warm foods and drink hot drinks to replace blood loss and to restore the balance of hot and cold in their bodies. These women may also wish to stay warm and avoid bathing, exercises, and hair washing for 7 to 30 days after childbirth. Self-care may not be a priority; care by family members is preferred. The woman has respect for elders and authority. These women may wear abdominal binders. They may prefer not to give their babies colostrum.
- *Arabic women* eat special meals designed to restore their energy. They are expected to stay at home for 40 days after childbirth to avoid illness resulting from exposure to the outside air.
- *Haitian women* may request to take the placenta home to bury or burn.
- *Muslim women* follow strict religious laws on modesty and diet. A Muslim woman must keep her hair, body, arms to the wrist, and legs to the ankles covered at all times. She cannot be alone in the presence of a man other than her husband or a male relative. Observant Muslims will not eat pork or pork products and are obligated to eat meat slaughtered according to Islamic laws (halal meat). If halal meat is not available, kosher meat, seafood, or a vegetarian diet is usually accepted.

FAMILY PLANNING

- Birth control is government mandated in mainland *China*. Most *Chinese women* will have an intrauterine device (IUD) inserted after the birth of their first child. Women do not want hormonal methods of contraception because they fear putting these medications in their bodies.
- *Hispanic women* will likely choose the rhythm method because most are Catholic.
- *(East) Indian men* are encouraged to have voluntary sterilization by vasectomy.
- *Muslim couples* may practice contraception by mutual consent as long as its use is not harmful to the woman. Acceptable contraceptive methods include foam and condoms, the diaphragm, and natural family planning.
- *Hmong women* highly value and desire large families, which limits birth control practices.
- *Arabic women* value large families, and sons are especially prized.

behaviors of other cultures may seem different or strange, they should be encouraged as long as the mother wants to conform to them and she and the baby suffer no ill effects. The nurse needs to determine whether a woman is using any folk medicine during the postpartum period because active ingredients in folk medicine may have adverse physiologic effects on the woman when ingested with prescribed

medicines. The nurse should not assume that a mother desires to use traditional health practices that represent a particular cultural group merely because she is a member of that culture. Many young women who are first- or second-generation Americans follow their cultural traditions only when older family members are present or not at all.

Evaluation

The nurse can be reasonably assured that care was effective if expected outcomes of care for psychosocial needs have been met.

DISCHARGE TEACHING ■

Self-Care, Signs of Complications

Discharge planning begins at the time of admission to the unit and should be reflected in the plan of care developed for each individual woman. For example, a great deal of time during the hospital stay is usually spent in teaching about maternal and newborn care, because all women must be capable of providing basic care for themselves and their infants at the time of discharge. It is also crucial that every woman be taught to recognize the physical signs and symptoms that might indicate problems and how to obtain advice and assistance quickly if these signs appear. Before discharge, women need basic instruction regarding the resumption of sexual intercourse, prescribed medications, routine mother-baby checkups, and contraception (Guidelines/Guías box).

Just before the time of discharge the nurse reviews the woman's chart to see that laboratory reports, medications, signatures, and other items are in order. Some hospitals have a checklist to use before the woman's discharge. The nurse verifies that medications, if ordered, have arrived on the unit; that any valuables kept secured during the woman's stay have been returned to her and that she has signed a receipt for them; and that the infant is ready to be discharged.

No medication that would make the mother sleepy should be administered if she is the one who will be holding the baby on the way out of the hospital. In most instances the woman is seated in a wheelchair and is given the baby to hold. Some families leave unescorted and ambulatory, depending on hospital protocol. The woman's possessions are gathered and taken out with her and her family. The woman's and the baby's identification bands are carefully checked. Babies must be secured in a car seat for the drive home (see Fig. 19-25).

Sexual Activity and Contraception

Many couples resume sexual activity before the traditional postpartum checkup 6 weeks after childbirth. The risk of hemorrhage or infection is minimal by approximately 2 weeks postpartum. Couples may be anxious about the topic but uncomfortable and unwilling to bring it up. It is important that the nurse discuss the physical and psychologic effects that

GUIDELINES/GUÍAS

Discharge Teaching

- When you go to the bathroom, always wipe from front to back.
- *Cuando vaya al baño, séquese siempre de adelante hacia atrás.*
- Sit in a warm tub to relieve discomfort.
- *Siéntese en una bañera con agua tibia para aliviarse.*
- You will have moderate amounts of vaginal discharge.
- *Usted tendrá cantidades moderadas de sangrado vaginal.*
- It may last from 4 to 6 weeks.
- *Puede durar desde 4 a 6 semanas.*
- The color may vary from dark brown to red to pink.
- *El color puede variar entre café oscuro a rojo a rosado.*
- It may contain blood clots.
- *Es probable que contenga coágulos.*
- Use a sanitary pad instead of a tampon.
- *Use una toalla sanitaria en vez de un tampón.*
- Your menstrual period will not resume for 4 to 10 weeks.
- *Su regla no regrasará hasta 4 a 10 semanas más tarde.*
- If you are breastfeeding, it may take a little longer.
- *Si está amamantando, puede demorar un poco más.*
- It is possible to become pregnant while you are breastfeeding.
- *Es posible quedar embarazada mientras amamanta.*
- Avoid having sexual relations for 2 to 4 weeks after birth.
- *Evite las relaciones sexuales por 2 a 4 semanas después del parto.*
- Gradually increase activity to incorporate everyday routines.
- *Aumente las actividades gradualmente hasta llegar a su rutina normal.*
- Do your Kegel exercises.
- *Haga los ejercicios Kegel.*
- Do not lift heavy objects (>10 pounds).
- *No levante objetos pesados (de más de 10 libras).*

- Rest as often as possible.
- *Descanse mucho.*
- Rest when your baby sleeps.
- *Descanse cuando duerma su bebé.*
- Eat daily:
- *Cómase diariamente:*
  - 4 servings of bread/cereals, fruits/vegetables (green), milk or foods made from milk, and 2 servings of meat. You need to drink 8 glasses of fluids a day to support breastfeeding.
  - *4 porciones de pan/cereal, frutas/vegetales (verduras), leche o comidas del grupo de leche, y 2 porciones de carne. Usted necesita tomar 8 vasos de líquidos diariamenta para soportar el dar de pecho.*
- Call your doctor (obstetrician) if you have:
- *Llame al médico de obstétricas si tenga cualquier de lo siguiente:*
  - Fever >38° C
  - *Fiebre >38° C*
  - Increased vaginal bleeding (more than a regular period)
  - *Aumento de desangre vaginal (más que una regla normal)*
  - Chills
  - *Escalofríos*
  - Painful, burning urination
  - *Orin que le duele o le quema*
  - Foul-smelling vaginal discharge
  - *Desangre vaginal de muy mal olor*
  - Increased pain or swelling
  - *Aumento de dolor o hinchazón*
  - Drainage or separation of incision (cesarean)
  - *Desangre o deshecho de la herida*

---

giving birth can have on sexual activity (Patient Instructions for Self-Care box). Contraceptive options should also be discussed with women (and their partners, if present) before discharge so that they can make informed decisions about fertility management before resuming sexual activity. Waiting to discuss contraception at the 6-week checkup may be too late. It is possible, particularly in women who bottle-feed, for ovulation to occur as soon as 1 month after birth. A woman who engages in unprotected sex risks becoming pregnant. Current contraceptive options are discussed in detail in Chapter 6. Women who are undecided about contraception at the time of discharge need information about using condoms with foam or creams until the first postpartum checkup.

Prescribed Medications

Women routinely continue to take their prenatal vitamins and iron during the postpartum period. It is especially important that women who are breastfeeding or who are discharged with a lower than normal hematocrit take these medications as prescribed. Women with extensive episiotomies or vaginal lacerations (third or fourth degree) are usually prescribed stool softeners to take at home. Pain relief medications (analgesics or nonsteroidal antiinflammatory medications) may be prescribed, especially for women who had cesarean birth. The nurse should make certain that the woman knows the route, dosage, frequency, and common side effects of all ordered medications.

Routine Mother and Baby Checkups

Women who have experienced uncomplicated vaginal births are still commonly scheduled for the traditional 6-week postpartum examination. Women who have had a cesarean birth are often seen in the physician's or nurse-midwife's office or clinic 2 weeks after hospital discharge. The date and time for the follow-up appointment should be included in the

PATIENT INSTRUCTIONS FOR SELF-CARE

Resumption of Sexual Intercourse

- You can safely resume sexual intercourse by the second to fourth week after birth when bleeding has stopped and the episiotomy has healed. For the first 6 weeks to 6 months, the vagina does not lubricate well.
- Your physiologic reactions to sexual stimulation for the first 3 months after birth will likely be slower and less intense. The strength of the orgasm may be reduced.
- A water-soluble gel, cocoa butter, or a contraceptive cream or jelly might be recommended for lubrication. If some vaginal tenderness is present, your partner can be instructed to insert one or more clean, lubricated fingers into the vagina and rotate them within the vagina to help relax it and to identify possible areas of discomfort. A position in which you have control of the depth of the insertion of the penis also is useful. The side-by-side or female-on-top position may be more comfortable.
- The presence of the baby influences postbirth lovemaking. Parents hear every sound made by the baby; conversely you may be concerned that the baby hears every sound you make. In either case, any phase of the sexual response cycle may be interrupted by hearing the baby cry or move, leaving both of you frustrated and unsatisfied. In addition, the amount of psychologic energy expended by you in child care activities may lead to fatigue. Newborns require a great deal of attention and time.
- Some women have reported feeling sexual stimulation and orgasms when breastfeeding their babies. Breastfeeding mothers often are interested in returning to sexual activity before nonbreastfeeding mothers.
- You should be instructed to correctly perform the Kegel exercises to strengthen your pubococcygeal muscle. This muscle is associated with bowel and bladder function and with vaginal feeling during intercourse.

discharge instructions. If an appointment has not been made before the woman leaves the hospital, she should be encouraged to call the physician's or nurse-midwife's office or clinic and schedule an appointment.

Parents who have not already done so need to make plans for newborn follow-up at the time of discharge. Most offices and clinics like to see newborns for an initial examination within the first week or by 2 weeks of age. If an appointment for a specific date and time was not made for the infant before leaving the hospital, the parents should be encouraged to call the office or clinic right away.

Follow-up after Discharge

Home visits

Home visits to new mothers and babies within a few days of discharge can help bridge the gap between hospital care and routine visits to health care providers. Nurses are able to assess the mother, infant, and home environment; answer questions and provide education; and make referrals to community resources if necessary. Home visits have been shown to reduce the need for more expensive health care, such as Emergency Department visits and rehospitalization. They can also help to improve the overall quality of care provided to infants and their parents (Paul, Phillips, Widome, & Hollenbeak, 2004). Immediate follow-up contact and home visits ideally are available 7 days a week.

Home nursing care may not be available even if needed because there are no agencies providing the service or there is no coverage for payment by third-party payers. If care is available, a referral form containing information about both mother and baby should be completed at hospital discharge and sent immediately to the home care agency. Fig. 16-9 is an example of such a referral form.

The home visit is most commonly scheduled on the woman's second day home from the hospital, but it may be scheduled on any of the first 4 days at home, depending on the individual family's situation and needs. Additional visits are planned throughout the first week, as needed. The home visits may be extended beyond that time if the family's needs warrant it and if a home visit is the most appropriate option for carrying out the follow-up care required to meet the specific needs identified.

During the home visit the nurse conducts a systematic assessment of mother and newborn to determine physiologic adjustment, identify any existing complications, and to answer any questions the mother has for herself and the mother or family has about the newborn or newborn care. Conducting the assessment in a separate room provides private time for the mother to ask questions on topics such as breast care, family planning, and constipation. The assessment focuses on the mother's emotional adjustment and her knowledge of self-care and infant care.

During the newborn assessment, the nurse can demonstrate and explain normal newborn behavior and capabilities and encourage the mother and family to ask questions or express concerns they may have. The home care nurse must verify if the newborn screen for phenylketonuria and other inborn errors of metabolism has been drawn. If the baby was discharged from the hospital before 24 hours of age, the newborn screen may be done by the home care nurse or the family will need to take the infant to the clinic or physician's office.

Telephone follow-up

As part of the routine follow-up of a woman and her infant after discharge from the hospital, many providers are implementing one or more postpartum telephone follow-up calls to their patients for assessment, health teaching, and identification of complications to effect timely intervention and referrals. Telephone follow-up may be among the services offered by the hospital, private physician or clinic, or a private agency; it may be either a separate service or combined with other strategies for extending postpartum care. Telephonic nursing assessments are frequently used after a postpartum home care visit to reassess a woman's knowledge about such

OB Homecare

**POSTPARTUM
HOME CARE REFERRAL**

Mother's Name:_____

Address/phone where mother will be staying:

Address:_____

City:_____

Phone #:_____

Language spoken: ☐ English ☐ Other:_____

Understands English: ☐ Well   ☐ Poor

        ☐ Mother Needs Interpreter   ☐ Hearing Impaired

Who interpreted in hospital:_____

Mom agrees to this referral: ☐ Yes   ☐ No

Currently being seen by PHN: ☐ Yes   ☐ No

Mom's M.D./Midwife:_____

Phone #:_____

Next Appt:_____

MOTHER:

Gravida_____ T_____ P_____ A_____ L_____

Marital Status: S   M   W   D   Sep

Normal Maternal Exam: ☐ Yes   ☐ No (explain below)

Epis/Incision:_____

Hgb pp:_____

Meds:_____

Allergies:_____

OTHER ISSUES:

Diabetic:_____

Other:_____

Psycho/Social Issues:

☐ Parent/Child Interaction   ☐ Adolescent Mother

☐ Mental Health Status   ☐ Drug Use/Dependency

☐ Previous Losses   ☐ Hx of Family Abuse

☐ Developmentally Delayed Parents ☐ Limited Support System

☐ Other:_____

Husband/Significant Other:_____

Baby's Name:_____ ☐ M ☐ F

DOB/Time:_____

Mother's Discharge Date/Time:_____

Newborn Discharge Date:(if different from mother's)_____

Baby's M.D. (Full Name):_____

Phone #:_____

Next Appt:_____

BABY:

Gestation:_____Weeks ☐ Fetal Loss

Birth Weight:_____ Discharge Weight:_____

Apgars: 1"_____ 5"_____

Feeding Issues:_____

Feedings: Breast _____ Bottle _____

Normal Infant Exam: ☐ Yes   ☐ No (explain below)

Circumcised: ☐ Yes   ☐ No

Cord Clamp Off: ☐ Yes   ☐ No

Voidings: ☐ Yes   ☐ No

Stooling: ☐ Yes   ☐ No

☐ Newborn screen was done in hospital—after baby 24
   hours of age.

☐ Newborn screen to be drawn at clinic.

☐ Newborn screen to be drawn at home.
   ☐ Lab slip sent home with family.

ADDITIONAL COMMENTS or ABNORMAL FINDINGS FOR MOTHER OR BABY: _____

_____

_____

Faxed to Home Care   ☐ *Facesheet* ☐ *Referral*   *Referral Completed By:* _____

Fig. 16-9 Referral form. (Courtesy OB Homecare of Allina Hospitals and Clinics, Minneapolis, MN.)

things as signs of adequate intake by the breastfeeding infant or, after initiating home phototherapy, to assess the caregiver's knowledge regarding equipment complications.

The warm line is another type of telephone link between the new family and concerned caregivers or experienced parent volunteers. A warm line is a help line or consultation service, not a crisis intervention line. The warm line is appropriately used for dealing with less extreme concerns that may seem urgent at the time the call is placed but are not actual emergencies. Calls to warm lines commonly relate to infant feeding, prolonged crying, or sibling rivalry. Warm line services may extend beyond the fourth trimester. Families need to call when concerns arise and be given phone numbers for easy access to answers to their questions.

Support groups

A special group experience is sometimes sought by the woman adjusting to motherhood. On occasion, postpartum women who have met earlier in prenatal clinics or on the hospital unit may begin to associate for mutual support. Members of childbirth classes who attend a postpartum reunion may decide to extend their relationship during the fourth trimester.

A postpartum support group enables mothers and fathers to share with and support each other as they adjust to parenting. Many new parents find it reassuring to discover that they are not alone in their feelings of confusion and uncertainty. An experienced parent can often impart concrete information that can be valuable to other members in a postpartum support group. Inexperienced parents may find themselves imitating the behavior of others in the group whom they perceive as particularly capable.

Referral to community resources

To develop an effective referral system, it is important that the nurse have an understanding of the needs of the woman and family and of the organization and community resources available for meeting those needs. Locating and compiling information about available community services contributes to the development of a referral system. It is important for the nurse to develop his or her own resource file of local and national services that are used commonly by health care providers (see Resources at the end of this chapter).

COMMUNITY ACTIVITY

Interview a home health care nurse regarding what such nurses teach expectant parents about postpartum care. How do they incorporate culture differences within their instructional material? Do they discuss topics that are specific to the woman's culture with regard to postpartum care? What concerns do they have about caring for women from different cultures? What are some topics that are taboo within certain cultures? How are these handled?

Key Points

- Postpartum care is modeled on the concept of health.
- Cultural beliefs and practices affect the patient's response to the puerperium.
- The nursing care plan includes assessments to detect deviations from normal, comfort measures to relieve discomfort or pain, and safety measures to prevent injury or infection.
- Teaching and counseling measures are designed to promote the woman's feelings of competence in self-care and baby care.
- Common nursing interventions in the postpartum period include evaluating and treating the boggy uterus and the full urinary bladder; providing for nonpharmacologic and pharmacologic relief of pain and discomfort associated with the episiotomy, lacerations, or breastfeeding; and instituting measures to promote or suppress lactation.
- Meeting the psychosocial needs of new mothers involves taking into consideration the composition and functioning of the entire family.
- Early postpartum discharge will continue to be the trend as a result of consumer demand, medical necessity, discharge criteria for low risk childbirth, and cost-containment measures.
- Early discharge classes, telephone follow-up, home visits, warm lines, and support groups are effective means of facilitating physiologic and psychologic adjustments in the postpartum period.

Answer Guidelines to Critical Thinking Exercises

Return to Nonpregnant Appearance

1 Yes, there is sufficient evidence to draw conclusions about counseling women with regard to regaining their nonpregnant appearance. Normal weight gain during pregnancy is approximately 25 pounds. Because Deidra gained almost twice that much weight during her pregnancy, she will need to make changes in her diet and exercise regularly in order to reach her prepregnant weight. There are multiple sources of information about diet and exercise during the postpartum period, including health care professionals, dietitians, web sites, television programs, and magazines available to Deidra. Although making changes in her diet and exercise regimen will not be easy, with determination and persistence Deidra can certainly succeed at regaining her prepregnant appearance.

2 a. The postpartum woman will lose weight gradually if she consumes a balanced diet that provides slightly fewer calories than her daily energy expenditure. Most women rapidly lose several pounds during the month after birth. Because fat is the most concentrated source of calories in the diet, the first step in weight reduction is to identify sources of fat in the diet and explore ways to reduce them.

b. Breastfeeding women are encouraged to follow the same well-balanced diet recommended for healthy pregnant women. The lactating woman needs to consume at least 1800 calories per day in order to produce an adequate milk supply. As a result of the caloric demands of lactation, the breastfeeding woman usually has a gradual but steady weight loss.

c. Women can begin exercising soon after birth, although they are encouraged to begin with simple exercises and gradually progress to more strenuous ones.

d. A woman's self esteem is often related to her perceived body image. How a new mother feels about herself and her body may affect her behavior and adaptation to parenting.

3 Priority for nursing care at this time is to educate Deidra regarding a weight reduction diet for a breastfeeding woman and a sensible exercise plan for a postpartum patient. She should be encouraged to follow the same balanced diet recommended during pregnancy and urged to avoid strenuous dieting. In addition, Deidra can be encouraged to eliminate "empty" calories, such as sugar-sweetened drinks, desserts, and chips from her diet. She will likely be surprised and pleased to learn that she will burn about 500 calories per day through milk production. Deidra's individual dietary preferences should also be considered. It is important to inform Deidra that dieting can cause her milk supply to decrease; she should monitor the baby's intake and output to see if the infant is receiving adequate nutrition. If her milk production is declining, she may need to add more calories to her diet.

Deidra can be encouraged to begin simple exercises immediately, since she is already 10 days postpartum. Taking the baby for a walk each day would provide both an opportunity for exercise and help in regaining a normal routine. Deidra should be encouraged to start with simple exercises and gradually progress to more strenuous ones.

In terms of body image and self-esteem, if Deidra voiced concerns about feeling unable to cope, having no support, or perceiving that things are now very different and will "never return to normal," a referral for more extensive evaluation and counseling would be warranted.

4 There is a significant amount of information available concerning diet and exercise for the postpartum woman who is breastfeeding. Data regarding self-esteem in new mothers also exist.

5 Most postpartum women are eager to regain their nonpregnant figures quickly. It can be discouraging when diet and exercise efforts fail to produce the desired results immediately.

Cultural Influences during the Postpartum Period

1 Yes, there is sufficient evidence to draw conclusions about the cultural beliefs of Asians as they relate to the postpartum period and breastfeeding. Potential sources of information include journal articles, books, and interviews with women who are members of that cultural group. Information regarding how traditional Asian beliefs may be adapted by women who emigrate to other countries is also available from these sources.

2 a. Asian women typically prefer warm foods and hot drinks after giving birth and refuse anything cold. In this culture, pregnancy is considered to be a "hot" state, and childbirth results in a sudden loss of this state. Warm food and drinks help to restore balance in the woman's body by facilitating the return of the "hot" state. Another typical Asian belief is that the mother and baby remain in a weak and vulnerable state for a period of several weeks following birth. During this time the mother may remain in a passive role, take no baths or showers, and stay in bed to prevent cold air from entering her body.

b. Because of the prevalent belief among Asians that the mother should rest and remain in bed to protect herself immediately after childbirth, routine baby care is usually provided by another female. In several cultures, including Asian cultures, colostrum is viewed as unnecessary and unhealthy for newborns. Breastfeeding is begun only several days after birth, when the "true milk" has come in. Before that time, babies may be fed prelacteal food. Asian parents often request infant formula for their infant while they are in the hospital.

c. In many cultures, female family members and friends play an essential role in providing care for the new mother and baby immediately after birth. In the Asian culture, new mothers observe specific diet and activity restrictions for several weeks. Following these traditional cultural practices in a different country may prove to be extremely difficult if family members or friends are not available. In the home country, males are often not expected to assist in caring for new mothers and babies. Even if a woman's husband is willing to do so, he may need much instruction and encouragement to provide even minimal care for his wife and baby.

d. Women are routinely taught that the ideal time to initiate breastfeeding is within the first hour after birth. During this time the baby is usually in the quiet alert state. However, women from cultures that wait hours or days to initiate breastfeeding are able to do so successfully.

3 The priority for nursing care at this time is to assist Terri in recovering from childbirth in a way that is congruent with her cultural beliefs. Every effort should be made to determine Terri's preferences with regard to diet, activity, and hygiene, and to honor them as much as possible. Although Terri's beliefs may seem unusual, they should be encouraged as long as she wants to conform to them and she and the baby suffer no ill effects. Culturally appropriate accommodations that can be made for Terri on the postpartum unit include providing a bedside bath if desired, offering only warm food and drink, and encouraging family members or friends to bring in especially desired foods if the hospital's dietary department is unable to provide them. If Terri desires, family members or friends can be encouraged to stay with her as much as possible to assist with her care and the baby's care.

Breastfeeding will also need to be addressed with Terri. A good way to determine the information Terri needs is to discover why she prefers to feed her baby infant formula. Discussing the benefits of colostrum for newborns may cause Terri to change her mind about delaying breastfeeding.

4 There is a significant amount of information available concerning culturally appropriate care during the postpartum period for Asian women. Women who receive culturally appropriate care during this time will likely be more satisfied with their care. They will also be better able to assume care for themselves and their babies in the future if their early needs for passive nurturing are met.

5 Not all women belonging to a particular cultural group will desire to use the traditional health practices that represent that group. Many young women who are first- or second-generation Americans follow their cultural traditions only when older family members are present or not at all. Adherents to the "melting pot" theory of acculturation in the United States would assert that women, regardless of their cultural heritage, should "act like Americans" if they live in America.

Resources

Child Welfare League of America
440 First St., NW, Third Floor
Washington, DC 20001-2085
202-638-2952
www.cwla.org/default.htm

Depression After Delivery
P.O. Box 59973
Renton, WA 98508
206-283-9278
www.depressionafterdelivery.com

HAND (Helping After Neonatal Death)
P.O. Box 341
Los Gatos, CA 95031
888-908-HAND
www.handonline.org

La Leche League
1400 N. Meacham Rd.
Schaumburg, IL 60168-4808
800-525-3243 (24-hour line)
www.lalecheleague.org

March of Dimes Birth Defects Foundation
National Foundation/March of Dimes
1275 Mamaroneck Ave.
White Plains, NY 10605
888-663-4637 (MODIMES)
www.marchofdimes.com

National Perinatal Association
2090 Linglestown Rd., Suite 107
Harrisburg, PA 17110
888-971-3295
www.nationalperinatal.org

Nursing Mothers Council
Consult telephone directory for local chapters

Parent Soup
www.parentsoup.com

Planned Parenthood Federation of America, Inc.
810 Seventh Ave.
New York, NY 10019
800-230-PLAN
www.plannedparenthood.org

Positive Parenting
www.positiveparenting.com

Postpartum Education for Parents
P.O. Box 6154
Santa Barbara, CA 93160
Warmline: 805-564-3888
www.sbpep.org

Special Supplemental Nutrition Program for Women, Infants, and Children (WIC)
Food and Consumer Service
3101 Park Center Dr., Room 819
Alexandria, VA 22302
703-305-2286
www.usda.gov/fns/wic.html

References

American Academy of Pediatrics (AAP) Committee on Fetus and Newborn. (2004). Hospital stay for healthy term infants. *Pediatrics, 113*(5), 1434-1436.

American Academy of Pediatrics (AAP) & American College of Obstetricians and Gynecologists (ACOG). (2002). *Guidelines for perinatal care* (5th ed.). Elk Grove Village, IL: AAP.

American College of Obstetricians and Gynecologists. (2002). ACOG Committee Opinion #281. Rubella vaccine. *Obstetrics and Gynecology, 100*(6), 1417.

Ayers, J. (2000). The use of alternative therapies in the support of breastfeeding. *Journal of Human Lactation, 16*(1), 52-56.

Benedetti, T. (2002). Obstetric hemorrhage. In S. Gabbe, J. Niebyl, & J. Simpson (Eds.), *Obstetrics: Normal and problem pregnancies* (4th ed.). New York: Churchill Livingstone.

Carter, A., Baker, C., & Brownell, K. (2000). Body mass index, eating attitudes, and symptoms of depression and anxiety in pregnancy and the postpartum period. *Psychosomatic Medicine, 62*(2), 264-270.

Davis, R. (2001). The postpartum experience for Southeast Asian women in the United States. *MCN American Journal of Maternal Child Nursing, 26*(4), 208-213.

Donnelly, A. et al. (2001). Commercial hospital discharge packs for breastfeeding women (Cochrane Review). In *The Cochrane Library,* Issue 2, 2004. Chichester, UK: John Wiley & Sons.

Indoria, S., & Wade, A. (2001). Support for breastfeeding women (Cochrane Review), 2001. In *The Cochrane Library,* Issue 2, 2004. Chichester, UK: John Wiley & Sons.

Jesse, D., & Graham, M. (2005). Are you often sad and depressed?: Brief measure to identify women at risk for depression in pregnancy. *MCN American Journal of Maternal Child Nursing, 30*(1), 40-45.

Kim-Godwin, Y. (2003). Postpartum beliefs and practices among non-western cultures. *MCN American Journal of Maternal Child Nursing, 28*(2), 74-78.

Luegenbiehl, D. (1997). Improving visual estimation of blood volume on peripads. *MCN American Journal of Maternal Child Nursing, 22*(6), 294-298.

Mass, S. (2004). Breast pain: Engorgement, nipple pain and mastitis. *Clinical Obstetrics and Gynecology, 47*(3), 676-682.

Meara, E., Kotagal, U., Atherton, H., & Lieu, T. (2004). Impact of early newborn discharge legislation and early follow-up visits on infant outcomes in a state Medicaid population. *Pediatrics, 113*(6), 1619-1627.

Paul, I., Phillips, T., Widome, M., & Hollenbeak, C. (2004). Cost-effectiveness of postnatal home nursing visits for prevention of hospital care for jaundice and dehydration. *Pediatrics, 114*(4), 1015-1022.

Sampselle, C., Wyman, J., Thomas, K., Newman, D., Gray, M., Dougherty, M., & Burns, P. (2000). Continence for women: A test of AWHONN's evidence-based protocol in clinical practice. *Journal of Obstetric, Gynecologic, and Neonatal Nursing, 29*(1), 18-26.

Sikorski, J. et al. (2001). Support for breastfeeding women (Cochrane Review). In *The Cochrane Library,* Issue 2, 2004. Chichester, UK: John Wiley & Sons.

Simpson, K., & Creehan, P. (Eds.) (2001). AWHONN's *Perinatal Nursing* (2nd ed.). Philadelphia: Lippincott.

Troy, N. (2003). Is the significance of postpartum fatigue being overlooked in the lives of women? *MCN American Journal of Maternal Child Nursing, 28*(4), 252-257.

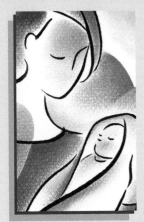

CHAPTER 17

Transition to Parenthood

BARBRA MANNING

LEARNING OBJECTIVES

- *Discuss ways to facilitate parent-infant adjustment.*
- *Describe sensual responses that strengthen attachment.*
- *Identify infant behaviors that facilitate and inhibit parental attachment.*
- *Differentiate three periods in parental role change after childbirth.*
- *Explain behaviors of the three phases of maternal adjustment.*

- *Discuss paternal adjustment.*
- *Examine the effects of the following on parental response: parental age (adolescence and over 35 years), culture, socioeconomic conditions, personal aspirations, and sensory impairment.*
- *Describe sibling adjustment.*
- *Explain grandparent adaptation.*

KEY TERMS AND DEFINITIONS

acquaintance Process used by parents to get to know or become familiar with their new infant; an important step in *attachment*

attachment A specific and enduring affective tie to another person

becoming a mother Transformation and growth of the mother identity

biorhythmicity Cyclic changes that occur with established regularity, such as sleeping and eating patterns

bonding A process by which parents, over time, form an emotional relationship with their infant

claiming process Process by which the parents identify their new baby in terms of likeness to other family members, differences, and uniqueness

en face Face-to-face position in which the parent's and infant's faces are approximately 20 cm apart and on the same plane

engrossment A parent's absorption, preoccupation, and interest in his or her infant; term typically used to describe the father's intense involvement with his newborn

entrainment Phenomenon observed in the microanalysis of sound films in which the speaker moves several parts of the body and the listener responds to the sounds by moving in ways that are coordinated with the rhythm of the sounds (infants have been observed to move in time to the rhythms of adult speech but not to random noises or disconnected words or vowels); believed to be an essential factor in the process of maternal-infant bonding

letting-go phase Interdependent phase after birth in which the mother and family move forward as a system with interacting members

mutuality Parent-infant interaction in which the infant's behaviors and characteristics call forth a corresponding set of maternal behaviors and characteristics

postpartum blues A let-down feeling, accompanied by irritability and anxiety, which usually begins 2 to 3 days after giving birth and disappears within a week or two; sometimes called "baby blues"

reciprocity Type of body movement or behavior that provides the observer with cues, such as the behavioral cues infants provide to parents and parents' responses to cues

sibling rivalry A sibling's jealousy of and resentment toward a new child in the family

synchrony Fit between the infant's cues and the parent's response

taking-hold phase Period after birth characterized by a woman becoming more independent and more interested in learning infant care skills; learning to be a competent mother is an important task

taking-in phase Period after birth characterized by the woman's dependency; maternal needs are dominant, and talking about the birth is an important task

transition to parenthood Period of time from the preconception parenthood decision through the first months after birth of the baby during which parents define their parental roles and adjust to parenthood

*B*ecoming a parent creates a period of change and instability for men and women who decide to have children. This occurs whether parenthood is biologic or adoptive and whether the parents are married husband-wife couples, cohabiting couples, single mothers, single fathers, lesbian couples with one woman as biologic mother, or gay male couples who adopt a child. Parenting may be described as a process of role attainment and role transition that begins during pregnancy. The transition ends when the parent develops a sense of comfort and confidence in performing the parental role.

PARENTAL ATTACHMENT, BONDING, AND ACQUAINTANCE

The process by which a parent comes to love and accept a child and a child comes to love and accept a parent is referred to as attachment. Using the terms *attachment* and *bonding*, Klaus and Kennell (1997) proposed that the period shortly after birth is important to mother-to-infant attachment. They defined the phenomenon of bonding as a sensitive period in the first minutes and hours after birth when mothers and fathers must have close contact with their infants for optimal later development (Klaus & Kennell, 1976). Klaus and Kennell (1982) later revised their theory of parent-infant bonding, modifying their claim of the critical nature of immediate contact with the infant after birth. They acknowledged the adaptability of human parents, stating that it took longer than minutes or hours for parents to form an emotional relationship with their infants. The terms *attachment* and *bonding* continue to be used interchangeably.

Attachment is developed and maintained by proximity and interaction with the infant, through which the parent becomes acquainted with the infant, identifies the infant as an individual, and claims the infant as a member of the family. Attachment is facilitated by positive feedback (i.e., social, verbal, and nonverbal responses, whether real or perceived, that indicate acceptance of one partner by the other). Attachment occurs through a mutually satisfying experience. A mother commented on her son's grasp reflex, "I put my finger in his hand, and he grabbed right on. It is just a reflex, I know, but it felt good anyway" (Fig. 17-1).

The concept of attachment has been extended to include mutuality; that is, the infant's behaviors and characteristics call forth a corresponding set of parental behaviors and characteristics. The infant displays signaling behaviors such as crying, smiling, and cooing that initiate the contact and bring the caregiver to the child. These behaviors are followed by executive behaviors such as rooting, grasping, and postural adjustments that maintain the contact. The caregiver is attracted to an alert, responsive, cuddly infant and repelled by an irritable, apparently disinterested infant. Attachment occurs more readily with the infant whose temperament, social capabilities, appearance, and gender fit the parent's expectations. If the infant does not meet these expectations, resolution of the parent's disappointment can delay the attachment process. A list of infant behaviors affecting parental attachment that continues to be a classic comprehensive reference is presented in Table 17-1. A corresponding list of parental behaviors that affect infant attachment is presented in Table 17-2.

An important part of attachment is acquaintance. Parents use eye contact (Fig. 17-2), touching, talking, and exploring to become acquainted with their infant during the immediate postpartum period. Adoptive parents undergo the same process when they first meet their new child. During this

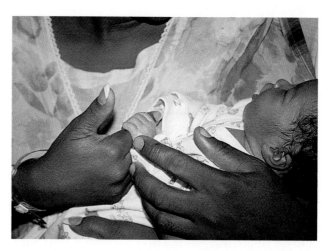

Fig. 17-1 *Hands. (Courtesy Marjorie Pyle, RNC, Lifecircle, Costa Mesa, CA.)*

TABLE 17-1

Infant Behaviors Affecting Parental Attachment

FACILITATING BEHAVIORS	INHIBITING BEHAVIORS
Visually alert; eye-to-eye contact; tracking or following of parent's face	Sleepy; eyes closed most of the time; gaze aversion
Appealing facial appearance; randomness of body movements reflecting helplessness	Resemblance to person parent dislikes; hyperirritability or jerky body movements when touched
Smiles	Bland facial expression; infrequent smiles
Vocalization; crying only when hungry or wet	Crying for hours on end; colicky
Grasp reflex	Exaggerated motor reflex
Anticipatory approach behaviors for feedings; sucks well; feeds easily	Feeds poorly; regurgitates; vomits often
Enjoys being cuddled, held	Resists holding and cuddling by crying, stiffening body
Easily consolable	Inconsolable; unresponsive to parenting, caretaking tasks
Activity and regularity somewhat predictable	Unpredictable feeding and sleeping schedule
Attention span sufficient to focus on parents	Inability to attend to parent's face or offered stimulation
Differential crying, smiling, and vocalizing; recognizes and prefers parents	Shows no preference for parents over others
Approaches through locomotion	Unresponsive to parent's approaches
Clings to parent; puts arms around parent's neck	Seeks attention from any adult in room
Lifts arms to parents in greeting	Ignores parents

From Gerson, E. (1973). *Infant behavior in the first year of life.* New York: Raven Press.

TABLE 17-2

Parental Behaviors Affecting Infant Attachment

FACILITATING BEHAVIORS	INHIBITING BEHAVIORS
Looks; gazes; takes in physical characteristics of infant; assumes en face position; eye contact	Turns away from infant; ignores infant's presence
Hovers; maintains proximity; directs attention to, points to infant	Avoids infant; does not seek proximity; refuses to hold infant when given opportunity
Identifies infant as unique individual	Identifies infant with someone parent dislikes; fails to discern any of infant's unique features
Claims infant as family member; names infant	Fails to place infant in family context or identify infant with family member; has difficulty naming
Touches; progresses from fingertip to fingers to palms to encompassing contact	Fails to move from fingertip touch to palmar contact and holding
Smiles at infant	Maintains bland countenance or frowns at infant
Talks to, coos, or sings to infant	Wakes infant when infant is sleeping; handles roughly; hurries feeding by moving nipple continuously
Expresses pride in infant	Expresses disappointment, displeasure in infant
Relates infant's behavior to familiar events	Does not incorporate infant into life
Assigns meaning to infant's actions and sensitively interprets infant's needs	Makes no effort to interpret infant's actions or needs
Views infant's behaviors and appearance in positive light	Views infant's behavior as exploiting, deliberately uncooperative; views appearance as distasteful, ugly

From Mercer, R. (1983). Parent-infant attachment. In L. Sonstegard, K. Kowalski, & B. Jennings (Eds.), *Women's health* (Vol. 2), *Childbearing.* New York: Grune & Stratton.

period families engage in the claiming process, which is the identification of the new baby (Fig. 17-3). The child is first identified in terms of "likeness" to other family members, then in terms of "differences," and finally in terms of "uniqueness." The unique newcomer is thus incorporated into the family. Mothers and fathers scrutinize their infant carefully and point out characteristics that the child shares with other family members and that are indicative of a relationship between them. The claiming process is revealed by maternal comments such as the following: "Russ held him close and said, 'He's the image of his father,' but I found one part like me—his toes are shaped like mine."

On the other hand, some mothers react negatively. They "claim" the infant in terms of the discomfort or pain the

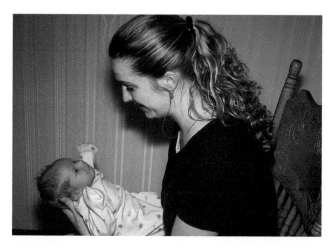

Fig. 17-2 Mother and baby make eye contact in *en face* position. (Courtesy Michael S. Clement, MD, Mesa, AZ.)

baby causes. The mother interprets the infant's normal responses as being negative toward her and reacts to her child with dislike or indifference. She does not hold the child close or touch the child to be comforting; for example, "The nurse put the baby into Marie's arms. She promptly laid him across her knees and glanced up at the television. 'Stay still until I finish watching; you've been enough trouble already.'"

Nursing interventions related to the promotion of parent-infant attachment are numerous and varied (Table 17-3). They can enhance positive parent-infant contacts by heightening parental awareness of an infant's responses and ability to communicate. As the parent attempts to become competent and loving in that role, nurses can bolster the parent's self-confidence and ego. Nurses are in prime positions to identify actual and potential problems and collaborate with other health care professionals who will provide care for the parents after discharge. Nursing considerations for fostering maternal-infant bonding among special populations may vary (Cultural Considerations box).

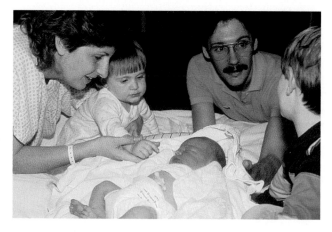

Fig. 17-3 Family members examine the new baby. They discuss how she resembles them and other family members. (Courtesy Marjorie Pyle, RNC, Lifecircle, Costa Mesa, CA.)

Cultural Considerations

Fostering Bonding in Women of Varying Ethnic and Cultural Groups

Childbearing practices and rituals of other cultures may not be congruent with standard practices associated with bonding in the Anglo-American culture. For example, Chinese families traditionally use extended family members to care for the newborn so that the mother can rest and recover, especially after a cesarean birth. Some Native-American, Asian, and Hispanic women do not initiate breastfeeding until their breast milk comes in. Haitian families do not name their babies until after the confinement month. Amount of eye contact varies among cultures, too. Yup'ik Eskimo mothers almost always position their babies so that eye contact can be made.

Nurses should become knowledgeable of the childbearing beliefs and practices of diverse cultural and ethnic groups. Because individual cultural variations exist within groups, nurses need to clarify with the patient and family members or friends what cultural norms the woman follows. Incorrect judgments may be made about mother-infant bonding if nurses do not practice culturally sensitive care.

Modified from D'Avanzo, C., & Geissler, E. (2003). *Pocket guide to cultural assessment* (3rd ed). St. Louis: Mosby.

Assessment of Attachment Behaviors

One of the most important areas of assessment is careful observation of those behaviors thought to indicate the formation of emotional bonds between the newborn and family, especially the mother. Unlike physical assessment of the neonate, which has concrete guidelines to follow, assessment of parent-infant attachment requires much more skill in terms of observation and interviewing. Rooming-in of mother and infant and liberal visiting privileges for father, siblings, and grandparents facilitate recognition of behaviors that demonstrate positive or negative attachment. An excellent opportunity exists during feeding. Guidelines for assessment of attachment behaviors are presented in Box 17-1.

During pregnancy, and often even before conception occurs, parents develop an image of the "ideal" or "fantasy" infant. At birth the fantasy infant becomes the real infant. How closely the dream child resembles the real child influences the bonding process. Assessing such expectations during pregnancy and at the time of the infant's birth allows identification of discrepancies in the parents' view of the fantasy child versus the real child.

The labor process significantly affects the immediate attachment of mothers to their newborn infants. Factors such as a long labor, feeling tired or "drugged" after birth, and problems with breastfeeding can delay the development of initial positive feelings toward the newborn.

TABLE 17-3

Examples of Parent-Infant Attachment Interventions

INTERVENTION LABEL AND DEFINITION	ACTIVITIES
ATTACHMENT PROMOTION Facilitation of development of parent-infant relationship	Provide opportunity for parent(s) to see, hold, and examine newborn immediately after birth Encourage parent(s) to hold infant close to body Assist parent(s) to participate in infant care
ENVIRONMENTAL MANAGEMENT: ATTACHMENT PROCESS Manipulation of individuals' surroundings to facilitate development of parent-infant relationship	Provide rooming-in in hospital Create environment that fosters privacy Individualize daily routine to meet parents' needs Permit father or significant other to sleep in room with mother Develop policies that permit presence of significant others as much as desired
FAMILY INTEGRITY PROMOTION: CHILDBEARING FAMILY Facilitation of growth of individuals or families who are adding infant to family unit	Prepare parent(s) for expected role changes involved in becoming a parent Prepare parent(s) for responsibilities of parenthood Monitor effects of newborn on family structure Reinforce positive parenting behaviors
LACTATION COUNSELING Use of interactive helping process to assist in maintenance of successful breastfeeding	Correct misconceptions, misinformation, and inaccuracies about breastfeeding Evaluate parents' understanding of infant's feeding cues (e.g., rooting, sucking, alertness) Determine frequency of feedings in relation to infant's needs Demonstrate breast massage and discuss its advantages to increasing milk supply
PARENT EDUCATION: INFANT Instruction on nurturing and physical care needed during first year of life	Determine parents' knowledge, readiness, and ability to learn about infant care Provide anticipatory guidance about developmental changes during first year of life Teach parent(s) skills to care for newborn Demonstrate ways in which parent(s) can stimulate infant's development Discuss infant's capabilities for interaction Demonstrate quieting techniques
RISK IDENTIFICATION: CHILDBEARING FAMILY Identification of individual or family likely to experience difficulties in parenting and assigning priorities to strategies to prevent parenting problems	Determine developmental stage of parent(s) Review prenatal history for factors that predispose individuals or family to complications Ascertain understanding of English or other language used in community Monitor behavior that may indicate problem with attachment Plan for risk-reduction activities in collaboration with individual or family

Modified from Dochterman, J., & Bulechek, G. (2004). *Nursing interventions classification (NIC)* (4th ed.). St. Louis: Mosby.

Assessing Attachment Behavior

- When the infant is brought to the parents, do they reach out for the infant and call the infant by name? (Recognize that in some cultures, parents may not name the infant in the early newborn period.)
- Do the parents speak about the infant in terms of identification—whom the infant looks like; what appears special about their infant over other infants?
- When parents are holding the infant, what kind of body contact is there—do parents feel at ease in changing the infant's position; are fingertips or whole hands used; are there parts of the body they avoid touching or parts of the body they investigate and scrutinize?
- When the infant is awake, what kinds of stimulation do the parents provide—do they talk to the infant, to each other, or to no one; how do they look at the infant—direct visual contact, avoidance of eye contact, or looking at other people or objects?
- How comfortable do the parents appear in terms of caring for the infant? Do they express any concern regarding their ability or disgust for certain activities, such as changing diapers?
- What type of affection do they demonstrate to the newborn, such as smiling, stroking, kissing, or rocking?
- If the infant is fussy, what kinds of comforting techniques do the parents use, such as rocking, swaddling, talking, or stroking?

PARENT-INFANT CONTACT

Early Contact

Early close contact may facilitate the attachment process between parent and child. This does not mean that a delay will inhibit this process (humans are too resilient for that), but additional psychologic energy may be needed to achieve the same effect. To date, no scientific evidence has demonstrated that immediate contact after birth is essential for the human parent-child relationship.

Parents who desire but are unable to have early contact with their newborn (e.g., the infant was transferred to the intensive care nursery) can be reassured that such contact is not essential for optimal parent-infant interactions. Otherwise, adopted infants would not form the usual affectionate ties with their parents. Nor does the mode of infant-mother contact after birth (skin-to-skin versus wrapped) appear to have any important effect. Nurses need to stress that the parent-infant relationship is a process that occurs over time.

Extended Contact

The provision of rooming-in facilities for the mother and her baby is common in family-centered care. The infant is transferred to the area from the transitional nursery (if the facility uses one) after showing satisfactory extrauterine adjustment. The father is encouraged to participate in the care of the infant, and siblings and grandparents are also encouraged to visit and become acquainted with the infant. Whether the method of family-centered care is rooming-in, mother-baby or couplet care, or a family birth unit, mothers and their partners are considered equal and integral parts of the developing family. Partners are encouraged to take as active a role as they wish.

Extended contact with the infant should be available for all parents but especially for those at risk for parenting inadequacies, such as adolescents and low-income women. Any activity that optimizes family-centered care is worthy of serious consideration by postpartum nurses.

COMMUNICATION BETWEEN PARENT AND INFANT

The parent-infant relationship is strengthened through the use of sensual responses and abilities by both partners in the interaction. The nurse should keep in mind that there may be cultural variations in these interactive behaviors.

The Senses
Touch

Touch, or the tactile sense, is used extensively by parents and other caregivers as a means of becoming acquainted with the newborn. Many mothers reach out for their infants as soon as they are born and the cord is cut. Mothers lift their infants to their breasts, enfold them in their arms, and cradle them. Once the infant is close, they begin the exploration process with their fingertips, one of the most touch-sensitive areas of the body. Within a short time the caregiver uses the palm to caress the baby's trunk and eventually enfolds the infant. Gentle stroking motions are used to soothe and quiet the infant; patting or gently rubbing the infant's back is a comfort after feedings. Infants also pat the mother's breast as they nurse. Both seem to enjoy sharing each other's body warmth. There is a desire in parents to touch, pick up, and hold the infant (Fig. 17-4). They

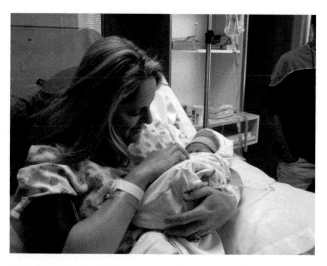

Fig. 17-4 Mother interacts with newborn. (Courtesy Tricia Olson, North Ogden, UT.)

comment on the softness of the baby's skin and are aware of milia and rashes. As parents become increasingly sensitive to the infant's like or dislike of different types of touch, they draw closer to the baby.

Variations in touching behaviors have been noted in mothers from different cultural groups (Galanti, 2003; Jiménez, 1995; Stewart & Jambunathan, 1996). For example, minimal touching and cuddling is a traditional Southeast Asian practice thought to protect the infant from evil spirits. Because of tradition and spiritual beliefs, women in India and Bali have practiced infant massage since ancient times (Miller, 2004; Zlotnick, 2000).

Eye contact

Interest in having eye contact with the baby has been demonstrated repeatedly by parents. Some mothers remark that once their babies have looked at them, they feel much closer to them. Parents spend much time getting their babies to open their eyes and look at them. In the United States, eye contact appears to cement the development of a trusting relationship and is an important factor in human relationships at all ages. In other cultures, eye contact may be perceived differently. For example, in Mexican culture, sustained direct eye contact is considered to be rude, immodest, and dangerous for some. This danger may arise from the *mal ojo* (evil eye), resulting from excessive admiration. Women and children are thought to be more susceptible to the *mal ojo* (D'Avanzo & Geissler, 2003).

As newborns become functionally able to sustain eye contact with their parents, time is spent in mutual gazing, often in the **en face** position, a position in which the parent's face and the infant's face are approximately 8 inches apart and on the same plane (see Fig. 17-2).

Nursing and medical practices that encourage this interaction should be implemented. Immediately after birth, for example, the infant can be positioned on the mother's abdomen or breasts with the mother's and the infant's faces on the same plane so that they can easily make eye contact. Lights can be dimmed so that the infant's eyes will open. Instillation of prophylactic antibiotic ointment in the infant's eyes can be delayed until the infant and parents have had some time together in the first hour after birth.

Voice

The shared response of parents and infants to each other's voices is also remarkable. Parents wait tensely for the first cry. Once that cry has reassured them of the baby's health, they begin comforting behaviors. As the parents talk in high-pitched voices, the infant is alerted and turns toward them.

Infants respond to higher-pitched voices and can distinguish their mother's voice from others soon after birth. Infants use their cries to signal hunger, pain, boredom, and tiredness. With experience, parents learn to distinguish among such cries.

Odor

Another behavior shared by parents and infants is a response to each other's odor. Mothers comment on the smell of their babies when first born and have noted that each infant has a unique odor. Infants learn rapidly to distinguish the odor of their mother's breast milk.

Entrainment

Newborns move in time with the structure of adult speech which is termed **entrainment.** They wave their arms, lift their heads, and kick their legs, seemingly "dancing in tune" to a parent's voice. Culturally determined rhythms of speech are ingrained in the infant long before spoken language is used to communicate. This shared rhythm also gives the parent positive feedback and establishes a positive setting for effective communication.

Biorhythmicity

The fetus is in tune with the mother's natural rhythms—**biorhythmicity**—such as heartbeats. After birth a crying infant may be soothed by being held in a position in which the mother's heartbeat can be heard or by hearing a recording of a heartbeat. One of the newborn's tasks is to establish a personal biorhythm. Parents can help in this process by giving consistent loving care and using their infant's alert state to develop responsive behavior and thereby increase social interactions and opportunities for learning (Fig. 17-5). The more quickly parents become competent in child care activities, the more quickly their psychologic energy can be directed toward observing the communication cues the infant gives them.

Reciprocity and Synchrony

Reciprocity is a type of body movement or behavior that provides the observer with cues. The observer or receiver interprets those cues and responds to them. Reciprocity often

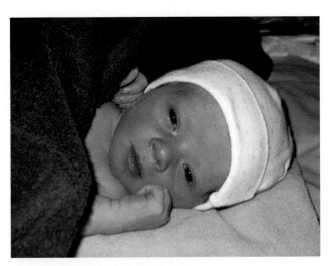

Fig. 17-5 Infant in alert state at one hour of age. (Courtesy Christine Brockett, Boulder, CO.)

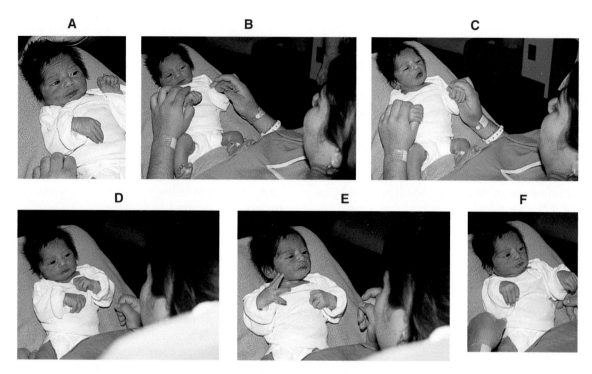

Fig. 17-6 Holding newborn in *en face* position, mother works to alert her daughter, 6 hours old. **A,** Infant is quiet and alert. **B,** Mother begins talking to daughter. **C,** Infant responds, opens mouth like her mother. **D,** Infant gazes at her mother. **E,** Infant waves hand. **F,** Infant glances away, resting. Hand relaxes. (Courtesy Marjorie Pyle, RNC, Lifecircle, Costa Mesa, CA.)

takes several weeks to develop with a new baby. For example, when the newborn fusses and cries, the mother responds by picking up and cradling the infant; the baby becomes quiet and alert and establishes eye contact; the mother verbalizes, sings, and coos while the baby maintains eye contact. The baby then averts the eyes and yawns; the mother decreases her active response (Fig. 17-6). If the parent continues to stimulate the infant, the baby may become fussy.

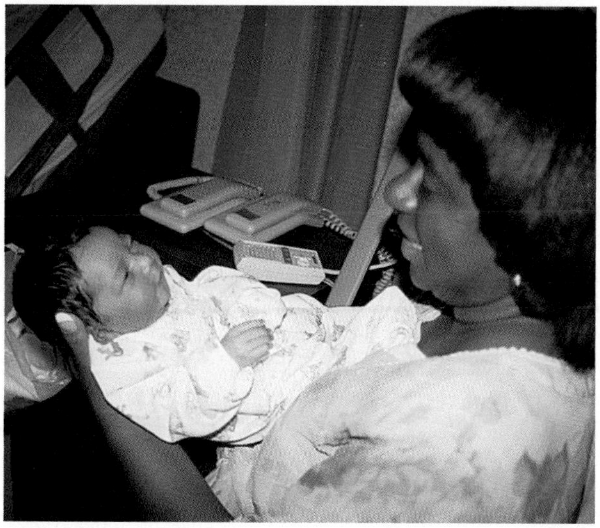

Fig. 17-7 Sharing a smile: example of synchrony. (Courtesy Marjorie Pyle, RNC, Lifecircle, Costa Mesa, CA.)

The term **synchrony** refers to the "fit" between the infant's cues and the parent's response. When parent and infant experience a synchronous interaction, it is mutually rewarding (Fig. 17-7). Parents need time to interpret the infant's cues correctly. For example, after a certain time the infant develops a specific cry in response to different situations such as boredom, loneliness, hunger, and discomfort. The parent may need assistance in deciphering these cries, along with trial and error interventions, before synchrony develops.

PARENTAL ROLE AFTER CHILDBIRTH

Adaptation involves a stabilizing of tasks, a coming to terms with commitments. Parents demonstrate growing competence in child care activities and are more attuned to their infant's behavior. Typically the period from the decision to conceive through the first months of having a child is termed the **transition to parenthood.**

Transition to Parenthood

Historically, the transition to parenthood was viewed as a crisis. The current perspective is that parenthood is a developmental transition (Tomlinson, 1996) rather than a major life crisis for the majority of families. The transition to parenthood is described as a time of disorder and disequilibrium, as well as satisfaction, for mothers and their partners (Rogan, Shmied, Barclay, Everitt, & Wyllie, 1997; Tomlinson, 1996).

Usual methods of coping often seem ineffective. Some parents can be so distressed that they are unable to be supportive of each other. Because men typically identify their spouses as their primary or only source of support, the transition can be harder for the fathers, who feel deprived when the mothers, who are also experiencing stress, cannot provide their usual level of support. Strong emotions such as helplessness, inadequacy, and anger that arise when dealing with a crying infant catch many parents unprepared. On the other hand, parenthood allows adults to develop and display a selfless, warm, and caring side of themselves, which may not be expressed in other adult roles.

For the majority of mothers and their partners, the transition to parenthood is viewed as an opportunity rather than a time of danger. Parents are stimulated to try new coping strategies as they work to master their new roles and reach new developmental levels. As they work through the transition, personal strength and resourcefulness are revealed (Rogan et al., 1997).

Parental Tasks and Responsibilities

Parents need to reconcile the actual child with the fantasy and dream child. This means coming to terms with the infant's physical appearance, sex, innate temperament, and physical status. If the real child differs greatly from the fantasy child, parents may delay acceptance of the child. In some instances they may never accept the child.

Some parents are startled by the normal appearance of the neonate—size, color, molding of the head, or bowed appearance of the legs. Many fathers have commented that they thought the odd shape of the infant's head (molding) meant the infant would be mentally retarded.

Many parents know the sex of the infant before birth because of the use of ultrasound assessments; for those who do not have this information, disappointment over the baby's sex can take time to resolve. The parents may provide adequate physical care but find it difficult to be sincerely involved with the infant until this internal conflict has been resolved. As one mother remarked, "I really wanted a boy. I know it is silly and irrational, but when they said, 'She's a lovely little girl,' I was so disappointed and angry—yes, angry—I could hardly look at her. Oh, I looked after her okay, her feedings and baths and things, but I couldn't feel excited. To tell the truth, I felt like a monster not liking my child. Then one day she was lying there and she turned her head and looked right at me. I felt a flooding of love for her come over me, and we looked at each other a long time. It's okay now. I wouldn't change her for all the boys in the world."

Parents need to become adept in the care of the infant, including care-giving activities, noting the communication cues given by the infant to indicate needs, and responding appropriately to the infant's needs. Self-esteem grows with competence. Breastfeeding makes mothers feel they are contributing in a unique way to the welfare of the infant. The infant's response to the parental care and attention may be interpreted by the parent as a comment on the quality of that care. Infant behaviors that are interpreted by parents as positive responses to their care include being consoled easily, enjoying being cuddled, and making eye contact. Spitting up frequently after feedings, crying, and being unpredictable may be perceived as negative responses to parental care. Continuation of these infant responses that are viewed as negative by the parent can result in alienation of parent and infant to the detriment of the infant.

Assistance, including advice by husbands, partners, wives, mothers, mothers-in-law, and professional workers, can either be seen as supportive or an indication of how inept these people have judged the new parents to be. Criticism, real or imagined, of the new parents' ability to provide adequate physical care, nutrition, or social stimulation for the infant can prove to be devastating. By providing encouragement and praise for parenting efforts, nurses can bolster the new parents' confidence.

Parents must establish a place for the newborn within the family group. Whether the infant is the firstborn or the last born, all family members must adjust their roles to accommodate the newcomer. The firstborn child needs support to accept a rival for parental affections. Children need help dealing with losing a favored position in the family hierarchy. The parents are expected to negotiate these changes.

Maternal Adjustment

Three phases are evident as the mother adjusts to her parental role (Table 17-4). These phases are characterized by dependent behavior, dependent-independent behavior, and interdependent behavior.

Dependent phase

During the first 24 to 48 hours after childbirth the mother's dependency needs predominate. To the extent that these needs are met by others, the mother is able to divert her psychologic energy to her infant rather than to focus on herself. She needs "mothering" herself to "mother." Rubin (1961) aptly described these few days as the taking-in phase, a time when nurturing and protective care are required by the new mother. In Rubin's classic description the taking-in phase lasted 2 to 3 days. Later studies found that women move more rapidly through the taking-in phase (Ament, 1990; Wrasper, 1996). Evans, Dick, Shields, Shook, & Smith (1998), in a study of women giving birth vaginally, found that both taking-in and taking-hold were present on the evening of birth. For 24 hours after the birth, mature and apparently healthy women appear to suspend their involvement in everyday responsibilities and activities. They rely on others to satisfy their needs for comfort, rest, nourishment and closeness to their families and the newborn.

This dependent phase is a time of great excitement during which parents need to verbalize their experience of pregnancy and birth. Focusing on, analyzing, and accepting these experiences help the parents move on to the next phase. Some parents use staff members or other mothers as

TABLE 17-4

Phases of Maternal Postpartum Adjustment

PHASE	CHARACTERISTICS

Dependent: Taking-in	• First 24 hr (range, 1 to 2 days)
	• Focus: self and meeting of basic needs
	  • Reliance on others to meet needs for comfort, rest, closeness, and nourishment
	  • Excited and talkative
	  • Desire to review birth experience

Dependent-independent: Taking-hold	• Starts second or third day; lasts 10 days to several weeks
	• Focus: care of baby and competent mothering
	  • Desire to take charge
	  • Still has need for nurturing and acceptance by others
	  • Eagerness to learn and practice—optimal period for teaching by nurses
	  • Handling of physical discomforts and emotional changes
	  • Possible experience with "blues"

Interdependent: Letting go	• Focus: forward movement of family as unit with interacting members
	  • Reassertion of relationship with partner
	  • Resumption of sexual intimacy
	  • Resolution of individual roles

From Rubin, R. (1961). Basic maternal behavior. *Nursing Outlook, 9,* 683-686.

an audience, whereas others are more comfortable talking with family and friends about the pregnancy and birth experience.

Because anxiety and preoccupation with her new role often narrow a mother's perceptions, information may have to be repeated. The new mother may require reminders to rest or, conversely, to ambulate enough to promote recovery.

Physical discomfort can interfere with the mother's need for rest and relaxation. The selective use of comfort measures and medication depends on the nurse. Many women hesitate to ask for medication, believing that any pain they experience is normal and to be expected; breastfeeding mothers may fear the effects of medication on the infant.

Dependent-independent phase

If the mother has received adequate nurturing in the first few hours or days, by the second or third day, her desire for independent action reasserts itself. In the dependent-independent phase, the mother alternates between a need for extensive nurturing and acceptance by others and the desire to "take charge" once again. She responds enthusiastically to opportunities to learn and practice baby care or, if she is an accomplished mother, to carry out or direct this care. Rubin (1961) described this phase as the taking-hold phase, noting that it lasts approximately 10 days. Several studies (Evans et al., 1998; Martell, 1996; Wrasper, 1996) found that contemporary women exhibit taking-hold behaviors sooner than did the women in Rubin's study; however, the peak and duration of the taking-hold phase were not determined. Evans and associates (1998) found that taking-hold behaviors began increasing between the evening of birth and the first morning despite high levels of sleep disturbance. Childbirth preparation classes, early contact with the newborn, rooming-in, and early discharge are some of the current ob-

stetric practices that seem to enhance taking-hold behaviors (Martell; Wrasper).

Most mothers are discharged home during this dependent-independent phase. Once home, mothers must continue to cope with physical adaptations and psychologic adjustments. Most mothers identify fatigue as their major physical concern. This problem is acute during the early postpartum period and may persist as long as 19 months after birth (Troy, 2003). This fatigue affects various aspects of their lives such as their relationships with their partners and other family members and household responsibilities. Maternity nurses working in hospital postpartum units, birth centers, obstetric offices and home care, as well as pediatric nurses who come in contact with mothers during newborn well-baby checkups, are in excellent positions to screen new mothers for fatigue and to offer suggestions for coping with their feelings.

Other physical concerns of mothers are loss of weight or figure, pain from the episiotomy or cesarean incision, sexual relations, and hemorrhoids. Although many women express enjoyment during the early postpartum period, most describe the period as hectic and a time of great adjustment. Primiparas report feeling uncertain, trapped, and overwhelmed by fatigue and lack of experience in infant care. Although many multiparas describe their current experience as being better than that with previous births, primarily because of their comfort with caring for an infant, O'Reilly (2004) found that achieving a new balance was very important.

Prenatally and postnatally, nurses can discuss common postpartal concerns that mothers experience and provide anticipatory guidance on coping strategies, such as resting when the infant sleeps and planning with an extended family member or friend to do the housework for the first week or two after the baby is born. Once a mother is home, periodic phone calls from a nurse who cared for her in the birth setting can provide the mother with an opportunity to vent her concerns and get support and advice from "her" nurse. Nurses can set up Web pages on a hospital or clinic website to provide information for new mothers. These pages can include information about a variety of topics. This would enable nurses to cover a host of topics that might be of interest to parents the first postpartum year. Additionally, a link to other helpful sites might be provided (O'Reilly, 2004). First-time mothers inexperienced in child care, women whose careers had provided outside stimulation, women who lack friends or family members with whom to share delights and concerns, substance-abusing mothers, and adolescent mothers may need additional supportive counseling. When possible, postpartum home visits are included in the plan of care.

Becoming a mother. Mercer (2004) has suggested that the concept *maternal role attainment,* introduced by Rubin in 1961, be replaced with becoming a mother to signify the transformation and growth of the mother identity. Becoming a mother implies more than attaining a role. It includes learning new skills and increasing her confidence in herself as she meets new challenges in caring for her child(ren).

Postpartum "blues." The "pink" period surrounding the first day or two after birth, characterized by heightened joy and feelings of well-being, is often followed by a "blue" period. Approximately 50% to 80% of women experience postpartum blues or "baby blues" (Beeber, 2002), which occur in women of all ethnic and racial groups (Campbell, 1992). When they have the blues, women are emotionally labile, often crying easily and for no apparent reason. This lability seems to peak around the fifth day and subside by the tenth day. Other symptoms of postpartum blues include depression, a let-down feeling, restlessness, fatigue, insomnia, headache, anxiety, sadness, and anger. Biochemical, psychological, social, and cultural factors have been explored as possible causes of the postpartum depressive state; however, the etiology remains unknown. Whatever the cause, the early postpartum period appears to be one of emotional and physical vulnerability for new mothers, who may be psychologically overwhelmed by the reality of parental responsibilities. The mother may feel deprived of the supportive care she received from family members and friends during pregnancy. Some mothers regret the loss of the mother–unborn child relationship and mourn its passing. Still others experience a let-down feeling when labor and birth are complete. Fatigue after childbirth is compounded by the around-the-clock demands of the new baby and can accentuate the feelings of depression. Postpartum depressive symptoms can have a negative effect on maternal role attainment (Fowles, 1998). To help mothers cope with postpartum blues, nurses can suggest various strategies (Patient Instructions for Self-Care box).

"Am I Blue?" (Johnson & Johnson, 1996), a self-administered questionnaire, can help mothers to assess their

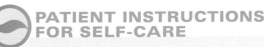

PATIENT INSTRUCTIONS FOR SELF-CARE

Coping with Postpartum Blues

- Remember that the "blues" are normal and that both the mother *and* father may experience them.
- Get plenty of rest; nap when the baby does if possible. Go to bed early, and let friends know when to visit and how they can help (remember, you are not "Supermom").
- Use relaxation techniques learned in childbirth classes (or ask the nurse to teach you and your partner some techniques).
- Do something for yourself. Take advantage of the time your partner or family members care for the baby— soak in the tub (a 20-minute soak can be the equivalent of a 2-hour nap) or go for a walk.
- Plan a day out of the house—go to the mall with the baby, being sure to take a stroller or carriage, or go out to eat with friends without the baby. Many communities have churches or other agencies that provide child care programs such as Mothers' Morning Out.
- Talk to your partner about the way you feel—for example, about feeling tied down, how the birth met your expectations, and things that will help you (don't be afraid to ask for specifics).
- If you are breastfeeding, give yourself and your baby time to learn.
- Seek out and use community resources such as La Leche League or community mental health centers.

level of "blues" and to decide when to seek advice from their nurse, nurse-midwife, or physician (Fig. 17-8). Home visits and telephone follow-up calls by the nurse are important to assess the mother's pattern of "blue" feelings and behavior over time.

Although the postpartum blues are usually mild and short lived, approximately half a million mothers in the United States each year experience a more severe syndrome termed *postpartum depression* (PPD) (Wisner, Parry, & Piontek, 2002). PPD symptoms can range from mild to severe, with women having "good days" and "bad days." Goodman (2004) noted that there is a high incidence of PPD in fathers (1% to 26%). Screening should be done in both the mother and father for PPD. PPD can go undetected because new parents generally do not voluntarily admit to this kind of emotional distress out of embarrassment, guilt, or fear. Nurses need to include teaching about how to differentiate symptoms of the "blues" and PPD and urge parents to report depressive symptoms promptly if they occur (see Chapter 25).

Interdependent phase

In this phase, interdependent behavior reasserts itself, and the mother and her family move forward as a unit with interacting members. The relationship of the partners, although altered by the introduction of a baby, resumes many of its former characteristics. A primary need is to establish a lifestyle that includes but in some respects also excludes

Am I Blue?

Many new mothers feel anxious, sad, or angry about the changes in their lives after the birth of their new baby. It is perfectly normal to feel this way, but sometimes the feelings grow so strong that they make life difficult. This quiz lists many feelings and experiences of "blue" or depressed mothers. Mark how strong each of these feelings or experiences is for you, compared with what is normal for you. For example: Do you feel no anger [0]; mild (very little) anger [1]; moderate (some) anger [2]; or severe (very strong) anger [3] compared with the way you usually feel? Add up your total score when you are finished, and discuss the results with your health care provider.

SCORE:

0 – 31 = MILD BLUES

This will probably pass, but pay attention to your feelings and needs.

32 – 64 = MODERATE BLUES

You may want to ask for help from a close friend or family member, or ask the advice of your health care provider.

65 – 98 = SEVERE BLUES

You could be depressed; see your health care provider for a check-up and advice as soon as possible.

If you are afraid you might harm yourself or your baby—ask a health care provider you trust for help— you don't have to be alone!

0 = Not there at all 1 = Mild 2 = Moderate 3 = Severe	0	1	2	3
Anger				
Anxiety attacks: periods of very strong fear, shortness of breath, rapid heartbeat				
Increased or decreased appetite and/or weight gain or loss that doesn't seem normal				
Strong feeling that you need to get away, need more time for your own interests				
Problems in a relationship with a family member, lover, close friend, etc.				
Crying spells				
Less interest in your personal appearance				
Less motivation—less energy or interest in accomplishing goals				
Depression				
Fatigue—feeling tired or exhausted				
Fear of harming yourself or your baby				
Loss of your sense of humor				
Nervousness, feeling tense or edgy				
Feelings of guilt				
Feelings of panic				
Feeling alone or lonely; without the support of others				
Feeling no love, or not enough love, for your baby				
Feeling forgetful, distracted, absent-minded—having trouble concentrating				
Frustration				
Hopelessness				
Insomnia				
Feeling irritable, bad-tempered				
Loss of sexual desire and/or pleasure in sex				
Loss of self-respect or confidence—feeling like you don't count or can't do anything right				
Feeling confused, uncertain				
Mood swings—your moods and emotions change all the time				
Obsessive thoughts—ideas or feelings you can't stop from repeating in your mind				
Odd or frightening thoughts—thoughts or images that scare you or that you can't control				
Thoughts of suicide, feeling like you want to die				
Feeling sad, unhappy				
TOTAL				

Fig. 17-8 "Am I Blue?" (Courtesy Johnson & Johnson Consumer Products, Skillman, NJ.)

the baby. The couple needs to share interests and activities that are adult in scope.

The couple may begin to engage in sexual intercourse during the second to fourth week after the baby is born. Some couples begin earlier, as soon as it can be accomplished without discomfort, depending on factors such as timing, amount of vaginal dryness, and breastfeeding status. Sexual intimacy enhances the adult aspect of the family, and the adult pair shares a closeness denied to other family members (see also Chapter 16). Changes in a woman's sexuality after childbirth are related to hormonal shifts, increased breast size, uneasiness with a body that has yet to return to a prepregnant size, chronic fatigue related to sleep deprivation, and physical exhaustion (Bitzer & Adler, 2000). Many new fathers speak of the alienation experienced when they observe the intimate mother-infant relationship, and some are frank in expressing feelings of jealousy toward the infant. The resumption of sexual intimacy seems to bring the parents' relationship back into focus. Before and after birth, nurses should review with new parents their plans for other pregnancies and their preferences for contraception.

The interdependent phase, termed the letting-go phase, is often stressful for the parental pair. Interests and needs often diverge during this time. Women and their partners must resolve the effects on their relationship of their individual roles related to childrearing, homemaking, and careers. Mothers (and partners) may take a more traditional role in an effort to adapt to parenthood; however, traditional women have reported more family disorganization months into parenthood. A special continuing effort has to be undertaken to strengthen the adult-adult relationship as a basis for the family unit.

Little is known about postpartum maternal adjustment in the lesbian couple. Relationship satisfaction in first-time lesbian parent couples appears related to egalitarianism, commitment, sexual compatibility, and communication skills, as well as the birth mother's decision for insemination by an anonymous sperm donor (Osterwell, 1991; Reimann, 1999). Similar to heterosexual parent couples, most lesbian parent couples voice concern about having less time and energy for their relationship after the arrival of the baby (Gartrell et al., 1996). Both partners consider themselves to be equal parents of the baby who share actively in child rearing (Brewaeys, Devroey, Helmerhorst, Van Hall, & Ponjaert, 1995). A primary concern of co-mothers is the legal vulnerability of lesbian families confounded by their social invisibility (Reimann).

Paternal Adjustment

Research on paternal adjustment to parenthood indicates that fathers go through predictable phases during their transition to parenthood (Henderson & Brouse, 1991; St. John, Cameron, & McVeigh, 2005) (Table 17-5). During this period, fathers experience intense emotions. Many fathers acknowledge that their expectations were of limited value once they were immersed in the reality of parenthood. Feelings that often accompany this reality are sadness, ambivalence, jealousy, frustration at not being able to participate in breastfeeding, and an overwhelming desire to be more involved, most of which are different from the feelings mothers report. On the other hand, some fathers are pleasantly surprised at the ease and fun of parenting. In their transition to mastery, fathers take control and become more actively involved in the infant's life.

First-time fathers perceive the first 4 to 10 weeks of parenthood in much the same way as mothers do, that is, as a period characterized by uncertainty, increased responsibility, disruption of sleep, and inability to control time needed to care for the infant and reestablish the marital dyad. Fathers express concern about decreased attention from their partners relative to their personal relationship, the mother's lack of recognition of the father's desire to participate in decision making for the infant, and limited time available to establish a relationship with their infants (Steinberg, Kruckman, & Steinberg, 2000). These concerns can precipitate feelings of jealousy of the infant. The father should discuss his individual concerns/needs with the mother/partner and become more involved with the infant. This can help alleviate feelings of jealousy in the father.

TABLE 17-5

Transition to Fatherhood: A Three-Stage Process

STAGES	CHARACTERISTICS
Stage 1: Expectations	Father has preconceptions about what life will be like after baby comes home
Stage 2: Reality	Father realizes that expectations are not always based on fact
	Common feelings experienced are as follows:
	Sadness
	Ambivalence
	Jealousy
	Frustration
	Overwhelming desire to be more involved
	Some fathers are pleasantly surprised at ease and fun of parenting
Stage 3: Transition to mastery	Father makes conscious decision to take control and become more actively involved with infant

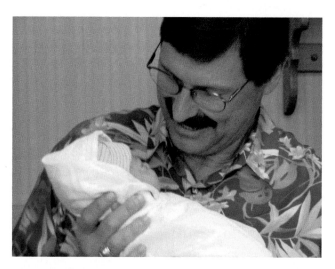

Fig. 17-9 Engrossment. Father is absorbed in looking at his newborn. (Courtesy Tricia Olson, North Ogden, UT.)

Father-infant relationship

In U.S. culture, neonates have a powerful impact on their fathers, who become intensely involved with their babies (Fig. 17-9). The term used for the father's absorption, preoccupation, and interest in the infant is engrossment. Characteristics of engrossment include some of the sensual responses relating to touch and eye contact that were discussed earlier and also the father's keen awareness of features that he and the baby share that validate his claim to the infant. An outstanding response is one of strong attraction to the newborn. Fathers spend considerable time "communicating" with the infant and taking delight in the infant's response to them. A sense of increased self-esteem and a sense of being proud, bigger, more mature, and older are all experienced by fathers after seeing their babies for the first time.

Fathers spend less time than mothers with infants, and fathers' interactions with infants tend to be characterized by stimulating social play rather than caretaking. The subtle and more open differences in stimulation from two sources, mother and father, provide a wider social experience for the infant.

Fathers can benefit from nursing interventions during the postpartum period just as mothers can. Nurses can arrange to teach infant care when the father is present and provide anticipatory guidance for fathers about the transition to parenthood. Separate prenatal and parenting classes and parenting support groups for fathers can provide them with an opportunity to discuss their concerns and have some of their needs met. Postpartum phone calls and home visits by the nurse should include time for assessment of the father's adjustment and needs.

FACTORS INFLUENCING PARENTAL RESPONSES ◼

How parents respond to the birth of a child is influenced by various factors, including age, social networks, socioeconomic conditions, and personal aspirations for the future.

Age

Maternal age has a definite effect on the outcome of pregnancy. The mother, fetus, and newborn are at highest risk when the mother is an adolescent or is more than 35 years old.

Adolescent mother

Although it is biologically possible for the adolescent female to become a parent, her egocentricity and concrete thinking interfere with her ability to parent effectively. The very young adolescent mother is inexperienced and unprepared to recognize the early signs of illness, potential danger, or household hazards. She may inadvertently neglect her child. The higher mortality rates among the infants of adolescent mothers are attributed to the inexperience, lack of knowledge, and immaturity of the mothers, causing them to be unable to recognize a problem and obtain the necessary resources to rectify the situation. Nevertheless, in most instances, with adequate support and developmentally appropriate teaching, adolescents can learn effective parenting skills.

The transition to parenthood may be difficult for adolescent parents. Coping with the developmental tasks of parenthood is often complicated by the unmet developmental needs and tasks of adolescence. Some young parents may experience difficulty accepting a changing self-image and adjusting to new roles related to the responsibilities of infant care. Other adolescent parents, however, may have higher self-concepts than their nonparenting peers (Alpers, 1998; Dalla & Gamble, 2000).

As adolescent parents move through the transition to parenthood, they may feel "different" from their peers, excluded from "fun" activities, and prematurely forced to enter an adult social role. The conflict between their own desires and the infant's demands, in addition to the low tolerance for frustration that is typical of adolescence, further contributes to the normal psychosocial stress of childbirth. Lower maternal education is associated with less favorable maternal responses to distress and infant behavior (Dalla & Gamble, 2000; Diehl, 1997).

Maintaining a relationship with the baby's father is beneficial for the teen mother and her infant. A close and satisfying relationship is positively correlated with maternal-fetal and maternal-infant attachment (Bloom, 1998). The involvement of the baby's father is related to appropriate maternal behaviors and positive mother-infant relationship (Diehl, 1997).

Adolescent mothers provide warm and attentive physical care; however, they use less verbal interaction than do older parents, and adolescents tend to be less responsive and to interact less positively with their infants than older mothers. Interventions emphasizing verbal and nonverbal communication skills between mother and infant are important. Such intervention strategies must be concrete and specific because of the cognitive level of adolescents. Although some observers suggest that some adolescents may use more aggressive behaviors, a higher incidence of child abuse has not been documented. In comparison with adult mothers, teenage mothers have a limited knowledge of child development. They tend to expect too much of their children too soon and often characterize their infants as being fussy. This limited knowledge may cause teenagers to respond to their infants inappropriately.

Many young mothers pattern their maternal role on what they themselves experienced. Therefore, nurses need to determine the type of support that people close to the young mother are able and prepared to give, as well as the kinds of community aid available to supplement this support. Many teen mothers can identify a source of social support, with the predominant source being their own mothers. Navajo adolescent mothers who had social support (emotional and instrumental) from their own mothers felt able to focus on both the adolescent and maternal roles without neglecting either role (Dalla & Gamble, 2000). Rural adolescent mothers who reported firm encouragement and resources to pursue their life aspirations had more resilient adjustments to parenthood than did adolescent mothers who did not have this type of support (Camarena et al., 1998).

The need for continued assessment of the new mother's parenting abilities during this postbirth period is essential.

Critical Thinking Exercise

Special Needs of Adolescent and Older First-Time Mothers

Emily is 42 years old, an ICU nurse, and the mother of a 1-week-old daughter, who was born by cesarean birth. Emily is breastfeeding. When the nurse calls to check on the new family, Emily says, "I can't seem to do anything right! I hurt, and I'm not getting any sleep. All the baby wants to do is cry, and so do I!"

Mia, age 16, lives at home with her mother and four siblings. She is bottle-feeding her new baby girl. Although the baby's father says that he wants to be involved, he has only seen the baby once since she was born. During a routine phone call 72 hours after discharge, Mia tells the nurse that the baby is "waking up all the time and eating a whole bottle every 2 or 3 hours. She looks just like her father and acts like him, too!" Mia's mother is helping her care for the baby but seems to want to take over and "do things her way."

1 Evidence—Is there sufficient evidence to draw conclusions about the teaching and care needed by these new parents?
2 Assumptions—What assumptions can be made about the following issues:
   a. Relationship between maternal age and postpartum adjustment
   b. Need for support during the postnatal period
   c. Need for perinatal education
   d. Long-term prognosis for positive outcomes for both mothers
3 What implications and priorities for nursing care can be drawn at this time?
4 Does the evidence objectively support your conclusion?
5 Are there alternative perspectives to your conclusion?

In addition, continued support should also be provided by involving the grandparents and other family members, as well as through home visits and group sessions for discussion of infant care and parenting problems. Outreach programs concerned with self-care, parent-child interactions, child injuries, and failure to thrive, in addition to programs that provide prompt and effective community intervention, prevent more serious problems from occurring. As the adolescent performs her mothering role within the framework of her family, she may need to address dependency versus independency issues. The adolescent's family members may also need help adapting to their new roles.

Adolescent father

The adolescent father and mother face immediate developmental crises, which include completing the developmental tasks of adolescence, making a transition to parenthood, and sometimes adapting to marriage. These transitions can be stressful. The nurse may initiate interaction with the adolescent father by asking him to be present when postpartum home visits are made and to accompany the mother and the baby to well-baby checkups at the clinic or pediatrician's office. With the adolescent mother's agreement the nurse may contact the father directly. Adolescent fathers need support to discuss their emotional responses to the pregnancy. The father's feelings of guilt, powerlessness, or bravado should be recognized because of their negative consequences for both the parents and the child. Counseling of adolescent fathers must be reality oriented. Topics such as finances, child care, parenting skills, and the father's role in the birth experience must be discussed. Teenage fathers also need to know about reproductive physiology and birth control options, as well as safer sex practices.

The adolescent father may continue to be involved in an ongoing relationship with the young mother and his baby. In many instances he also plays an important role in the decisions about child care and raising the child. He may need help to develop realistic perceptions of his role as "father to a child." He is encouraged to use coping mechanisms that are not detrimental to his own, his partner's, or his child's well-being. The nurse enlists support systems, parents, and professional agencies on his behalf.

Maternal age greater than 35 years

Adjustment of older mothers to changes involved in becoming a parent and seeing themselves as competent is aided by support from their partners. Support from other family members and friends is also important for positive self-evaluation of parenting, a sense of well-being and satisfaction, and help in dealing with stress.

Changes in the sexual aspect of a relationship can be a stressor for new midlife parents. Mothers report that finding time and energy for a romantic rendezvous is more difficult. They attribute much of this to the reality of caring for an infant, but the decreasing libido that normally accompanies getting older also contributes.

Work and career issues are sources of conflict for older mothers (Reese & Harkless, 1996). Conflicts emerge over being disinterested, worrying about giving enough attention to work with the distractions of a new baby, and anticipating what it will be like to return to work. Child care is a major factor causing stress about work.

Another major issue for older mothers with careers is the perception of loss of control (Reese & Harkless, 1996). Mothers older than 35, when compared with younger mothers, are at a different stage in their careers, having attained high levels of education, career, and income. The loss of control experienced when going from the consistency of a work role to the inconsistency of the parent role comes as a surprise to many. Helping the older mother have realistic expectations of herself and of parenthood is essential.

New mothers who are also perimenopausal may find it hard to distinguish fatigue, loss of sleep, decreased libido, or other physiologic symptoms as the cause of the changes in their lives. Although many women view menopause as a natural stage of life, for midlife mothers this cessation of menstruation coincides with the state of parenthood. The changes of midlife and menopause can add more emotional and physical stress to older mothers' lives because of the time- and energy-consuming aspects of raising a young child. Resources that older parents may find helpful are listed under Resources at the end of this chapter.

Paternal age older than 35 years

Older fathers describe their experience of midlife parenting as wonderful but not without drawbacks. What they see as positive aspects of parenthood in older years include increased love and commitment between the spouses, a reinforcement of why one married in the first place, a feeling of being complete, experiencing of "the child" again in oneself, more financial stability than in younger years, and more freedom to focus on parenting rather than on career. A common theme expressed is *sharing:* sharing joy, sharing in raising the child, sharing as a family. The main drawback of midlife parenting is the change that it makes in the relationships with their partners.

Culture

Cultural beliefs and practices are important determinants of parenting behaviors. Culture defines what is socially acceptable in terms of eye contact, touch, and space (Lipson, Dibble, & Minarik, 1996). Culture influences the interactions with the baby, as well as the parents' or family's caregiving style. For example, the provision for a period of rest and recuperation for the mother after birth is prominent in several cultures. Asian mothers must remain at home with the baby at least 30 days after birth and are not supposed to engage in household chores, including care of the baby. Many times the grandmother takes over the baby's care immediately, even before discharge from the hospital (D'Avanzo & Geissler, 2003; Kim-Godwin, 2003). Likewise, Jordanian mothers have a 40-day lying-in after birth during

which their mothers or sisters care for the baby (D'Avanzo & Geissler). Hispanics practice an intergenerational family ritual, *la cuarentena.* For 40 days after birth the mother is expected to recuperate and get acquainted with her infant. Traditionally, this involves many restrictions concerning food (e.g., spicy or cold foods, fish, pork, and citrus are avoided; tortillas and chicken soup are encouraged); exercise; and activities, including sexual intercourse. Abdominal binding is a traditional practice, and many women avoid tub bathing and washing their hair. Traditional Hispanic husbands do not expect to see their wives or infants until both have been cleaned and dressed after birth. *La cuarentena* incorporates individuals into the family, instills parental responsibility, and integrates the family during a critical life event (D'Avanzo & Geissler, Niska, Snyder, & Lia-Hoagberg, 1998).

Desire for and valuing of children is salient in all cultures. In Asian families, children are valued as a source of family strength and stability, are perceived as wealth, and are objects of parental love and affection. Infants almost always are given an affectionate "cradle" name that is used during the first years of life; for example, a Filipino girl might be called "Ling-Ling" and a boy "Bong-Bong." See Table 2-2 for examples of some traditional cultural beliefs that may be important to parents from African-American, Asian, and Hispanic cultures.

Knowledge of cultural beliefs can help the nurse make more accurate assessments and diagnoses of observed parenting behaviors. For example, nurses may become concerned when they observe cultural practices that appear to reflect poor maternal-infant bonding. Algerian mothers may not unwrap and explore their infants as part of the acquaintance process because in Algeria, babies are wrapped tightly in swaddling clothes to protect them physically and psychologically (D'Avanzo & Geissler, 2003). The nurse may observe a Vietnamese woman who gives minimal care to her infant but refuses to cuddle or further interact with her baby. This apparent lack of interest in the newborn is this cultural group's attempt to ward off "evil spirits" and actually reflects an intense love and concern for the infant (Galanti, 2003). An Asian mother might be criticized for almost immediately relinquishing the care of the infant to the grandmother and not even attempting to hold her baby when the infant is brought to her room. However, in Asian extended families, members show their support for a new mother's rest and recuperation by assisting with the care of the baby. Contrary to the guidance given to mothers in the United States about "nipple confusion," a mix of breastfeeding and bottle-feeding is standard practice for Japanese mothers. This is out of concern for the mother's rest during the first 2 to 3 months and does not lead to any problems with lactation; breastfeeding is widespread and successful among Japanese women (Sharts-Hopko, 1995).

Cultural beliefs and values give perspective to the meaning of childbirth and parenting for a new mother. Nurses can provide an opportunity for a new mother to talk about her perception of the meaning of childbearing. In helping new families adjust to parenthood, nurses must provide culturally sensitive care by following principles that enhance nursing practice within transcultural situations.

Socioeconomic Conditions

Socioeconomic conditions often determine access to available resources. Parents whose economic condition is made worse with the birth of each child and who are unable to use an effective method of fertility management may find childbirth complicated by concern for their own health and a sense of helplessness. Mothers who are single, separated, or divorced from their husbands or without a partner, family, and friends for whatever reason may view the birth of a child with dread. Serious financial problems may override any desire to mother the infant.

Personal Aspirations

For some women, parenthood interferes with or blocks their plans for personal freedom or advancement in their careers. Resentment concerning this loss may not have been resolved during the prenatal period, and if it remains unresolved, it will spill over into caregiving activities. This may result in indifference and neglect of the infant or in excessive concerns; the mother may set impossibly high standards for her own behavior or the child's performance.

Nursing interventions include providing opportunities for mothers to express their feelings freely to an objective listener, to discuss measures to permit personal growth, and to learn about the care of their infant. Referring the woman to a support group of other mothers "in the same situation" may also be helpful.

Nurses also can be proactive in influencing changes in work policies related to maternity and paternity leaves, varying models of work sharing and "family friendly" work environments. Some corporations already structure their work sites to support new mothers (e.g., by providing on-site day care facilities and breastfeeding rooms).

PARENTAL SENSORY IMPAIRMENT

In the early dialogue between the parent and child, all senses—sight, hearing, touch, taste, and smell—are used by each to initiate and sustain the attachment process. A parent who has an impairment of one of the senses needs to maximize use of the remaining senses.

Visually Impaired Parent

Visual impairment alone does not seem to have a negative effect on mothers' early parenting experiences. These mothers, just as sighted mothers, express the wonders of parenthood and encourage other visually impaired persons to become parents (Conley-Jung & Olkin, 2001). Mothers with disabilities tend to value the importance of performing parenting tasks in the perceived culturally usual way. Their maternal engagement also is facilitated by self-acceptance of

their own unique differences in performing parenting tasks (Farber, 2000).

Although visually impaired mothers initially feel a pressure to conform to traditional, sighted ways of parenting, they soon adapt these ways and develop methods better suited to themselves (Conley-Jung & Olkin, 2001). Examples of activities that visually impaired mothers do differently include preparation of the infant's nursery, clothes, and supplies. Mothers may put an entire clothing outfit together and hang it in the closet rather than keeping items separate in drawers. They might develop a labeling system for the infant's clothing and put diapering, bathing, and other care supplies where they will be easy to locate with minimal searching (Conley-Jung & Olkin). A strength that visually impaired parents have is a heightened sensitivity to other sensory outputs. A visually impaired mother can tell when her infant is facing her because she notices the baby's breath on her face.

One of the major difficulties that visually impaired parents experience is the skepticism, open or hidden, of health care professionals. Visually impaired people sense reluctance on the part of others to acknowledge that they have a right to be parents. All too often, nurses and doctors lack the experience to deal with the childbearing and childrearing needs of visually impaired mothers, as well as mothers with other disabilities (such as the hearing impaired, physically impaired, and mentally challenged). The best approach by the nurse is to assess the mother's capabilities. From that basis, the nurse can make plans to assist the woman, often in much the same way as for a mother without impairments. Visually impaired mothers have made suggestions for providing care for women such as themselves during childbearing (Box 17-2). Such approaches by the nurse can help avoid a sense of increased vulnerability on the mother's part.

Eye contact is considered important in U.S. culture. With a parent who is visually impaired, this critical factor in the parent-child attachment process is obviously missing. However, the blind parent, who may never have experienced this method of strengthening relationships, does not miss it. The infant will need other sensory input from that parent. An infant looking into the eyes of a mother who is blind may not be aware that the eyes are unseeing. Other people in the newborn's environment can also participate in active eye-to-eye contact to supply this need. A problem may arise, however, if the visually impaired parent has an impassive facial expression. Her infant, after making repeated unsuccessful attempts to engage in face play with the mother, will abandon the behavior with her and intensify it with the father or other people in the household. Nurses can provide anticipatory guidance regarding this situation and help the mother learn to nod and smile while talking and cooing to the infant.

Hearing-Impaired Parent

The parent who has a hearing impairment faces another set of problems, particularly if the deafness dates from birth or early childhood. The mother and her partner are likely to

BOX 17-2

Nursing Approaches for Working with Visually Impaired Parents

1 Parents who are blind need oral teaching by health care providers because maternity information is not accessible to blind people.
2 A visually impaired parent needs an orientation to the hospital room that allows the parent to move about the room independently. For example, "Go to the left of the bed and trail the wall until you feel the first door. That is the bathroom."
3 Parents who are blind need explanations of routines.
4 Parents who are blind need to feel devices (e.g., monitors, pelvic models) and to hear descriptions of the devices.
5 Visually impaired parents need "a chance to ask questions."
6 Visually impaired parents need the opportunity to hold and touch the baby after birth.
7 Nurses need to demonstrate baby care by touch and to follow with, "Now show me how you would do it."
8 Nurses need to give instructions such as, "I'm going to give you the baby. The head is to your left side."

have established an independent household. A number of devices that transform sound into light flashes are now marketed and can be fitted into the infant's room to permit immediate detection of crying. Even if the parent is not speech trained, vocalizing can serve as both a stimulus and a response to the infant's early vocalizing. Deaf parents can provide additional vocal training by use of recordings and television so that from birth the child is aware of the full range of the human voice. Sign language is acquired readily by young children, and the first sign used is as varied as the first word.

Section 504 of the Rehabilitation Act of 1973 requires that hospitals and other institutions receiving funds from the U.S. Department of Health and Human Services use various communication techniques and resources with the deaf, including having staff members or certified interpreters who are proficient in sign language. For example, provision of written materials with demonstrations and having nurses stand where the parent can read their lips (if the parent practices lip reading) are two techniques that can be used. A creative approach is for the nursing unit to develop videotapes in which information on postpartum care, infant care, and parenting issues is signed by an interpreter and spoken by a nurse. A videotape in which a nurse signs while speaking would be ideal. With the advent of the Internet, many resources are available to the deaf parent (see Resources at the end of the chapter).

SIBLING ADAPTATION

Because the family is an interactive, open unit, the addition of a new family member affects everyone in the family. Siblings have to assume new positions within the family hier-

archy. The older child's goal is to maintain the lead position. Parents are faced with the task of caring for a new child while not neglecting the others. Parents need to distribute their attention in an equitable manner.

Reactions of siblings may result from temporary separation from the mother, changes in the mother's or father's behavior, or the siblings' response to the infant's coming home. Positive behavioral changes of siblings include interest in and concern for the baby and increased independence. Regression in toileting and sleep habits, aggression toward the baby, and increased seeking of attention and whining are examples of negative behaviors.

The parents' attitudes toward the arrival of the baby can set the stage for the other children's reactions (Fig. 17-10). Because the baby absorbs the time and attention of the important people in the other children's lives, jealousy **(sibling rivalry)** is to be expected once the initial excitement of having a new baby in the home is over. However, sibling rivalry, or negative behaviors in siblings, may have been overemphasized in the past and exists for a comparatively short time. Developmentally appropriate behaviors in siblings are similar before and after the baby arrives. Firstborn children seem to continue their usual routines and are more pleased with newborns and more understanding of the baby's need for care than the parents predict.

Parents, especially mothers, spend much time and energy promoting sibling acceptance of a new baby. Participating in sibling preparation classes makes a difference in the ability of mothers to cope with sibling behavior. Older children are actively involved in preparing for the infant, and this involvement intensifies after the birth of the child. Parents have to manage the feeling of guilt that the older children are being deprived of parental time and attention. Parents have to monitor the behavior of older children toward the

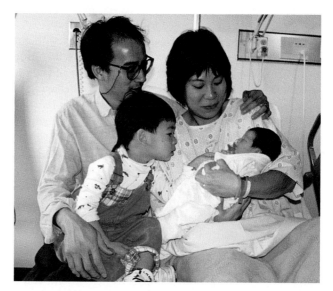

Fig. 17-10 Parents introducing "big" brother to infant daughter. (Courtesy Kim Molloy, Knoxville, IA.)

Strategies for Facilitating Sibling Acceptance of a New Baby

1 Take your firstborn child on a tour of your hospital room and point out similarities between this birth and his or her birth. "This is like the room I was in with you, and the baby is in the same kind of bassinet that you were in."

2 Have a small gift from the baby to give to your older child each day.

3 Give the older child a T-shirt that says "I'm a big brother" (or "sister").

4 Arrange for your children to be in the first group (grandparents, sister) to see the newborn. Let them hold the baby in the hospital. One mother and father arranged for their firstborn son to be present at the births of his three brothers and to be the first one to hold them.

5 Plan time for both children. "When I get home, I'll arrange my day so that I can have the baby's care done in the morning while Sam (first child) is at school. Maybe the baby will sleep part of the afternoon and I can spend some time with Sam."

6 Fathers can spend time with the older sibling while mothers are taking care of the baby and vice versa. Siblings like to have time and attention from both parents.

7 Give preschool and early school-age siblings a newborn doll as "their baby" to care for. Give sibling a photograph of the new baby to take to school to show off "his" or "her" baby. Older siblings may enjoy the responsibility of helping care for the newborn, such as learning how to give the baby a bottle or change a diaper. Remember to supervise interactions between the siblings and new baby.

more vulnerable infant and divert aggressive behavior. Strategies that parents have used to facilitate acceptance of a new baby by siblings are presented in Box 17-3.

Siblings demonstrate acquaintance behaviors with the newborn. The acquaintance process depends on the information given to the child before the baby is born and on the child's cognitive development level. The initial behaviors of siblings with the newborn include looking at the infant and touching the head (Fig. 17-11). The initial adjustment of older children to a newborn takes time, and children should be allowed to interact at their own pace rather than being forced to do so. To expect a young child to accept and love a rival for the parents' affection assumes an unrealistic level of maturity. Sibling love grows as does other love—that is, by being with another person and sharing experiences (Fig. 17-12). The relationship that develops between siblings has been conceptualized as sibling attachment. This bond between siblings involves a secure base in which one child provides support for the other, is missed when absent, and is looked to for comfort and security.

GRANDPARENT ADAPTATION

Grandparents experience a transition to grandparenthood. Intergenerational relationships shift, and grandparents must deal with changes in practices and attitudes toward childbirth, childrearing, and men's and women's roles at home and in the workplace. The degree to which grandparents understand and accept current practices can influence how supportive they are perceived to be by their adult children.

At the same time that they are adjusting to grandparenthood, the majority of grandparents are experiencing normative middle- and old-age life transition issues, such as retirement and a move to smaller housing, and need support from their adult children. Some may feel regret about their limited involvement because of poor health or geographic distance. Maternal grandmothers, more so than the other three grandparents, may have high expectations of themselves that cause them to be very self-critical.

The extent of grandparent involvement in the care of the newborn depends on many factors, for example, the willingness of the grandparents to become involved, the proximity of the grandparents, and ethnic and cultural expectations of the grandparents' role. If the new parents live in the United States, Asian grandparents typically are asked to come to the United States to care for the baby and the mother after birth and to care for the children once the parents return to work. In the United States, paternal grandparents, in contrast to those in other cultures, frequently consider themselves secondary to the maternal grandparents. Less seems expected of them and they are initially less involved. Nevertheless, these grandparents are eager to help and express great pleasure in their son's fatherhood and his involvement with the baby (Fig. 17-13).

For first-time parents, pregnancy and parenthood can reawaken old issues related to dependence versus independence. Couples often do not plan on their parents' help immediately after the baby arrives. They want time "to be a family," implying a couple-baby unit, not the intergenerational family network. Contrary to their expectations, however, new parents do call on their parents for help, especially the maternal grandmother (Steinberg, Kruckman, & Steinberg, 2000). Many grandparents are aware of their adult children's wishes for autonomy, respect these wishes, and remain available to help when asked.

A simple technique to help people span the generation gap is through a printed "letter to new parents" (written from the grandparents' perspective), which can be included in prenatal kits distributed in childbirth preparation classes and made available to all family members in the postpartum unit. Grandparents' classes can be used to bridge the generation gap and help the grandparents understand their adult children's parenting concepts. The classes include information on up-to-date childbearing practices, family-centered care, infant care, feeding, and safety (car seats), as

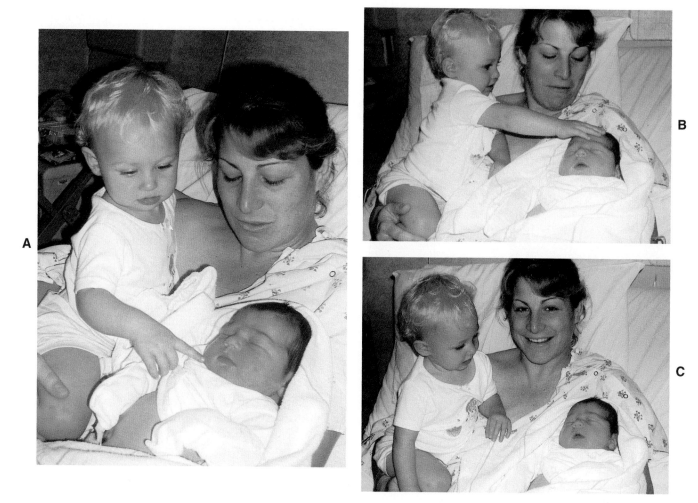

Fig. 17-11 First meeting. **A,** Sister touching new sibling with fingertip. **B,** Touching with whole hand. **C,** Smiles indicate acceptance. (Courtesy Sara Kossuth, Los Angeles, CA.)

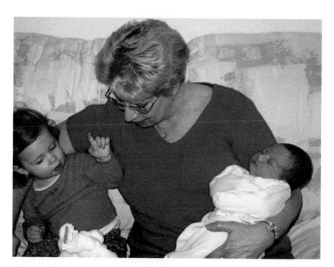

Fig. 17-12 Grandmother with newborn and older sibling. Family contacts are important for newborn and siblings. (Courtesy Susan McGuire, Lexington, IL.)

well as exploration of roles that grandparents play in the family unit.

The 2000 Census reported that 2.4 million grandparents had primary responsibility for grandchildren who lived with them. Of this number, 39% had cared for their grandchildren more than 5 years (Simmons & Dye, 2003). Increasing numbers of grandparents are providing permanent care to their grandchildren as a result of divorce, substance abuse, child abuse and/or neglect, abandonment, teenage pregnancy, death, human immunodeficiency virus (HIV) and acquired immunodeficiency syndrome (AIDS), unemployment, incarceration, and/or mental health problems (Pebley & Rudkin, 1999). This emerging trend requires the nurse to evaluate the role of the grandparent in parenting the infant. Educational and financial considerations must be addressed and available support systems identified for these families (see Resources at the end of the chapter).

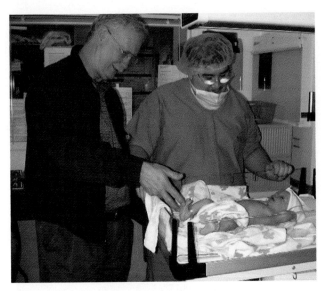

Fig. 17-13 Father, grandfather, and new grandson get acquainted. Note fingertip touch by grandfather. (Courtesy Sharon Johnson, Petaluma, CA.)

CD: Critical Thinking Exercise—Postpartum Home Care

CARE MANAGEMENT— PRACTICAL SUGGESTIONS FOR THE FIRST WEEKS AT HOME

Numerous changes occur during the first weeks of parenthood. Care management should be directed toward helping parents cope with infant care, role changes, altered lifestyle, and change in family structure resulting from the addition of a new baby. Parents may have inadequate or incorrect understanding of what to expect in the early postpartum weeks. Developing skill and confidence in caring for an infant can be especially anxiety provoking.

Nurses, especially those making postpartum visits to parents' homes, are in a prime position to help new families. The nurse's role becomes primarily one of teacher-supporter, focusing on enabling new parents to become capable of self-care and infant care and of meeting the needs of the family unit.

Assessment and Nursing Diagnoses

Assessment should include a psychosocial assessment focusing on parent-infant attachment, adjustment to the parental role, sibling adjustment, social support, and education needs, as well as mother's and baby's physical adaptation. Early home visits are an excellent opportunity for the nurse to assess beginnings of successful or harmful parenting behaviors and provide positive reinforcement for loving and nurturing behaviors with the infant. Parents who interact in inappropriate or abusive ways with the infant should be followed more closely, and an appropriate mental health practitioner or professional social worker should be notified.

Nursing diagnoses pertinent to transition to parenthood include the following:

- *Readiness for enhanced family coping related to*
  —positive attitude and realistic expectations for newborn and adapting to parenthood
  —nurturing behaviors with newborn
  —verbalizing positive factors in lifestyle change
- *Risk for impaired parenting related to*
  —lack of knowledge of infant care
  —feelings of incompetence or lack of confidence
  —unrealistic expectations of newborn or infant
  —fatigue from interrupted sleep
- *Parental role conflict related to*
  —role transition and role attainment
  —unwanted pregnancy
  —lack of resources to support parenting (e.g., no paid leave)
- *Risk for impaired parent-infant attachment related to*
  —difficult labor and birth
  —postpartum complications
  —neonatal complications or anomalies

Expected Outcomes of Care

A plan of care is formulated in collaboration with the family, incorporating their priorities and preferences, to meet their specific needs. Expected outcomes for effective transition to parenthood include that the parents will do the following:

- Demonstrate behaviors that reflect appreciation of sensory and behavioral capacities of the infant
- Verbalize increasing confidence and competence in feeding, diapering, dressing, and sensory stimulation of the infant
- Identify deviations from normal in the infant that should be brought to the immediate attention of the primary health care provider
- Relate effectively to the newborn's siblings and grandparents

Plan of Care and Interventions
Instructions for the first days at home

Parents, especially first-time parents, must be helped to anticipate what the transition from hospital to home will be like. Anticipatory guidance can help prevent a shock of reality that might negate the parents' joy or cause them undue stress. Even the simplest strategies can provide enormous support. Written information reinforcing education topics is helpful to provide to parents, as is a list of available community resources, both local and national (see Resources at end of chapter). Classes in the prenatal period or during the postpartum stay are helpful. Instructions for the first days at home should minimally include activities of daily living, dealing with visitors, and activity and rest.

BACKGROUND

- Emotional and behavioral problems in young children are predictive of later depression, substance abuse, poor work and marital outcomes, delinquency, and criminal behavior. These outcomes are frequently associated with harsh and inconsistent discipline, little positive parental involvement, and poor supervision. Parenting practices can account for 30% to 40% of the antisocial behavior in children. Praise, encouragement, and loving involvement with a child have a protective effect against later disruptive behavior and substance abuse. Social learning and attachment theories both claim that caregiving accounts for behavior problems in early childhood. Specific behavior problems include low sociability, poor peer relationships, anger, poor self-control, adolescent anxiety, and dissociation. Poor maternal-infant relationships result in cognitive deficits and poor achievement in school. Primary prevention is aimed at stopping the problem before it develops. Secondary prevention screens for early detection and treatment of the problem. Group parenting programs have a dual preventive role, since some of the children already demonstrate troubled behavior, even by 3 to 4 years of age. Group parenting programs have been found effective in improving behaviors in 3- to 10-year-olds and in reducing anxiety, depression, and poor self-esteem.

OBJECTIVES

- In the review authors wished to determine whether group-based parenting programs are effective at improving the emotional and behavioral outcomes of children, 0 to 3 years of age. The intervention was any group-based parenting program. The outcomes could be at least one measure of emotional and behavioral adjustment.

METHODS
Search Strategy

- The reviewers searched Cochrane, MEDLINE, EMBASE, Biological Abstracts, British Nursing Index, CINAHL, PsycINFO, Sociological Abstracts, Social Science Citation Index, ASSIA, National Research Registry, Dissertation Abstracts, ERIC, and bibliographies. Search keywords were *parent, training, preschool, toddler, infant, baby, babies* and combinations of these terms. Five randomized or quasi-randomized, controlled trials met the criteria, representing 417 parents. Some studies included both mother and father or grandparent/caretaker of the child, and some participants had more than one child in that age group. It is not clear how many children are represented in the studies. The trials, dated 1995 to 2000, were conducted in the United States and the United Kingdom.

Statistical Analyses

- Similar data were pooled. The treatment effect for each outcome was calculated and metaanalyzed, where appropriate. The authors accepted differences between groups that exceeded the 95% confidence interval to be significant.

FINDINGS

- The five studies measured many outcomes. Some measured child-only behaviors (e.g., parent and teacher questionnaires about behaviors such as inattentiveness, aggression, or excessive crying), while others addressed observable parent-child interactions (e.g., parent affect with child, physical negative behavior causing pain, praise, or critical statements). There was a significant improvement in the observed behavior of the children in the parenting group when compared with the controls. Parents' report of children's behavior trended in favor of the intervention group, but not to the level of significance. This was interesting, because parents frequently report behavior more favorably than independent observers. Follow-up data showed that improvement in the intervention group persisted, although it no longer reached the level of significance.

LIMITATIONS

- The reviewers had to compare a variety of scales to measure similar outcomes, which was a challenge. The limited number of studies, their small sizes, and some randomization problems (e.g., using volunteers and cluster data) limit generalizability. The dropout rate, 30% from two trials, was significant. In one of these studies, the dropouts were already using less harsh discipline. In another study, the dropout parents rated their children as significantly less problematic than the group that stayed. In prior studies, dropout rates were higher among subjects with more severe psychosocial problems and stress, and those who dropped out were more likely to be from a lower social class or an ethnic minority. Dropout rates introduce bias; therefore researchers have to account for the dropouts and evaluate the studies' outcomes on "intention-to-treat" basis (i.e., their original randomized allocation), or the remaining data will be skewed.

CONCLUSIONS

- There is some support for group-based programs for parents of children up to 3 years of age, but conclusions regarding whether benefits are long term are equivocal. Anecdotally, parenting groups provide peer modeling for parents and networking that can provide support through future stages.

IMPLICATIONS FOR PRACTICE

- Two trials used 10-week Webster-Stratton programs, one called "Incredible Years," and one used a videotape modeling program called "Parent and Child Series." These programs might be useful in parenting programs. Parenting classes during pregnancy and in the postpartum period can help parents know what to expect and can prepare them for the challenges of parenting.

IMPLICATIONS FOR FURTHER RESEARCH

- The trials did not address the question of primary prevention of mental health problems, and further longer-term research is necessary. Early childhood parenting may provide greater benefits later. The researchers' challenge is to capture those follow-up outcomes. Specific programs should be tested for effectiveness, so that the research is reproducible. Therapist credentials and training may account for variable results. (For more information, see "Parenting Groups for Teenage Parents," the Evidence-Based Practice box in Chapter 3).

Reference: Barlow, J., & Parsons, J. (2003). Group-based parent-training programmes for improving emotional and behavioral adjustment in 0-3 year old children (Cochrane Review). In *The Cochrane Library*, Issue 2, 2004. Chichester, UK: John Wiley & Sons.

Activities of daily living. Given the demands of a newborn, the mother's discomfort or fatigue associated with giving birth, and a busy homecoming day, even small details of daily life can become stressful. Such things as using disposable diapers, preparing frozen or microwave dinners during pregnancy, or getting takeout meals can decrease stress by eliminating at least one or two parental responsibilities during the first few days at home.

Planning for discharge soon after an infant feeding ensures that the couple will have adequate time to get home and relatively settled before the next feeding. Offering a sample carton of premixed bottles for the formula-fed infant prevents need for rushed preparation of formula.

Visitors. New parents are often inadequately prepared for the reality of bringing a new infant home because they romanticize the homecoming. One mother stated, "By the time we drove an hour through traffic, my stitches were hurting and all I wanted was a warm sitz bath and some private time with Bill and the baby, in that order. Instead a carload of visitors pulled into the driveway as we were unbuckling the baby from his car seat. I thought I would surely cry."

The nurse can help parents to explore ways, in advance, to assert their need to limit visitors. When family and friends ask what they can do to help, new parents can suggest they prepare and bring them a meal (which might be used immediately or frozen for later) or pick up items at the store. Parents can work out a signal for alerting the partner that the mother is getting tired or uncomfortable and needs the partner to invite the visitors to another room or to leave. Some mothers find that wearing a robe and not appearing ready for company leads visitors to stay a shorter time. A sign on the front door saying "Mother and baby resting—Please do not disturb" may be useful.

Activity and rest. Because mothers have reported fatigue to be a major problem during the first few weeks after giving birth, mothers need to be encouraged to limit their activities and be realistic about their level of fatigue. Activities should not be sustained for long periods of time. Family, friends, and neighbors can be solicited for support and help with meals, housecleaning, picking up other children, and so on. Rest periods throughout the day are important. Mothers can nap when the baby sleeps. Adequate nutrition is also important for postpartum recovery and in dealing with fatigue.

Infant care.

Providing practical suggestions for infant care can help parents adjust to parenthood. Mothers and fathers want to feel capable and confident in the physical care of their infant. The nurse should assess each parent's need for instruction on care such as bathing, clothing, and safety (Guidelines/Guías box).

Infant bathing. The infant bath time provides a wonderful opportunity for parent-infant social interaction. Some fathers consider this their own special time with their

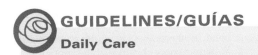

GUIDELINES/GUÍAS
Daily Care

BATHING

- Bathing two or three times a week is enough, using a mild soap like Johnson's, Dove, Tone, or Purpose. Sponge bathe the baby until the umbilical cord falls off and the belly button looks healed. Never leave the baby alone in the tub or sink!

BAÑAR A SU BEBÉ

- *Es suficiente bañar a su bebé dos o tres veces por semana. Use un jabón suave como Johnson's, Dove, Tone, o Purpose. Lave al bebé con una esponja suave hasta que se caiga el cordón umbilical y parezca que el ombligo esté curado. ¡Nunca deje sólo al bebé en la bañera o en el lavabo!*

CLOTHING

- The best clothing is soft and made of cotton. Dress your baby lightly when indoors and on hot days. Too many layers of clothing or blankets can make the baby too hot. On cold days, cover the baby's head when you go outdoors.

LA ROPA DEL BEBÉ

- *La mejor ropa para su bebé debe ser suave y hecha de algodón. No vista al bebé con mucha ropa cuando está dentro de la casa o cuando hace calor afuera. Demasiada ropa o cobijas pueden hacer que el bebé tenga demasiado calor. Cuando hace frío, cubra la cabeza del bebé al ir afuera.*

CAR SEATS

- Use a real car seat (not a baby carrier for the house). It should face the rear of the car until the baby is 1 year old. Always place the car seat in the back seat of the car. Make sure the shoulder straps are snug enough that they don't fall off the baby's shoulders. Car seats are required until age 4.

EL ASIENTO DE BEBÉ PARA EL COCHE

- *Use un asiento de bebé que sea adecuado para el coche. Ponga el asiento de bebé para que el bebé vea la parte de atrás del coche hasta que el bebé tenga un año. Siempre ponga el asiento de bebé en el asiento de atrás del coche. Los cinturones deben estar suficientemente ajustados para que no se caigan de los hombros del bebé. Se requiere por ley usar los asientos de bebé para el coche hasta que el niño tenga 4 años.*

babies. While bathing the baby, parents can talk to the infant, caress and cuddle the infant, and engage in arousal and imitation of facial expressions and smiling (Fig. 17-14).

Sponge baths are recommended until the infant's umbilical cord falls off and the umbilicus is healed (see Chapter 19, Teaching Guidelines box on sponge bathing). At approximately 10 to 14 days, tub baths can be started (Box 17-4). Newborns do not need a bath every day. The diaper area and creases under the arms and neck need more attention.

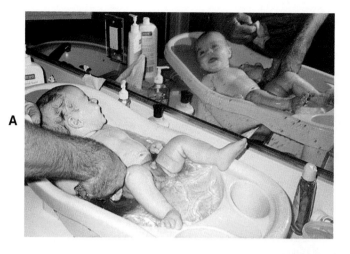

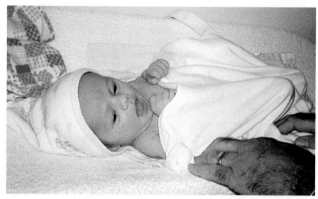

Fig. 17-14 **A,** Baths can be special times for babies and parents. **B,** After the bath, the baby is gently dried to minimize heat loss. (Courtesy Leslie Canerday, Phoenix, AZ.)

BOX 17-4

Tub Bathing

- See guidelines for sponge bathing (see Chapter 19).
- Place liner on bottom of tub to prevent infant from slipping.
- Add 3 inches of comfortably warm water (97.9° F to 99° F—pleasantly warm to your inner wrist). Many babies like to be immersed to their shoulders in water during a bath. If you do this, remember to never let go of the baby or turn your back).
- Wash face and shampoo hair as for sponge bath. Undress baby. Lower infant slowly into water.
- Hold baby safely with fingers under the baby's armpit, with your thumb around the shoulder. The other hand supports the baby's bottom and legs.
- Wash the front of the baby.
- Go from front to back between the legs. Rinse with a wet washcloth.
- Wash the baby's back with your free hand lathered with soap.
- Rinse well with the wet washcloth.
- Remove infant from the water and gently pat dry.

Parents can pick a time for the bath that is easy for them and when the baby is awake, usually before a feeding.

An important consideration in skin cleansing is preservation of the skin's acid mantle. The acid mantle is formed from the uppermost horny layer of the epidermis, sweat, superficial fat, metabolic products, and external substances such as amniotic fluid, microorganisms, and cosmetics. By 4 days of age, the newborn skin surface becomes more acidic, falling to within the bacteriostatic range (pH 5). Therefore only plain, warm water should be used in the early newborn period. Alkaline soaps (such as Ivory), oils, powders, and many lotions alter the acid mantle and provide a medium for bacterial growth (Lund et al., 2001). Powders are not recommended, because the infant can inhale powder.

Infant clothing. A simple rule of thumb for dressing infants is to dress them as the parents would dress themselves, adding or subtracting clothes and wraps for the infant as necessary. A shirt and diaper may be sufficient clothing for the young infant. A bonnet is needed to protect the scalp and to minimize heat loss if it is cool or to protect against sunburn and to shade the infant's eyes if it is sunny and hot. Sunglasses for infants are available. Wrapping the infant snugly in a blanket maintains body temperature and promotes a feeling of security. Overdressing in warm temperatures can cause discomfort and prickly heat rash. Underdressing in cold weather also can cause discomfort; cheeks, fingers, and toes can easily become frostbitten.

Infants have sensitive skin; therefore new clothes should be washed before they are put on the infant. Baby clothes should be washed with a mild detergent and hot water. A double rinse usually removes traces of the potentially irritating cleansing agent or acid residue from urine or stool. If possible, the clothing and bed linens are dried in the sun to neutralize residue. Parents who use coin-operated machines in self-service laundries to wash and dry clothes may find it expensive or impossible to wash and rinse the baby's clothes well.

Bedding requires frequent changing. The top of a plastic-coated mattress should be washed frequently, and the crib or bassinet should be dusted with a damp cloth. The infant's toilet articles may be kept in a box, basket, or plastic carrier for convenience.

Infant safety. Providing for the safety of an infant is not a matter of common sense. There are many things new parents may not be aware of that are potential dangers to their infant (e.g., window blind cords near the crib or a parent throwing an infant in the air during play). Nurses should provide parents with concrete instructions on infant safety (Box 17-5).

Anticipatory guidance regarding the newborn

Anticipatory guidance helps prepare new parents for what to expect as their newborn grows and develops. Parents with realistic expectations of infant needs and behavior are

BOX 17-5

Tips for Keeping Your Baby Safe

- Never leave your baby alone on a bed, couch, or table. Even newborns can move enough to eventually reach the edge and fall off.
- Never put your baby on a cushion, pillow, beanbag, or waterbed to sleep. Your baby may suffocate. Also, do not keep pillows, large floppy toys, or loose plastic sheeting in the crib.
- Do not place your infant on his or her stomach to sleep during the first few months of life. The American Academy of Pediatrics advises against this prone position because it has been associated with an increased incidence of sudden infant death syndrome (SIDS). The back-lying position is preferable.
- When using an infant carrier, stay within arm's reach when the carrier is on a high place, such as a table, sofa, or store counter. If at all possible, place the carrier on the floor near you.
- Infant carriers do not keep your baby safe in a car. Always place your baby in an approved car safety seat when traveling in a motor vehicle (car, truck, bus, or van). Car safety seats are recommended for travel on trains and airplanes as well. Use the car seat for *every* ride. Your baby should be in a rear-facing infant car seat from birth to 20 pounds, and the car seat should be in the back seat of the car (see Fig. 19-25). This is especially important in vehicles with front passenger air bags, because when air bags inflate they can be fatal for infants and toddlers.

- When bathing your baby, never leave him or her alone. Newborns and infants can drown in 1 to 2 inches of water.
- Be sure that your hot water heater is set at 120° F or less. Always check bathwater temperature with your elbow before putting your baby in the bath.
- Do not tie anything around your baby's neck. Pacifiers, for example, tied around the neck with a ribbon or string may strangle your baby.
- Check your baby's crib for safety. Slats should be no more than 2½ inches apart. The space between the mattress and sides should be less than 2 fingerwidths. There should be no decorative knobs on the bedposts.
- Keep crib or playpen away from window blind and drapery cords; your baby could strangle on them.
- Keep crib and playpen well away from radiators, heat vents, and portable heaters. Linens in crib or playpen could catch fire if in contact with these heat sources.
- Install smoke detectors on every floor of your home. Check them once a month to be sure they work. Change batteries once a year.
- Avoid exposing your baby to cigarette or cigar smoke in your home or other places. Passive exposure to tobacco smoke greatly increases the likelihood that your infant will have respiratory symptoms and illnesses.
- Be gentle with your baby. Do not pick your baby up or swing your baby by the arms or throw him or her up in the air.

---

better prepared to adjust to the demands of a new baby and to parenthood itself (Guidelines/Guías box).

New parents can be overwhelmed by a large volume of information and become anxious. Anticipatory guidance should include the following: newborn sleep-wake cycles, interpretation of crying and quieting techniques, infant developmental milestones, sensory enrichment and infant stimulation, recognizing signs of illness, and well-baby follow-up and immunizations. Printed materials and audiotapes or videotapes for parents to take home are helpful. With more and more use of the Internet, parents may also be given a list of websites that might be accessed for information.

Development of day-night routines. Nurses can help prepare new parents for the fact that most newborns cannot tell the difference between night and day and must learn the rhythm of day-night routines. Nurses should provide basic suggestions for settling a newborn and for helping him or her develop a predictable routine. Examples of such suggestions include the following:

- In the late afternoon, bring the baby out to the center of family activity. Keep the baby there for the rest of the evening. If the baby falls asleep, let the baby do so in the infant seat or in someone's arms. Save the crib or bassinet for nighttime sleep.
- Give the baby a bath right before bedtime. This soothes the baby and helps him or her expend energy.

- Feed the baby for the last evening time around 11 PM and put him or her to bed in the crib or bassinet.
- For nighttime feedings and diaper changes, keep a small night-light on to avoid turning on bright lights. Talk in soft whispers (if at all) and handle the baby gently and only as absolutely necessary to feed and diaper. Nighttime feedings should be all business and no play! Babies usually go back to sleep if the room is quiet and dark.

A predictable, stable routine gradually develops for *most* babies; however, some babies *never* develop one. New parents will find it easier if they are willing to be flexible and to give up some control during the early weeks.

Interpretation of crying and quieting techniques. Crying is an infant's first social communication. Some babies cry more than others, but all babies cry. They cry to communicate that they are hungry, uncomfortable, wet, ill, or bored, and sometimes for no apparent reason at all. The longer parents are around their infants, the easier it becomes to interpret what a cry means. Many infants have a fussy period during the day, often in the late afternoon or early evening when everyone is naturally tired. Environmental tension adds to the length and intensity of crying spells. Babies also have periods of vigorous crying when no comforting can help. These periods of crying may last for long stretches until the infants seem to cry themselves to

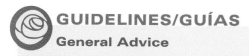

GUIDELINES/GUÍAS
General Advice

CRYING

- Babies cry when they are hungry; need to burp; have a wet diaper; feel cold, hot, tired, bored, or overstimulated; and (rarely) when they are sick or in pain. After a while you will learn the meaning of your baby's different cries. Be careful not to feed him every time he cries, since overfeeding causes tummy aches. Check to see if he needs burping or a new diaper. It is not harmful to let a baby cry for short periods (5 to 10 minutes). This may be what he needs to fall asleep.

LLORAR

- *Todos los bebés lloran cuando tienen hambre; cuando necesitan eructar; cuando necesitan que les cambie el pañal; cuando tienen calor o frío; cuando están cansados, aburridos o sobreestimulados; y (raras veces) cuando están enfermos o tienen algún dolor. Después de un tiempo, usted aprenderá a distinguir los significados diferentes entre los gritos de su bebé y sabrá lo que él necesite. Tenga cuidado de no darle de comer cada vez que llora ya que demasiada comida puede causar un dolor de estómago. Compruebe si el bebé necesita eructar o si está mojado el pañal. No le hará ningún daño al bebé si llora por un ratito (cinco a diez minutos). Eso puede ser lo que necesita para dormirse.*

SLEEPING

- Most babies can sleep through most of the night without a feeding by 4 to 5 months of age. You can help your baby sleep by keeping things quiet and dark at night. Both you and he will usually sleep better and wake up less often if he is sleeping in a separate bed. If your baby stirs at night but doesn't fully wake up, give him a chance to fall back asleep by himself. Only get him up if he stays wide awake and seems hungry. The baby should sleep on his side or back for safety. Babies sleeping on their tummies seem to be more prone to crib death.

DORMIR

- *La mayoría de los bebés puede dormir por casi toda la noche sin comer a los cuatro o cinco meses de edad. Un cuarto tranquilo y oscuro ayuda que su bebé duerma tranquilamente. Ambos usted y su bebé dormirán mejor y se despertarán menos si usted y el bebé duermen en camas separadas. Si se despierta el bebé durante la noche, déle la oportunidad de dormirse de nuevo. Pero si se queda despierto y tiene hambre, atiéndale. El bebé debe estar acostado sobre un costado o de espalda para su seguridad. Los bebés que duermen acostados de estómago con boca abajo tienen un riesgo más grande de muerte de cuna.*

SPITTING UP

- Most babies spit up a little after feedings. If your baby is gaining weight, this is normal. It helps to keep your baby upright and quiet for a few minutes after feedings. If your baby seems to be spitting up a lot, bring him to your doctor for a weight check.

ESCUPIR

- *La mayoría de los bebés escupe un poquito de la leche después de comer o de eructar. Esto es normal si su bebé está aumentando de peso. Es bueno poner a su bebé en una posición vertical y calmarlo por unos minutos después de darle de comer. Si parece que su bebé escupe mucha leche o si lo hace con mucha frecuencia, llévelo al doctor para verificar el peso del bebé.*

---

sleep. Possibly the infants are trying to discharge enough energy that they can settle themselves down. The nurse needs to reinforce for new parents that time and infant maturation will take care of these types of cries.

Crying because of colic is a common concern of new parents. Babies with colic cry inconsolably for several hours, pull their legs up to their stomach, and pass large amounts of gas. No one really knows what colic is or why babies get it. Parents can be encouraged to contact their nurse-practitioner or pediatrician if they are concerned that their baby has colic.

Certain types of sensory stimulation can calm and quiet infants and help them get to sleep. Important characteristics of this sensory stimulation—whether tactile, vestibular, auditory, or visual—appear to be that the stimulation is mild, slow, and rhythmic, and consistently and regularly presented. Tactile stimulation can include warmth, patting, back rubbing, and covering the skin with textured cloth. Swaddling (Box 17-6) to keep arms and legs close to the body (as in utero) provides widespread and constant tactile stimulation and a sense of security. Vestibular stimulation is especially effective and can be accomplished by mild rhythmic

movement such as rocking or by holding the infant upright, as on the parent's shoulder.

The nurse can teach parents a number of strategies that help quiet a fussy baby, prevent crying, and induce quiet attention or sleep (Box 17-7).

Developmental milestones. Knowledge of infant growth and development helps parents have realistic expectations of what an infant can do. When parents understand and appreciate the limitations and developing abilities of their infant, adjustment to parenthood can go more smoothly. Emphasizing the individuality of the infant enhances the capacity of the family to offer their infant an optimally nurturing environment (Brazelton, 1995).

Brazelton (1995) suggests the concept of "touch-points" for intervention, that is, points at which a change in the system (baby, parent, and family) is brought about by the baby's spurts in development (cognitive, motor, or emotional). Immediately before each spurt in development, there is a predictable short period of disorganization in the baby. Parents are likely to feel disorganized and stressed as well. Because these periods of disorganization are predictable, nurses can offer parents anticipatory guidance to help them understand

CD: Skill —Swaddling

BOX 17-6

How to Swaddle an Infant

1 Fold down the top corner of the blanket. Position the infant on the blanket with the infant's neck near the fold.
2 Bring the blanket around the infant's right side and across the infant, tucking the corner under the left side.
3 Bring the bottom of the blanket up to the infant's chest.
4 Bring the remaining corner of the blanket across the infant, tucking the corner under the infant's right side. The infant should be wrapped securely but not tightly; some room should be left for the infant to move.

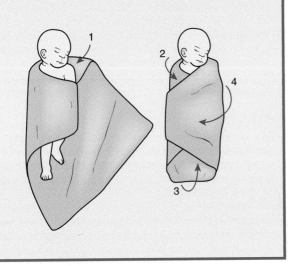

what happens with infant development and to prepare them for the subsequent spurts in development.

Two touch-points occur during the early postpartum-newborn period: one soon after birth and another at 2 to 3 weeks (Brazelton, 1995). In the hospital or at a home visit during the first week, the nurse can use Brazelton's Neonatal Behavioral Assessment Scale (Brazelton & Nugent, 1996) to demonstrate to parents their baby's amazing repertoire of abilities. In this way, parents begin to appreciate their baby's individuality and become more sensitive to their baby's behavioral cues. At 2 to 3 weeks the home care nurse or pediatric office nurse should assess for the regular end-of-the-day fussy period that most infants have between 3 and 12 weeks of age. Helpful topics to include in the anticipatory guidance are the normalcy and positive value of the fussy period, how to settle a fussy baby, and ways to help a baby develop a predictable schedule.

It is also helpful for nurses to provide parents with information on month-by-month infant growth and development. Written information that parents can refer to later is especially helpful. See Table 17-6 for a summary of infant growth and development during the first 2 to 3 months.

Infant stimulation. Interacting with their parents is an important way in which infants learn about themselves and their environment. Nurses can teach parents a variety of ways to stimulate their infant's development and to enrich the infant's learning environment. Home health nurses are in a prime position to evaluate the home environment

BOX 17-7

Infant Quieting Techniques

- Many newborns feel insecure in the center of a large crib. They prefer a small, warm, soft space that reminds them of intrauterine life. Try a smaller bed, such as a bassinet, portable crib, buggy, or cradle, or use a rolled-up blanket to turn a corner of the big crib into a smaller place.
- Carry your baby in a frontpack or backpack.
- Swaddle your newborn snugly in a receiving blanket. Swaddling keeps your newborn's arms and legs close to his or her body, similar to the intrauterine position. It makes the newborn feel more secure.
- Prewarm the crib sheets with a hot water bottle or heating pad that you remove before putting your baby to bed. Some babies startle when placed on a cold sheet.
- Some newborns need extra sucking to soothe themselves to sleep. Breastfeeding mothers may prefer to let their infant suckle at the breast as a soothing technique. Other mothers choose to use a pacifier. Stroke the pacifier against the roof of the baby's mouth to encourage him or her to suck it during the first 2 weeks. Around 3 months of age, infants become able to consistently find and suck their thumbs as a way of self-consoling.
- A rhythmic, monotonous noise simulating the intrauterine sounds of your heartbeat and blood flow may help

your infant settle down. Some parents have found that putting the baby in a portable crib beside the dishwasher or washing machine helps settle a fussy baby.
- Movement often helps quiet a baby. Take your baby for a ride in the car, or take your baby for an outing in a stroller or carriage. Rock your baby in a rocking chair or cradle.
- Place your baby on his or her stomach across your lap; pat and rub his or her back while gently bouncing your legs or swaying them from left to right.
- Babies enjoy close skin-to-skin contact. A combination of this and warm water often helps soothe a fussy baby. Fill your tub with warm water. Get in and let the baby lie on your chest so that the baby is immersed in the water up to his or her neck. Cuddle the baby close.
- Let your baby see your face. Talk to your baby in a soothing voice.
- Your baby may simply be bored. Bring him or her into the room where you and the rest of the family are. Change your baby's position; many babies like to be upright, for example, by being held up on your shoulder.

TABLE 17-6

Growth and Development during Infancy

1 MONTH	2 MONTHS	3 MONTHS
PHYSICAL		
Weight gain of 5 to 7.5 oz (150 to 210 g) weekly for first 6 mo	Posterior fontanel closed	Primitive reflexes fading
Height gain of 1 in (2.5 cm) monthly for first 6 mo	Crawling reflex disappears	
Head circumference increases by 0.6 in (1.5 cm) monthly for first 6 mo		
Primitive reflexes present and strong		
Doll's eye reflex and dance reflex fading		
Preferential nose breathing (most infants)		
GROSS MOTOR		
Assumes flexed position with pelvis high but knees not under abdomen when prone (at birth, knees flexed under abdomen)[†]	Assumes less flexed position when prone—hips flat, legs extended, arms flexed, head to side[†]	Able to hold head more erect when sitting, but still bobs forward
Can turn head from side to side when prone, lifts head momentarily from bed[†]	Less head lag when pulled to sitting position	Has only slight head lag when pulled to sitting position
Has marked head lag, especially when pulled from lying to sitting position	Can maintain head in same plane as rest of body when held in ventral suspension	Assumes symmetric body positioning
Holds head momentarily parallel and in midline when suspended in prone position	When prone, can lift head almost 45 degrees off table	Able to raise head and shoulders from prone position to a 45- to 90-degree angle from table; bears weight on forearms
Assumes asymmetric tonic neck reflex position when supine	When held in sitting position, head is held up but bobs forward	When held in standing position, able to bear slight fraction of weight on legs
When held in standing position, body limp at knees and hips	Assumes asymmetric tonic neck reflex position intermittently	Regards own hand
In sitting position, back is uniformly rounded; absence of head control		
FINE MOTOR		
Hands predominantly closed	Hands often open	Actively holds rattle but will not reach for it[†]
Grasp reflex strong	Grasp reflex fading	Grasp reflex absent
Hand clenches on contact with rattle		Hands kept loosely open
		Clutches own hand; pulls at blanket and clothes
SENSORY		
Able to fixate on moving object in range of 45 degrees when held at a distance of 8-10 in. Visual acuity approaches 20/100*[†]	Binocular fixation and convergence to near objects beginning	Follows object to periphery (180 degrees)[†]
Follows light to midline	When supine, follows dangling toy from side to point beyond midline	Locates sound by turning head to side and looking in same direction[†]
Quiets when hears a voice	Visually searches to locate sounds	Begins to have ability to coordinate stimuli from various sense organs
	Turns head to side when sound is made at level of ear	
VOCALIZATION		
Cries to express displeasure	Vocalizes, distinct from crying[†]	Squeals aloud to show pleasure[†]
Makes small throaty sounds	Crying becomes differentiated	Coos, babbles, chuckles
Makes comfort sounds during feeding	Coos	Vocalizes when smiling
	Vocalizes to familiar voice	"Talks" a great deal when spoken to
		Less crying during periods of wakefulness
SOCIALIZATION AND COGNITION		
Is in sensorimotor phase—stage I, use of reflexes (birth-1 mo), and stage II, primary circular reactions (1-4 mo)	Demonstrates social smile in response to various stimuli[†]	Displays considerable interest in surroundings
Watches parent's face intently as she or he talks to infant		Ceases crying when parent enters room
		Can recognize familiar faces and objects, such as feeding bottle
		Shows awareness of strange situations

From Hockenberry, M. (2003). *Wong's nursing care of infants and children* (7th ed.). St. Louis: Mosby.
† Milestones that represent essential integrative aspects of development that lay the foundation for the achievement of more advanced skills.
*Degree of visual acuity varies according to vision measurement procedure used.

and to make suggestions to parents for promotion of their baby's physical, cognitive, and emotional development. Suggestions for teaching infants during the first few months are presented in Boxes 17-8 and 17-9. Table 17-7 presents suggestions for visual, auditory, tactile, and kinetic stimulation.

Another method of sensory enrichment that parents can learn to use is infant massage. This type of nurturing touch can help create a loving bond between the infant and parent and has been shown to contribute to the physical and emotional well-being of the massage giver and receiver (Miller, 2004; Zlotnick, 2000). Infant massage is a gentle, warm communication done with the infant, not to the infant. The focus is on reciprocal interaction between infant and parent; the parent talks to the infant, asks permission to start the massage, questions the infant, and facilitates dialogue. Massage produces a deep relaxation, increasing the baby's ability to self-console and release tension. Soothing

techniques aid in the child's self-regulation. Improved sleep patterns mean that the baby's disposition tends to be better when awake (Miller).

It is not just the baby that enjoys infant massage; the parent or caregiver also benefits. Massage can be a concrete way for parents to learn about their baby, gain self-confidence, and become more proficient in their nurturing abilities. Spending time massaging the baby helps parents develop sensitivity to the baby's cues and provides insight into the wants and needs of this child. Parents also become more aware of changes in the growth, development, and health of their child (Miller, 2004).

Well-baby follow-up and immunizations. Parents should be advised to plan for their infant's health follow-up care at the following ages: 2 to 4 weeks, then every 2 months until 6 to 7 months, then every 3 months until 18 months, at 2 years, at 3 years, at preschool, and every 2 years

---

BOX 17-8

Teaching Your Newborn

- Newborns learn things every day. You can teach your newborn by playing with him or her and giving your newborn toys that help him or her to learn.
- Talk to your baby a lot. Tell your baby what is going on in the room ("Listen to the dog barking."). Label objects that you see or use ("Here's the washcloth.") and describe things you are doing ("Let's put the shirt over Kerry's head!").
- Look at your baby's face and make eye contact. Play face-making games: smile, stick out your tongue, open your eyes wide. As your baby gets older, he or she will try to imitate these facial expressions.
- Babies like music and rhythmic movement. Rock or swing your baby as you sing to him or her in a gentle voice.

- Acknowledge your baby's attempts to "answer" your talking and singing. He or she will respond to you by looking in your direction, making eye contact, moving his or her arms and legs, and/or making sounds.
- Babies like bright colors and vivid contrasts. Show your baby pictures and objects that are black and white, are bright primary colors (red, blue, yellow, green), and/or have large patterns. Keep colorful mobiles and toys where your baby can see them.
- Babies like to be held upright. Holding your newborn on your shoulder lets your baby look around his or her world and provides vestibular stimulation. Let your baby lift his or her head for a few seconds. Keep your hand ready to support your baby's head.

BOX 17-9

Teaching Your 1- to 2-Month-Old Infant

At 1 to 2 months of age, your infant is gaining more control of his or her movements: the infant has more head control, and even may hold an object briefly in his or her hand. Your baby also is becoming more social. He or she demonstrates behaviors to engage you in interaction: smiling, cooing, making longer eye contact, and following you with his or her eyes.

During these months you can help your baby learn if you:

- Put your baby on his or her stomach on a blanket on the floor. Lie on your stomach facing your baby. Talk to your baby to get him or her to raise his or her head to see you.
- Roll your baby onto his or her back and play with your baby's legs. Move the legs in a bicycle-riding motion. Try to get your baby to kick his or her legs.
- Play hand games, such as pat-a-cake, with your baby; kiss your baby's fingers; place your baby's hands on your face.

Bring your baby's hands in front of his or her eyes as you play; get your baby to look at his or her hands.
- Encourage your baby to watch and follow things with his or her eyes. Use a noise-making toy, such as a rattle or a chime, or a brightly colored object about 12 inches from his or her eyes; move it slowly to one side and then the other. Objects hanging from a play frame are good for your baby to watch while he or she is on his or her back or sitting in an infant seat.
- Continue to talk and sing a lot to your baby. Continue to tell your baby what you are doing with him or her and what is going on in the immediate environment.
- Keep your baby near you during times when the family usually is together, such as at mealtimes. Infant seats, especially ones that bounce or rock, and infant swings are good to use at these times.

TABLE 17-7

Play during Infancy: Suggested Activities for Birth through 3 Months

AGE (MONTHS)	VISUAL STIMULATION	AUDITORY STIMULATION	TACTILE STIMULATION	KINETIC STIMULATION
Birth-1	Look at infant at close range Hang bright, shiny object within 9 to 10 inches of infant's face and in midline Hang mobiles with black-and-white contrast designs	Talk to infant, sing in soft voice Play music box, radio, television Have ticking clock or metronome nearby	Hold, caress, cuddle Keep infant warm Infant may like to be swaddled	Rock infant, place in cradle Use carriage for walks
2-3	Provide bright objects Make room bright with pictures or mirrors on walls Take infant to various rooms while doing chores Place infant in infant seat for vertical view of environment	Talk to infant Include in family gatherings Expose to various environmental noises other than those of home Use rattles, wind chimes	Caress infant while bathing, at diaper change Comb hair with a soft brush	Use infant swing Take in car for rides Exercise body by moving extremities in swimming motion Use cradle gym

From Hockenberry, M. (2003). *Wong's nursing care of infants and children* (7th ed.). St. Louis: Mosby.

thereafter. These well-baby follow-up visits with a nurse-practitioner or pediatrician are important for the parents, as well as the infant. They provide a time for parents to have questions answered, to get reassurance about their adaptation to parenthood, and to receive anticipatory guidance for the ensuing weeks before the next well-baby visit.

The schedule for immunizations should be reviewed with parents (Table 17-8). Nurses should become familiar with this schedule and should provide written instructions to the parents about when and where to obtain immunizations. Immunization schedules change periodically and the nurse can update any information needed by checking with the website www.cdc.gov. An infant's ability to protect himself or herself against antigens by the formation of antibodies develops

sequentially; therefore the infant must be developmentally capable of responding to these antibodies. This is the reason for planning sequential immunizations for infants.

Recognizing signs of illness. As well as explaining the need for well-baby follow-up visits, the nurse should discuss with parents the signs of illness in newborns (Box 17-10). Parents should be advised to call their nurse-practitioner or pediatrician immediately if they notice such signs and to ask about over-the-counter medications, such as Tylenol for infants, to keep at home (Plan of Care).

Evaluation

Evaluation is based on the expected outcomes of care. The plan is revised as needed based on the evaluation findings.

TABLE 17-8

Immunization Schedule—2005*

IMMUNIZATION	AGE GIVEN
DTaP (diphtheria, tetanus, acellular pertussis)	2, 4, 6 mo
Hib (*Haemophilus influenzae* b conjugate vaccine)	2, 4, 6 mo
IPV (inactivated polio vaccine—injectable)	2, 4, 6 to 18 mo
MMR (measles, mumps, rubella)	12 to 15 mo (12 mo if community outbreak)
HBIG (hepatitis B immunoglobulin—if mother is HBsAg positive)	Within 12 hours after birth
HBV (hepatitis B)	Before hospital discharge, 1 to 6 mo, 6 to 18 mo
PCV (*Pneumococcal* conjugate vaccine)	2, 4, 6, 12 to 18 mo
Varicella (chicken pox)	12 to 18 mo
Influenza ("flu shot")	Yearly after 6 mo if at risk and/or in day care
Tuberculin skin test (not an immunization)	12 to 15 mo

U.S. Department of Health and Human Services, Centers for Disease Control and Prevention. (2005). *Childhood and adolescent immunization schedule.* Internet document available at http://www.cdc.gov/nip/recs/child-schedule.pdf (accessed May 30, 2005).
*This is the schedule for the first 18 months. For the full schedule, go to www.cdc.gov.

BOX 17-10

Signs of Illness to Report Immediately

- Fever: temperature above 38° C (100.4° F) axillary (under arm for 3 to 4 minutes); also, a continual rise in temperature
- Hypothermia: temperature below 36.5° (97.7° F) axillary
- Poor feeding or little interest in food: refusal to eat for two feedings in a row
- Vomiting: more than one episode of forceful vomiting or frequent vomiting (over a 6-hour period)
- Diarrhea: two consecutive green, watery stools (NOTE: Stools of breastfed infants are normally looser than stools of formula-fed infants. Diarrhea will leave a water ring around the stool, whereas breastfed stools will not.)
- Decreased bowel movement: less than two soiled diapers per day after 48 hours or less than three soiled diapers per day by the fifth day of life
- Decreased urination: no wet diapers for 18 to 24 hours or less than six to eight wet diapers per day

- Breathing difficulties: labored breathing with flared nostrils or absence of breathing for more than 15 seconds (NOTE: A newborn's breathing is normally irregular and between 30 to 40 breaths per minute. Count the breaths for a full minute.)
- Cyanosis whether accompanying a feeding or not
- Lethargy: sleepiness, difficulty waking, or periods of sleep longer than 6 hours (Most newborns sleep for short periods, usually from 1 to 4 hours, and wake to be fed.)
- Inconsolable crying (attempts to quiet not effective) or continuous high-pitched cry
- Bleeding or purulent drainage from umbilical cord or circumcision
- Drainage developing in the eyes

⊘ PLAN OF CARE | *Home Care Follow-up: Transition to Parenthood*

NURSING DIAGNOSIS Deficient knowledge of infant care related to lack of experience or lack of support

Expected Outcomes *Infant care routines are adequate, and infant appears healthy.*

Nursing Interventions/Rationales

- Observe infant care routines (bathing, diapering, feeding, play) *to evaluate parental ease with care and adequacy of techniques.*
- Observe infant appearance (height-weight ratio, head circumference, fontanels, skin tone and turgor); assess infant's vital signs, overall tone, reflexes, and age-appropriate developmental skills *to evaluate for signs indicative of inadequate care.*
- Explore available support systems for infant care *to determine adequacy of existing system.*
- Demonstrate troublesome care routines and have involved family members return demonstration *to facilitate improvements in care.*
- Provide ongoing follow-up as needed *to ensure that identified potential and actual care deficits are addressed and resolved.*

NURSING DIAGNOSIS Disturbed sleep patterns related to infant demands and environmental interruptions

Expected Outcomes *Woman sleeps for uninterrupted periods and feels rested on waking.*

Nursing Interventions/Rationales

- Discuss woman's routine and specify things that interfere with sleep *to determine scope of problem and direct interventions.*
- Explore ways woman and significant others can make environment more conducive to sleep (e.g., privacy, darkness, quiet, back rubs, soothing music, warm milk); teach use of guided imagery and relaxation techniques *to promote optimal conditions for sleep.*
- Eliminate things or routines (e.g., caffeine, foods that induce heartburn, strenuous mental or physical activity) *that may interfere with sleep.*
- Advise family to limit visitors and activities *to avoid further stress and fatigue.*
- Have family plan specific times to care for the newborn to allow mother time to sleep; have mother learn to use infant nap time as a time for her to nap as well *to replenish energy and decrease fatigue.*

NURSING DIAGNOSIS Risk for impaired home maintenance related to addition of new family member, inadequate resources, or inadequate support systems

Expected Outcome *Home exhibits signs of safe and functional environment.*

Nursing Interventions/Rationales

- Observe the home environment (e.g., available living space and sleeping arrangements; adequacy of facilities for food preparation and storage, hygiene and toileting; overall state of repair; cleanliness; presence of safety hazards) *to determine adequacy and effective use of resources.*
- Observe arrangements for the newborn, such as sleeping space, care equipment and supplies (bathing, changing, feeding, transportation) *to determine adequacy of resources.*
- Explore who is responsible for cooking, cleaning, child care, and newborn care and determine whether the mother seems adequately rested *to determine adequacy of support systems.*
- Identify and arrange referrals to needed social agencies (e.g., Temporary Assistance for Needy Families [TANF], Women, Infants, and Children [WIC] program, food pantries) *to address resource deficits (finances, supplies, equipment).*

NURSING DIAGNOSIS Risk for interrupted family processes related to inclusion of new family member

Expected Outcome *Infant is successfully incorporated into family structure.*

Nursing Interventions/Rationales

- Explore with family the ways that the birth and neonate have changed family structure and function *to evaluate functional and role adjustment.*
- Observe family interaction with the newborn and note degree of bonding, evidence of sibling rivalry, and involvement in newborn care *to evaluate acceptance of newest family member.*
- Clarify identified misinformation and misperceptions *to promote clear communication.*
- Assist family to explore options for solutions to identified problems *to promote effective problem resolution.*
- Support family efforts as they move toward adjusting and incorporating the new member *to reinforce new functions and roles.*
- If needed, make referrals to appropriate social services or community agencies *to ensure ongoing support and care.*

Fathers, as well as mothers, can suffer from postpartum depression. Unfortunately, they are seldom identified and their needs are often overlooked. Interview a nurse working in a pediatric clinic or office. How often does the nurse identify symptoms of postpartum depression in fathers? Are the needs of fathers with postpartum depression similar to or different from those of depressed mothers? Is a father more likely to develop postpartum depression if his wife is also depressed? What support is available in the community for this group of men? What type of support would fathers with postpartum depression consider most helpful?

Key Points

- The birth of a child necessitates changes in the existing interactional structure of a family.
- Attachment is the process by which the parent and infant come to love and accept each other.
- Attachment is strengthened through the use of sensual responses or interactions by both partners in the parent-infant interaction.
- In adjusting to the parental role, the mother moves from a dependent state (taking in) to an interdependent state (letting go).
- Mothers may exhibit signs of postpartum blues (baby blues).
- Fathers experience emotions and adjustments during the transition to parenthood that are similar to, and also distinctly different from, those of mothers.

- Modulation of rhythm, modification of behavioral repertoires, and mutual responsivity facilitate infant-parent adjustment.
- Many factors influence adaptation to parenthood (e.g., age, culture, socioeconomic level, and expectations of what the child will be like).
- Parents face a number of tasks related to sibling adjustment that require creative parental interventions.
- Grandparents can have a positive influence on the postpartum family.
- Providing practical suggestions for infant care can help parents adjust to parenthood.
- Anticipatory guidance helps prepare new parents for what to expect as their newborn grows and develops.

Answer Guidelines to Critical Thinking Exercise

Special Needs of Adolescent and Older First-Time Mothers

1 Yes, both new mothers have stated what they perceive as their current priority needs. Nurses should address the needs identified by parents as important. Emily is an older mother who is used to being in control. She is upset about not being able to control the baby's behavior (eating and sleeping routines). She may be experiencing postpartum blues and needs further assessment in this area. Physical concerns after a cesarean birth and breastfeeding should be explored also. The adolescent mother often needs additional family support in caring for her infant. However, there may be conflict between the mother and grandmother about what is best. Further exploration of the relationships between Mia and her mother and Mia and the baby's father is indicated. An increased incidence of abuse may occur when one parent attributes negative characteristics of a partner to the infant. Mia has a knowledge deficit with regard to infant sleeping patterns and nutrition.

2 a. Both the adolescent and older woman may have difficulty adjusting to motherhood. Adolescents may have unrealistic expectations about newborn behavior and their relationship with the father of the infant. Intergenerational conflicts regarding childcare may also develop. The older mother may need to adjust to the loss of freedom and interruption in her career caused by the new baby.

b. Support from the father is very important to most new mothers. The adolescent mother may look to the father for both financial and emotional support. She may dream about becoming an "ideal" family. At this point, Mia is likely not receiving as much support as she desires from the baby's father. On the surface, Emily appears to have more support. However, in an attempt to regain control by showing everyone she can "do it by herself," she may refuse all offers of assistance.

c. Education about parenting, infant care, and realistic expectations for the postpartum period should have begun during pregnancy. Teaching should be individualized and continued in the hospital after delivery and beyond.

d. Adolescents who become parents have an increased likelihood of dropping out of school and are more likely to be single parents, have less income, and experience repeat pregnancies. With support from families and the community this outcome can be changed. With time, older mothers can adjust to the changes in their lives caused by the baby. Support from significant others and increasing competency can ease the transition to parenthood.

3 Priority nursing care at this time is to address Mia's knowledge deficit regarding infant behavior and nutrition. Emily needs prompt attention because of her possible postpartum blues or depression. Additionally, Emily needs education about

breastfeeding and physical recovery after cesarean birth. More information on infant care and development should be given to both mothers.

4 Yes, there is evidence that meeting the new mother's information needs regarding her care and care for the baby will increase her knowledge and skill and assist her in adapting to the role of mother. Adolescent and older women are two groups of new mothers that can especially benefit from individualized teaching.

5 Mia's daughter might have an increased risk for child abuse because of her mother's unrealistic expectations and negative feelings. Follow-up care should be arranged to assist Mia with her transition to parenthood. Mia might benefit from participating in a support group for adolescent mothers, where child care, infant development, and needs of the adolescent mother or parent are discussed. Including the grandmother in planning care for Mia and her baby will also be very important. Emily needs to be continually assessed at each visit for postpartum blues or depression.

Resources

At-Home Dad (newsletter for fathers who stay at home)
61 Brightwood Ave.
North Andover, MA 01845-1702
email: athomedad@aol.com

Baby-Friendly USA
www.babyfriendly-usa.org

Deafparent.com (website with message board and support for parents who are deaf)
www.deafparent.com

The Fatherhood Project at the Families and Work Institute
330 Seventh Ave.
New York, NY 10001
212-465-2044
www.fww.org

FEMALE (Formerly Employed Mother at the Leading Edge)
P.O. Box 31
Elmhurst, IL 60126
630-941-3553
www.mainstreetmom.com/jm_female.htm

Grandparents Place (support information for grandparents and others caring for children)
www.grandsplace.com

Institute for Responsible Fatherhood and Family Revitalization
9500 Arena Dr., Suite 400
Largo, MD 20744
301-773-2044
http://www.ncoff.gse.upenn.edu/

International Association of Infant Massage (IAIM)
P.O. Box 1045
Oak View, CA 93022
800-248-5432
www.iaim-us.com

La Leche League International (local La Leche League groups are usually listed in city and town phone books)
1400 North Meacham Rd.
Schaumburg, IL 60168-4079
847-519-7730
www.lalecheleague.org

Motherhood Maternity Health and Fitness Program
SBI Corporation
1106 Stratford Dr.
Carlisle, PA 17103
717-258-4641

Mothers at Home
9493-C Silver King Ct.
Fairfax, VA 22031
703-352-1072
www.family&home.org

National Council for Adoption
202-328-8072
www.ncfa-usa.org

National Organization of Mothers of Twins Clubs
Executive Office
P.O. Box 700860
Plymouth, MI 48170
www.nomtc.org

Postpartum Support International
927 North Kellogg Ave.
Santa Barbara, CA 93111
805-967-7636
www.postpartum.net

Single Parent Resource Center
141 West 28th St. Suite 302
New York, NY 10001
212-947-0221
www.singleparentusa.com

U.S. Department of Health and Human Services (source for up-to-date information on immunizations, childhood illnesses)
Centers for Disease Control and Prevention
www.cdc.gov

U.S. Department of Transportation (source for child safety seat information)
National Highway Traffic Safety Administration (NHTSA)
Auto Safety Hotline 800-424-9393
www.nhtsa.gov

www.babycenter.com
(good website for answers to parents' questions)

www.estronaut.com
(great website for information on women's health and pregnancy; also includes a useful search engine)

www.slowlane.com
(excellent website for both mothers and fathers)

References

Alpers, R. (1998). The changing self-concept of pregnant and parenting teens. *Journal of Professional Nursing, 14*(2), 111-118.

Ament, L. (1990). Maternal tasks of the puerperium re-identified. *Journal of Obstetric, Gynecologic, and Neonatal Nursing, 19*(4), 330-335.

Barlow, J., & Parsons, J. (2003). Group-based parent-training programmes for improving emotional and behavioral adjustment in 0-3 year old children. (Cochrane Review). In *The Cochrane Library*, Issue 2, 2004. Chichester, UK: John Wiley & Sons.

Beeber, L. (2002). The pinks and the blues. *American Journal of Nursing, 102*(11), 91-98.

Bitzer, J., & Adler, J. (2000). Sexuality during pregnancy and the postpartum period. *Journal of Sex Education and Therapy, 25*(1), 49-58.

Bloom, K. (1998). Perceived relationship with the father of the baby and maternal attachment in adolescents. *Journal of Obstetric, Gynecologic, and Neonatal Nursing, 27*(4), 420-430.

Brazelton, T. (1995). Working with families: Opportunities for early intervention. *Pediatric Clinics of North America, 42*(1), 1.

Brazelton, T., & Nugent, J. (1996). *Neonatal behavioural assessment scale* (3rd ed.). London: MacKeith.

Brewaeys, A., Devroey, P., Helmerhorst, F., Van Hall, E., & Ponjaert, I. (1995). Lesbian mothers who conceived after donor insemination: A follow-up study. *Human Reproduction, 10*(10), 2731-2735.

Camarena, P. et al. (1998). The nature and support of adolescent mothers' life aspirations. *Family Relations, 47*(2), 129-137.

Campbell, J. (1992). Maternity blues: A model for biological research. In J. Hamilton & P. Harberger (eds), *Postpartum psychiatric illness: A picture puzzle*, Philadelphia: University of Pennsylvania Press.

Conley-Jung, C., & Olkin, R. (2001). Mothers with visual impairments who are raising young children. *Journal of Visual Impairment and Blindness, 95*(1), 14-30.

Dalla R., & Gamble, E. (2000). Mother, daughter, teenager—who am I? Perceptions of adolescent maternity in a Navajo reservation community. *Journal of Family Issues, 21*(2), 225-245.

D'Avanzo, C., & Geissler, E. (2003). *Pocket guide to cultural assessment* (3rd ed.). St. Louis: Mosby.

Diehl, K. (1997). Adolescent mothers: What produces positive mother-infant interaction? *MCN American Journal of Maternal Child Nursing, 22*(2), 89-95.

Dochterman, J., & Bulechek, G. (2004). *Nursing interventions classification* (4th ed.). St. Louis: Mosby.

Evans, M., Dick, M., Shields, D., Shook, D., & Smith M. (1998). Postpartum sleep in the hospital: Relationship to taking-in and taking-hold. *Clinical Nursing Research, 7*(4), 379-389.

Farber, R. (2000). Mothers with disabilities: In their own voice. *American Journal of Occupational Therapy, 54*(3), 260-268.

Fowles, E. (1998). The relationship between maternal role attainment and postpartum depression. *Health Care of Women International, 19*(1), 83-94.

Galanti, G. (2003). *Caring for patients of different cultures* (3rd ed.). Philadelphia: University of Pennsylvania Press.

Gartrell, N., Hamilton, J., Banks, A., Mosbacher, D., Reed, N., Sparks, C., & Bishop, H. (1996). The National Lesbian Family Study: Interview with prospective mothers. *American Journal of Orthopsychiatry, 66*(2), 272-281.

Gerson, E. (1973). *Infant behavior in the first year of life*. New York: Raven Press.

Goodman, J. (2004). Paternal postpartum depression, its relationship to maternal postpartum depression and implications for family health. *Journal of Advanced Nursing, 45*(1), 26-35.

Henderson, A., & Brouse, A. (1991). The experiences of new fathers during the first three weeks of life. *Journal of Advanced Nursing, 16*(3), 293-298.

Hockenberry, M. (2003). *Wong's nursing care of infants and children* (7th ed.). St. Louis: Mosby.

Jiménez, S. (1995). The Hispanic culture, folklore, and perinatal health. *Journal of Perinatal Education, 4*(1), 9.

Johnson & Johnson. (1996). *Compendium of postpartum care*. Skillman, NJ: Johnson & Johnson Consumer Products.

Kim-Godwin, Y. (2003). Beliefs and practices among non-Western cultures. *MCN American Journal of Maternal Child Nursing, 28*(2), 74-78.

Klaus, M., & Kennell, J. (1976). *Maternal-infant bonding*. St. Louis: Mosby.

Klaus, M., & Kennell, J. (1982). *Parent-infant bonding* (2nd ed.). St. Louis: Mosby.

Klaus, M., & Kennell, J. (1997). The doula: An essential ingredient of childbirth rediscovered. *Acta Paediatrica, 86*, 1034-1036.

Lipson, J., Dibble, S., & Minarik, P. (1996). *Culture and nursing care: A pocket guide*. San Francisco: UCSF Nursing Press.

Lund, C., Kuller, J. Lane, A., Lott, J., Raines, D., Thomas, K. (2001). Neonatal skin care: Evaluation of the AWHONN/NANN research-based practice project on knowledge and skin care practices. *Journal of Obstetric, Gynecologic, and Neonatal Nursing, 30*(1), 30-40.

Martell, L. (1996). Is Rubin's "taking-in" and "taking-hold" a useful paradigm? *Health Care of Women International, 17*(1), 1-13.

Mercer, R. (1983). Parent-infant attachment. In L. Sonstegard, K. Kowalski, & B. Jennings, (Eds.), *Women's health* (Vol. 2), *Childbearing*. New York: Grune & Stratton.

Mercer, R. (2004). Becoming a mother versus maternal role attainment. *Journal of Nursing Scholarship, 36*(3), 226-232.

Miller, E. (2004). Infant massage: A nurturing welcome to the world. *New Life Journal*, August-September.

Niska, K., Snyder, M., & Lia-Hoagberg, B. (1998). Family ritual facilitates adaptation to parenthood. *Public Health Nursing, 15*(5), 329-337.

O'Reilly, M. (2004). Achieving a new balance: Women's transition to second-time parenthood. *Journal of Obstetric, Gynecologic, and Neonatal Nursing, 33*(4), 455-462.

Osterwell, D. (1991). *Correlates of relationship satisfaction in lesbian couples who are parenting their first child together*. Doctoral dissertation, Berkeley, California, School of Professional Psychology.

Pebley, A., & Rudkin, L. (1999). Grandparents caring for grandchildren: What do we know? *Journal of Family Issues, 20*(2), 218-242.

Reese, S., & Harkless, G. (1996). Divergent themes in maternal experience in women older than 35 years of age. *Applied Nursing Research, 9*(3), 148-153.

Reimann, R. (1999). *Becoming lesbian mothers: Lesbian couples' transition to parenthood*. American Sociological Association proceedings: Washington, DC.

Rogan, F., Shmied, V., Barclay, L., Everitt, L., & Wyllie, A. (1997). Becoming a mother: Developing a new theory of early motherhood. *Journal of Advanced Nursing, 25*(5), 877-885.

Rubin, R. (1961). Basic maternal behavior. *Nursing Outlook, 9*, 683-686.

Sharts-Hopko, N. (1995). Birth in the Japanese context. *Journal of Obstetric, Gynecologic, and Neonatal Nursing, 24*(14), 343-351.

Simmons, T., & Dye, J. (2003). *Grandparents living with grandchildren: 2000*. Internet document available at http://www.census.gov/prod/2003pubs/c2kbr-32.pdf (accessed May 30, 2005).

St. John, W., Cameron, C., & McVeigh, C. (2005). Meeting the challenges of new fatherhood during the early weeks. *Journal of Obstetric, Gynecologic, and Neonatal Nursing, 34*(2), 180-190.

Steinberg, S., Kruckman, L., & Steinberg, S. (2000). Reinventing fatherhood in Japan and Canada. *Social Science & Medicine, 50*(9), 1257-1272.

Stewart, S., & Jambunathan, J. (1996). Hmong women and postpartum depression. *Health Care of Women International, 17*(4), 319-330.

Tomlinson, P. (1996). Marital relationship change in the transition to parenthood: A reexamination as interpreted through transition theory. *Journal of Family Nursing, 2*(3), 286-305.

Troy, N. (2003). Is the significance of postpartum fatigue being overlooked in the lives of women? *MCN American Journal of Maternal Child Nursing, 28*(4), 252-257.

U.S. Department of Health and Human Services, Centers for Disease Control and Prevention. (2005). *Childhood and adolescent immunization schedule.* Internet document available at http://www.cdc.gov/nip/recs/child-schedule.pdf (accessed May 30, 2005).

Wisner, K., Parry, B., & Piontek, C. (2002). Clinical practice: Postpartum depression. *New England Journal of Medicine, 347*(3), 194-199.

Wrasper, C. (1996). Discharge timing and Rubin's concept of puerperal change. *Journal of Perinatal Education, 5*(2), 13-23.

Zlotnick, M. (2000). Infant massage: Building relationships through touch. *International Journal of Childbirth Education*, March.

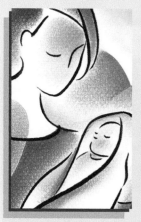

CHAPTER 18

Physiologic and Behavioral Adaptations

KATHRYN RHODES ALDEN

LEARNING OBJECTIVES

- *Discuss the physiologic adaptations that the neonate must make during the period of transition from the intrauterine to the extrauterine environment.*
- *Describe the behavioral adaptations that are characteristic of the newborn during the transition period.*
- *Explain thermoregulation in the neonate and the rationale for preventing heat loss.*
- *Recognize newborn reflexes and differentiate characteristic responses from abnormal responses.*
- *Discuss the sensory and perceptual functioning of the neonate.*

KEY TERMS AND DEFINITIONS

acrocyanosis Peripheral cyanosis; blue color of hands and feet in most infants at birth that may persist for 7 to 10 days

brown fat Source of heat unique to neonates that is capable of greater thermogenic activity than ordinary fat; deposits are found around the adrenals, kidneys, and neck, between the scapulae, and behind the sternum for several weeks after birth

caput succedaneum Swelling of the tissue over the presenting part of the fetal head caused by pressure during labor

cephalhematoma Extravasation of blood from ruptured vessels between a skull bone and its external covering, the periosteum; swelling is limited by the margins of the cranial bone affected (usually parietals)

cold stress Excessive loss of heat that results in increased respirations and nonshivering thermogenesis to maintain core body temperature

erythema toxicum Innocuous pink papular neonatal rash of unknown cause, with superimposed vesicles appearing within 24 to 48 hours after birth and resolving spontaneously within a few days

habituation Psychologic and physiologic phenomenon whereby the response to a constant or repetitive stimulus is decreased

hyperbilirubinemia Elevation of unconjugated serum bilirubin concentrations

meconium Greenish black, viscous first stool formed during fetal life from the amniotic fluid and its constituents, intestinal secretions (including bilirubin), and cells (shed from the mucosa).

milia Small, white sebaceous glands, appearing as tiny, white, pinpoint papules on the forehead, nose, cheeks, and chin of the neonate

mongolian spots Bluish gray or dark nonelevated pigmented areas usually found over the lower back and buttocks present at birth in some infants, primarily nonwhite; usually fade by school age

physiologic jaundice Yellow tinge to skin and mucous membranes in response to increased serum levels of unconjugated bilirubin; not usually apparent until after 24 hours; also called *neonatal jaundice, physiologic hyperbilirubinemia*

sleep-wake states Variation in states of newborn consciousness from deep sleep to extreme irritability

surfactant Phosphoprotein necessary for normal respiratory function that prevents alveolar collapse (atelectasis)

thermogenesis Creation or production of heat, especially in the body

thermoregulation Control of temperature; a balance between heat loss and heat production

transition period Period from birth to 4 to 6 hours later; infant passes through period of reactivity, sleep, and second period of reactivity

vernix caseosa Protective gray-white fatty substance of cheesy consistency covering the fetal skin

The neonatal period includes the time from birth through day 28 of life. During this time the neonate must make many physiologic and behavioral adaptations to extrauterine life. Physiologic adjustment tasks are those that involve (1) establishing and maintaining respirations; (2) adjusting to circulatory changes; (3) regulating temperature; (4) ingesting, retaining, and digesting nutrients; (5) eliminating waste; and (6) regulating weight. Behavioral tasks include (1) establishing a regulated behavioral tempo independent of the mother, which involves self-regulation of arousal, self-monitoring of changes in state, and patterning of sleep; (2) processing, storing, and organizing multiple stimuli; and (3) establishing a relationship with caregivers and the environment. The term infant usually makes these adjustments with little or no difficulty.

TRANSITION TO EXTRAUTERINE LIFE

Infants undergo phases of instability during the first 6 to 8 hours after birth. These phases are collectively called the transition period between intrauterine and extrauterine existence. To detect disorders in adaptation soon after birth, nurses must be aware of normal features of the transition period. Labor and immediate neonatal events stimulate a sympathetic response reflected by changes in heart rate, color, respiration, motor activity, gastrointestinal function, and temperature of the infant. Behavioral characteristics also change during this transition period.

The first phase of the transition period lasts up to 30 minutes after birth and is called the *first period of reactivity*. The newborn's heart rate increases rapidly to 160 to 180 beats/min but gradually decreases after 30 minutes or so to a baseline rate of between 100 and 120 beats/min. Respirations are irregular, with a rate between 60 and 80 breaths/min. Crackles may be present on auscultation; audible grunting, nasal flaring, and retractions of the chest also may be noted. In addition, brief periods of apnea (periodic breathing) may occur. Coincident with these changes in heart rate and respiratory rate, the infant is alert. The infant's behavior is marked by spontaneous startle reactions, tremors, crying, and movement of the head from side to side. This characteristic exploratory behavior is accompanied by a decrease in body temperature and a generalized increase in motor activity, with an increase in muscle tone. Gastrointestinal manifestations of this first period of reactivity include the onset of bowel sounds, passage of meconium, and production of saliva.

Between 30 minutes and 2 hours after birth, the neonate enters a period of decreased responsiveness, characterized by a marked decrease in motor activity and/or sleep. Respirations are rapid and shallow with a rate of up to 60 breaths/ minute. The heart rate averages 100 to 120 beats/min. At this time the infant's color is pink. This period lasts for 60 to 100 minutes and is followed by a second period of reactivity.

The second period of reactivity occurs roughly between 2 and 8 hours after birth. This period of reactivity lasts from 10 minutes to several hours. The infant becomes more responsive to all types of stimuli. Periods of tachycardia and tachypnea occur, associated with increased muscle tone, skin color, and mucous production. Meconium is commonly passed at this time. As this period diminishes, the infant is relatively stable.

All well newborns experience this transition, regardless of gestational age or type of birth. The length of time the periods last will vary depending on the amount and kind of stress experienced by the neonate before or after birth.

PHYSIOLOGIC ADAPTATIONS

Respiratory System

With the cutting of the umbilical cord, the infant must undergo rapid and complex changes. The most critical adjustment of a newborn at birth is the establishment of respirations. At term the lungs hold approximately 20 ml of fluid per kilogram. Air must be substituted for the fluid that filled the respiratory tract. During normal vaginal birth, some lung fluid is squeezed or drained from the newborn's trachea and lungs. With the first breath of air, the newborn begins a sequence of cardiopulmonary changes.

Initiation of breathing

Initial breathing is probably the result of a reflex triggered by pressure changes, chilling, noise, light, and other sensations related to the birth process. In addition, the chemoreceptors in the aorta and carotid bodies initiate neurologic reflexes when arterial oxygen pressure (PO_2) decreases from

80 to 15 mm Hg, arterial carbon dioxide pressure (P_{CO_2}) increases from 40 to 70 mm Hg, and arterial pH declines. In most cases, an exaggerated respiratory reaction follows within 1 minute of birth, and the infant takes a first gasping breath and cries.

Certain respiratory patterns are characteristic of the normal term newborn. After respirations are established, breaths are shallow and irregular, ranging from 30 to 60 breaths/min, with short periods of apnea (less than 15 seconds). These short periods of apnea occur most often during the active (rapid eye movement [REM]) sleep cycle and decrease in frequency and duration with age. Apneic periods longer than 20 seconds should be evaluated.

NURSE ALERT *Newborn infants are preferential nose breathers. The reflex response to nasal obstruction is to open the mouth to maintain an airway. This response is not present in most infants until 3 weeks after birth; therefore cyanosis or asphyxia may occur with nasal blockage.*

Signs of respiratory distress

Most term infants breathe spontaneously and continue to have normal respirations (Fig. 18-1, *A*). However, infants can manifest other problems through respiratory distress. Signs of respiratory distress may include nasal flaring, retractions (indrawing of tissue between the ribs, below the rib cage, or above the sternum and clavicles), or grunting with expirations. Any increased use of the intercostal muscles may be a sign of distress. Seesaw respirations, instead of normal abdominal respirations, are not normal and should be reported (Fig. 18-1, *B*). Within the first hour after birth the respiratory rate is between 40 and 60 breaths/min and should thereafter range from 30 to 60 breaths/min. A respiratory rate that is less than 30 or greater than 60 breaths/min with the infant at rest must be reported to the pediatrician. The respiratory rate of the infant may be slowed or depressed by the analgesics or anesthetics administered to the mother during labor and birth. Apneic episodes may be related to a number of events (rapid increase in body temperature; hypothermia, low blood glucose, and sepsis) that require careful evaluation. Tachypnea may result from inadequate clearance of lung fluid, or it may be an indication of newborn respiratory distress syndrome (RDS).

Maintaining adequate oxygen supply

During the first hour of life, the pulmonary lymphatics continue to remove large amounts of fluid. Removal of fluid also is a result of the pressure gradient from alveoli to interstitial tissue to blood capillary. Reduced vascular resistance accommodates this flow of lung fluid. Retention of lung fluid may interfere with the infant's ability to maintain adequate oxygenation, especially if other factors (meconium aspiration, congenital diaphragmatic hernia, esophageal atresia with fistula, choanal atresia, congenital cardiac defect, immature alveoli) that compromise respirations are present.

Auscultation of the chest reveals loud, clear breath sounds that seem very near, because little chest tissue intervenes. The ribs of the infant articulate with the spine at a horizontal rather than a downward slope; consequently, the rib cage cannot expand with inspiration as readily as that of an adult. Because neonatal respiratory function is largely a matter of diaphragmatic contraction, abdominal breathing is characteristic of newborns. The newborn infant's chest and abdomen rise simultaneously with inspiration (Fig. 18-1, *A*). Characteristics of the respiratory system of the neonate and the effects of these characteristics on respiratory function are listed in Table 18-1.

The alveoli of the term infant's lungs are lined with surfactant, a protein manufactured in type II cells of the lungs. Lung expansion is largely dependent on chest wall contraction and adequate presence of secretion of surfactant. Surfactant reduces surface tension, therefore reducing the pressure required to keep the alveoli open with inspiration, and prevents total alveolar collapse on exhalation, thereby maintaining alveolar stability.

Cardiovascular System

The cardiovascular system changes markedly after birth. The infant's first breaths, combined with increased alveolar capillary distention, inflate the lungs and reduce pulmonary vascular resistance to the pulmonary blood flow from the pulmonary arteries. Pulmonary artery pressure drops, and pressure in the right atrium declines. Increased pulmonary blood flow from the left side of the heart increases pressure in the left atrium, which causes a functional closure of the foramen ovale. During the first few days of life, crying may

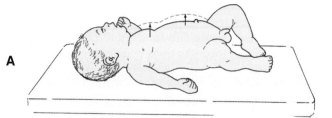
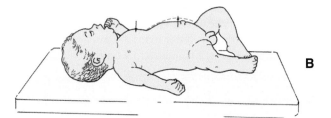

Fig. 18-1 Comparison of normal and seesaw respirations. **A,** Normal respiration. Chest and abdomen rise with inspiration. **B,** Seesaw respiration. Chest wall retracts and abdomen rises with inspiration. (Courtesy Mead Johnson & Co., Evansville, IN.)

Characteristics of the Respiratory System of the Neonate

CHARACTERISTIC	EFFECT ON FUNCTION
Decreased lung elastic tissue and recoil	Decreased lung compliance requiring higher pressures and more work to expand; increased risk of atelectasis
Reduced diaphragm movement and maximal force potential	Less effective respiratory movement; difficulty generating negative intrathoracic pressures; risk of atelectasis
Tendency to nose breathe; altered position of larynx and epiglottis	Enhanced ability to synchronize swallowing and breathing; risk of airway obstruction; possibly more difficult to intubate
Small compliant airway passages with higher airway resistance; immature reflexes	Risk of airway obstruction and apnea
Increased pulmonary vascular resistance with sensitive pulmonary arterioles	Risk of ductal shunting and hypoxemia with events such as hypoxia, acidosis, hypothermia, hypoglycemia, and hypercarbia
Increased oxygen consumption	Increased respiratory rate and work of breathing; risk of hypoxia
Increased intrapulmonary right-left shunting	Increased risk of atelectasis with wasted ventilation; lower P_{CO_2}
Immaturity of pulmonary surfactant system in immature infants	Increased risk of atelectasis and respiratory distress syndrome; increased work of breathing
Immature respiratory control	Irregular respirations with periodic breathing; risk of apnea; inability to rapidly alter depth of respirations

From Blackburn, S. (2003). *Maternal, fetal, & neonatal physiology: A clinical perspective* (2nd ed.). St. Louis: Saunders.

reverse the flow through the foramen ovale temporarily and lead to mild cyanosis.

The ductus arteriosus begins to constrict as pulmonary circulation increases and arterial oxygen tension increases. In term infants the ductus arteriosus functionally closes within 24 hours; permanent closure may take several weeks. With the clamping and severing of the cord, the umbilical arteries, umbilical vein, and ductus venosus are functionally closed and are converted into ligaments within 2 to 3 months (Kliegman, 2002). Table 18-2 summarizes the cardiovascular changes at birth.

Heart rate and sounds

The term newborn has a resting heart rate between 100 and 160 beats/min, with brief fluctuations above and below these values, usually noted during sleeping and waking states. Shortly after the first cry the infant's heart rate may accelerate as high as 180 beats/min. The range of the heart rate in the term infant is about 85 to 100 beats/min during deep sleep and 120 to 160 beats/min while the infant is awake. A heart rate of 180 beats/min is not unusual when the infant cries. A heart rate that is either high (more than 160 beats/min) or low (fewer than 100 beats/min) should be reevaluated within 30 minutes to 1 hour or when the activity of the infant changes. Immediately after birth the heart rate can be palpated by grasping the base of the umbilical cord.

By term the infant's heart lies midway between the crown of the head and the buttocks, and the axis is more transverse than that in an adult (Fig. 18-2). The apical impulse (point of maximal impulse [PMI]) in the newborn is at the fourth intercostal space and to the left of the midclavicular line. The PMI is often visible because of the thin chest wall.

Apical pulse rates should be determined for all infants. Auscultation should be for a full minute, preferably when the infant is asleep. An irregular heart rate is not uncommon in the first few hours of life. After this time an irregular heart rate not attributed to changes in activity or respiratory pattern should be further evaluated.

Heart sounds during the neonatal period are of higher pitch, shorter duration, and greater intensity than those during adult life. The first sound is typically louder and duller than the second sound, which is sharp. Transient murmurs are common during the first few hours after birth. Most heart murmurs heard during the first few days of life have no pathologic significance; they usually result from a patent ductus arteriosus, tricuspid regurgitation, or the acute angle of the pulmonary artery bifurcation (Lissauer, 2002). If a murmur is present, it is important to note the presence of other signs of cardiovascular dysfunction such as tachypnea, tachycardia, pallor, cyanosis, absence of peripheral pulses, or poor perfusion (Miller & Newman, 2005).

Blood pressure

The newborn infant's average systolic blood pressure (BP) is 60 to 80 mm Hg, and the average diastolic pressure is 40 to 50 mm Hg. A decrease in systolic BP of approximately 15 mm Hg during the first hour of life is common. Neonates are considered hypotensive if the mean BP is less than the gestational age. Hypertension is present if the mean pressure exceeds 50 to 70 mm Hg (Sniderman & Taeusch, 2005). Crying and movement result in changes in BP,

TABLE 18-2

Cardiovascular Changes at Birth

PRENATAL STATUS	POSTBIRTH STATUS	ASSOCIATED FACTORS
PRIMARY CHANGES		
Pulmonary circulation: high pulmonary vascular resistance, increased pressure in right ventricle and pulmonary arteries	Low pulmonary vascular resistance; decreased pressure in right atrium, ventricle, and pulmonary arteries	Expansion of collapsed fetal lung with air
Systemic circulation: low pressures in left atrium, ventricle, and aorta	High systemic vascular resistance; increased pressure in left atrium, ventricle, and aorta	Loss of placental blood flow
SECONDARY CHANGES		
Umbilical arteries: patent, carrying of blood from hypogastric arteries to placenta	Functionally closed at birth; obliteration by fibrous proliferation possibly taking 2-3 mo, distal portions becoming lateral vesicoumbilical ligaments, proximal portions remaining open as superior vesicle arteries	Closure preceding that of umbilical vein, probably accomplished by smooth muscle contraction in response to thermal and mechanical stimuli and alteration in oxygen tension, mechanically severed with cord at birth
Umbilical vein: patent, carrying of blood from placenta to ductus venosus and liver	Closed, becoming ligamentum teres hepatis after obliteration	Closure shortly after umbilical arteries, hence blood from placenta possibly entering neonate for short period after birth, mechanically severed with cord at birth
Ductus venosus: patent, connection of umbilical vein to inferior vena cava	Closed, becoming ligamentum venosum after obliteration	Loss of blood flow from umbilical vein
Ductus arteriosus: patent, shunting of blood from pulmonary artery to descending aorta	Functionally closed almost immediately after birth, anatomic obliteration of lumen by fibrous proliferation requiring 1-3 mo, becoming ligamentum arteriosum	High systemic resistance increasing aortic pressure; low pulmonary resistance reducing pulmonary arterial pressure Increased oxygen content of blood in ductus arteriosus creating vasospasm of its muscular wall
Foramen ovale: formation of a valve opening that allows blood to flow directly to left atrium (shunting of blood from right to left atrium)	Functionally closed at birth, constant apposition gradually leading to fusion and permanent closure within a few months or years in majority of persons	Increased pressure in left atrium and decreased pressure in right atrium causing closure of valve over foramen

especially in the systolic pressure. BP also is sensitive to the changes in blood volume that occur with the adaptations in circulation. The measurement of BP is best accomplished with a Doppler device and while the infant is at rest. The correct-size BP cuff must be used for accurate measurement of an infant's BP.

Blood volume

The blood volume of the newborn depends on the amount of blood transferred placentally. The blood volume of the term infant is about 80 to 85 ml/kg of body weight. Immediately after birth the total blood volume averages 300 ml, but this volume can increase by as much as 100 ml, depending on the length of time the infant is attached to the placenta. The preterm infant has a proportionately greater blood volume than that of the term newborn. This occurs because the preterm infant has a greater plasma volume, not a greater red blood cell (RBC) mass (Hockenberry, 2003; Luchtman-Jones, Schwartz, & Wilson, 2002).

Early or late clamping of the umbilical cord changes circulatory dynamics of the newborn. Early clamping of the cord reduces the mean blood volume, whereas late clamping expands the blood volume from the so-called *placental transfusion*. This, in turn, causes an increase in heart size, higher systolic BP, and increased respiratory rate.

Signs of risk for cardiovascular problems

Close monitoring of the infant's vital signs is important for early detection of impending problems. Persistent tachycardia (more than 160 beats/min) may indicate RDS, whereas persistent bradycardia (less than 120 beats/min) may be a sign of a congenital heart block. Any prolonged cyanosis other than in the hands or feet may indicate respiratory

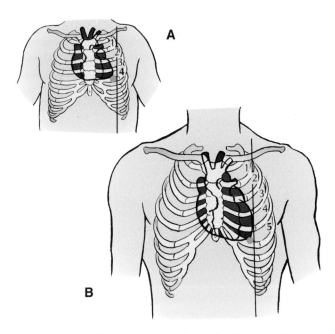

Fig. 18-2 Differences in locations of apical pulse in newborn versus in adult. **A,** Neonate. **B,** Adult.

and/or cardiac problems. A difference between upper and lower extremity BP may be an early sign of coarctation of the aorta. The presence of jaundice may indicate ABO or Rh factor problems (see Chapter 27).

Hematopoietic System

The hematopoietic system of the newborn exhibits certain variations from that of the adult. Levels of RBCs and leukocytes differ, but platelet levels are relatively the same.

Red blood cells

Because fetal circulation is less efficient at oxygen exchange than the lungs, the fetus needs additional RBCs for transport of oxygen in utero. Therefore at birth the average levels of RBCs and hemoglobin are higher than those in the adult. Cord blood of the term newborn may have a hemoglobin concentration of 14 to 24 g/dl (mean, 17 g/dl). The hematocrit ranges from 44% to 64% (mean, 55%). The RBC count is correspondingly elevated, ranging from 4.8 to 7.1 mm^3 (mean, 5.14). By 2 weeks of age, slight decreases in hemoglobin (mean, 16.5 g/dl), hematocrit (mean, 50%), and RBC count (mean, 4.2 mm^3) are found. At 3 months, hemoglobin ranges from 9.5 g/dl to 14.5 g/dl (mean, 12), and hematocrit ranges from 31% to 41% (mean, 36%) (Luchtman-Jones, Schwartz, & Wilson, 2002; Scott, 2002).

The initial blood values may be affected by delayed clamping of the cord, which results in an increase in hemoglobin level, RBC count, and hematocrit value. The source of the sample is another important factor because capillary blood yields higher values than venous blood. The time after birth when the blood sample was obtained also is significant; the slight increase in RBC numbers after birth is followed by a substantial decrease. At birth 80% of the infant's blood contains fetal hemoglobin, but because of the shorter life span of the cells containing fetal hemoglobin, the percentage decreases to 55% by 5 weeks and to 5% by 20 weeks. Iron stores are generally sufficient to sustain normal RBC production for 5 months, and therefore mild, brief anemia is not serious.

Leukocytes

Leukocytosis, with a white blood cell (WBC) count of approximately 18,000/mm^3 (range, 9000 to 30,000/mm^3), is normal at birth. The number of WBCs, predominantly polymorphonuclear leukocytes, increases to 23,000 to 24,000/mm^3 during the first day after birth. This early high WBC count of the newborn decreases rapidly, and a resting level of 12,000/mm^3 is normally maintained during the neonatal period (Scott, 2002). Serious infection is not well tolerated by the newborn, and a marked increase in the WBC count is unlikely, even in critical sepsis (infection). In most instances, sepsis is accompanied by a decline in WBCs, particularly in neutrophils. The activity of the bone marrow is accurately reflected by the number of circulating cells, both RBCs and WBCs.

Platelets

The platelet count ranges between 150,000 and 300,000/mm^3 and is essentially the same in newborns as in adults. The levels of factors II, VII, IX, and X, found in the liver, are decreased during the first few days of life because the newborn cannot synthesize vitamin K. However, bleeding tendencies in the newborn are rare, and unless the vitamin K deficiency is great, clotting is sufficient to prevent hemorrhage (Kliegman, 2002).

Blood groups

The infant's blood group is genetically determined and established early in fetal life. However, during the neonatal period, a gradual increase occurs in the strength of the agglutinogens present in the RBC membrane. Cord blood samples may be used to identify the infant's blood type and Rh status.

Thermogenic System

Next to establishing respirations, heat regulation is most critical to the newborn's survival. Thermoregulation is the maintenance of balance between heat loss and heat production. Newborns attempt to stabilize their internal body temperatures within a narrow range. Hypothermia from excessive heat loss is a common and dangerous problem in neonates. The newborn infant's ability to produce heat (thermogenesis) often approaches that of the adult; however, the tendency toward rapid heat loss in a cold environment is increased in the newborn and poses a hazard.

Thermogenesis

The shivering mechanism of heat production is rarely operable in the newborn. Nonshivering thermogenesis is accomplished primarily by metabolism of brown fat, which is unique to the newborn, and by increased metabolic activity in the brain, heart, and liver. Brown fat is located in superficial deposits in the interscapular region and axillae, as well as in deep deposits at the thoracic inlet, along the vertebral column, and around the kidneys. Brown fat has a richer vascular and nerve supply than does ordinary fat. Heat produced by intense lipid metabolic activity in brown fat can warm the newborn by increasing heat production as much as 100%. Reserves of brown fat, usually present for several weeks after birth, are rapidly depleted with cold stress. The less mature the infant, the less reserve of this essential fat is available at birth.

Heat loss

Heat loss in the newborn occurs by four modes:

- *Convection* is the flow of heat from the body surface to cooler ambient air. Because of heat loss by convection, the ambient temperatures in the nursery are kept at approximately 24° C, and newborns are wrapped to protect them from the cold.
- *Radiation* is the loss of heat from the body surface to a cooler solid surface not in direct contact but in relative proximity. Nursery cribs and examining tables are placed away from outside windows to prevent this type of heat loss.
- *Evaporation* is the loss of heat that occurs when a liquid is converted to a vapor. In the newborn, heat loss by evaporation occurs as a result of vaporization of moisture from the skin. The process is invisible and is known as *insensible water loss* (IWL). This heat loss can be intensified by failure to dry the newborn directly after birth or by too-slow drying of the infant after a bath.
- *Conduction* is the loss of heat from the body surface to cooler surfaces in direct contact. When admitted to the nursery, the newborn is placed in a warmed crib to minimize heat loss.

Loss of heat must be controlled to protect the infant. Control of such modes of heat loss is the basis of caregiving policies and techniques.

Temperature regulation

Anatomic and physiologic differences among the newborn, child, and adult are notable. The newborn's thermal insulation is less than that of an adult. The blood vessels are closer to the surface of the skin. Changes in environmental temperature alter the temperature of the blood, thereby influencing temperature regulation centers in the hypothalamus. Newborns have larger body surface–to–body weight (mass) ratios than do children and adults. The flexed position of the newborn helps guard against heat loss because it diminishes the amount of body surface exposed to the environment. Infants also can reduce the loss of internal heat through the body surface by constricting peripheral blood vessels.

Changes in environmental temperature can disturb body temperature. This may lead to serious consequences in the newborn. Brown fat metabolism is activated in response to changes in environmental temperature perceived by the thermal sensors in the newborn's skin, even when the temperature of the newborn is unchanged. When exposed to cold, the newborn may cry, become restless, and increase muscular activity to generate heat. However, crying increases workload and energy expenditure. Newborns also may increase their respiratory rates in an attempt to stimulate muscular activity.

Cold stress imposes metabolic and physiologic demands on all infants, regardless of gestational age and condition. The respiratory rate increases in response to the increased need for oxygen. In the cold-stressed infant, oxygen consumption and energy are diverted from maintaining normal brain and cardiac function and growth to thermogenesis for survival. If the infant cannot maintain an adequate oxygen tension, vasoconstriction jeopardizes pulmonary perfusion. As a consequence, the partial pressure of arterial oxygen (PO_2) is decreased, and the blood pH declines. These changes aggravate existing RDS. Moreover, decreased pulmonary perfusion and oxygen tension may maintain or reopen the right-to-left shunt across the patent ductus arteriosus.

The basal metabolic rate increases with cold stress (Fig. 18-3). If cold stress is protracted, anaerobic glycolysis occurs, resulting in increased production of acids. Metabolic acidosis develops, and if a defect in respiratory function is present,

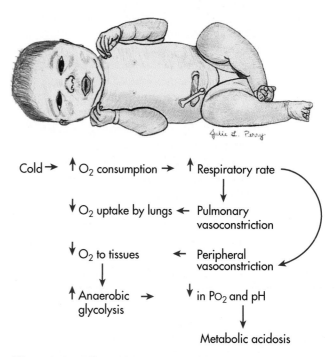

Cold → ↑ O_2 consumption → ↑ Respiratory rate

↓ O_2 uptake by lungs ← Pulmonary vasoconstriction

↓ O_2 to tissues ← Peripheral vasoconstriction

↑ Anaerobic glycolysis → ↓ in PO_2 and pH

Metabolic acidosis

Fig. 18-3 Effects of cold stress. When an infant is stressed by cold, oxygen consumption increases and pulmonary and peripheral vasoconstriction occur, thereby decreasing oxygen uptake by the lungs and oxygen to the tissues; anaerobic glycolysis increases; and there is a decrease in PO_2 and pH, leading to metabolic acidosis.

CD: Skill—Thermoregulation

respiratory acidosis also develops. Excessive fatty acids displace the bilirubin from the albumin-binding sites. The resulting increased level of circulating unbound bilirubin heightens the risk of kernicterus even at serum bilirubin levels of 10 mg/dl or less.

Hyperthermia develops more rapidly in the newborn than in the adult because of the larger surface area of an infant. Although newborns have six times as many sweat glands per unit area as adults, these glands do not function. Serious overheating of the newborn can cause cerebral damage from dehydration or heat stroke and death.

Renal System

At term gestation, the kidneys occupy a large portion of the posterior abdominal wall. The bladder lies close to the anterior abdominal wall and is an abdominal as well as a pelvic organ. In the newborn, almost all palpable masses in the abdomen are renal in origin.

A small quantity (approximately 40 ml) of urine is usually present at birth in the bladder of a term infant. Newborns usually void within the first 24 hours of life.

NURSE ALERT *Noting and recording the first voiding is important. An infant who has not voided by 24 hours of age should be assessed for adequacy of fluid intake, bladder distention, restlessness, and symptoms of pain. The pediatrician also should be notified.*

The frequency of voiding varies according to the amount of fluid intake. It is expected that infants will void at least once during the first 24 hours, twice during the second 24 hours, and three times during the third 24 hours. Formula-fed infants may void more frequently; however, in breastfed infants, the urine output increases after the third or fourth day when the mother's milk has "come in." After the fourth day of life, all newborns should have at least six to eight voidings of straw-colored urine every 24 hours.

Term infants are unable to concentrate urine; therefore the specific gravity of the urine may range from 1.001 to 1.020 (Pagana & Pagana, 2002). The ability to concentrate urine fully is attained by about age 3 months. After the first voiding, the infant's urine may appear cloudy (because of mucos content) and have a much higher specific gravity, which decreases as fluid intake increases. Normal urine during early infancy is usually straw colored and almost odorless. Sometimes pink-tinged stains (brick dust) appear on the diaper. These stains are caused by uric acid crystals and are normal during the first few days, but if seen later can be a sign of dehydration. Blood may be found on a diaper of a female infant. This *pseudomenstruation* is caused by the withdrawal of maternal hormones. Male infants may have some minimal bloody spotting from a circumcision. If there is no apparent cause of bleeding, the physician should be notified.

Loss of fluid through urine, feces, lungs, increased metabolic rate, and limited fluid intake results in a 5% to 10% loss of the birth weight (weight loss greater than 7% should be evaluated by the health care provider). This usually occurs during the first 3 to 5 days of life. If the mother is breastfeeding and her milk supply has not come in yet (which happens on the third or fourth day after birth), the neonate is usually protected from dehydration by its increased extracellular fluid volume. The neonate should regain the birth weight within 14 days after birth.

Because renal thresholds are low in the infant, bicarbonate concentration and buffering capacity are decreased, which may lead to acidosis and electrolyte imbalance.

Fluid and electrolyte balance

Approximately 40% of the body weight of the newborn is extracellular fluid. Each day the newborn takes in and excretes roughly 600 to 700 ml of fluid, which is 20% of the total body fluid or 50% of the extracellular fluid. The glomerular filtration rate of a newborn is approximately 30% to 50% that of the adult. This results in a decreased ability to remove nitrogenous and other waste products from the blood.

Sodium reabsorption is decreased as a result of a reduced sodium- or potassium-activated adenosine triphosphatase (ATPase) activity. The decreased ability to excrete excessive sodium results in hypotonic urine compared with plasma, with a higher concentration of sodium, phosphates, chloride, and organic acids and a lower concentration of bicarbonate ions. The infant has a higher renal threshold for glucose.

Signs of risk for renal system problems

The renal system has a wide range of functions, and dysfunction can result from physiologic abnormalities ranging from the lack of a steady stream of urine to gross anomalies. Gross anomalies such as hypospadias and exstrophy of the bladder can be identified easily at birth. Enlarged or cystic kidneys may be identified as masses during abdominal palpation. Some kidney anomalies also can be detected in utero by ultrasound examination of the pregnant woman.

Gastrointestinal System

The term newborn is capable of swallowing, digesting, metabolizing, and absorbing proteins and simple carbohydrates, and emulsifying fats. With the exception of pancreatic amylase, the characteristic enzymes and digestive juices are present even in low-birth-weight neonates.

In the adequately hydrated infant the mucous membrane of the mouth is moist and pink. The hard and soft palates are intact. Retention cysts, small whitish areas (Epstein's pearls), may be found on the gum margins and at the juncture of the hard and soft palate. The cheeks are full because of well-developed sucking pads. These, like the labial tubercles (sucking calluses) on the upper lip, disappear when the sucking period is over, around the age of 12 months.

Even though sucking motions in utero have been recorded by ultrasonography, these motions are not coordinated in any infant who weighs less than 1500 g at birth or is born before 32 weeks of gestation. Sucking behavior is

BACKGROUND

- Early, continuous maternal-infant contact after birth is our evolutionary norm. Until comparatively recently, separation of mothers and infants at birth was routine within the Western medical model. For the mother, touch, warmth, and odor are vagal stimulants that release oxytocin, which increases social responsiveness, decreases anxiety, and increases the temperature around the breasts. The newborn in the first awake-alert period has a heightened response to maternal smell. During the sensitive minutes and hours after birth, close contact primes the synchronicity between mother and infant. Skin-to-skin contact (SSC) for more than 50 minutes after birth leads to an eightfold increase in spontaneous nursing and may be a critical component in breastfeeding success. Mothers of premature infants benefit from SSC by improved bonding and confidence, and thus duration of breastfeeding is increased. (See "Kangaroo Care for Low-Birth-Weight Infants," Evidence-Based Practice box in Chapter 27.)

OBJECTIVES

- Reviewers sought to examine whether early SSC results in beneficial or adverse maternal and infant outcomes. Specific outcomes to be examined included:
  1 Breastfeeding duration and problems
  2 Maternal bonding and attachment behaviors (en face position [eye-to-eye contact while being held], kissing, smiling, holding, and encompassing)
  3 Maternal psychologic changes (anxiety, self-efficacy, parenting competence)
  4 Infant physiologic changes (temperature, respiratory rate, heart rate, and blood glucose)
  5 Infant behavioral changes (crying and grimacing)
  6 Other outcomes, such as length of stay, cost, and long-term morbidity

METHODS
Search Strategy

- The reviewers searched MEDLINE and Cochrane Central Register of Controlled Trials (CENTRAL). Search keywords were *baby, infant, newborn, neonate, infant care, mother-child relations, mothers, maternal behavior, infant behavior, neonatal, nursing, breastfeeding, lactation, monitoring physiologic, heart rate, respiration, skin temperature, object attachment, touch, therapeutic touch, early contact, immediate contact, kangaroo,* and *skin-to-skin.* Reviewers selected 17 studies, involving a total of 806 women from both upper and lower socioeconomic classes. The studies, dating from 1977 to 1999, were from Canada, Guatemala, Spain, Sweden, Taiwan, and the United States. All were controlled trials. The intervention was some protocol for SSC, with the naked or diapered infant placed on the mother's chest and covered with a warmed blanket. The controls received standard postpartum care. Sixteen studies used random assignments, while one was quasi-random (assignment not based on patient or clinician preference).

Statistical Analyses

- Reviewers performed meta\analyses of studies with comparable outcomes. The reviewers then compared outcomes to see if the outcomes influenced one another.

FINDINGS

- There seemed to be a "golden 2 hours," beginning immediately after birth, that resulted in maximum benefit. Spontaneous, effective suckling occurred at about 55 minutes and lasted through the following hour. More effective suckling was associated with long-term breastfeeding success. Significantly less breast engorgement occurred in the SSC group than with standard care. The SSC group was twice as likely as controls to still be breastfeeding at 3 months. Breastfeeding was also more likely in the SSC group at 1 year, but not significantly so. The benefits to breastfeeding were significant even if SSC was delayed by up to 24 hours, but they were most notable when SSC was instituted immediately after birth. Mothers in the SSC group showed significantly more maternal attachment behavior than controls. Studies found that mothers in the SSC group practiced more affectionate love touch during breastfeeding at 36 to 48 hours, kissed the infant more at 3 months, and increased en face positioning, holding, and touching—effects that persisted up to a year later. Newborns in the SSC group had significantly higher temperatures, with less variability, and remained in the thermoneutral zone. Blood glucose was significantly higher and respiratory rate was significantly lower in the SSC group, demonstrating conservation of energy. Heart rate was also decreased with SSC, but not significantly. Infants in the SCC group showed significantly less crying and grimacing than the controls. This is important for the preterm infant, for whom crying causes hypoxemia, fluctuating cerebral blood flow and risk for hemorrhage, intracranial pressure, and wasted calories.

LIMITATIONS

- It would be difficult to blind a randomization such as SSC from the staff and patients. Measured outcomes in the studies varied, making comparison challenging. Protocols also varied. Some SSC was initiated immediately, whereas in other studies SSC was delayed as long as 24 hours. Infant physiologic measurements were done on examination tables instead of in the SSC intervention.

CONCLUSIONS

- By all measures studied, SSC was a beneficial intervention for maternal and infant well-being. No adverse effects of SSC were noted. Our evolutionary norm is strengthened.

IMPLICATIONS FOR PRACTICE

- In particular, SSC during the "golden 2 hours" immediately after birth seems to strengthen bonding and increase success and duration of breastfeeding. Infant physiology is also more favorable with SSC. Effective latching-on and early bonding can strengthen the confidence and decrease the anxiety of a new mother.

IMPLICATIONS FOR FURTHER RESEARCH

- More research on SSC effects with preterm and cesarean births would be useful. There is a need to standardize the measures in future trials, especially of maternal emotional well-being and attachment behaviors.

Reference: Anderson, G., Moore, E., Hepworth, J., & Bergman, N. (2003). Early skin-to-skin contact for mothers and their healthy newborn infants. *The Cochrane Database of Systematic Reviews,* Issue 2, 2003. Art.No.: CD003519.

influenced by neuromuscular maturity, maternal medications and anesthetics received during labor and birth, and the type of initial feeding.

A special mechanism present in normal newborns coordinates the breathing, sucking, and swallowing reflexes necessary for oral feeding. Sucking in the newborn takes place in small bursts of three to eight sucks at a time. In the term newborn, longer and more efficient sucking attempts occur a few hours after birth. The infant is unable to move food from the lips to the pharynx; therefore placing the nipple (breast or bottle) well inside the baby's mouth is necessary. Peristaltic activity in the esophagus is uncoordinated in the first few days of life. It quickly becomes a coordinated pattern in normal infants, and they swallow easily.

Teeth begin developing in utero, with enamel formation continuing until about age 10 years. Tooth development is influenced by neonatal or infant illnesses, medications, and illnesses of or medications taken by the mother during pregnancy. The fluoride level in the water supply also influences tooth development. Occasionally an infant may be born with one or more teeth. Native American infants are commonly born with teeth.

Bacteria are not present in the infant's gastrointestinal tract at birth. Soon after birth, oral and anal orifices permit entry of bacteria and air. Generally the highest bacterial concentration is found in the lower portion of the intestine, particularly in the large intestine. Normal colonic bacteria are established within the first week after birth, and normal intestinal flora help synthesize vitamin K, folate, and biotin. Bowel sounds can usually be heard shortly after birth.

The capacity of the stomach varies from 30 to 90 ml, depending on the size of the infant. The emptying time for the stomach is highly variable. Several factors, such as time and volume of feedings or type and temperature of food, may affect the emptying time. The cardiac sphincter is immature, and nervous control of the stomach is not well established, so some regurgitation may occur. Regurgitation during the first day or two of life can be decreased by avoiding overfeeding, by burping the infant, and by positioning the infant with the head slightly elevated.

Digestion

The infant's ability to digest carbohydrates, fats, and proteins is regulated by the presence of certain enzymes. Most of these enzymes are functional at birth. One exception is amylase, produced by the salivary glands after about 3 months and by the pancreas at about 6 months of age. This enzyme is necessary to convert starch into maltose. The other exception is lipase, also secreted by the pancreas; it is necessary for the digestion of fat. Therefore the normal newborn is capable of digesting simple carbohydrates and proteins but has a limited ability to digest fats.

Further digestion and absorption of nutrients occur in the small intestine in the presence of pancreatic secretions, secretions from the liver through the common bile duct, and secretions from the duodenal portion of the small intestine.

Stools

At birth the lower intestine is filled with meconium. Meconium is formed during fetal life from the amniotic fluid and its constituents, intestinal secretions (including bilirubin), and cells (shed from the mucosa). Meconium is greenish black and viscous and contains occult blood. The first meconium passed is sterile, but within hours, all meconium passed contains bacteria. The majority of normal term infants pass meconium within the first 12 hours of life, and almost all do so by 24 hours. Stools change in color and consistency over the first 2 to 3 days as the infant feeds. Breast milk stools are generally more frequent and more liquid than formula stools. They contain small yellow curds, whereas formula stools are more pasty in appearance, with larger green-brown curds. Progressive changes in the appearance of stools and in the stooling pattern indicate a properly functioning gastrointestinal system (Box 18-1). Stooling also is an indicator of the adequacy of nutritional intake. For example, breastfed infants should have at least three stools per 24 hours after day 3 or 4 of life when the mother's milk is in.

Feeding behaviors

Variations occur among infants regarding interest in food, symptoms of hunger, and amount ingested at one time. The amount of food that the infant takes in at any feeding depends on the size, hunger level, and alertness of the infant. When put to breast, some infants feed immediately, whereas others require a longer learning period before breastfeeding is completely effective. Random hand-to-mouth movement and sucking of fingers are well developed at birth and intensified when the infant is hungry. Caregivers should be alert and responsive to these hunger cues.

BOX 18-1

Change in Stooling Patterns of Newborns

MECONIUM
- Infant's first stool is composed of amniotic fluid and its constituents, intestinal secretions, shed mucosal cells, and possibly blood (ingested maternal blood or minor bleeding of alimentary tract vessels)
- Passage of meconium should occur within first 24 to 48 hours, although it may be delayed up to 7 days in very low-birth-weight infants

TRANSITIONAL STOOLS
- Usually appear by third day after initiation of feeding; greenish brown to yellowish brown, thin, and less sticky than meconium; may contain some milk curds

MILK STOOL
- Usually appears by fourth day
- Breastfed infants: stools yellow to golden, pasty in consistency, with an odor similar to that of sour milk
- Formula-fed infants: stools pale yellow to light brown, firmer in consistency, with a more offensive odor

Signs of risk for gastrointestinal problems

The time, color, and character of the infant's first stool should be noted. A lack of passage of stool could indicate bowel obstruction related to conditions such as an inborn error of metabolism (e.g., cystic fibrosis) or a congenital disorder (e.g., Hirschsprung disease or an imperforate anus). An active rectal "wink" reflex (contraction of the anal sphincter muscle in response to touch) usually is a good sign of sphincter tone.

Some infants do not digest specific formulas well. If an infant is allergic to or unable to digest a formula, the stools may become very soft with a high water content that is seen as a distinct water ring around the stool on the diaper. Forceful ejection of stool and a water ring around the stool are signs of diarrhea. Care must be taken to avoid misinterpreting transitional stools for diarrhea. The loss of fluid in diarrhea can rapidly lead to fluid and electrolyte imbalance. Passage of meconium from the vagina or urinary meatus is a sign of a possible fistulous tract from the rectum.

Abdominal distention at birth usually indicates a serious disorder such as a ruptured viscus (from abdominal wall defects) or tumors. Distention that occurs later may be the result of overfeeding or may signal gastrointestinal disorders. A scaphoid (sunken) abdomen with bowel sounds heard in the chest and signs of respiratory distress indicate a diaphragmatic hernia.

The amount and frequency of regurgitation ("spitting up") after feedings must be recorded. Color change, gagging, and projectile (very forceful) vomiting occur in association with esophageal and tracheoesophageal anomalies.

Hepatic System

In the newborn the liver can be palpated about 1 cm below the right costal margin because it is enlarged and occupies about 40% of the abdominal cavity. The infant's liver plays an important role in iron storage, carbohydrate metabolism, conjugation of bilirubin, and coagulation.

Iron storage

The infant's iron store in the liver is proportional to the body weight and, for the term infant, should be sufficient for the first 4 to 6 months. Preterm and small-for-date infants have lower iron stores, which are sufficient for only 2 to 3 months.

Carbohydrate metabolism

At birth the newborn is cut off from its maternal glucose supply and, as a result, has an initial decrease in serum glucose levels. The newborn's increased energy needs, decreased hepatic release of glucose from glycogen stores, increased RBC volume, and increased brain size may initially contribute to the rapid depletion of stored glycogen within the first 24 hours after birth. In most healthy term newborns, blood glucose levels stabilize at 40 to 60 mg/dl during the first several hours after birth; by the third day of life the blood glucose levels should be approximately 60 to 70 mg/dl. The initiation of feedings assists in the stabilization of the newborn's blood glucose levels. If the infant appears to be jittery or has tremors, the blood glucose level should be determined to rule out hypoglycemia.

Conjugation of bilirubin

Bilirubin is a yellow pigment derived from the hemoglobin released with the breakdown of RBCs and the myoglobin in muscle cells. The hemoglobin is phagocytized by the reticuloendothelial cells, converted to bilirubin, and released in an unconjugated form. Unconjugated bilirubin, termed *indirect bilirubin*, is relatively insoluble and almost entirely bound to circulating albumin, a plasma protein. The unbound bilirubin can leave the vascular system and permeate other extravascular tissues (e.g., the skin, sclera, and oral mucous membranes). The resultant yellow coloring is termed *jaundice*.

In the liver the unbound bilirubin is conjugated with glucuronide in the presence of the enzyme glucuronyl transferase. The conjugated form of bilirubin is excreted from liver cells as a constituent of bile. This form is termed *direct bilirubin* and is water soluble. Along with other components of bile, direct bilirubin is excreted into the biliary tract system that carries the bile into the duodenum. Bilirubin is converted to urobilinogen and stercobilinogen within the duodenum by the action of the bacterial flora. Urobilinogen is excreted in urine and feces; stercobilinogen is excreted in the feces (Fig. 18-4). The total serum bilirubin level is the sum

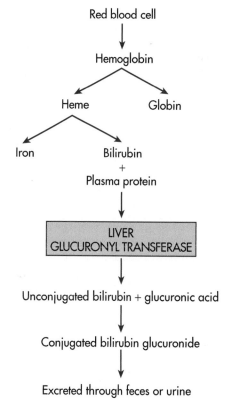

Fig. 18-4 Formation and excretion of bilirubin. (From Hockenberry, M. [2003]. *Wong's nursing care of infants and children* [7th ed.]. St. Louis: Mosby.)

of the levels of both conjugated (direct) and unconjugated (indirect) bilirubin.

Adequate serum albumin-binding sites are available unless the infant has asphyxia neonatorum (respiratory failure in the newborn), cold stress, or hypoglycemia. A mother's prebirth ingestion of medications such as sulfa drugs and aspirin can reduce the amount of serum albumin-binding sites in the newborn. Although the neonate has the functional capacity to convert bilirubin, physiologic hyperbilirubinemia commonly occurs in infants.

Physiologic jaundice

Physiologic jaundice or neonatal jaundice or hyperbilirubinemia occurs in as many as 60% of newborn infants but is more severe in preterm infants (Frank, Cooper, & Merenstein, 2002; Reiser, 2004). The incidence and severity of physiologic jaundice is increased in Asian and Native American infants (Hockenberry, 2003). Although neonatal jaundice is considered benign, bilirubin may accumulate to hazardous levels and lead to a pathologic condition. Physiologic jaundice results from characteristics of normal newborn physiology, such as increased bilirubin production resulting from increased RBC mass, shortened life span of the fetal RBCs, and liver immaturity. Newborns also tend to reabsorb bilirubin from the small intestine.

The infant who is diagnosed with physiologic jaundice appears to be otherwise well and exhibits signs of jaundice after age 24 hours. Jaundice is clinically visible when bilirubin levels reach 5 to 7 mg/dl. Clinically the indirect-reacting bilirubin (unconjugated) is no more than 12 mg/dl by 3 days of age. In preterm infants the peak is higher (15 mg/dl) and tends to occur later. The peak indirect bilirubin level may be higher in breastfed infants (15 to 17 mg/dl). Jaundice is considered to be pathologic if it appears before 24 hours of age, increases more than 0.5 mg/dl/hr, peaks at greater than 13 mg/dl in a term infant, or is associated with anemia and hepatosplenomegaly. Jaundice that appears before 24 hours of age always warrants immediate attention. Pathologic jaundice is usually caused by blood group incompatibility or infection but may rarely be the result of RBC enzyme defects (glucose-6-phosphate dehydrogenase [G6PD], pyruvate kinase), RBC membrane disorders (spherocytosis, ovalocytosis), or hemoglobinopathy (thalassemia) (Frank, Cooper, & Merenstein, 2002).

NURSE ALERT *At any serum bilirubin level, the appearance of jaundice during the first 24 hours of life or persistence beyond day 7 usually indicates a pathologic process.*

Jaundice appears in a cephalocaudal manner. It is generally first noticed in the head, especially the sclera and mucous membranes, and then progresses gradually to the thorax, abdomen, and extremities. It dissipates in the reverse order.

Feeding practices may influence the appearance and degree of physiologic hyperbilirubinemia. Early (within the first hour) and frequent feeding tends to keep the serum bilirubin level low by stimulating intestinal activity (the gastrocolic reflex) and passage of meconium.

Cold stress of the newborn may result in acidosis and increase the level of free fatty acids. In the presence of acidosis, albumin binding of bilirubin is weakened, and bilirubin is freed.

Kernicterus, or bilirubin encephalopathy, is the most serious complication of neonatal hyperbilirubinemia. It occurs when bilirubin is deposited in the basal ganglia and brainstem, disrupting neuronal function and metabolism. Kernicterus usually occurs when bilirubin levels are higher than 25 mg/dl but may be noted with levels that are lower than 20 mg/dl in the presence of sepsis, meningitis, hypothermia, hypoglycemia, prematurity, and bilirubin-displacing drugs. In the acute stage of kernicterus, the infant is lethargic and hypotonic and has a poor suck. If untreated, the infant becomes hypertonic (with backward arching of the neck and trunk), has a high-pitched cry, and may develop fever. If an infant survives kernicterus, there may be residual cerebral palsy, epilepsy, and mental retardation. Although neonatal jaundice is common and kernicterus is rare, in recent years, there has been a resurgence in the number of infants with kernicterus. This may be related to the shortened hospital stays after birth, an increase in the incidence of neonatal jaundice, and a lack of concern and attention to infants exhibiting

? Critical Thinking Exercise

Near Term Infant with Physiologic Jaundice

Veronica gave birth vaginally with the assistance of vacuum extraction to a 7-lb baby boy 36 hours ago. The baby was estimated to be at 35 to 36 weeks of gestation. As a result of the vacuum extraction, the baby's occiput is bruised and slightly edematous (it looked much worse yesterday). For the first 24 hours, he was very sleepy and difficult to arouse for feedings, but for the last 12 hours he has breastfed every 2 to 3 hours for approximately 15 minutes. He has voided twice and passed only one small meconium stool since birth. Randy was holding his baby this morning and stated, "Look at his handsome skin tones! Why, he looks like he has been on vacation and started to get his suntan."

1 Evidence—Is there sufficient evidence to draw conclusions about the baby's skin color?
2 Assumptions—What assumptions can be made about the following?
   a. The baby's skin color
   b. Baby's intake and output since birth
   c. The parents' understanding of physiologic jaundice
3 What implications and priorities for nursing care can be drawn at this time?
4 Does the evidence objectively support your conclusion?
5 Are there alternative perspectives to your conclusion?

signs of jaundice (Maisels, 2001) (see Chapters 19 and 27). The Joint Commission on Accreditation of Healthcare Organizations (2001) issued a sentinel event alert with guidelines for the prevention of neonatal kernicterus by health care workers and institutions.

Noninvasive monitoring of bilirubin by means of cutaneous reflectance measurements (transcutaneous bilirubinometry [TcB]) allows for repetitive estimations of bilirubin levels. These devices work well on dark- and light-skinned infants and correlate fairly well with serum measurements of bilirubin levels in term infants. With shorter maternity stays, the transcutaneous bilirubin measurement can be valuable as an assessment tool for home care follow-up. Transcutaneous bilirubin meters have been significantly improved in the last two decades and may reduce or obviate the need for blood sampling in certain healthy neonates (Briscoe, Clark, & Yoxall, 2002). The TcB monitors provide accurate measurements within 2 to 3 mg/dl in most neonatal populations at serum levels less than 15 mg/dl (American Academy of Pediatrics [AAP], 2004). After phototherapy has been initiated, TcB is no longer useful as a screening tool. It is important to note that the intensity of jaundice is not always related to the degree of hyperbilirubinemia.

The use of hour-specific serum bilirubin levels to predict newborns at risk for rapidly rising levels has now become an official recommendation of the AAP Subcommittee on Hyperbilirubinemia (2004), for the monitoring of healthy neonates at 35 weeks of gestation or greater before discharge from the hospital. A nomogram with three levels (high, intermediate, or low risk) of rising total serum bilirubin may be used at the same time as the routine newborn profile (phenylketonuria [PKU], galactosemia, and others). In many institutions the hour-specific bilirubin risk nomogram is used to determine the infant's risk for development of hyperbilirubinemia requiring medical treatment or closer screening. Risk factors recognized to place infants in the high risk category include gestational age less than 38 weeks, breastfeeding, previous sibling with significant jaundice, and jaundice appearing before discharge. It is now recommended that healthy infants (35 weeks or greater) receive follow-up care and assessment of bilirubin within 3 days of discharge if discharged at less than 24 hours and a risk assessment with tools such as the hour-specific nomogram; likewise, newborns discharged at 24 to 47.9 hours should receive follow-up evaluation within 4 days (96 hours), and those discharged between 48 and 72 hours should receive follow-up within 5 days. (AAP, 2004).

NURSE ALERT *In cases in which the infant is discharged from the hospital before 48 hours after birth or the infant is born at home, a professional attendant may not be available to assess pathologic increases in circulating unbound bilirubin. Therefore all parents need instruction in how to assess jaundice and when to call the health care provider.*

Jaundice associated with breastfeeding

Breastfeeding is associated with an increased incidence of jaundice. Two types have been identified; however, nomenclature may vary among experts. Breastfeeding-associated jaundice (early-onset jaundice) begins at 2 to 4 days of age and occurs in approximately 10% to 25% of breastfed newborns. The jaundice is related to the process of breastfeeding and probably results from decreased caloric and fluid intake by breastfed infants before the milk supply is well established; this is related to decreased hepatic clearance of bilirubin (Blackburn, 2003; Porter & Dennis, 2002). Breast milk jaundice (late-onset jaundice) has been defined as a progressive indirect hyperbilirubinemia beyond the first week of life; it typically occurs after 3 to 5 days of age and peaks by about 2 weeks. Despite high levels of bilirubin that may persist for 3 to 12 weeks, these infants are well. The jaundice may be caused by factors in the breast milk that either inhibit the conjugation or decrease the excretion of bilirubin. Less frequent stooling by breastfed infants may allow for extended time for reabsorption of bilirubin from stools (Blackburn, 2003). (See Chapter 20 for a discussion of this topic.)

Coagulation

The liver plays an important role in blood coagulation. Coagulation factors, which are synthesized in the liver, are activated by vitamin K. The lack of intestinal bacteria needed to synthesize vitamin K results in a transient blood coagulation deficiency between days 2 and 5 of life. The levels of coagulation factors slowly increase to reach adult levels by age 9 months. An injection of vitamin K soon after birth helps prevent clotting problems. Any bleeding problems noted in an infant should be reported immediately, and tests for clotting ordered.

Signs of risk for hepatic system problems

Some problems such as kernicterus and hypoglycemia have already been discussed. The infant's hemoglobin levels must be assessed for anemia. Because infants may develop a coagulation deficiency, a male child who has been circumcised must be observed closely for signs of hemorrhage. Hemorrhage also could be caused by a clotting defect, indicating a serious problem such as hemophilia.

Immune System
Immunity

The cells that provide the infant with immunity are developed early in fetal life; however, they are not activated for several months. For the first 3 months of life the infant is protected by passive immunity received from the mother. Natural barriers such as the acidity of the stomach and the production of pepsin and trypsin, which maintain sterility of the small intestine, are not fully developed until age 3 to

4 weeks. The membrane-protective immunoglobulin A (IgA) is missing from the respiratory and urinary tracts, and unless the newborn is breastfed, it also is absent from the gastrointestinal tract. The infant begins to synthesize IgG, and about 40% of adult levels are reached by age 1 year. Significant concentrations of IgM are produced at birth, and adult levels are reached by age 9 months. The production of IgA, IgD, and IgE is much more gradual, and maximal levels are not attained until early childhood. The infant who is breastfed receives passive immunity through the colostrum and breast milk. The protection provided varies with the age and maturity of the infant and the mother's level of immunity.

Signs of risk for immune system problems

All newborns and preterm newborns especially are at high risk for infection during the first several months of life. During this period, infection is one of the leading causes of morbidity and mortality. The newborn cannot limit the invading pathogen to the portal of entry because of the generalized hypofunctioning of the inflammatory and immune mechanisms. Any unusual discharges from the infant's eyes, nose, mouth, or other orifice must be investigated. If a rash appears, it must be evaluated closely; many normal rashes in the newborn are not associated with any infection. When an infant is in a septic state, the usual response is respiratory distress. Infants must be protected from infections by the use of good handwashing techniques.

Integumentary System

All skin structures are present at birth. The epidermis and dermis are loosely bound and extremely thin. Vernix caseosa (a cheeselike, whitish substance) is fused with the epidermis and serves as a protective covering. The infant's skin is very sensitive and can be easily damaged. The term infant has an erythematous (red) skin for a few hours after birth, after which it fades to its normal color. The skin often appears blotchy or mottled, especially over the extremities. The hands and feet appear slightly cyanotic (acrocyanosis); this is caused by vasomotor instability, capillary stasis, and a high hemoglobin level. Acrocyanosis is normal and appears intermittently over the first 7 to 10 days, especially with exposure to cold.

The healthy term newborn is plump. Subcutaneous fat accumulated during the last trimester acts as insulation. The newborn's skin may be slightly tight, suggesting fluid retention. Fine lanugo hair may be noted over the face, shoulders, and back. Actual edema of the face and ecchymosis (bruising) or petechiae may be present as a result of face presentation or forceps-assisted birth.

Creases can be found on the palms of the hands. The simian line, a single palmar crease, is often found in Asian infants or in infants with Down syndrome. The soles of the feet should be inspected for the number of creases. Premature newborns have few if any creases. Increasing numbers of creases correlate with a greater maturity rating.

Caput succedaneum

Caput succedaneum is a generalized, easily identifiable edematous area of the scalp, most commonly found on the occiput (Fig. 18-5, *A*). With vertex presentation the sustained pressure of the occiput against the cervix results in compression of local vessels, thereby slowing venous return. The slower venous return causes an increase in tissue fluids within the skin of the scalp, and an edematous swelling develops. This boggy edematous swelling, present at birth, extends across suture lines of the fetal skull and disappears spontaneously within 3 to 4 days. Infants who are born with the assistance of vacuum extraction usually have a caput (and bruising) in the area where the cup was applied.

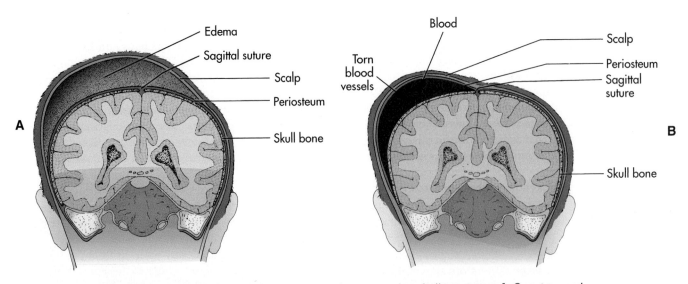

Fig. 18-5   Differences between caput succedaneum and cephalhematoma. **A,** Caput succedaneum: edema of scalp noted at birth; crosses suture lines. **B,** Cephalhematoma: bleeding between periosteum and skull bone appearing within first 2 days; does not cross suture lines.

Cephalhematoma

Cephalhematoma is a collection of blood between a skull bone and its periosteum; therefore a cephalhematoma does not cross a cranial suture line (Fig. 18-5, *B*). Caput succedaneum and cephalhematoma often occur simultaneously.

Bleeding resulting in cephalhematoma may occur with spontaneous birth from pressure against the maternal bony pelvis. Low forceps birth and difficult forceps rotation and extraction also may cause bleeding. This soft, fluctuating, irreducible fullness of cephalhematoma does not pulsate or bulge when the infant cries. It appears several hours or the day after birth and may not become apparent until a caput succedaneum is absorbed. A cephalhematoma is usually largest on the second or third day, by which time the bleeding stops. The fullness of a cephalhematoma spontaneously resolves in 3 to 6 weeks. It is not aspirated because infection may develop if the skin is punctured. As the hematoma resolves, hemolysis of RBCs occurs, and jaundice may result. Hyperbilirubinemia may occur after the newborn is home.

Subgaleal hemorrhage

Subgaleal hemorrhage is bleeding into the subgaleal compartment. The subgaleal compartment is a potential space that contains loosely arranged connective tissue; it is located beneath the galea aponeurosis, the tendinous sheath that connects the frontal and occipital muscles and forms the inner surface of the scalp. The injury occurs as a result of forces that compress and then drag the head through the pelvic outlet (Paige & Carney, 2002). There have been reports of concern regarding the increased use of the vacuum extractor at birth and an association with cases of subgaleal hemorrhage and neonatal mortality (Garas et al., 2001; Ross, Fresquez, & El-Haddad, 2001); however, the rates of such outcomes are reportedly declining (Putta & Spencer, 2000). The bleeding extends beyond bone, often posteriorly into the neck, and continues after birth, with the potential for serious complications such as anemia or hypovolemic shock.

Early detection of the hemorrhage is vital; serial head circumference measurements and inspection of the back of the neck for increasing edema and a firm mass are essential. A boggy scalp, pallor, tachycardia, and increasing head circumference may also be early signs of a subgaleal hemorrhage (Putta & Spencer, 2000). Computerized tomography or magnetic resonance imaging is useful in confirming the diagnosis. Replacement of lost blood and clotting factors is required in acute cases of hemorrhage. Another possible sign of subgaleal hemorrhage is a forward and lateral positioning of the infant's ears because the hematoma extends posteriorly. Monitoring the newborn for changes in level of consciousness and a decrease in the hematocrit are also key to early recognition and management. An increase in serum bilirubin levels may be seen as a result of the degrading blood cells within the hematoma.

Desquamation

Desquamation (peeling) of the skin of the term infant does not occur until a few days after birth. Its presence at birth is an indication of postmaturity.

Sweat and oil glands

Sweat glands are present at birth but do not respond to increases in ambient or body temperature. Some fetal sebaceous (oil) gland hyperplasia and secretion of sebum result from the hormonal influences of pregnancy. Vernix caseosa is a product of the sebaceous glands. Removal of the vernix is followed by desquamation of the epidermis in most infants. Distended, small, white sebaceous glands (milia) may be noticeable on the newborn face.

Mongolian spots

Mongolian spots, bluish-black areas of pigmentation, may appear over any part of the exterior surface of the body, including the extremities. They are more commonly noted on the back and buttocks (Fig. 18-6). These pigmented areas are most frequently noted in babies whose ethnic origins are in the Mediterranean area, Latin America, Asia, or Africa. They are more common in dark-skinned individuals, regardless of race. They fade gradually over months or years. Mongolian spots have no clinical significance but can be mistaken for bruises.

Nevi

Known as "stork bites" or "angel kisses," telangiectatic nevi are pink and easily blanched (Fig. 18-7, *A*). They may appear on the upper eyelids, nose, upper lip, lower occipital area, and nape of the neck. They have no clinical significance and fade by the second year of life.

The strawberry mark, or nevus vasculosus, is a common type of capillary hemangioma. It consists of dilated, newly formed capillaries occupying the entire dermal and subdermal layers, with associated connective tissue hypertrophy. The typical lesion is a raised, sharply demarcated, bright or

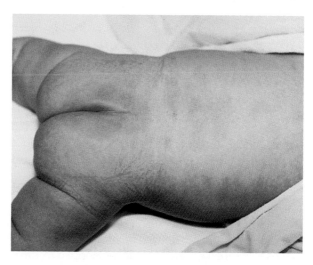

Fig. 18-6 Mongolian spot.

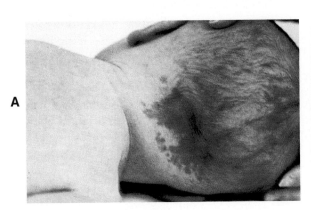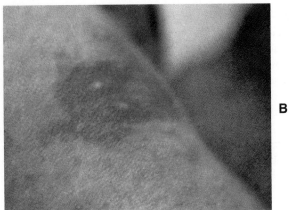

Fig. 18-7 **A,** Telangiectatic nevi (stork bite). **B,** Erythema toxicum (flea bite). (Courtesy Mead Johnson & Co., Evansville, IN.)

dark red, rough-surfaced swelling that resembles a strawberry. Lesions usually are single but may be multiple, with 75% occurring on the head. These lesions can remain until the child is of school age or sometimes even longer.

A port-wine stain, or nevus flammeus, is usually observed at birth and is composed of a plexus of newly formed capillaries in the papillary layer of the corium. It is red to purple; varies in size, shape, and location; and is not elevated. True port-wine stains do not blanch on pressure or disappear. They are most frequently found on the face.

Erythema toxicum

A transient rash, erythema toxicum, is also called *erythema neonatorum, newborn rash,* or *flea bite dermatitis.* It has lesions in different stages: erythematous macules, papules, and small vesicles (Fig. 18-7, *B*). The lesions may appear suddenly anywhere on the body. The rash is thought to be an inflammatory response. Eosinophils, which help decrease inflammation, are found in the vesicles. The rash is found in term neonates (gestational age of 36 weeks or more) during the first 3 weeks after birth. Although the appearance is alarming, the rash has no clinical significance and requires no treatment.

Signs of risk for integumentary problems

Close observation of the newborn's skin color can lead to early detection of potential problems. Any pallor, plethora (deep purplish color from increased circulating RBCs), petechiae, central cyanosis, or jaundice should be noted and described. The skin should be examined for signs of birth injuries, such as forceps marks and lesions related to fetal monitoring. Bruises or petechiae may be present on the head, neck, and face of an infant born with a nuchal cord (cord around the neck) or in an infant who had a face presentation at birth. When bruises are present, the infant's bilirubin levels may become elevated. Petechiae may be present if increased pressure was applied to an area. Petechiae scattered over the infant's body should be reported to the pediatrician because their presence may indicate underlying

problems such as low platelet count or infection. Unilateral or bilateral periauricular papillomas (skin tags) occur fairly frequently. Their occurrence is usually a family trait and of no consequence.

Reproductive System
Female

At birth the ovaries contain thousands of primitive germ cells. These represent the full complement of potential ova; no oogonia form after birth in term infants. The ovarian cortex, which is made up primarily of primordial follicles, occupies a larger portion of the ovary in the female newborn than in the female adult. From birth to sexual maturity the number of ova decreases by approximately 90%.

An increase of estrogen during pregnancy followed by a decrease after birth results in a mucoid vaginal discharge and even some slight bloody spotting (pseudomenstruation). External genitals are usually edematous with increased pigmentation. In term newborn infants the labia majora and minora cover the vestibule (Fig. 18-8, *A*). In preterm infants, the clitoris is prominent, and the labia majora are small and widely separated. Vaginal or hymenal tags are common findings and have no clinical significance. Vernix caseosa may be present between the labia.

If the female was born in the breech position, the labia may be edematous and bruised. The edema and bruising resolve in a few days; no treatment is necessary.

Male

The testes descend into the scrotum by birth in 90% of newborn boys. Although this percentage decreases with premature birth, by 1 year of age the incidence of undescended testes in all boys is less than 1%.

A tight prepuce (foreskin) is common in newborns. The urethral opening may be completely covered by the prepuce, which may not be retractable for 3 to 4 years. Smegma, a white, cheesy substance, is commonly found under the foreskin. Small, white, firm lesions called *epithelial pearls* may be seen at the tip of the prepuce. By 28 to 36 weeks of gestation,

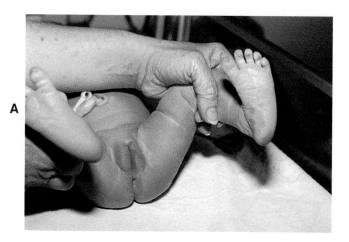 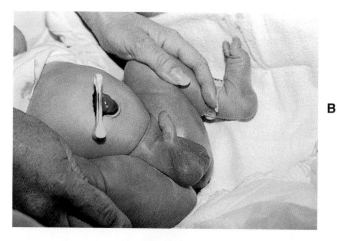

Fig. 18-8   External genitalia. **A**, Genitals in female term infant. Note mucoid vaginal discharge. **B**, Genitals in male infant. Uncircumcised penis. Rugae cover scrotum, indicating term gestation. Cord has been swabbed with ethylene blue to prevent infection. (Courtesy Marjorie Pyle, RNC, Lifecircle, Costa Mesa, CA.)

the testes can be palpated in the inguinal canal, and a few rugae appear on the scrotum. At 36 to 40 weeks of gestation, the testes are palpable in the upper scrotum, and rugae appear on the anterior portion. After 40 weeks, the testes can be palpated in the scrotum, and rugae cover the scrotal sac. The postterm neonate has deep rugae and a pendulous scrotum. The scrotum is usually more deeply pigmented than the rest of the skin (Fig. 18-8, *B*), particularly in darker-skinned infants. Hydroceles, caused by an accumulation of fluid around the testes, may be present. They can be easily transilluminated with a light and usually decrease in size without treatment.

If the male infant was born in a breech presentation, the scrotum may appear very edematous and bruised. The swelling and discoloration resolve within a few days.

Swelling of breast tissue

Swelling of the breast tissue in infants of both sexes is caused by the hyperestrogenism of pregnancy. In a few infants a thin discharge (witch's milk) can be seen. This condition has no clinical significance, requires no treatment, and subsides as the maternal hormones are eliminated from the infant's body within a few days.

The nipples should be symmetric on the chest. Breast tissue and areola size increase with gestation. The areola appears slightly elevated at 34 weeks of gestation. By 36 weeks, a breast bud of 1 to 2 mm is palpable and increases to 12 mm by 42 weeks.

Signs of risk for reproductive system problems

The infant must be closely inspected for ambiguous genitalia and other abnormalities. Normally in a female infant the urethral opening is located behind the clitoris. Any deviation from this may incorrectly suggest that the clitoris is a small penis, which can occur in conditions such as adrenal hyperplasia. Nearly all female infants are born with

hymenal tags; absence of such tags could indicate vaginal agenesis. Fecal discharge from the vagina indicates a rectovaginal fistula. Any of these findings must be reported to the physician for further evaluation.

The male infant's scrotum should always be palpated for the presence of testes. Inguinal hernias may be present and become more obvious when the infant cries. If the urinary meatus is not at the tip of the glans penis, hypospadias (urethral meatus opening on the underside of the penis) or epispadias (urethral meatus opening on the top of the penis) may be present. These problems are usually associated with other anomalies.

Skeletal System

The infant's skeletal system undergoes rapid development during the first year of life. At birth, more cartilage is present than ossified bone. Because of cephalocaudal (head-to-rump) development, the newborn looks somewhat out of proportion.

At term the head is one fourth the total body length. The arms are slightly longer than the legs. In the newborn, the legs are one third the total body length, but only 15% of the total body weight. As growth proceeds, the midpoint in head-to-toe measurements gradually descends from the level of the umbilicus at birth to the level of the symphysis pubis at maturity.

The face appears small in relation to the skull, which appears large and heavy. Cranial size and shape can be distorted by molding (the shaping of the fetal head by the overlapping of cranial bones to facilitate movement through the birth canal during labor) (Fig. 18-9).

The bones in the vertebral column of the newborn form two primary curvatures—one in the thoracic region and one in the sacral region (Fig. 18-10, *A*). Both are forward, concave curvatures. As the infant gains head control at approximately age 3 months, a secondary curvature appears in the cervical region (Fig. 18-10, *B*).

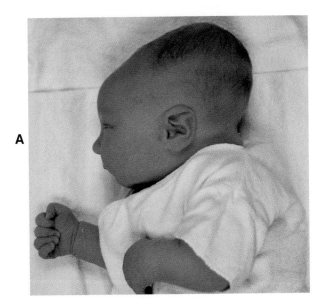

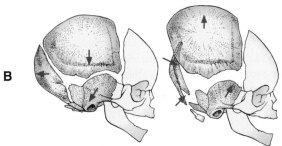

Fig. 18-9 Molding. **A,** Significant molding, soon after birth. **B,** Schematic of bones of skull when molding is present. (**A,** Courtesy Kim Molloy, Knoxville, IA.)

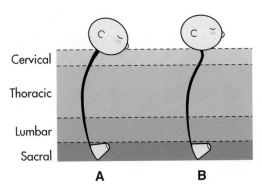

Fig. 18-10 Development of spinal curvatures. **A,** Newborn. **B,** Cervical secondary curvature. (From Wong, D. [1999]. *Whaley and Wong's nursing care of infants and children* [6th ed.]. St. Louis: Mosby.)

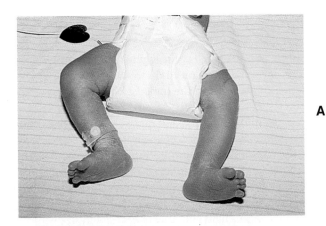

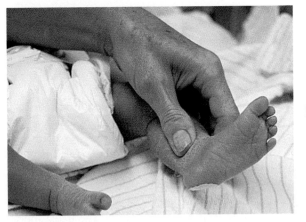

Fig. 18-11 Extremities. **A,** Bowed appearance of legs. **B,** Normal absence of arch in newborn's foot. (Courtesy Marjorie Pyle, RNC, Lifecircle, Costa Mesa, CA.)

In some newborns, a significant separation of the knees occurs when the ankles are held together, resulting in an appearance of bowlegs (Fig. 18-11, *A*). If an infant was in the frank breech position in utero, the legs may be extended and remain in this position for several weeks. The newborn is also very flat footed because no clearly apparent arch to the foot is present (Fig. 18-11, *B*).

The infant's extremities should be symmetric and of equal length. Fingers and toes should be equal in number and should have nails present. Extra digits (polydactyly) are sometimes found on hands or feet. Fingers or toes may be fused (syndactyly).

The infant's hips should be inspected for symmetry. Skin folds should be equal and symmetric. Hip integrity is assessed by using the Ortolani maneuver (Fig. 18-12). The examiner places the index and middle fingers of each hand over the greater trochanters of the hips at the same time. Downward pressure is exerted on the hips while the neonate's knees are flexed. The hips are flexed at least 70 degrees and then abducted. The motion should be smooth without any unusual clicks. The presence of a click, unequal movement, or uneven gluteal skin folds is considered a positive response, indicating that the hip is dislocated, and the physician should be notified.

The newborn's spine appears straight and can be easily flexed. The newborn can lift the head and turn it from side to side when prone. The vertebrae should appear straight and flat. The base of the spine should not have a dimple. If a dimple is noted, further inspection is required to determine whether a sinus is present. A pilonidal dimple, especially with a sinus and nevus pilosis (hairy nevus), is significant because it can be associated with spina bifida.

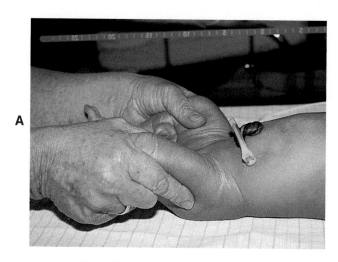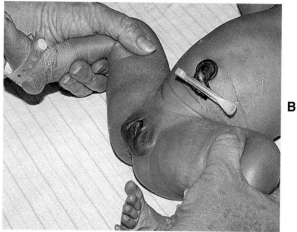

Fig. 18-12 Method of assessing for hip dysplasia or dislocation using the Ortolani maneuver. **A,** Examiner's middle fingers are placed over greater trochanter, and thumbs are placed over inner thigh opposite lesser trochanter. **B,** Gentle pressure is exerted to flex thigh on hip further, and thighs are rotated outward. If hip dysplasia is present, head of femur can be felt to slip forward in acetabulum and flip back when pressure is released and legs are returned to their original position. A click is sometimes heard (Ortolani sign). (Courtesy Marjorie Pyle, RNC, Lifecircle, Costa Mesa, CA.)

Signs of risk for skeletal problems

Skeletal deformities may be congenital or drug induced. Clubfoot (talipes equinovarus), a deformity in which the foot turns inward and is fixed in a plantar-flexion position, and any absence of a limb or digit should be recorded and reported. Signs of congenital hip dislocation, additional digits or webbing of digits, and any other abnormality should be recorded and reported to the health care provider.

Neuromuscular System

Unlike the skeletal system, the neuromuscular system is almost completely developed at birth. The term newborn is a responsive and reactive being with remarkable sensory development and an amazing ability for self-organization and social interaction.

Growth of the brain after birth follows a predictable pattern of rapid growth during infancy and early childhood, more gradual growth during the remainder of the first decade, and minimal growth during adolescence. The cerebellum ends its growth spurt, which began at about 30 gestational weeks, by the end of the first year. This may be the reason the brain is vulnerable to nutritional deficiencies and trauma in early infancy.

The brain requires glucose as a source of energy and a relatively large supply of oxygen for adequate metabolism. Such requirements signal a need for careful assessment of the infant's respiratory status. The necessity for glucose requires attentiveness to those neonates who may have hypoglycemic episodes.

Spontaneous motor activity may be seen as transient tremors of the mouth and chin, especially during crying episodes, and of the extremities, notably the arms and hands. Transient tremors are normal and can be observed in nearly every newborn. These tremors should not be present when the infant is quiet and should not persist beyond 1 month of age. Persistent tremors or tremors involving the total body may indicate pathologic conditions. Marked tonicity, clonicity, and twitching of facial muscles are signs of seizure activity. Normal tremors, tremors of hypoglycemia, and central nervous system (CNS) disorders must be differentiated so that diagnostic workups and corrective care can be instituted as necessary.

Although it is limited, some neuromuscular control is present in the newborn. If newborns are placed face down on a firm surface, they will turn their heads to the side to maintain an airway. They attempt to hold their heads in line with their bodies if they are raised by their arms.

Newborn reflexes

The newborn has many primitive reflexes. The times at which these reflexes appear and disappear reflect the maturity and intactness of the developing nervous system. The most common reflexes found in the normal newborn are described in Table 18-3. The physical assessment includes a neurologic assessment of the newborn's reflexes. This provides useful information about the infant's nervous system and state of neurologic maturation. Many reflex behaviors are important for survival, for example, sucking and rooting. Other reflexes act as safety mechanisms, for instance, gagging, coughing, and sneezing. The assessment must be carried out as early as possible because abnormal signs present in the early neonatal period may disappear. They may reappear months or years later as abnormal functions.

TABLE 18-3

Assessment of Newborn's Reflexes

REFLEX	ELICITING THE REFLEX	CHARACTERISTIC RESPONSE	COMMENTS
Sucking and rooting	Touch infant's lip, cheek, or corner of mouth with nipple	Infant turns head toward stimulus, opens mouth, takes hold, and sucks	Response is difficult if not impossible to elicit after infant has been fed; if response weak or absent, consider prematurity or neurologic defect Parental guidance: Avoid trying to turn head toward breast or nipple, allow infant to root; response disappears after 3 to 4* mo but may persist up to 1 yr
Swallowing	Feed infant; swallowing usually follows sucking and obtaining fluids	Swallowing is usually coordinated with sucking and usually occurs without gagging, coughing, or vomiting	If response is weak or absent, may indicate prematurity or neurologic defect Sucking and swallowing are often uncoordinated in preterm infant

Grasp
  Palmar
  Plantar
	Place finger in palm of hand
	Place finger at base of toes
		Infant's fingers curl around examiner's fingers, toes curl downward	Palmar response lessens by 3 to 4 mo; parents enjoy this contact with infant; plantar response lessens by 8 mo

Extrusion	Touch or depress tip of tongue	Newborn forces tongue outward	Response disappears about fourth month of life
Glabellar (Myerson's)	Tap over forehead, bridge of nose, or maxilla of newborn whose eyes are open	Newborn blinks for first four or five taps	Continued blinking with repeated taps is consistent with extrapyramidal disorder
Tonic neck or "fencing"	With infant falling asleep or sleeping, turn head quickly to one side	With infant facing left side, arm and leg on that side extend; opposite arm and leg flex (turn head to right, and extremities assume opposite postures)	Responses in leg are more consistent Complete response disappears by 3 to 4 mo, incomplete response may be seen until third or fourth year After 6 wk, persistent response is sign of possible cerebral palsy

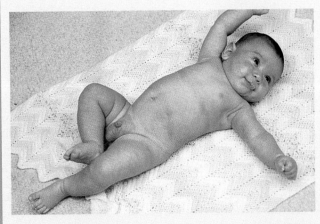

Classic pose in spontaneous tonic neck reflex. (Courtesy Marjorie Pyle, RNC, Lifecircle, Costa Mesa, CA.)

*All durations for persistence of reflexes are based on time elapsed after 40 wk of gestation, that is, if this newborn was born at 36 wk of gestation, add 1 mo to all time limits given.

TABLE 18-3

Assessment of Newborn's Reflexes—cont'd

REFLEX	ELICITING THE REFLEX	CHARACTERISTIC RESPONSE	COMMENTS
Moro	Hold infant in semisitting position, allow head and trunk to fall backward to an angle of at least 30 degrees Place infant on flat surface, strike surface to startle infant	Symmetric abduction and extension of arms are seen; fingers fan out and form a C with thumb and forefinger; slight tremor may be noted; arms are adducted in embracing motion and return to relaxed flexion and movement Legs may follow similar pattern of response Preterm infant does not complete "embrace"; instead, arms fall backward because of weakness	Response is present at birth; complete response may be seen until 8 wk; body jerk is seen only between 8 and 18 wk; response is absent by 6 mo if neurologic maturation is not delayed; response may be incomplete if infant is deeply asleep; give parental guidance about normal response Asymmetric response may connote injury to brachial plexus, clavicle, or humerus Persistent response after 6 mo indicates possible brain damage

Moro reflex. (From Dickason, E., Silverman, B., & Kaplan, J. [1998]. *Maternal-infant nursing care* [3rd ed.]. St. Louis; Mosby.)

REFLEX	ELICITING THE REFLEX	CHARACTERISTIC RESPONSE	COMMENTS
Stepping or "walking"	Hold infant vertically, allowing one foot to touch table surface	Infant will simulate walking, alternating flexion and extension of feet; term infants walk on soles of their feet, and preterm infants walk on their toes	Response is normally present for 3 to 4 wk

Stepping reflex. (From Dickason, E., Silverman, B., & Kaplan, J. (1998). *Maternal-infant nursing care* [3rd ed.]. St. Louis: Mosby.)

Continued

Assessment of Newborn's Reflexes—cont'd

REFLEX	ELICITING THE REFLEX	CHARACTERISTIC RESPONSE	COMMENTS
Crawling	Place newborn on abdomen	Newborn makes crawling movements with arms and legs	Response should disappear about 6 wk of age
Deep tendon	Use finger instead of percussion hammer to elicit patellar, or knee jerk, reflex; newborn must be relaxed	Reflex jerk is present; even with newborn relaxed, nonselective overall reaction may occur	
Crossed extension	Infant should be supine; extend one leg, press knee downward, stimulate bottom of foot; observe opposite leg	Opposite leg flexes, adducts, and then extends	

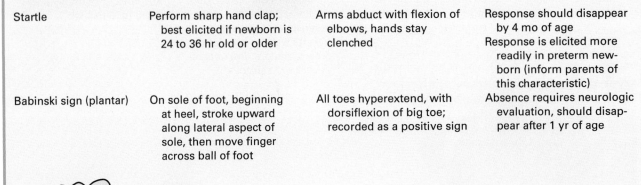

Crossed extension reflex. With the infant in supine position, examiner extends one leg of the infant and presses the knee down. Stimulation of sole of foot of fixated limb should cause free leg to flex, adduct, and extend as if attempting to push away stimulating agent. This reflex should be present during newborn period. (Courtesy Marjorie Pyle, RNC, Lifecircle, Costa Mesa, CA.)

REFLEX	ELICITING THE REFLEX	CHARACTERISTIC RESPONSE	COMMENTS
Startle	Perform sharp hand clap; best elicited if newborn is 24 to 36 hr old or older	Arms abduct with flexion of elbows, hands stay clenched	Response should disappear by 4 mo of age Response is elicited more readily in preterm newborn (inform parents of this characteristic)
Babinski sign (plantar)	On sole of foot, beginning at heel, stroke upward along lateral aspect of sole, then move finger across ball of foot	All toes hyperextend, with dorsiflexion of big toe; recorded as a positive sign	Absence requires neurologic evaluation, should disappear after 1 yr of age

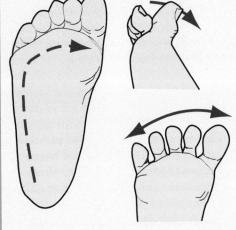

Babinski reflex. (From Hockenberry, M. [2003]. *Wong's nursing care of infants and children* [7th ed.]. St. Louis: Mosby.)

TABLE 18-3

Assessment of Newborn's Reflexes—cont'd

REFLEX	ELICITING THE REFLEX	CHARACTERISTIC RESPONSE	COMMENTS
Pull-to-sit (traction)	Pull infant up by wrists from supine position with head in midline	Head will lag until infant is in upright position, then head will be held in same plane with chest and shoulder momentarily before falling forward; infant will attempt to right head	Response depends on general muscle tone and maturity and condition of infant
Trunk incurvation (Galant)	Place infant prone on flat surface, run finger down back about 4 to 5 cm lateral to spine, first on one side and then down other	Trunk is flexed, and pelvis is swung toward stimulated side With transverse lesions of cord, no response below the level of the lesion is present.	Response disappears by fourth week Absence suggests general depression of nervous system Response may vary but should be obtainable in all infants, including preterm ones.

(Courtesy Marjorie Pyle, RNC, Lifecircle, Costa Mesa, CA.)

Magnet	Place infant in supine position, partially flex both lower extremities, and apply pressure to soles of feet	Both lower limbs should extend against examiner's pressure	Absence suggests damage to spinal cord or malformation Reflex may be weak or exaggerated after breech birth

(Courtesy Michael S. Clement, M.D., Mesa, AZ)

Additional newborn responses: Yawn, stretch, burp, hiccup, sneeze	These are spontaneous behaviors	May be slightly depressed temporarily because of maternal analgesia or anesthesia, fetal hypoxia, or infection	Parental guidance: most of these behaviors are pleasurable to parents Parents need to be assured that behaviors are normal Sneeze is usually response to lint, etc., in nose and not an indicator of a cold No treatment is needed for hiccups; sucking may help

Signs of risk for neuromuscular problems

Any absence of a newborn reflex could indicate major neurologic problems. Birth trauma may cause nerve damage that results in facial asymmetry and paralysis. CNS depression resulting from maternal medications received during labor and birth also will influence neuromuscular functioning. Observation of the neonate for any abnormalities must be documented. A thorough physical examination of the newborn assists in detecting any potential complications (see Table 19-2).

BEHAVIORAL CHARACTERISTICS ■

The healthy infant must achieve behavioral and biologic tasks to develop normally. Behavioral characteristics form the basis of the social capabilities of the infant. Normal newborns differ in their activity levels, feeding patterns, sleeping patterns, and responsiveness. Parents' reactions to their newborns often are determined by these differences. Showing parents the unique characteristics of their infant assists parents to develop a more positive perception of the infant with increased interaction between infant and parent.

Behavioral responses, as well as physical characteristics, change during the period of transition. The Brazelton Neonatal Behavioral Assessment Scale (BNBAS) can be used to assess the infant's behavior systematically (Brazelton, 1999; Brazelton & Nugent, 1996). The BNBAS is an interactive examination that assesses the infant's response to 28 areas organized according to the clusters in Box 18-2. It is generally used as a research or diagnostic tool and requires special training.

In addition to use as initial and ongoing tools to assess neurologic and behavioral responses, the scales can be used to assess initial parent-infant relationships and as a guide for parents to help them focus on their infant's individuality and to develop a deeper attachment to their child. See Chapter 17 for further discussion of attachment.

BOX 18-2

Clusters of Neonatal Behaviors in the Brazelton Neonatal Behavioral Assessment Scale (BNBAS)

Habituation—Ability to respond to and then inhibit responding to discrete stimuli (light, rattle, bell, pinprick) while asleep
Orientation— Quality of alert states and ability to attend to visual and auditory stimuli while alert
Motor performance—Quality of movement and tone
Range of state—Measure of general arousal level or arousability of infant
Regulation of state—How infant responds when aroused
Autonomic stability—Signs of stress (tremors, startles, skin color) related to homeostatic (self-regulator) adjustment of the nervous system
Reflexes—Assessment of several neonatal reflexes

Sleep-Wake States

Variations in the state of consciousness of infants are called sleep-wake states (Brazelton, 1999). The six states form a continuum from deep sleep to extreme irritability (Fig. 18-13): two sleep states (deep sleep and light sleep) and four wake states (drowsy, quiet alert, active alert, and crying). Each state has specific characteristics and state-related behaviors. The optimal state of arousal is the quiet alert state. During this state infants smile, vocalize, move in synchrony with speech, watch their parents' faces, and respond to people talking to them. The infants' reactions to internal and external stimuli and ability to control their responses while in these sleep-wake states reflect their ability to organize behavior.

Infants use purposeful behavior to maintain the optimal arousal state: (1) actively withdrawing by increasing physical distance, (2) rejecting by pushing away with hands and feet, (3) decreasing sensitivity by falling asleep or breaking eye contact by turning head, or (4) using signaling behaviors, such as fussing and crying. These behaviors permit infants to quiet themselves and reinstate readiness to interact.

The first 6 weeks of life involve a steady decrease in the proportion of active REM sleep to total sleep. A steady increase in the proportion of quiet sleep to total sleep also occurs. Periods of wakefulness increase. For the first few weeks the wakeful periods seem dictated by hunger, but soon a need for socializing appears as well. The newborn sleeps approximately 17 hours a day, with periods of wakefulness gradually increasing. By the fourth week of life, some infants stay awake from one feeding to the next.

Other Factors Influencing Newborn Behavior
Gestational age

The gestational age of the infant and level of CNS maturity affect the observed behavior. In an infant with an immature CNS, the entire body responds to a pinprick of the foot. The mature infant withdraws only the foot. CNS immaturity is reflected in reflex development and sleep-wake cycles. Preterm infants have brief periods of alertness but have difficulty maintaining this state. Premature or sick infants show fatigue or stress sooner than do term healthy infants.

Time

The time elapsed since birth affects the behavior of infants as they attempt to become organized initially. Time elapsed since the previous feeding and time of day also may influence infants' responses.

Stimuli

Environmental events and stimuli affect the behavioral responses of infants. The newborn responds differently to animate and inanimate stimuli. Nurses in intensive care nurseries observe that infants respond to loud noises, bright lights, monitor alarms, and tension in the unit. If a mother is tense and has a fast heart beat while feeding an infant, the infant will have an increase in heart rate that is similar to the mother's.

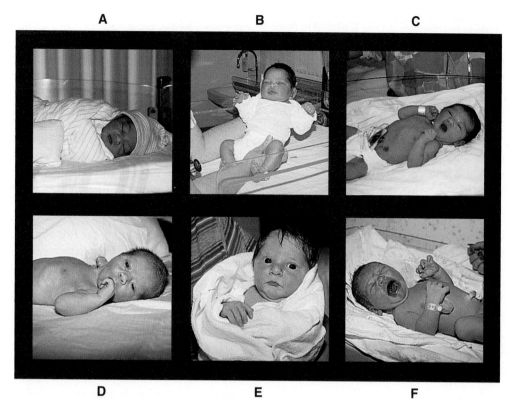

Fig. 18-13 Summary of newborn sleep-wake states. States of consciousness: **A,** Deep sleep. **B,** Light sleep. **C,** Drowsy. **D,** Quiet alert. **E,** Active alert. **F,** Crying. (Courtesy Marjorie Pyle, RNC, Lifecircle, Costa Mesa, CA.)

Medication

Analgesic and anesthetic medications administered to the mother during labor may affect the newborn's neurologic status and behavior. Narcotics are likely to cause CNS depression and hypotonia and may even cause apnea (Kliegman, 2002). These medications also can affect the infant's sucking ability, at the breast or from a bottle.

Sensory Behaviors

From birth, infants possess sensory capabilities that indicate a state of readiness for social interaction. Infants effectively use behavioral responses in establishing their first dialogues. These responses, coupled with the newborns' "baby appearance" (e.g., facial proportions of forehead and eyes larger than the lower portion of the face) and their small size and helplessness, rouse feelings of wanting to hold, protect, and interact with them.

Vision

Compared with other sensory systems, the visual system is the least mature at term gestation. Development of the visual system continues for the first 6 months. The pupils react to light, the blink reflex is easily stimulated, and the corneal reflex is activated by light touch. Infants are sensitive to light, preferring low illumination. If the room is darkened, they will open their eyes wide and look about. Newborns respond to a flash of bright light by frowning, blinking, and withdrawing the head by arching the entire body.

Newborns have the ability to fixate and will track a high-contrast object horizontally and vertically. Infants seem attentive to the human face and will track their parents' eyes. Parents often comment on how exciting this behavior is.

Visual acuity is difficult to determine, although it appears that the clearest visual distance for the newborn is approximately 19 cm, which is about the distance the infant's face is from the mother's face as she breastfeeds or cuddles. Newborns prefer to look at patterns rather than plain surfaces, even if the latter are brightly colored, and they prefer more complex patterns to simple ones (Brazelton, 1999; Gupta, Hamming, & Miller, 2002).

Hearing

As soon as the amniotic fluid drains from the ear, the infant's hearing is similar to that of an adult. This may occur as early as 1 minute after birth. Loud sounds of about 90 decibels cause the infant to respond with a startle reflex. The newborn responds to low-frequency sounds such as a heartbeat or lullaby by decreasing motor activity or stopping crying. High-frequency sound elicits an alerting reaction.

The infant responds readily to the mother's voice. Studies indicate a selective listening to maternal voice sounds and rhythms during intrauterine life that prepares newborns for recognition and interaction with their primary caregivers—their mothers. Newborns are accustomed in the uterus to hearing the regular rhythm of the mother's heartbeat. As a result, they respond by relaxing and ceasing to fuss and cry if a regular heartbeat simulator is placed in their cribs.

The internal and middle portions of the ear are larger at birth, but the external canal is small. The mastoid process and bony parts of the external canal have not developed; therefore the tympanic membrane and facial nerve are very close to the surface and can be easily damaged. Hearing loss is common at birth; 1 to 3 of every 1000 well newborn infants have bilateral hearing loss. Routine hearing screening is recommended for all newborns before hospital discharge (AAP Task Force on Newborn and Infant Hearing, 1999) (see Fig. 19-9).

Smell

Newborns have a highly developed sense of smell and are responsive to odors that facilitate adaptation to the extrauterine environment. Newborns react to strong odors such as alcohol or vinegar by turning their heads away but are attracted to sweet smells. By the fifth day of life, newborn infants can recognize their mother's smell (Brazelton, 1999). Breastfed infants are able to smell breast milk and can differentiate their mothers from other lactating women (Lawrence & Lawrence, 2005).

Taste

The newborn can distinguish among tastes, and various types of solutions elicit differing facial expressions. A tasteless solution produces no response; a sweet solution elicits eager sucking. A sour solution causes a puckering of the lips, and a bitter liquid produces a grimace. Newborns prefer glucose water to plain water.

Young infants are particularly oriented toward the use of their mouths, both for meeting their nutritional needs for rapid growth and for releasing tension through sucking. The early development of circumoral sensation, muscle activity, and taste would seem to be preparation for survival in the extrauterine environment.

Touch

The infant is responsive to touch on all parts of the body. The face (especially the mouth), the hands, and the soles of the feet appear to be the most sensitive. Reflexes can be elicited by stroking the infant. The newborn's responses to touch suggest that this sensory system is well prepared to receive and process tactile messages. Touch and motion are essential to normal growth and development; however, each infant is unique, and variations can be seen in newborns' responses to touch. Birth trauma or stress and depressant drugs taken by the mother decrease the infant's sensitivity to touch or painful stimuli.

Response to Environmental Stimuli
Temperament

Classic studies identified individual variations in the primary reaction pattern of newborns and described them as temperament. Their style of behavioral response to stimuli is guided by the temperament affecting the newborn's sensory threshold, ability to habituate, and response to maternal behaviors. The newborn possesses individual characteristics that affect selective responses to various stimuli present in the internal and external environment.

Habituation

Habituation is a protective mechanism that allows the infant to become accustomed to environmental stimuli. Habituation is a psychologic and physiologic phenomenon whereby the response to a constant or repetitive stimulus is decreased. In the term newborn this can be demonstrated in several ways. Shining a bright light into a newborn's eyes will cause a startle or squinting the first two or three times. The third or fourth flash will elicit a diminished response, and by the fifth or sixth flash, the infant ceases to respond (Brazelton, 1999). The same response pattern holds true for the sounds of a rattle or a pinprick to the heel. A newborn presented with new stimuli becomes wide eyed and alters his or her gaze for a time but will eventually show a diminished interest.

The ability to habituate also allows the newborn to select stimuli that promote continued learning about the social world, thereby avoiding overload. The intrauterine experience seems to have programmed the newborn to be especially responsive to human voices, soft lights, soft sounds, and sweet tastes.

The newborn quickly learns the sounds in a newborn nursery and the home and is able to sleep in their midst. The selective responses of the newborn indicate cerebral organization capable of remembering and making choices. The ability to habituate depends on state of consciousness, hunger, fatigue, and temperament. These factors also affect consolability, cuddliness, irritability, and crying.

Consolability

Newborns vary in their ability to console themselves or to be consoled. In the crying state, most newborns initiate one of several methods for reducing their distress. Hand-to-mouth movements are common, with or without sucking, as well as alerting to voices, noises, or visual stimuli.

Cuddliness

Cuddliness is especially important to parents because they often gauge their ability to care for the child by the child's responses to their actions. There is variability in the degree to which newborns will mold into the contours of the persons holding them. Babies are soothed and become alert with the vestibular stimulation of being picked up and moved.

Irritability

Some newborns cry longer and harder than others. For some the sensory threshold seems low. They are readily upset by unusual noises, hunger, wetness, or new experiences, and therefore respond intensely. Others with a high sensory threshold require a great deal more stimulation and variation to reach the active, alert state.

Crying

Crying in an infant may signal hunger, pain, desire for attention, or fussiness. Most mothers learn to distinguish among the cries. The duration of crying is highly variable in each infant; newborns may cry for as little as 5 minutes or as much as 2 hours or more per day. The amount of crying peaks in the second month and then decreases. The diurnal rhythm of crying typically includes more crying in the evening hours. Crying does not seem to differ with different caregivers.

COMMUNITY ACTIVITY

Determine whether or not newborn classes are available in your community. Interview the instructor to determine what is included in the class content. Is there attention to normal physical characteristics of the neonate? What information do parents receive related to newborn behaviors? What suggestions would you make in including content related to physiologic and behavioral adaptations of the newborn? What is the value of providing expectant parents with this information?

Key Points

- By term the infant's various anatomic and physiologic systems have reached a level of development and functioning that permits a physical existence apart from the mother. The infant has sensory capabilities that indicate a state of readiness for social interaction.
- Several significant differences exist between the respiratory, renal, and thermogenic systems of the newborn and those of an adult.
- At any serum bilirubin level, the appearance of jaundice during the first 24 hours of life or persistence of jaundice for more than 7 days usually indicates a pathologic process in term infants.

- Loss of heat in a newborn, even a healthy newborn, may result in acidosis and increase the level of free fatty acids, leading to cold stress.
- Many reflex behaviors are important for the newborn's survival.
- Individual personalities and behavioral characteristics of infants play major roles in their ultimate relationships with their parents.
- Sleep-wake states and other factors influence the newborn's behavior.
- Each newborn has a predisposed capacity to handle the multitude of stimuli in the external world.

Answer Guidelines to Critical Thinking Exercise

Near Term Infant with Physiologic Jaundice

1 The nurse can assess the newborn for the presence of jaundice by blanching the skin over the baby's forehead, chest, abdomen, and legs. At this point, the baby is over 24 hours of age and would likely be experiencing physiologic jaundice.

2 a. At 36 hours of age, the newborn is likely exhibiting physiologic jaundice. He is at risk for development of physiologic jaundice because of the bruising of his head and because he is preterm.

   b. The baby has not been feeding well thus far and has had only one stool. Because bilirubin is excreted primarily through the stool, it is important that his bowel movements increase. Because he is preterm, he may be more difficult to awaken for feedings than a full-term infant. The more he feeds, the greater his output will be.

   c. Randy noted the appearance of his son's skin color as evidenced by his comment. The nurse can explain why the baby appears somewhat "yellow" and describe physiologic jaundice in terms that the parents can understand.

3 The infant's level of jaundice should be assessed and the health care provider notified. The nurse may be able to determine a transcutaneous measurement of hyperbilirubinemia if equip-

ment is available. The health care provider may order a serum bilirubin measurement to establish a baseline and reassess bilirubin levels periodically to determine if hyperbilirubinemia is increasing. It is important to closely monitor the infant and to intervene to prevent the development of kernicterus.

Feeding is important in order for the newborn to excrete excess bilirubin. The parents may need to be encouraged to awaken the baby for feedings, and breastfeeding should be observed to determine the mother's ability to feed and to assess for milk transfer. Assistance is given as needed. The baby's output is closely monitored; parents may be instructed to keep a log of feedings, urination, and stooling.

The parents will likely need some explanation about physiologic jaundice. First, the nurse will assess their knowledge and proceed to provide needed information. They are encouraged to ask questions of the nurse and the health care provider.

4 If bilirubin levels are measured, there may be evidence to support the conclusion that the baby is experiencing physiologic jaundice. If this is the case, the baby will appear more jaundiced over the next two or three days.

5 Jaundice could also be caused by blood incompatibilities or liver anomalies; however, this type of jaundice is considered pathologic and usually appears within the first 24 hours of life.

Resources

Academy of Neonatal Nursing
2777 Yulupa Ave., No. 166
Santa Rosa, CA 94505-8584
707-568-2168
www.academyonline.org

Advances in Neonatal Care
Elsevier
The Curtis Center
Independence Square West
Philadelphia, PA 19106-3399
800-654-2452
www.advancesinneonatalcare.org

American Academy of Pediatrics (AAP)
141 Northwest Point Blvd.
Elk Grove, IL 60007-1098
www.aap.org

Journal of Perinatal and Neonatal Nursing
Aspen Publishers, Inc.
7201 McKinney Circle
Frederick, MD 21701
800-234-1660

National Association of Neonatal Nurses (NANN)
4700 W. Lake Ave.
Glenview, IL 60025-1485
800-451-3795
888-477-6266 (fax)
www.nann.org
E-mail: info@nann.org

Neonatal Network
1410 Neotomas Ave., Suite 107
Santa Rosa, CA 95405-7533
www.neonatalnetwork.com

References

American Academy of Pediatrics (AAP), Subcommittee on Hyperbilirubinemia. (2004). Clinical practice guideline: Management of hyperbilirubinemia in the newborn infant 35 or more weeks of gestation. *Pediatrics, 114*(1), 297-316.

American Academy of Pediatrics (AAP) Task Force on Newborn and Infant Hearing. (1999). Newborn and infant hearing loss: Detection and intervention. *Pediatrics, 103*(2), 527-530.

Anderson, G., Moore, E., Hepworth, J., & Bergman, N. (2003). Early skin-to-skin contact for mothers and their healthy newborn infants. *The Cochrane Database of Systematic Reviews* Issue 2, 2003, Art. No.: CD003519.

Blackburn, S. (2003). *Maternal, fetal, & neonatal physiology: A clinical perspective* (2nd ed.). St. Louis: Saunders.

Brazelton, T. (1999). Behavioral competence. In G. Avery, M. Fletcher, & M. MacDonald (Eds.), *Neonatology: Pathophysiology and management of the newborn* (5th ed.). Philadelphia: Lippincott Williams & Wilkins.

Brazelton, T., & Nugent, K. (1996). *Neonatal behavioural assessment scale* (3rd ed.). London: MacKeith.

Briscoe, L., Clark, S., & Yoxall, C. (2002). Can transcutaneous bilirubinometry reduce the need for blood tests in jaundiced full term babies? *Archives of Disease in Childhood. Fetal and Neonatal Edition, 85*(3), F190-192.

Dickason, E., Silverman, B., & Kaplan, J. (1998). *Maternal-infant nursing care* (3rd ed.). St. Louis: Mosby.

Frank, C., Cooper, S., & Merenstein, G. (2002). Jaundice. In G. Merenstein & S. Gardner (Eds.), *Handbook of neonatal intensive care* (5th ed.). St. Louis: Mosby.

Garas, T. et al. (2001). Perinatal morbidity: A comparison of vacuum delivery and spontaneous delivery. *Obstetrics and Gynecology, 97* (4 Suppl 1), S64.

Gupta, B., Hamming, N., & Miller, M. (2002). The eye: Diagnosis and evaluation. In A. Fanaroff & R. Martin (Eds.), *Neonatal-perinatal medicine: Diseases of the fetus and infant* (7th ed.). St. Louis: Mosby.

Hockenberry, M. (2003). *Wong's nursing care of infants and children* (7th ed.). St. Louis: Mosby.

Joint Commission on Accreditation of Healthcare Organizations. (2001). *Sentinel event alert: Kernicterus threatens healthy newborns,* Issue 18, April. Internet document available at www.jcaho.org (accessed September 6, 2005).

Kliegman, R. (2002). Fetal and neonatal medicine. In R. Behrman & R. Kliegman (Eds.), *Nelson essentials of pediatrics* (4th ed.). Philadelphia: Saunders.

Lawrence, R., & Lawrence R. (2005). *Breastfeeding: A guide for the medical profession* (6th ed.). St. Louis: Mosby.

Lissauer, T. (2002). Physical examination and care of the newborn. In A. Fanaroff & R. Martin (Eds.), *Neonatal-perinatal medicine: Diseases of the fetus and infant* (7th ed.). St. Louis: Mosby.

Luchtman-Jones, L., Schwartz, A., & Wilson, D. (2002). The blood and hematopoietic system. In A. Fanaroff & R. Martin (Eds.), *Neonatal-perinatal medicine: Diseases of the fetus and infant* (7th ed.). St. Louis: Mosby.

Maisels, M. (2001). Neonatal jaundice and kernicterus. *Pediatrics, 108,* 763-765.

Miller, C., & Newman, T. (2005). Routine newborn care. In H. Taeusch, R. Ballard, & C. Gleason (Eds.). *Avery's diseases of the newborn* (8th ed.). Philadelphia: Saunders.

Pagana, K., & Pagana, T. (2002). *Mosby's manual of diagnostic and laboratory tests* (2nd ed.). St. Louis: Mosby.

Paige, P., & Carney, P. (2002). Neurologic disorders. In G. Merenstein & S. Gardner (Eds.), *Handbook of neonatal intensive care* (5th ed.). St. Louis: Mosby.

Porter, M., & Dennis, B. (2002). Hyperbilirubinemia in the term newborn. *American Family Physician, 65*(4), 599-606, 613-614.

Putta, L., & Spencer, J. (2000). Assisted vaginal delivery using the vacuum extractor. *American Family Physician, 62*(6), 1316-1320.

Reiser, D. (2004). Neonatal jaundice: Physiologic variation or pathologic process. *Critical Care Clinics of North America, 16*(2), 257-269.

Ross, M., Fresquez, M., El-Haddad, M. (2001). Impact of FDA advisory on reported vacuum-assisted delivery and morbidity. *Journal of Fetal and Maternal Medicine, 9*(6), 321-326.

Scott, J. (2002). Hematology. In R. Behrman & R. Kliegman (Eds.), *Nelson essentials of pediatrics* (4th ed.). Philadelphia: Saunders.

Sniderman, S., & Taeusch, H. (2005). Initial evaluation: History and physical examination of the newborn. In H. Taeusch, R. Ballard, & C. Gleason (Eds.). *Avery's diseases of the newborn* (8th ed.). Philadelphia: Saunders.

Wong, D. (1999). *Whaley and Wong's nursing care of infants and children* (6th ed.). St. Louis: Mosby.

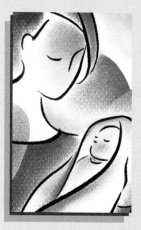

CHAPTER *19*

Assessment and Care of the Newborn

KATHRYN RHODES ALDEN

LEARNING OBJECTIVES

- Describe the purpose and components of the Apgar score.
- Describe the method for estimating the gestational age of a newborn.
- Explain the procedure for assessment of the newborn.
- Describe common deviations from normal physiologic findings during examination of the newborn.
- Discuss nursing care management of the newborn in transition to extrauterine life.
- Explain what is meant by a protective environment.

- Discuss phototherapy and the guidelines for teaching parents about this treatment.
- Explain purposes for and methods of circumcision, the postoperative care of the circumcised infant, and parent teaching regarding circumcision.
- Describe procedures for doing a heel stick, collecting urine specimens, assisting with venipuncture, and restraining the newborn.
- Evaluate pain in the newborn based on physiologic changes and behavioral observations.
- Discuss parent education related to caring for the infant during the first weeks at home.

KEY TERMS AND DEFINITIONS

Apgar score Numeric expression of the condition of a newborn obtained by rapid assessment at 1 and 5 minutes of age; developed by Dr. Virginia Apgar
circumcision Excision of the prepuce (foreskin) of the penis, exposing the glans
hypothermia Temperature that falls below normal range, that is, below 35° C, usually caused by exposure to cold

ophthalmia neonatorum Infection in the neonate's eyes usually resulting from gonorrheal, chlamydial, or other infection contracted when the fetus passes through the birth canal (vagina)
phototherapy Use of lights to reduce serum bilirubin levels by oxidation of bilirubin into water-soluble compounds that are processed in the liver and excreted in bile and urine

ELECTRONIC RESOURCES

Additional information related to the content in Chapter 19 can be found on

the companion website at *evolve*
http://evolve.elsevier.com/Lowdermilk/Maternity/
- NCLEX Review Questions
- Case Study—Normal Newborn
- WebLinks

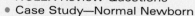
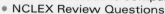

or on the interactive companion CD
- NCLEX Review Questions
- Case Study—Normal Newborn
- Critical Thinking Exercise—Circumcision
- Critical Thinking Exercise—Jaundice
- Plan of Care—Normal Newborn
- Skill—Changing a Diaper
- Skill—Infant Bathing
- Skill—Pain Assessment
- Video—Assessment of the Newborn

*T*he numerous biologic changes the neonate makes during the transition to extrauterine life are discussed in the preceding chapter. The first 24 hours are critical because respiratory distress and circulatory failure can occur rapidly and with little warning. Although most infants make the necessary biopsychosocial adjustment to extrauterine existence without undue difficulty, their well-being depends on the care they receive from others. This chapter describes assessment and care of the infant immediately after birth until discharge, as well as important parent education related to ongoing infant care. A discussion of pain in the neonate and its management is included.

CARE MANAGEMENT: FROM BIRTH THROUGH THE FIRST 2 HOURS

Care begins immediately after birth and focuses on assessing and stabilizing the newborn's condition. The nurse has primary responsibility for the infant during this period, because the physician or nurse-midwife is involved with delivery of the placenta and caring for the mother. The nurse must be alert for any signs of distress and must initiate appropriate interventions.

With the possibility of transmission of viruses such as hepatitis B virus (HBV) and human immunodeficiency virus (HIV) through maternal blood and blood-stained amniotic fluid, the traditional timing of the newborn's bath has been questioned. The newborn must be considered a potential contamination source until proved otherwise. As part of Standard Precautions, nurses should wear gloves when handling the newborn until blood and amniotic fluid are removed by bathing.

Assessment and Nursing Diagnoses

The initial assessment of the neonate is done at birth by using the Apgar score (Table 19-1) and a brief physical examination (Box 19-1). A gestational age assessment is done within 2 hours of birth (Fig. 19-1). A more comprehensive physical assessment is completed within 24 hours of birth (Table 19-2).

BOX 19-1

Initial Physical Assessment by Body System

CNS	[ ] moves extremities, muscle tone good
	[ ] symmetric features, movement
	[ ] suck, rooting, Moro response, grasp reflexes good
	[ ] anterior fontanel soft and flat
CV	[ ] heart rate strong and regular
	[ ] no murmurs heard
	[ ] pulses strong and equal bilaterally
RESP	[ ] lungs clear to auscultation bilaterally
	[ ] no retractions or nasal flaring
	[ ] respiratory rate, 30-60 breaths/min
	[ ] chest expansion symmetric
	[ ] no upper airway congestion
GU	[ ] male: urethral opening at tip of penis; testes descended bilaterally
	[ ] female: vaginal opening apparent
GI	[ ] abdomen soft, no distention
	[ ] cord attached and clamped
	[ ] anus appears patent
ENT	[ ] eyes clear
	[ ] palates intact
	[ ] nares patent
SKIN	Color [ ] pink [ ] acrocyanotic
	[ ] no lesions or abrasions
	[ ] no peeling
	[ ] birthmarks _____
	[ ] caput and molding
	[ ] vacuum "cap"
	[ ] forceps marks
	[ ] other

Comments: _____
_____
_____
_____

Apgar score

The Apgar score permits a rapid assessment of the need for resuscitation based on five signs that indicate the physiologic state of the neonate: (1) heart rate, based on auscultation with a stethoscope; (2) respiratory rate, based on observed movement of the chest wall; (3) muscle tone, based on degree of flexion and movement of the extremities;

TABLE 19-1

Apgar Score

	SCORE		
SIGN	0	1	2
Heart rate	Absent	Slow (<100)	>100
Respiratory rate	Absent	Slow, weak cry	Good cry
Muscle tone	Flaccid	Some flexion of extremities	Well flexed
Reflex irritability	No response	Grimace	Cry
Color	Blue, pale	Body pink, extremities blue	Completely pink

NEUROMUSCULAR MATURITY

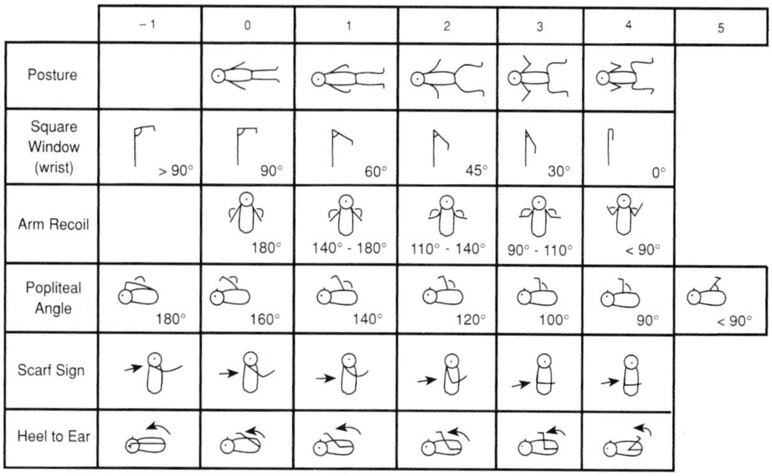

	−1	0	1	2	3	4	5
Posture							
Square Window (wrist)	> 90°	90°	60°	45°	30°	0°	
Arm Recoil		180°	140° - 180°	110° - 140°	90° - 110°	< 90°	
Popliteal Angle	180°	160°	140°	120°	100°	90°	< 90°
Scarf Sign							
Heel to Ear							

A

PHYSICAL MATURITY

Skin	sticky friable transparent	gelatinous red, translucent	smooth pink, visible veins	superficial peeling or rash, few veins	cracking pale areas rare veins	parchment deep cracking no vessels	leathery cracked wrinkled
Lanugo	none	sparse	abundant	thinning	bald areas	mostly bald	
Plantar Surface	heel-toe 40-50 mm: -1 <40 mm: -2	>50 mm no crease	faint red marks	anterior transverse crease only	creases ant. 2/3	creases over entire sole	
Breast	imperceptible	barely perceptible	flat areola no bud	stippled areola 1-2 mm bud	raised areola 3-4 mm bud	full areola 5-10 mm bud	
Eye/Ear	lids fused loosely: -1 tightly: -2	lids open pinna flat stays folded	sl. curved pinna; soft; slow recoil	well-curved pinna; soft but ready recoil	formed & firm instant recoil	thick cartilage ear stiff	
Genitals (male)	scrotum flat, smooth	scrotum empty faint rugae	testes in upper canal rare rugae	testes descending few rugae	testes down good rugae	testes pendulous deep rugae	
Genitals (female)	clitoris prominent labia flat	prominent clitoris small labia minora	prominent clitoris enlarging minora	majora & minora equally prominent	majora large minora small	majora cover clitoris & minora	

MATURITY RATING

score	weeks
-10	20
-5	22
0	24
5	26
10	28
15	30
20	32
25	34
30	36
35	38
40	40
45	42
50	44

Fig. 19-1 Estimation of gestational age. **A,** New Ballard Scale for newborn maturity rating. Expanded scale includes extremely premature infants and has been refined to improve accuracy in more mature infants. (From Ballard, J. et al. [1991]. New Ballard Score, expanded to include extremely premature infants. *Journal of Pediatrics, 119*[3], 417-423.)

Continued

(4) reflex irritability, based on response to gentle slaps on the soles of the feet; and (5) generalized skin color, described as pallid, cyanotic, or pink. Each item is scored as a 0, 1, or 2. Evaluations are made 1 and 5 minutes after birth. Scores of 0 to 3 indicate severe distress; scores of 4 to 6 indicate moderate difficulty; and scores of 7 to 10 indicate that the infant is having no difficulty adjusting to extrauterine life. Apgar scores do not predict future neurologic outcome but are useful for describing the newborn's transition to extrauterine environment (Box 19-2). Should resuscitation be required, it should be initiated before the 1-minute Apgar score (American Academy of Pediatrics [AAP] and American College of Obstetricians and Gynecologists [ACOG], 2002).

Initial Physical Assessment

The initial physical assessment includes a brief review of systems (see Box 19-1):

1. *External:* Note skin color, general activity, position; assess nasal patency by covering one nostril at a time while observing respirations; skin: peeling, or lack of subcutaneous fat (dysmaturity or postterm); note meconium staining of cord, skin, fingernails, or amniotic fluid (staining may indicate fetal release of meconium, often related to hypoxia; offensive odor may indicate intrauterine infection); note length of nails and creases on soles of feet.

2. *Chest:* Auscultate apical heart for rate and rhythm, heart tones and presence of abnormal sounds; note character of respirations and presence of crackles or

CLASSIFICATION OF NEWBORNS—
BASED ON MATURITY AND INTRAUTERINE GROWTH
Symbols: X - 1st Examination O - 2nd Examination

Fig. 19-1, cont'd Estimation of gestational age. **B,** Newborn classification based on maturity and intrauterine growth. (Modified from Lubchenco, L., Hansman, C., & Boyd, E. [1966]. Intrauterine growth in length and head circumference as estimated from live births at gestational ages from 26 to 42 weeks. *Journal of Pediatrics, 37*[3], 403-408; and Battaglia, F., & Lubchenco, L. [1967]. A practical classification of newborn infants by weight and gestational age. *Journal of Pediatrics, 71*[2], 159-167.)

other adventitious sounds; note equality of breath sounds by auscultation.

3. *Abdomen:* Observe characteristics of abdomen (rounded, flat, concave) and absence of anomalies; auscultate bowel sounds; note number of vessels in cord.

4. *Neurologic:* Check muscle tone; assess Moro and suck reflexes; palpate anterior fontanel; note by palpation the presence and size of the fontanels and sutures.

5. *Genitourinary:* Note external sex characteristics and any abnormality of genitalia; check anal patency, presence of meconium; note passage of urine.

6. *Other observations:* Note gross structural malformations obvious at birth that may require immediate medical attention.

The nurse responsible for the care of the newborn immediately after birth verifies that respirations have been

Text continued on p. 575.

TABLE 19-2

Physical Assessment of Newborn

AREA ASSESSED	NORMAL FINDINGS	DEVIATIONS FROM NORMAL RANGE	ETIOLOGY
POSTURE			
Inspect newborn before disturbing Refer to maternal chart for fetal presentation, position, and type of birth (vaginal, surgical), because newborn readily assumes prenatal position	Vertex: arms, legs in moderate flexion; fists clenched Normal spontaneous movement bilaterally asynchronous but equal extension in all extremities Frank breech: legs straighter and stiff	Hypotonia Hypertonia Opisthotonos Limitation of motion in any of extremities (see p. 573)	Prematurity or hypoxia in utero, maternal medications Drug dependence, central nervous system (CNS) disorder CNS disturbance
VITAL SIGNS			

Heart rate and pulses:
  Inspection
  Palpation
  Auscultation
	Visible pulsations in left midclavicular line, fifth intercostal space
	Apical pulse, fourth intercostal space 100-160 beats/min
	80-100 beats/min (sleeping) to 180 beats/min (crying)
	Quality: *first sound* (closure of mitral and tricuspid valves) and *second sound* (closure of aortic and pulmonic valves) sharp and clear
	Possible murmur
		Tachycardia: persistent, ≥180 beats/min
		Bradycardia: persistent, ≤80 beats/min
		Murmurs
		Arrhythmias: irregular rate
		Sounds distant, poor quality, extra
		Heart on right side of chest
			Respiratory distress syndrome (RDS)
			Congenital heart block, maternal lupus
			Possibly functional
			
			Pneumomediastinum
			
			Dextrocardia, often accompanied by reversal of intestines

Peripheral pulses: femoral, brachial, popliteal, posterior tibial	Peripheral pulses equal and strong Femoral pulses equal and strong	Weak or absent peripheral Weak or absent femoral pulses; unequal	Decreased cardiac output, thrombus Hip dysplasia, coarctation of aorta if weak on left and strong on right, thrombophlebitis
Temperature	Axillary: 36.5° C to 37.2° C Temperature stabilized by 8-10 hr of age	Subnormal Increased Temperature not stabilized by 6-8 hr after birth	Prematurity, infection, low environmental temperature, inadequate clothing, dehydration Infection, high environmental temperature, excessive clothing, proximity to heating unit or in direct sunshine, drug addiction, diarrhea and dehydration If mother received magnesium sulfate, maternal analgesics
Check respiratory rate and effort when infant is at rest Count respirations for full minute	30-60 breaths/min Shallow and irregular in rate, rhythm, and depth when infant is awake Crackles may be heard after birth	Apneic episodes: >15 sec Bradypnea: <25/min	Preterm infant: "periodic breathing," rapid warming or cooling of infant Maternal narcosis from analgesics or anesthetics, birth trauma

Continued

TABLE 19-2

Physical Assessment of Newborn—cont'd

AREA ASSESSED	NORMAL FINDINGS	DEVIATIONS FROM NORMAL RANGE	ETIOLOGY
VITAL SIGNS—cont'd			
Respirations—cont'd	Breath sounds loud, clear, near	Tachypnea: >60/min	RDS, congenital diaphragmatic hernia, transient tachypnea of the newborn
		Crackles, rhonchi, wheezes	Fluid in lungs
		Expiratory grunt	Narrowing of bronchi
		Distress evidenced by nasal flaring, retractions, chin tug, labored breathing	RDS, fluid in lungs
Measure blood pressure (BP) using oscillometric monitor BP cuff; palpate brachial, popliteal, or posterior tibial pulse (depending on measurement site)	80-90s/40s-50s	Difference between upper and lower extremity pressures	Coarctation of aorta
		Hypotension	Sepsis, hypovolemia
Check electronic monitor BP cuff: BP cuff width affects readings, use cuff 2.5 cm wide and palpate radial pulse		Hypertension	Coarctation of aorta, renal involvement, thrombus
WEIGHT*			
Weigh at same time each day	2500-4000 g	Weight ≤2500 g	Prematurity, small for gestational age, rubella syndrome
	Acceptable weight loss: ≤10%		
	Second baby weighs more than first	Weight ≥4000 g	Large for gestational age, maternal diabetes, heredity—normal for these parents
	Birth weight regained within first 2 weeks		
		Weight loss >10% to 15%	Dehydration

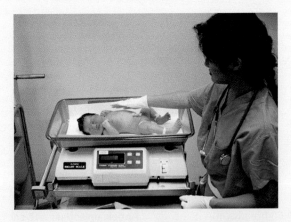

Weighing the infant. Note that a hand is held over the infant as a safety measure. The scale is covered to protect against cross-infection. (Courtesy Kim Molloy, Knoxville, IA.)

*Note: Weight, length, and head circumference all should be close to the same percentile for any newborn.

TABLE 19-2

Physical Assessment of Newborn—cont'd

AREA ASSESSED	NORMAL FINDINGS	DEVIATIONS FROM NORMAL RANGE	ETIOLOGY
LENGTH			
Length from top of head to heel	45-55 cm	<45 cm or >55 cm	Chromosomal abnormality, heredity—normal for these parents

Length, crown to rump. To determine total length, include length of legs. If measurements are taken before the infant's initial bath, wear gloves. (Courtesy Marjorie Pyle, RNC, Lifecircle, Costa Mesa, CA.)

AREA ASSESSED	NORMAL FINDINGS	DEVIATIONS FROM NORMAL RANGE	ETIOLOGY
HEAD CIRCUMFERENCE			
Measure head at greatest diameter: occipitofrontal circumference	32-36.8 cm Circumference of head and chest approximately the same for first 1 or 2 days after birth	Small head ≤32 cm: micro-cephaly	Maternal rubella, toxoplas-mosis, cytomegalic inclu-sion disease, fused cranial sutures (craniosynostosis)
		Hydrocephaly: sutures widely separated, circum-ference ≥4 cm more than chest circumference	Maldevelopment, infection
		Increased intracranial pressure	Hemorrhage, space-occupying lesion

Circumference of head. (Courtesy Marjorie Pyle, RNC, Lifecircle, Costa Mesa, CA.)

Continued

TABLE 19-2

Physical Assessment of Newborn—cont'd

AREA ASSESSED	NORMAL FINDINGS	DEVIATIONS FROM NORMAL RANGE	ETIOLOGY
CHEST CIRCUMFERENCE			
Measure at nipple line	2-3 cm less than head circumference, averages between 30 and 33 cm	≤30 cm	Prematurity

Circumference of chest. (Courtesy Marjorie Pyle, RNC, Lifecircle, Costa Mesa, CA.)

ABDOMINAL CIRCUMFERENCE			
Measure above umbilicus Not usually measured unless specific indication	Same size as chest	Enlarging abdomen between feedings	Abdominal mass or blockage in intestinal tract

Abdominal circumference. (Courtesy Marjorie Pyle, RNC, Lifecircle, Costa Mesa, CA.)

SKIN			
Color	Generally pink	Dark red	Prematurity, polycythemia
	Varying with ethnic origin	Gray	Hypotension, poor perfusion
	Acrocyanosis, especially if chilled	Pallor	Cardiovascular problem, CNS damage, blood dyscrasia, blood loss, twin-to-twin transfusion, nosocomial infection
	Mottling		
	Harlequin sign		
	Plethora		
	Telangiectases ("stork bites" or capillary hemangiomas)	Cyanosis	Hypothermia, infection, hypoglycemia, cardiopulmonary diseases, cardiac, neurologic, or respiratory malformations
	Erythema toxicum or neonatorum ("newborn rash")		
	Milia		

TABLE 19-2

Physical Assessment of Newborn—cont'd

AREA ASSESSED	NORMAL FINDINGS	DEVIATIONS FROM NORMAL RANGE	ETIOLOGY
SKIN—cont'd			
	Petechiae over presenting part	Petechiae over any other area	Clotting factor deficiency, infection
	Ecchymoses from forceps in vertex births or over buttocks, genitalia, and legs in breech births	Ecchymoses in any other area	Hemorrhagic disease, traumatic birth
Jaundice	None at birth	Jaundice within first 24 hr	Increased hemolysis, Rh isoimmunization, ABO incompatibility
	Physiologic jaundice in up to 50% of term infants in first week of life		
Birthmarks	Mongolian spot (see Fig. 18-6)	Hemangiomas	
	Infants of African-American, Asian, and Native American origin: 70%-85%	Nevus flammeus: port-wine stain	
		Nevus vasculosus: strawberry mark	
	Infants of Caucasian origin: 5%-13%	Cavernous hemangiomas	
Check condition	No skin edema	Edema on hands, feet; pitting over tibia	Overhydration
	Opacity: few large blood vessels visible indistinctly over abdomen	Texture thin, smooth, or of medium thickness; rash or superficial peeling visible	Prematurity, postmaturity
		Numerous vessels very visible over abdomen	Prematurity
		Texture thick, parchment-like; cracking, peeling	Postmaturity
		Skin tags, webbing	
		Papules, pustules, vesicles, ulcers, maceration	Impetigo, candidiasis, herpes, diaper rash
Gently pinch skin between thumb and forefinger over abdomen and inner thigh to check for turgor	Dehydration: loss of weight best indicator	Loose, wrinkled skin	Prematurity, postmaturity, dehydration: fold of skin persisting after release of pinch
	After pinch released, skin returns to original state immediately	Tense, tight, shiny skin	Edema, extreme cold, shock, infection
	Normal weight loss after birth: ≤10% of birth weight	Lack of subcutaneous fat, prominence of clavicle or ribs	Prematurity, malnutrition
	Possibly puffy		
Vernix caseosa: Color and odor	Whitish, cheesy, odorless; usually more found in creases, folds	Absent or minimal	Postmaturity
		Excessive	Prematurity
		Green color	Possible in utero release of meconium or presence of bilirubin
		Odor	Possible intrauterine infection
Lanugo	Over shoulders, pinnas of ears, forehead	Absent	Postmaturity
		Excessive	Prematurity, especially if lanugo abundant and long and thick over back

Continued

Physical Assessment of Newborn—cont'd

AREA ASSESSED	NORMAL FINDINGS	DEVIATIONS FROM NORMAL RANGE	ETIOLOGY
HEAD			
	Making up one fourth of body length	Cephalhematoma	
	Molding	Severe molding	Birth trauma
	Caput succedaneum, possibly showing some ecchymosis	Indentation	Fracture from trauma Tumor, hemorrhage, infection
Fontanels Open vs closed	Anterior fontanel 5 cm diamond, increasing as molding resolves	Full, bulging Large, flat, soft Depressed	Malnutrition, hydrocephaly, retarded bone age, hypothyroidism Dehydration
	Posterior fontanel triangle, smaller than anterior		
Sutures	Palpable and unjoined sutures	Widely spaced	Hydrocephaly
	Possible overlap of sutures with molding	Premature closure	Craniosynostosis
Hair	Silky, single strands lying flat; growth pattern toward face and neck, variation in amount	Fine, woolly Unusual swirls, patterns, hairline or coarse, brittle	Prematurity Endocrine or genetic disorders
EYES			
Eyeballs	Both present and of equal size, both round, firm	Agenesis or absence of one or both eyeballs	
	Eyes and space between eyes each one third the distance from outer-to-outer canthus	Epicanthal folds when present with other signs Discharge: purulent	Chromosomal disorders such as Down, cri-du-chat syndromes Infection
	Epicanthal folds: normal racial characteristic Symmetric in size, shape Blink reflex	Small eyeball Lens opacity or absence of red reflex	Rubella syndrome Congenital cataracts, possibly from rubella
	No discharge	Discharge (purulent) Chemical conjunctivitis	Infection Eye medication (requires no treatment)
	No tears Subconjunctival hemorrhage	Lesions: coloboma, absence of part of iris Pink color of iris Jaundiced sclera	Congenital Albinism Hyperbilirubinemia

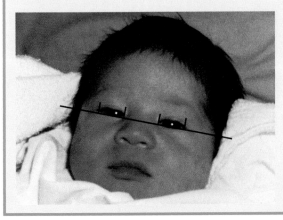

Eyes. In pseudostrabismus, inner epicanthal folds cause the eyes to appear misaligned; however, corneal light reflexes are perfectly symmetric. Eyes are symmetric in size and shape and are well placed.

TABLE 19-2

Physical Assessment of Newborn—cont'd

AREA ASSESSED	NORMAL FINDINGS	DEVIATIONS FROM NORMAL RANGE	ETIOLOGY
EYES—cont'd			
Pupils	Present, equal in size, reactive to light	Pupils: unequal, constricted, dilated, fixed	Intracranial pressure, medications, tumors
Eyeball movement	Random, jerky, uneven, focus possible briefly, following to midline	Persistent strabismus	
		Doll's eyes	Increased intracranial pressure
	Transient strabismus or nystagmus until third or fourth month	Sunset	Increased intracranial pressure
Eyebrows	Distinct (not connected in midline)	Connection in midline	Cornelia de Lange syndrome
NOSE			
	Midline	Copious drainage, with or without regular periods of cyanosis at rest and return of pink color with crying	Choanal atresia, congenital syphilis
	Some mucus but no drainage		
	Preferential nose breather		
	Sneezing to clear nose		
	Slight deformity (flat or deviated to one side) from passage through birth canal	Malformed	Congenital syphilis, chromosomal disorder
		Flaring of nares	Respiratory distress
EARS			
Pinna	Correct placement: line drawn through inner and outer canthi of eyes reaching to top notch of ears (at junction with scalp)	Agenesis	
		Lack of cartilage	Prematurity
		Low placement	Chromosomal disorder, mental retardation, kidney disorder
		Preauricular tags	
	Well-formed, firm cartilage	Size: possibly overly prominent or protruding ears	
Hearing	Responds to voice and other sounds	No response to sound	Deaf, rubella syndrome
	State (e.g., alert, asleep) influences response		

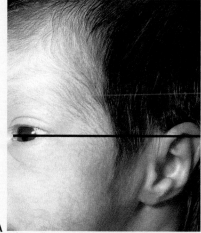 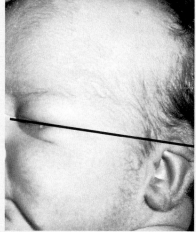 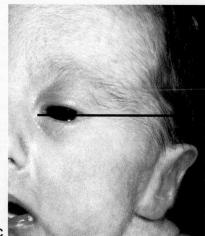

Placement of ears on the head in relation to a line drawn from the inner to the outer canthus of the eye. **A,** Normal position. **B,** Abnormally angled ear. **C,** True low-set ear. (Courtesy Mead Johnson Nutritionals, Evansville, IN.)

Continued

TABLE 19-2

Physical Assessment of Newborn—cont'd

AREA ASSESSED	NORMAL FINDINGS	DEVIATIONS FROM NORMAL RANGE	ETIOLOGY
FACIES			
	"Normal" appearance, well-placed, proportionate, symmetric features	Infant appearance "odd" or "funny"	
	Positional deformities	Usually accompanied by other features such as low-set ears, other structural disorders	Hereditary, chromosomal aberration
MOUTH			
Lips	Symmetry of lip movement	Gross anomalies in placement, size, shape	Cleft lip and/or palate, gums
Buccal mucosa	Dry or moist		
	Pink	Cyanosis, circumoral pallor	Respiratory distress, hypothermia
	Transient circumoral cyanosis	Asymmetry in movement of lips	Cranial nerve VII paralysis
Gums	Pink gums	Teeth: predeciduous or deciduous	Hereditary
	Inclusion cysts (Epstein pearls—Bohn nodules, whitish, hard nodules on gums or roof of mouth)		
Tongue	Tongue not protruding, freely movable, symmetric in shape, movement	Macroglossia	Prematurity, chromosomal disorder
		Short lingual frenulum	
		Thrush: white plaques on cheeks or tongue that bleed if touched	*Candida albicans*
	Sucking pads inside cheeks		
Palate (soft, hard): Arch	Soft and hard palates intact	Cleft hard or soft palate	
Uvula	Uvula in midline		
	Epstein pearls		
Chin	Distinct chin	Micrognathia	Pierre Robin or other syndrome
Saliva	Mouth moist	Excessive saliva	Esophageal atresia, tracheoesophageal fistula
Reflexes: Rooting	Reflexes present	Absent	Prematurity
Sucking	Reflex response dependent on state of wakefulness and hunger		
Extrusion			
NECK			
Sternocleidomastoid muscles	Short, thick, surrounded by skin folds; no webbing	Webbing	Turner syndrome
	Head held in midline (sternocleidomastoid muscles equal), no masses	Restricted movement, holding of head at angle	Torticollis (wryneck), opisthotonos
	Transient positional deformity	Absence of head control	Prematurity, Down syndrome
	Freedom of movement from side to side and flexion and extension, no movement of chin past shoulder		
Thyroid gland	Thyroid not palpable	Masses	Enlarged thyroid
		Distended veins	Cardiopulmonary disorder
CHEST			
Thorax	Almost circular, barrel shaped	Bulging of chest, unequal movement	Pneumothorax, pneumomediastinum
	Tip of sternum possibly prominent	Malformation	Funnel chest—pectus excavatum

TABLE 19-2

Physical Assessment of Newborn—cont'd

AREA ASSESSED	NORMAL FINDINGS	DEVIATIONS FROM NORMAL RANGE	ETIOLOGY
CHEST—cont'd			
Respiratory movements	Symmetric chest movements, chest and abdominal movements synchronized during respirations Occasional retractions, especially when crying	Retractions with or without respiratory distress	Prematurity, RDS
Clavicles	Clavicles intact	Fracture of clavicle; crepitus	Trauma
Ribs	Rib cage symmetric, intact; moves with respirations	Poor development of rib cage and musculature	Prematurity
Nipples	Prominent, well formed; symmetrically placed	Supernumerary, along nipple line Malpositioned or widely spaced	
Breast tissue	Breast nodule: approximately 3-10 mm in term infant		Prematurity
	Secretion of witch's milk	Lack of breast tissue	Maternal hormones
ABDOMEN			
Umbilical cord	Two arteries, one vein	One artery	Renal anomalies
	Whitish gray	Meconium stained	Intrauterine distress
	Definite demarcation between cord and skin, no intestinal structures within cord	Bleeding or oozing around cord	Hemorrhagic disease
	Dry around base, drying Odorless	Redness or drainage around cord	Infection, possible persistence of urachus
	Cord clamp in place for 24 hr	Herniation of abdominal contents into area of cord (e.g., omphalocele); defect covered with thin, friable membrane, possibly extensive	
	Reducible umbilical hernia		
Abdomen	Rounded, prominent, dome shaped because abdominal musculature not fully developed	Gastroschisis: fissure of abdominal cavity	
	Some diastasis of abdominal musculature		
	Liver possibly palpable 1-2 cm below right costal margin		
	No other masses palpable		
	No distention	Distention at birth	Ruptured viscus, genitourinary masses or malformations: hydronephrosis, teratomas, abdominal tumors
		Mild	Overfeeding, high gastrointestinal tract obstruction
		Marked	Lower gastrointestinal tract obstruction, imperforate anus
		Intermittent or transient	Overfeeding
		Partial intestinal obstruction	Stenosis of bowel
		Visible peristalsis	Obstruction
		Malrotation of bowel or adhesions	
		Sepsis	Infection

Continued

TABLE 19-2

TABLE 19-2

Physical Assessment of Newborn—cont'd

AREA ASSESSED	NORMAL FINDINGS	DEVIATIONS FROM NORMAL RANGE	ETIOLOGY
ABDOMEN—cont'd			
Bowel sounds	Sounds present within minutes after birth in healthy term infants	Scaphoid, with bowel sounds in chest and respiratory distress	Diaphragmatic hernia
Stools	Meconium stool passing within 24-48 hr after birth	No stool	Imperforate anus
Color	Linea nigra possibly apparent		Hormone influence during pregnancy
Movement with respiration	Respirations primarily diaphragmatic, abdominal and chest movement synchronous	Decreased abdominal breathing "Seesaw"	Intrathoracic disease, phrenic nerve palsy, diaphragmatic hernia Respiratory distress
GENITALIA			
Female	Female genitals	Ambiguous genitals— enlarged clitoris with urinary meatus on tip, fused labia	Chromosomal disorder, maternal drug ingestion
Clitoris	Usually edematous	Virilized female; extremely large clitoris	Congenital adrenal hyperplasia
Labia majora	Usually edematous, covering labia minora in term newborns		
	Increased pigmentation		Pregnancy hormones
	Edema and ecchymosis		Breech birth
Labia minora	Possible protrusion over labia majora	Labia majora widely separated and labia minora prominent	Prematurity
Discharge	Smegma		
Vagina	Open orifice	Absence of vaginal orifice	
	Some vernix caseosa between labia possible		
	Blood-tinged discharge from pseudomenstruation caused by pregnancy hormones	Fecal discharge	Fistula
	Mucoid discharge		
	Hymenal or vaginal tag	Stenosed meatus	
Urinary meatus	Beneath clitoris, difficult to see (to watch for voiding)	Bladder extrophy	
Male	Male genitals	Increased size and pigmentation caused by pregnancy hormones	Ambiguous genitals
Penis			
Urinary meatus as slit	Meatus at tip of penis	Urinary meatus not on tip of glans penis	Hypospadias, epispadias
Prepuce	Prepuce (foreskin) covering glans penis and not retractable	Prepuce removed if circumcised	Round meatal opening
		Wide variation in size of genitals	

TABLE 19-2

Physical Assessment of Newborn—cont'd

AREA ASSESSED	NORMAL FINDINGS	DEVIATIONS FROM NORMAL RANGE	ETIOLOGY
GENITALIA—cont'd			
Male—cont'd			
Scrotum	Large, edematous, pendulous in term infant; covered with rugae	Scrotal edema and ecchymosis if breech birth	
Rugae (wrinkles)		Scrotum smooth and testes undescended	Prematurity, cryptorchidism
		Hydrocele, small, noncommunicating	
		Inguinal hernia	
		Bulge palpable in inguinal canal	Prematurity
Testes	Palpable on each side	Undescended	
Check urination	Voiding within 24 hr, stream adequate, amount adequate	Uric acid crystals*	
Check reflex	Rust-stained urine		
Cremasteric	Testes retracted, especially when newborn is chilled		
EXTREMITIES			
Degree of flexion	Assuming of position maintained in utero	Limited motion	Malformations
Range of motion		Poor muscle tone	Prematurity, maternal medications, CNS anomalies
Symmetry of motion	Transient (positional) deformities	Positive scarf sign	
	Attitude of general flexion	Asymmetry of movement	
Muscle tone	Full range of motion, spontaneous movements		Fracture or crepitus, brachial nerve trauma, malformations
Arms and hands	Longer than legs in newborn period	Asymmetry of contour	Malformations, fracture
Intactness		Amelia or phocomelia	Teratogens
Appropriate placement	Contours and movement symmetric	Palmar creases	
	Slight tremors sometimes apparent	Simian line with short, incurved little fingers	Down syndrome
Color	Some acrocyanosis, especially when chilled		
Fingers	Five on each hand	Webbing of fingers: syndactyly	Familial trait
	Fist often clenched with thumb under fingers	Absence or excess of fingers	
		Strong, rigid flexion; persistent fists; positioning of fists in front of mouth constantly	CNS disorder
Joints	Full range of motion, symmetric contour	Increased tonicity, clonus, prolonged tremors	CNS disorder
Grasp (palmar and plantar)			
Humerus	Intact	Fractured humerus	Trauma
Legs and feet	Appearance of bowing because lateral muscles more developed than medial muscles	Amelia (absence of limbs), phocomelia (shortened limbs)	Chromosomal deficiency, teratogenic effect
	Feet appearing to turn in but can be easily rotated externally, positional defects tending to correct while infant is crying	Temperature of one leg different from that of the other	Circulatory deficiency CNS disorder
	Acrocyanosis		

*To determine whether rust color is caused by uric acid or blood, rinse diaper under running warm tap water; uric acid washes out, blood does not.

TABLE 19-2

Physical Assessment of Newborn—cont'd

AREA ASSESSED	NORMAL FINDINGS	DEVIATIONS FROM NORMAL RANGE	ETIOLOGY
EXTREMITIES—cont'd			
Toes	Five on each foot	Webbing, syndactyly	Chromosomal defect
		Absence or excess of digits	Chromosomal defect, familial trait
Femur	Intact femur	Femoral fracture	Difficult breech birth
	No click heard, femoral head not overriding acetabulum	Developmental dysplasia or dislocation	
	Major gluteal folds even		
Soles of feet	Soles well lined (or wrinkled) over two thirds of foot in term infants	Soles of feet	
		Few lines	Prematurity
		Covered with lines	Postmaturity
	Plantar fat pad giving flat-footed effect	Congenital clubfoot	
Joints	Full range of motion, symmetric contour	Hypermobility of joints	Down syndrome
		Asymmetric movement	Trauma, CNS disorder
BACK			
Spine	Spine straight and easily flexed	Limitation of movement	Fusion or deformity of vertebra
Shoulders	Infant able to raise and support head momentarily when prone		
Scapulae			
Iliac crests			
	Temporary minor positional deformities, correction with passive manipulation		
	Shoulders, scapulae, and iliac crests lining up in same plane		
Base of spine—pilonidal area		Spina bifida cystica	Meningocele, myelomeningocele
		Pigmented nevus with tuft of hair	Often associated with spina bifida occulta
ANUS			
Patency	One anus with good sphincter tone	Low obstruction: anal membrane	
Sphincter response (active "wink" reflex)	Passage of meconium within 24-48 hr after birth	High obstruction: anal or rectal atresia	
	Good "wink" reflex of anal sphincter	Absence of anal opening	
		Drainage of fecal material from vagina in female or urinary meatus in male	Rectal fistula
STOOLS			
Frequency, color, consistency	Meconium followed by transitional and soft yellow stools	No stool	Obstruction
		Frequent watery stools	Infection, phototherapy

BOX 19-2

Significance of the Apgar Score

The Apgar score was developed to provide a systematic method of assessing an infant's condition at birth. Researchers have tried to correlate Apgar scores with various outcomes such as development, intelligence, and neurologic development. In some instances, researchers have attempted to attribute causality to the Apgar score, that is, to suggest that the low Apgar score caused or predicted later problems. This is an inappropriate use of the Apgar score. Instead the score should be used to ensure that infants are systematically observed at birth to ascertain the need for immediate care. Either a physician or a nurse may assign the score; however, to avoid the real or perceived appearance of bias, the person assisting with the birth should not assign the score. Lack of consistency in the assigned scores limits studies of the Apgar's long-term predictive value. Prospective parents and the public need education on the significance of the Apgar score, as well as its limits. Because infants often do not receive the maximum score of 10, parents need to know that scores of 7 to 10 are within normal limits. Attorneys involved in litigation related to injury of an infant at birth or negative outcomes, either short term or long term, also need education about the Apgar score, its significance, and its limits. This useful tool needs to be used appropriately; health care providers, parents, and the public may need education to ensure appropriate use of the score.

Data from Montgomery, K. (2000). Apgar scores: Examining the long-term significance. *Journal of Perinatal Education, 9*(3), 5-9.

BOX 19-3

Routine Admission Orders

- Vital signs on admission and q30min × 2, q1hr × 2, then q8hr
- Weight, length, and head and chest circumference on admission; then weigh daily
- Tetracycline or erythromycin ophthalmic ointment 5 mg 1 to 2 cm line in lower conjunctiva of each eye after initial parent-infant contact (but within 2 hr of birth)
- Vitamin K 0.5 to 1 mg intramuscularly
- Breastfeeding on demand may be initiated immediately after birth
- If formula feeding, give formula of mother's choice q3-4 hr on demand
- Allow rooming-in as desired and infant's condition permits
- Newborn screening panel per state health department protocol (phenylketonuria [PKU], thyroxine [T_4], and galactosemia or other newborn screening tests as ordered at least 24 hr after first feeding)
- Perform hearing screening and document results before discharge
- Serum bilirubin measurement if clinical jaundice evident
- Hepatitis B injection if indicated

established, dries the infant, assesses temperature, and places identical identification bracelets on the infant and the mother. In some settings, the father or partner also wears an identification bracelet. The infant may be wrapped in a warm blanket and placed in the arms of the mother, given to the partner to hold, or kept partially undressed under a radiant warmer. In some settings, immediately after birth the infant is placed on the mother's abdomen to allow skin-to-skin contact. This contributes to maintenance of the infant's optimum temperature and parental bonding. The infant may be admitted to a nursery or may remain with the parents throughout the hospital stay.

The initial examination of the newborn can occur while the nurse is drying and wrapping the infant, or observations can be made while the infant is lying on the mother's abdomen or in her arms immediately after birth. Efforts should be directed to minimizing interference in the initial parent-infant acquaintance process. If the infant is breathing effectively, is pink in color, and has no apparent life-threatening anomalies or risk factors requiring immediate attention (e.g., infant of a diabetic mother), further examination can be delayed until after the parents have had an opportunity to interact with the infant. Routine procedures and the admission process can be carried out in the mother's room or in a separate nursery. Box 19-3 shows an example of newborn routine orders.

Nursing diagnoses are established after analysis of the findings of the physical assessment and may include the following:

- *Ineffective airway clearance related to*
  —airway obstruction with mucus, blood, and amniotic fluid
- *Impaired gas exchange related to*
  —airway obstruction
- *Ineffective thermoregulation related to*
  —excess heat loss
- *Risk for infection related to*
  —intrauterine or extrauterine exposure to virulent virus or bacteria
  —multiple sites for opportunistic bacterial and viral entry (e.g., umbilical cord, lesions from fetal scalp electrode or vacuum extraction)

Expected Outcomes of Care

Expected outcomes can apply to both the infant and the caregiver. The expected outcomes for the newborn during the immediate recovery period include that the infant will achieve the following:

- Maintain effective breathing pattern
- Maintain effective thermoregulation
- Remain free from infection
- Receive necessary nutrition for growth

Expected outcomes for the parents include that they will do the following:

- Attain knowledge, skill, and confidence relevant to infant care activities

Procedure

Suctioning with a Bulb Syringe

The mouth is suctioned first to prevent the infant from inhaling pharyngeal secretions by gasping as the nares are touched.

The bulb is compressed (see Fig. 19-2) and inserted into one side of the mouth. The center of the infant's mouth is avoided because this could stimulate the gag reflex.

The nasal passages are suctioned one nostril at a time.

When the infant's cry does not sound as though it is through mucus or a bubble, suctioning can be stopped. The bulb syringe should always be kept in the infant's crib.

The parents should be given demonstrations on how to use the bulb syringe and asked to perform a return demonstration.

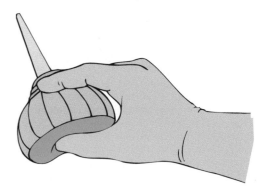

Fig. 19-2 Bulb syringe. Bulb must be compressed before insertion.

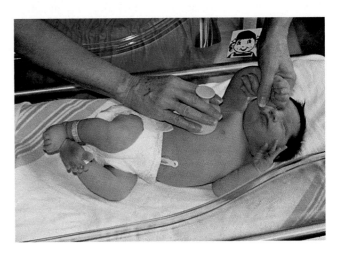

Fig. 19-3 Chest percussion. Nurse performs gentle percussion over the chest wall by using a percussion cup to aid in loosening secretions before suctioning. (Courtesy Shannon Perry, Phoenix, AZ.)

- State understanding of biologic and behavioral characteristics of the newborn
- Begin to integrate the infant into the family

Plan of Care and Interventions

Changes can occur rapidly in newborns immediately after birth. Assessment must be followed quickly by the implementation of appropriate care.

Identification

Information on the matching identification bracelets applied immediately after birth to the newborn and mother (and in some institutions, the father or significant other) should include name, sex, date and time of birth, and identification number, according to hospital protocol. Infants also are footprinted by using a form that includes the mother's fingerprints, name, and date and time of birth. These identification procedures must be performed before the mother and infant are separated after birth.

Stabilization

Generally, the normal term infant born vaginally has little difficulty clearing the airway. Most secretions are moved by gravity and brought to the oropharynx by the cough reflex. The infant is often maintained in a side-lying position (head stabilized, not in Trendelenburg) with a rolled blanket at the back to facilitate drainage.

If the infant has excess mucus in the respiratory tract, the mouth and nasal passages may be suctioned with the bulb syringe (Procedure box and Fig. 19-2). The nurse may perform gentle percussion over the chest wall using a soft circular mask or a percussion cup to aid in loosening secretions before suctioning (Fig. 19-3). Routine chest percussion is avoided, especially in preterm newborns, because this may cause more harm than good; the head should be kept steady during the procedure and the infant's tolerance to the procedure carefully evaluated (Hagedorn, Gardner, & Abman,

2002). The infant who is choking on secretions should be supported with the head to the side. The mouth is suctioned first to prevent the infant from inhaling pharyngeal secretions by gasping as the nares are touched. The bulb is compressed and inserted into one side of the mouth. The center of the mouth is avoided because this could stimulate the gag reflex. The nasal passages are suctioned one nostril at a time. The bulb syringe should always be kept in the infant's crib. The parents should be given a demonstration of how to use the bulb syringe and asked to perform a return demonstration.

Use of nasopharyngeal catheter with mechanical suction apparatus. Deeper suctioning may be needed to remove mucus from the newborn's nasopharynx or posterior oropharynx. Proper tube insertion and suctioning for 5 seconds or less per tube insertion helps prevent vagal stimulation and hypoxia (Niermeyer, 2005) (Procedure box).

Relieving airway obstruction. A choking infant needs immediate attention. Often, simply repositioning the infant and suctioning the mouth and nose with the bulb sy-

Procedure

Suctioning with a Nasopharyngeal Catheter with Mechanical Suction Apparatus

To remove excessive or tenacious mucus from the infant's nasopharynx:

If wall suction is used, adjust the pressure to <80 mm Hg. Proper tube insertion and suctioning for 5 sec per tube insertion help prevent laryngospasms and oxygen depletion.

Lubricate the catheter in sterile water and then insert either orally along the base of the tongue or up and back into the nares.

After the catheter is properly placed, create suction by placing your thumb over the control as the catheter is carefully rotated and gently withdrawn.

Repeat the procedure until the infant's cry sounds clear and air entry into the lungs is heard by stethoscope.

---

signs of
POTENTIAL COMPLICATIONS

Abnormal Newborn Breathing

- Bradypnea: respirations (≤25/min)
- Tachypnea: respirations (≥60/min)
- Abnormal breath sounds: crackles, rhonchi, wheezes, expiratory grunt
- Respiratory distress: nasal flaring, retractions, chin tug, labored breathing

---

ringe eliminates the problem. The infant should be positioned with the head slightly lower than the body to facilitate gravity drainage. The nurse also should listen to the infant's respiration and lung sounds with a stethoscope to determine whether there are crackles, rhonchi, or inspiratory stridor. Fine crackles may be auscultated for several hours after birth. If air movement is adequate, the bulb syringe may be used to clear the mouth and nose. If the bulb syringe does not clear mucus interfering with respiratory effort, mechanical suction can be used.

If the newborn has an obstruction that is not cleared with suctioning, further investigation must be performed to determine if there is a mechanical defect (e.g., tracheoesophageal fistula, choanal atresia) causing the obstruction (see Emergency: Relieving Airway Obstruction, p. 612).

Maintaining an adequate oxygen supply. Four conditions are essential for maintaining an adequate oxygen supply:

- A clear airway
- Effective establishment of respirations
- Adequate circulation, adequate perfusion, and effective cardiac function
- Adequate thermoregulation (exposure to cold stress increases oxygen and glucose needs)

Signs of potential complications related to abnormal breathing are listed in the Signs of Potential Complications box.

Maintenance of body temperature

Effective neonatal care includes maintenance of an optimal thermal environment. Cold stress increases the need for oxygen and may deplete glucose stores. The infant may react to exposure to cold by increasing the respiratory rate and may become cyanotic. Ways to stabilize the newborn's body temperature include placing the infant directly on the mother's abdomen and covering with a warm blanket (skin-to-skin contact); drying and wrapping the newborn in warmed blankets immediately after birth; keeping the head well covered; and keeping the ambient temperature of the nursery at 23.8° to 26.1° C (AAP & ACOG, 2002).

If the infant does not remain with the mother during the first 1 to 2 hours after birth, the nurse places the thoroughly dried infant under a radiant warmer until the body temperature stabilizes. The infant's skin temperature is used as the point of control in a warmer with a servocontrolled mechanism. The control panel usually is maintained between 36° and 37°C. This setting should maintain the healthy newborn's skin temperature at approximately 36.5° to 37°C. A thermistor probe (automatic sensor) is taped to the right upper quadrant of the abdomen immediately below the right intercostal margin (never over a bone). A reflector adhesive patch may be used over the probe to provide adequate warming. This will ensure detection of minor changes resulting from external environmental factors or neonatal factors (peripheral vasoconstriction, vasodilation, or increased metabolism) before a dramatic change in core body temperature develops. The servocontroller adjusts the warmer temperature to maintain the infant's skin temperature within the present range. The sensor must be checked periodically to make sure it is securely attached to the infant's skin. The axillary temperature of the newborn is checked every hour (or more often as needed) until the newborn's temperature stabilizes. The time to stabilize and maintain body temperature varies; each newborn should therefore be allowed to achieve thermal regulation as necessary, and care should be individualized.

During all procedures, heat loss must be avoided or minimized for the newborn; therefore examinations and activities are performed with the newborn under a heat panel. The initial bath is postponed until the newborn's skin temperature is stable and can adjust to heat loss from a bath. The exact and optimal timing of the bath for each newborn remains unknown.

Even a normal term infant in good health can become hypothermic. Birth in a car on the way to the hospital, a cold birthing room, or inadequate drying and wrapping immediately after birth may cause the newborn's temperature to fall below the normal range (**hypothermia**). Warming the hypothermic infant is accomplished with care. Rapid warming may cause apneic spells and acidosis in an infant. The warming process is monitored to progress slowly over a period of 2 to 4 hours.

Therapeutic interventions

It is the nurse's responsibility to perform certain interventions immediately after birth to provide for the safety of the newborn.

Eye prophylaxis. The instillation of a prophylactic agent in the eyes of all neonates is mandatory in the United States as a precaution against ophthalmia neonatorum (Fig. 19-4). This is an inflammation of the eyes resulting from gonorrheal or chlamydial infection contracted by the newborn during passage through the mother's birth canal. The agent used for prophylaxis varies according to hospital protocols, but the usual agent is erythromycin, tetracycline, or silver nitrate. In some institutions, eye prophylaxis is delayed until an hour or so after birth so that eye contact and parent-infant attachment and bonding are facilitated. The Centers for Disease Control and Prevention specifies that it should be given as soon as possible after birth; if instillation is delayed, there should be a monitoring process in place to ensure that all newborns are treated (Workowski & Levine, 2002) (Medication Guide). In the United States, if parents object to eye prophylaxis, they may be asked to sign an informed refusal form, and their refusal will be noted in the infant's record.

Topical antibiotics such as tetracycline and erythromycin, silver nitrate, and a 2.5% povidone-iodine solution (currently unavailable in commercial form in the United States) have not proved to be effective in the treatment of chlamydial conjunctivitis.

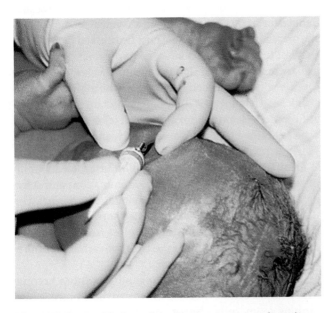

Fig. 19-4 Instillation of medication into eye of newborn. Thumb and forefinger are used to open the eye; medication is placed in the lower conjunctiva from the inner to the outer canthus. (Courtesy Marjorie Pyle, RNC, Lifecircle, Costa Mesa, CA.)

Medication Guide

Eye Prophylaxis: Erythromycin Ophthalmic Ointment, 0.5%, and Tetracycline Ophthalmic Ointment, 1%

ACTION
- These antibiotic ointments are both bacteriostatic and bactericidal. They provide prophylaxis against *Neisseria gonorrhoeae* and *Chlamydia trachomatis*.

INDICATION
- These medications are applied to prevent ophthalmia neonatorum in newborns of mothers who are infected with gonorrhea, conjunctivitis, and chlamydia.

NEONATAL DOSAGE
- Apply a 1- to 2-cm ribbon of ointment to the lower conjunctival sac of each eye; also may be used in drop form.

ADVERSE REACTIONS
- May cause chemical conjunctivitis that lasts 24 to 48 hours; vision may be blurred temporarily.

NURSING CONSIDERATIONS
- Administer within 1 to 2 hr of birth. Wear gloves. Cleanse eyes if necessary before administration. Open eyes by putting a thumb and finger at the corner of each lid and gently pressing on the periorbital ridges. Squeeze the tube and spread the ointment from the inner canthus of the eye to the outer canthus. Do not touch the tube to the eye. After 1 min, excess ointment may be wiped off. Observe eyes for irritation. Explain treatment to parents.
- Eye prophylaxis for ophthalmia neonatorum is required by law in all states of the United States.

A 14-day course of oral erythromycin or an oral sulfonamide may be given for chlamydial conjunctivitis (AAP & ACOG, 2002) (see Medication Guide).

Vitamin K administration. For the first few days after birth the newborn is at risk for prolonged clotting and bleeding because of vitamin K deficiency. Vitamin K is poorly transferred across the placenta or through breast milk, and the infant's intestines are not yet colonized by microflora that synthesize vitamin K. Administering vitamin K intramuscularly is routine in the newborn period. A single parenteral dose of 0.5 to 1 mg of vitamin K is given soon after birth to prevent hemorrhagic disorders (Kliegman, 2002; Miller & Newman, 2005). By day 8, term newborns are able to produce their own vitamin K (Medication Guide).

NURSE ALERT *Vitamin K is never administered by the intravenous route for prevention of hemorrhagic disease of the newborn except in some cases of a preterm infant who has no muscle mass. In such cases, the medication should be diluted and given over 10 to 15 minutes, with the infant being closely monitored with a cardiorespiratory monitor. Rapid bolus administration of vitamin K may cause cardiac arrest.*

Medication Guide

Vitamin K: Phytonadione (AquaMEPHYTON, Konakion)

ACTION
- This intervention provides vitamin K because the newborn does not have the intestinal flora to produce this vitamin in the first week after birth. It also promotes formation of clotting factors (II, VII, IX, X) in the liver.

INDICATION
- Vitamin K is used for prevention and treatment of hemorrhagic disease in the newborn.

NEONATAL DOSAGE
- Administer a 0.5- to 1-mg (0.25- to 0.5-ml) dose intramuscularly within 2 hr of birth; may be repeated if newborn shows bleeding tendencies.

ADVERSE REACTIONS
- Edema, erythema, and pain at injection site may occur rarely; hemolysis, jaundice, and hyperbilirubinemia have been reported, particularly in preterm infants.

NURSING CONSIDERATIONS
- Wear gloves. Administer in the middle third of the vastus lateralis muscle by using a 25-gauge, ⅝-inch needle. Inject into skin that has been cleaned, or allow alcohol to dry on puncture site for 1 min to remove organisms and prevent infection. Stabilize leg firmly, and grasp muscle between the thumb and fingers. Insert the needle at a 90-degree angle; release muscle; aspirate, and inject medication slowly if there is no blood return. Massage the site with a dry gauze square after removing needle to increase absorption. Observe for signs of bleeding from the site.

Umbilical cord care. The cord is clamped immediately after birth. The goal of cord care is to prevent or decrease the risk of hemorrhage or infection. The umbilical cord stump is an excellent medium for bacterial growth and can easily become infected (Miller & Newman, 2005).

NURSE ALERT *If bleeding from the blood vessels of the cord is noted, the nurse checks the clamp (or tie) and applies a second clamp next to the first one. If bleeding is not stopped immediately, the nurse calls for assistance.*

Hospital protocol directs the time and technique for routine cord care. Many hospitals have subscribed to the practice of "dry care" consisting of cleaning the periumbilical area with soap and water and wiping it dry. Others apply an antiseptic solution such as Triple Dye or alcohol to the cord (Janssen, Selwood, Dobson, Peacock, & Thiessen, 2003). Current recommendations for cord care by the Association of Women's Health, Obstetric and Neonatal Nurses (AWHONN) include cleaning the cord with sterile water or a neutral pH cleanser. Subsequent care entails cleansing the cord with water (AWHONN, 2001). The stump and base of

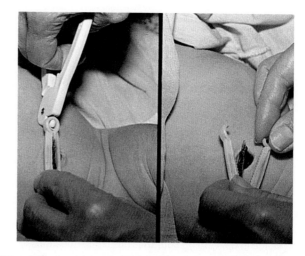

Fig. 19-5 With special scissors, remove clamp after cord dries (about 24 hours). (Courtesy Marjorie Pyle, RNC, Lifecircle, Costa Mesa, CA.)

the cord should be assessed for edema, redness, and purulent drainage with each diaper change. The cord clamp is removed after 24 hours when the cord is dry (Fig. 19-5). Cord separation time is influenced by a number of factors, including type of cord care, type of birth, and other perinatal events. The average cord separation time is 10 to 14 days.

Promoting parent-infant interaction

Today's childbirth practices strive to promote the family as the focus of care. Parents generally desire to share in the birth process and have early contact with their infants. Early contact between mother and newborn can be important in developing future relationships. It also has a positive effect on the duration of breastfeeding. The physiologic benefits of early mother-infant contact include increased oxytocin and prolactin levels in the mother and activation of sucking reflexes in the infant. The infant can be put to breast soon after birth. The process of developing active immunity begins as the infant ingests flora from the mother's colostrum.

Evaluation

Evaluation of the effectiveness of immediate care of the newborn is based on the previously stated outcomes.

CARE MANAGEMENT: FROM 2 HOURS AFTER BIRTH UNTIL DISCHARGE

The infant's admission to the nursery may be delayed, or it may never actually occur. Depending on the routine of the hospital, the infant frequently remains in the labor area and is then transferred to either the nursery or the postpartum unit with the mother. Many hospitals have adopted variations of single-room maternity care (SRMC) or mother-baby care in which one nurse provides care for the mother and newborn. SRMC allows the infant to remain with the parents after the birth. Many of the procedures, such as

EVIDENCE-BASED PRACTICE

Optimum Duration of Exclusive Breastfeeding: Systematic World Health Organization Review

BACKGROUND

- Breastfeeding provides many documented health benefits and can be lifesaving in developing countries. Breastfeeding has a protective effect against gastrointestinal and respiratory infection, sudden infant death syndrome (SIDS), atopic disease, obesity, diabetes, Crohn's disease, and lymphoma. Breastfeeding may accelerate neurocognitive development and achievement. Maternal health benefits include possible protection against breast cancer, ovarian cancer, and osteoporosis.
- An observation of "growth faltering" at about 3 months of age in developing countries has led to questions about the nutritional and energy content of breast milk after 3 or 4 months, the nutritional quality of supplemental foods introduced at about 3 to 4 months, and the risk of infection-caused energy deficit in infants. A debate about the "weanling's dilemma" stemmed from questions about inadequate breast milk nutrition versus nutritionally inadequate or contaminated weaning foods. WHO requested this review of available evidence regarding the optimum duration of breastfeeding.

OBJECTIVES

- All agreed that exclusive breastfeeding was best for 3 to 4 months. The reviewers compared health, growth, and development outcomes for those who continued exclusive breastfeeding until 6 months, versus those who gradually added supplemental liquid or food to breastfeeding. The participants could all be healthy, singleton, term infants (low birth weight accepted, as long as gestationally full term). Infant outcome measures could include weight, length, head circumference, infections, morbidity, mortality, micronutrient status, neuromotor and cognitive developmental milestones, atopic disease, type 1 diabetes, blood pressure, adult chronic illnesses, and inflammatory and autoimmune diseases. Maternal outcome measures include postpartum weight loss, lactational amenorrhea, breast and ovarian cancer, and osteoporosis.

METHODS

Search Strategy

- A search of world literature included Cochrane, MEDLINE, EMBASE, CINAHL, HealthSTAR, EBM Reviews—Best Evidence, SocioFile, CAB Abstracts, EMBASE—Psychology, EconLit, Index Medicus for the WHO Eastern Mediterranean, African Index Medicus, and LILACS Latin American and Caribbean literature. Search keywords included *exclusive breastfeeding* and *growth.*
- Twenty studies were reviewed, nine from developing countries (including the Philippines, Peru, Chile, Honduras, Bangladesh, Belarus, East India, and Senegal) and eleven from developed countries (the United States, Sweden, Finland, Australia, and Italy). The studies were published from 1980 to 2000. Two were controlled trials from Honduras, and the rest were observational studies.

Statistical Analyses

- Statistical analyses were possible in only the two controlled trials. The observational studies were too heterogeneous and limited by design to pool data.

FINDINGS

- The authors found no significant difference in weight, length, or atopic disease in the two groups. Exclusively breastfed infants had significantly decreased gastrointestinal infections. There was a marginally significant decrease in the iron stores of exclusively breastfed infants in developing countries at 6 months, unless they were receiving an iron supplement. Maternal weight loss was accelerated in exclusive breastfeeding, and lactational amenorrhea was prolonged.

LIMITATIONS

- Observational studies are subject to bias. *Confounding by indication* refers to statistical errors that occur because the reason for the treatment (i.e., food supplementation given to a growth-faltering breastfed infant) affects the outcome. Bias can also occur because of reverse causality. For example, an infant with an infection becomes anorectic and reduces milk intake to the point of loss of milk production. The infection might be blamed on the weaning, instead of the reverse.

CONCLUSIONS

- The researchers found no evidence of a "weanling's dilemma," and no benefits from adding supplemental food between 4 and 6 months. The iron deficit of exclusively breastfed babies in developing countries can be corrected with infant drops and does not warrant the loss of protection against gastrointestinal and respiratory infections that exclusive breastfeeding confers. Maternal lactational amenorrhea provides contraceptive benefit for child spacing. Rapid postpartum weight loss may not benefit women with marginal nutritional status. The policy statements of WHO and the World Health Assembly were modified to reflect the recommendation for exclusive breastfeeding for the first 6 months of life.

IMPLICATIONS FOR PRACTICE

- Exclusive breastfeeding should be recommended. Iron supplements for breastfeeding infants are beneficial. The contraceptive benefits of lactational amenorrhea are important.

IMPLICATIONS FOR FURTHER RESEARCH

- Public health policy demands information about breastfeeding beyond the observational stage. Large, randomized trials are needed, especially in developing countries, to confirm infection morbidity and infant nutritional status in exclusively breastfed infants of 6 months' duration or longer. Costs are not addressed in these studies. More information on long-term outcomes is needed.

Reference: Kramer, M., & Kakuma, R. (2001). Optimal duration of exclusive breastfeeding (Cochrane Review). In *The Cochrane Library,* Issue 2, 2004. Chichester, UK: John Wiley & Sons.

assessment of weight and measurement (i.e., circumference of head and chest, length), instillation of eye medications, intramuscular administration of vitamin K, and physical assessment, may be carried out in the labor and birth unit. Nurses who work in an SRMC unit; labor, delivery, and recovery (LDR) room; or labor, delivery, recovery, and postpartum (LDRP) room must be knowledgeable and competent in intrapartal, neonatal, and postpartum nursing care. If an infant is transferred to the nursery, the infant's identification is verified by the nurse receiving the infant, who places the baby in a warm environment and begins the admission process.

Regardless of the physical organization for care, many hospitals have a small holding nursery, which is available for procedures or on the request of the mother who wishes her infant to be placed there. This arrangement promotes parent-infant bonding while still allowing the new parents some time to be alone.

Assessment and Nursing Diagnoses
Gestational age assessment

Assessment of gestational age is an important criterion because perinatal morbidity and mortality rates are related to gestation age and birth weight. The simplified Assessment of Gestational Age (Ballard, Novak, & Driver, 1979) is commonly used to assess gestational age of infants between 35 and 42 weeks. It assesses six external physical and six neuromuscular signs. Each sign has a number score, and the cumulative score correlates with a maturity rating of 26 to 44 weeks of gestation. The score is accurate to plus or minus 2 weeks and is accurate for infants of all races.

The New Ballard Score, a revision of the original scale, can be used with newborns as young as 20 weeks of gestation. The tool has the same physical and neuromuscular sections but includes -1 to -2 scores that reflect signs of extremely premature infants, such as fused eyelids; imperceptible breast tissue; sticky, friable, transparent skin; no lanugo; and square-window (flexion of wrist) angle greater than 90 degrees (see Fig. 19-1, *A*). The examination of infants with a gestational age of 26 weeks or less should be performed at a postnatal age of less than 12 hours. For infants with a gestational age of at least 26 weeks, the examination can be performed up to 96 hours after birth. To ensure accuracy, it is recommended that the initial examination be performed within the first 48 hours of life. Neuromuscular adjustments after birth in extremely immature neonates require that a follow-up examination be performed to further validate neuromuscular criteria. The scale overestimates gestational age by 2 to 4 days in infants younger than 37 weeks of gestation, especially at gestational ages of 32 to 37 weeks (Ballard et al., 1991).

Classification of newborns by gestational age and birth weight

Classification of infants at birth by both birth weight and gestational age provides a more satisfactory method for predicting mortality risks and providing guidelines for management of the neonate than estimating gestational age or birth weight alone. The infant's birth weight, length, and head circumference are plotted on standardized graphs that identify normal values for gestational age. A normal range of birth weights exists for each gestational week (see Fig. 19-1, *B*), but the birth weights of preterm, term, postterm, or postmature newborns also may be outside these normal ranges. Birth weights are classified in the following ways:

- *Large for gestational age (LGA)*—Weight is above the 90th percentile (or two or more standard deviations above the norm) at any week.
- *Appropriate for gestational age (AGA)*—Weight falls between the 10th and 90th percentile for infant's age.
- *Small for gestational age (SGA)*—Weight is below the 10th percentile (or two or more standard deviations below the norm) at any week.
- *Low birth weight (LBW)*—Weight of 2500 g or less at birth. These newborns have had either less than the expected rate of intrauterine growth or a shortened gestation period. Preterm birth and LBW commonly occur together (e.g., less than 32 weeks of gestation and birth weight of less than 1200 g).
- *Very low birth weight (VLBW)*—Weight of 1500 g or less at birth.
- *Intrauterine growth restriction (IUGR)*—Term applied to the fetus whose rate of growth does not meet expected norms.

Newborns are classified according to their gestational ages in the following ways:

- *Preterm or premature*—Born before completion of 37 weeks of gestation, regardless of birth weight
- *Term*—Born between the beginning of week 38 and the end of week 42 of gestation
- *Postterm (postdate)*—Born after completion of week 42 of gestation
- *Postmature*—Born after completion of week 42 of gestation and showing the effects of progressive placental insufficiency

Maternal effects on gestational age assessment and birth weight. Some maternal conditions can affect the results of the gestational assessment. For instance, any infant who has had oxygen deprivation during labor will show poor muscle tone. Infants in respiratory distress tend to be flaccid and assume a "frog-leg" posture. Even though an infant may look large, such as the infant of a diabetic mother, it may respond more like a premature infant. The infant of a mother who has been receiving magnesium sulfate will tend to be somewhat lethargic.

Physical assessment

A complete physical examination is performed within 24 hours after birth. The parents' presence during this examination encourages discussion of parental concerns and actively involves the parents in the health care of their infant from birth. It also affords the nurse an opportunity to observe parental interactions with the infant.

The area used for the examination should be well lighted, warm, and free from drafts. The infant is undressed as needed and placed on a firm, warmed, flat surface or under a radiant warmer. The physical assessment should begin with a review of the maternal history and prenatal and intrapartal records. This provides a background for the recognition of any potential problems.

The assessment includes general appearance, behavior, vital signs measurement, and parent-infant interactions. The assessment should progress systematically from head to toe, with assessment and evaluation of each system (i.e., cardiovascular, respiratory, and so on). Descriptions of any variations from normal findings and all abnormal findings are included. The findings provide a database for implementing the nursing process with newborns and providing anticipatory guidance for the parents. (Table 19-2 summarizes the newborn assessment.) Ongoing assessments of the newborn are made throughout the hospital stay, and an evaluation is performed before discharge.

Nursing considerations in assessment. The neonate's maturity level can be gauged by assessment of general appearance. Features to assess in the general survey include skin color, posture, state of alertness, cry, head size, lanugo, vernix caseosa, breast tissue, and sole creases. The normal resting posture of the neonate is one of general flexion. The neck is short, and the abdomen is prominent.

The temperature, heart rate, and respiratory rate are always obtained. Blood pressure (BP) is not routinely assessed unless cardiac problems are suspected. An irregular, very slow, or very fast heart rate may indicate a need for BP measurements.

The axillary temperature is a safe, accurate substitute for the rectal temperature. Electronic thermometers have expedited this task and provide a reading within 1 minute. Taking an infant's temperature may cause the infant to cry and struggle against the placement of the thermometer in the axilla. Tympanic thermometers may be used after the newborn's ear canals are free of vernix and fluid. Before taking the temperature, the examiner may want to determine the apical heart rate and respiratory rate while the infant is quiet and at rest. The normal axillary temperature averages 37° C with a range from 36.5° C to 37.2° C.

The respiratory rate varies with the state of alertness after birth. Respirations are abdominal and can easily be counted by observing or lightly feeling the rise and fall of the abdomen. Neonatal respirations are shallow and irregular. It is important to count the respirations for a full minute to obtain an accurate count because of normal short periods of apnea. The examiner also should observe for symmetry of chest movements (see Table 19-2 for normal respiratory rates).

Apical pulse rates should be obtained for all infants. Auscultation should be for a full minute, preferably when the infant is asleep. The infant may need to be held and comforted during assessment. Auscultation of the heart sounds is difficult because of the rapid rate and effective transmission of respiratory sounds. However, the first (S_1) and second (S_2) sounds should be clear and well defined; the second sound is somewhat higher in pitch and sharper than the first. Murmurs are often heard in the newborn, especially over the base of the heart or at the left sternal border in the third or fourth interspace. These are usually functional murmurs resulting from incomplete closure of fetal shunts. Any murmur or other unusual sounds should be recorded and reported. See Table 19-2 for normal heart rates.

If BP is measured, a Doppler (electronic) monitor facilitates this procedure. It is important to use the correct size BP cuff. Neonatal BP usually is highest immediately after birth and decreases to a minimum by 3 hours after birth. It then begins to increase steadily and reaches a plateau between 4 and 6 days after birth. This measurement is usually equal to that of the immediate postbirth BP. BP may be measured in both arms and legs to detect any discrepancy between the two sides or between the upper and lower body. A discrepancy of 10 mm Hg or more between the arms and legs may signal a cardiac defect such as coarctation of the aorta.

Molding may give the neonate's head an asymmetric appearance (see Fig. 18-9). Parents should be reassured that this will go away and that nothing need be done to the head. Facial asymmetry may occur from fetal positioning in utero; asymmetry usually disappears spontaneously over time. The hard and soft palates are assessed with the gloved little finger of the examiner. At the same time the suck reflex can be assessed.

A gross assessment of hearing can be done by watching the neonate's response to voices or other sounds; a loud noise should elicit a startle reflex. Formal hearing screening of all infants is conducted in the newborn nursery.

The nose is examined for size, shape, mucous membrane integrity, and discharge. The nose should be midline on the face. The nares are checked for patency by occluding one nostril at a time and observing for respirations.

When palpating the clavicles, the examiner moves the fingers slowly over the anterior clavicular surface. If a mass or lump is detected, the examiner tries to move the neonate's arm gently while palpating with the other hand. A crepitant, grating sensation and uneven movement of two juxtaposed bone fragments indicate a fracture. If a fractured clavicle is present, the infant will usually have limited movement of the arm on the affected side.

Breast tissue is assessed through observation and palpation. To measure breast tissue, palpate the nipple gently with one finger or place the second and third fingers on either side of the nipple. The amount of breast tissue is measured between the two fingers. Breast tissue and areola size increase with gestational age.

Movement of the arms should be assessed. Trauma to the brachial plexus during a difficult birth may result in brachial palsy. The most common type, Duchenne-Erb paralysis, involves the fifth and sixth cervical nerve roots (see Fig. 27-2). The affected arm is held in a position of tight adduction and internal rotation at the shoulder. The grasp reflex on the affected side may be intact; however, the Moro reflex is absent on that side. With treatment, most neonates have complete recovery. Surgery may be necessary in some instances.

A neurologic assessment of the newborn's reflexes (see Table 18-3) provides useful information about the infant's nervous system and state of neurologic maturation. The assessment must be carried out as early as possible because abnormal signs present in the early neonatal period may disappear. They may reappear months or years later as abnormal functions.

Common problems in the newborn

Physical injuries.   Birth trauma includes any physical injury sustained by a newborn during labor and birth. Although most injuries are minor and resolve during the neonatal period without treatment, some types of trauma require intervention. A few are serious enough to be fatal.

Factors that may predispose the neonate to birth trauma include prolonged or precipitous labor, preterm labor, fetal macrosomia, cephalopelvic disproportion, abnormal presentation, and congenital anomalies. Injury can be the result of obstetric birth techniques such as forceps-assisted birth, vacuum extraction, version and extraction, and cesarean birth (Efird & Hernandez, 2005).

Soft tissue injuries.   Cephalhematoma is the most common type of cranial injury in newborns and can be associated with an underlying skull fracture. Caput succeda-

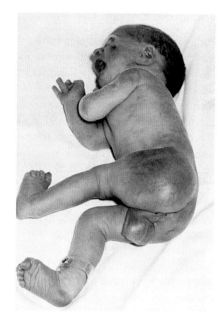

Fig. 19-7   Swelling of the genitals and bruising of the buttocks after a breech birth. (From O'Doherty, N. [1986]. *Neonatology: Micro atlas of the newborn.* Nutley, NJ: Hoffman-LaRoche.)

neum is diffuse swelling of the soft tissues of the scalp and is a result of pressure of the uterus or vaginal wall on the fetal head (Efird & Hernandez, 2005). Caput succedaneum and cephalhematoma are described in Chapter 18 (see Fig. 18-5).

Subconjunctival and retinal hemorrhages result from rupture of capillaries caused by increased pressure during birth (see Chapter 18). These hemorrhages usually clear within 5 days after birth and present no further problems. Parents need explanation and reassurance that these injuries will resolve without sequelae.

Erythema, ecchymoses, petechiae, abrasions, lacerations, or edema of buttocks and extremities may be present. Localized discoloration may appear over presenting parts and may result from the application of forceps or the vacuum extractor. Ecchymoses and edema may appear anywhere on the body.

Bruises over the face may be the result of face presentation (Fig. 19-6). In a breech presentation, bruising and swelling may be seen over the buttocks or genitalia (Fig. 19-7). The skin over the entire head may be ecchymotic and covered with petechiae caused by a tight nuchal cord. Petechiae (pinpoint hemorrhagic areas) acquired during birth may extend over the upper trunk and face. These lesions are benign if they disappear within 2 or 3 days of birth and no new lesions appear. Ecchymoses and petechiae may be signs of a more serious disorder, such as thrombocytopenic purpura.

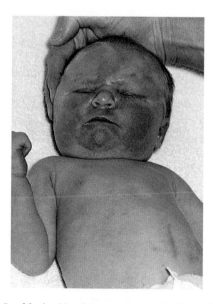

Fig. 19-6   Marked bruising on the entire face of an infant born vaginally after face presentation. Less severe ecchymoses were present on the extremities. Phototherapy was required for treatment of jaundice resulting from the breakdown of accumulated blood. (From O'Doherty, N. [1986]. *Neonatology: Micro atlas of the newborn.* Nutley, NJ: Hoffman-LaRoche.)

NURSE ALERT   *To differentiate hemorrhagic areas from skin rashes and discolorations, try to blanch the skin with two fingers. Petechiae and ecchymoses do not blanch because extravasated blood remains within the tissues, whereas skin rashes and discolorations do.*

Trauma resulting from dystocia occurs to the presenting fetal part. Forceps injury and bruising from the vacuum cup occur at the site where the instruments were applied. In a forceps injury, commonly a linear mark appears across both sides of the face in the shape of the forceps blades. The affected areas are kept clean to minimize the risk of infection. With the increased use of the vacuum extractor and the use of padded forceps blades, the incidence of these lesions may be significantly reduced (Mangurten, 2002).

Accidental lacerations may be inflicted with a scalpel during a cesarean birth. These cuts may occur on any part of the body but are most often found on the face, scalp, buttocks, and thighs. Usually they are superficial and only need to be kept clean. Liquid skin adhesive or butterfly adhesive strips can hold together the edges of more serious lacerations. Rarely are sutures needed.

Skeletal injuries. Fracture of the clavicle (collarbone) is the most common birth injury. This injury is often associated with macrosomia and is a result of compression of the shoulder or manipulation of the affected arm during birth. A fractured clavicle usually heals without treatment, although the arm and shoulder may be immobilized for comfort (Efird & Hernandez, 2005).

Fractures of the humerus and femur may occur during a difficult birth, but such fractures in newborns generally heal rapidly. Immobilization is accomplished with slings, splints, swaddling, and other devices.

The infant's immature, flexible skull can withstand a great deal of molding before fracture results. Fractures may occur during difficult births and result from the head pressing on the bony pelvis or from the injudicious application of forceps (Fig. 19-8). The location of a skull fracture determines

whether it is insignificant or fatal. Spontaneous or nonsurgical elevation of the indentation using a hand breast pump or vacuum extractor has been reported.

Nerve injuries may result in temporary or permanent paralysis. Brachial plexus injuries can affect movement of the shoulder, arm, wrist, or hand. Phrenic nerve palsy can occur because of hyperextension of the neck during difficult birth and can cause respiratory distress. Facial palsy affects one side of the face and is usually self-limiting (Efird & Hernandez, 2005).

Parents need emotional support when it comes to handling a newborn with birth injuries because they are often fearful of hurting their newborn. Parents are encouraged to practice handling, changing, and feeding the injured newborn under the guidance of the nursing staff. This increases the parents' knowledge and confidence, in addition to facilitating attachment. A plan for follow-up therapy is developed with the parents so that the times and arrangements for therapy are convenient for them.

Physiologic problems

Physiologic jaundice. The majority of term newborns have some degree of physiologic jaundice (become yellowish) during the first 3 days of life (see Chapter 18). Jaundice is clinically visible when serum bilirubin levels reach 5 to 7 mg/dl.

Every newborn is assessed for jaundice. The blanch test helps differentiate cutaneous jaundice from skin color. To do the test, apply pressure with a finger over a bony area (e.g., the nose, forehead, sternum) for several seconds to empty all the capillaries in that spot. If jaundice is present, the blanched area will look yellow before the capillaries refill. The conjunctival sacs and buccal mucosa also are assessed, especially in darker-skinned infants. It is better to assess for jaundice in daylight, because artificial lighting and reflection from nursery walls can distort the actual skin color.

Jaundice is noticeable first in the head and then progresses gradually toward the abdomen and extremities because of the newborn infant's circulatory pattern (cephalocaudal developmental progression). If jaundice is suspected, evaluation of serum bilirubin level is needed. Jaundice that appears before the infant is 24 hours old is likely to be pathologic instead of physiologic, and the primary health care provider should be notified.

Hypoglycemia. Hypoglycemia during the early newborn period of a term infant is defined as a blood glucose concentration of less than 35 mg/dl or as a plasma concentration of less than 40 mg/dl. When the neonate is born and abruptly disconnected from the continuous supply of maternal glucose, there is a period of adjustment as the newborn begins to regulate blood glucose concentration in accordance with intermittent feedings. Hypoglycemia can result if this metabolic adaptation is delayed, if early feedings result in limited intake, or if the neonate is stressed. The glucose level normally declines during the first hours after birth. Not all newborns are routinely screened for hypoglycemia. Instead, those who are symptomatic and those considered

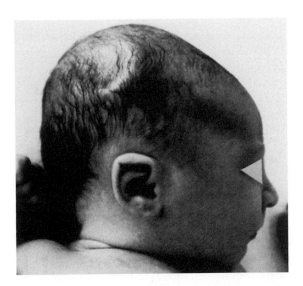

Fig. 19-8 Depressed skull fracture in a term male after rapid (1-hour) labor. The infant was delivered by occiput-anterior position after rotation from occiput-posterior position. (From Mangurten, H. (2002), Birth injuries. In A. Fanaroff & R. Martin, *Neonatal-perinatal medicine: Diseases of the fetus and infant* [7th ed.]. St. Louis: Mosby.)

to be at risk for hypoglycemia are tested. Risk factors for hypoglycemia include birth weight less than 2500 g or greater than 4000 g, gestational age less than 37 weeks or greater than 42 weeks, LGA infant, SGA infant, maternal diabetes, and 5-minute APGAR of 5 or less. Blood glucose levels should be checked initially between 30 minutes and 2 hours of life, and repeated every 30 minutes to 1 hour until the levels are consistently within normal limits. Glucose levels may be measured every 4 hours until the risk period has passed (Townsend, 2005).

Signs of hypoglycemia include jitteriness; an irregular respiratory effort; cyanosis; apnea; a weak, high-pitched cry; feeding difficulty; hunger; lethargy; twitching; eye rolling; and seizures. The signs may be transient and recurrent.

Hypoglycemia in the low risk term infant is usually eliminated by feeding the infant. Occasionally the intravenous administration of glucose is required for newborns with persistently high insulin levels or those with depleted glycogen stores.

Hypocalcemia. Hypocalcemia (serum calcium levels of less than 7.8 to 8 mg/dl in term infants and 7 mg/dl in preterm infants) may occur in newborns of diabetic mothers or in those who had perinatal asphyxia or trauma, and in LBW and preterm infants. Early-onset hypocalcemia occurs within the first 72 hours after birth. Signs of hypocalcemia include jitteriness, high-pitched cry, irritability, apnea, intermittent cyanosis, abdominal distention, and laryngospasm, although some hypocalcemic infants are asymptomatic (Blackburn, 2003).

In most instances, early-onset hypocalcemia is self-limiting and resolves within 1 to 3 days. Treatment includes early feeding and, occasionally, the administration of calcium supplements. Preterm or asphyxiated infants may require intravenous elemental calcium.

Jitteriness is a symptom of both hypoglycemia and hypocalcemia; therefore hypocalcemia must be considered if the therapy for hypoglycemia proves ineffective. In many newborns, jitteriness remains despite therapy and cannot be explained by hypoglycemia or hypocalcemia (DeMarini & Tsang, 2002).

Laboratory and diagnostic tests

Because newborns experience many transitional events in the first 28 days of life, laboratory samples are often gathered to determine adequate physiologic adaptation and to identify disorders that may adversely affect the child's life beyond the neonatal period. Tests that are commonly performed include blood glucose levels, bilirubin levels, complete blood count (CBC), newborn screening tests, and drug tests. Standard laboratory values for a term newborn are given in Box 19-4.

Newborn genetic screening. Before hospital discharge, a heel-stick blood sample is obtained to detect a variety of congenital conditions. Mandated by U.S. law, newborn genetic screening is an important public health program that is aimed at early detection of genetic diseases that re-

sult in severe health problems if not treated early. All states screen for phenylketonuria (PKU) and hypothyroidism, but each state determines whether other tests are performed. Other genetic defects that are included in some screening programs include galactosemia, cystic fibrosis, maple syrup urine disease, and sickle cell disease. It is recommended that the screening test be repeated at age 1 to 2 weeks if the initial specimen was obtained when the infant was younger than 24 hours (Albers & Levy, 2005; Zinn, 2002).

Newborn hearing screening. Universal newborn hearing screening is required by law in over 30 states and is performed routinely in other states. Infants in the neonatal intensive care unit (NICU) and those with other risk factors are screened in many settings where universal screening is not routinely done. Newborn hearing screening is completed before hospital discharge, and infants who do not pass are referred for repeated testing within the next 2 to 8 weeks. The practice of universal hearing screening reduces the age at which infants with hearing loss are identified and treated (Joint Committee on Infant Hearing, 2000) (Fig. 19-9).

Collection of specimens. Ongoing evaluation of a newborn often requires obtaining blood by the heel-stick or venipuncture method or the collection of a urine specimen.

Heel stick. Most blood specimens are drawn by laboratory technicians. Nurses, however, may be required to perform heel sticks to obtain blood for glucose monitoring and

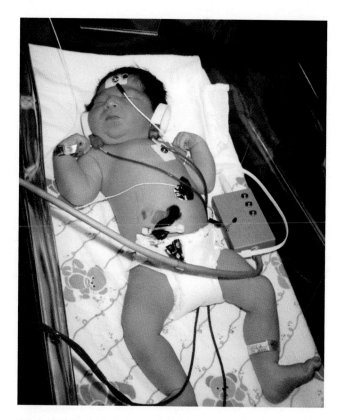

Fig. 19-9 Hearing screening in the newborn nursery. (Courtesy Dee Lowdermilk, Chapel Hill, NC.)

BOX 19-4

Standard Laboratory Values in the Neonatal Period

	NEONATAL
1. HEMATOLOGIC VALUES	
Clotting factors	
Activated clotting time (ACT)	2 min
Bleeding time (Ivy)	2 to 7 min
Clot retraction	Complete 1 to 4 hr
Fibrinogen	125 to 300 mg/dl*

	TERM	PRETERM
Hemoglobin (g/dl)	14 to 24	15 to 17
Hematocrit (%)	44 to 64	45 to 55
Reticulocytes (%)	0.4 to 6	Up to 10
Fetal hemoglobin (% of total)	40 to 70	80 to 90
Red blood cells (RBCs)/mcl[†]	4.8×10^6 to 7.1×10^6	
Platelet count/mm^3	150,000 to 300,000	120,000 to 180,000
White blood cells (WBCs)/mcl	9000 to 30,000	10,000 to 20,000
Neutrophils (%)	54 to 62	47
Eosinophils and basophils (%)	1 to 3	
Lymphocytes (%)	25 to 33	33
Monocytes (%)	3 to 7	4
Immature WBCs (%)	10	16

*dl refers to deciliter (1 dl = 100 ml); this conforms to the SI system (standardized international measurements).
†mcl refers to microliter.

			NEONATAL
2. BIOCHEMICAL VALUES			
Bilirubin, direct			0 to 1 mg/dl
Bilirubin, total	Cord:		<2 mg/dl
	Peripheral blood:	0 to 1 day	6 mg/dl
		1 to 2 days	8 mg/dl
		2 to 5 days	12 mg/dl
Blood gases	Arterial:		pH 7.31 to 7.49
			P_{CO_2} 26 to 41 mm Hg
			P_{O_2} 60 to 70 mm Hg
	Venous:		pH 7.31 to 7.41
			P_{CO_2} 40 to 50 mm Hg
			P_{O_2} 40 to 50 mm Hg
Serum glucose			40 to 60 mg/dl

	NEONATAL
3. URINALYSIS	
Color	Clear, straw
Specific gravity	1.001 to 1.020
pH	5 to 7
Protein	Negative
Glucose	Negative
Ketones	Negative
RBCs	0 to 2
WBCs	0 to 4
Casts	None

Volume: 24 to 72 ml/kg excreted daily in the first few days; by week 1, 24-hr urine volume close to 200 ml.
Protein: may be present in first 2 to 4 days.
Osmolarity (mOsm/L): 100 to 600.

Some data from Hockenberry, M. (2003). *Wong's nursing care of infants and children* (7th ed.). St. Louis: Mosby; Pagana, K., & Pagana, T. (2003). *Mosby's diagnostic and laboratory test reference* (6th ed.). St. Louis: Mosby.

to measure hematocrit levels. The same technique is used to obtain a blood sample for newborn genetic screening tests.

It may be helpful to warm the heel before the sample is taken, because the application of heat for 5 to 10 minutes helps dilate the vessels in the area. A cloth soaked with warm water and wrapped loosely around the foot can effectively warm the foot (Fig. 19-10, *A*). Disposable heel warmers also are available from a variety of companies but should be used with care to prevent burns. Nurses should wear gloves when collecting any specimen. The nurse first cleanses the area with alcohol, restrains the infant's foot with his or her free hand, and then punctures the site. A spring-loaded automatic puncture device causes less pain and requires fewer punctures than a manual lance blade.

The most serious complication of an infant heel stick is necrotizing osteochondritis resulting from lancet penetration of the bone. To prevent this, the stick should be made at the outer aspect of the heel and should penetrate no deeper than 2.4 mm (Hockenberry, 2003). To identify the appropriate puncture site, the nurse should draw an imaginary line from between the fourth and fifth toes that runs parallel to the lateral aspect of the heel, where the stick should be made; a line can also be drawn from the great toe that runs parallel to the medial aspect of the heel, another site for a stick (Fig. 19-10, *B*). Repeated trauma to the walking surface of the heel can cause fibrosis and scarring that may lead to problems with walking later in life.

After the specimen has been collected, pressure should be applied with a dry gauze square, but no further alcohol should be applied because this will cause the site to continue to bleed. The site is then covered with an adhesive bandage. The nurse ensures proper disposal of equipment used, reviews the laboratory slip for correct identification, and checks the specimen for accurate labeling and routing.

A heel stick is traumatic for the infant and causes pain. After several heel sticks, infants often withdraw their feet when they are touched. To reassure the infant and promote feelings of safety, the neonate should be cuddled and comforted when the procedure is complete and appropriate pain management measures taken to minimize the pain.

Venipuncture. A venipuncture may be less painful than a heel stick for blood sampling. Venous blood samples can be drawn from antecubital, saphenous, superficial wrist, and rarely, scalp veins. If an intravenous site is used to

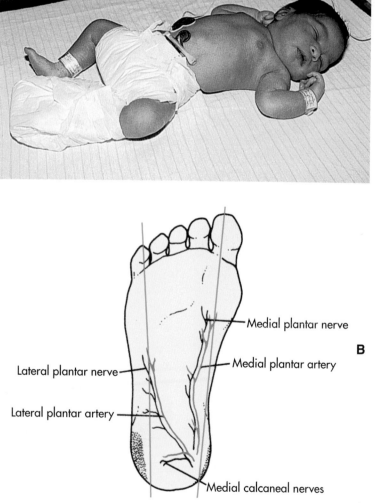

Fig. 19-10 Heel stick. **A,** Newborn with foot wrapped for warmth to increase blood flow to extremity before heel stick. **B,** Heel-stick sites (*shaded areas*) on infant's foot for obtaining samples of capillary blood. (**A,** Courtesy Marjorie Pyle, RNC, Lifecircle, Costa Mesa, CA.)

obtain a blood specimen, it is important to consider the type of infusion fluid, because mixing of the blood sample with the fluid can alter the results.

When venipuncture is required, positioning of the needle is extremely important. Although regular venipuncture needles may be used, some prefer butterfly needles. A 25-gauge needle is adequate for blood sampling in neonates, with minimal hemolysis occurring when the proper procedure is followed. It is necessary to be very patient during the procedure, because the blood return in small veins is slow,

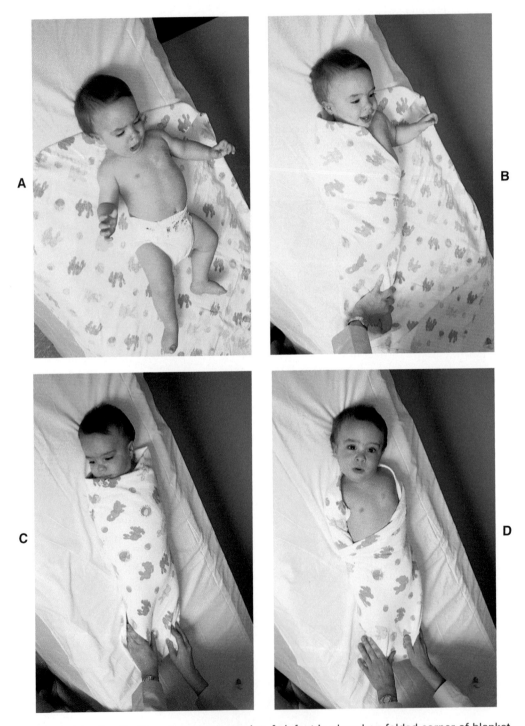

Fig. 19-11 Application of mummy restraint. **A,** Infant is placed on folded corner of blanket. **B,** One corner of blanket is brought across body and secured beneath the body. **C,** Second corner is brought across body and secured, and lower corner is folded and tucked or pinned in place. **D,** Modified mummy restraint with chest uncovered. (From Hockenberry, M. [2003]. *Wong's nursing care of infants and children* [7th ed.]. St. Louis: Mosby.)

and consequently the small needle must remain in place longer. The mummy restraint commonly is used to help secure the infant (Fig. 19-11).

For external jugular venipuncture, "mummy" the infant as necessary, and then lower the infant's head over a rolled towel, the edge of a table, or your knee, and stabilize. For femoral venipuncture, place your hands over the infant's knees, but avoid pressing your fingers over the inner aspect of the thigh (Fig. 19-12, *A*). Both of these positions ensure the safety of the infant and exposure of the puncture sites. If the radial vein is used, the infant's arm is exposed and held securely in place.

If venipuncture or arterial puncture is being performed for blood gas studies, crying, fear, and agitation will affect the values; therefore every effort must be made to keep the infant quiet during the procedure. For blood gas studies, the blood sample tubes are packed in ice (to reduce blood cell metabolism) and are taken immediately to the laboratory for analysis.

Pressure must be maintained over an arterial or femoral vein puncture with a dry gauze square for at least 3 to 5 min-

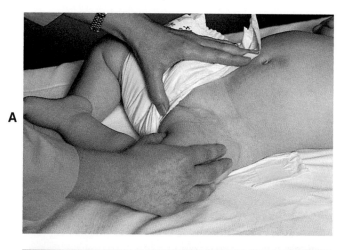

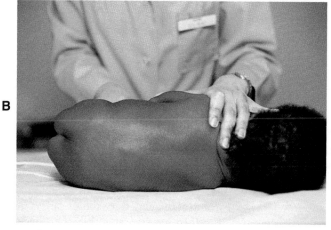

Fig. 19-12 **A,** Restraining infant for femoral vein puncture. **B,** Modified side-lying position for lumbar puncture. (From Hockenberry, M. [2003]. *Wong's nursing care of infants and children* [7th ed.]. St. Louis: Mosby.)

utes to prevent bleeding from the site. For an hour after any venipuncture, the nurse should then observe the infant frequently for evidence of bleeding or hematoma formation at the puncture site. The infant's tolerance of the procedure also should be recorded. The infant should be cuddled and comforted when the procedure is completed.

Obtaining a urine specimen. Examination of urine is a valuable laboratory tool for infant assessment; the way in which the urine specimen is collected may influence the results. The urine sample should be fresh and analyzed within 1 hour of collection.

A variety of urine collection bags are available, including the Hollister U-Bag (Fig. 19-13). These are clear plastic, single-use bags with an adhesive material around the opening at the point of attachment.

To prepare the infant, the nurse removes the diaper and places the infant in a supine position. The genitalia, perineum, and surrounding skin are washed and thoroughly dried because the adhesive on the bag will not stick to moist, powdered, or oily skin surfaces. The protective paper is removed to expose the adhesive (Fig. 19-13, *A*). In female infants, the perineum is first stretched to flatten skin folds, and then the adhesive area on the bag is pressed firmly onto the skin all around the urinary meatus and vagina. (*NOTE:* Start with the narrow portion of the butterfly-shaped adhesive patch.) Starting the application at the bridge of skin separating the rectum from the vagina and working upward is most effective (Fig. 19-13, *B*). In male infants, the penis and scrotum are tucked through the opening into the collection bag before the protective paper is removed from the adhesive and it is pressed firmly onto the perineum, making sure the entire adhesive is firmly attached to skin and the edges of the opening do not pucker (Fig. 19-13, *C*). This helps ensure a leakproof seal and decreases the chance of contamination from stool. Cutting a slit in the diaper and pulling the bag through the slit also may help prevent leaking.

The diaper is carefully replaced, and the bag is checked frequently. When a sufficient amount of urine (this amount varies according to the test done) appears, the bag is removed. The infant's skin is observed for signs of irritation while the bag is in place. The specimen can be aspirated with a syringe or drained directly from the bag.

Collection of a 24-hour specimen can be a challenge; the infant may need to be restrained. The 24-hour urine bag is applied in the manner just described, and the urine is drained into a receptacle. During the collection, the infant's skin is observed closely for signs of irritation and for lack of a proper seal.

For some types of urine tests, urine can be aspirated directly from the diaper by means of a syringe without a needle. If the diaper has absorbent gelling material that traps urine, a small gauze dressing or some cotton balls can be placed inside the diaper and the urine aspirated from them (Hockenberry, 2003).

Restraining the infant. Infants may need to be restrained to (1) protect the infant from injury, (2) facilitate

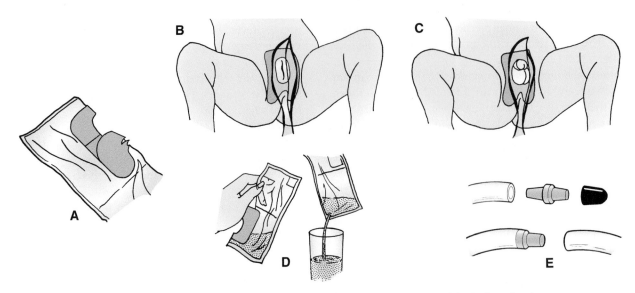

Fig. 19-13 Collection of urine specimen. **A,** Protective paper is removed from the adhesive surface. **B,** Applied to girls. **C,** Applied to boys. **D,** Cut to drain urine. **E,** Collection tube. (Permission to use and/or reproduce this copyrighted material has been granted by the owner, Hollister, Inc., Libertyville, IL.)

examinations, and (3) limit discomfort during tests, procedures, and specimen collections (see Figs. 19-11 and 19-12). The following special considerations must be kept in mind when restraining an infant:

- Apply restraints and check them to make sure they are not irritating the skin or impairing circulation.
- Maintain proper body alignment.
- Apply restraints without using knots or pins if possible. If knots are necessary, make the kind that can be released quickly. Use pins with care so that there is no danger of their puncturing or pressing against the infant's skin.
- Check the infant hourly, or more frequently if indicated.

Restraint without appliance. The nurse may restrain the infant by using the hands and body. Figure 19-12, *B* illustrates ways to restrain an infant in this manner.

Possible nursing diagnoses for the newborn from 2 hours after birth until discharge include the following:

- *Ineffective breathing pattern related to*
  —obstructed airway
- *Impaired gas exchange related to*
  —ineffective breathing pattern
- *Ineffective thermoregulation related to*
  —excess heat loss to the environment
- *Acute pain related to*
  —circumcision
  —heel stick, venipuncture

Possible nursing diagnoses for the parents are as follows:

- *Readiness for enhanced family coping related to*
  —knowledge of newborn's social capabilities

  —knowledge of newborn's dependency needs
  —knowledge of newborn's biologic characteristics
- *Situational low self-esteem related to*
  —misinterpretation of newborn's behavioral cues

Examples of nursing diagnoses derived from specific assessment findings are listed in the Plan of Care.

Expected Outcomes of Care

The expected outcomes for newborn care relate to the infant and parents. The outcomes for the infant are that the infant will do the following:

- Maintain an effective breathing pattern
- Maintain effective thermoregulation
- Remain free from infection
- Establish adequate elimination patterns
- Experience minimal pain

For the parents, expected outcomes include the following:

- Attain knowledge, skill, and confidence relevant to infant care activities
- State understanding of biologic and behavioral characteristics of their newborn
- Have opportunities to intensify their relationship with the infant
- Begin to integrate the infant into the family

Plan of Care and Interventions

In the inpatient setting, priorities of care must be established and a systematic teaching plan devised for infant care. One way to accomplish this is to use critical path case management. A care path may be developed to cover the changes expected in the infant during the first several days of life (Care Path). When variations from the care path occur, further assessment and intervention may be necessary.

PLAN OF CARE *Normal Newborn*

NURSING DIAGNOSIS **Risk for ineffective airway clearance related to excess mucus production or improper positioning**

Expected Outcomes *Neonate's airway remains patent; breath sounds are clear, and no respiratory distress is evident.*

Nursing Interventions/*Rationales*

- Teach parents that gagging, coughing, and sneezing are normal neonatal responses *that assist the neonate in clearing airways.*
- Teach parents feeding techniques that prevent overfeeding and distention of the abdomen and to burp neonate frequently *to prevent regurgitation and aspiration.*
- Position neonate on back when sleeping *to prevent suffocation.*
- Suction mouth and nasopharynx with bulb syringe as needed; clean nares of crusted secretions *to clear airway and prevent aspiration and airway obstruction.*

NURSING DIAGNOSIS **Risk for imbalanced body temperature related to larger body surfaces in relationship to mass**

Expected Outcome *Neonate temperature remains in range of 36.5° C to 37.2° C.*

Nursing Interventions/*Rationales*

- Maintain neutral thermal environment *to identify any changes in neonate's temperature that may be related to other causes.*
- Monitor neonate's axillary temperature frequently *to identify any changes promptly and ensure early interventions.*
- Bathe neonate efficiently when temperature is stable, using warm water, drying carefully, and avoiding exposing neonate to drafts *to avoid heat losses from evaporation and convection.*
- Report any alterations in temperature findings promptly *to assess and treat for possible infection.*

NURSING DIAGNOSIS **Risk for infection related to immature immunologic defenses and environmental exposure**

Expected Outcome *The neonate will be free from signs of infection.*

Nursing Interventions/*Rationales*

- Review maternal record for evidence of any risk factors *to ascertain whether the neonate may be predisposed to infection.*
- Monitor vital signs *to identify early possible evidence of infection, especially temperature instability.*
- Have all care providers, including parents, practice good handwashing techniques before handling newborn *to prevent spread of infection.*

- Provide prescribed eye prophylaxis *to prevent infection.*
- Keep genital area clean and dry using proper cleansing techniques *to prevent skin irritation, cross-contamination, and infection.*
- Keep umbilical stump clean and dry and keep exposed to air *to allow to dry and minimize chance of infection.*
- If infant is circumcised, keep site clean and apply diaper loosely *to prevent trauma and infection.*
- Teach parents to keep neonate away from crowds and environmental irritants *to reduce potential sources of infection.*

NURSING DIAGNOSIS **Risk for injury related to sole dependence on caregiver**

Expected Outcome *Neonate remains free of injury.*

Nursing Interventions/*Rationales*

- Monitor environment for hazards such as sharp objects, long fingernails of caretaker and neonate, and jewelry of caretaker that may be sharp *to prevent injury.*
- Handle neonate gently and support head, ensure use of car seat by parents, teach parents never to place neonate on high surface unsupervised, and to supervise pet and sibling interactions *to prevent injury.*
- Assess neonate frequently for any evidence of jaundice *to identify rising bilirubin levels, treat promptly, and prevent kernicterus.*

NURSING DIAGNOSIS **Readiness for enhanced family coping related to anticipatory guidance regarding responses to neonate's crying**

Expected Outcome *Parents will verbalize understanding of methods of coping with neonate's crying and describe increased success in interpreting neonate's cries.*

Nursing Interventions/*Rationales*

- Alert parents to crying as neonate's form of communication and that cries can be differentiated to indicate hunger, wetness, pain, and loneliness *to provide reassurance that crying is not indicative of neonate's rejection of parents and that parents will learn to interpret the different cries of their child.*
- Differentiate self-consoling behaviors from fussing or crying *to give parents concrete examples of interventions.*
- Discuss methods of consoling a neonate who has been crying, such as checking and changing diapers, talking softly to neonate, holding neonate's arms close to body, swaddling, picking neonate up, rocking, using a pacifier, feeding, or burping *to provide anticipatory guidance.*

Protective environment

The provision of a protective environment is basic to the care of the newborn. The construction, maintenance, and operation of nurseries in accredited hospitals are monitored by national professional organizations such as the AAP, Joint Commission on Accreditation of Healthcare Organizations, Occupational Health and Safety Administration, and local or state governing bodies. In addition, hospital personnel develop their own policies and procedures for protecting the newborns under their care. Prescribed standards cover areas such as the following:

- Environmental factors: Provision of adequate lighting, elimination of potential fire hazards, safety of electrical appliances, adequate ventilation, and controlled temperature (i.e., warm and free of drafts) and humidity (lower than 50%).
- Measures to control infection: Adequate floor space to permit the positioning of bassinets at least 3 feet

Text continued on p. 595

CARE PATH Healthy Term Newborn

CARE ASPECTS	FIRST HOUR	2-3 HR	6 HR	12 HR	18 HR	24 HR	36-48 HR TO DISCHARGE
Safety	ID band on and verified matching parents'; bulb syringe (for suction) at bedside; newborn safety alarm system activated.*	ID band on Parent teaching regarding bulb syringe; NB alarm system active	ID band on Bulb syringe in crib; NB alarm system active	ID band on Bulb syringe in crib; NB alarm system active	ID band on Bulb syringe in crib; NB alarm system active	ID band on Bulb syringe in crib; NB alarm system active	ID band on† Remove at discharge only Parents verbalize appropriate car seat in place Discuss and reinforce home safety, including abduction prevention, infection prevention, car seat safety, and falls prevention Reinforce teaching for use of bulb syringe Discuss sleep position—on back, always; sleep environment (mattress, crib rails) Reinforce smoke-free environment around infant Deactivate NB alarm system at discharge
Temperature (axillary)	36.5° - 37.2° C	36.5° - 37.2° C	36.5° - 37.2° C	36.5° - 37.2° C	36.5° - 37.2° C	36.5° - 37.2° C	36.5° - 37.2° C Reinforce teaching for taking axillary temperature and when to take Thermometer type Normal ranges Discuss home environment temperature
Vital signs	Blood pressure on admission per protocol (not usual unless indicated)						
Heart rate	100-180 beats/min	80-180 beats/min	120-140 beats/min	120-140 beats/min	120-140 beats/min VS stable	VS stable: 120-140 beats/min	VS stable and documented If murmur present, document Monitor blood pressure per protocol
Respiratory rate	30-50 breaths/min (may be less if asleep)	30-50 breaths/min	30-50 breaths/min	30-50 breaths/min	30-50 breaths/min	30-50 breaths/min	
Feeding Breast	Initiated—latch-on		1 latch-on‡	1 latch-on‡	2 latch-ons verified	3-4 successful latch-ons verified‡	Feeding successfully 8-10 times/day; discuss and reinforce feeding cues and associated behaviors

•Formula	Sips to verify suck, swallow, and breathing	Sips to verify suck, swallow, and breathing	2 feedings— 15-25 ml each	3 successful feedings verified—15-30 ml each	4-5 feedings verified; adequate suck, swallow, and breathing coordination	Feeding successfully 5-6 times/day; discuss and reinforce feeding cues and associated behaviors
Elimination •Voiding	Check		1 void		Minimum of 3 voids/24 hr in first few days	2-3 voids minimum; or number of voids = number of days old Reinforce teaching and care—minimum of 5 to 6 voids/day
•Stooling	Verify anal patency Check for stool	Check for stool	Check for stool		1 meconium documented	1 meconium documented Reinforce teaching and care—approximately 1-2 stools/72-96 hr after first week of life depending on feeding method; more if breastfeeding
Parent interaction	Initiated eye contact and verbalization	Exhibit newborn care interest and involvement	Involvement in newborn care		Continued involvement in newborn care	Demonstrates interest in newborn care; participates in newborn care; asks appropriate questions regarding home care; follow-up time and location provided
Cord care	Cord clamped	Cord care per institutional protocol	Clamped; no drainage		Cord drying; no drainage	Cord drying; care reinforced to parents; clamp removed before discharge
Circumcision				Pain management—recommend topical anesthesia with DPNB or regional and oral sucrose; verify after procedure	Pain management—recommend topical anesthesia with DPNB or regional and oral sucrose; verify after procedure	Continued evaluation for absence of bleeding and presence of voiding Dressing applied with each diaper change depending on method (Gomco and Mogen clamp) Ring intact if PlastiBell Reinforce teaching on care of circumcision at home; pain management care
Bilirubin	<5-6 mg/dl		<5-6 mg/dl		≤5-6 mg/dl; color pink; note if jaundice present and documented; transcutaneous bilirubin check per protocol	Note skin color; transcutaneous jaundice meter reading per protocol AND check serum bilirubin at 24-36 hr: <7 mg/dl—low risk 7 to 11 mg/dl—low intermediate risk 11-13 mg/dl—high intermediate risk >13 mg/dl—high risk

CARE PATH   *Healthy Term Newborn—cont'd*

CARE ASPECTS	FIRST HOUR	2-3 HR	6 HR	12 HR	18 HR	24 HR	36-48 HR TO DISCHARGE
Bilirubin—cont'd	No visible jaundice; pink	No visible jaundice; pink		No visible jaundice; pink		Check for jaundice	Note color—document; Provide parent instruction regarding jaundice and follow-up visit with primary care practitioner within 3-4 days
Newborn screening				Hearing screening completed and documented		Newborn screening completed after 24 hr—document time and method	Verify newborn screening completed, including PKU after 24 hr of oral intake—reschedule if needed
Medications		Eye prophylaxis; Vitamin K; Maternal HBsAg status verified and documented	Hepatitis B vaccine within 12 hr of birth if mother positive; document			Check eye status; verify free of drainage	Reinforce hepatitis B vaccination at follow-up if not given in birth hospital
Activity	Active, flexed, primitive reflexes present (Moro, suck, tonic neck, Babinski)	May be drowsy but arousable	Active and alert; Flexed, strong suck reflex		Active and alert; Sleep periods noted; Reflexes present; Neurologic status intact		Discuss and reinforce sleep-wake patterns with parents; reinforce cues to active engagement with infant (eye contact, socialization); potential signs of danger (decreased activity; not arousable for feedings; color changes [not acrocyanosis], central cyanosis, apnea)

Prepared by David Wilson, MS, RNC.
DPNB, Dorsal penile nerve block; *HBsAg,* hepatitis B surface antigen; *ID,* identification; *PKU,* phenylketonuria; *VS,* vital signs.
*NB alarm system is the hospital protocol designed to protect infant from abduction.
†If still in hospital.
‡Minimum observed and documented.

apart in all directions, handwashing facilities, and areas for cleaning and storing equipment and supplies.

Only those personnel directly involved in the care of mothers and infants are allowed in these areas, thereby reducing the opportunities for the transmission of pathogenic organisms.

NURSE ALERT *Personnel are instructed to use good handwashing techniques. Handwashing between each infant handling is the single most important measure in the prevention of neonatal infection.*

Health care personnel must wear gloves when handling the infant until blood and amniotic fluid have been removed from the infant's skin, when drawing blood (e.g., heel stick), when caring for a fresh wound (e.g., circumcision), and during diaper changes.

Visitors and health care providers such as nurses, physicians, physicians, parents, brothers and sisters, department supervisors, electricians, and housekeepers are expected to wash their hands before having contact with infants or equipment. Cover gowns are not necessary.

Individuals with infectious conditions are excluded from contact with newborns or must take special precautions when working with infants. This includes persons with upper respiratory tract infections, gastrointestinal tract infections, and infectious skin conditions. Most agencies have now coupled this day-to-day self-screening of personnel with yearly health examinations.

- Safety factors: Health care institutions must be proactive in protecting newborns from abductions. Examples of the measures include placing identification bracelets on infants and their parents, using identification bands with radiofrequency transmitters that set off an alarm if the bracelet is removed or if a certain threshold is crossed (doorway to exit unit or building), and footprinting or taking identification pictures immediately after birth, before the infant leaves the

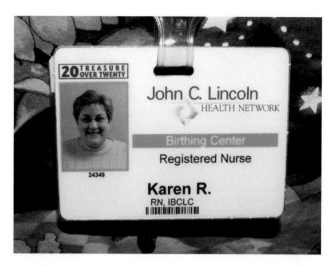

Fig. 19-15 Photo ID for personnel working in maternity settings. (Courtesy Shannon Perry, Phoenix, AZ.)

mother's side (Fig. 19-14). Personnel wear picture identification badges or other badges that identify them as newborn unit personnel (Fig. 19-15). Mother-baby units may have infant tracking systems that will set off an alarm if a baby is left alone or is with unauthorized personnel. Mothers are instructed to be certain they know the identity of anyone who cares for the infant and never to release the infant to anyone who is not wearing the appropriate identification.

Supporting parents in the care of their infant

The sensitivity of the caregiver to the social responses of the infant is basic to the development of a mutually satisfying parent-child relationship. Sensitivity increases over time as parents become more aware of their infant's social capabilities (Cultural Considerations box).

Social interaction. The activities of daily care during the neonatal period are the best times for infant and family interactions. While caring for their baby, the mother and father can talk to the infant, play baby games, caress and cuddle the child, and perhaps use infant massage. Too much stimulation should be avoided after feeding and before a sleep period. Older children's contact with a newborn is encouraged and supervised based on the developmental level of the child (Fig. 19-16).

Infant feeding. The infant is put to breast as soon as possible after birth or at least within 4 hours. If the infant is to be bottle-fed, a nurse may first offer a few sips of sterile water to make certain the sucking and swallowing reflexes are intact and that there are no anomalies such as a tracheoesophageal fistula. Most infants are on demand feeding schedules and are allowed to feed when they awaken. Ordinarily mothers are encouraged to feed their infants every 3 to 4 hours during the day and only when the infant awakens during the night in the first few days after birth. Formula-fed infants usually eat approximately every 3 to 4 hours.

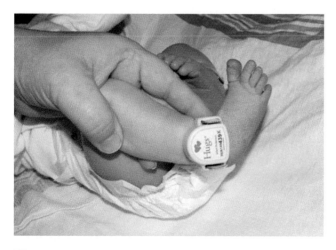

Fig. 19-14 Neonatal safety device. (Courtesy Shannon Perry, Phoenix, AZ.)

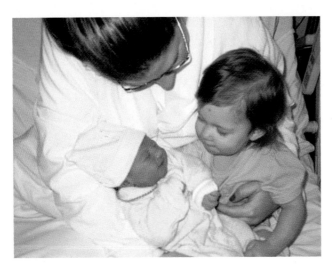

Fig. 19-16 Mother supervising contact of older sibling with newborn. (Courtesy Rebekah Vogel, Fort Collins, CO.)

Breastfed babies nurse more often (every 2 to 3 hours) than bottle-fed babies because breast milk is digested faster than formulas made from cow's milk, and the stomach empties sooner as a result. Water supplements are not recommended. For a thorough discussion of infant feeding, see Chapter 20.

Therapeutic and surgical procedures

Intramuscular injection. As discussed previously, it is routine to administer a single dose of 0.5 to 1 mg of vitamin K intramuscularly to an infant soon after birth (see Medication Guide box on p. 579).

Hepatitis B (Hep B) vaccination is recommended for all infants. Infants at highest risk for contracting hepatitis B are those born to women who come from Asia, Africa, South America, the South Pacific, or southern or eastern Europe (Medication Guide). If the infant is born to an infected mother or to a mother who is a chronic carrier, hepatitis vaccine and hepatitis B immune globulin (HBIG) should be administered within 12 hours of birth (Medication Guide). The hepatitis

Cultural Considerations

Cultural Beliefs and Practices

Nurses working with childbearing families from other cultures and ethnic groups must be aware of cultural beliefs and practices that are important to individual families. People with a strong sense of heritage may hold on to traditional health beliefs long after adopting other U.S. lifestyle practices. These health beliefs may involve practices regarding the newborn. For example, some Asians, Hispanics, eastern Europeans, and Native Americans delay breastfeeding because they believe that colostrum is "bad." Some Hispanics and African-Americans place a belly band over the infant's navel. The birth of a male child is generally preferred by Asians and Indians, and some Asians and Haitians delay naming their infants (D'Avanzo & Geissler, 2003).

Medication Guide

Hepatitis B Vaccine (Recombivax HB, Engerix-B)

ACTION
- Hepatitis B vaccine induces protective antihepatitis B antibodies in 95% to 99% of healthy infants who receive the recommended three doses. The duration of protection of the vaccine is unknown.

INDICATION
- Hepatitis B vaccine is for immunization against infection caused by all known subtypes of hepatitis B virus (HBV).

NEONATAL DOSAGE
- The usual dosage is Recombivax HB, 5 mg/0.5 ml, or Engerix-B, 10 mg/0.5 ml, at 0, 1, and 6 mo. An alternate dosing schedule is 0, 1, 2, and 12 mo and is usually for newborns whose mothers were hepatitis B surface antigen (HBsAg)–positive.

ADVERSE REACTIONS
- Common adverse reactions are rash, fever, erythema, swelling, and pain at injection site.

NURSING CONSIDERATIONS
- Parental consent must be obtained before administration. Wear gloves. Administer in the middle third of the vastus lateralis muscle by using a 25-gauge, ⅝-inch needle. Inject into skin that has been cleaned, or allow alcohol to dry on puncture site for 1 min to remove organisms and prevent infection. Stabilize leg firmly and grasp muscle between the thumb and fingers. Insert the needle at a 90-degree angle; aspirate, and inject medication slowly if there is no blood return. Massage the site with a dry gauze square after removing needle to increase absorption. If the infant was born to HBsAg-positive mother, hepatitis B immune globulin (HBIG) should be given within 12 hr of birth in addition to the HB vaccine. Separate sites must be used.

vaccine is given in one site and the HBIG in another. For infants born to healthy women, the first dose of the vaccine may be given at birth or at age 1 or 2 months. Parental consent should be obtained before these vaccines are administered.

In most cases, a 25-gauge, ⅝-inch needle should be used for the vitamin K and hepatitis vaccine injections. A 22-gauge needle may be necessary if thicker medications such as some penicillins are to be given.

Selection of the site for injection is important. Injections must be given in muscles large enough to accommodate the medication, and major nerves and blood vessels must be avoided. The muscles of newborns may not tolerate more than a 0.5 ml per intramuscular injection. The injection site for newborns is the vastus lateralis (Fig. 19-17). The dorsogluteal muscle is very small, poorly developed, and dangerously close to the sciatic nerve, which occupies a larger area in infants compared with older children. Therefore it

Medication Guide

Hepatitis B Immune Globulin

ACTION

- Hepatitis B immune globulin (HBIG) provides a high titer of antibody to hepatitis B surface antigen (HBsAg).

INDICATION

- The HBIG vaccine provides prophylaxis against infection in infants born of HBsAg-positive mothers.

NEONATAL DOSAGE

- Administer one 0.5-ml dose intramuscularly within 12 hr of birth.

ADVERSE REACTIONS

- Hypersensitivity may occur.

NURSING CONSIDERATIONS

- Must be given within 12 hr of birth. Wear gloves. Administer in the middle third of the vastus lateralis muscle by using a 25-gauge, ⅝-inch needle. Inject into skin that has been cleaned, or allow alcohol to dry on puncture site for 1 min to remove organisms and prevent infection. Stabilize leg firmly, and grasp muscle between the thumb and fingers. Insert the needle at a 90-degree angle; release muscle; aspirate, and inject medication slowly if there is no blood return. Massage the site with a dry gauze square after removing needle to increase absorption. May be given at same time as hepatitis B vaccine but at a different site.

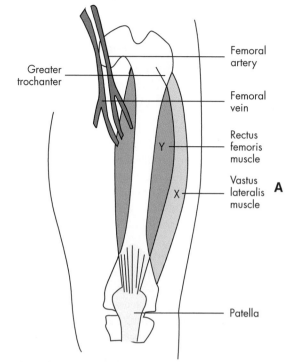

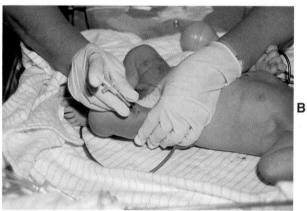

Fig. 19-17 Intramuscular injection. **A,** Acceptable intramuscular injection site for newborn infant. *X,* Injection site. **B,** Infant's leg stabilized for intramuscular injection. Nurse is wearing gloves to give injection. (**B,** Courtesy Marjorie Pyle, RNC, Lifecircle, Costa Mesa, CA.)

is not recommended that it be used as an injection site until the child has been walking for at least 1 year. The newborn's deltoid muscle has an inadequate amount of muscle for intramuscular injection.

The neonate's leg should be stabilized. Gloves should be worn by the person giving the injection. The nurse cleanses the injection site with an appropriate skin antiseptic (e.g., alcohol), then pinches up the infant's muscle between the thumb and forefinger. The needle is inserted into the vastus lateralis at a 90-degree angle. The muscle is released and the plunger of the syringe gently withdrawn. If no blood is aspirated, the medication is injected. If blood is aspirated, the needle is withdrawn and the injection is given in another site. After the injection has been given, the needle is withdrawn quickly and the site massaged with a gauze square to hasten absorption, unless contraindicated. A small amount of bleeding at the injection site is not uncommon, but it is not necessary to cover the site with an adhesive bandage. Pressure should be applied until bleeding stops.

The nurse should always remember to comfort the infant after an injection and to discard equipment properly. It is important to record the name of the medication, date and time of administration, amount, route, and site of injection on the newborn's chart.

Therapy for hyperbilirubinemia. The best therapy for hyperbilirubinemia is prevention. Because bilirubin is excreted primarily through stooling, prevention can be facilitated by early feeding, which stimulates the passage of meconium. However, despite early passage of meconium, the term infant may have trouble conjugating the increased amount of bilirubin derived from disintegrating fetal red blood cells. As a result, the serum levels of unconjugated bilirubin may increase beyond normal limits, causing hyperbilirubinemia (see Chapter 18). The goal of treatment of hyperbilirubinemia is to help reduce the newborn's serum levels of unconjugated bilirubin. The two principal ways of doing this are phototherapy and, rarely, exchange blood transfusion. Exchange transfusion treats those infants whose increased levels of bilirubin cannot be controlled by phototherapy (Ip et al., 2004).

Phototherapy. During phototherapy the unclothed infant is placed beneath a bank of lights. The distance may vary based on unit protocol and the type of light used. There should always be a Plexiglas panel or shield between the lights and the infant when conventional lighting is used. The most effective therapy is achieved with lights at 400 to 500 manometers, and blue light spectrum is the most efficient. The lamp energy should be monitored routinely during treatment with a photometer to ensure efficacy of therapy. Phototherapy is carried out until the infant's serum bilirubin level decreases to within an acceptable range. The decision to discontinue therapy is based on the observation of a definite downward trend in the bilirubin values. After therapy has been terminated, the infant may have a rebound in bilirubin levels, which is usually harmless (Kliegman, 2002).

Several precautions must be taken while the infant is undergoing phototherapy. The infant's eyes must be protected by an opaque mask to prevent overexposure to the light. The eye shield should cover the eyes completely but not occlude the nares. Before the mask is applied, the infant's eyes should be closed gently to prevent excoriation of the corneas. The mask should be removed during infant feedings so that the eyes can be checked and the parents can have visual contact with the infant (Fig. 19-18).

To promote optimal skin exposure during phototherapy, the diaper may be left off, or a "string bikini" made from a disposable face mask may be used to cover the infant's gen-

ital area. Before placing the mask on the infant, the metal strip must be removed from the face mask to prevent burning the infant. Lotions and ointments should not be used during phototherapy because they absorb heat, and this can cause burns.

Phototherapy may cause changes in the infant's temperature depending partially on the bed used: bassinet, isolette, or radiant warmer. The infant's temperature is closely monitored. Phototherapy lights may increase insensible water loss, placing the infant at risk for fluid loss and dehydration; therefore it is important that the infant be adequately hydrated. Hydration maintenance in the healthy newborn is accomplished with human milk or infant formula; there is no reason to administer glucose water or plain water because these do not promote excretion of bilirubin in the stools and may actually perpetuate enterohepatic circulation, thus delaying bilirubin excretion. Urine output may be decreased or unaltered; the urine may have a brown or gold appearance. All aspects of the phototherapy treatment should be accurately recorded in the infant's chart.

The number and consistency of stools are monitored. Bilirubin breakdown increases gastric motility, which results in the formation of loose stools that can cause skin excoriation and breakdown. The infant's buttocks are cleaned after each stool to help maintain skin integrity. A fine maculopapular rash may appear during phototherapy, but this is transient. Because visualization of the infant's skin color is difficult with blue light, appropriate cardiorespiratory monitoring should be implemented based on the infant's overall condition.

An alternative device for phototherapy that is safe and effective is a fiberoptic panel attached to an illuminator. This fiberoptic blanket may be wrapped around the newborn's torso or flat in the bed, thus delivering continuous phototherapy. Although the fiberoptic lights do not produce heat as do conventional lights, staff should ensure that there is a covering pad between the infant's skin and the fiberoptic device. This helps to prevent burns, especially in preterm infants. During treatment with the fiberoptic blanket the newborn can remain in the mother's room in an open crib or in her arms (Fig. 19-18, *C*); follow unit protocol for the use of eye patches. The blanket also may be used for home care. In certain instances the infant's bilirubin levels may be increasing rapidly and intensive phototherapy is required; this involves the use of a combination of conventional lights and fiberoptic blankets.

Exchange transfusion.   Exchange transfusion is usually reserved for infants at risk for kernicterus because of high bilirubin levels. Small amounts of cross-matched whole blood are transfused into the infant as equivalent amounts of the infant's blood are withdrawn and discarded. This is most often accomplished through an umbilical venous catheter. Potential complications of exchange transfusion include transfusion reaction, infection, metabolic instability, and complications related to placement of the umbilical catheter (Kliegman, 2002) (see Chapter 27).

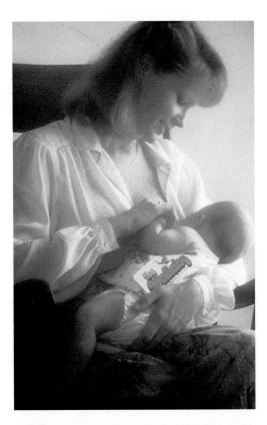

Fig. 19-18   A mother can breastfeed her baby without interrupting phototherapy. Eye patches are worn when infant is under bililights but not when a BiliBlanket is used. (Courtesy Respironics, Inc., Pittsburgh, PA.)

Parent education. Serum levels of bilirubin in the newborn continue to increase until the fifth day of life. Many parents leave the hospital within 24 hours, and some as early as 6 hours after birth. Therefore parents must be able to assess the newborn's degree of jaundice. They should have written instructions for assessing the infant's condition and the name of the contact person to whom to report their findings and concerns. Some health care agencies have a nurse make a home visit to evaluate the infant's condition. If it proves necessary to measure the infant's bilirubin levels after discharge from the hospital, either the home care nurse may draw the blood specimen or the parents may take the baby to a laboratory for the determination.

Home phototherapy. Healthy term infants may at times be discharged home and need phototherapy for hyperbilirubinemia. Candidates for home phototherapy include those infants who are healthy and active with no signs and symptoms of other complications; the parents or other caregivers must be willing and able to assume responsibility for therapy maintenance and monitoring, and the home environment should be adequate with a telephone, heat, and electricity (University of California San Francisco Home Health Care [UCSF], 2001). Home health care nurses are usually responsible for assessing the parents' or other caregivers' willingness to use the equipment and monitor the infant and making home visits to assess the infant's response to therapy, including obtaining blood specimens for measuring bilirubin levels. The company that provides the home therapy equipment is responsible for setting up the phototherapy unit and teaching the parents or caregivers how to use the equipment. The home care nurse schedules home visits to assess the infant's response to therapy including weight, feeding, output, and temperature stability. Additional education of parents may be necessary; their understanding of the therapy and their responsibilities is assessed. Blood may be drawn for laboratory work, and results reported to the primary health care provider. When therapy is discontinued, follow-up visits for monitoring may be ordered. The equipment company is called to arrange for pick-up of the phototherapy unit (UCSF Home Health Care, 2001).

Circumcision. Circumcision of newborn males is commonly performed in the United States, although there is controversy over its value. The AAP Task Force on Circumcision (1999) noted that, although there is scientific evidence of potential medical benefits of circumcision, the data are not sufficient to recommend routine circumcision. The Task Force further recommended that if circumcision is performed, analgesia should be used. ACOG (2001) and the American Medical Association (2005) have issued similar recommendations regarding newborn circumcision.

Circumcision is a matter of personal parental choice. Parents usually decide to have their newborn circumcised for one or more of the following reasons: hygiene, religious conviction, tradition, culture, or social norms. Regardless of the reason for the decision, parents should be given unbiased information and the opportunity to discuss the benefits and risks of the procedure. Suggested medical benefits of circumcision for the infant include decreased incidence of urinary tract infection and decreased risk for sexually transmitted infection, penile cancer, and human papilloma virus (HPV) infection. There may be a lower risk of cervical cancer among female partners of circumcised men (Alanis & Lucidi, 2004). Although there may be potential benefits, none of these are deemed sufficient to suggest that newborn males be routinely circumcised (AAP Task Force on Circumcision, 1999). Risks and potential complications associated with circumcision include hemorrhage, infection, and penile injury (removal of excessive skin, damage to the meatus or glans) (Alanis & Lucidi, 2004).

Expectant parents should begin learning about circumcision during the prenatal period, but circumcision often is not discussed with the parents before labor. In many instances, it is only when the mother is being admitted to the hospital or birth unit that parents are first confronted with the decision regarding circumcision. Because the stress of the intrapartum period makes this a difficult time for parental decision making, this is not an ideal time to broach the topic of circumcision and expect a well-thought-out decision.

Procedure. Circumcision involves removing the prepuce (foreskin) of the glans. The procedure is usually not done immediately after birth because of the danger of cold stress but is performed in the hospital before the infant's discharge. The circumcision of a Jewish male is commonly performed on the eighth day after birth and is done at home, in a ceremony called a *bris*. This timing is logical from a physiologic standpoint because clotting factors decrease somewhat immediately after birth and do not return to prebirth levels until the end of the first week.

Formula feedings are usually withheld up to 4 hours before the circumcision to prevent vomiting and aspiration; breastfed infants may be allowed to nurse up until the procedure is done; this varies with unit protocol. To prepare the infant for the circumcision, he is positioned on a plastic restraint form (Fig. 19-19), and his penis is cleansed with soap and water or a preparatory solution such as povidone-iodine. The infant is draped to provide warmth and a sterile field, and the sterile equipment is readied for use.

Although some circumcision procedures require no special equipment or appliances (Fig. 19-20), numerous instruments have been designed for this purpose. Use of the Gomco, Yellen, or Mogen clamp (Fig. 19-21) may make this an almost bloodless operation. The procedure itself takes only a few minutes. After it is completed, a small petrolatum gauze dressing or a generous amount of petrolatum may be applied for the first day or two to prevent the diaper from adhering to the site. A PlastiBell also may be used for the circumcision. The advantages to its use are that it applies constant direct pressure to prevent hemorrhage during the procedure and afterward protects against infection, keeps the site from sticking to the diaper, and prevents pain with urination. To use the bell for circumcision, first fit it over the glans, tie the suture around the rim of the bell, and then cut away

CD: Critical Thinking Exercise—Circumcision

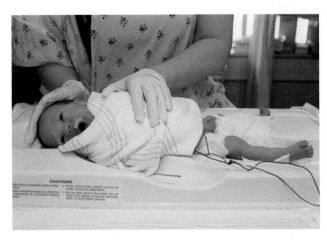

Fig. 19-19 Proper positioning of infant in Circumstraint. (Photo by Paul Vincent Kuntz, Texas Children's Hospital, Houston, TX.)

excess prepuce. The plastic rim remains in place for about a week until it falls off, after healing has taken place (Fig. 19-22). Petrolatum need not be applied when the PlastiBell is used (Glass, 2005).

Discomfort. Circumcision is painful, and the pain is manifested by both physiologic and behavioral changes in

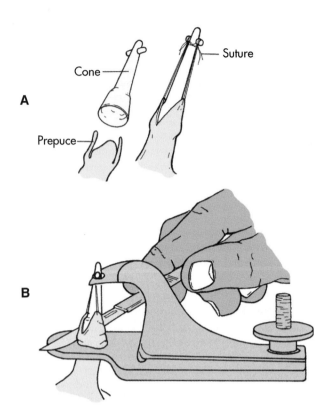

Fig. 19-21 Circumcision with Yellen clamp. **A,** Prepuce drawn over cone. **B,** Yellen clamp is applied, hemostasis occurs, and then prepuce (over cone) is cut away.

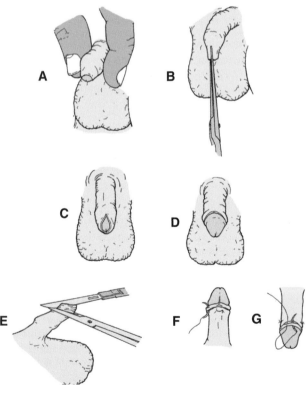

Fig. 19-20 Technique of circumcision. **A to D,** Prepuce is stripped and slit to facilitate its retraction behind glans penis. **E,** Prepuce is clamped and excessive prepuce cut off. **F and G,** A very small needle and plain 2-0 or 3-0 catgut are used for suture material; some physicians prefer silk.

the infant. The AAP Task Force on Circumcision (1999) recommends the use of environmental, nonpharmacologic, and pharmacologic pain interventions to prevent, decrease, or alleviate pain during neonatal circumcision.

Three types of anesthesia and analgesia are used in newborns who undergo circumcisions. These include (from most effective to less effective) ring block, dorsal penile nerve block (DPNB), and topical anesthetic (AAP Task Force on Circumcision, 1999). Nonpharmacologic methods such as nonnutritive sucking, containment, and swaddling may be used in addition to pharmacologic use of oral acetaminophen and a concentrated oral glucose solution. A combination of ring block or DPNB, topical anesthetic, nonnutritive sucking, oral acetaminophen, concentrated oral sucrose solution (2 ml of a 24% concentration given during the procedure on a pacifier, with a syringe or nipple), and swaddling has been shown to be the most effective at decreasing the pain associated with circumcision.

A ring block is the injection of buffered lidocaine administered subcutaneously on each side of the penile shaft. A DPNB includes subcutaneous injections of buffered lidocaine at the 2 o'clock and 10 o'clock positions at the base of the penis. The circumcision should not be done for at least 5 minutes after these injections.

A topical cream containing prilocaine-lidocaine such as EMLA can be applied to the base of the penis at least 1 hour before the circumcision. The area where the prepuce attaches

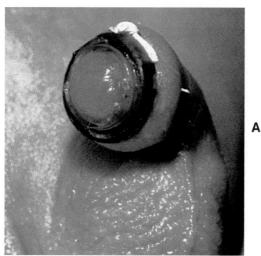

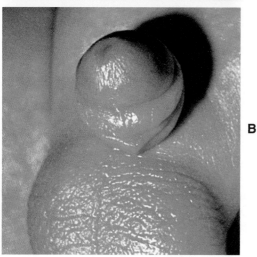

Fig. 19-22 Circumcision by using Hollister PlastiBell. **A,** Suture around rim of PlastiBell controls bleeding. **B,** Plastic rim and suture drop off in 7 to 10 days. (Permission to use and/or reproduce this copyrighted material has been granted by the owner, Hollister, Inc., Libertyville, IL.)

to the glans is well coated with 1 g of the cream and then covered with a transparent occlusive dressing or finger cot. Just before the procedure, the cream is removed. Blanching or redness of the skin may occur (Taddio, Ohlsson, & Ohlsson, 2001).

After the circumcision, the infant is comforted until he is quieted. If the parents were not present during the procedure, the infant is returned to them. The infant may be fussy for several hours, or he may be sleepy and difficult to awaken for feedings. Oral acetaminophen may be administered after the procedure every 4 hours (as ordered by the practitioner) for a maximum of five doses in 24 hours or a maximum of 75 mg/kg/day (Alanis & Lucidi, 2004).

Nurses are instrumental in implementing changes in health care practices to effectively manage the pain of neonatal circumcision (Razmus, Dalton, & Wilson, 2004).

Care of the newly circumcised infant. Bleeding is the most common complication of circumcision (AAP Task Force on Circumcision, 1999). The nurse checks the infant hourly for the 12 hours after the procedure to make sure no bleeding is occurring and that voiding is normal. If bleeding is noted from the circumcision, the nurse applies gentle pressure to the site of bleeding with a folded sterile gauze square; absorbable gelatin sponge (Gelfoam) powder or sponge may be applied to stop bleeding. If bleeding is not easily controlled, a blood vessel may require ligation. In this event, one nurse notifies the physician and prepares the necessary equipment (circumcision tray and suture material), while another nurse maintains intermittent pressure until the physician arrives. If the parents take the baby home before the end of the 12-hour observation period, they must be instructed about postcircumcision care and when to notify the physician (Teaching Guidelines box). Before the infant is discharged, the nurse checks to see that the parents have the physician's telephone number.

If the PlastiBell technique was used, the parents are instructed to observe the position of the plastic ring on the glans; it should remain on the glans (not on the shaft of the penis) and should fall off within 5 to 7 days. No petrolatum is used in caring for the penis circumcised with the PlastiBell technique. Otherwise, care is the same as for the other types of circumcision.

Evaluation

Evaluation is based on the expected outcomes of care. The plan is revised as needed, based on the evaluation findings.

NEONATAL PAIN

Until recent years, pain in the neonate was unrecognized and untreated. A common myth was that because newborns are developmentally immature, they do not experience pain, nor do they recall having felt pain. Fortunately, care providers now acknowledge that newborns actually do feel pain. Much attention has been drawn to assessment of that pain as well as to interventions that alleviate discomfort and return the newborn to a state of equilibrium (Clifford, Stringer, Christensen, & Mountain, 2004).

Pain has physiologic and psychologic components. The psychologic component of pain and the diffuse total body response to pain exhibited by the neonate led many health care providers to believe that infants, especially preterm infants, do not experience pain. The central nervous system is well developed, however, as early as 24 weeks of gestation. The peripheral and spinal structures that transmit pain information are present and functional between the first and second trimester. The pituitary-adrenal axis also is well developed at this time, and a fight-or-flight reaction is observed in response to the catecholamines released in response to stress (AAP & Canadian Paediatric Society, 2000; Walden & Franck, 2003).

The physiologic response to pain in neonates can be life threatening. Pain response can decrease tidal volume, increase demands on the cardiovascular system, increase metabolism, and cause neuroendocrine imbalance. The hormonal-metabolic response to pain in a term infant has greater magnitude and shorter duration than that in adults. The newborn's sympathetic response to pain is less mature and therefore less predictable than an adult's.

Assessment

Pain can be assessed in behavioral, physiologic or autonomic, and metabolic categories (Walden & Franck, 2003).

Behavioral responses

The most common behavioral sign of pain is a vocalization or crying, ranging from a whimper to a distinctive high-pitched, shrill cry. Facial expressions of pain include grimacing, eye squeeze, brow contraction, deepened nasolabial furrows, a taut and quivering tongue, and open mouth. The infant will flex and adduct the upper body and lower limbs in an attempt to withdraw from the painful stimulus (Clifford et al., 2004). The preterm infant has a lower threshold for initiation of this flex response. An infant who receives a muscle-paralyzing agent such a vecuronium will be unable to mount a behavioral or visible pain response.

Physiologic or autonomic responses

Significant changes in heart rate, BP (increased or decreased), intracranial pressure, vagal tone, respiratory rate, and oxygen saturation occur during noxious stimulation (Walden & Franck, 2003).

Metabolic responses

Infants release epinephrine, norepinephrine, glucagon, corticosterone, cortisol, 11-deoxycorticosterone, lactate, pyruvate, and glucose (Walden & Franck, 2003).

In assessing pain, the care provider needs to consider the health of the neonate, the type and duration of the painful stimulus, environmental factors, and the infant's state of alertness. For example, severely compromised neonates may be unable to generate a pain response, although they are, in fact, experiencing pain.

Every patient should have an initial pain assessment as well as a pain management plan; this includes newborns. The National Association of Neonatal Nurses (NANN) (1999) developed practice guidelines stating that all nurses who care for newborns should have education and competency validation in pain assessment. Pain should be assessed and documented on a regular basis.

Several pain assessment tools have been developed for use with neonates. A combination of behavioral and physiologic indicators of pain are used to diagnose and differentiate infant pain levels. Tools that have been shown to have validity and reliability include the Neonatal Infant Pain Scale (NIPS) (Lawrence et al., 1993) and the Premature Infant Pain Profile (PIPP) (Stevens, Johnston, Petryshen, & Taddio, 1996). A pain assessment tool used by nurses in the NICU is the CRIES (Krechel & Bildner, 1995) (Table 19-3). This tool was developed for use by nurses who work with preterm and term infants. CRIES is an acronym for the physiologic and behavioral indicators of pain used in the tool: crying, requiring increased oxygen, increased vital signs, expression, and sleeplessness. Each indicator is scored from 0 to 2. The total possible pain score, which represents the worst pain, is 10. A pain score greater than 4 should be considered significant. This tool can be used on infants between ages 32 weeks of gestation and 20 weeks after birth (Pasero, 2002).

Management of neonatal pain

The goals of the management of neonatal pain are to (1) minimize the intensity, duration, and physiologic cost of the pain; and (2) maximize the neonate's ability to cope with and

CD: Skill—Pain Assessment

TABLE 19-3

CRIES Neonatal Postoperative Pain Scale

	0	1	2
Crying	No	High pitched	Inconsolable
Requires O_2 for saturation >95%	No	<30%	>30%
Increased vital signs	Heart rate and blood pressure equal to or less than preoperative state	Heart rate and blood pressure <20% of preoperative state	Heart rate and blood pressure >20% of preoperative state
Expression	None	Grimace	Grimace and grunt
Sleepless	No	Wakes at frequent intervals	Constantly awake

CODING TIPS FOR USING CRIES

Crying	The characteristic cry of pain is high pitched.
	If no cry or cry that is not high pitched, score 0.
	If cry is high pitched but infant is easily consoled, score 1.
	If cry is high pitched and infant is inconsolable, score 2.
Requires O_2 for saturation >95%	Look for changes in oxygenation. Infants experiencing pain manifest decreases in oxygenation as measured by tCO_2 or oxygen saturation. (Consider other causes of changes in oxygenation, such as atelectasis, pneumothorax, oversedation.)
	If no oxygen is required, score 0.
	If <30% O_2 is required, score 1.
	If >30% O_2 is required, score 2.
Increased vital signs	NOTE: Measure blood pressure last because this may wake child, causing difficulty with other assessments. Use baseline preoperative parameters from a nonstressed period.
	Multiply baseline heart rate (HR) $\times$ 0.2, then add this to baseline HR to determine the HR that is 20% over baseline. Do likewise for blood pressure (BP). Use mean BP.
	If HR and BP are both unchanged or less than baseline, score 0.
	If HR or BP is increased but increase is <20% of baseline, score 1.
	If either one is increased >20% over baseline, score 2.
Expression	The facial expression most often associated with pain is a grimace. This may be characterized by brow lowering, eyes squeezed shut, deepening of the nasolabial furrow, open lips and mouth.
	If no grimace is present, score 0.
	If grimace alone is present, score 1.
	If grimace and noncry vocalization grunt is present, score 2.
Sleepless	This is scored based on the infant's state during the hour preceding this recorded score.
	If the child has been continuously asleep, score 0.
	If he or she has awakened at frequent intervals, score 1.
	If he or she has been awake constantly, score 2.

Neonatal pain assessment tool developed at the University of Missouri-Columbia. From Krechel, S., & Bildner, J. (1995). CRIES: A new neonatal postoperative pain measurement score: Initial testing of validity and reliability. *Paediatric Anaesthesia, 5*(1), 53-61.

recover from the pain (Walden & Franck, 2003). Nonpharmacologic and pharmacologic strategies are used.

Nonpharmacologic management

Containment, also known as *swaddling*, is effective in reducing excessive immature motor responses. This may provide comfort through other senses, such as thermal, tactile, and proprioceptive senses. Nonnutritive sucking on a pacifier, with or without sucrose, is a common comfort measure used with newborns. Skin-to-skin contact with the mother during a painful procedure can help to reduce pain. Combining these nonpharmacologic methods results in greater pain reduction. Distraction with visual, oral, auditory, or tactile stimulation may be helpful in term or older infants (Clifford et al., 2004; Walden & Franck, 2003).

Pharmacologic management

Pharmacologic agents are used to alleviate pain in neonates related to procedures. Local anesthesia has become routine during procedures such as chest tube insertion and circumcision. Topical anesthesia has been used for circumcision, lumbar puncture, venipuncture, and heel sticks. Nonopioid analgesia (acetaminophen) is effective for mild to moderate pain from inflammatory conditions. Morphine and fentanyl are the most widely used opioid analgesics for pharmacologic management of neonatal pain. Continuous or bolus intravenous infusion of opioids provides effective and safe pain control (AAP Committee on Fetus and Newborn, 2000). Ketorolac (Toradol) has been shown to be effective in the management of postoperative neonatal pain (Burd & Tobias, 2002). Postoperative neonatal pain should be managed with around-the-clock dosing or use of a continual drip. Dosing as needed (prn) is not considered to be an effective management of chronic or postoperative pain (Hummel & Puchalski, 2001). Traditional belief holds that the continued use of opioids for neonates in the postoperative period results in prolonged intubation. Consequently, traditional practice is to discontinue all opioids several hours before and after extubation, preventing pain relief. Furdon and colleagues (1998) found that continuous opioid infusion in infants without an underlying pulmonary or neurologic pathologic condition actually shortened the time to extubation and caused no problems of respiratory depression that required reintubation.

Other methods for managing neonatal pain are epidural infusion, local and regional nerve blocks, and intradermal or topical anesthetics (AAP Committee on Fetus and Newborn, 2000; Anand & International Evidence-Based Group for Neonatal Pain, 2001). A concentrated sucrose solution, especially when administered with a pacifier, can decrease pain associated with heel lance and venipuncture (Blass & Watt, 1999; Gradin et al., 2002; Stevens, Yamada, & Ohlsson, 2004). Oral acetaminophen may be administered for painful procedures such as circumcision, venous puncture, and heel stick.

CARE MANAGEMENT: DISCHARGE PLANNING AND TEACHING

Infant care activities can cause much anxiety for the new parent (see Plan of Care). Support from nursing staff members can be an important factor in determining whether new mothers seek and accept help in the future. Whether this is the woman's or couple's first newborn or an adolescent whose mother will be the primary caregiver, and whether or not the parents attended parenthood preparation classes, parents appreciate anticipatory guidance in the care of their infant. The nurse should not try to cover all the content at one time because the parents can be overwhelmed by too much information and become anxious. However, because early discharge of new mothers is currently common practice, it may be a problem for the nurse to teach all the content that is necessary. As a result, many institutions have developed home visitation programs that take the necessary teaching to the new parents, although the hospital nurse still provides most of the essential information for newborn care (see Community Activity box).

To set priorities for teaching, the nurse follows parental cues. Deficient knowledge should be identified before the nurse begins to teach. The nurse can use a tool such as the Infant Teaching/Discharge Record (Fig. 19-23) to identify parental needs. Normal growth and development and the changing needs of the infant (e.g., for stimulation, exercise, and social contacts), as well as the topics that follow, should be included during discharge planning with parents.

Temperature

The following topics should be reviewed:
- The causes of elevation in body temperature (e.g., overwrapping, cold stress with resultant vasoconstriction, or minimal response to infection) and the body's response to extremes in environmental temperature
- Signs to be reported, such as high or low temperatures with accompanying fussiness, lethargy, irritability, poor feeding, and crying
- Ways to promote normal body temperature, such as dressing the infant appropriately for the environmental air temperature and protecting the infant from exposure to direct sunlight
- Use of warm wraps or extra blankets in cold weather
- Technique for taking the newborn's axillary temperature

Respirations

Review the following points:
- Normal variations in the rate and rhythm
- Reflexes such as sneezing to clear the airway
- Need to protect the infant from the following:
  - Exposure to people with upper respiratory tract infections and respiratory syncytial virus (RSV)
  - Exposure to secondhand tobacco smoke
  - Suffocation from loose bedding, water beds, and beanbag chairs; drowning (in bath water); entrapment under excessive bedding or in soft bedding; anything tied around the infant's neck; poorly constructed playpens, bassinets, or cribs
- Sleep position—on back when put to sleep
- Aspiration pneumonia; symptoms of the common cold
  - A commonly aspirated substance is baby powder, which usually is a mixture of talc (hydrous magnesium silicate) and other silicates. Parents are advised that, if they prefer to use a powder, a cornstarch preparation can be substituted. Whenever a powder is used, it should be placed in the caregiver's hand and then applied to the skin, never sprinkled directly onto the skin.
  - Symptoms of the common cold include nasal congestion and excess drainage of mucus, coughing, sneezing, difficulty in swallowing or breathing, decreased vigor in feeding, and low-grade fever. Advise the parents on measures to help the infant, such as the following:
    - Feeding smaller amounts more often to prevent overtiring the infant
    - Holding the baby in an upright position to feed
    - For sleeping, raising the infant's head and chest by raising the mattress 30 degrees (do not use pillow)
    - Avoiding drafts; not overdressing the baby
    - Using only medications prescribed by a physician
    - Using nasal saline drops in each nostril and suctioning well with bulb syringe to decrease and relieve secretions

INFANT TEACHING/DISCHARGE RECORD

Our nursing staff wish to give you the information you want and need most during your stay with us. Please look over the following list of educational topics and complete the form by putting a check in the column that most applies to you, using the following scale:

IMPRINT AREA

1 = Most important to learn before I go home   2 = I would like to review   3 = I already know or am comfortable with

SELF-ASSESSMENT CHECKLIST		1	2	3	PATENT EDUCATION	
					Date/Time	Nurse Int.
BABY CARE						
Crying as Communication	Hunger, pain from not burping or gas, need for diaper change, too warm, too cold.					
Hiccoughs and Sneezing	Normal.					
Bath Sponge/Tub	Bath as needed.					
Soaps	Mild (Dove, Neutrogena, baby care products.)					
Nail Care	Emery board.					
Cord Care	Keep dry. Fold diaper below cord. Cord falls off 1–2 weeks.					
Skin Care/Diaper Rash	Air dry, zinc oxide. Call advice if no improvement in 2 days.					
Diaper Change	Wash girls front to back.					
Genitals	Vaginal care—white or pink discharge, cheesy material, normal.					
Circumcision Care	Remove Vaseline gauze after 4° if present. Vaseline applied to diaper as needed for 24°.					
Uncircumcised Baby Care	No need to retract foreskin.					
Elimination	Meconium first, then seedy soft yellow. Urinates 6–8 times/day.					
Axillary Temperature	Normal axillary temp. 97.6° F. Call advice if over 100° F.					
Clothing	Flame retardant. Dress comfortably. Do not overdress.					
Positioning	Side or back, **NOT STOMACH.**					
Bulb Syringe/Choking	Keep within reach/use to clear nose and mouth.					
Handwashing	Viruses and bacteria easily transmitted through hands. Wash frequently.					
Environment	Smoke free, smoke detector.					
Car Seat	Calif. Vehicle Code #27365.5. Follow manufacturer's directions for installation.					
BREASTFEEDING	See Breastfeeding Information Guide.					
Latching on	Breastfeeding. Demand feed, usually every 1½–3 hours around the clock. Be flexible.					
Positioning Mom/Baby	• Frequency: 8–12 times in 24 hours.					
Frequency & Lengths of	• Duration: 10–15 minutes of swallowing at each breast each feeding.					
Care of Breasts/Nipples	• Sore nipples: check latch, vary positions; air dry; shorter, more frequent nursing.					
Breast Pump/Pumping Storage	• Breast engorgement: hot soaks or hot showers, hand express, frequent nursing.					
	• Supplements: not necessary.					
BOTTLE FEEDING	Bottle feeding. Demand feed, usually every 3–4 hours. Be sure tongue is under nipple.					
Latching on & Positioning	• Clean bottles and nipples with hot, soapy water or dishwasher.					
Positioning	• No need to sterilize.					
	• May use tap or bottled water to mix formula.					
Frequency & Lengths of	• Refrigerate extra feeding in quantities taken per feeding.					
	• Do not microwave formula.					
Formula Preparation	• Do not prop bottle.					

SEEK MEDICAL ADVICE FOR THE FOLLOWING:
• Redness, discharge or foul odor from circumcision or umbilical cord.
• Less than 4 wet diapers/day by 4 days old.
• Less than 6–8 wet diapers/day by 6 days old.
• Frequent, explosive, watery stools that soak through the diaper.
• Axillary temperature of less than 97.4° F or greater than 100° F.
• Poor feeding, weak suck, no interest in eating.
• Yellow coloring of skin (jaundice) or whites of eyes.
• Vomiting forcefully several times (not just spitting up).
• Very irritable or excessive sleepiness.

Special instructions or comments:_____

_____

_____

☐ Home Health referral:_____
☐ Mother verbalizes understanding of discharge instructions.

MOTHER'S SIGNATURE   DATE

RN INITIALS	RN SIGNATURE		RN INITIALS	RN SIGNATURE

ID BAND #		M.R. #	*Staple 1 Infant ID Band Here.*

I acknowledge receipt of my baby and have received educational instructions and materials.   MOTHER'S SIGNATURE

DISCHARGE Date_____ Time_____	DISCHARGE To_____ With_____	CARRIED OUT BY ☐	☐ Mother ☐ Nurse	NURSE'S SIGNATURE

01737-2 (REV. 12-96)   DISTRIBUTION: WHITE = MOTHER'S CHART • CANARY = BABY'S CHART • PINK = MOTHER

Fig. 19-23   Infant Teaching/Discharge Record. (Courtesy Kaiser Permanente, Redwood City, CA.)

Feeding Schedules

Feeding practices and schedules for newborns are discussed in Chapter 20.

Elimination

A review includes the following reminders:

- Color of normal urine and number of voidings (6 to 8) to expect each day
- Changes to be expected in the color of the stool (i.e., meconium to transitional to soft yellow or golden yellow) and the number of bowel evacuations, plus the odor of stools for breastfed or bottle-fed infants (see Chapter 20)
- Expected pattern of stools in formula-fed infants may be as few as one stool every other day after first few weeks of life

Positioning and Holding

The AAP Task Force on Infant Sleep Position and Sudden Infant Death Syndrome (2000), recommends placing the infant in the supine position during the first few months of life to prevent sudden infant death syndrome (SIDS). The prone position has been associated with an increased incidence of SIDS. Death rates from SIDS have decreased by more than 40% in the United States since the original sleep position statement recommending supine sleeping for all newborns was made in 1992.

Anatomically, the infant's shape—a barrel chest and flat, curveless spine—makes it easy for the infant to roll from the side to the prone position; therefore the side-lying position for sleep is not recommended. Care must also be taken to prevent the infant from rolling off flat, unguarded surfaces. When an infant is on such a surface, the parent or nurse who

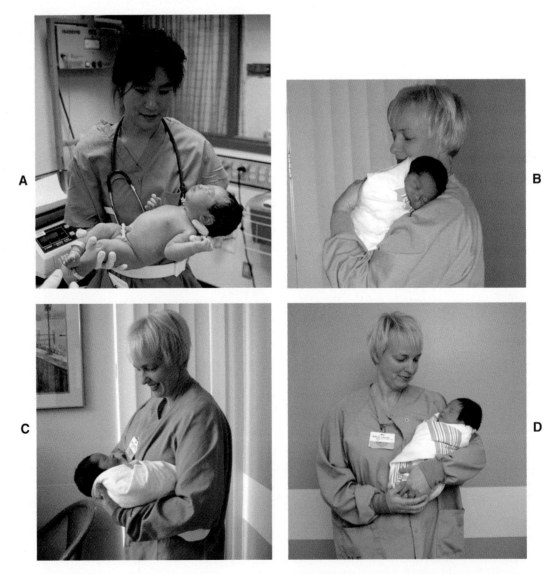

Fig. 19-24 Holding baby securely with support for head. **A,** Holding infant while moving infant from one place to another. Baby is undressed to show posture. **B,** Holding baby upright in "burping" position. **C,** "Football" hold. **D,** Cradling hold. (**A,** Courtesy Kim Molloy, Knoxville, IA; **B, C,** and **D,** courtesy Julie Perry Nelson, Gilbert, AZ.)

must turn away from the infant even for a moment should always keep one hand placed securely on the infant. The infant is always held securely with the head supported because newborns are unable to maintain an erect head posture for more than a few moments. Fig. 19-24 illustrates various positions for holding an infant with adequate support.

Rashes

Diaper rash

The warm, moist atmosphere in the diaper area provides an optimal environment for *Candida albicans* growth; dermatitis appears in the perianal area, inguinal folds, and lower abdomen. The affected area is intensely erythematous with a sharply demarcated, scalloped edge, often with numerous satellite lesions that extend beyond the larger lesion. The usual source of infection is from handling by persons who do not practice adequate handwashing. It may also appear 2 to 3 days after an oral infection (thrush).

Therapy consists of applications of an anticandidal ointment, such as clotrimazole or miconazole, with each diaper change. Sometimes the infant also is given an oral antifungal preparation such as nystatin or fluconazole to eliminate any gastrointestinal source of infection.

Washing and drying the wet and soiled area and changing the diaper immediately after voiding or stooling will prevent and help treat diaper rash. Parents can be taught to expose the buttocks to air to help dry up diaper rash. Because bacteria thrive in moist dark areas, exposing the skin to dry air decreases bacterial proliferation. A skin barrier ointment such as zinc oxide may be effective in preventing further excoriation, especially in the presence of loose stools or systemic gastrointestinal candidiasis; the latter will require treatment with a systemic antifungal drug.

Other rashes

A rash on the cheeks may result from the infant's scratching with long unclipped fingernails or from rubbing the face against the crib sheets, particularly if regurgitated stomach contents are not washed off promptly. The newborn's skin begins a natural process of peeling and sloughing after birth. Dry skin may be treated with a neutral pH lotion, but this should be used sparingly. Newborn rash, erythema toxicum, is a common finding (see Chapter 18) and needs no treatment.

Nail Care

Fingernails and toenails should not be cut immediately after birth, but should be allowed to grow out far enough to avoid cutting the attached skin. If needed, the infant's hands can be covered with loose-fitting mittens to prevent scratching the face. However, this should be avoided if possible, because mittens inhibit the infant from sucking on fingers for self-consolation. Nails can be safely trimmed with manicure scissors or infant nail clippers, cutting nails straight across. Emery boards can be used to file nails. Nail care is most easily accomplished after bathing, when the nails are soft, or when the infant is sleeping.

Clothing

Parents commonly ask how warmly they should dress their infant. A simple rule of thumb is to dress the child as they dress themselves, adding or subtracting clothes and wraps for the child as necessary. A cotton shirt and diaper may be sufficient clothing for the young infant. A cap or bonnet is needed to protect the scalp and minimize heat loss if the weather is cool, or to protect against sunburn and shade the eyes if it is sunny and hot. Wrapping the infant snugly in a blanket maintains body temperature and promotes a feeling of security. Overdressing in warm temperatures can cause discomfort, as can underdressing in cold weather. Parents are encouraged to dress the infant at all times in flame-retardant clothing. Infant sunglasses are available to protect the infant's eyes when outdoors.

Infants have sensitive skin; therefore new clothes should be washed before putting them on the infant. Baby clothes should be washed separately with a mild detergent and hot water. A double rinse usually removes traces of the potentially irritating cleansing agent or acid residue from urine or stool. If possible, the clothing and bed linens are dried in the sun to neutralize residue. Parents who have to use coin-operated machines in commercial laundries to wash and dry clothes may find it expensive or impossible to wash and rinse the baby's clothes well.

Bedding requires frequent changing. The top of a plastic-coated mattress should be washed frequently, and the crib or bassinet should be dusted with a damp cloth. The infant's toilet articles may be kept convenient for use in a box, basket, or plastic carrier.

Sleeping

Since 1992, the AAP has recommended that infants be placed on their backs to sleep. This supine position is associated with a decreased risk of SIDS. Loose bedding should be kept away from the infant's face and head to avoid the risk of suffocation (Pollack & Frohna, 2002).

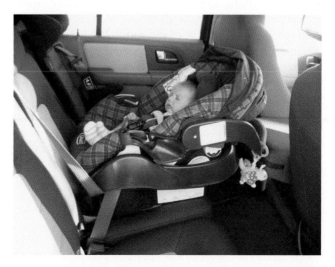

Fig. 19-25 Rear-facing car seat in rear seat of car. Infant is placed in seat when going home from the hospital. (Courtesy Brian and Mayannyn Sallee, Las Vegas, NV.)

Critical Thinking Exercise

Sudden Infant Death Syndrome and Infant Sleep Position

Marlys gave birth to a full-term infant; she and Daniel are being discharged today. The nurse has given her instructions about placing the baby on his back for sleep. Marlys said that she had noticed that the nurses placed Daniel on his side in the nursery and wondered why they did that when she was instructed to place Daniel on his back.

Michelle gave birth to Michael at 32 weeks. During the stay in the nursery the nurses placed Michael on his abdomen to sleep. At discharge, Michelle was instructed to place Michael on this back to sleep. Michelle asked why she had to place Michael on his back to sleep when he was used to sleeping on his abdomen. How should the nurses respond to these questions?

1 Evidence—Is there sufficient evidence to draw conclusions about the safety and efficacy of the supine position for sleep in reducing the incidence of sudden infant death syndrome (SIDS)?

2 Assumptions—What assumptions can be made about the following factors related to infant positioning?
   a. Role modeling by nurses
   b. Sleep position in the nursery versus sleep position at home
   c. Sleep position for preterm versus term infants
   d. Nurses' knowledge and use of research evidence

3 What implications and priorities for nursing care can be drawn at this time?

4 Does the evidence objectively support your conclusion?

5 Are there alternative perspectives to your conclusion?

Safety: Use of Car Seat

Infants should travel only in federally approved, rear-facing safety seats that meet Federal Motor Vehicle Safety Standard (FMVSS) 213 and that are secured in the rear seat (Fig. 19-25). Parents should bring the car seat to the hospital before discharge for training on positioning and securing the infant as well as proper installation of the car seat. Many hospitals have staff that are specially trained and certified in car seat safety; parents can also check with local fire, police, or highway patrol agencies for assistance with proper installation of car seats.

The safest area of the car is the back seat. A car seat that faces the rear gives the best protection for the disproportionately weak neck and heavy head of an infant. In this position, the force of a frontal crash is spread over the head, neck, and back; the back of the car seat supports the spine.

NURSE ALERT *Infants should use a rear-facing car seat from birth to 20 pounds and to 1 year of age. If the infant reaches the weight limit before the first birthday, the rear-facing position should still be used. In cars equipped with air bags, rear-facing infant seats must not be placed in the front seat. Serious injury can occur if the air bag inflates because these types of infant seats fit closer to the dashboard.*

The car seat is secured using the vehicle seat belt; the infant is secured using the harness system in the car seat. If the infant must ride in the front seat, the air bag must be turned off to prevent injury from the air bag (AAP Committee on Injury and Poison Prevention, 2002).

Infants are positioned at a 45-degree angle in a car seat to prevent slumping and subsequent airway obstruction. Many seats allow for adjustment of seat angle. For seats that are not adjustable, a tightly rolled newspaper, a solid-core Styrofoam roll, or a firm roll of fabric can be placed under the car safety seat to place the infant at a 45-degree angle (AAP Committee on Injury and Poison Prevention, 2002).

Infants born at less than 37 weeks of gestation and with birth weight less than 2500 g should be observed in a car seat for a period of time (equal to the length of the car ride home) before discharge. The infant is monitored for apnea, bradycardia, and a decrease in oxygen saturation. It may be necessary to place blanket rolls on either side of the infant for support of the head and trunk. To prevent slumping, the back-to-crotch strap distance should be 14 cm.

Nonnutritive Sucking

Sucking is the infant's chief pleasure. However, sucking needs may not be satisfied by breastfeeding or bottle-feeding alone. In fact, sucking is such a strong need that infants who are deprived of sucking, such as those with a cleft lips, will suck on their tongues. Some newborns are born with sucking pads on their fingers that developed during in utero sucking. Several benefits of nonnutritive sucking have been demonstrated, such as an increased weight gain in preterm infants, increased ability to maintain an organized state, and decreased crying.

Problems arise when parents are concerned about the sucking of fingers, thumb, or pacifier and try to restrain this natural tendency. Before giving advice, nurses should investigate the parents' feelings and base the guidance they give on the information solicited. For example, some parents may see no problem with the use of a finger but may find the use of a pacifier objectionable. In general, there is no need to restrain either practice, unless thumb sucking persists past 4 years of age or past the time when the permanent teeth erupt. Parents are advised to consult with their pediatrician, pediatric dentist, or pediatric nurse practitioner about this topic.

A parent's excessive use of the pacifier to calm the child should also be explored, however. It is not unusual for parents to place a pacifier in their infant's mouth as soon as the infant begins to cry, thus reinforcing a pattern of distress-relief.

If parents choose to let their child use a pacifier, they need to be aware of certain safety considerations before purchasing one. A homemade or poorly designed pacifier can be dangerous because the entire object may be aspirated if it is small, or a portion may become lodged in the pharynx. Improvised pacifiers, such as those commonly made in hospitals from a padded nipple, also pose dangers because the nipple may separate from the plastic collar and be aspirated. Safe pacifiers are made of one piece that includes a shield

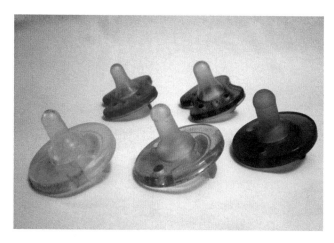

Fig. 19-26 Safe pacifiers for term and preterm infants. Note one-piece construction, easily grasped handle, and large shield with ventilation holes. (Courtesy Julie Perry Nelson, Gilbert, AZ.)

or flange large enough to prevent entry into the mouth and a handle that can be grasped (Fig. 19-26).

Sponge Bathing, Cord Care, and Skin Care

Bathing serves a number of purposes. It provides opportunities for (1) completely cleansing the infant, (2) observing the infant's condition, (3) promoting comfort, and (4) parent-child-family socializing.

An important consideration in skin cleansing is a preservation of the skin's acid mantle, which is formed from the uppermost horny layer of the epidermis, sweat, superficial fat, metabolic products, and external substances such as amniotic fluid and microorganisms. At birth the skin has a pH of 6.4. Within 4 days the pH of the newborn's skin surface falls to within the bacteriostatic range (pH less than 5) (Krebs, 1998). Consequently, only plain, warm water should be used for the bath during that 4-day period. Alkaline soaps (such as Ivory) and oils, powder, and lotions should not be used during this time because they alter the acid mantle, thus providing a medium for bacterial growth. Although the sponging technique is generally used, bathing the newborn by immersion has been found to allow less heat loss and provoke less crying; this is not advised, however, until the umbilical cord falls off. A daily bath is not necessary for achieving cleanliness and may do more harm by disrupting the integrity of the newborn's skin; cleansing the perineum after a soiled diaper and daily cleansing of the face may suffice.

The umbilical cord begins to dry, shrivel, and blacken by the second or third day of life depending in part on the cleansing method used. The umbilicus should be inspected often for signs of infection (e.g., foul odor, redness, and purulent discharge), granuloma (i.e., small, red, raw-appearing polyp where the umbilical cord separates), bleeding, and discharge. The cord clamp is removed when the cord is dry, in about 24 to 36 hours (see Fig. 19-5). The cord normally falls off in 10 to 14 days after birth but may remain attached for as long as 3 weeks in some cases.

Parents are instructed in appropriate home cord care (per practitioner or institution protocol) and the expected time of cord separation.

The Teaching Guidelines box contains information regarding sponge bathing, skin care, cord care, cutting nails, and dressing the infant.

Infant Follow-up Care

With shorter hospital stays, the focus and site of infant care are changing. Home care may be provided either by a nurse as part of the routine follow-up care of patients, or through a visiting nurse or community health nurse referral service. For infants discharged early, newborn home care is essential (Teaching Guidelines box) (see also Chapter 3).

Parents should plan for their infant's follow-up health care at the following ages: within 3 days if early discharge to check for status of jaundice, feeding, and elimination (see also Physiologic Jaundice, pp. 542 to 543 for follow-up guidelines); 2 to 4 weeks of age; then every 2 months until 6 to 7 months of age; then every 3 months until 18 months; at 2 years; at 3 years; at preschool; and every 2 years thereafter.

Immunizations

The schedule for immunizations should be reviewed with the parents. Hepatitis B vaccine is currently administered to newborns before hospital discharge (depending on maternal hepatitis B status) with parental permission.

Cardiopulmonary resuscitation

All personnel working with infants must have current infant cardiopulmonary resuscitation (CPR) certification. Parents should receive instruction in relieving airway obstruction (Emergency box) and CPR (Emergency box). Often classes are offered in hospitals and clinics during the prenatal period or to parents of newborns. Such instruction is especially important for parents whose infants were preterm or had cardiac or respiratory problems. Babysitters also should learn CPR.

COMMUNITY ACTIVITY

Investigate infant car seat safety laws in your state. Find out age and weight guidelines for the various types of safety seats. Where can parents go to have their infant car seats checked for proper installation?

Are there programs in your community to provide car seats for low income families? What are hospitals in your area doing to promote infant safety?

TEACHING GUIDELINES
Sponge Bathing

FIT BATHS INTO FAMILY'S SCHEDULE

- Give a bath at any time convenient to you but not immediately after a feeding period because the increased handling may cause regurgitation.

PREVENT HEAT LOSS

- The temperature of the room should be 24° C (75° F), and the bathing area should be free of drafts.
- Control heat loss during the bath to conserve the infant's energy. Bathing the infant quickly, exposing only a portion of the body at a time, and drying thoroughly are all parts of the bathing technique.

GATHER SUPPLIES AND CLOTHING BEFORE STARTING

- Clothing suitable for wearing indoors: diaper, shirt; stretch suit or nightgown optional
- Unscented, mild soap
- Pins, if needed for diaper, closed and placed well out of baby's reach
- Cotton balls
- Towels for drying infant and a clean washcloth
- Receiving blanket
- Tub for water; fill only to 3 to 4 inches of water

BATHE THE BABY

- Bring infant to bathing area when all supplies are ready.
- ***Never leave the infant alone on bath table or in bath water, not even for a second!*** If you have to leave, take the infant with you or put back into crib.
- Test temperature of the water. It should feel pleasantly warm to the inner wrist—36.6° to 37.2°C (98° to 99° F).
- Do not hold infant under running water—water temperature may change, and infant may be scalded or chilled rapidly. Baby may be tub bathed after the cord drops off and umbilicus and circumcised penis are completely healed.
- If sponge bathing is to be done, undress the baby and wrap in a towel with the head exposed. Uncover the parts of the body you are washing, taking care to keep the rest of the baby covered as much as possible to prevent heat loss.
- Begin by washing the face with water; do not use soap on the face. Cleanse the eyes from the inner canthus outward, using separate parts of a clean washcloth for each eye. For the first 2 to 3 days, a discharge may result from the reaction of the conjunctiva to the substance (erythromycin) used as a prophylactic measure against infection. Any discharge should be considered abnormal and reported to the health care provider.
- Cleanse ears and nose with twists of moistened cotton or a corner of the washcloth. Do not use cotton-tipped swabs because they may cause injury. The areas behind the ears need daily cleansing.
- Wash the body with mild soap; rinse and dry to decrease heat loss. Place your hand under the shoulders and lift gently to expose the neck, lift the chin, and wash the neck, taking to care to cleanse between the skin folds. Wash between the fingers and toes, rinse and dry thoroughly. Wash the genital area last.

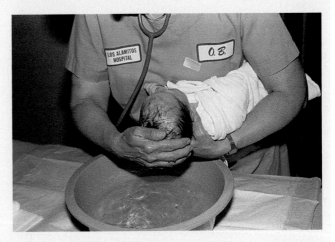

Wash hair with baby wrapped to limit heat loss. (Courtesy Marjorie Pyle, RNC, Lifecircle, Costa Mesa, CA.)

- If the hair is to be washed, begin by wrapping the infant in a towel with the head exposed. Hold the infant in a football position with one hand, using the other hand to wash the hair. Wash the scalp with water and mild soap and a soft brush; rinse well and dry thoroughly. Scalp desquamation, called *cradle cap*, often can be prevented by removing any scales with a fine-toothed comb or brush after washing. If condition persists, the health care provider may prescribe an ointment to massage into the scalp. A blow dryer is never used on an infant because the temperature is too hot for a baby's skin.

SKIN CARE

- The skin of a newborn is sensitive and should be cleaned only with water between baths. Soap is drying and its use is limited to bathing. Creams, lotions, ointments, or powders are not recommended. If the skin seems excessively dry during the first 2 to 3 weeks after birth, an unscented, non–alcohol-based lotion may be used; it is best to check with the health care provider for suggestions on skin care products. It may be advisable to launder baby clothes separately, using a mild laundry detergent (Dreft or Ivory Snow); clothes should be rinsed twice with plain water.
- The fragile skin can be injured by too vigorous cleansing. If stool or other debris has dried and caked on the skin, soak the area to remove it. Do not attempt to rub it off, because abrasion may result. Gentleness, patting dry rather than rubbing, and use of a mild soap without perfumes or coloring are recommended. Chemicals in the coloring and perfume can cause rashes on sensitive skin.
- Babies are very prone to sunburn and should be kept out of direct sunlight. Use of sunscreens should be discussed with the health care provider.
- Babies often develop rashes that are normal. Neonatal acne resembles pimples and may appear at 2 to 4 weeks of age, resolving without treatment by 6 to 8 months. Heat rash is common in warm weather; this appears as a fine red rash around creases or folds where the baby sweats.

TEACHING GUIDELINES—cont'd
Sponge Bathing

CARE OF THE CORD

• Cleanse around base of the cord where it joins the skin with soap and water. If the use of alcohol on the cord is suggested, use cotton-tipped swabs dipped in alcohol to cleanse the cord at the base where the cord meets the skin; this should be done with each diaper change. Notify the health care provider of any odor, discharge, or skin inflammation around the cord. The clamp is removed when the cord is dry (approximately 24 hr). The diaper should not cover the cord because a wet or soiled diaper will slow or prevent drying of the cord and foster infection. When the cord drops off after a 10 to 14 days, small drops of blood may be seen when the baby cries. This will heal by itself. It is not dangerous.

NAIL CARE

• Do not cut fingernails and toenails immediately after birth. The nails have to grow out far enough from the skin so that the skin is not cut by mistake. If the baby scratches himself or herself, apply loosely fitted mitts over each of the baby's hands. Do so as a last resort, however, because it interferes with the baby's ability for self-consolation sucking on thumb or finger. When the nails have grown, the fingernails and toenails can be trimmed with manicure scissors or clippers; nails should be cut straight across. The ideal time to do this is when the infant is sleeping. Soft emery boards may be used to file the nails. Nails should be kept short.

CLEANSE GENITALS

• Cleanse the genitals of infants daily and after voiding or defecating. For girls the genitals may be cleansed by separating the labia and gently washing from the pubic area to the anus. For uncircumcised boys, gently pull back (retract) the foreskin. Stop when resistance is felt. Wash and rinse the tip (glans) with soap and warm water, and replace the foreskin. The foreskin must be returned to its original position to prevent constriction and swelling. In most newborns, the inner layer of the foreskin adheres to the glans, and the foreskin cannot be retracted. By age 3 years in 90% of boys, the foreskin can be retracted easily without causing pain or trauma. For others, the foreskin is not retractable until adolescence. As soon as the foreskin is partly retractable and the child is old enough, he can be taught self-care. Once healed, the circumcised penis does not require any special care other than cleansing with diaper changes.

TEACHING GUIDELINES
Newborn Home Care after Early Discharge*

• Wet diapers: 6 to 8 per day
• Breastfeeding: successful latch-on and feeding every 1.5 to 3 hours daily
• Formula-feeding: successfully, voiding as noted above, taking approximately 3 to 4 ounces every 3 to 4 hours daily
• Circumcision: wash with warm water only; yellow exudate forming, nonbleeding, PlastiBell intact for 48 hours
• Stools: at least one every 48 hours (bottle-feeding) or two to three per day (breastfeeding)
• Color: pink to ruddy when crying; pink centrally when at rest or asleep
• Activity: has four or five wakeful periods per day and alerts to environmental sounds and voices
• Jaundice: physiologic jaundice (not appearing in first 24 hours), feeding, voiding, and stooling as noted above, or practitioner notification for suspicion of pathologic jaundice (appears within 24 hours of birth, ABO/Rh problem suspected; hemolysis); decreased activity; poor feeding; dark orange skin color persisting beyond fifth day in light-skinned newborn
• Cord: kept above diaper line; drying; periumbilical area skin pink (erythematous circle at umbilical site may be sign of omphalitis)
• Vital signs: heart rate 120 to 140 beats/min at rest; respiratory rate 30 to 55 breaths/min at rest without evidence of retractions, grunting, or nasal flaring; temperature 36.5° to 37.2° C axillary
• Position of sleep: back

From Hockenberry, M. (2003). *Wong's nursing care of infants and children* (7th ed.). St. Louis: Mosby.
*Any deviation from the above or suspicion of poor newborn adaptation should be reported to the practitioner at once.

Relieving Airway Obstruction

- Back blow and chest thrusts are used to clear an airway obstructed by a foreign body.

BACK BLOWS

- Position the infant prone over forearm with the head down and the infant's jaw firmly supported.
- Rest the supporting arm on the thigh.
- Deliver four back blows forcefully between the infant's shoulder blades with the heel of the free hand.

TURN INFANT

- Place the free hand on the infant's back to sandwich the baby between both hands; one hand supports the neck, jaw, and chest, while the other supports the back.
- Turn the infant over, and place the head lower than the chest, supporting the head and neck.
- Alternative position: Place the infant face down on your lap with the head lower than the trunk; firmly support the head. Apply back blows, and then turn the infant as a unit.

CHEST THRUSTS

- Provide four downward chest thrusts on the lower third of the sternum.
- Remove foreign body, if it is visible.

OPEN AIRWAY

- Open airway with the head tilt–chin lift maneuver, and attempt to ventilate.
- Repeat the sequence of back blows, turning, and chest thrusts.
- Continue these emergency procedures until signs of recovery occur:
  - Palpable peripheral pulses return.
  - The pupils become normal in size and are responsive to light.
  - Mottling and cyanosis disappear.
- Record the time and duration of the procedure and the effects of this intervention.

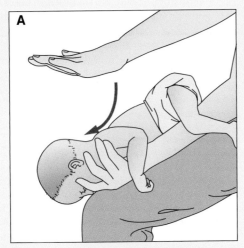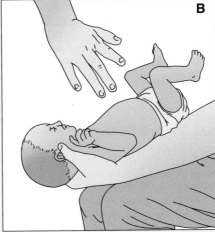

Back blows and chest thrust in infant to clear airway obstruction. **A,** Back blow. **B,** Chest thrust.

EMERGENCY

Cardiopulmonary Resuscitation (CPR)

- Wash hands before and after touching infant and equipment. Wear gloves, if possible.

ASSESS RESPONSIVENESS

- Observe color; tap or gently shake shoulders.
- Yell for help; if alone, perform CPR for 1 min before calling for help again.

POSITION INFANT

- Turn the infant onto back, supporting the head and neck.
- Place the infant on firm, flat surface.

AIRWAY

- Open the airway with the head tilt-chin lift method.
- Place one hand on the infant's forehead, and tilt the head back.
- Place the fingers of other hand under the bone of the lower jaw at the chin.

BREATHING

- Assess for evidence of breathing:
- Observe for chest movement.
- Listen for exhaled air.
- Feel for exhaled air flow.
- To breathe for infant:
  - Take a breath.
  - Place mouth over the infant's nose and mouth to create a seal. *NOTE:* When available, a mask with a one-way valve should be used.
  - Give two slow breaths (1 to 1.5 sec/breath), pausing to inhale between breaths. *Note:* Gently puff the volume of air in your cheeks into infant. Do not force air.
  - The infant's chest should rise slightly with each puff; keep fingers on the chest wall to sense air entry.

CIRCULATION

- Assess circulation:
  - Check pulse of the brachial artery while maintaining the head tilt.
  - If the pulse is present, initiate rescue breathing. Continue doing once every 3 sec or 20 times/min until spontaneous breathing resumes.
  - If the pulse is absent, initiate chest compressions and coordinate them with breathing.
- Chest compression
  - There are two systems of chest compression. Nurses should know both methods.
    - Maintain the head tilt and
      1. Place thumbs side-by-side in the middle third of the sternum with fingers around the chest and supporting the back.
         - Compress the sternum 1.25 to 2 cm.
      2. Place index finger of hand just under an imaginary line drawn between the nipples. Place the middle and ring fingers on the sternum adjacent to the index finger.
         - Using the middle and ring fingers, compress the sternum approximately 1.25 to 2.5 cm.
- Avoid compressing the xiphoid process.
- Release the pressure without moving the thumbs and fingers from the chest.
- Repeat at least 100 times/min, doing five compressions in 3 sec or less.
- Perform 10 cycles of five compressions and one ventilation.
- After the cycles, check the brachial artery to determine whether there is a pulse.
- Discontinue compressions when the infant's spontaneous heart rate reaches or exceeds 80 beats/min.
- Record the time and duration of the procedure and the effects of intervention.

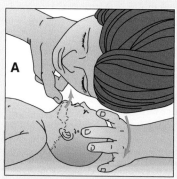 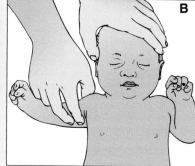 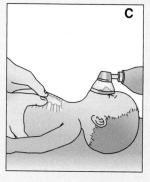

A, Opening airway with head tilt–chin lift method. **B,** Checking pulse of brachial artery. **C,** Side-by-side thumb placement for chest compression in newborn.

Source: Stapleton, E. et al. (2001). *Fundamentals of BLS for healthcare providers.* Dallas, TX: American Heart Association.

Key Points

- Assessment of the newborn requires data from the prenatal, intrapartal, and postnatal periods.
- The newborn assessment should proceed systematically so that each system is thoroughly evaluated.
- Gestational assessment should be completed within 12 hours of birth for infants with less than 26 weeks of gestation and within 48 hours of birth for infants with at least 26 weeks of gestation.
- The immediate nursing assessment of the newborn includes Apgar scoring and a general evaluation of physical status.
- Nursing care of the newborn immediately after birth includes maintaining a patent airway, preventing heat loss, stabilizing the infant, and promoting parent-infant interaction.
- Nursing care of the newborn may include diagnostic and therapeutic procedures.
- Providing a protective environment is a key responsibility of the nurse and includes such measures as careful identification procedures, support of physiologic functions, measures to prevent infection, and restraining techniques.
- Circumcision is an elective surgical procedure.
- Pain in neonates must be assessed and managed.
- Anticipatory guidance helps prepare new parents for what to expect after hospital discharge.
- Instruction in infant CPR is often provided to new parents.

Answer Guidelines to Critical Thinking Exercise

Sudden Infant Death Syndrome and Infant Sleep Position

1 Yes, there is ample evidence that the supine position for sleep reduces the incidence of sudden infant death syndrome (SIDS). The nurses should cite the evidence as well as explain that in preterm infants, use of the prone position can assist breathing in the early phases of recovery from respiratory distress. However, as the infant matures, he should be placed on his back to sleep.

2 a. Role modeling by nurses is a powerful teacher. Stastny and colleagues (2004) found that only 30% of nursery staff placed babies on their backs to sleep and cited fear of aspiration as the reason. Continued staff education is necessary to promote the use of the supine position for sleep.

  b. In the newborn nursery, nurses may place an infant on his or her side to promote drainage of secretions, although there is no evidence that this is effective. In the neonatal intensive care unit (NICU), infants in respiratory distress may breathe more easily in the prone position. As the distress lessens and the infant matures, the infant should be placed on his or her back for sleep. Parents should be counseled to place infants on their backs for sleep. During waking hours, while the parent is supervising, the infant can be placed on his or her side or abdomen.

  c. Discuss sleep position for preterm versus term infants. Preterm infants may be placed in prone position to facilitate respiration; however, they should be on a cardiorespiratory monitor.

  d. Not all nurses read research reports and use research evidence in their practices. Therefore they do not place infants on their backs to sleep and do not instruct parents in sleep positioning. Continuing education programs for nurses working in nurseries should address the latest findings related to the prevention of SIDS by use of positioning infants on their backs to sleep.

3 The nurse needs to reinforce the importance of placing the infant on his or her back to sleep and discuss with the parents the acceptability of placing the infant on the side or abdomen while the infant is awake. The nurse can also advocate for continuing education programs for the nurses to update their clinical knowledge. Signs could be posted in the nursery to remind nurses of the correct positioning.

4 There is ample evidence of the efficacy of sleeping on the back in prevention of SIDS. There is also documentation that many nurses do not follow these recommendations. Stastny and colleagues (2004) found that Latina and Pacific Islander mothers were less likely than Caucasian mothers to be instructed in positioning the infant on his or her back to sleep.

5 Nursery nurses may have had experience with babies choking on mucus and used the prone or side-lying position to promote drainage of mucus. Based on that experience, they may fear that the back-lying position will promote aspiration. They may rely on experience rather than research evidence in their care of infants. Continuing education programs should address research findings. Nurse managers can implement programs of reward for those nurses who base their practice on evidence.

Resources

American Academy of Pediatrics (AAP)
Air Bag Safety Sheets
141 Northwest Point Blvd.
Elk Grove, IL 60007
847-228-5005
www.aap.org

National Healthy Mothers, Healthy Babies Coalition
121 North Washington St., Suite 300
Alexandria, VA 22314
703-836-6110
www.hmhb.org

National Institute of Child Health and Human Development
(NICHD)
National Institutes of Health
9000 Rockville Pike
Bldg. 31, Room 2A32
Bethesda, MD 20892
301-496-4000
www.nih.gov

Neonatal Network
1410 Neotomas Ave., Suite 107
Santa Rosa, CA 95405
www.neonatalnetwork.com

Resources for Parents

At-Home Dad (newsletter for fathers who stay at home)
61 Brightwood Ave.
North Andover, MA 01845-1702
E-mail: athomedad@aol.com

The Fatherhood Project at the Families and Work Institute
330 Seventh Ave.
New York, NY 10001
212-465-2044

Infant Massage: A Handbook for Loving Parents
Vimala McClure
International Association of Infant Massage (IAIM)
800-248-5432

The Institute for Responsible Fatherhood and Family Revitalization
1146 19th St., NW
Suite 800
Washington, DC 20036
800-732-8437 or 800-7-FATHER

La Leche League International (Local La Leche League groups are
usually listed in city and town phone books)
1400 North Meacham Rd.
Schaumburg, IL 60168-4079
847-519-7730

Motherhood Maternity Health and Fitness Program
SBI Corporation
1106 Stratford Dr.
Carlisle, PA 17013
717-258-4641

Pink Inc! Publishing
P.O. Box 866
Atlantic Beach, FL 32233-0866
904-731-7120

Postpartum Support International
927 North Kellogg Ave.
Santa Barbara, CA 93111
805-967-7636

Protecting Your Newborn, Video and Instructor's Guide (1997)
Ford Motor Company and the U.S. Department of Transportation
National Highway Traffic Safety Administration (NHTSA)
Auto Safety Hotline 800-424-9393
www.nhtsa.dot.gov

Single Parent Resource Center
141 West 28th St.
Suite 302
New York, NY 10001
212-947-0221

References

Alanis, M., & Lucidi, R. (2004). Neonatal circumcision: A review of the world's oldest and most controversial operation. *Obstetrical and Gynecological Survey, 59*(5), 379-395.

Albers, S., & Levy, H. (2005). Newborn screening. In H. Taeusch, R. Ballard, & C. Gleason (Eds.), *Avery's diseases of the newborn* (8th ed.). Philadelphia: Saunders.

American Academy of Pediatrics (AAP) Committee on Fetus and Newborn, Committee on Drugs, Section on Anesthesiology, Section on Surgery, and Canadian Pediatric Society, Fetus and Newborn Committee. (2000). Prevention and management of pain and stress in the neonate. *Pediatrics, 105*(2), 454-460.

American Academy of Pediatrics (AAP) Committee on Injury and Poison Prevention. (1999). Safe transportation of newborns at hospital discharge. *Pediatrics, 104*(4), 986-987.

American Academy of Pediatrics (AAP) Committee on Injury and Poison Prevention. (2002). Selecting and using the most appropriate car safety seats for growing children: Guidelines for counseling parents. *Pediatrics, 109*(3), 550-553.

American Academy of Pediatrics (AAP) Task Force on Circumcision. (1999). Circumcision policy statement. *Pediatrics, 103*(3), 686-693.

American Academy of Pediatrics (AAP) Task Force on Infant Sleep Position and Sudden Infant Death Syndrome. (2000). Changing concepts of sudden infant death syndrome: Implications for infant sleeping environment and sleep position. *Pediatrics, 105*(3), 650-656.

American Academy of Pediatrics (AAP) & American College of Obstetricians and Gynecologists (ACOG). (2002). *Guidelines for perinatal care* (5th ed.). Elk Grove Village, IL: AAP.

American Academy of Pediatrics (AAP) & Canadian Paediatric Society. (2000). Prevention and management of pain and stress in the neonate. *Pediatrics, 105*(2), 454-461.

American College of Obstetricians and Gynecologists (ACOG). (2001). Circumcision. ACOG Committee Opinion No. 260. *Obstetrics & Gynecology, 98*(4), 707-708.

American Medical Association Council on Scientific Affairs. (2005). *Report 10 of the Council on Scientific Affairs (1-99): Neonatal circumcision.* Internet document available at http:// www.ama-assn.org/ ama/pub/category/13585.html (accessed September 12, 2005).

Anand, K., & International Evidence-Based Group for Neonatal Pain. (2001). Consensus statement for the prevention and management of pain in the newborn. *Archives in Pediatric and Adolescent Medicine, 155*(2), 173-180.

Association of Women's Health, Obstetric and Neonatal Nurses (AWHONN). (2001). *Evidence-based clinical practice guideline: Neonatal skin care.* Washington, DC: AWHONN.

Ballard, J., Khoury, J., Wedig, K., Wang, L., Eilers-Walsman, B., & Lipp, R. (1991). New Ballard score, expanded to include extremely premature infants. *Journal of Pediatrics, 119*(3), 417-423.

Ballard, J., Novak, K., & Driver, M. (1979). A simplified score for assessment of fetal maturity of newly born infants. *Journal of Pediatrics, 95*(5 Pt 1), 769-774.

Battaglia, F., & Lubchenco, L. (1967). A practical classification of newborn infants by weight and gestational age. *Journal of Pediatrics, 71*(2), 159-163.

Blackburn, S. (2003). *Maternal, fetal, and neonatal physiology: A clinical perspective* (2nd ed.). St. Louis: Saunders.

Blass, E., & Watt, L. (1999). Suckling- and sucrose-induced analgesia in human newborns. *Pain, 83*(3), 611-623.

Burd, R., & Tobias, J. (2002). Ketorolac for pain management after abdominal surgical procedures in infants. *Southern Medicine, 95*(3), 331-333.

Clifford, P., Stringer, M., Christensen, H., & Mountain, D. (2004). Pain assessment and intervention for term newborns. *Journal of Midwifery & Women's Health, 49*(6), 514-519.

D'Avanzo, C., & Geissler, E. (2003). *Pocket guide to cultural assessment* (3rd ed.). St. Louis: Mosby.

DeMarini, S., & Tsang, R. (2002). Disorders of calcium, phosphorus, and magnesium metabolism. In A. Faranoff & R. Martin (Eds.), *Neonatal-perinatal medicine: Diseases of the fetus and infant* (7th ed.). St. Louis: Mosby.

Efird, M., & Hernandez, J. (2005). Birth injuries. In P. Thureen, J. Deacon, J. Hernandez, & D. Hall, (Eds.), *Assessment and care of the well newborn* (2nd ed.). St. Louis: Saunders.

Furdon, S., Eastman, M., Benjamin, K., & Horgan, M. (1998). Outcome measures after standardized pain management strategies in postoperative patients in the NICU. *Journal of Perinatal and Neonatal Nursing, 12*(1), 58-69.

Glass, S. (2005). Circumcision. In P. Thureen, J. Deacon, J. Hernandez, & D. Hall (Eds.), *Assessment and care of the well newborn* (2nd ed.). St. Louis: Saunders.

Gradin, M., Eriksson, M., Holmquist, G., Holstein, A., & Schollin, J. (2002). Pain reduction at venipuncture in newborns: Oral glucose compared with local anesthetic cream. *Pediatrics, 110*(6), 1053-1057.

Hagedorn, M., Gardner, S., & Abman, S. (2002). Common systemic diseases of the neonate: Respiratory diseases. In G. Merenstein & S. Gardner (Eds.), *Handbook of neonatal intensive care* (5th ed.). St. Louis: Mosby.

Hockenberry, M. (2003). *Wong's nursing care of infants and children* (7th ed.). St. Louis: Mosby.

Hummel, P., & Puchalski, M. (2001). Assessment and management of pain in infancy. *Newborn Infant Nursing Review, 1*(2), 114-122.

Ip, S., Chung, M., Kulig, J., O'Brien, R., Sege, R. et al. (2004). An evidence-based review of important issues concerning neonatal hyperbilirubinemia. *Pediatrics, 114*(1), e130-153. Available at pediatrics.aappublications/org. (accessed September 12, 2005).

Janssen, P., Selwood, B., Dobson, S., Peacock, D., & Thiessen, P. (2003). To dye or not to dye: A randomized, clinical trial of a triple dye/alcohol regime versus dry cord care. *Pediatrics, 111*(1), 15-20.

Joint Committee on Infant Hearing. (2000). Year 2000 position statement: Principles and guidelines for early hearing detection and intervention programs. *Pediatrics, 106*(4), 798-817.

Kliegman, R. (2002). Fetal and neonatal medicine. In R. Behrman & R. Kliegman (Eds.), *Nelson essentials of pediatrics* (4th ed.). Philadelphia: Saunders.

Kramer, M., & Kakuma, R. (2001). Optimal duration of exclusive breastfeeding (Cochrane Review). In *The Cochrane Library*, Issue 2, 2004. Chichester, UK: John Wiley & Sons.

Krebs, T. (1998). Cord care: Is it necessary? *Mother Baby Journal, 3*(2), 5-12, 18-20.

Krechel, S., & Bildner, J. (1995). CRIES: A new neonatal postoperative pain measurement score–Initial testing of validity and reliability. *Paediatric Anaesthesia, 5*(1), 53-61.

Lawrence, J., Alcock, D., McGrath, P., Kay, J., MacMurray, S., & Dulberg, C. (1993). The development of a tool to assess neonatal pain. *Neonatal Network, 12*(6), 59-66.

Lubchenco, L., Hansman, C., & Boyd, E. (1966). Intrauterine growth in length and head circumference as estimated from live births at gestational ages from 26-42 weeks. *Journal of Pediatrics, 37*(3), 403-408.

Mangurten, H. (2002). Birth injuries. In A. Faranoff & R. Martin (Eds.), *Neonatal-perinatal medicine: Diseases of the fetus and infant* (7th ed.). St. Louis: Mosby.

Miller, C., & Newman, T. (2005). Routine newborn care. In H. Taeusch, R. Ballard, & C. Gleason, (Eds.), *Avery's diseases of the newborn* (8th ed.). Philadelphia: Saunders.

National Association of Neonatal Nurses (NANN). (1999). *Position statement on pain management in infants*. Internet document available at http://www.nann.org/i4a/store/category.cfm?category_id=75#pain. (accessed March 31, 2005).

Niermeyer, S. (2005). Resuscitation of the newborn. In H. Taeusch, R. Ballard, & C. Gleason (Eds.), *Avery's diseases of the newborn* (8th ed.). Philadelphia: Saunders.

O'Doherty, N. (1986). *Neonatology: Micro atlas of the newborn*. Nutley, N.J.: Hoffman-LaRoche.

Pagana, K., & Pagana, T. (2003). *Mosby's diagnostic and laboratory test reference* (6th ed.). St. Louis: Mosby.

Pasero, C. (2002). Pain assessment in infants and young children: Neonates. *American Journal of Nursing, 102*(8), 61, 63, 65.

Pollack, H., & Frohna, J. (2002). Infant sleep after the Back to Sleep campaign. *Pediatrics, 109*(4), 608-614.

Razmus, I., Dalton, M., & Wilson, D. (2004). Pain management for newborn circumcision. *Pediatric Nursing, 30*(5), 414-417, 427.

Stapleton, E. et al. (2001). *Fundamentals of BLS for healthcare providers*. Dallas, TX: American Heart Association.

Stastny, P., Ichinose, T., Thayer, S., Olson, R., & Keens, T. (2004). Infant sleep positioning by nursery staff and mothers in newborn hospital nurseries. *Nursing Research, 53*(2), 122-129.

Stevens, B., Johnston, C., Petryshen, P., & Taddio, A. (1996). Premature infant pain profile: Development and initial validation. *Clinical Journal of Pain, 12*(1), 13-22.

Stevens, B., Yamada, J., & Ohlsson, A. (2004). Sucrose for analgesia in newborn infants undergoing procedures, *The Cochrane Database of Systematic Reviews*, No. CD001069. DOI: 10.1002/14651858.CD001069.pub2.

Taddio, A., Ohlsson, I., & Ohlsson, A. (2001). Lidocaine-prilocaine cream for analgesia during circumcision of newborn boys. *The Cochrane Library*, Issue 1. Oxford: Update Software.

Townsend, S. (2005). Approach to the infant at risk for hypoglycemia. In P. Thureen, J. Deacon, J. Hernandez, & D. Hall (Eds.), *Assessment and care of the well newborn* (2nd ed.). St. Louis: Saunders.

University of California San Francisco (UCSF) Home Health Care. (2001). *Guidelines for home therapy*. San Francisco: University of California.

Walden, M., & Franck, L. (2003). Identification, management, and prevention of newborn/infant pain. In C. Kenner & J. Lott (Eds.), *Comprehensive neonatal nursing: A physiologic perspective* (3rd ed.). St. Louis: Saunders.

Workowski, K., & Levine, W. (2002). Sexually transmitted disease treatment guidelines, 2002. *Morbidity and Mortality Weekly Report, 51*(RR-6), 1-78.

Zinn, A. (2002). Inborn errors of metabolism. In A. Faranoff & R. Martin (Eds.), *Neonatal-perinatal medicine: Diseases of the fetus and infant* (7th ed.). St. Louis: Mosby.

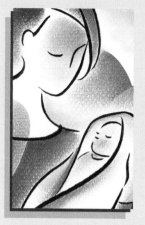

CHAPTER 20

Newborn Nutrition and Feeding

KATHRYN RHODES ALDEN

LEARNING OBJECTIVES

- *Describe current recommendations for infant feeding.*
- *Explain the nurse's role in helping families to choose an infant feeding method.*
- *Describe nutritional needs of infants.*
- *Recognize newborn feeding-readiness cues.*
- *Explain maternal and infant indicators of effective breastfeeding.*
- *Discuss benefits of breastfeeding for infants, mothers, families, and society.*
- *Describe the anatomy and physiology of breastfeeding.*

- *Examine nursing interventions to facilitate and promote successful breastfeeding.*
- *Analyze common problems associated with breastfeeding and nursing interventions to help resolve them.*
- *Compare powdered, concentrated, and ready-to-use forms of commercial infant formula.*
- *Develop a teaching plan for the formula-feeding family.*

KEY TERMS AND DEFINITIONS

colostrum The fluid in the breast from pregnancy into the early postpartal period; rich in antibodies, which provide protection from many diseases; high in protein, which binds bilirubin; and laxative acting, which speeds the elimination of meconium and helps loosen mucus

demand feeding Feeding a newborn when feeding cues are exhibited by the baby, indicating that hunger is present

engorgement Swelling of breast tissue brought about by an increase in blood and lymph supply to the breast, which precedes true lactation; lasts approximately 48 hours and usually reaches a peak between the third and fifth postbirth days

feeding-readiness cues Infant responses (mouthing motions, sucking fist, awakening, and crying) that indicate optimal times to begin a feeding

growth spurts Times of increased neonatal growth that usually occur at approximately 6 to 10 days, 6 weeks, 3 months, and 4 to 5 months; increased caloric needs necessitate more frequent feedings to increase the amount of milk produced

inverted nipples Nipples invert rather than evert when stimulated; interferes with latch-on

lactation consultant Health care professional who has specialized training in breastfeeding

lactogenesis Beginning of milk production

latch-on Attachment of the infant to the breast for feeding

let-down reflex Release of milk caused by the contraction of the myoepithelial cells within the milk glands in response to oxytocin; also called *milk ejection reflex (MER)*

mastitis Infection in a breast, usually confined to a milk duct, characterized by influenza-like symptoms and redness and tenderness in the affected breast

nipple confusion Difficulty experienced by some infants in mastering breastfeeding after having been given a pacifier or bottle

plugged milk ducts Milk ducts blocked by small curds of dried milk

rooting reflex Normal response of the newborn to move toward whatever touches the area around the mouth and to attempt to suck; usually disappears by 3 to 4 months of age

supply-meets-demand system Physiologic basis for determining milk production; the volume of milk produced equals the amount removed from the breast

617

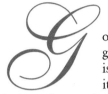

ood nutrition in infancy fosters optimal growth and development. Infant feeding is more than the provision of nutrition; it is an opportunity for social, psychologic, and even educational interaction between parent and infant. It also can establish a basis for developing good eating habits that last a lifetime. Health supervision of infants requires knowledge of their nutritional needs.

Through preconception and prenatal education and counseling, nurses play an instrumental role in assisting parents with the selection of an infant feeding method, which ideally will be breastfeeding. Whether the parents choose to breastfeed or to give their infant artificial breast milk (formula), nurses provide support and ongoing education. Education of parents is necessarily based on current research findings and standards of practice.

This chapter focuses on meeting nutritional needs for normal growth and development from birth to age 6 months, with emphasis on the neonatal period, when feeding practices and patterns are being established. Both breastfeeding and formula feeding are addressed.

RECOMMENDED INFANT NUTRITION

The American Academy of Pediatrics (AAP) recommends exclusive breastfeeding or human milk feeding for the first 6 months of life and that breastfeeding or human milk feeding continue as the sole source of milk for the next 6 months. During the second 6 months of life, appropriate complementary foods (solids) are added to the infant diet. If infants are weaned from breast milk before 12 months of age, they should receive iron-fortified infant formula, not cow's milk (Gartner et al., 2005)

BREASTFEEDING RATES

Breastfeeding rates in the United States have risen steadily over the past decade, reaching record levels with 70.1% of mothers initiating breastfeeding in the hospital. When their babies are 6 months old, 33.2% of mothers are still breast-

feeding (Abbott Laboratories, 2003). If breastfeeding rates continue to rise at their current rate, it is likely that the breastfeeding goals of *Healthy People 2010* will be attained; the goals are for breastfeeding initiation rates to reach 75% and continuance rates at 6 months to reach 50% (U.S. Department of Health and Human Services, 2000).

Although breastfeeding rates have increased across all demographic groups, certain trends still remain. Women least likely to breastfeed typically are younger than 25 years of age, have a lower income, are African-American, are primiparas, have a high-school education or less, are employed full time outside the home, and participate in the Special Supplemental Nutrition Program for Women, Infants, and Children (WIC) (Abbott Laboratories, 2003; Ryan, Wenjun, & Acosta, 2002).

BENEFITS OF BREASTFEEDING

Human milk is designed specifically for human infants and is nutritionally superior to any alternative. It is bacteriologically safe and always fresh. The nutrients in breast milk are ideally balanced and more easily absorbed than are those in formula. Breast milk changes over time to meet changing needs as infants grow. It contains growth factors that promote development of the brain and gastrointestinal (GI) system. Breast milk provides immune factors that fight illnesses and allergens within the maternal-infant environment (Gartner et al., 2005; Lawrence & Lawrence, 2005).

Numerous research studies have identified the beneficial effects of human milk for infants during the first year of life. Long-term epidemiologic studies have shown that these benefits do not cease when the infant is weaned, but instead extend into childhood and beyond. Breastfeeding has many advantages for mothers, for families, and for society in general. In discussing the benefits of breastfeeding with parents, it is critical that nurses and other health care professionals have a thorough understanding of these benefits from both a physiologic and a psychosocial perspective (Gartner et al., 2005; Lawrence & Lawrence, 2005). Benefits of breastfeeding are listed in Table 20-1.

TABLE 20-1

Benefits of Breastfeeding

BENEFITS FOR THE INFANT	BENEFITS FOR THE MOTHER	BENEFITS TO FAMILIES AND SOCIETY
• Decreased incidence and severity of infectious diseases: bacterial meningitis, bacteremia, diarrhea, respiratory infection, necrotizing enterocolitis, otitis media, urinary tract infection, late onset sepsis in preterm infants • Reduced postneonatal infant mortality • Decreased rates of SIDS • Decreased incidence of type I and type 2 diabetes • Decreased incidence of lymphoma, leukemia, Hodgkin disease • Reduced risk of obesity, and hypercholesterolemia • Decreased incidence and severity of asthma and other allergies • Slightly enhanced cognitive development • Enhances jaw development, decreasing problems with malocclusions and malalignment of teeth • Analgesic effect for infants undergoing painful procedures such as venipuncture	• Decreased postpartum bleeding and more rapid uterine involution • Reduced risk of breast cancer, uterine cancer, and ovarian cancer • Earlier return to prepregnancy weight • Decreased risk of postmenopausal osteoporosis • Unique bonding experience • Increases maternal role attainment	• Convenient; ready to feed • No bottles or other necessary equipment • Less expensive than infant formula • Reduced annual health care costs • Less parental absence from work due to ill infant • Reduced environmental burden related to disposal of formula cans

(From Gartner, L. et al. (2005). Breastfeeding and the use of human milk. *Pediatrics, 115*(2), 496-506; Lawrence, R., & Lawrence, R. (2005). *Breastfeeding: A guide for the medical profession* (6th ed.). St. Louis: Mosby.)

CHOOSING AN INFANT FEEDING METHOD

Breastfeeding is a natural extension of pregnancy and childbirth; it is much more than simply a means of supplying nutrition for infants. Women most often breastfeed their babies because they are aware of the benefits to the infant. Many seek the unique bonding experience between mother and infant that is characteristic of breastfeeding. The support of the partner and family is a major factor in the mother's decision to breastfeed and in her ability to do so successfully. Prenatal preparation ideally includes the father of the baby, giving him information about benefits of breastfeeding and how he can participate in infant care and nurturing (Pollock, Bustamante-Forest, & Giarrantano, 2002).

Parents who choose to formula-feed often make this decision without complete information and understanding of the benefits of breastfeeding and the potential hazards of formula feeding. Even women who are educated about the advantages of breastfeeding may still decide to formula-feed. Cultural beliefs, as well as myths and misconceptions about breastfeeding, influence women's decision making. Many women see bottle-feeding as more convenient or less embarrassing than breastfeeding. Formula feeding is often viewed as a way to ensure that the father, other family members, and day-care providers can feed the baby. Some women lack confidence in their ability to produce breast milk of an adequate quantity or quality. Women who have had previous unsuccessful breastfeeding experiences may choose to formula feed subsequent infants. Breastfeeding is seen by some women as incompatible with an active social life, or they think that it will prevent them from going back to work. Modesty issues and societal barriers exist against breastfeeding in public. A major barrier for many women is the influence of family and friends.

There are situations in which breastfeeding is contraindicated. Newborns who have galactosemia should not be breastfed. Mothers with active tuberculosis or human immunodeficiency virus (HIV) infection and those who are positive for human T-cell lymphotropic virus type I or type II should not breastfeed. Breastfeeding is not recommended when mothers are receiving chemotherapy or radioactive isotopes (e.g., with diagnostic procedures). Maternal use of drugs of abuse ("street drugs") is incompatible with breastfeeding (Gartner et al., 2005; Kline et al., 2003).

CD: Skill—Infant Feeding

Critical Thinking Exercise

Breastfeeding: Engorgement and Nipple Soreness

Mary was discharged from the birthing center at 48 hours postpartum with her newborn son, Matthew. He is now 4 days old, and she has brought him to the clinic for a follow-up visit. She states that her milk came in yesterday, and her breasts have been hard and painful ever since. It has been difficult to latch the baby on. She reports that breastfeeding is very painful and that her nipples are cracked and so sore she "can hardly stand to feed the baby." Matthew has had only one wet diaper and no bowel movements in the last 24 hours. He is crying most of the time and never seems to settle down to sleep for very long. Mary states, "I am ready to give up on this breastfeeding thing and just switch to formula."

1 Evidence—Is there sufficient evidence to draw conclusions about the feeding difficulties experienced by this mother and infant?
2 Assumptions—What assumptions can be made about the following issues?
   a. Mary's milk supply
   b. Mary's sore nipples
   c. Matthew's urinary output and bowel elimination pattern
   d. Mary's commitment to breastfeeding
3 What implications and priorities for nursing care can be identified at this time?
4 Does the evidence objectively support your conclusion?
5 Are there alternative perspectives to your conclusion?

The key to encouraging mothers to breastfeed is education, beginning as early as possible during pregnancy and even before pregnancy. Each encounter with an expectant mother is an opportunity to educate, dispel myths, clarify misinformation, and address personal concerns. It may be helpful to connect expectant mothers with women from similar backgrounds who are breastfeeding or have successfully breastfed. Peer counseling programs, such as those instituted by Special Supplemental Nutrition Program for Women, Infants, and Children (WIC) programs, are beneficial.

For those women with limited access to health care, the postpartum period may provide the first opportunity for education about breastfeeding. Even women who have indicated the desire to bottle-feed may benefit from information about the differences in formula and breast milk for their infants. Offering these women the chance to try breastfeeding with the assistance of a nurse may influence a change in infant feeding practices.

It is the responsibility of the nurse and other health care professionals to promote feelings of competence and confidence in the breastfeeding mother and to reinforce the unequaled contribution she is making toward the health and well-being of her infant. Evidence-based guidelines for supporting breastfeeding are available for use by health care professionals (Association of Women's Health, Obstetric and Neonatal Nurses [AWHONN], 1998; International Lactation Consultant Association [ILCA], 1999) (Box 20-1).

Cultural Influences on Infant Feeding

Cultural beliefs and practices are significant influences on infant feeding methods. Although recognized cultural norms exist, one cannot assume that generalized observations about any cultural group hold true for all members of that group. Within the United States many regional and ethnic cultures are found. Dealing effectively with these groups requires that the nurse be knowledgeable about and sensitive to the cultural factors influencing infant feeding practices.

Persons who have immigrated to the United States from poorer countries often choose to formula-feed their infants because they believe it is a better, more "modern" method or because they want to adapt to U.S. culture and perceive that it is the custom to bottle-feed.

Among some cultural groups within the United States, breastfeeding rates have declined. As increasing numbers of families leave Native American reservations to reside in urban areas, the traditional practice of breastfeeding often shifts to formula feeding. The separation from female relatives who lend childbirth and lactation support may be a factor in the change in feeding practices (Houghton, 2001).

The onset of breastfeeding varies among cultures. Because of beliefs about the harmful nature of colostrum, there may be restrictions on breastfeeding for a period of days after birth; this is true for many cultures in Southern Asia, the Pacific Islands, and parts of sub-Saharan Africa (Holman &

BOX 20-1

AWHONN's Guidelines for Breastfeeding Support

- During pregnancy a breast assessment is performed that includes a breastfeeding history, a breast examination, and a medication-use history.
- A prenatal plan of care is developed to prepare the woman for lactation.
- Immediately after birth, the newborn is kept with the mother when possible so that breastfeeding can be initiated when the newborn is most receptive.
- After birth:
  —Assistance with latch-on and positioning are given as needed.
  —Encouragement of frequent feedings is reinforced.
  —Discharge instructions for knowing criteria for successful breastfeeding are given.
  —Information about community resources for breastfeeding is given.
- Especially for premature and low-birth-weight infants, breastfeeding is encouraged.

Adapted from Association of Women's Health, Obstetric and Neonatal Nurses (AWHONN). (1998). *Standards and guidelines for professional nursing practice in the care of women and newborns* (5th ed.). Washington, DC: AWHONN.

TABLE 20-2

The Advised First Food for Newborn Babies in Countries of Africa, Asia, and Latin America

	COUNTRY	PEOPLE	FIRST FOOD	RATIONALE
Africa	Ghana	Asante	Gin, rum, lime-juice	To clear the infant's throat
	Nigeria	Yoruba	Palm wine	
	South Africa	Pedi, Zulu, Sotho	Watery porridge, cow's milk, water, dextrose/water mixture	To clear the infant's throat
	Zambia	Lozi, Mbunda	Light beer (mahel)	To clear the infant's bowel of meconium
Asia	Bangladesh		Mustard oil	To clean intestine of meconium
			Honey, sugar (gur or talmisri)	
			Sugar water	For ritual and/or medicinal purpose
	India		Honey, water	To clean and purify the body
			Castor oil, herbs	To remove the fluids of the womb ingested by the newborn during birth
	Thailand	Karen	Rice	To learn the taste
	Indonesia	Minangkabau	Honey, coconut water	
			Rice water	To learn the taste
	Iran Jaya			
	Lowland		Sago, sago-porridge	To learn the taste
	Highland		Taro (yam), pork fat	To learn the taste
Latin America	Jamaica		Mint tea, castor oil	To cough up mucus
	Haiti		Castor oil	To get the meconium out
	Guatemala	Maya, Ladinos	Tea, boiled with anise, sugar, onion stalk, garlic, salt, tea of chicoria	To cough up mucus / To get the meconium out
	Bolivia		Wine, cow's milk, water with herbs or salt, coffee	To cough up mucus / To get the meconium out

From Lefeber, Y., & Voorhoeve, H. (1999). Indigenous first feeding practices in newborn babies. *Midwifery, 15*(2), 97-100.

Grimes, 2003; Morse, Jehle, & Gamble, 1990). Before the mother's milk is deemed to be "in," babies are fed prelacteal food (Lefeber & Voorhoeve, 1999) (Table 20-2). Other cultures begin breastfeeding immediately and offer the breast each time the infant cries. Cultural attitudes regarding modesty and breastfeeding are important considerations.

Some cultures have specific beliefs and practices related to the mother's intake of foods that foster milk production. Korean mothers often eat seaweed soup and rice to enhance milk production. Hmong women believe that boiled chicken, rice, and hot water are the only appropriate nourishments during the first postpartum month. The balance between energy forces, hot and cold, or yin and yang is integral to the diet of the lactating mother. Hispanics, Vietnamese, Chinese, East Indians, and Arabs often use this belief in choosing foods. "Hot" foods are considered best for new mothers; this does not necessarily relate to the temperature or spiciness of foods. For example, chicken and broccoli are considered "hot," whereas many fresh fruits and vegetables are considered "cold." Families often bring desired foods into the health care setting.

NUTRIENT NEEDS

Fluids

The fluid requirement for normal infants is 100 to 140 ml of water per kilogram of body weight per 24 hours; however, during the first 24 hours after birth, most infants need only 60 to 80 ml/kg/24 hours (Kliegman, 2002). In general, neither breastfed nor formula-fed infants need to be fed water, not even those living in very hot climates. Breast milk contains 87% water, which easily meets fluid requirements. Feeding water to infants may only decrease caloric consumption at a time when infants are growing rapidly.

Infants have room for little fluctuation in fluid balance and should be monitored closely for fluid intake and water loss. Infants lose water through excretion of urine and insensibly through respiration. Under normal circumstances, infants are born with some fluid reserve, and some of the weight loss during the first few days is related to fluid loss. In some cases, however, infants do not have this fluid reserve, possibly because of inadequate maternal hydration during labor or birth.

Energy

Infants require adequate caloric intake to provide energy for growth, digestion, physical activity, and maintenance of organ metabolic function. For the first 3 months, the infant needs 110 kcal/kg/day. From 3 months to 6 months, the requirement is 100 kcal/kg/day. This decreases slightly to 95 kcal/kg/day from 6 to 9 months and increases to 100 kcal/kg/day from 9 months to 1 year (AAP, 1998).

Human milk provides 67 kcal/100 ml or 20 kcal/oz; the greatest amount of energy is provided by the fat content of breast milk. Infant formulas are made to simulate the caloric content of human milk; standard formulas contain 20 kcal/oz, with differences in composition varying among brands.

During the first 3 months, formula-fed infants consume more energy than breastfed infants and therefore tend to grow more rapidly (Ziegler, Fomon, & Carlson, 2003).

Carbohydrate

The average daily intake of carbohydrates for infants is 10 to 30 g/kg. Because newborns have only small hepatic glycogen stores, carbohydrates should provide at least 40% to 50% of the total calories in the diet. Moreover, newborns may have a limited ability to carry out gluconeogenesis (the formation of glucose from amino acids and other substrates) and ketogenesis (the formation of ketone bodies from fat), the mechanisms that provide alternative sources of energy.

As the primary carbohydrate in human milk and cow's milk formula, lactose is the most abundant carbohydrate in the diet of infants up to age 6 months. Lactose provides calories in an easily available form. Its slow breakdown and absorption also increase calcium absorption. Corn syrup solids or glucose polymers are added to infant formulas to supplement the lactose in the cow's milk and thereby provide sufficient carbohydrates.

Oligosaccharides, another form of carbohydrates found in breast milk, are critical in the development of microflora in the intestinal tract of the newborn. These prebiotics promote an acidic environment in the intestines, preventing the growth of gram-negative and other pathogenic bacteria, thus increasing the infant's resistance to GI illness (Uauy & Araya, 2004; Ziegler, Fomon, & Carlson, 2003).

Fat

The daily fat intake for infants should be approximately 5 to 7 g/kg/day. For infants to acquire adequate calories from human milk or formula, at least 15% of the calories provided must come from fat (triglycerides). This fat must therefore be easily digestible. The fat in human milk is easier to digest and absorb than that in cow's milk because of the arrangement of the fatty acids on the glycerol molecule. Fat absorption also is related to the natural lipase activity present in human milk.

Cow's milk is used in most infant formulas, but the milk fat is removed, and another fat source such as corn oil, which can be digested and absorbed by the infant, is added in its place. If whole milk or evaporated milk without added carbohydrate is fed to infants, the resulting fecal loss of fat (and therefore loss of energy) may be excessive because the milk moves through the infant's intestines too quickly for adequate absorption to take place. This can lead to poor weight gain.

Human milk contains the essential fatty acids (EFAs), linoleic acid and linolenic acid, as well as the long chain polyunsaturated fatty acids arachidonic acid (ARA) and docosahexaenoic acid (DHA). Fatty acids are important in the development of cellular membranes and are particularly important in eye and brain development. Cow's milk contains fewer of the EFAs and no polyunsaturated fatty acids. Most formula companies are now adding DHA and ARA to their products (Preedy, Grimble, & Watson, 2001).

Protein

The protein requirement per unit of body weight is greater in the newborn than at any other time of life. The recommended daily allowance (RDA) for protein during the first 6 months is 2.25 to 4g/kg.

The protein content of human milk, which is lower than that of unmodified cow's milk, is ideal for the newborn. The primary protein in human milk is whey, mainly consisting of lactoalbumin, lactoferrin, secretory immunoglobulin A (IgA), and enzymes (e.g., lysozyme and lipase). The major protein in cow's milk is casein, which is more difficult to digest. Lactoglobulins in cow's milk are responsible for much of the cow's milk protein intolerance that is widely recognized (Preedy, Grimble, & Watson, 2001).

Vitamins

Human milk contains all of the vitamins required for infant nutrition, with individual variations based on maternal diet and genetic differences. Vitamins are added to cow's-milk formulas to resemble levels found in breast milk. Although cow's milk contains adequate amounts of vitamin A and vitamin B complex, vitamin C (ascorbic acid), vitamin E, and vitamin D must be added. Infants of mothers who are strict vegans also should receive vitamin B_{12} supplements (Tershakovec & Stallings, 2002).

Human milk contains small amounts of vitamin D, and therefore it is recommended that breastfeeding infants receive 200 international units of oral vitamin D drops daily starting during the first 2 months and continuing until the infant is consuming at least 500 ml per day of vitamin D–fortified formula or milk. Vitamin K, required for blood coagulation, is produced by intestinal bacteria. However, the gut is sterile at birth, and a few days are needed for intestinal flora to become established and produce vitamin K. To prevent hemorrhagic problems in the newborn, an injection of vitamin K is given at birth to all newborns, regardless of feeding method (Gartner et al., 2005).

Minerals

The mineral content of commercial infant formula is designed to reflect that of breast milk. Unmodified cow's milk is much higher in mineral content than is human milk, which also makes it unsuitable for infants during the first year of life. Minerals are typically highest in human milk during the first few days after birth and decrease slightly throughout lactation.

The ratio of calcium to phosphorus in human milk is 2:1, a proportion optimal for bone mineralization. Although cow's milk is high in calcium, the calcium-to-phosphorus ratio is low, resulting in decreased calcium absorption. Consequently, young infants fed unmodified cow's milk are at risk for hypocalcemia, seizures, and tetany. The calcium-to-phosphorus ratio in commercial infant formula is between that of human milk and cow's milk.

Iron levels are low in all types of milk; however, iron from human milk is better absorbed (50%) than that from cow's milk, iron-fortified formula, or infant cereals. Breastfed infants draw on iron reserves deposited in utero and benefit from the high lactose and vitamin C levels in human milk that facilitate iron absorption. The infant who is entirely breastfed normally maintains adequate hemoglobin levels for the first 6 months. After that time, iron-fortified cereals and other iron-rich foods are added to the diet. Infants who are weaned from the breast before 6 months of age and all formula-fed infants should receive an iron-fortified commercial infant formula until 12 months of age.

Fluoride levels in human milk and commercial formulas are low. This mineral, which is important in the prevention of dental caries, may cause spotting of the permanent teeth (fluorosis) in excess amounts. It is recommended that no fluoride supplements be given to infants under 6 months of age; from 6 months to 3 years, fluoride supplements are based on the concentration of fluoride in the water supply (Gartner et al., 2005).

ANATOMY AND PHYSIOLOGY OF LACTATION

Breast Development

Each female breast is composed of approximately 15 to 20 segments (lobes) embedded in fat and connective tissues and well supplied with blood vessels, lymphatic vessels, and nerves (Fig. 20-1). Within each lobe are alveoli, the milk-producing cells, surrounded by myoepithelial cells, which contract to send the milk forward into the ductules. Each ductule enlarges into lactiferous ducts and sinuses where milk collects just behind the nipple. Each nipple has 15 to 20 pores through which milk is transferred to the suckling infant.

The size of the breast is not an accurate indicator of its ability to produce milk. Although nearly every woman can lactate, a small number have insufficient mammary gland development to breastfeed their infants exclusively. Typically, these women experience few breast changes during puberty or early pregnancy. In some cases, women may still be able to breastfeed and offer supplemental nutrition to support optimal infant growth. Devices are available to allow mothers to offer supplements while the baby is nursing at the breast (Fig. 20-2).

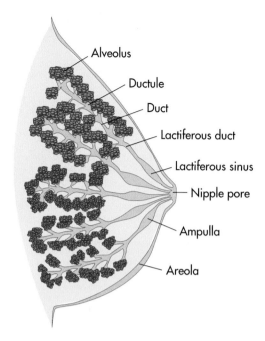

Fig. 20-1 Detailed structural features of human mammary gland.

Because of the effects of estrogen and progesterone during pregnancy, the lobular components of the breast enlarge while the ductal system proliferates and differentiates. The nipples become more erect, and pigmentation of the areola increases. Nipples and areola may enlarge. The breasts increase in size and sensitivity and exhibit more prominent veins. Around week 16 of gestation, the alveoli begin producing colostrum (early milk) in response to human placental lactogen.

Lactogenesis

After the mother gives birth, a precipitate decrease in estrogen and progesterone levels triggers the release of prolactin from the anterior pituitary gland. During pregnancy, prolactin prepares the breasts to secrete milk and, during lactation, to synthesize and secrete milk. Prolactin levels are highest during the first 10 days after birth, gradually declining over time, but remaining above baseline levels for the duration of lactation. Prolactin is produced in response to infant suckling and emptying of the breasts (lactating breasts are never completely empty; milk is constantly being produced by the alveoli as the infant feeds) (Fig. 20-3, *A*). Milk production is a **supply-meets-demand system;** that is, as milk is removed from the breast, more is produced. Incomplete emptying of the breasts with feedings can lead to a decreased milk supply.

Oxytocin is the other hormone essential to lactation. As the nipple is stimulated by the suckling infant, the posterior pituitary is prompted by the hypothalamus to produce oxytocin. This hormone is responsible for the **milk ejection reflex (MER), or let-down reflex** (Fig. 20-3, B). The myoepithelial cells surrounding the alveoli respond to oxytocin by

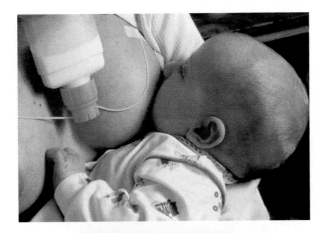

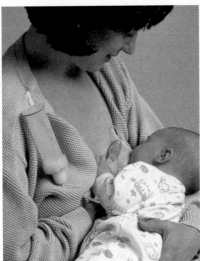

Fig. 20-2 Supplemental nursing system. (Courtesy Medela, Inc., McHenry, IL.)

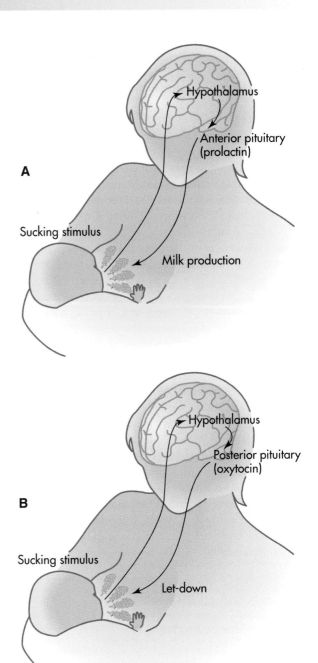

Fig. 20-3 Maternal breastfeeding reflexes. **A,** Milk production. **B,** Let-down.

contracting and sending the milk forward through the ducts to the nipple. Many "let-downs" can occur with each feeding session. The MER can be triggered by thoughts, sights, sounds, or odors that the mother associates with her baby (or other babies), such as hearing the baby cry. Many women report a tingling "pins and needles" sensation in the breasts as let-down occurs, although some mothers can detect milk ejection only by observing the sucking and swallowing of the infant. Let-down also may occur during sexual activity, because oxytocin is released during orgasm.

Oxytocin is the same hormone that stimulates uterine contractions during labor. Consequently, the laboring woman can experience let-downs that may be evidenced by leakage of colostrum. This readies the breast for immediate feeding by the infant after birth. Oxytocin has the important function of contracting the mother's uterus after birth to control postpartum bleeding and promote uterine involution. Thus mothers who breastfeed are at decreased risk for postpartum hemorrhage. These uterine contractions or "afterpains" that occur with breastfeeding can be painful during and after feeding for the first 3 to 5 days, particularly in multiparas.

Prolactin and oxytocin have been referred to as the "mothering hormones," because they are known to affect the postpartum woman's emotions, as well as her physical state. Many women report feeling thirsty or very relaxed during breastfeeding, probably as a result of these hormones.

The nipple-erection reflex is an important part of lactation. When the infant cries, suckles, or rubs against the breast, the nipple becomes erect. This assists in the propulsion of milk through the lactiferous sinuses to the nipple pores. Nipple sizes, shapes, and ability to become erect vary with individuals. Some women have flat or **inverted nipples** that do not become erect with stimulation. Babies are usually able to learn to breastfeed successfully with any nipple. It is important that these infants not be offered bottles or pacifiers until breastfeeding is well established.

Uniqueness of Human Milk

Human milk is a highly complex, species-specific fluid uniquely designed to meet the needs of the human infant. It is a dynamic substance whose composition changes to meet the changing nutritional and immunologic needs of the infant as growth and development ensue. Breast milk is specific to the needs of each newborn; for example, the milk of preterm mothers differs in composition from that of mothers who give birth at term.

Human milk contains antimicrobial factors (antibodies) that provide some protection against a broad spectrum of bacterial, viral, and protozoan infections. Secretory IgA is the major antibody in human milk. Other factors in human milk that help protect against infection include lactoferrin, the bifidus factor, oligosaccharides, milk lipids, and milk leukocytes. Antiinflammatory agents, growth factors, hormones, and enzymes are found in human milk, many of which contribute to the maturation of the infant's intestine. Immunomodulating agents found in human milk are instrumental in preventing disease after infancy (Table 20-3).

Human milk composition and volumes vary according to the stage of lactation. In **lactogenesis** stage I, beginning

TABLE 20-3

Summary of Immune Properties of Breast Milk

COMPONENT	ACTION
WHITE BLOOD CELLS	
B lymphocytes	Give rise to antibodies targeted against specific microbes
Macrophages	Kill microbes outright in baby's gut, produce lysozyme, and activate other components of the immune system
Neutrophils	May act as phagocytes, ingesting bacteria in baby's digestive system
T lymphocytes	Kill infected cells directly or send out chemical messages to mobilize other defenses
	Proliferate in the presence of organisms that cause serious illness in infants
	Manufacture compounds that can strengthen an infant's own immune response
MOLECULES	
Antibodies of secretory immunoglobulin A (IgA) class	Bind to microbes in infant's digestive tract and thereby prevent them from passing through walls of the gut into body tissues
B_{12}-binding protein	Reduces amount of vitamin B_{12}, which bacteria need to grow
Bifidus factor	Promotes growth of *Lactobacillus bifidus,* a harmless bacterium, in infant's gut; growth of such nonpathogenic bacteria helps crowd out dangerous varieties
Fatty acids	Disrupts membranes surrounding certain viruses and destroys them
Fibronectin	Increases antimicrobial activity of macrophages; helps repair tissues that have been damaged by immune reactions in infant's gut
Gamma-interferon	Enhances antimicrobial activity of immune cells
Hormones and growth factors	Stimulates infant's digestive tract to mature more quickly. Once the initially "leaky" membranes lining the gut mature, infants become less vulnerable to microorganisms
Lactoferrin	Binds to iron, a mineral many bacteria need to survive. By reducing the available amount of iron, lactoferrin thwarts growth of pathogenic bacteria
Lysozyme	Kills bacteria by disrupting their cell walls
Mucins	Adheres to bacteria and viruses, thus keeping such microorganisms from attaching to mucosal surfaces
Oligosaccharides	Binds to microorganisms and bars them from attaching to mucosal surfaces

From Newman, J. (1995). How breast milk protects newborns. *Scientific American, 273*(6), 76-79.

in pregnancy, the breasts prepare for milk production by producing colostrum. Colostrum, a clear yellowish fluid, is more concentrated than mature milk and is extremely rich in immunoglobulins. It has higher concentrations of protein and minerals but less fat than mature milk. The high protein level of colostrum facilitates binding of bilirubin, and the laxative action of colostrum promotes early passage of meconium. Colostrum gradually changes to mature milk; this is referred to as "the milk coming in" or as lactogenesis stage II. By day 3 to 5 after birth, most women have had this onset of copious milk secretion. Breast milk continues to change in composition for approximately 10 days, when the mature milk is established in stage III of lactogenesis (Lawrence & Lawrence, 2005).

Composition of mature milk changes during each feeding. As the infant nurses, the fat content of breast milk increases. Initially, a bluish-white foremilk is released that is part skim milk (about 60% of the volume) and part whole milk (about 35% of the volume). It provides primarily lactose, protein, and water-soluble vitamins. The hindmilk, or cream (about 5%), is usually let down 10 to 20 minutes into the feeding, although it may occur sooner. It contains the denser calories from fat necessary for ensuring optimal growth and contentment between feedings. Because of this changing composition of human milk during each feeding, it is important to breastfeed the infant long enough to supply a balanced feeding.

Milk production gradually increases as the baby grows. Babies have fairly predictable growth spurts (at about 10 days, 3 weeks, 6 weeks, 3 months, and 6 months), when more frequent feedings stimulate increased milk production. These growth spurts usually last 24 to 48 hours, and then the infants resume their usual feeding pattern.

CARE MANAGEMENT—THE BREASTFEEDING MOTHER AND INFANT

Effective management of the breastfeeding mother and infant requires that the caregivers be knowledgeable about the benefits of breastfeeding, as well as about basic anatomy and the physiology of breastfeeding, how to assist the mother with feeding, and interventions for common problems. Ongoing support of the mother enhances her self-confidence and promotes a satisfying and successful breastfeeding experience. Planning care for the breastfeeding couplet is based on thorough assessment of both the mother and infant.

Assessment and Nursing Diagnoses
Infant

Before the initiation of breastfeeding, the nurse must consider the following in preparing to assist the breastfeeding infant effectively:

- Maturity level: gestational age, term or preterm, birth weight (small for gestational age [SGA], large for gestational age [LGA])

- Labor and birth: length of labor, maternal medications (narcotics, magnesium sulfate [MgSO$_4$]); type of birth: vaginal (with or without use of vacuum extraction or forceps) or cesarean; type of anesthesia
- Birth trauma: fractured clavicle, bruising of face or head
- Maternal risk factors: diabetes, preeclampsia, infection, HIV, herpes, hepatitis B
- Congenital defects: cleft lip or palate, cardiac anomalies, Down syndrome, or other genetic anomalies
- Physical stability: vital signs within normal limits, unlabored respirations, bowel sounds present
- State of alertness: awake, sleepy, crying

Feeding readiness. Term neonates are born with reflexes that facilitate feeding: rooting, sucking, and swallowing. However, coordination of sucking, swallowing, and breathing in order to feed requires adaptation by the infant. Although the majority of newborns experience minimal hunger or thirst in the first hours after birth, they will suckle when given the opportunity.

Physical assessment of the newborn reveals signs that the baby is physiologically ready to begin feeding:
- Vital signs within normal limits
- Unlabored respirations; nares patent; no cyanosis
- Active bowel sounds
- No abdominal distention

When newborns feel hunger, they usually cry vigorously until their needs are met. Some infants, however, will withdraw into sleep because of discomfort associated with hunger. Babies exhibit feeding-readiness cues that can be recognized by a knowledgeable caregiver. Instead of waiting to feed until the infant is crying in a distraught manner or withdrawing into sleep, it is better to begin a feeding when the baby exhibits some of these cues (even during light sleep):
- Hand-to-mouth or hand-to-hand movements
- Sucking motions
- Rooting reflex—infant moves toward whatever touches the area around the mouth and attempts to suck
- Mouthing

Babies normally consume small amounts of milk during the first 3 days of life. As the baby adjusts to extrauterine life and the digestive tract is cleared of meconium, milk intake increases from 15 to 30 ml per feeding in the first 24 hours to 60 to 90 ml by the end of the first week.

At birth and for several months thereafter, all of the secretions of the infant's digestive tract contain enzymes especially suited to the digestion of human milk. The ability to digest foods other than milk depends on the physiologic development of the infant. The capacities for salivary, gastric, pancreatic, and intestinal digestion increase with age, indicating that the natural time for introduction of solid foods may be around 6 months of age.

Babies are born with a tongue extrusion reflex that causes them to push out of the mouth anything placed on the tongue. This reflex disappears by 6 months—another indication of physiologic readiness for solids.

Evolve/CD: Case Study—Breastfeeding

Early introduction of solids may make the infant more prone to food allergies. Regular feeding of solids can lead to decreased intake of breast milk or formula and may be associated with early cessation of breastfeeding.

The infant is assessed for latch-on (attachment of the infant to the breast for feeding), position, alignment, and sucking and swallowing by direct observation while breastfeeding. Behavior after feedings (contented, sleepy) is noted. Elimination patterns and the presence of jaundice; weight loss of less than 10%; and regaining of birth weight by age 10 to 14 days are important data.

Before breastfeeding is begun, the mother's knowledge of breastfeeding, as well as her physical and psychologic readiness to breastfeed, are assessed. Factors to consider include previous experience with breastfeeding, cultural factors, feelings about breastfeeding, physical development of the breasts, physical limitations, time since giving birth, type of birth, complications, discomfort, energy level, and support.

During the time in the hospital, the nurse can help the mother to view each breastfeeding session as a "feeding lesson" or "practice session" that will foster maternal confidence and a satisfying breastfeeding experience for mother and baby.

Nursing diagnoses for the breastfeeding woman include the following:

- *Effective breastfeeding related to*
  - —mother's knowledge of breastfeeding techniques
  - —mother's appropriate response to infant's feeding-readiness cues
  - —mother's ability to facilitate efficient breastfeeding
  - —mother's adequate fluid and caloric intake for breastfeeding
- *Risk for ineffective breastfeeding related to:*
  - —insufficient knowledge regarding newborn's reflexes and breastfeeding techniques
  - —lack of support from father of baby, family, friends
  - —lack of maternal self-confidence; anxiety, fear of failure
  - —poor infant sucking reflex
  - —difficulty waking sleepy baby

Expected Outcomes of Care

In planning care, the nurse discusses the desired outcomes with the parents. The expected outcomes include that the infant will do the following:
- Latch on and feed effectively at least eight times per day
- Gain weight appropriately
- Remain well hydrated (have six to eight wet diapers and at least three bowel movements every 24 hours after day 4)
- Sleep or seem contented between feedings

Examples of expected outcomes for the mother include that she will do the following:
- Verbalize or demonstrate understanding of breastfeeding techniques, including positioning and latch-on, signs of adequate feeding, self-care
- Report no nipple discomfort with breastfeeding
- Express satisfaction with the breastfeeding experience
- Consume a nutritionally balanced diet with appropriate caloric and fluid intake to support breastfeeding

Plan of Care and Interventions

Interventions are based on the expected outcomes and are influenced by the resources and time available to achieve the desired goals. In the early days after birth, interventions focus on helping the mother and the newborn initiate breastfeeding and achieve some degree of success and satisfaction before discharge from the hospital or birthing center. Interventions to promote successful breastfeeding include basics such as latch-on and positioning, signs of adequate feeding, and self-care measures such as prevention of engorgement. An important intervention is to provide the parents with a list of resources that they may contact after discharge from the hospital. Guidelines for Spanish-speaking patients are in the accompanying Guidelines/Guías box.

The ideal time to begin breastfeeding is immediately after birth. Newborns without complications should be allowed to remain in direct skin-to-skin contact with the mother until the baby is able to breastfeed for the first time (Gartner et al., 2005). Each mother should receive instruction, assistance, and support in positioning and latching on until she is able to do so independently (see Guidelines/Guías box).

GUIDELINES/GUÍAS

Breastfeeding: Latching On

- Do you want to breastfeed your baby?
- *¿Desea amamantar a su bebé?*

- I will help you.
- *Yo le ayudaré.*

- Hold your baby's head close to your breast.
- *Sostenga la cabeza del bebé cerca del pecho.*

- Lightly touch your nipple to the baby's lower lip until he opens his mouth.
- *Con el pezón, toque suavemente el labio inferior del bebé hasta que abra la boca.*

- Lift your breast to the baby's mouth.
- *Levante el seno hasta la boca del bebé.*

- Center your nipple and areola as far in the baby's mouth as possible.
- *Centre el pezón y la areola lo más que se pueda dentro de la boca del bebé.*

- Make sure the baby's tongue is under the nipple and the gums close around the areola.
- *Asegúrese de que la lengua del bebé esté debajo del pezón y que sus encías se cierren sobre la areola.*

- To change breasts, push one of your fingers into the corner of the baby's mouth.
- *Para cambiar al otro seno, métase un dedo en la comisura de los labios del bebé.*

- This will break the suction and prevent the baby from biting the nipple.
- *Esto interrumpe la aspiración e impide que el bebé muerda el pezón.*

Positioning

The four basic positions for breastfeeding are the football hold, cradle, modified cradle or across-the-lap, and side-lying position (Fig. 20-4). Initially it is advantageous to use the position that most easily facilitates latch-on while allowing maximal comfort for the mother. The football hold is often recommended for early feedings because the mother can easily see the baby's mouth as she guides the infant onto the nipple. The football hold is usually preferred by mothers who gave birth by cesarean. The modified cradle or across-the-lap hold also works well for early feedings, especially with smaller babies. The side-lying position allows the mother to rest while breastfeeding and is often preferred by women with perineal pain and swelling. Cradling is the most common breastfeeding position for infants who have learned to latch on easily and feed effectively. Before discharge from the hospital, the nurse should assist the mother to try all of the positions so that she will feel confident in her ability to vary positions at home.

Whichever position is used, the mother should be comfortable. The infant is placed at the level of the breast, supported by pillows or folded blankets, turned completely on his or her side, and facing the mother so that the infant is "belly to belly," with the arms "hugging" the breast. The baby's mouth is directly in front of the nipple. It is important that the mother support the baby's neck and shoulders with her hand and not push on the occiput. The baby's body is held in correct alignment (ears, shoulders, and hips are in a straight line) during latch-on and feeding.

Latch-on

In preparation for latch-on, it may be helpful for the mother to manually express a few drops of colostrum or milk and spread it over the nipple. This lubricates the nipple and may entice the baby to open the mouth as the milk is tasted.

To facilitate latch-on, the mother supports her breast in one hand with the thumb on top and four fingers underneath at the back edge of the areola. The breast is compressed slightly, as one might compress a large sandwich in preparing to take a bite, so that an adequate amount of breast tissue is taken into the mouth with latch-on (Weissinger, 1998). Most mothers need to support the breast during feeding for at least the first days until the infant is adept at feeding.

With the baby held close to the breast with the mouth directly in front of the nipple, the mother tickles the baby's lower lip with the tip of her nipple, stimulating the mouth to open. When the mouth is open wide and the tongue is down, the mother quickly pulls the baby onto the nipple (Fig. 20-5).

The amount of areola in the baby's mouth with correct latch-on depends on the size of the baby's mouth and the size of the areola and the nipple. In general, the baby's mouth should cover the nipple and an areolar radius of approximately 2 to 3 cm all around the nipple.

When latched on correctly, the baby's cheeks and chin are touching the breast (Fig. 20-6). Depressing the breast tissue around the baby's nose is not necessary. If she is worried

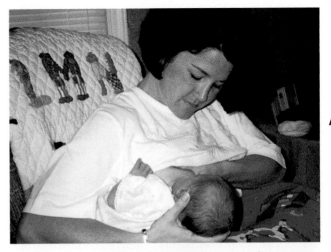

A

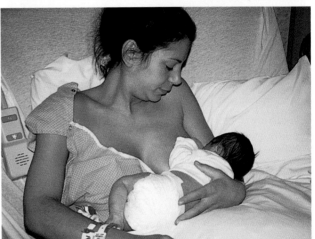

B

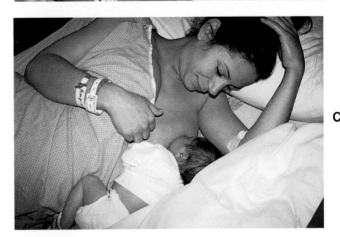

C

Fig. 20-4 Breastfeeding positions. **A,** Football hold. **B,** Cradling. **C,** Lying down. (**B** and **C** courtesy Marjorie Pyle, RNC, Lifecircle, Costa Mesa, CA.)

about the baby's breathing, the mother can raise the baby's hips slightly to change the angle of the baby's head at the breast. The nurse should reassure the mother that if the baby cannot breathe, innate reflexes will prompt the baby to move the head and pull back to breathe.

When the baby is latched on correctly and sucking appropriately, (1) the mother reports a firm tugging sensation

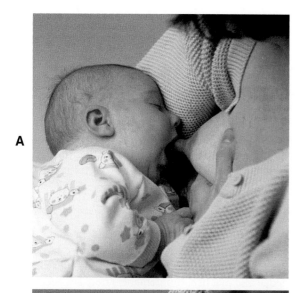

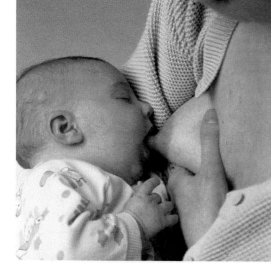

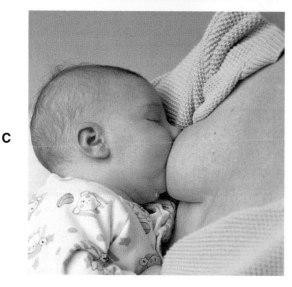

Fig. 20-5 Latching on. **A,** Tickle baby's lower lip with your nipple until he or she opens wide. **B,** Once baby's mouth is opened wide, quickly pull baby onto breast. **C,** Baby should have as much areola (dark area around nipple) in his or her mouth as possible, not just the nipple. (Courtesy Medela, Inc., McHenry, IL.)

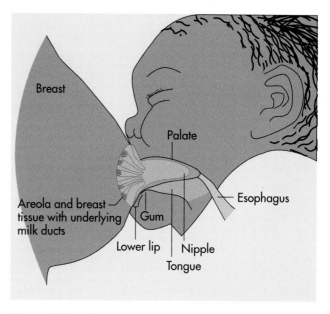

Fig. 20-6 Correct attachment (latch-on) of infant at breast.

on her nipples, but no pinching or pain; (2) the baby sucks with cheeks rounded, not dimpled; (3) the baby's jaw glides smoothly with sucking; and (4) swallowing is audible. Sucking creates a vacuum in the intraoral cavity as the breast is compressed between the tongue and the palate. If the mother feels pinching or pain after the initial sucks or does not feel a strong tugging sensation on the nipple, the latch-on and positioning should be evaluated. Any time the signs of adequate latch-on and sucking are not present, the baby should be taken off the breast and latch-on attempted again. To prevent nipple trauma as the baby is taken off the breast, the mother is instructed to break the suction by inserting a finger in the side of the baby's mouth between the gums and leaving it there until the nipple is completely out of the baby's mouth (Fig. 20-7).

Milk ejection or let-down

As the baby begins sucking on the nipple, the let-down, or milk ejection, reflex is stimulated (see Fig. 20-3, *B*). The following signs indicate that let-down has occurred:
- The mother may feel a tingling sensation in the nipples, although many women never feel their milk let down.
- The baby's suck changes from quick, shallow sucks to a slower, more drawing, sucking pattern.
- Swallowing is heard as the baby sucks.
- The mother feels uterine cramping and may have increased lochia during and after feedings.
- The mother feels relaxed, even sleepy, during feedings.
- The opposite breast may leak.

Frequency of feedings

Newborns need to breastfeed 8 to 12 times in a 24-hour period. Feeding patterns are variable because every baby is unique. Some infants will breastfeed every 2 to 3 hours

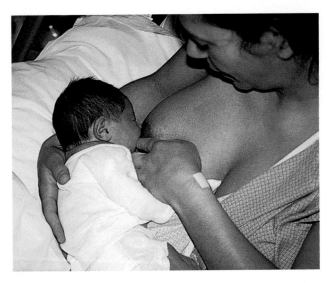

Fig. 20-7 Removing infant from the breast. (Courtesy Marjorie Pyle, RNC, Lifecircle, Costa Mesa, CA.)

throughout a 24-hour period. Others may cluster-feed, breastfeeding every hour or so for three to five feedings and then sleeping for 3 to 4 hours between clusters. During the first 24 to 48 hours after birth, most babies do not awaken this often to feed. It is important that parents understand that they should awaken the baby to feed at least every 3 hours during the day and at least every 4 hours at night. (Feeding frequency is determined by counting from the beginning of one feeding to the beginning of the next.) Once the infant is feeding well and gaining weight adequately, it is more appropriate to go to **demand feeding,** in which the infant determines the frequency of feedings. (With demand feeding, the infant should still receive at least eight feedings in 24 hours.) Parents should be cautioned about attempting to place newborn infants on strict feeding schedules.

Infants should be fed whenever they exhibit feeding cues. Crying is a late sign of hunger, and babies may become frantic when they have to wait too long to feed. Some infants will go into a deep sleep when their hunger needs are not met. Keeping the baby close is the best way to observe and respond to infant feeding cues. Newborns should remain with mothers during the recovery period after birth and room-in during the hospital stay. At home, babies should be kept nearby so that parents can observe signs that the baby is ready to feed.

Duration of feedings

The duration of breastfeeding sessions is highly variable because the timing of milk transfer differs for each mother-baby pair. The average time for feeding is 30 to 40 minutes, or approximately 15 to 20 minutes per breast. Some mothers do one-sided nursing, in which the baby nurses only one breast at each feeding. The first breast offered should be alternated at each feeding to ensure that each breast receives equal stimulation and emptying. In reality, instructing mothers to feed for a set number of minutes is inappropriate. Mothers can determine when a baby has finished a feeding:

the baby's suck and swallow pattern has slowed, the breast is softened, and the baby appears content and may fall asleep or release the nipple.

If a baby seems to be feeding effectively and the urine output is adequate but the weight gain is not satisfactory, the mother may be switching to the second breast too soon. The high-lactose, low-fat foremilk may cause the baby to have explosive stools, gas pains, and inconsolable crying. Feeding on the first breast until it softens ensures that the baby will receive the hindmilk, which usually results in increased weight gain.

Supplements, bottles, and pacifiers

The AAP (2005) recommends that, unless a medical indication exists, no supplements should be given to breastfeeding infants (Gartner et al., 2005). With sound breastfeeding knowledge and practice, supplements rarely are needed.

Situations that may necessitate supplementary feeding include such things as low birth weight, hypoglycemia, dehydration, or inborn errors of metabolism. Mothers may be unable to breastfeed because of severe illness or complications of birth, or they may be taking medications incompatible with breastfeeding (Table 20-4).

Offering formula to a baby after breastfeeding just to "make sure the baby is getting enough" is normally unnecessary and should be avoided. This can contribute to low milk supply because the baby becomes overly full and does not breastfeed often enough. Supplementation interferes with the supply-meets-demand system of milk production. The parents may interpret the baby's willingness to take a bottle to mean that the mother's milk supply is inadequate. They need to know that a baby will automatically suck from a bottle, as the easy flow of milk from the nipple triggers the suck and swallow reflex.

Babies who receive supplementary feedings in the early days of breastfeeding may develop **nipple confusion** (i.e., difficulty knowing how to latch-on to the breast). This is because breastfeeding and bottle feeding require different skills. If supplementation is needed, devices such as supplemental nursing systems may be used, in which the baby can be supplemented while breastfeeding (see Fig. 20-2). Syringe feeding, finger feeding, and cup feeding are other methods for offering supplements to breastfed infants. If parents choose to use bottles, a slow-flow nipple is recommended. Although some parents combine breastfeeding and bottle feeding, many babies never take a bottle and go directly from the breast to a cup as they grow.

Pacifiers are not recommended until breastfeeding is well established. Their use has been associated with shorter duration of breastfeeding, sore nipples, and insufficient milk supply (Howard et al., 2003).

Special considerations

Sleepy baby. During the first few days of life, some babies need to be awakened for feedings. Parents are instructed to be alert for behavioral signs or feeding cues such

TABLE 20-4

Selected Drugs Excreted in Milk

Drug	AAP Rating
Acetaminophen (Datril, Tylenol, Darvocet, Excedrin)	6
Alcohol (ethanol)	6
Aspirin (Bayer, Anacin, Bufferin, Excedrin, Fiorinal, Empirin)	5
Caffeine	6
Cocaine	2
Codeine	6
Heroin	2
Ibuprofen (Advil, Nuprin, Motrin)	6
Indomethacin (Indocin)	6
Ketorolac tromethamine (Toradal)	6
Marijuana	2
Medroxyprogesterone acetate (Depo-Provera)	6
Meperidine (Demerol, Mepergan)	6
Methadone	6
Morphine	6
Naproxen (Naproxyn, Anaprox, Naprosyn, Aleve)	6
Oxycodone	Not rated
Phenobarbitol (Luminal, Donnatal, Tedral)	5
Phenytoin (Dilantin)	6
Propylthiouracil	6
Thyroid and thyroxine	6
Tolbutamide (Orinase)	6

American Academy of Pediatrics (AAP) Committee on Drugs rated drugs that transfer into human milk. The ratings are as follows:
1. Drugs that are contraindicated during breastfeeding
2. Drugs of abuse that are contraindicated during breastfeeding
3. Radioactive compounds that require temporary cessation of breastfeeding
4. Drugs with unknown effects on breastfeeding but may be of concern
5. Drugs that have been associated with significant effects on some breastfeeding infants and should be given to breastfeeding mothers with caution
6. Maternal medication usually compatible with breastfeeding
7. Food and environmental agents that have an effect of breastfeeding

BOX 20-2

Waking the Sleepy Newborn

- Lay the baby down and unwrap.
- Change the diaper.
- Hold the baby upright, turn from side to side.
- Talk to the baby.
- Gently, but firmly, massage the chest and back.
- Rub the baby's hands and feet.
- Do baby "sit-ups." Gently rock the baby from a lying to sitting position and back again until the eyes open.
- Adjust lighting up for stimulation or down to encourage the baby to open the eyes.
- Apply cool cloth to face.

BOX 20-3

Calming the Fussy Baby

- Swaddle the baby.
- Hold closely.
- Move or rock gently.
- Talk soothingly.
- Reduce environmental stimuli.
- Allow baby to suck on adult finger.
- Place baby skin-to-skin with mother.

as rapid eye movements under the eyelids, sucking movements, or hand-to-mouth motions. When these signs are present, it is a good time to attempt breastfeeding. If the infant is awakened from a sound sleep, attempts at feeding are more likely to be unsuccessful. Unwrapping the baby, changing the diaper, sitting the baby upright, talking to the baby with variable pitch, gently massaging the baby's chest or back, and stroking the palms or soles may bring the baby to an alert state (Box 20-2).

Fussy baby. Babies sometimes awaken from sleep crying frantically. Although they may be hungry, they cannot focus on feeding until they are calmed. The nurse can encourage parents to swaddle the baby, hold the baby close, talk soothingly, and allow the baby to suck on a clean finger until calm enough to latch on to the breast (Box 20-3).

Infant fussiness during feeding may be the result of birth injury such as bruising of the head or fractured clavicle. Changing the feeding position may alleviate this problem.

Infants who were suctioned extensively or intubated at birth may demonstrate an aversion to oral stimulation. The baby may scream and stiffen if anything approaches the mouth. Parents may need to spend time holding and cuddling the baby before attempting to breastfeed.

An infant may become fussy and appear discontented when sucking if the nipple does not extend far enough into the mouth. The feeding may begin with well-organized sucks and swallows, but the infant soon begins to pull off the breast and cry. It may be helpful for the mother to support her breast throughout the feeding so that the nipple stays in the same position as the feeding proceeds and the breast softens.

Fussiness may be related to GI distress (i.e., cramping and gas pains). This may occur in response to an occasional feeding of infant formula, or it may be related to something the mother has ingested. Although most mothers can consume their normal diet without affecting the baby, foods such as broccoli, cabbage, or onions may irritate some babies. Others may react to cow's milk protein ingested by the mother. No standard foods should be avoided by all mothers when breastfeeding; each mother-baby couple responds individually. If gas is a problem, the physician may suggest giving the baby liquid simethicone drops before feeding.

Parents should be taught that persistent crying or refusing to breastfeed can indicate illness, and the health care provider should be notified. Ear infections, sore throat, or oral thrush may cause the infant to be fussy and not breastfeed well.

Slow weight gain. Newborn infants typically lose 5% to 10% of body weight before they begin to show weight gain. Weight loss of 7% in a breastfeeding infant during the first 3 days of life should be investigated (Lawrence & Lawrence, 2005). Thereafter they should begin to show a weight gain of 110 to 200 g/week or 20 to 28 g/day for the first 3 months. (Breastfed infants usually do not gain weight as quickly as formula-fed infants.) The infant who continues to lose weight after 5 days, who does not regain birth weight by 14 days, or whose weight is below the 10th percentile by 1 month should be evaluated and closely monitored by a health care provider.

Most often, slow weight gain is related to inadequate breastfeeding. Feedings may be short or infrequent, or the infant may be latching on incorrectly or sucking ineffectively or inefficiently. Other possibilities are illness or infection, malabsorption, or circumstances that increase the baby's energy needs such as congenital heart disease, cystic fibrosis, or simply being SGA.

Maternal factors may be the cause of slow weight gain. There may be a problem with inadequate emptying of the breasts, pain with feeding, or inappropriate timing of feedings. Inadequate glandular breast tissue or previous breast surgery may affect milk supply. Severe intrapartum or postpartum hemorrhage, illness, or medications may decrease milk supply. Stress and fatigue also may negatively affect milk production.

Usually the solution to slow weight gain is to improve the feeding technique. Positioning and latch-on are evaluated, and adjustments made. It may help to add a feeding or two in a 24-hour period. If the problem is a sleepy baby, parents are taught waking techniques.

Using alternate breast massage during feedings may help increase the amount of milk going to the infant. With this technique, the mother massages her breast from the chest wall to the nipple whenever the baby has sucking pauses. Some think this technique also may increase the fat content of the milk, which aids in weight gain.

When babies are calorie deprived and need supplementation, expressed breast milk or formula can be given with a nursing supplementer (see Fig. 20-2), cup, syringe, or bottle. In most cases, supplementation is needed only for a short time until the baby gains weight and is feeding adequately.

If the baby's slow weight gain is related to the mother's milk supply, it must be determined if this is an actual or perceived problem and whether it is related to milk production or milk transfer to the infant. Maternal health habits should be assessed because such things as medications, smoking, stress, fatigue, or infection can decrease milk supply.

Jaundice. Jaundice (hyperbilirubinemia) in the newborn is discussed in detail in Chapter 18. Physiologic jaundice usually occurs after age 24 hours and peaks by the third day. This has been referred to as *early-onset jaundice* or *breast-feeding jaundice,* which in the breastfed infant may be associated with insufficient feeding and infrequent stooling. Colostrum has a natural laxative effect and promotes early passage of meconium. Bilirubin is excreted from the body primarily through the intestines. Infrequent stooling allows bilirubin in the stool to be reabsorbed into the infant's system, thus promoting hyperbilirubinemia. Infants who receive water or glucose water supplements are more likely to have hyperbilirubinemia, because only small amounts of bilirubin are excreted through the kidneys. Decreased caloric intake (less milk) is associated with decreased stooling and increased jaundice.

To prevent early-onset breastfeeding jaundice from occurring, babies should be breastfed frequently during the first several days of life. More frequent feedings are associated with lower bilirubin levels.

To treat early-onset jaundice, breastfeeding is evaluated in terms of frequency and length of feedings, positioning and latch-on, and the infant's ability to empty the breast. Factors such as a sleepy or lethargic baby or breast engorgement may interfere with effective breastfeeding and should be corrected. If the infant's intake of milk needs to be increased, a supplemental feeding device may be used to deliver additional breast milk or formula while the infant is nursing. Hyperbilirubinemia may reach levels that require treatment with phototherapy administered with a light or a fiberoptic blanket (see Chapter 19).

Late-onset jaundice or *breast milk jaundice* affects a few breastfed infants and develops in the second week of life, peaking at about age 10 days. Affected infants are typically thriving, gaining weight, and stooling normally; all pathologic causes of jaundice have been ruled out. It was once postulated that an enzyme in the milk of some mothers caused the bilirubin level to increase. It now appears that a factor in human milk increases the intestinal absorption of bilirubin. In most cases, no intervention is necessary, although some experts recommend temporary interruption of breastfeeding for 12 to 24 hours to allow bilirubin levels to decrease. During this time, the mother pumps her breasts, and the baby is offered alternative nutrition, usually formula (Lawrence & Lawrence, 2005).

Preterm infants. Human milk is the ideal food for preterm infants, with benefits that are unique and in addition to those received by term, healthy infants. Breast milk enhances retinal maturation in the preterm infant and improves neurocognitive outcome. It also decreases the risk of necrotizing enterocolitis. Greater physiologic stability occurs with breastfeeding as compared with bottle feeding (Lawrence & Lawrence, 2005).

Depending on gestational age and physical condition, many preterm infants are capable of breastfeeding for at least some feedings each day. Mothers of preterm infants who are not able to breastfeed their infants should begin pumping their breasts as soon as possible after birth with a hospital-grade electric pump (Fig. 20-8). To establish an optimal milk supply, the mother should use a dual collection kit and pump 8 to 10 times daily for 10 to 15 minutes and/or until the milk flow has ceased for a few minutes. These women are taught proper handling and storage of breast milk to

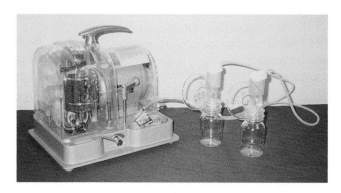

Fig. 20-8 Hospital-grade electric breast pump.

minimize bacterial contamination and growth (Riordan, 2005).

The mothers of preterm infants often receive specific emotional benefits in breastfeeding or providing breast milk for their babies. They find rewards in knowing they can provide the healthiest nutrition for the infant and believe that breastfeeding enhances feelings of closeness to the infant.

Breastfeeding multiple infants. Breastfeeding is especially beneficial to twins, triplets, and other higher order multiples because of the immunologic and nutritional advantages, as well as the opportunity for the mother to interact with each baby frequently. Most mothers are capable of producing an adequate milk supply for multiple infants. Parenting multiples may be overwhelming, and mothers, as well as fathers, need extra support and assistance learning how to manage feedings (Fig. 20-9).

Expressing breast milk

In some situations, expression of breast milk is necessary or desirable, such as when engorgement occurs, the mother and baby are separated (e.g., preterm or sick infant), the mother is employed outside the home and needs to maintain her milk supply, the nipples are severely sore or damaged, or the mother is leaving the infant with a caregiver and will not be present for feeding.

Because pumping and hand expression are rarely as efficient as a baby in removing milk from the breast, the milk supply should never be judged based on the volume expressed.

Hand expression. After her hands are thoroughly washed, the mother places one hand on her breast at the edge of the areola. With her thumb above and fingers below, she presses in toward her chest wall and gently compresses the breast while rolling her thumb and fingers forward toward the nipple. These motions are repeated rhythmically until the milk begins to flow. The mother simply maintains steady, light pressure while the milk is flowing easily. The thumb and fingers should not pinch the breast or slip down to the nipple, and the mother should rotate her hand to reach all sections of the breast.

Pumping. For most women, it is advisable to initiate pumping only after the milk supply is well established and the infant is latching on and breastfeeding well. However, when breastfeeding is delayed after birth, pumping is started as soon as possible and continued regularly until the infant is able to breastfeed effectively.

Numerous ways exist to approach pumping. Some women pump on awakening in the morning, or when the baby has fed but did not completely empty the breast. Others choose to pump after feedings or may pump one breast while the baby is feeding from the other. Double pumping (pumping both breasts at the same time) saves time and may stimulate the milk supply more effectively than single pumping (Fig. 20-10).

The amount of milk obtained when pumping depends on the type of pump being used, the time of day, how long it has been since the baby breastfed, the mother's milk supply, how practiced she is at pumping, and her comfort level (pumping is uncomfortable for some women). Breast milk may vary in color and consistency, depending on the time of day, the age of the baby, and foods the mother has eaten.

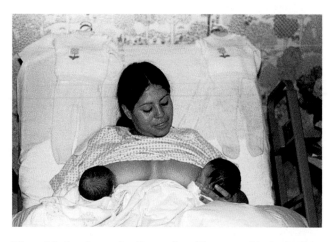

Fig. 20-9 Breastfeeding twins. (Courtesy Marjorie Pyle, RNC, Lifecircle, Costa Mesa, CA.)

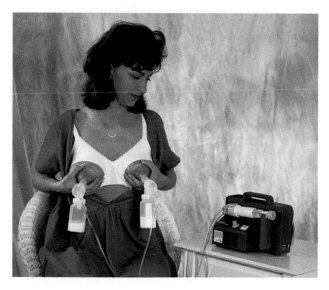

Fig. 20-10 Bilateral breast pumping. (Courtesy Medela, Inc., McHenry, IL.)

Types of pumps. Many types of breast pumps are available, varying in price and effectiveness. Before purchasing or renting a breast pump, the mother would benefit from counseling by a nurse or lactation consultant to determine which pump best suits her needs.

Manual or hand pumps are least expensive and may be the most appropriate where portability and quietness of operation are important. These are most often used by mothers who are pumping for an occasional bottle (Fig. 20-11).

Full-service electric pumps, or hospital-grade pumps (see Fig. 20-8) most closely duplicate the sucking action and pressure of the breastfeeding infant. When breastfeeding is delayed after birth (e.g., preterm or ill newborn), or when mother and baby are separated for lengthy periods, these pumps are most appropriate. Because hospital-grade breast pumps are very heavy and expensive, portable versions of these pumps can be rented for home use.

Electric, self-cycling double pumps are efficient and easy to use. These pumps were designed for working mothers. Some of these pumps come with carry bags containing coolers to store pumped milk.

Smaller electric or battery-operated pumps also are available. Some have automatic suck/release cycling, and others require use of a finger to regulate strength and speed of suction. These are typically used when pumping is done occasionally, but some models are satisfactory for working mothers or others who pump on a regular basis.

Storage of breast milk. Breast milk can be safely stored in any clean glass or plastic container. Plastic bags especially designed for freezing breast milk can be purchased.

For full-term, healthy infants, freshly expressed breast milk can be stored at room temperature for up to 8 hours and can be refrigerated safely for 5 days. Milk can be frozen for 3 to 6 months in the freezer section of a refrigerator with a separate door, and for 6 to 12 months in a deep freeze (0° C). When breast milk is stored, the container should be dated, and the oldest milk should be used first (Eglash, Chantry, & Howard, 2004).

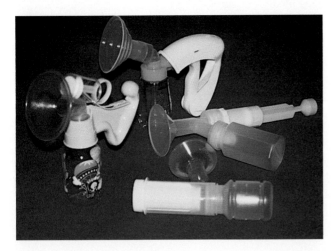

Fig. 20-11 Manual breast pumps. (Courtesy Marjorie Pyle, RNC, Lifecircle, Costa Mesa, CA.)

Frozen milk is thawed by placing the container in the refrigerator for gradual thawing or in warm water for faster thawing. It cannot be refrozen and should be used within 24 hours. After thawing, the container should be shaken to mix the layers that have separated (Patient Instructions for Self-Care box).

Frozen milk is never thawed or heated in a microwave oven. Microwaving does not heat evenly and can cause encapsulated boiling bubbles to form in the center of the liquid. This may not be detected when drops of milk are checked for temperature. Babies have sustained severe burns to the mouth, throat, and upper GI tract as a result of microwaved milk (Lawrence & Lawrence, 2005).

PATIENT INSTRUCTIONS FOR SELF-CARE

Breast Milk Storage Guidelines for Home Use

- Before expressing breast milk, wash your hands.
- Containers for storing milk should be washed in hot, soapy water and rinsed thoroughly; they can also be washed in a dishwasher. Plastic bags designed specifically for breast milk storage can be used.
- Write the date of expression on the container before storing the milk.
- It is acceptable to store breast milk in the refrigerator or freezer with other food items.
- When storing milk in a refrigerator or freezer, place the containers in the middle or back of the freezer, not on the door.
- Freeze milk in serving sizes of 2 to 4 ounces to avoid waste.
- When filling a storage container that will be frozen, allow space at the top of the container for expansion.
- To thaw frozen breast milk, place the container in the refrigerator for gradual thawing or place the container under warm, running water for quicker thawing. Never boil or microwave.
- Milk thawed in the refrigerator can be stored for 24 hours. Milk thawed in warm water can be refrigerated for use within 4 hours.
- Thawed breast milk should never be refrozen.
- Shake the milk container before feeding baby, and test the temperature of the milk on the inner aspect of your wrist.
- Any unused milk left in the bottle after feeding must be discarded.
- Freshly expressed breast milk can be stored at room temperature (less than 77° F [25° C]) for up to 8 hours.
- Breast milk can be stored in the refrigerator for 5 days.
- Frozen breast milk can be stored for 2 weeks in a freezer compartment within a refrigerator.
- Frozen breast milk can be stored for up to 6 months in a freezer section with a separate door.
- Frozen breast milk can be stored for 6 to 12 months in a deep freeze (32° F [0° C] or lower).

From Lawrence, R., & Lawrence, R. (2005). *Breastfeeding: A guide for the medical profession* (6th ed.). St. Louis: Mosby; Eglash, A., Chantry, C., & Howard, C. (2004). *Protocol #8: Human milk storage information for home use for healthy term infants*. The Academy of Breastfeeding Medicine. Available at http://www.abm.org. Accessed 9/11/2005.

Being away from the baby

Many women are able to combine breastfeeding successfully with employment, attending school, or other commitments. If feedings are missed, the milk supply may be affected. Some women's bodies adjust the milk supply to the times she is with the baby for feedings, whereas other women find they must pump or the supply diminishes quickly. Employers are becoming increasingly more aware of the importance of supporting breastfeeding mothers who return to work; some businesses provide rooms where mothers can nurse their infants or use breast pumps (see Fig. 1-4 on p. 6).

Weaning

Weaning is initiated when babies are introduced to foods other than breastmilk and concludes with the last breastfeeding. Gradual weaning, over a period of weeks or months, is easier for mothers and infants. Abrupt weaning is likely to be distressing for both mother and baby, as well as physically uncomfortable for the mother.

With infant-led weaning the infant moves at his or her own pace in omitting feedings. This usually facilitates a gradual decrease in the mother's milk supply.

Mother-led weaning means that the mother decides which feedings to drop. This is most easily done by omitting the feeding of least interest to the baby or the one the infant is most likely to sleep through. Every few days thereafter, another feeding is dropped, and so on, until the infant is gradually weaned from the breast.

Infants can be weaned directly from the breast to a cup. Bottles are usually offered to infants younger than 6 months. If the infant is weaned before age 1 year, formula should be fed to the infant instead of cow's milk.

If abrupt weaning is necessary, breast engorgement often occurs. The mother is instructed to take mild analgesics, wear a supportive bra, apply ice packs or cabbage leaves to the breasts, and pump small amounts if needed to increase comfort. It is best to avoid pumping because the breasts should remain full enough to promote a decrease in the milk supply.

Weaning can be a very emotional time for mothers. Many women feel that weaning is the end to a special, satisfying relationship with the infant and benefit from time to adapt to the changes. Sudden weaning may evoke feelings of guilt and disappointment; some women go through a grieving period after weaning. The nurse can assist the mother by discussing other ways to continue this nurturing relationship with the infant, such as skin-to-skin contact while bottle feeding, or holding and cuddling the baby. Support from the father of the baby and other family members is essential at this time.

Milk banking

For those infants who cannot be breastfed but who also cannot survive except on human milk, banked donor milk is critically important. Because of the antiinfective and growth-promoting properties of human milk, as well as its superior nutrition, donor milk is used in many neonatal intensive care units for preterm or sick infants when the mother's own milk is not available. Donor milk also is used therapeutically for a variety of medical conditions, such as in transplant recipients who are immunocompromised.

The Human Milk Banking Association of North America (HMBANA) has established annually reviewed guidelines for the operation of donor human milk banks. Donor milk banks collect, screen, process, and distribute the milk donated by breastfeeding mothers who are feeding their own infants and pumping a few ounces extra each day for the milk bank. All donors are screened both by interview and serologically for communicable diseases. Donor milk is stored frozen until it is heat processed to kill potential pathogens; then it is refrozen for storage until it is dispensed for use. The heat processing adds a level of protection for the recipient that is not possible with any other donor tissue or organ. Banked milk is dispensed only by prescription. A per-ounce fee is charged by the bank to pay for the processing costs, but the HMBANA guidelines prohibit payment to donors (see the Resource list at the end of this chapter).

Diet. The breastfeeding mother should eat a healthy, well-balanced diet that includes an extra 200 to 500 calories per day. Prenatal vitamins are continued throughout breastfeeding. Fluid intake of at least 2 to 3 quarts per day is recommended.

There are no specific foods for the mother to avoid while breastfeeding. In most cases, the mother can consume a normal diet, according to her personal preferences and cultural practices.

Rest. It is important for the breastfeeding mother to rest as much as possible, especially in the first 1 or 2 weeks after birth. Fatigue, stress, and worry can negatively affect milk production and let-down. The nurse can encourage the mother to sleep when the baby sleeps. Breastfeeding in a side-lying position promotes rest for the mother. Assistance with household chores and caring for other children can be done by the father, grandparents or other relatives, and friends.

Breast care. The breastfeeding mother's normal routine bathing is all that is necessary to keep her breasts clean. Soap can have a drying effect on nipples, so she should be instructed to avoid washing the nipples with soap.

Breast creams should not be used routinely because they may block the natural oil secreted by the Montgomery glands on the areola. Some breast creams contain alcohol, which may dry the nipples. Vitamin E oil or cream is not recommended for use on nipples because it is a fat-soluble vitamin, and a breastfeeding infant might consume enough vitamin E from the nipple to reach toxic levels. In addition, some people are allergic to vitamin E oil.

Modified lanolin with reduced allergens can be used safely on dry or sore nipples. Lanolin is beneficial in moist wound healing of sore nipples. Because lanolin is made from wool, the nurse should ask the mother if she is allergic to wool before applying the lanolin.

The mother with flat or inverted nipples will likely benefit from wearing breast shells in her bra. These hard plastic devices exert mild pressure around the base of the nipple to encourage nipple eversion. It is advisable for women with flat or inverted nipples to begin wearing breast shells during the last month of pregnancy. Breast shells also are useful for sore nipples to keep the mother's bra or clothing from touching the nipples (Fig. 20-12).

If a mother needs breast support, she will likely be uncomfortable unless she wears a bra, because the ligament that supports the breast (Cooper's ligament) will otherwise stretch and be painful. Bras should fit well and provide nonbinding support.

If leakage of milk between feedings is a problem, breast pads (disposable or washable) may be worn inside the bra. Plastic-lined breast pads are not recommended because they trap moisture and may contribute to sore nipples.

Sexual sensations. Some women experience rhythmic uterine contractions during breastfeeding. Such sensations are not unusual because uterine contractions and milk ejection are both triggered by oxytocin. Occasionally, these uterine contractions may provoke sensations resembling an orgasmic response, which is disturbing to some mothers.

Breastfeeding during pregnancy. It is possible for a breastfeeding woman to conceive and continue breastfeeding throughout the pregnancy if there are no medical contraindications (e.g., risk of preterm labor). When the baby is born, colostrum is produced. The practice of breastfeeding a newborn and an older child is called *tandem nursing*. The nurse should remind the mother always to feed the infant first to ensure that the newborn is receiving adequate nutrition. The supply-meets-demand principle works in this situation, just as with breastfeeding multiples.

Medications and breastfeeding. Although there is much concern about the compatibility of drugs and breastfeeding, few drugs are absolutely contraindicated during lactation (see Box 20-4). In evaluating the safety of a specific medication during breastfeeding, the health care provider considers the pharmacokinetics of the drug in the maternal system, as well as the absorption, metabolism, distribution, storage, and excretion in the infant. The gestational and chronologic age of the infant, body weight, and breast-

feeding pattern also are considered. Breastfeeding mothers should be cautioned about taking any medications except those that are deemed essential; they should be advised to check with their physician before taking any medication. If a breastfeeding mother is taking a medication that has questionable effect on the infant, she can be advised to take the medication just after nursing the baby or just before the infant is expected to sleep for a long time. References are available with specific information about medications and breastfeeding (Hale, 2004; Hale & Berens, 2002; Ward, Bates, Benitz, Burchfield, Ring et al., 2001).

Alcohol consumed by the breastfeeding mother is transferred to the infant in significant amounts, although it is not deemed harmful if the amount and duration are limited (Hale, 2004). If a mother chooses to consume alcohol, she should be advised to minimize its effects by having only an occasional drink, and not to breastfeed for two hours after the drink. The mother who is pumping for a sick or preterm infant should avoid alcohol entirely until her infant is healthy (Lawrence & Lawrence, 2005).

Women who smoke are less likely to breastfeed than nonsmokers; smokers who choose to breastfeed tend to do so for shorter durations than nonsmokers (Amir & Donath, 2003). Nicotine is transferred to the infant in breast milk, whether the mother smokes or uses a nicotine patch, although the effect on the infant is uncertain. Exposing the infant to second-hand smoke is of concern, and breastfeeding mothers are encouraged to stop smoking. Mothers who smoke should be advised to limit smoking, to smoke after feeding the infant, and to consider switching to the nicotine patch (Hale, 2004).

Maternal intake of caffeine may cause infant irritability and poor sleeping patterns. For most women, two servings of caffeine a day does not cause untoward effects; however, some infants are sensitive to even small amounts of caffeine. Mothers of such infants should limit caffeine intake. Caffeine is found in coffee, tea, chocolate, and many soft drinks.

Herbs and herbal teas are becoming more widely used during lactation. Although some are considered safe, others contain pharmacologically active compounds that may have detrimental effects. A thorough maternal history should include the use of any herbal remedies. Each remedy should then be evaluated for its compatibility with breastfeeding. The regional poison control center may provide information on the active properties of herbs.

Environmental contaminants. Except under unusual circumstances, breastfeeding is not contraindicated because of exposure to environmental contaminants such as DDT (an insecticide) and tetrachloroethylene (used in dry cleaning plants) (Lawrence & Lawrence, 2005).

Common problems of the breastfeeding mother

Engorgement. Engorgement, characterized by painful overfilling of the breasts, can occur as a result of infrequent or ineffective emptying of the breasts. It typically

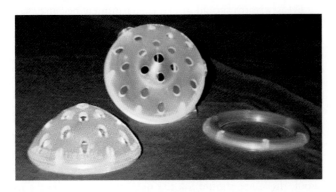

Fig. 20-12 Breast shells.

occurs 3 to 5 days after birth when the milk "comes in" and lasts about 24 hours. There is vascular congestion and increased vascularity, accumulation of milk in the breast tissue, and edema related to swelling and obstruction of lymphatic drainage (Mass, 2004). The breasts are firm, tender, and hot and may appear shiny and taut. The areolae are firm, and the nipples may flatten. The unyielding areolae make it difficult for the infant to latch on. Because back pressure on full milk glands inhibits milk production, if milk is not removed from the breasts, the milk supply may diminish.

Breastfeeding the baby frequently, at least every 2 to 3 hours, as the milk is coming in may help prevent engorgement. The baby should be encouraged to feed at least 15 to 20 minutes on each breast or until one breast softens per feeding.

When engorgement occurs, the mother is instructed to feed every 2 hours, massaging the breasts as the baby is feeding. The baby should feed on the first breast until it softens before switching to the other side. If the infant does not soften the second breast, the mother may use a breast pump to empty the breast. Pumping during engorgement will not cause a problematic increase in milk supply. A warm shower just before feeding or pumping can aid in relaxation and let-down.

Cold compresses (ice packs) may reduce swelling, vascularity, and pain. Cold compresses are usually applied after feeding or pumping. Raw cabbage leaves placed over the breasts between feedings may help reduce the swelling. The cabbage leaves are washed, placed in the refrigerator until they are cool, and then crushed. The leaves are placed over the breasts for 15 to 20 minutes. This can be repeated for two or three sessions; frequent application of cabbage leaves can decrease milk supply. Cabbage leaves should not be used if the mother is allergic to cabbage or sulfa drugs or develops a skin rash. Antiinflammatory medications, such as ibuprofen, may help reduce the pain and swelling associated with engorgement.

Sore nipples. Mild nipple tenderness during the first few days of breastfeeding is common. Severe soreness and abraded, cracked, or bleeding nipples are not normal and most often result from poor positioning, incorrect latch-on, improper suck, or a monilial infection. The key to preventing sore nipples is correct breastfeeding technique.

To make the initial sucks less painful, the mother can express a few drops of colostrum or milk to moisten the nipple and areola before latch-on. If the mother continues to experience nipple pain or discomfort after the first few sucks, it is necessary to help the mother evaluate the latch-on and baby's position at the breast. The nurse helps the mother to reposition as necessary to try to resolve the nipple discomfort. If the nipple pain continues, the mother needs to remove the baby from the breast, breaking suction with her finger in the baby's mouth. She then proceeds to attempt latch-on again, making sure the baby's mouth is open wide before the baby is pulled quickly to the breast (see Fig. 20-5). Often sore nipples are the result of the mother latching the baby onto the breast before the mouth is open wide.

The infant's suck can be assessed by inserting a clean gloved finger into the baby's mouth and stimulating the baby to suck. If the baby is not extruding the tongue over the lower gum, and the mother reports pain or pinching with sucking, the baby may have a short frenulum (commonly referred to as being "tongue-tied"). Sometimes this is corrected surgically to free the tongue for less painful, more effective breastfeeding (Griffiths, 2004; Messner, Lalakea, Aby, Macmahon, & Bair, 2000).

The treatment for sore nipples is first to correct the cause. Once the problem is identified and corrected, sore nipples should heal within a few days, even though the baby continues to breastfeed regularly. When sore nipples occur, it is more comfortable to start the feeding on the least sore nipple. After feeding, the nipples are wiped with water to remove the baby's saliva. A few drops of milk can be expressed, rubbed into the nipple, and allowed to air dry. Sore nipples should be open to air as much as possible. Breast shells worn inside the bra allow air to circulate while keeping clothing off sore nipples (see Fig. 20-12).

Rapid healing of sore nipples is critical to relieve the mother's discomfort, maintain breastfeeding, and prevent mastitis. Although numerous creams, ointments, and gels have been used to treat sore nipples, warm water, purified lanolin, and hydrogel are the only treatments that have been studied and shown to have some effect (Riordan, 2005). Purified lanolin helps sore nipples by retaining the skin's natural moisture and protecting the nipple from further abrasion. It is applied to nipples after feeding and need not be removed for the next feeding. (Mothers with history of wool allergy should not use lanolin until a skin test is done.) Hydrogel dressings, applied to nipples after feeding, create a soothing, moist healing environment by using a glycerin-based gel or saline-based hydrophilic polymer to promote healing. An antibiotic ointment may be recommended if nipples are cracked, abraded, or bleeding; this must be washed off before the feeding (Riordan, 2005).

If nipples are extremely sore or damaged, and the mother cannot tolerate breastfeeding, she may be advised to use an electric breast pump for 24 to 48 hours to allow the nipples to begin healing before resuming breastfeeding. It is important that the mother use a pump that will effectively empty the breasts; a rental pump is likely the best choice (see Fig. 20-10).

Monilial infections. Nipple soreness that is not resolved by the previously mentioned methods may be caused by a monilial (yeast) infection. Sore nipples that occur after the newborn period are often the result of a yeast infection. The mother usually reports sudden onset of severe nipple pain and tenderness, burning, or stinging and may have sharp, shooting, burning pains into the breasts during and after feedings. The nipples appear somewhat pink and shiny or may be scaly or flaky; there may be a visible rash, small blisters, or thrush. Most often, the pain is out of proportion to the appearance of the nipple. Yeast infections of the nipples and breast can be excruciatingly painful and can lead to early cessation of breastfeeding if not recognized and treated promptly.

Babies may or may not exhibit symptoms of monilial infection. Oral thrush and a red, raised diaper rash are common indications of a yeast infection.

Mothers and babies must be treated simultaneously with antifungal medication, even if the infant has no visible signs of infection (Hoover, 2001).

Plugged milk ducts. A milk duct may become plugged or clogged, causing a red, tender area or small lump in the breast, which may or may not be tender. Plugged milk ducts are most often the result of inadequate emptying of the breast. This may occur because of poor breastfeeding, delayed or missed feedings, always using the same position for feeding, clothing that is too tight, or a poorly fitting or underwire bra.

Application of warm compresses to the affected area and to the nipple before feeding helps promote emptying of the breast and release of the plug. (A disposable diaper filled with warm water makes an easy compress.) Soaking in a warm bath before feeding may be helpful.

Frequent feeding is recommended, with the baby beginning the feeding on the affected side to foster more complete emptying. The mother is advised to massage the affected area while the baby nurses or while she is pumping. Varying feeding positions and feeding without wearing a bra may be useful in resolving a plugged duct.

Mastitis. A breast infection, or mastitis, is characterized by the sudden onset of flulike symptoms such as fever, chills, body aches, and headache. Localized breast pain and tenderness usually is accompanied by a warm, reddened area on the breast, often resembling the shape of a pie wedge. Mastitis most commonly occurs in the upper outer quadrant of the breast; it may affect one or both breasts (see Fig. 25-4).

Certain factors may predispose a woman to mastitis. Inadequate emptying of the breasts is common, related to engorgement, plugged ducts, a sudden decrease in the number of feedings, abrupt weaning, or wearing underwire bras. Sore, cracked nipples may lead to mastitis by providing a portal of entry for causative organisms (*Staphylococcus*, *Streptococcus*, and *Escherichia coli* are most common). Stress and fatigue, ill family members, breast trauma, and poor maternal nutrition also are predisposing factors for mastitis (Mass, 2004; Osterman & Rahm, 2000).

Breastfeeding mothers should be taught the signs of mastitis before they are discharged from the hospital after birth, and they need to know to call the health care provider promptly if the symptoms occur. Treatment includes antibiotics such as cephalexin or dicloxacillin for 10 to 14 days, and analgesic and antipyretic medications such as ibuprofen. The mother is advised to rest as much as possible, and she should feed the baby or pump frequently, striving to empty the affected side adequately. Warm compresses to the breast before feeding or pumping may be useful. Adequate fluid intake and a balanced diet are important for the mother with mastitis (Hale & Berens, 2002).

Complications of mastitis include breast abscess, chronic mastitis, or fungal infections of the breast. Most complications can be prevented by early recognition and treatment (Mass, 2004).

Follow-up after hospital discharge

Problems with sore nipples, engorgement, and jaundice are likely to occur after discharge. It is the role of the nurse to educate and prepare the mother for problems she may encounter once she is home. It is important that the mother be given a list of resources for help with breastfeeding concerns and that she realize when to call for assistance. Community resources for breastfeeding mothers include lactation consultants in hospitals, physician offices, or in private practice; nurses in pediatric or obstetric offices; support groups such as La Leche League; and peer counseling programs (e.g., those offered through WIC) (see Resources at end of chapter.)

Telephone follow-up by hospital, birth center, or office nurses within the first day or two after discharge can provide a means to identify any problems and offer needed advice and support. The AAP (2005) recommends that breastfeeding infants should be seen by a health care provider at 3 to 5 days of age and again at 2 to 3 weeks to assess weight gain and offer encouragement and support to the mother (Gartner et al., 2005).

Evaluation

Evaluation is based on the expected outcomes, and the plan of care is revised as needed based on the evaluation (Plan of Care).

FORMULA FEEDING

The vast majority of infants in the United States receive infant formula at some point during their first year of life (Ryan, Wenjun, & Acosta, 2002). Although some parents may choose to exclusively formula feed, formula also may be used to supplement breastfeeding if the mother's milk supply appears to be inadequate, or it may be fed to the baby when the mother is away and leaves a bottle of formula instead of expressed breast milk.

Parent Education

Mothers and fathers who are formula feeding their infants need teaching, counseling, and support, particularly if they are first time parents or if they have never formula fed. Parents are likely to have questions related to feeding frequency, the appropriate amount of formula to give the infant at each feeding, formula intolerance, weight gain, and "spitting up" (Borghese-Lang, Morrison, Ogle, & Wright, 2003). They may need assistance with the feeding process and with any problems they may have. Emphasis on the beneficial use of feeding times for close contact and socializing with the infant can help promote bonding and infant interaction.

The alarming increase in childhood and adolescent obesity in the United States is prevalent among low-income, mi-

PLAN OF CARE *Breastfeeding and Infant Nutrition*

NURSING DIAGNOSIS Ineffective breastfeeding related to knowledge deficit of mother as evidenced by ongoing incorrect latch-on technique

Expected Outcomes *Mother will demonstrate correct latch-on technique. Infant will latch on and suck with gliding jaw movements and audible swallowing. Mother will report no nipple pain with infant suckling. Mother will express increased satisfaction with breastfeeding, and neonate will exhibit satisfaction of hunger and sucking needs.*

Nursing Interventions/*Rationales*

- Assess mother's knowledge and motivation for breastfeeding *to acknowledge patient's desire for effective outcome and provide starting point for teaching.*
- Observe a breastfeeding session *to provide database for positive reinforcement and problem identification.*
- Describe and demonstrate ways to stimulate the sucking reflex, various positions for breastfeeding, and the use of pillows during a session *to promote maternal and neonatal comfort and effective latch-on.*
- Monitor neonatal position of mouth on areola and position of head and body *to give positive reinforcement for correct latch-on position or to correct poor latch-on position.*
- Teach mother ways to stimulate neonate to maintain an awake state by diapering, unwrapping, massaging, or burping *to complete a breastfeeding thoroughly and satisfactorily.*
- Give mother information regarding lactation diet, expression of milk by hand or pump, and storage of expressed breast milk *to provide basic information.*
- Make sure mother has written information on all aspects of breastfeeding *to reinforce verbal instructions and demonstrations.*
- Refer to support groups and lactation consultant if needed *to provide further information and group support.*

NURSING DIAGNOSIS Ineffective infant feeding pattern related to inability to coordinate sucking and swallowing

Expected Outcome *Neonate will coordinate sucking and swallowing in order to accomplish an effective feeding pattern.*

Nursing Interventions/*Rationales*

- Assess for factors that may contribute to ineffective sucking and swallowing *to provide a basis for plan of care.*
- Teach mother to observe feeding readiness cues *to enhance effective feeding.*
- Modify feeding methods as needed *to maintain hydration status and nutritional requirements.*
- Promote a calm, relaxed atmosphere *to provide a pleasant breastfeeding experience for mother and neonate.*
- Refer to lactation consultant *to provide specialized support.*

NURSING DIAGNOSIS Anxiety related to ineffective infant feeding pattern

Expected Outcome *Mother will report a decrease in anxiety level.*

Nursing Interventions/*Rationales*

- Monitor maternal anxiety level during feeding sessions *to provide a basis for care planning.*
- Provide positive reinforcement for feeding pattern improvement *to decrease anxiety.*
- Monitor weight, intake, and output of neonate *to provide information regarding effective feeding.*
- Enlist assistance of support persons *to provide positive feedback for increasing skill.*
- Provide information for lactation support *to decrease anxiety after discharge.*
- Initiate follow-up of telephone calls *to assess progress and detect problems.*

---

norities, who receive WIC benefits. Many of these mothers believe that heavier infants are healthier, which is indicative of successful parenting. Parents who bottle feed are more likely to feed on a regular schedule, without attending to infant feeding readiness cues (Birch & Davison, 2001; Borghese-Lang et al., 2003). Teaching parents to observe for signs that the infant is hungry and how to tell if the baby is full can help decrease the likelihood of overfeeding.

Readiness for feeding

The first feeding of formula is ideally given after the initial transition to extrauterine life is made. Feeding-readiness cues include such things as stability of vital signs, presence of bowel sounds, an active sucking reflex, and those described earlier for breastfed infants. The type of formula is usually determined by the pediatrician. Parents are advised to avoid switching formulas unless instructed to do so by the physician.

Before the first formula feeding, some institutions have the policy of offering sips of water to the newborn to assess patency of the GI tract and absence of tracheoesophageal fistula. If the infant sucks and swallows the water without difficulty, formula is then offered.

Feeding patterns

Typically, a newborn will drink 15 to 30 ml of formula per feeding during the first 24 hours, with the intake gradually increasing during the first week of life. Most newborn infants should be fed every 3 to 4 hours, even if that requires waking the baby for the feedings. The infant showing an adequate weight gain can be allowed to sleep at night and fed only on awakening. Most newborns need six to eight feedings in 24 hours, and the number of feedings decreases as the infant matures. Usually by 3 to 4 weeks after birth, a fairly predictable feeding pattern has developed. Scheduling feedings arbitrarily at predetermined intervals may not meet a baby's needs, but initiating feedings at convenient times often moves the baby's feedings to times that work for the family.

Mothers will usually notice increases in the infant's appetite at 7 to 10 days, 3 weeks, 6 weeks, 3 months, and 6 months. These appetite spurts correspond to growth spurts. The amount of formula per feeding should be increased by about 30 ml to meet the baby's needs at these times.

Feeding technique

Parents who choose formula feeding often need education regarding feeding techniques. Babies should be held for all feedings. During feedings, parents are encouraged to sit comfortably, holding the infant closely in a semiupright position with good head support. Feedings provide opportunities to bond with the baby through touching, talking, singing, or reading to the infant. Parents should consider feedings as a time of peaceful relaxation with the baby.

A bottle should never be propped with a pillow or other inanimate object and left with the infant. This practice may result in choking, and it deprives the infant of important interaction during feeding. Moreover, propping the bottle has been implicated in causing nursing bottle caries, or decay of the first teeth resulting from continuous bathing of the teeth with carbohydrate-containing fluid as the infant sporadically sucks the nipple.

The bottle should be held so that fluid fills the nipple and none of the air in the bottle is allowed to enter the nipple (Fig. 20-13). When the infant falls asleep, turns aside the head, or ceases to suck, it is usually an indication that enough formula has been taken to satisfy the baby. Parents should be taught to look for these cues and avoid overfeeding, which can contribute to obesity.

Most infants swallow air when fed from a bottle and should be given a chance to burp several times during a feeding (Fig. 20-14) (see Guidelines/Guías box).

Common concerns

Parents need to know what to do if the infant is spitting up. They may need to decrease the amount of feeding, or feed smaller amounts more frequently. Burping the infant

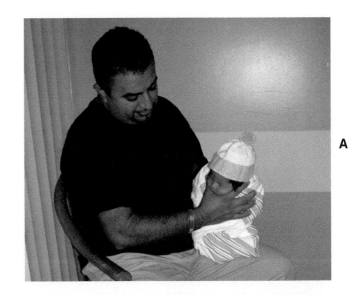

A

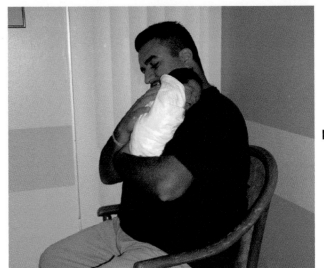

B

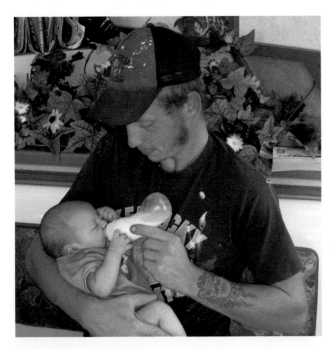

Fig. 20-13 Father bottle feeding infant son. Note angled bottle that ensures that milk covers nipple area. (Courtesy Eugene Doerr, Leitchfield, KY.)

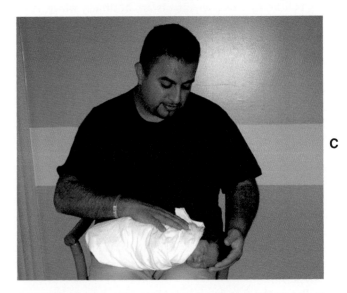

C

Fig. 20-14 Positions for burping an infant. **A,** Sitting. **B,** On the shoulder. **C,** Across the lap. (Courtesy Julie Perry Nelson, Gilbert, AZ.)

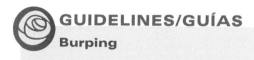

GUIDELINES/GUÍAS
Burping

POSITION #1 (SEE FIG. 20-14, *B*)
POSICIÓN #1

- Hold your baby up, head on your shoulder.
- *Ponga su bebé con la cabeza muy alta sobre su hombro.*

- Put one arm under the baby's bottom.
- *Ponga un brazo debajo de las nalgas del bebé.*

- With the other hand, pat or rub the baby's back.
- *Con la otra mano, dé leves palmaditas o sobe la espalda del bebé.*

POSITION #2 (SEE FIG. 20-14, *A*)
POSICIÓN #2

- Sit your baby up in your lap.
- *Siente al bebé sobre su regazo.*

- Hold the head and back with one hand.
- *Con una mano, sostenga la cabeza y la espalda del bebé.*

- Hold the chin and front with the other.
- *Con la otra mano, sostenga la barbilla y la parte delantera del bebé.*

- Rock the baby's upper body back and forth.
- *Mueva la parte superior del bebé hacia adelante y hacia atrás.*

- Or pat the baby's back.
- *O dé suaves palmaditas a la espalda del bebé.*

POSITION #3 (SEE FIG. 20-14, *C*)
POSICIÓN #3

- Lay your baby face down on your lap.
- *Coloque al bebé boca abajo sobre su regazo.*
- Hold the baby's head with one hand.
- *Con una mano, sostenga la cabeza del bebé.*
- Rub or pat the baby's back.
- *Sobe o dé suaves palmaditas a la espalda del bebé.*

several times during a feeding, such as when the infant's sucking slows down or stops, may decrease spitting. It may help to hold the baby upright for 30 minutes after feeding, and to avoid bouncing or placing the infant on the abdomen soon after the feeding is finished. Spitting may be a result of overfeeding or may be symptomatic of gastroesophageal reflux. Vomiting one third or more of the feeding at most feeding sessions or projectile vomiting should be reported to the health care provider. Parents should be cautioned not to change the infant's formula without consulting the health care provider.

Bottles and nipples

Various brands and styles of bottles and nipples are available to parents. Most babies will feed well with any bottle and nipple. It is important that the bottles and nipples be washed in warm soapy water, using a bottle and nipple brush to facilitate thorough cleansing. Careful rinsing is necessary.

Boiling of bottles and nipples is not needed unless there is some question about the safety of the water supply.

Infant formulas

Commercial formulas. Because human milk is species specific to meet the needs of the human infant, it is used as the "gold standard" for all infant formulas. Commercial infant formulas are designed to resemble human milk as closely as possible, although none has ever duplicated it. The exact composition of infant formula varies with the manufacturer, but all must meet specific standards.

In an effort to make formula as similar to breast milk as possible, formula manufacturers have added a variety of ingredients including iron and nucleotides. Recently, manufacturers have added long-chain polyunsaturated fatty acids (LCPUFAs), consisting of arachidonic acid (ARA) and docosahexaenoic acid (DHA); the rationale for the addition of these substances is to enhance brain growth and retinal development. Research is ongoing to determine if, in fact, this is true (Morin, 2004). Other possible additives are currently under consideration such as probiotics to promote the development of fecal flora and enhance the intestinal immune response (Agostoni & Haschke, 2003; Institute of Medicine, 2004).

Infants who are not breastfed should be given commercial formulas. If this is too expensive, the family would likely be eligible for services through the WIC program, which provides iron-fortified commercial infant formula. Cow's milk is the basis for most infant formulas, although soy-based and other specialized formulas are available for the infant who cannot tolerate cow's milk. Parents should be encouraged to use infant formulas that are fortified with iron.

Commercial formulas are available in three forms: powder, concentrate, and ready-to-feed. All are equivalent in terms of nutritional content, but they vary considerably in cost.

- Powdered formula is the least expensive type. It is easily mixed by using one scoop for every 60 ml of water.
- Concentrated formula is more expensive than powder. It is diluted with equal parts of water and can be stored in the refrigerator for 48 hours after opening.
- Ready-to-feed formula is the most expensive but easiest to use. The desired amount is poured into the bottle. The opened can is safely refrigerated for 48 hours. This type of formula can be purchased in individual disposable bottles for the most convenient feeding.

Special formulas. Some infants have an allergic reaction to cow's milk formula. They may have diarrhea, rash, colic, or vomiting, and, in extreme cases, failure to thrive. Some of these infants may better tolerate a soy-milk formula; however, some may be allergic to soy protein. If hypersensitivity to cow's milk protein is suspected, a hydrolyzed casein formula may be recommended; however, special formulas are very expensive. Some women may be able to begin breastfeeding or, in life-threatening cases, obtain human milk through a milk bank, at least temporarily. Other special formulas are available for infants with a variety of disorders such as protein allergy, malabsorption syndromes, and inborn errors of metabolism.

CD: Critical Thinking Exercise—Formula Preparation

EVIDENCE-BASED PRACTICE
Hydrolyzed Protein Infant Formula for Prevention of Allergies

BACKGROUND

- Allergies are the specific immunoglobulin E (IgE) response to normally benign substances (allergens). Twenty percent of the population suffer from allergies, including allergic rhinitis (hay fever), asthma, eczema or atopic dermatitis, and food allergies. Half of all childhood asthma and 80% of all hay fever persists into adulthood. The risk of atopy (inherited allergy) is 33% if one parent has allergies and 70% if both parents are atopic. There is evidence that the longer the duration of exclusive breastfeeding, the less likely the baby will suffer childhood allergies. Food intolerance is an adverse reaction that is to the result of an enzyme error, irritation, toxicity, or pharmacologic effect. It is diagnosed when the cause is eliminated from the diet with subsequent symptom relief, and recurs with a challenge of the substance. Cow's milk allergy is often associated with exposure to cow's milk in the first month of life. Prevention of allergies can include maternal avoidance of allergens during pregnancy and lactation, and avoidance of infant sensitization to allergens. Cow's milk and soy milk infant formulas may have their allergenic properties decreased by partially or completely hydrolyzing the protein. This may decrease childhood allergies in vulnerable children.

OBJECTIVES

- The reviewers sought to compare allergy and food intolerance in infants fed hydrolyzed formula. Of interest was whether there was a difference among partially or completely hydrolyzed milk or soy formula, the most effective onset and duration of feeding, and the type of infant likely to benefit from hydrolyzed formula. The intervention was the hydrolyzed formula. The control group received human breast milk or cow's milk–based infant formula. The subjects were infants up to 6 months of age without evidence of allergy. The outcomes could include any type of diagnosed atopy (asthma, eczema, allergic rhinitis, and food allergy), food intolerance, growth parameters, cost, and infant refusal.

METHODS

Search Strategy

- The authors searched Cochrane, MEDLINE, CINAHL, EMBASE, references, and conferences. Search keywords were *infant, newborn, neonatal, pediatric, paediatric, plus feed, food, formula, hydrolysed, allergies, diet, protein,* and *milk.* Eighteen randomized or quasirandomized trials were included in the review, dated 1989 to 2001, representing 7453 infants. Countries were not always noted in the review, but included Canada, Belgium, The Netherlands, and the United Kingdom.

Statistical Analyses

- Similar data were pooled. Reviewers calculated relative risks for categoric data and weighted mean differences for continuous data, all with a 95% confidence interval. Results outside the confidence interval represent significant differences.

FINDINGS

- None of the trials compared the development of allergies in infants fed human milk with prolonged hydrolyzed formula-fed infants. Short-term hydrolyzed formula groups showed no significant difference in allergies with human milk–fed groups in two trials. In high risk infants, meta-analysis revealed a significant reduction in infant and childhood allergies, including asthma, eczema, allergic rhinitis, and cow's milk allergy in the hydrolyzed formula group when compared with the cow's milk–formula group. These benefits seem to persist at least until 5 years of age. When completely hydrolyzed formula was compared with partially hydrolyzed formula, the differences in allergy symptoms were equivocal. The reviewers found no adverse effects from hydrolyzed formulas, and no difference in weight gain or length at 6 months of age.

LIMITATIONS

- The trial criteria limited studies to less than a 10% loss to follow-up or dropout rate, which is a strength. Some trials were quasirandomized, limiting generalizability. Some trials did not address allocation concealment, suggesting the possibility of bias by the clinical allergy assessors. Several trials were sponsored by infant formula manufacturers, suggesting possible conflict of interest.

CONCLUSIONS

- For prevention of allergies and many other reasons, breast milk is still best. For high risk infants who cannot breastfeed, the prolonged use of hydrolyzed formula seems to be less allergenic than cow's milk formula. Partially hydrolyzed formula is more cost-effective than completely hydrolyzed formula, but evidence about their allergenic differences is inconclusive.

IMPLICATIONS FOR PRACTICE

- Breastfeeding should be encouraged, especially among infants at risk for allergies. When breastfeeding is not possible, hydrolyzed formula should be used.

IMPLICATIONS FOR FURTHER RESEARCH

- Much more research is needed about allergies beyond childhood. Cost, which was not addressed in these trials, can be a daily struggle for parents trying to provide the more expensive hydrolyzed formula. The question of the benefits of partially versus completely hydrolyzed formula persists.

Reference: Osborn, D., & Sinn, J. (2003). Formulas containing hydrolysed protein for prevention of allergy and food intolerance in infants (Cochrane Review). In *The Cochrane Library,* Issue 2, 2004. Chichester, UK: John Wiley & Sons.

Formulas for preterm infants contain higher calorie concentration (22 to 24 cal/oz) and higher concentrations of some nutrients such as protein, vitamin A, folic acid, and zinc (Morrow, 2004).

Evaporated milk. Although evaporated milk is concentrated and less expensive than commercial formula, the mixing of evaporated milk and water to feed a baby is no longer recommended because evaporated milk does not provide adequate nutrition for an infant.

Unmodified cow's milk. Unmodified cow's milk is not suited to the nutritional needs of the human infant in the first year of life. Specific concerns include the excessive amounts of calcium, phosphorus, and other minerals it contains; an imbalance of calcium and phosphorus; its excessive protein content; the poor absorption of the fat it contains; and its low iron concentration. In addition, its use in infants is apt to cause microscopic hemorrhages that lead to GI blood loss. This blood loss, as well as the low levels of iron in the milk, increases the likelihood of iron-deficiency anemia.

Formula preparation

The commercial infant formula must include directions for preparation and use with pictures and symbols for the benefit of persons who cannot read. Some manufacturers are translating the directions into various languages, such as Spanish, French, Vietnamese, Chinese, and Arabic to prevent misunderstanding and errors in formula preparation.

NURSE ALERT *It is important to impress on families that the proportions must not be altered—neither diluted to expand the amount of formula nor concentrated to provide more calories.*

Although manufacturers of commercial formula include directions for preparing their products, the nurse should review formula preparation with the parents. It is especially important that formula be mixed properly. The newborn's kidneys are immature, and giving the infant overly concentrated formula may provide protein and minerals in amounts that exceed the kidney's excretory ability. In contrast, if the formula is diluted too much (sometimes done in an effort to save money), the infant does not consume enough calories and does not grow well (Renfrew, Ansell, & Macleod, 2003).

Sterilization of formula rarely is recommended for those families with access to a safe public water supply. Instead, the formula is prepared with attention to cleanliness. When water from a private well is used, parents should be advised to contact the health department to have a chemical and bacteriologic analysis of the water done before using the water in formula preparation. The presence of nitrates, excess fluoride, or bacteria may be harmful to the infant.

If the sanitary conditions in the home appear unsafe, it would be better to recommend the use of ready-to-feed formula or to teach the mother to sterilize the formula. The two traditional methods for sterilization are terminal heating and the aseptic method. In the terminal-heating method, the prepared formula is placed in the bottles, which are topped with the nipples placed upside down and covered with the caps, and then sealed loosely with the rings. The bottles are then boiled together in a water bath for 25 minutes. In the aseptic method, the bottles, rings, caps, nipples, and any other necessary equipment, such as a funnel, are boiled separately, after which the formula is poured into the bottles. Any formula left in the bottle after the feeding should be discarded because the baby's saliva has mixed with it. Instructions for formula preparation and feeding are provided in the Teaching Guidelines box.

Vitamin and mineral supplementation

Commercial iron-fortified formula has all of the nutrients the infant needs for the first 6 months of life. After 6 months, the only mineral supplementation required is fluoride if the local water supply is not fluoridated.

Weaning

The bottle-fed infant will gradually learn to use a cup, and the parents will find that they are preparing fewer bottles. Often the bottle feeding before bedtime is the last one to remain. Babies have a strong need to suck, and the baby who has the bottle taken away too early or abruptly will compensate with nonnutritive sucking on his or her fingers, thumb, a pacifier, or even his or her own tongue. Weaning from a bottle should therefore be done gradually because the baby has learned to rely on the comfort that sucking provides.

Introducing solid foods

The infant receives the right balance of nutrients from breast milk or formula during the first 4 to 6 months. It is not true that the feeding of solids will help the infant sleep through the night. Cereal should not be put into the infant's bottle. Introduction of solid foods before the infant is 4 to 6 months of age may result in overfeeding and decreased intake of breast milk or formula. The infant cannot communicate feeling full as can an older child, who is able to turn the head away. The proper balance of carbohydrate, protein, and fat for an infant to grow properly is in the breast milk or formula.

The infant's individual growth pattern should help determine the right time to start solids. The primary health care provider will advise when to introduce solid foods. The schedule for introducing solid foods and the types of foods to serve will be discussed during well-baby supervision visits with the pediatrician or pediatric nurse practitioner.

TEACHING GUIDELINES
Formula Preparation and Feeding

FORMULA PREPARATION

- Wash your hands and clean the bottle, nipple, and can opener carefully before preparing formula.
- If new nipples seem too firm or stiff, they can be softened by boiling them in water for 5 minutes before use.
- Read the label on the container of formula and mix it exactly according to the directions.
- Use tap water to mix concentrated or powdered formula unless directed otherwise by your baby's physician or nurse.
- Test the size of the nipple hole by holding a prepared bottle upside down. The formula should drip from the nipple. If it runs in a stream, the hole is too big and should not be used. If it has to be shaken for the formula to come out, the hole is too small. You can either buy a new nipple or enlarge the hole by boiling the nipple for 5 minutes with a sewing needle inserted in the hole.
- If a nipple collapses when your baby sucks, loosen the nipple ring a little to let in air.
- Opened cans of ready-to-feed or concentrated formula should be covered and refrigerated. Any unused portions must be discarded after 48 hours.
- Bottles or cans of unopened formula can be stored at room temperature.
- If the formula is refrigerated, warm it by placing the bottle in a pan of hot water. Never use a microwave to warm any food to be given to a baby. Test the temperature of the formula by letting a few drops fall on the inside of your wrist. If the formula feels comfortably warm to you, it is the correct temperature.

FEEDING TECHNIQUES AND TIPS

- Newborns should be fed at least every 3 to 4 hours and should never go longer than 4 hours without feeding until a satisfactory pattern of weight gain is established. This may take 2 weeks. If a baby cries or fusses between feedings, check to see if the diaper should be changed, and if the baby needs to be picked up and cuddled. If the baby continues to cry and acts hungry, go ahead and feed. Babies do not get hungry on a regular schedule.
- Babies gradually increase the amount of milk they drink with each feeding. The first day or so, most newborns consume 15 to 30 ml (one-half to 1 ounce) with each feeding. This amount increases as the infant grows. If any formula remains in the bottle as the feeding ends, that milk must be thrown away, because saliva from the baby's mouth can cause the formula to spoil.
- It is a good idea to keep a feeding diary, writing down the amount of formula the baby drinks with each feeding for the first week or so. Also record the wet diapers and bowel movements the baby is having. Take this "diary" with you when you take the baby for the first pediatrician visit.
- For feeding, hold the baby close in a semireclining position. Talk to the baby during the feeding. This is a great time for social interaction and cuddling.
- Place the nipple in the baby's mouth on the tongue. It should touch the roof of the mouth to stimulate the baby's sucking reflex. Hold the bottle like a pencil. Keep the bottle tipped so that the nipple stays filled with milk and the baby does not suck in air.
- It is normal for babies to take a few sucks and then pause briefly before continuing to suck again. Some newborns take longer to feed than others. Be patient. It may be necessary to keep the baby awake and to encourage sucking. Moving the nipple gently in the baby's mouth may stimulate sucking.
- Newborns are apt to swallow air when sucking. Give the baby opportunities to burp several times during a feeding. As the baby gets older, you will know better when it is necessary to stop for burping.
- After the first 2 or 3 days, the stools of a formula-fed infant are yellow and soft, but formed. The baby may have a stool with each feeding in the first 2 weeks, although this may decrease to one or two stools each day.

SAFETY TIPS

- Babies should be held and never left alone while feeding. Never prop the bottle. The baby might inhale formula or choke on any that was spit up. Babies who fall asleep with a propped bottle of milk or juice may be prone to cavities when the first teeth come in.
- Know how to use the bulb syringe and how to help a baby who is choking.

COMMUNITY ACTIVITY

Explore the resources in your community for breastfeeding mothers after they are discharged from the hospital. Find out if there are lactation consultants in hospitals, pediatricians' offices, health departments, or in private practice who are accessible to mothers. What services are provided (e.g., phone consultations, one-on-one consultations)? Is there a charge to the patient for these services? Are there peer counselors for nursing mothers through the local WIC program? Are there nursing support groups in the community, such as La Leche League, where mothers can attend meetings to gain information and support? What supports are available for formula feeding mothers? Are there groups similar to the ones for breastfeeding mothers?

Key Points

- Human breast milk is species specific and is the recommended form of infant nutrition. It provides immunologic protection against many infections and diseases.
- Breast milk changes in composition with each stage of lactation, during each feeding, and as the infant grows.
- During the prenatal period, parents should be informed of the benefits of breastfeeding for infants, mothers, families, and society.
- Infants should be breastfed as soon as possible after birth and at least 8 to 12 times per day thereafter.
- Specific, measurable indicators show that the infant is breastfeeding effectively.

- Breast milk production is based on a supply-meets-demand principle: the more the infant nurses, the greater the milk supply.
- Commercial infant formulas provide satisfactory nutrition for most infants.
- All infants should be held for feedings.
- Parents should be instructed about the types of commercial infant formulas, proper preparation for feeding, and correct feeding technique.
- Solid foods should be started after age 4 to 6 months.
- Nurses must be knowledgeable about feeding methods and provide education and support for families.

Answers Guidelines to Critical Thinking Exercise

Breastfeeding: Engorgement and Nipple Soreness

1 Mary is experiencing a crisis that involves physical discomfort from engorged breasts and sore nipples, physical exhaustion from the demands of a fussy infant who is not sleeping well, frustration in being unable to successfully latch her baby on and provide milk to satisfy him, such that she is questioning her commitment to breastfeeding and considering formula for her infant.

2 a. This mother has experienced the onset of mature milk production at the expected time, approximately 3 days after birth. Her breasts are engorged, the tissues surrounding the milk glands and milk ducts are edematous, and the milk is not flowing well from the breasts because of the compression of the milk ducts. She is producing mature milk, but has a problem with milk transfer to the baby.

   b. The sore nipples are likely to be the result of a problem with latching the baby onto the breast. This most likely began during the first 2 days after birth and has grown more severe with the increased pressure in the breasts because of fullness, which tends to flatten the nipple and make it more difficult for the baby to latch on. She is experiencing pain with latch-on, which can inhibit her milk ejection or let-down reflex.

   c. The urinary output and number of stools are signs that the baby has not received sufficient feeding. After the milk has come in, from about the fourth day of life, the baby should have at least six to eight wet diapers and at least three or four bowel movements every 24 hours. His fussiness and lack of sleep are evidence that he is not being satisfied when he nurses; he is hungry and needs more milk to feel satiated.

   d. Mary's frustration, fatigue, and mental exhaustion are causing her to question her desire to breastfeed. She is tired and her breasts are painful. The discomfort intensifies when the baby tries to breastfeed on the very sore nipples. She may be wondering, is breastfeeding worth all this?

3 The major priority at this time is to feed the baby. He is at risk of becoming dehydrated because of inadequate intake. If the engorgement can be treated quickly, he may be able to breastfeed. Otherwise, he needs to be fed some infant formula via syringe or slow flow bottle until she can express milk or get him to nurse. Mary needs help with her engorgement; ice packs can be applied to the breasts for 20 minutes to help reduce the tissue swelling. She can also take an anti-inflammatory medication such as ibuprofen. After the ice is applied, Mary can use a hospital grade electric breast pump to try to express milk to begin softening the breasts. Even with the pumping of just a half ounce or so, the nipples may soften enough for the baby to latch on and continue softening the breasts. Ideally, the infant will latch on and the milk will flow sufficiently to provide him with enough milk to feel satisfied and to allow Mary's breasts to feel more comfortable. If the ice and pumping do not result in milk flow, cabbage leaves may be used on the breasts for 20 minutes, followed by pumping. The cracked, sore nipples need to be treated. Hydrogel pads can be applied after feeding or pumping. If the nipples are too uncomfortable for the baby to nurse, Mary may pump her breasts with an electric breast pump for 24 hours to allow the nipples some time to begin healing; the expressed breast milk can be syringe fed or fed with a slow flow nipple or bottle. As the nipples improve, the baby can be gradually reintroduced to the breast, with a nurse or lactation consultant assisting Mary with proper latch-on technique.

Mary needs emotional support at this time. The nurse can provide her an opportunity to express her frustrations and concerns. It is important that Mary is aware that what she is experiencing is not uncommon; the breasts of many women become engorged. It is a temporary condition, usually lasting no more than 24 to 48 hours. She may be feeling as if she is failing as a mother. Empathetic concern from the nurse can help to boost Mary's self-esteem and increase her confidence as a mother.

4 Yes, according to the AAP (2005) guidelines for breastfeeding, the infant is not receiving adequate feedings. Mary is experiencing primary engorgement, a common problem that is temporary and should resolve with appropriate interventions.

5 Mary could have a history of breast surgery, in which case the milk ducts may have been severed, and there is no outlet for the milk to be emptied from the breasts. The baby may be the source of the latch problem because of some physical characteristic such as a tight frenulum ("tongue-tied"). The baby needs to be assessed to determine if there are factors that may inhibit successful latch-on. In addition, Mary may be lacking in her commitment to breastfeed and may be looking for an excuse to stop. In her mind, the difficulties she is experiencing may provide her with enough reason to switch to formula.

Resources

American Academy of Pediatrics (AAP)
141 Northwest Point Blvd.
Elk Grove Village, IL 60007-1098
800-422-4784
www.aap.org

The Breastfeeding and Human Lactation Study Center
University of Rochester School of Medicine and Dentistry
Department of Pediatrics, Box 777
601 Elmwood Ave.
Rochester, NY 14642
716-275-0088
716-461-3614 (fax)

Breastfeeding resources
www.parentsplace.com/expert/lactation/

Bright Future Lactation Resource Centre
www.bflrc.com

Dr. Thomas Hale (medications and breastfeeding)
neonatal.ttuhsc.edu/lact/

International Lactation Consultant Association (ILCA)
4101 Lake Boone Trail, Suite 201
Raleigh, NC 27607
919-787-5181
919-787-4916 (fax)
www.ilca.org

Journal of Human Lactation
Sage Publications
2455 Teller Rd.
Thousand Oaks, CA 91320
805-499-9774
805-375-1700
www.sagepub.com

Lact-Aid (provides information and services to promote
   breastfeeding)
P.O. Box 1066
Athens, TN 37303
614-744-9090

La Leche League
1400 N. Meacham Rd.
Schaumburg, IL 60168-4079
800-525-3243 (24-hour line)
www.lalecheleague.org

Lactation Education Resources
www.leron-line.com

Human Milk Banking Association of North America
1500 Sunday Drive
Suite 102
Raleigh, NC 27607
919 861 4530
919 787-4916 (FAX)
www.hmbana.org

Mothers' Milk Banks

Lactation Support Service
   Children's and Women's Milk Bank
   British Columbia Children's Hospital
   Vancouver, British Columbia, Canada V6H 3V4
   604-875-2345, ext. 7607

Mothers' Milk Bank
Presbyterian/St. Luke's Medical Center
Denver, CO 80218
303-869-1888

Mothers' Milk Bank
Valley Medical Center
San Jose, CA 95128
408-998-4550

Mothers' Milk Bank
WakeMed
3000 New Bern Ave.
Raleigh, NC 27610
919-350-8599
919-350-8923 (fax)

Special Care Nursery Mothers' Milk Bank
Christiana Care Health Services
4755 Ogletown Stanton Rd.
P.O. Box 6001
Newark, DE 19718
302-733-2340

Nursing Mothers Advisory Council
www.nursingmoms.net
E-mail: nmac@phillyburbs.com

Special Supplemental Nutrition Program for Women, Infants, and
   Children (WIC)
Food and Consumer Service
3103 Park Center Dr., Room 819
Alexandria, VA 22302
703-305-2286

References

Abbott Laboratories. (2003). *New data show U.S. breastfeeding rates at all-time recorded high.* News release, 11/25/03, Abbott Park, IL: Ross Products Division.

Agostoni, C., & Haschke, F. (2003). Infant formulas: Recent developments and new issues. *Minerva Pediatrics, 55*(3), 181-194.

American Academy of Pediatrics (AAP). (1998). *Pediatric nutrition handbook* (4th ed.). Elk Grove Village, IL: AAP.

American Academy of Pediatrics Section on Breastfeeding (AAP). (2005). Breastfeeding and the use of human milk, Policy Statement. *Pediatrics, 115*(23) 496-506.

Amir, L., & Donath, S. (2003). Does maternal smoking have a negative physiological effect on breastfeeding? The epidemiological evidence. *Breastfeeding Review, 11*(2), 19-29.

Association of Women's Health, Obstetric, and Neonatal Nurses (AWHONN). (1998). *Standards and guidelines for professional nursing practice in the care of women and newborns* (5th ed.). Washington, DC: AWHONN.

Bachrach, V., Schwarz, E., & Bachrach, L. (2003). Breastfeeding and the risk of hospitalization for respiratory disease in infancy. *Archives of Pediatric and Adolescent Medicine, 157*(3), 237-243.

Birch, L., & Davison, K. (2001). Family environmental factors influencing the developing behavioral controls of food intake and childhood overweight. *Pediatric Clinics of North America, 48*(4), 893-907.

Borghese-Lang, T., Morrison, L., Ogle, A., & Wright, A. (2003). Successful bottle feeding of the young infant. *Journal of Pediatric Health Care, 17*(2), 94-101.

Eglash, A., Chantry, C., & Howard, C. (2004). *Protocol #8: Human milk storage information for home use for healthy term infants.* The Academy of Breastfeeding Medicine. Available at http://www.abm.org. (Accessed 9/11/2005).

Gartner, L., Morton, J., Lawrence, R., Naylor, A., O'Hare, D., Schanler, R., & Eidelman, R. (2005). Breastfeeding and the use of human milk. *Pediatrics, 115*(2), 496-506.

Griffiths, D. (2004). Do tongue ties affect breastfeeding? *Journal of Human Lactation, 20*(4), 409-414.

Hale, T. (2004). Maternal medications during breastfeeding. *Clinical Obstetrics and Gynecology, 47*(3), 696-711.

Hale, T., & Berens, P. (2002). *Clinical therapy in breastfeeding patients.* Amarillo, TX: Pharmasoft Publishing.

Holman, D., & Grimes, M. (2003). Patterns for the initiation of breastfeeding in humans. *American Journal of Human Biology, 15*(6), 765-780.

Hoover, K. (2001). Yeast infections of the nipples and breasts. *Medela Messenger, 18*(3), 11-12.

Houghton, M. (2001). Breastfeeding practices of Native-American mothers participating in WIC. *Journal of the American Dietetic Association, 101*(2), 245-247.

Howard, C., Howard, F., Lanphear, B., Eberly, S., deBlieck, E., Oakes, D., & Lawrence, R. (2003). Randomized clinical trial of pacifier use and bottle-feeding or cupfeeding and their effect on breastfeeding. *Pediatrics, 111*(3), 511-518.

Institute of Medicine. (2004). *Infant formula: Evaluating the safety of new ingredients.* Washington, DC: National Academies Press.

International Lactation Consultant Association (ILCA). (1999). *Evidence-based guidelines for breastfeeding management during the first fourteen days.* Raleigh, NC: ILCA.

Kliegman, R. (2002). Fetal and neonatal medicine. In R. Behrman & R. Kliegman (Eds.), *Nelson essentials of pediatrics* (4th ed.). Philadelphia: Saunders.

Kline, M., Boyle, R., Futterman, D., Havens, P., Henry-Reid, L., King, S., & Read, J. (2003). Human milk, breastfeeding, and transmission of human immunodeficiency virus type 1 in the United States. *Pediatrics, 112*(5), 1196-1205.

Larson-Meyer, D. (2002). Effect of postpartum exercise on mothers and their offspring: A review of the literature. *Obstetric Research, 10*, 841-853.

Lawrence, R., & Lawrence, R. (2005). *Breastfeeding: A guide for the medical profession* (6th ed.). St. Louis: Mosby.

Lefeber, Y., & Voorhoeve, H. (1999). Indigenous first feeding practices in newborn babies. *Midwifery, 15*(2), 97-100.

Mass, S. (2004). Breast pain: Engorgement, nipple pain, and mastitis. *Clinical Obstetrics and Gynecology, 47*(3), 676-682.

Messner, A., Lalakea, M., Aby, J., Macmahon, J., & Bair, E. (2000). Ankyloglossia: Incidence and associated feeding difficulties. *Archives of Otolaryngology: Head and Neck Surgery, 126*(1), 36-39.

Morin, K. (2004). Current thoughts on healthy term infant nutrition: The first twelve months. *MCN American Journal of Maternal Child Nursing, 29*(5), 312-317.

Morrow, A. (2004). Choosing an infant or pediatric formula. *Journal of Pediatric Health Care, 18*(1), 49-52.

Morrow, A., Ruiz-Palacios, M., Altaye, M., Jiang, X. et al. (2004). Human milk oligosaccharides are associated with protection against diarrhea in breast-fed infants. *Journal of Pediatrics, 145*(3), 297-303.

Morse, J., Jehle, C., & Gamble, D. (1990). Initiating breastfeeding: A world survey of the timing of postpartum breastfeeding. *International Journal of Nursing Studies, 27*(3), 303-313.

Newman, J. (1995). How breast milk protects newborns. *Scientific American, 273*(6), 76-79.

Osborn, D., & Sinn, J. (2003). Formulas containing hydrolysed protein for prevention of allergy and food intolerance in infants (Cochrane Review). In *The Cochrane Library,* Issue 2, 2004. Chichester, UK: John Wiley & Sons.

Osterman, K., & Rahm, V. (2000). Lactation mastitis: Bacterial cultivation of breast milk, symptoms, treatment, and outcome. *Journal of Human Lactation, 16*(4), 297-302.

Pollock, C., Bustamante-Forest, R., & Giarrantano, G. (2002). Men of diverse cultures: Knowledge and attitudes about breastfeeding. *Journal of Obstetric, Gynecologic, and Neonatal Nursing, 31*(6), 673-679.

Preedy, V., Grimble, G., & Watson, R. (2001). *Nutrition in the infant.* London: Greenwich Medical Media.

Renfrew, M., Ansell, P., & Macleod, K. (2003). Formula feed preparation: Helping reduce the risks; a systematic review. *Archives of Diseases in Childhood, 88*(10), 855-858.

Riordan, J. (2005). *Breastfeeding and human lactation* (3rd ed.). Boston: Jones & Bartlett.

Ryan, A., Wenjun, Z., & Acosta, A. (2002). Breastfeeding continues to increase into the new millennium. *Pediatrics, 110*(6), 1103-1109.

Tershakovec, A., & Stallings, V. (2002). Pediatric nutrition and nutritional disorders. In R. Behrman & R. Kliegman (Eds.), *Nelson essentials of pediatrics* (4th ed.). Philadelphia: Saunders.

Uauy, R., & Araya, M. (2004). Novel oligosaccharides in human milk: Understanding mechanisms may lead to better prevention of enteric and other infections. *Journal of Pediatrics, 145*(3), 283-285.

U.S. Department of Health and Human Services. (2000). *Healthy People 2010.* (Conference edition) (Vol. 2). Washington, DC: Department of Health and Human Services. Internet document available at www.health.gov/healthypeople/document/ default.htm.

Ward, R., Bates, B., Benitz, W., Burchfield, D., Ring, J. et al. (2001). The transfer of drugs and other chemicals into human milk. *Pediatrics, 108*(3), 776-789.

Weissinger, D. (1998). A breastfeeding teaching tool using a sandwich analogy for latch-on. *Journal of Human Lactation, 14*(1), 51-56.

Ziegler, E., Fomon, S., & Carlson, S. (2003). The term infant. In W. Walker, J. Watkins, & C. Duggan (Eds.), *Nutrition in pediatrics* (3rd ed.). London: BC Decker.

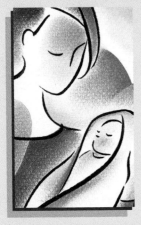

CHAPTER *21*

Assessment for Risk Factors

DEITRA LEONARD LOWDERMILK

LEARNING OBJECTIVES

- *Explore physiologic and psychologic aspects of high risk pregnancy.*
- *Discuss regionalization of health care services.*
- *Examine risk factors identified through history, physical examination, and diagnostic techniques.*
- *Differentiate among diagnostic techniques, including when they are used in pregnancy and for what purposes.*
- *Develop a teaching plan to explain diagnostic techniques and implications of findings to patients and their families.*

KEY TERMS AND DEFINITIONS

acoustic stimulation test Antepartum test to elicit fetal heart rate response to sound; performed by applying sound source (laryngeal stimulator) to maternal abdomen over the fetal head

alpha-fetoprotein (AFP) Fetal antigen; elevated levels in amniotic fluid and maternal blood are associated with neural tube defects

amniocentesis Procedure in which a needle is inserted through the abdominal and uterine walls to obtain amniotic fluid; used for assessment of fetal health and maturity

amniotic fluid index (AFI) Estimation of amount of amniotic fluid by means of ultrasound to determine excess or decrease

biophysical profile (BPP) Noninvasive assessment of the fetus and its environment using ultrasonography and fetal monitoring; includes fetal breathing movements, gross body movements, fetal tone, reactive fetal heart rate, and qualitative amniotic fluid volume

chorionic villus sampling (CVS) Removal of fetal tissue from placenta for genetic diagnostic studies

contraction stress test (CST) Test to stimulate uterine contractions for the purpose of assessing fetal response; a healthy fetus does not react to contractions, whereas a compromised fetus

demonstrates late decelerations in the fetal heart rate that are indicative of uteroplacental insufficiency

daily fetal movement count (DFMC) Maternal assessment of fetal activity; the number of fetal movements within a specified time are counted; also called "kick count"

Doppler blood flow analysis Use of ultrasound for noninvasive measurement of blood flow in the fetus and placenta

magnetic resonance imaging (MRI) Noninvasive nuclear procedure for imaging tissues with high fat and water content; in obstetrics, uses include evaluation of fetal structures, placenta, and amniotic fluid volume

nonstress test (NST) Evaluation of fetal response (fetal heart rate) to natural contractile uterine activity or to an increase in fetal activity

percutaneous umbilical blood sampling (PUBS) Procedure during which a fetal umbilical vessel is accessed for blood sampling or for transfusions

uteroplacental insufficiency (UPI) Decline in placental function (exchange of gases, nutrients, and wastes) leading to fetal hypoxia and acidosis; evidenced by late decelerations of the fetal heart rate in response to uterine contractions

ELECTRONIC RESOURCES

Additional information related to the content in Chapter 21 can be found on

the companion website at **evolve**
http://evolve.elsevier.com/Lowdermilk/Maternity/
- NCLEX Review Questions
- WebLinks

or on the interactive companion CD
- NCLEX Review Questions

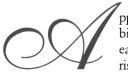pproximately 500,000 of the 4 million births that occur in the United States each year will be categorized as high risk because of maternal or fetal complications. Identification of the risks, together with appropriate and timely intervention during the perinatal period, can prevent morbidity and mortality among mothers and infants.

With the changing demographics in the United States, more women and families can be identified as at risk because of factors other than biophysical criteria. The increasing numbers of homeless, single, or uninsured pregnant women who have no access to prenatal care during any stage of pregnancy and the behaviors and lifestyles that pose a risk to the health of the mother and fetus contribute to the problem (U.S. Department of Health and Human Services [USDHHS], 2000).

Care of these high risk patients requires the unified efforts of medical and nursing personnel. The high risk patient and the factors associated with a diagnosis of high risk are identified in this chapter; diagnostic techniques used to monitor the maternal-fetal unit are emphasized.

DEFINITION AND SCOPE OF THE PROBLEM

A high risk pregnancy is one in which the life or health of the mother or fetus is jeopardized by a disorder coincidental with or unique to pregnancy. For the mother, the high risk status arbitrarily extends through the puerperium (30 days after childbirth). Postbirth maternal complications are usually resolved within 1 month of birth, but perinatal morbidity may continue for months or years.

High risk pregnancy is a critical problem for modern medical and nursing care. The new social emphasis on the quality of life and the wanted child has resulted in a reduction of family size and the number of unwanted pregnancies. At the same time, technologic advances have facilitated pregnancies in previously infertile couples. As a consequence, emphasis is on the safe birth of normal infants who can develop to their potential. Scientific and technologic advances have allowed perinatal health care to reach a level far beyond that previously available.

The diagnosis of high risk imposes a situational crisis on the family (e.g., loss of pregnancy before the anticipated date, development of gestational diabetes mellitus with its potential complications, or birth of a neonate who does not meet cultural, societal, or familial norms and expectations).

Maternal Health Problems

The leading causes of maternal death attributable to pregnancy differ over the world. In general, three major causes have persisted for the last 50 years: hypertensive disorders, infection, and hemorrhage. The three leading causes of maternal mortality today are gestational hypertension, pulmonary embolism, and hemorrhage. Factors that are strongly related to maternal death include age (younger than 20 years and 35 years or older), lack of prenatal care, low educational attainment, unmarried status, and nonwhite race. African-American maternal mortality rates are more than three times higher than those for Caucasian women (Kochanek, Murphy, Anderson, & Scott, 2004). Reaching the goal set by *Healthy People 2010* of no more than 3.3 maternal deaths per 100,000 live births (USDHHS, 2000) will be a significant challenge.

Although the overall number of maternal deaths is small, maternal mortality remains a significant problem because a high proportion of deaths are preventable, primarily through improving the access to and use of prenatal care services. Nurses can be instrumental in educating the public about the importance of obtaining early and regular care during pregnancy.

Fetal and Neonatal Health Problems

The leading cause of death in the neonatal period is congenital anomalies (Arias, MacDorman, Strobino, & Guyer, 2003). Other causes of neonatal death include disorders related to short gestation and low birth weight, sudden infant death, respiratory distress syndrome, and the effects of maternal complications. Racial differences in the infant mortality rates continue to challenge public health experts. Increased rates of survival during the neonatal period have resulted largely from high quality prenatal care and the improvement in perinatal services, including technologic advances in neonatal intensive care and obstetrics.

What can be done to prevent antepartum fetal deaths? Some factors are presumed avoidable, such as failure to respond appropriately to abnormalities of pregnancy and labor. Such abnormalities may include results of fetal growth or fetal well-being assessments, significant maternal weight loss, or decreased fetal movements (Druzin, Gabbe, & Reed, 2002). In addition, commitment at national, state, and local levels is required to reduce the infant mortality rate. More research is needed to identify the extent to which financial, educational, sociocultural, and behavioral factors individually and collectively affect perinatal morbidity and mortality. Barriers to care must be removed and perinatal services modified to meet contemporary health care needs.

Regionalization of Health Care Services

Early and ongoing risk assessment is a crucial component of perinatal care. Conditions associated with perinatal morbidity and mortality can be prevented, treated, or referred to more skilled health care providers. Factors to consider when determining a patient's risk status include resources available locally to treat the condition, availability of appropriate facilities for transport if needed, and determination of the best match for the patient's needs.

Not all facilities develop and maintain the full spectrum of services required for high risk perinatal patients. As a consequence, regionalization of hospital-based perinatal health care services—facilities within a geographic region organized to provide different levels of care—emerged. This system of coordinated care was also applied to preconception and ambulatory prenatal care services.

Guidelines have been established regarding the level of care that could be expected at any given facility. In ambulatory settings, providers must distinguish themselves by the level of care they provide. *Basic care* is provided by obstetricians, family physicians, certified nurse-midwives, and other advanced practice clinicians approved by local governance. Routine risk-oriented prenatal care, education, and support is provided. Providers offering *specialty care* are obstetricians who must provide fetal diagnostic testing and management of obstetric and medical complications in addition to basic care. *Subspecialty care* is provided by maternal-fetal medicine specialists and includes the aforementioned in addition to genetic testing, advanced fetal therapies, and management of severe maternal and fetal complications (American Academy of Pediatrics [AAP] & American College of Obstetricians and Gynecologists [ACOG], 2002).

In hospital settings, perinatal services also are designated as basic, specialty, or subspecialty. Criteria for basic perinatal services include care of all patients admitted to the service, with an established triage system for high risk patients who should be transferred to a higher level of care; ability to perform a cesarean birth within 30 minutes of a decision to do so; availability of blood and blood products; availability of radiology, anesthesia, and laboratory services on a 24-hour basis; presence of nursery and postpartum care; resuscitation and stabilization of all neonates born in the hospital; availability of transport for all sick neonates; family visitation; and data collection and retrieval (AAP & ACOG, 2002).

Specialty hospital care includes these requirements in addition to care of high risk mothers and fetuses, stabilization of ill neonates before transfer, and care of preterm infants with a birth weight of 1500 g or more. Women in preterm labor or those with impending births at 32 weeks of gestation or less should be transferred for subspecialty care. Additional criteria for subspecialty care include provision of comprehensive perinatal care for women and infants of all risk categories, evaluation and use of new high risk technologies and therapies, and data collection and retrieval. Collaboration among providers to meet the patient's needs is the key in reducing perinatal morbidity and mortality (AAP & ACOG, 2002).

Assessment of Risk Factors

Pregnancies can be designated as high risk for any of several undesirable outcomes. Those considered to be at risk for **uteroplacental insufficiency** (UPI; the gradual decline in delivery of needed substances by the placenta to the fetus) carry a serious threat for fetal growth restriction, intrauterine fetal death, intrapartum death, intrapartum fetal distress, and various types of neonatal morbidity.

In the past, risk factors were evaluated only from a medical viewpoint; therefore only adverse medical, obstetric, or physiologic conditions were considered to place the woman at risk. Today, a more comprehensive approach to high risk pregnancy is used, and the factors associated with

GUIDELINES/GUÍAS
High Risk Factors

HIGH RISK ASSESSMENT	POTENTIAL PROBLEM
• Have you had any problems with this pregnancy? • ¿Ha tenido problemas con este embarazo?	General assessment
• Have you had blurred vision? • ¿Ha tenido visión borrosa?	Preeclampsia
• Have you had severe headaches? • ¿Ha tenido dolores fuertes de cabeza?	Preeclampsia
• Have you had difficulty breathing? • ¿Ha tenido dificultad para respirar?	Cardiac disease
• Have you had heart palpitations? • ¿Ha tenido palpitaciones del corazón?	Cardiac disease
• Have you been vomiting? • ¿Ha tenido vómitos?	Hyperemesis gravidarum
• Have you had any infections? • ¿Ha tenido alguna infección?	Sexually transmitted infections or vaginal infections
• Have you had swelling? • ¿Ha tenido hinchazón?	Preeclampsia
• Were all your pregnancies term? • ¿Llegaron a las cuarenta semanas todos sus embarazos?	Preterm labor
• Have you ever had diabetes? • ¿Ha tenido diabetes?	Diabetes
• Have you ever had high blood pressure? • ¿Ha tenido alta presión sanguínea?	Gestational hypertension/ Chronic hypertension
• Have you ever had anemia? • ¿Ha estado anémica?	Anemia
• Do you take drugs? Prescription medicine? • ¿Usa drogas? ¿Medicina recetada?	Substance abuse
• Do you drink alcohol? Smoke? • ¿Toma bebidas alcohólicas? ¿Fuma?	Substance abuse

high risk childbearing are grouped into broad categories based on threats to health and pregnancy outcome (see Guidelines/Guías box). Categories of risk are biophysical,

BOX 21-1

Categories of High Risk Factors

BIOPHYSICAL FACTORS

- *Genetic considerations.* Genetic factors may interfere with normal fetal or neonatal development, result in congenital anomalies, or create difficulties for the mother. These factors include defective genes, transmissible inherited disorders and chromosomal anomalies, multiple pregnancy, large fetal size, and ABO incompatibility.
- *Nutritional status.* Adequate nutrition, without which fetal growth and development cannot proceed normally, is one of the most important determinants of pregnancy outcome. Conditions that influence nutritional status include the following: young age; three pregnancies in the previous 2 years; tobacco, alcohol, or drug use; inadequate dietary intake because of chronic illness or food fads; inadequate or excessive weight gain; and hematocrit value less than 33%.
- *Medical and obstetric disorders.* Complications of current and past pregnancies, obstetric-related illnesses, and pregnancy losses put the patient at risk (see Box 21-2).

PSYCHOSOCIAL FACTORS

- *Smoking.* A strong, consistent, causal relation has been established between maternal smoking and reduced birth weight. Risks include low-birth-weight infants, higher neonatal mortality rates, increased miscarriages, and increased incidence of premature rupture of membranes. These risks are aggravated by low socioeconomic status, poor nutritional status, and concurrent use of alcohol.
- *Caffeine.* Birth defects in humans have not been related to caffeine consumption. High intake (three or more cups of coffee per day) has been related to a slight decrease in birth weight.
- *Alcohol.* Although its exact effects in pregnancy have not been quantified and its mode of action is largely unexplained, alcohol exerts adverse effects on the fetus, resulting in fetal alcohol syndrome, fetal alcohol effects, learning disabilities, and hyperactivity.
- *Drugs.* The developing fetus may be adversely affected by drugs through several mechanisms. They can be teratogenic, cause metabolic disturbances, produce chemical effects, or cause depression or alteration of central nervous system function. This category includes medications prescribed by a health care provider or bought over the counter, as well as commonly abused drugs such as heroin, cocaine, and marijuana. (See Chapter 22 for more information about drug and alcohol abuse.)
- *Psychologic status.* Childbearing triggers profound and complex physiologic, psychologic, and social changes, with evidence to suggest a relation between emotional distress and birth complications. This risk factor includes conditions such as specific intrapsychic disturbances and addictive lifestyles; a history of child or spouse abuse; inadequate support systems; family disruption or dissolution; maternal role changes or conflicts; noncompliance with cultural norms; unsafe cultural, ethnic, or religious practices; and situational crises.

SOCIODEMOGRAPHIC FACTORS

- *Low income.* Poverty underlies many other risk factors and leads to inadequate financial resources for food and prenatal care, poor general health, increased risk of medical complications of pregnancy, and greater prevalence of adverse environmental influences.
- *Lack of prenatal care.* Failure to diagnose and treat complications early is a major risk factor arising from financial barriers or lack of access to care; depersonalization of the system resulting in long waits, routine visits, variability in health care personnel, and unpleasant physical surroundings; lack of understanding of the need for early and continued care or cultural beliefs that do not support the need; and fear of the health care system and its providers.
- *Age.* Women at both ends of the childbearing age spectrum have a higher incidence of poor outcomes; however, age may not be a risk factor in all cases. Both physiologic and psychologic risks should be evaluated.
  a. *Adolescents.* More complications are seen in young mothers (younger than 15 years), who have a 60% higher mortality rate than those older than 20 years, and in pregnancies occurring less than 6 years after menarche. Complications include anemia, preeclampsia, prolonged labor, and contracted pelvis and cephalopelvic disproportion. Long-term social implications of early motherhood are lower educational status, lower income, increased dependence on government support programs, higher divorce rates, and higher parity.
  b. *Mature mothers.* The risks to older mothers are not from age alone but from other considerations such as number and spacing of previous pregnancies; genetic disposition of the parents; and medical history, lifestyle, nutrition, and prenatal care. The increased likelihood of chronic diseases and complications that arises from more invasive medical management of a pregnancy and labor combined with demographic characteristics put an older woman at risk. Medical conditions more likely to be experienced by mature women include hypertension and preeclampsia, diabetes, extended labor, cesarean birth, placenta previa, abruptio placentae, and mortality. Her fetus is at greater risk for low birth weight and macrosomia, chromosomal abnormalities, congenital malformations, and neonatal mortality.
- *Parity.* The number of previous pregnancies is a risk factor associated with age and includes all first pregnancies, especially a first pregnancy at either end of the childbearing age continuum. The incidence of preeclampsia and dystocia is higher with a first birth.
- *Marital status.* The increased mortality and morbidity rates for unmarried women, including a greater risk for preeclampsia, are often related to inadequate prenatal care and a younger childbearing age.
- *Residence.* The availability and quality of prenatal care varies widely with geographic residence. Women in metropolitan areas have more prenatal visits than do those in rural areas, who have fewer opportunities for

Continued

Categories of High Risk Factors—cont'd

SOCIODEMOGRAPHIC FACTORS–cont'd

specialized care and consequently a higher incidence of maternal mortality. Health care in the inner city, where residents are usually poorer and begin childbearing earlier and continue for longer, may be of lower quality than in a more affluent neighborhood.

- *Ethnicity.* Although ethnicity by itself is not a major risk, race is an indicator of other sociodemographic risk factors. Nonwhite women are more than 3 times as likely as Caucasian women to die of pregnancy-related causes. African-American babies have the highest rates of prematurity and low birth weight, with the infant mortality rate among African-Americans being more than double that among Caucasians.

ENVIRONMENTAL FACTORS

- Various environmental substances can affect fertility and fetal development, the chance of a live birth, and the child's subsequent mental and physical development. Environmental influences include infections, radiation, chemicals such as pesticides, therapeutic drugs, illicit drugs, industrial pollutants, cigarette smoke, stress, and diet. Paternal exposure to mutagenic agents in the workplace has been associated with an increased risk of miscarriage.

psychosocial, sociodemographic, and environmental (Gilbert & Harmon, 2003) (Box 21-1).

Biophysical risks include factors that originate within the mother or fetus and affect the development or functioning of either one or both. Examples include genetic disorders, nutritional and general health status, and medical or obstetric-related illnesses.

Psychosocial risks consist of maternal behaviors and adverse lifestyles that have a negative effect on the health of the mother or fetus. These risks may include emotional distress and disturbed interpersonal relationships, as well as inadequate social support and unsafe cultural practices.

Sociodemographic risks arise from the mother and her family. These risks may place the mother and fetus at risk. Examples include lack of prenatal care, low income, marital status, and ethnicity (see Box 21-1). Environmental factors include hazards in the workplace and the woman's general environment and may include environmental chemicals (e.g., pesticides, lead, and mercury), radiation, and pollutants (Silbergeld & Patrick, 2005).

Risk factors are interrelated and cumulative in their effects. Box 21-2 lists specific pregnancy problems and risk factors. Risk factors for the postpartum woman and newborn are shown in Box 21-3.

The development of a comprehensive database for pregnancy risk assessment will help generate appropriate nursing diagnoses. For example, use of functional health patterns can be the basis for an assessment tool (Box 21-4).

ANTEPARTUM TESTING: BIOPHYSICAL ASSESSMENT

The major expected outcome of all antepartum testing is the detection of potential fetal compromise. Ideally the technique used identifies fetal compromise before intrauterine asphyxia of the fetus so that the health care provider can take measures to prevent or minimize adverse perinatal outcomes. No single test can provide this information. Assessment tests should be selected based on their effectiveness, and the results must be interpreted in light of the complete clinical picture. The most reliable evidence for effectiveness is provided by randomized controlled trials. Nurses can be informed about the most recent research on fetal assessment by using an up-to-date systematic review such as the Cochrane Database of Systematic Reviews (Enkin et al., 2001). Table 21-1 lists the evidence for recommending care for fetal assessment screening based on this database.

Daily Fetal Movement Count

Assessment of fetal activity by the mother is a simple yet valuable method for monitoring the condition of the fetus. The **daily fetal movement count (DFMC)** (also called "kick counts") can be done at home, is noninvasive, is simple to understand, and usually does not interfere with a daily routine. The DMFC is frequently used to monitor the fetus in pregnancies complicated by conditions that may affect fetal oxygenation. These conditions include but are not limited to gestational hypertension or chronic hypertension and diabetes. The presence of movements is generally a reassuring sign of fetal health.

Several protocols are used for counting. One recommendation is to count once a day for 60 minutes and another common recommendation is that mothers count fetal activity two or three times daily for 60 minutes each time. Except for establishing a very low number of daily fetal movements or a trend toward decreased motion, the clinical value of the absolute number of fetal movements has not been established, except in the situation in which fetal movements cease entirely for 12 hours (the so-called *fetal alarm signal*). A count of fewer than three fetal movements within 1 hour warrants further evaluation by a nonstress test (NST) or contraction stress test (CST), biophysical profile (BPP), or a combination of these (see later discussion). Women should be taught the significance of the presence and/or absence of fetal movements, the procedure for counting that is to be used, how to record findings on a DFM record, and when to notify the health care provider.

BOX 21-2

Specific Pregnancy Problems and Related Risk Factors

PRETERM LABOR
Age younger than 16 or older than 35 years
Low socioeconomic status
Maternal weight below 50 kg
Poor nutrition
Previous preterm birth
Incompetent cervix
Uterine anomalies
Smoking
Drug addiction and alcohol abuse
Pyelonephritis, pneumonia
Multiple gestation
Anemia
Abnormal fetal presentation
Preterm rupture of membranes
Placental abnormalities
Infection
Abdominal surgery in current pregnancy
History of cervical surgery

POLYHYDRAMNIOS
Diabetes mellitus
Multiple gestation
Fetal congenital anomalies
Isoimmunization (Rh or ABO)
Nonimmune hydrops
Abnormal fetal presentation

INTRAUTERINE GROWTH RESTRICTION (IUGR)
Multiple gestation
Poor nutrition

Maternal cyanotic heart disease
Prior pregnancy with IUGR
Maternal collagen diseases
Chronic hypertension
Preeclampsia
Recurrent antepartum hemorrhage
Smoking
Maternal diabetes with vascular problems
Fetal infections
Fetal cardiovascular anomalies
Drug addiction and alcohol abuse
Fetal congenital anomalies
Hemoglobinopathies

OLIGOHYDRAMNIOS
Renal agenesis (Potter's syndrome)
Prolonged rupture of membranes
IUGR
Intrauterine fetal death

POSTTERM PREGNANCY
Anencephaly
Placental sulfatase deficiency
Perinatal hypoxia, acidosis
Placental insufficiency

CHROMOSOMAL ABNORMALITIES
Maternal age 35 years or older
Balanced translocation (maternal and paternal)

Reference: Gillem-Goldstein, J. et al. (2003). Methods of assessment for pregnancy at risk. In A. DeCherney, A., & L. Nathan (Eds.), *Current obstetric and gynecologic diagnosis and treatment* (9th ed.). New York: Lange Medical Books/McGraw-Hill.

BOX 21-3

Factors That Place the Postpartum Woman and Neonate at High Risk

MOTHER
Hemorrhage
Infection
Abnormal vital signs
Traumatic labor or birth
Psychosocial factors

INFANT (FOR ADMISSION TO NICU)
High Risk
Infants who continue with or develop signs of RDS or
  other respiratory distress
Asphyxiated infants (Apgar score less than 6 at 5 min),
  resuscitation required at birth
Preterm infants, dysmature infants
Infants with cyanosis or suspected cardiovascular dis-
  ease, persistent cyanosis
Infants with major congenital malformations requiring
  surgery, chromosomal anomalies
Infants with convulsions, sepsis, hemorrhagic diathesis,
  or shock
Meconium aspiration syndrome

CNS depression for more than 24 hr
Hypoglycemia
Hypocalcemia
Hyperbilirubinemia

Moderate Risk
Dysmaturity
Prematurity (weight between 2000 and 2500 g)
Apgar score less than 5 at 1 min
Feeding problems
Multifetal birth
Transient tachypnea
Hypomagnesemia or hypermagnesemia
Hypoparathyroidism
Failure to gain weight
Jitteriness or hyperactivity
Cardiac anomalies not requiring immediate catheteriza-
  tion
Heart murmur
Anemia
CNS depression for less than 24 hr

CNS, Central nervous system; *NICU,* neonatal intensive care unit; *RDS,* respiratory distress syndrome.

BOX 21-4

Assessment for High Risk Pregnancy with Functional Health Patterns

For each of the following functional health patterns, the nurse includes questions that will provide data about the woman, her family, her community, and her cultural practices and beliefs:

- *Health perception or health management pattern.* Current health, medical history, family medical history, environmental or chemical exposure, family decision making about health, community resources, beliefs about health care during pregnancy
- *Nutritional-metabolic pattern.* Nutritional status, knowledge of pregnancy needs, pregnancy discomforts, community resources (WIC), cultural eating practices
- *Elimination pattern.* Urinary and bowel patterns, family or cultural practices (laxatives), community waste and sanitation services
- *Activity-exercise pattern.* Usual exercise, recreation, community resources, cultural practices or taboos for activities during pregnancy
- *Sleep-rest pattern.* Usual sleep patterns, use of remedies, family sleep arrangements, cultural beliefs about sleep and rest in pregnancy

- *Cognitive-perceptual pattern.* Communication problems, knowledge deficits about pregnancy and birth (individual and family), community resources for support for high risk pregnant patients, cultural beliefs about pain and its management
- *Self-perception or self-concept pattern.* Body image, responses of family to high risk pregnancy, housing conditions, cultural practices about parenting
- *Role-relationship pattern.* Feelings of security, occupation, hobbies, family living arrangements, community resources
- *Sexuality-reproductive pattern.* Sexual activities, problems, restrictions, obstetric history, current obstetric status, cultural beliefs about sexual practices during pregnancy
- *Coping-stress pattern.* Life stressors, losses experienced, coping mechanisms, support systems, community resources, spiritual or religious practices or beliefs that are important

References: Gilbert, E., & Harmon, J. (2003). *Manual of high risk pregnancy and delivery* (3rd ed.). St. Louis: Mosby; Gordon, M. (2002). *Manual of nursing diagnosis* (10th ed.). St. Louis: Mosby.
WIC, special Supplemental Nutrition Program for Women, Infants, and Children.

TABLE 21-1

Fetal Assessment Screening: Recommendations for Care

FETAL ASSESSMENT TEST	RECOMMENDATION OR CONCLUSION
• Doppler ultrasound use in pregnancy at high risk for fetal compromise	Beneficial effects
• Ultrasound use to estimate gestational age in first and early second trimesters	Effects likely to be beneficial
• Ultrasound use to confirm suspected multiple pregnancy	
• Ultrasound use for placental location in suspected placenta previa	
• Ultrasound use to assess amniotic fluid volume	
• Early second trimester amniocentesis for identification of chromosomal abnormalities	
• Transabdominal instead of transvaginal chorionic villus sampling (CVS)	
• Formal systems of risk scoring	Trade-off between beneficial and adverse effects
• Routine use of early ultrasound	
• CVS versus amniocentesis for diagnosing chromosomal abnormalities	
• Serum alpha-fetoprotein screening for neural tube defects	
• Triple screen test for Down syndrome and neural tube defects	
• Placental grading by ultrasound to improve perinatal outcome	Unknown effectiveness
• Biophysical profile for fetal surveillance	
• Routine fetal movement counts to improve perinatal outcome	
• Routine use of ultrasound for fetal anthropometry (body measurements) in late pregnancy	Unlikely to be beneficial
• Use of Doppler ultrasound screening in all pregnancies	
• Measurement of placental hormones (estriol and human placental lactogen)	
• Nipple stimulation test to improve perinatal outcome	Likely to be ineffective or harmful
• Nonselective nonstress test to improve perinatal outcome	
• Contraction stress test to improve perinatal outcome	

Source: Enkin, M. et al. (2001). Effective care in pregnancy and childbirth: A synopsis. *Birth, 28*(1), 41-51.

NURSE ALERT *In assessing fetal movements, it is important to remember that they are usually not present during the fetal sleep cycle; they may be temporarily reduced if the woman is taking depressant medications, drinking alcohol, or smoking a cigarette. They do not decrease as the woman nears term. Obesity decreases the ability of the mother to perceive fetal movement.*

Ultrasonography

Sound is a form of wave energy that causes small particles in a medium to oscillate. The frequency of sound, which refers to the number of peaks or waves that move over a given point per unit of time, is expressed in hertz (Hz). Sound with a frequency of 1 cycle, or one peak per second, has a frequency of 1 Hz. When directional beams of sound strike an object, an echo is returned. The time delay between the emission of the sound and the return of the echo and the direction of the echo are noted. From these data, the distance and location of an object can be calculated. Ultrasound is sound frequency higher than that detectable by humans (greater than 20,000 Hz). Diagnostic ultrasound instruments operate within a frequency range of 2 to 10 million Hz (or 2 to 10 MHz), which is below the range used by sonar and radar equipment. Ultrasound images are a reflection of the strength of the sending beam, the strength of the returning echo, and the density of the medium (e.g., muscle [uterus], bone, tissue [placenta], fluid, or blood through which the beam is sent and returned) (Chervenak & Gabbe, 2002).

Diagnostic ultrasonography is an important, safe technique in antepartum fetal surveillance. It provides critical information to health care providers regarding fetal activity and gestational age, normal versus abnormal fetal growth curves, visual assistance with which invasive tests may be performed more safely, fetal and placental anatomy, and fetal well-being (Chervenak & Gabbe, 2002). Ultrasound examination can be done abdominally or transvaginally during pregnancy. Both produce a three-dimensional view from which a pictorial image is obtained. Abdominal ultrasonography is more useful after the first trimester when the pregnant uterus becomes an abdominal organ. For the procedure, the woman usually should have a full bladder to displace the uterus upward to get a better image of the fetus. Transmission gel or paste is applied to the woman's abdomen before a transducer is moved over the skin to enhance transmission and reception of the sound waves. She is positioned with small pillows under her head and knees. The display panel is positioned so that the woman and/or her partner can observe the images on the screen if they desire.

Transvaginal ultrasonography, in which the probe is inserted into the vagina, allows pelvic anatomy to be evaluated in greater detail and intrauterine pregnancy to be diagnosed earlier (Manning, 2004). A transvaginal ultrasound examination is well tolerated by most patients because it alleviates the need for a full bladder. It is especially useful in obese women whose thick abdominal layers cannot be penetrated adequately with an abdominal approach. A transvaginal ultrasound may be performed with the woman in a lithotomy position or with her pelvis elevated by towels, cushions, or a folded pillow. This pelvic tilt is optimal to image the pelvic structures. A protective cover such as a condom, the finger of a clean rubber surgical glove, or a special probe cover provided by the manufacturer is used to cover the transducer probe. The probe is lubricated with a water-soluble gel and placed in the vagina either by the examiner or by the woman herself. During the examination, the position of the probe or the tilt of the examining table may be changed so that the complete pelvis is in view. The procedure is not physically painful, although the woman will feel pressure as the probe is moved. Transvaginal ultrasonography is optimally used in the first trimester to detect ectopic pregnancies, monitor the developing embryo, help identify abnormalities, and help establish gestational age. In some instances it may be used as an adjunct to abdominal scanning to evaluate preterm labor in second- and third-trimester pregnancies.

Levels of ultrasonography

Perinatal care providers and ultrasonographers have come to a tentative agreement on terminology describing two different levels of ultrasonography. The basic screening or limited examination is used most frequently and can be performed by ultrasonographers or other health care professionals, including nurses, who have had special training. Indications for limited ultrasonography are described in detail in the next section; its primary use is to detect fetal viability, determine the presentation of the fetus, assess gestational age, locate the placenta, examine the fetal anatomy for malformations, and determine amniotic fluid volume (AFV). Targeted or comprehensive examinations are performed if a woman is suspected of carrying an anatomically or a physiologically abnormal fetus. Indications for a comprehensive examination include abnormal findings on clinical examination, especially with polyhydramnios or oligohydramnios, elevated alpha-fetoprotein (AFP) levels, and a history of offspring with anomalies that can be detected by ultrasound examination. Comprehensive ultrasonography is performed by highly trained and experienced personnel.

Indications for use

Major indications for obstetric sonography appear by trimester in Table 21-2. During the first trimester, ultrasound examination is performed to obtain information regarding (1) number, size, and location of gestational sacs; (2) presence or absence of fetal cardiac and body movements; (3) presence or absence of uterine abnormalities (e.g., bicornuate uterus or fibroids) or adnexal masses (e.g., ovarian cysts or an ectopic pregnancy); (4) date of pregnancy (by measuring the crown-rump length); and (5) presence and location of an intrauterine contraceptive device.

During the second and third trimesters, information regarding the following conditions is sought: (1) fetal viability, number, position, gestational age, growth pattern, and anomalies; (2) AFV; (3) placental location and maturity;

TABLE 21-2

Major Uses of Ultrasonography during Pregnancy

FIRST TRIMESTER	SECOND TRIMESTER	THIRD TRIMESTER
Confirm pregnancy	Establish or confirm dates	Confirm gestational age
Confirm viability	Confirm viability	Confirm viability
Determine gestational age	Detect polyhydramnios, oligohy-	Detect macrosomia
Rule out ectopic pregnancy	dramnios	Detect congenital anomalies
Detect multiple gestation	Detect congenital anomalies	Detect IUGR
Use for visualization during chori-	Detect intrauterine growth restric-	Determine fetal position
onic villus sampling	tion (IUGR)	Detect placenta previa or abruptio
Detect maternal abnormalities such	Confirm placenta placement	placentae
as bicornuate uterus, ovarian	Use for visualization during amnio-	Use for visualization during amnio-
cysts, fibroids	centesis	centesis, external version
		Biophysical profile
		Amniotic fluid volume assessment
		Doppler flow studies
		Detect placental maturity

(4) uterine fibroids and anomalies; (5) adnexal masses; and (6) cervical length.

Ultrasonography provides earlier diagnoses, allowing therapy to be instituted early in the pregnancy, thereby decreasing the severity and duration of morbidity, both physical and emotional, for the family. For instance, early diagnosis of a fetal anomaly gives the family choices such as (1) intrauterine surgery or other therapy for the fetus, (2) termination of the pregnancy, or (3) preparation for the care of an infant with a disorder.

Fetal heart activity. Fetal heart activity can be demonstrated as early as 6 to 7 weeks by real-time echo scanners and at 10 to 12 weeks by Doppler mode. By 9 to 10 weeks, gestational trophoblastic disease can be diagnosed. Fetal death can be confirmed by lack of heart motion, the presence of fetal scalp edema, and maceration and overlap of the cranial bones.

Gestational age. Gestational dating by ultrasonography is indicated for conditions such as (1) uncertain dates for the last normal menstrual period, (2) recent discontinuation of oral contraceptives, (3) bleeding episode during the first trimester, (4) uterine size that does not agree with dates, and (5) other high risk conditions.

During the first 20 weeks of gestation, ultrasonography provides an accurate assessment of gestational age because most normal fetuses grow at the same rate. Accuracy is increased as the fetus ages because more than one variable is measured. The four methods of fetal age estimation used include (1) determination of gestational sac dimensions (at about 8 weeks), (2) measurement of crown-rump length (between 7 and 12 weeks), (3) measurement of the biparietal diameter (BPD) (after 12 weeks), and (4) measurement of femur length (after 12 weeks). Fetal BPD at 36 weeks should be approximately 8.7 cm. Term pregnancy and fetal maturity can be diagnosed with some confidence if the biparietal measurement by ultrasound examination is greater than 9.8 cm (Fig. 21-1), especially when this is combined with appropriate femur length measurement.

In later gestational periods, serial measurements can provide a more accurate determination of fetal age. Two and preferably three composite measurements are recommended, at least 2 weeks apart, and these are plotted against standard fetal growth curves. This method, when applied between 24 and 32 weeks of gestation, yields an estimation error of 10 days more or less than the actual age (Manning, 2004).

Fetal growth. Fetal growth is determined by both intrinsic growth potential and environmental factors. Conditions that require ultrasound assessment of fetal growth include (1) poor maternal weight gain or pattern of weight gain, (2) previous intrauterine growth restriction (IUGR), (3) chronic infections, (4) ingestion of drugs (tobacco, alcohol, over-the-counter, and street drugs), (5) maternal diabetes mellitus, (6) hypertension, (7) multifetal pregnancy, and (8) other medical or surgical complications.

Serial evaluations of BPD, limb length, and abdominal circumference (AC) (Fig. 21-2) can allow differentiation among size discrepancy resulting from inaccurate dates, true IUGR, and macrosomia. IUGR may be symmetric (the fe-

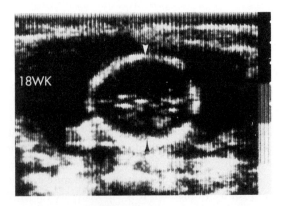

Fig. 21-1 Real-time image of fetal biparietal diameters at 18 weeks. (From Athey, P., & Hadlock, F. [1985]. *Ultrasound in obstetrics and gynecology* [2nd ed.]. St. Louis: Mosby.)

mother is obese without glucose intolerance results in symmetric changes—excessive growth of abdominal and head circumferences (Chervenak & Gabbe, 2002).

Fetal anatomy. Anatomic structures that can be identified by ultrasonography (depending on the gestational age) include the following: head (including ventricles and blood vessels) (Fig. 21-3), neck, spine, heart, stomach, small bowel, liver, kidneys, bladder, and limbs. Ultrasonography permits the confirmation of normal anatomy, as well as the detection of major fetal malformations. The presence of an anomaly may influence the location of birth (e.g., a delivery room versus a labor-delivery-recovery room or a subspecialty center versus a basic care center) and the method of birth (vaginal versus cesarean) to optimize neonatal outcomes.

The number of fetuses and their presentations also may be assessed by ultrasonography, allowing plans for therapy and method of birth to be made in advance.

Fetal genetic disorders and physical anomalies. A prenatal screening technique called *fetal nuchal*

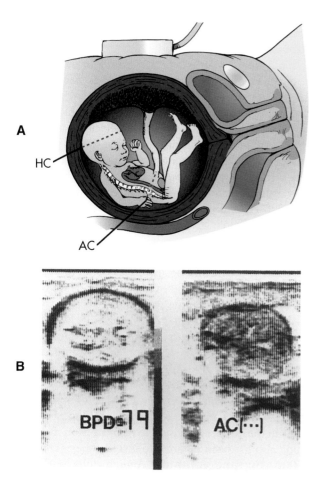

Fig. 21-2 **A,** Appropriate planes of sections *(dotted lines)* for head circumference *(HC)*, and abdominal circumference *(AC)*. **B,** Real-time ultrasound image demonstrates typical head and body images that correspond to planes in **A**. By use of these two images, biparietal diameter (BPD) (7.9 cm), head circumference (30 cm), abdominal circumference (28 cm), and estimated fetal weight (1840 g) in this normal 32-week fetus can be determined. (From Athey, P., & Hadlock, F. [1985]. *Ultrasound in obstetrics and gynecology* [2nd ed.]. St. Louis: Mosby.)

tus is small in all parameters) or asymmetric (head and body growth vary). Symmetric IUGR reflects a chronic or long-standing insult and may be caused by low genetic growth potential, intrauterine infection, undernutrition, heavy smoking, or chromosomal aberration. Asymmetric growth suggests an acute or late-occurring deprivation, such as placental insufficiency resulting from hypertension, renal disease, or cardiovascular disease. Reduced fetal growth is still one of the most frequent conditions associated with stillbirth.

Macrosomic infants (those weighing 4000 g or more) are at increased risk for traumatic injury, and asphyxia during birth. In addition, fetal macrosomia associated with maternal glucose intolerance or diabetes carries an increased risk of intrauterine fetal death. Macrosomia in the infant of a diabetic mother is asymmetric and characterized by increases in fat and muscle in the abdomen and shoulders, while head circumference remains normal. Macrosomia in an infant whose

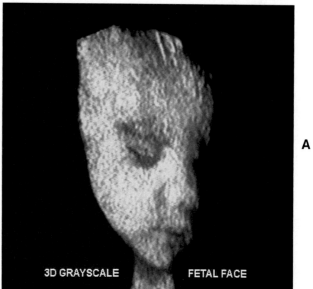

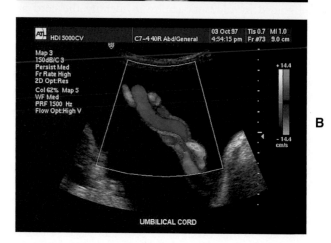

Fig. 21-3 Two views of the fetus during ultrasonography. **A,** Fetal face (20 weeks). **B,** Umbilical cord (26 weeks). (Courtesy Advanced Technology Laboratories, Bothell, WA.)

translucency (FNT) screening uses ultrasound measurement of fluid in the nape of the fetal neck between 10 and 14 weeks of gestation to identify possible fetal abnormalities. A finding of abnormal fluid collection that is greater than 2.5 mm is considered abnormal, whereas a measurement of 3 mm or greater is highly indicative of genetic disorders and/or physical anomalies. If the FNT is abnormal, diagnostic genetic testing is recommended (ACOG, 2004).

Placental position and function. The pattern of uterine and placental growth and the fullness of the maternal bladder influence the apparent location of the placenta by ultrasonography. During the first trimester, differentiation between the endometrium and small placenta is difficult. By 14 to 16 weeks, the placenta is clearly defined; but if it is seen to be low lying, its relation to the internal cervical os can sometimes be dramatically altered by varying the fullness of the maternal bladder. In approximately 15% to 20% of all pregnancies in which ultrasound scanning is performed during the second trimester, the placenta seems to be overlying the os, but the incidence of placenta previa at term is only 0.5%. Therefore the diagnosis of placenta previa can seldom be confirmed before 27 weeks, primarily because of the elongation of the lower uterine segment as pregnancy advances.

Another use for ultrasonography is grading of placental maturation. Calcium deposits are of significance in postterm pregnancies because as they increase, the available surface area that can be adequately bathed by maternal blood decreases. The point at which this results in fetal wastage and hypoxia cannot be determined precisely; however, the effects are usually observable by 42 weeks and are progressive (Gilbert & Harmon, 2003).

Adjunct to other invasive tests. The safety of amniocentesis is increased when the positions of the fetus, placenta, and pockets of amniotic fluid can be identified accurately. Ultrasound scanning has reduced risks previously associated with amniocentesis, such as fetomaternal hemorrhage from a pierced placenta. Percutaneous umbilical blood sampling (PUBS) and chorionic villus sampling also are guided by ultrasonography to identify the cord and chorion frondosum accurately (see Fig. 21-3, *B*).

Fetal well-being

Physiologic parameters of the fetus that can be assessed with ultrasound scanning include AFV, vascular waveforms from the fetal circulation, heart motion, fetal breathing movements (FBMs), fetal urine production, and fetal limb and head movements. Assessment of these parameters, singly or in combination, yields a fairly reliable picture of fetal well-being. The significance of these findings is discussed in the following sections.

Doppler blood flow analysis. One of the major advances in perinatal medicine is the ability to study blood flow noninvasively in the fetus and placenta with ultrasound. Doppler blood flow analysis is a helpful adjunct in the management of pregnancies at risk because of hypertension, IUGR, diabetes mellitus, multiple fetuses, or preterm labor.

When a sound wave is reflected from a moving target, there is a change in frequency of the reflected wave relative to the transmitted wave. This is called the *Doppler effect.* An ultrasound beam scattered by a group of red blood cells (RBCs) is an example of this effect. The velocity of the RBCs can be determined by measuring the change in the frequency of the sound wave reflected off the cells (Fig. 21-4).

The shifted frequencies can be displayed as a plot of velocity versus time, and the shape of these waveforms can be analyzed to give information about blood flow and resistance in a given circulation. Velocity waveforms from umbilical and uterine arteries, reported as systolic/diastolic (S/D) ratios, can be first detected at 15 weeks of pregnancy. Because of the progressive decline in resistance in both the umbilical and uterine arteries, this ratio decreases as pregnancy advances. Most fetuses will achieve an S/D ratio of 3 or less by 30 weeks. Persistent elevation of S/D ratios after 30 weeks is associated with IUGR, usually resulting from UPI (Druzin, Gabbe, & Reed, 2002). In postterm pregnancies evaluated by Doppler umbilical flow studies, an elevated S/D ratio indicates a poorly perfused placenta. Abnormal results also are seen with certain chromosome abnormalities (trisomy 13 and 18) in the fetus and with lupus erythematosus in the mother. Exposure to nicotine from maternal smoking also has been reported to increase the S/D ratio.

Amniotic fluid volume. Abnormalities in AFV are frequently associated with fetal disorders. Subjective determinants of oligohydramnios (decreased fluid) include the absence of fluid pockets in the uterine cavity and the impression of crowding of small fetal parts. An objective criterion of decreased AFV is met if the largest pocket of fluid measured in two perpendicular planes is less than 2 cm (Manning, 2004). In polyhydramnios (increased fluid), subjective criteria include multiple large pockets of fluid, the impression of a floating fetus, and free movement of fetal limbs. The diagnosis may be made when the largest pocket of fluid exceeds 8 cm in two perpendicular planes (Chervenak & Gabbe, 2002).

The total AFV can be evaluated by a method in which the depths (in centimeters) of the amniotic fluid in all four quad-

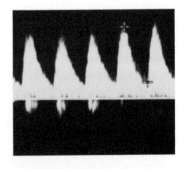

Fig. 21-4 Umbilical artery velocity waveform in a 17-week fetus with S/D ratio of 4.4, which is normal for this stage. (Courtesy Michael S. Clement, MD, Mesa, AZ.)

rants surrounding the maternal umbilicus are totaled, providing an amniotic fluid index (AFI). An AFI less than 5 cm indicates oligohydramnios; 5 to 19 cm is considered a normal measurement; and a measurement greater than 20 cm reflects polyhydramnios (Chervenak & Gabbe, 2002). Oligohydramnios is associated with congenital anomalies (such as renal agenesis), growth restriction, and fetal distress during labor. Polyhydramnios is associated with neural tube defects (NTDs), obstruction of the fetal gastrointestinal tract, multiple fetuses, and fetal hydrops.

Biophysical profile. Real-time ultrasound permits detailed assessment of the physical and physiologic characteristics of the developing fetus and cataloging of normal and abnormal biophysical responses to stimuli. The biophysical profile (BPP) is a noninvasive dynamic assessment of a fetus that is based on acute and chronic markers of fetal disease. The BPP includes FBMs, fetal movements, fetal tone, fetal heart rate (FHR) patterns by means of an NST, and AFV. The BPP may therefore be considered a physical examination of the fetus, including determination of vital signs. The fetal response to central hypoxia is alteration in movement, muscle tone, breathing, and heart rate patterns. The presence of normal fetal biophysical activities indicates that the central nervous system (CNS) is functional, and the fetus therefore is not hypoxemic (Harman, 2004). BPP variables and scoring are detailed in Table 21-3.

The BPP is an accurate indicator of impending fetal death. Fetal acidosis can be diagnosed early with a nonreactive NST and absent FBMs. An abnormal BPP score and oligohydramnios are indications that labor should be induced (Harman, 2004). Fetal infection in women whose membranes rupture prematurely (at less than 37 weeks of gestation) can be diagnosed early by changes in biophysical activity that precede the clinical signs of infection and indicate the necessity for immediate birth. When the BPP score is normal and the risk of fetal death low, intervention is indicated only for obstetric or maternal factors.

Nursing role

Although a growing number of nurses perform ultrasound scans and BPPs in certain centers, the main role of nurses is in counseling and educating women about the procedure (Garcia et al., 2002). Providing accurate information regarding the procedure is imperative to allay the mother's anxiety. Although ultrasound scanning has become a widely used diagnostic tool, recommendations for the procedure are based on expectations of a fetal problem and therefore may cause concern. Women should be provided ample opportunity to

---

TABLE 21-3

Biophysical Profile

VARIABLES	NORMAL (SCORE = 2)	ABNORMAL (SCORE = 0)
Fetal breathing movements	One or more episodes in 30 min, each lasting ≥30 sec	Episodes absent or no episode ≥30 sec in 30 min
Gross body movements	Three or more discrete body or limb movements in 30 min (episodes of active continuous movement are considered as a single movement)	Less than three episodes of body or limb movements in 30 min
Fetal tone	One or more episodes of active extension with return to flexion of fetal limb(s) or trunk; opening and closing of hand is considered normal tone	Slow extension with return to flexion, movement of limb in full extension, or fetal movement absent
Reactive fetal heart rate	Two or more episodes of acceleration (≥15 beats/min) in 20 min, each lasting ≥15 sec and associated with fetal movement	Less than two episodes of acceleration or acceleration of <15 beats/min in 20 min
Qualitative amniotic fluid volume	One or more pockets of fluid measuring ≥1 cm in two perpendicular planes	Pockets absent or pocket <1 cm in two perpendicular planes
SCORE		
Normal	8-10 (if amniotic fluid index is adequate)	
Equivocal	6	
Abnormal	<4	

Reference: Harman, C. (2004). Assessment of fetal health. In R. Creasy, R. Resnik, & J. Iams (Eds.), *Maternal-fetal medicine: Principles and practice* (5th ed.). Philadelphia: Saunders.

ask questions and be reassured that the procedure is safe. In the 30 years that diagnostic ultrasonography has been used, no conclusive evidence of any harmful effects on humans has emerged. Although the possibility of unidentified biologic effects exists, the benefits to the patient of prudent use of diagnostic ultrasonography appear to outweigh any possible risk (Chervenak & Gabbe, 2002).

> **LEGAL TIP** **Performance of Limited Ultrasound Examinations**
>
> *Nurses who have the training and competence may perform limited ultrasound examinations if it is within the scope of practice in their state or area and consistent with regulations of the agencies in which they practice (Menihan, 2000). Limited ultrasound examinations include identification of fetal number, fetal presentation, fetal cardiac activity, location of the placenta, and BPP, including AFV assessment. Women should be informed about the limited information provided by these examinations. They are not meant to evaluate or identify fetal anomalies, assess fetal age, or estimate fetal weight (Stringer, Miesnik, Brown, Menei, & Macones, 2003). The obstetric health care provider is responsible for obtaining a more comprehensive ultrasound examination when complete patient assessment is necessary (Association of Women's Health, Obstetric and Neonatal Nurses [AWHONN], 1998).*

Magnetic Resonance Imaging

Magnetic resonance imaging (MRI) is a noninvasive radiologic technique used for obstetric and gynecologic diagnosis. Like computed tomography (CT), MRI provides excellent pictures of soft tissue. Unlike CT, ionizing radiation is not used; therefore vascular structures within the body can be visualized and evaluated without injection of an iodinated contrast medium, thus eliminating any known biologic risk. Like sonography, MRI is noninvasive and can provide images in multiple planes, but there is no interference from skeletal, fatty, or gas-filled structures, and imaging of deep pelvic structures does not require a full bladder.

With MRI, the examiner can evaluate (1) fetal structure (CNS, thorax, abdomen, genitourinary tract, musculoskeletal system) and overall growth; (2) placenta (position, density, and presence of gestational trophoblastic disease); (3) quantity of amniotic fluid; (4) maternal structures (uterus, cervix, adnexa, and pelvis); (5) biochemical status (pH, adenosine triphosphate content) of tissues and organs; and (6) soft-tissue, metabolic, or functional anomalies.

The woman is placed on a table in the supine position and slid into the bore of the main magnet, which is similar in appearance to a CT scanner. Depending on the reason for the study, the procedure may take from 20 to 60 minutes, during which time the woman must be perfectly still except for short respites. Because of the long time needed to produce MRIs, the fetus will probably move, which will obscure anatomic details. The only way to ensure that this does not occur is to administer a sedative to the mother, but this ap-

proach should be reserved for selected cases in which visualization of fetal detail is critical.

MRI has little effect on the fetus; concerns that the FHR or fetal movement would decrease have not been supported.

BIOCHEMICAL ASSESSMENT

Biochemical assessment involves biologic examination (e.g., as chromosomes in exfoliated cells) and chemical determinations (e.g., lecithin/sphingomyelin [L/S] ratio and bilirubin level) (Table 21-4). Procedures used to obtain the needed specimens include amniocentesis, PUBS, chorionic villus sampling, and maternal sampling (Box 21-5).

Amniocentesis

Amniocentesis is performed to obtain amniotic fluid, which contains fetal cells. Under direct ultrasonographic visualization, a needle is inserted transabdominally into the uterus, amniotic fluid is withdrawn into a syringe, and the various assessments are performed (Fig. 21-5). Amniocentesis is possible after week 14 of pregnancy, when the uterus becomes an abdominal organ, and sufficient amniotic fluid is available for testing. Indications for the procedure include prenatal diagnosis of genetic disorders or congenital anomalies (NTDs in particular), assessment of pulmonary maturity, and diagnosis of fetal hemolytic disease.

Complications in the mother and fetus occur in fewer than 1% of the cases and include the following:

- Maternal: Hemorrhage, fetomaternal hemorrhage with possible maternal Rh isoimmunization, infection, labor, abruptio placentae, inadvertent damage to the intestines or bladder, and amniotic fluid embolism. Because of the possibility of fetomaternal hemorrhage, it is standard practice after an amniocentesis to administer Rh₀D immune globulin to the woman who is Rh negative.
- Fetal: Death, hemorrhage, infection (amnionitis), direct injury from the needle, miscarriage or preterm labor, and leakage of amniotic fluid

Many of the complications have been minimized or eliminated by using ultrasonography to direct the procedure.

> **BOX 21-5**
>
> *Fetal Rights*
>
> Amniocentesis, percutaneous umbilical blood sampling (PUBS), and chorionic villus sampling (CVS) are prenatal tests used for diagnosing fetal defects in pregnancy. They are invasive and carry risks to the mother and fetus. A consideration of induced abortion is linked to the performance of these tests because there is no treatment for genetically affected fetuses; therefore the issue of fetal rights is a key ethical concern in prenatal testing for fetal defects.

TABLE 21-4

Summary of Biochemical Monitoring Techniques

TEST	POSSIBLE FINDINGS	CLINICAL SIGNIFICANCE
MATERNAL BLOOD		
Coombs' test	Titer of 1:8 and increasing	Significant Rh incompatibility
AFP	See below	
AMNIOTIC FLUID ANALYSIS		
Color	Meconium	Possible hypoxia or asphyxia
Lung profile		Fetal lung maturity
L/S ratio	>2:1	
Phosphatidylglycerol	Present	
Creatinine	>2 mg/dl	Gestational age >36 weeks
Bilirubin (ΔOD, 450/nm)	<0.015	Gestational age >36 weeks, normal pregnancy
	High levels	Fetal hemolytic disease in Rh isoimmunized pregnancies
Lipid cells	>10%	Gestational age >35 weeks
AFP	High levels after 15-week gestation	Open neural tube or other defect
Osmolality	Decline after 20-week gestation	Advancing gestational age
Genetic disorders	Dependent on cultured cells for	Counseling possibly required
Sex-linked	karyotype and enzymatic activity	
Chromosomal		
Metabolic		

AFP, Alpha-fetoprotein; *L/S*, lecithin-sphingomyelin.

Indications for use

Genetic concerns. Prenatal assessment of genetic disorders is indicated in women older than 35 years (Box 21-6), with a previous child with a chromosomal abnormality, or with a family history of chromosomal anomalies. Inherited errors of metabolism (such as Tay-Sachs disease,

hemophilia, and thalassemia) and other disorders for which marker genes are known also may be detected. Fetal cells are cultured for karyotyping of chromosomes (see Chapter 7). Karyotyping also permits determination of fetal sex, which is important if an X-linked disorder (occurring almost always in a male fetus) is suspected.

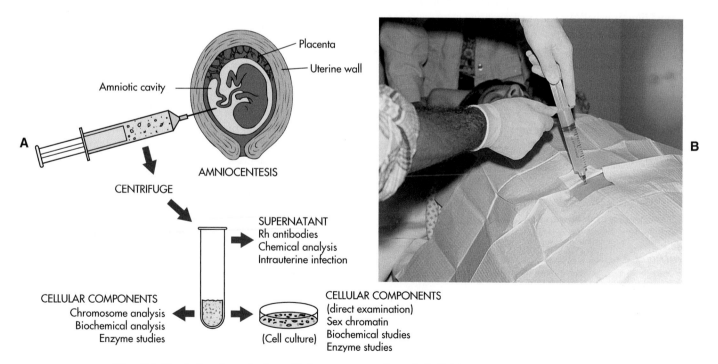

Fig. 21-5 **A,** Amniocentesis and laboratory use of amniotic fluid aspirant. **B,** Transabdominal amniocentesis. (**B,** Courtesy Marjorie Pyle, RNC, Lifecircle, Costa Mesa, CA.)

Biochemical analysis of enzymes in amniotic fluid can detect inborn errors of metabolism. For example, AFP levels in amniotic fluid are assessed as a follow-up for elevated levels in maternal serum. High AFP levels in amniotic fluid help confirm the diagnosis of an NTD such as spina bifida or anencephaly or an abdominal wall defect such as omphalocele. The elevation results from the increased leakage of cerebrospinal fluid into the amniotic fluid through the closure defect. AFP levels may also be elevated in a normal multifetal pregnancy and with intestinal atresia, presumably caused by lack of fetal swallowing.

A concurrent test that finds the presence of acetylcholinesterase almost always indicates a fetal defect (Jenkins & Wapner, 2004). In such instances, follow-up ultrasound examination is recommended.

Fetal maturity. Accurate assessment of fetal maturity is possible through examination of amniotic fluid or its exfoliated cellular contents. The laboratory tests described are determinants of term pregnancy and fetal maturity (see Table 21-4). A quick means of determining an approximate L/S ratio is the *shake test* foam test, or bubble stability test. Serial dilutions of fresh amniotic fluid are mixed with ethanol and shaken. After 15 minutes, the amount of bubbles present at different dilutions indicates the presence of surfactant.

Fetal hemolytic disease. Another indication for amniocentesis is the identification and follow-up of fetal hemolytic disease in cases of isoimmunization. The procedure is usually not done until the mother's antibody titer reaches 1:8 and is increasing. Currently PUBS is the procedure of choice to evaluate and treat fetal hemolytic disease.

Meconium. The presence of meconium in the amniotic fluid is usually determined by visual inspection of the sample. The significance of meconium in the fluid varies depending on when it is found.

Antepartal period. Meconium in the amniotic fluid before the beginning of labor is not usually associated with an adverse fetal outcome. The finding may be the result of acute and subsequently corrected fetal stress, chronic continuing stress, or simply the physiologic passage of meconium. Because there has been some association between meconium in amniotic fluid in the third trimester and hypertensive disorders and postmaturity, the fetus should undergo further antepartum evaluation if the birth is not imminent (Glantz & Woods, 2004).

Intrapartal period. Intrapartal meconium-stained amniotic fluid is an indication for more careful evaluation by electronic fetal monitoring (EFM) and perhaps fetal scalp blood sampling. The presence of meconium, however, should not be the sole indicator for intervention.

Three possible reasons for the passage of meconium during the intrapartal period are as follows: (1) it is a normal physiologic function that occurs with maturity (meconium passage being infrequent before weeks 23 or 24, with an increased incidence after 38 weeks); (2) it is the result of hypoxia-induced peristalsis and sphincter relaxation; and (3) it may be a sequel to umbilical cord compression–induced vagal stimulation in mature fetuses. Thick, fresh meconium passed for the first time in late labor and in association with nonremediable severe variable or late FHR decelerations is an ominous sign.

NURSE ALERT *The birth team should be ready to suction the nasopharynx of the neonate carefully at the time of birth, ideally before the first breath is taken. Suctioning at this time may reduce the incidence and severity of meconium aspiration in the neonate, however the practice is being challenged. At least one study has found no difference in suctioned versus unsuctioned infants.*

Chorionic Villus Sampling

The combined advantages of earlier diagnosis and rapid results have made chorionic villus sampling (CVS) a popular technique for genetic studies, although some risks to the fetus exist. Although indications for CVS are similar to those for amniocentesis, second-trimester amniocentesis appears to be safer than CVS (Alfirevic, Sundberg, & Brigham, 2003). The benefits of earlier diagnosis must be weighed against the increased risk of pregnancy loss and risk of anomalies.

The procedure is performed between 10 and 12 weeks of gestation and involves the removal of a small tissue specimen from the fetal portion of the placenta (Fig. 21-6). Because chorionic villi originate in the zygote, this tissue reflects the genetic makeup of the fetus.

CVS procedures can be accomplished either transcervically or transabdominally. In transcervical sampling, a sterile catheter is introduced into the cervix under continuous ultrasonographic guidance, and a small portion of the chorionic villi is aspirated with a syringe. The aspiration cannula and obturator must be placed at a suitable site, and rupture of the amniotic sac must be avoided.

If the abdominal approach is used, an 18-gauge spinal needle with stylet is inserted under sterile conditions through the abdominal wall into the chorion frondosum under ultrasound guidance. The stylet is then withdrawn, and the chorionic tissue is aspirated into a syringe (see Fig. 21-6).

Complications of the procedure include vaginal spotting or bleeding immediately afterward, miscarriage (in 0.3% of

---

BOX 21-6

Elimination of Maternal Age as an Indication for Invasive Prenatal Diagnosis

Maternal age of 35 years and older has been a standard indication for invasive prenatal testing since 1979 despite a sensitivity of only 30%. The importance of age as a single indication for testing is being reevaluated, as serum screening has evolved. The most effective use of resources involves screening the whole population of pregnant women. Presently many centers offer the option of screening before invasive testing for women over 35 years of age (Jenkins & Wapner, 2004).

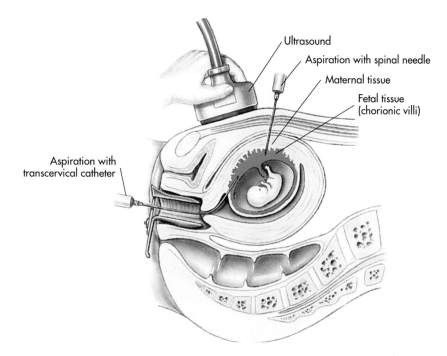

Fig. 21-6   Chorionic villus sampling. (Courtesy Medical and Scientific Illustration, Crozet, VA.)

cases), rupture of membranes (in 0.1% of cases), and chorioamnionitis (in 0.5% of cases). Because of the possibility of fetomaternal hemorrhage, women who are Rh negative should receive immune globulin to avoid isoimmunization (Gilbert & Harmon, 2003). An increased risk of limb anomalies (transverse digital anomalies) has been noted when CVS is done before 10 weeks of gestation (Wilson, 2000).

Use of amniocentesis and CVS is declining because of advances in noninvasive screening techniques. These techniques include measurement of nuchal translucency, maternal serum screening tests in the first and second trimesters, and ultrasonography in the second trimester (Benn, Egan, Fang, & Smith-Bindman, 2004).

Percutaneous Umbilical Blood Sampling

Direct access to the fetal circulation during the second and third trimesters is possible through **percutaneous umbilical blood sampling** (PUBS), or cordocentesis, which is the most widely used method for fetal blood sampling and transfusion. PUBS involves the insertion of a needle directly into a fetal umbilical vessel under ultrasound guidance. Ideally, the umbilical cord is punctured 1 to 2 cm from its insertion into the placenta (Fig. 21-7) (Simpson, 2002). At this point the cord is well anchored and will not move, and the risk of maternal blood contamination (from the placenta) is slight. Generally, 1 to 4 ml of blood is removed and tested immediately by the Kleihauer-Betke procedure to ensure that it is fetal in origin. Indications for use of PUBS include prenatal diagnosis of inherited blood disorders, karyotyping of malformed fetuses, detection of fetal infection, determination of the acid-base status of fetuses with IUGR, and assessment and treatment of isoimmunization and throm-

bocytopenia in the fetus (Jenkins & Wapner, 2004). Complications that can occur include leaking of blood from the puncture site, cord laceration, thromboembolism, preterm labor, premature rupture of membranes, and infection (Simpson, 2002).

In fetuses at risk for isoimmune hemolytic anemia, PUBS permits precise identification of fetal blood type and RBC count and may prevent the need for further intervention. If the fetus is positive for the presence of maternal antibodies, a direct blood test can confirm the degree of anemia resulting from hemolysis. Intrauterine transfusion of severely anemic fetuses can be done 4 to 5 weeks earlier than through the intraperitoneal route.

Follow-up includes continuous FHR monitoring for several minutes to 1 hour and a repeated ultrasound examination 1 hour later to ensure that no further bleeding or hematoma formation has occurred.

Maternal Assays
Alpha-fetoprotein

Maternal serum **alpha-fetoprotein** (AFP) (MSAFP) levels have been used as a screening tool for NTDs in pregnancy. Through this technique, approximately 80% to 85% of all open NTDs and open abdominal wall defects can be detected early in pregnancy. Screening is recommended for all pregnant women.

The cause of NTDs is not well understood, but 95% of all affected infants are born to women with no family history of similar anomalies (Jenkins & Wapner, 2004). The defect occurs in 1 to 2 per 1000 births in most parts of the United States. The birth of one affected child increases the risk of NTD recurrence in future pregnancies to 1% to 5% (Fanaroff, Martin, & Rodriguez, 2004).

EVIDENCE-BASED PRACTICE
Prenatal Diagnostics: Amniocentesis and Chorionic Villus Sampling

BACKGROUND

- Women requesting prenatal genetic diagnostic testing may have anxiety while waiting, receive false-positive results (abnormal results but a normal fetus), and have a lack of options if the test is abnormal. Many women want the testing done early enough that they may consider pregnancy termination if the results are abnormal.

- Amniocentesis is conventionally done around 16 weeks of gestation. Genetic results are returned after 18 weeks, in time for the woman to choose a second-trimester termination. The wait is agonizing for parents, and second-trimester abortion is not always a personal option, nor is it always available.

- There is pressure for earlier diagnostic procedures, such as chorionic villus sampling (CVS) of the placenta, accessed either transabdominally or transcervically. Most clinicians delay this procedure until after 9 weeks gestation because of some limb reduction (missing or hypoplastic limbs) seen after early CVS. Early amniocentesis is another option, requiring skillful removal of amniotic fluid from the inner amniotic sac only, filtering for fetal cells, and replacing the fluid. Both early procedures may cause pregnancy loss.

OBJECTIVE

- The reviewers' goal was to compare early and late amniocentesis and chorionic villus sampling (both transabdominal and transcervical) for safety and accuracy. Outcomes were the technical difficulties encountered in sampling, problems with the genetic analysis, pregnancy complications such as bleeding, leaking fluid, preterm labor, any pregnancy losses and still births, and neonatal abnormalities, such as talipes (clubfoot), hemangiomas, limb reduction, respiratory distress syndrome, low birth weight, and admission to special care nursery.

METHODS
Search Strategy

- The reviewers searched Cochrane, MEDLINE, 30 journals, and a weekly awareness search that covered 37 journals. Search keywords included *amniocentesis* and *chorionic villus sampling.*

- There were 14 randomized studies that were accepted into this review, ranging in publication dates from 1986 to 1999. The number of women was not reported for every study but totaled more than 15,000. The countries of origin included Denmark, Sweden, Finland, Italy, the United States, and Canada.

Statistical Analyses

- Statistical analyses allowed a weighted estimate of risk for each outcome, and the results were pooled from the studies.

FINDINGS

- The incidence of pregnancy loss after second-trimester amniocentesis was 3%, which was not significantly increased over the general population risk of 2%. However,

FINDINGS cont'd

amniocentesis was associated with an increased risk of spontaneous miscarriage and amniotic fluid leakage. Second-trimester amniocentesis was safer and easier than early amniocentesis, with fewer fetal anomalies, fewer needle inserts, fewer lab failures (because of inadequate fetal cells), and fewer false negatives. Transcervical CVS was associated with significantly more pregnancy loss, more lab failures, and more vaginal bleeding than second-trimester amniocentesis. Transabdominal CVS appears to be safer than the transcervical procedure. Early amniocentesis appeared to cause more spontaneous miscarriage than transabdominal CVS. The incidence of anomalies was not increased significantly.

LIMITATIONS

- The expertise of the operators varied, as CVS was fairly new in 1991. This, however, may not necessarily be a limitation, because it reflects the reality that there are always practitioners of varying skill levels practicing. Some studies "randomized" by giving women the choice of procedures. During the course of some of the trials, information became publicized about CVS leading to limb reduction (never replicated in later, larger studies), and so recruitment and dropouts became a problem. None of the trials assessed the laboratory accuracy adequately. One large trial excluded 70% of potential CVS-randomized women because of placental position, thus reducing generalizability.

CONCLUSIONS

- Second-trimester amniocentesis appears to be the safest and most accurate prenatal diagnostic procedure. Amniocentesis should never be done before 15 weeks of gestation. Transabdominal CVS is preferable if an early procedure is warranted. If the transabdominal procedure is contraindicated, then transcervical CVS is preferred in the first trimester and amniocentesis is preferred in the second trimester.

IMPLICATIONS FOR PRACTICE

- Women presented with the possibility of fetal anomalies need to know the risks and benefits of the diagnostic procedures offered. They also need to consider the therapeutic options available, should the results be abnormal, including the availability and acceptability of second-trimester abortion.

IMPLICATIONS FOR FURTHER RESEARCH

- Much more research needs to focus on the acceptability and satisfaction of women with the procedures, and their decision making. The unavailability of second-trimester abortion in some areas creates hardships that deserve research. All new prenatal procedures should be rigorously tested before general use. Outcomes should include antenatal and neonatal loss, details about anomalies, and diagnostic accuracy. Neonatal assessors should be blinded as to procedure used.

Reference: Alfirevic, Z., Sundberg, K., & Brigham, S. (2003). Amniocentesis and chorionic villi sampling for prenatal diagnosis (Cochrane Review). In *The Cochrane Library*, Issue 4, 2005. Chichester, UK: John Wiley & Sons.

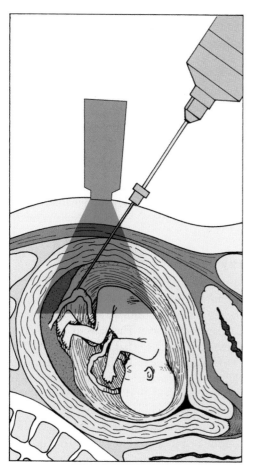

Fig. 21-7 Technique for percutaneous umbilical blood sampling guided by ultrasound.

AFP is produced by the fetal liver, and increasing levels are detectable in the serum of pregnant women from 14 to 34 weeks. Although amniotic fluid AFP is diagnostic for NTD, MSAFP is a screening tool only and identifies candidates for the more definitive procedures of amniocentesis and ultrasound examination. MSAFP screening can be done with reasonable reliability any time between 15 and 22 weeks of gestation (16 to 18 weeks being ideal) (Jenkins & Wapner, 2004).

Once the maternal level of AFP is determined, it is compared with normal values for each week of gestation. Values also should be correlated with maternal age, weight, race, and whether the woman has insulin-dependent diabetes. If findings are abnormal, follow-up procedures include genetic counseling for families with a history of NTD, repeated AFP, ultrasound examination, and possibly, amniocentesis.

Down syndrome and probably other autosomal trisomies are associated with lower-than-normal levels of MSAFP and amniotic fluid AFP. The triple-marker test also is performed at 16 to 18 weeks of gestation and uses the levels of three maternal serum markers, MSAFP, unconjugated estriol, and human chorionic gonadotropin (hCG), in combination with maternal age, to calculate a new risk level. In the presence

? Critical Thinking Exercise

Down Syndrome

Patty and David, both 37 years old, are expecting their first baby. Patty is 8 weeks pregnant and is worried about the risk of their baby being born with Down syndrome. She tells the nurse that she is relieved to be having an ultrasound done today because the procedure will show whether or not the baby has Down syndrome and she won't have to have other tests. What response by the nurse to Patty's statement would be appropriate?

1 Evidence—Is there sufficient evidence to draw conclusions about what response the nurse should give?
2 Assumptions—Describe underlying assumptions about the following issues:
   a. Maternal age and risk of Down syndrome
   b. Ultrasound use by trimester
   c. Screening versus diagnosis for Down syndrome
3 What implications and priorities for nursing care can be made at this time?
4 Does the evidence objectively support your conclusion?
5 Are there alternative perspectives to your conclusion?

of a fetus with Down syndrome, the MSAFP and unconjugated estriol levels are low, whereas the hCG level is elevated. With these two additional screening tests, approximately 60% of cases of Down syndrome can be identified. Other maternal markers are being investigated as predictors of fetal abnormalities as well. Serum pregnancy-associated placental protein A (PAPP-A) is low in Down syndrome, whereas another substance, inhibin-A, is elevated in Down syndrome and other trisomies (Simpson, 2002).

As with MSAFP, these tests are screening procedures only and are not diagnostic. A definitive examination of amniotic fluid for AFP and chromosomal analysis combined with ultrasound visualization of the fetus is necessary for diagnosis.

Coombs' Test

The indirect Coombs' test is a screening for Rh incompatibility. If the maternal titer for Rh antibodies is greater than 1:8, amniocentesis for determination of bilirubin in amniotic fluid is indicated to establish the severity of fetal hemolytic anemia. Coombs' test also can detect other antibodies that may place the fetus at risk for incompatibility with maternal antigens.

ANTEPARTAL ASSESSMENT USING ELECTRONIC FETAL MONITORING
Indications

First- and second-trimester antepartal assessment is directed primarily at the diagnosis of fetal anomalies. The goal of third-trimester testing is to determine whether the intrauterine environment continues to be supportive to the fetus. The testing is often used to determine the timing of childbirth for women at risk for UPI. Gradual loss of placental function results first in inadequate nutrient delivery to the fetus, leading to IUGR. Subsequently, respiratory function also is compromised, resulting in fetal hypoxia. Common indications for both the NST and the CST are listed in Box 21-7.

No clinical contraindications exist for the NST, but results may not be conclusive if gestation is 26 weeks or less. Absolute contraindications for the CST are the following: rupture of membranes, previous classic incision for cesarean birth, preterm labor, placenta previa, and abruptio placentae. Other conditions in which the CST may be contraindicated are multifetal pregnancy, previous preterm labor, hydramnios, more than 36 weeks of gestation, and incompetent cervix. As a rule, reactive patterns with the NST or negative results with the CST are associated with favorable outcomes.

Fetal Responses to Hypoxia and Asphyxia

Observable fetal responses to hypoxia or asphyxia are the clinical basis for testing with EFM. Hypoxia or asphyxia elicits a number of responses in the fetus. Blood flow is redistributed to certain vital organs. This series of responses (redistribution of blood flow favoring vital organs, decrease in total oxygen consumption, and switch to anaerobic glycolysis) is a temporary mechanism that enables the fetus to survive up to 30 minutes of limited oxygen supply without decompensation of vital organs. However, during more severe asphyxia or sustained hypoxemia, these compensatory responses are no longer maintained, and a decrease in the cardiac output, arterial blood pressure, and blood flow to the brain and heart occurs with characteristic FHR patterns reflecting these changes (Parer & Nageotte, 2004).

Variability

Considerable evidence supports the clinical belief that FHR variability indicates an intact nervous pathway through the cerebral cortex, midbrain, vagus nerve, and cardiac conduction system. With 98% accuracy in predicting fetal well-being, the presence of normal FHR variability is a reassuring indicator. Inputs from various areas of the brain decrease after cerebral asphyxia, leading to a decrease in variability after failure of the fetal hemodynamic compensatory mechanisms to maintain cerebral oxygenation (Parer & Nageotte, 2004).

Nonstress Test

The nonstress test (NST) is the most widely applied technique for antepartum evaluation of the fetus. It is an ideal screening test and is the primary method of antepartum fetal assessment at most sites. The basis for the NST is that the normal fetus will produce characteristic HR patterns in response to fetal movement. In the healthy fetus with an intact CNS, 90% of gross fetal body movements are associated with accelerations of the FHR. The acceleration with movement response may be blunted by hypoxia, acidosis, drugs (analgesics, barbiturates, and beta-blockers), fetal sleep, and some congenital anomalies (Tucker, 2004). The NST can be performed easily and quickly in an outpatient setting because it is noninvasive, is relatively inexpensive, and has no known contraindications. Disadvantages center around the high rate of false-positive results for nonreactivity as a result of fetal sleep cycles, chronic tobacco smoking, medications, and fetal immaturity. The test also is slightly less sensitive in detecting fetal compromise than are the CST or BPP.

Procedure

The woman is seated in a reclining chair (or in semi-Fowler position) with a slight left tilt to optimize uterine perfusion and avoid supine hypotension. The FHR is recorded with a Doppler transducer, and a tocodynamometer is applied to detect uterine contractions or fetal movements. The tracing is observed for signs of fetal activity and a concurrent acceleration of FHR. If evidence of fetal movement is not apparent on the tracing, the woman may be asked to depress a button on a hand-held event marker connected to the monitor when she feels fetal movement. The movement is then noted on the tracing. Because almost all accelerations are accompanied by fetal movement, the movements need not be recorded for the test to be considered reactive. The test is usually completed within 20 to 30 minutes, but it may take longer if the fetus must be awakened from a sleep state.

It has been suggested that the woman drink orange juice or be given glucose to increase her blood sugar level and thereby stimulate fetal movements. This practice is common; however, research has not proven this practice to be effec-

---

> ### BOX 21-7
>
> #### Indications for Electronic Fetal Monitoring Assessment Using NST and CST
>
> - Maternal diabetes mellitus
> - Chronic hypertension
> - Hypertensive disorders in pregnancy
> - Intrauterine growth restriction
> - Sickle cell disease
> - Maternal cyanotic heart disease
> - Postmaturity
> - History of previous stillbirth
> - Decreased fetal movement
> - Isoimmunization
> - Meconium-stained amniotic fluid at third-trimester amniocentesis
> - Hyperthyroidism
> - Collagen disease
> - Older pregnant woman
> - Chronic renal disease

NST, nonstress test; *CST,* contraction stress test.

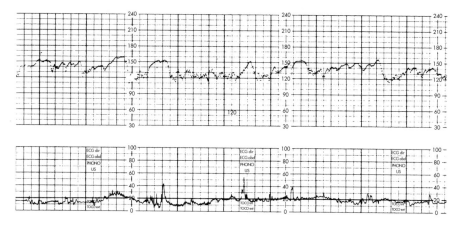

Fig. 21-8 Reactive nonstress test (fetal heart rate acceleration with movement). (From Tucker, S. [2004]. *Pocket guide to fetal monitoring and assessment* [5th ed.]. St. Louis: Mosby.)

tive (Tan & Sabapathy, 2001). Some sources suggest that fetal movements increase when maternal glucose levels are low. Other methods that have been used to stimulate fetal activity, such as manipulating the woman's abdomen or using a transvaginal light, have not been very effective either. Only vibroacoustic stimulation has had some impact (Tan & Smyth, 2001).

Interpretation

Generally accepted criteria for a reactive tracing are as follows:

- Two or more accelerations of 15 beats/min lasting for 15 seconds over a 20-minute period
- Normal baseline rate
- Long-term variability amplitude of 10 or more beats/min

If the test does not meet the criteria after 40 minutes, it is considered nonreactive (Fig. 21-8 and Table 21-5), in which case further assessments are needed with a CST or BPP. The current recommendation is that the NST be performed twice weekly (after 28 weeks of gestation) with women who have diabetes or are at risk for having a fetal death (Druzin, Gabbe, & Reed, 2002).

Vibroacoustic Stimulation

Vibroacoustic stimulation (also called *fetal acoustic stimulation test*) is another method of testing antepartum FHR response and is sometimes used in conjunction with the NST. The test takes approximately 15 minutes to complete, with the fetus monitored for 5 to 10 minutes before stimulation to obtain a baseline FHR. If the fetal baseline pattern is nonreactive, the sound source (usually a laryngeal stimulator) is then activated for 3 seconds on the maternal abdomen over the fetal head. Monitoring continues for another 5 minutes, after which the monitor tracing is assessed. A test is considered reactive if there is an immediate and sustained increase in long-term variability and HR accelerations. The accelerations produced may have a significant increase in duration. The test may be repeated at 1-minute intervals up to 3 times when there is no response. Further evaluation

---

TABLE 21-5

Interpretation of the Nonstress Test

RESULT	INTERPRETATION	CLINICAL SIGNIFICANCE
Reactive	Two or more accelerations of FHR of 15 beats/min lasting ≥ 15 sec, associated with each fetal movement in 20-min period	As long as twice-weekly NSTs remain reactive, most high risk pregnancies are allowed to continue
Nonreactive	Any tracing with either no FHR accelerations or accelerations <15 beats/min or lasting <15 sec throughout any fetal movement during testing period	Further indirect monitoring may be attempted with abdominal fetal electrocardiography in effort to clarify FHR pattern and quantitate variability; external monitoring should continue, and CST or BPP should be done
Unsatisfactory	Quality of FHR recording not adequate for interpretation	Test is repeated in 24 hr or CST is done, depending on clinical situation

Reference: Tucker, S. (2004). *Pocket guide to fetal monitoring and assessment* (5th ed.). St. Louis: Mosby.
BPP, Biophysical profile; *CST,* contraction stress test; *FHR,* fetal heart rate; *NST,* nonstress test.

is needed with BPP or CST if the pattern is still nonreactive (Druzin, Gabbe, & Reed, 2002).

Contraction Stress Test

The contraction stress test (CST) is one of the first electronic methods to be developed for assessment of fetal health. It was devised as a graded stress test of the fetus, and its purpose was to identify the jeopardized fetus that was stable at rest but showed evidence of compromise after stress. Uterine contractions decrease uterine blood flow and placental perfusion. If this decrease is sufficient to produce hypoxia in the fetus, a deceleration in FHR will result, beginning at the peak of the contraction and persisting after its conclusion (late deceleration).

NURSE ALERT *In a healthy fetoplacental unit, uterine contractions usually do not produce late decelerations, whereas if there is underlying uteroplacental insufficiency, contractions will produce late decelerations.*

The CST provides an earlier warning of fetal compromise than the NST and with fewer false-positive results. In addition to the contraindications described earlier, the CST is more time consuming and expensive than the NST. It also is an invasive procedure if oxytocin stimulation is required. It is infrequently used.

Procedure

The woman is placed in semi-Fowler position or sits in a reclining chair with a slight left tilt to optimize uterine perfusion and avoid supine hypotension. She is monitored electronically with the fetal ultrasound transducer and uterine tocodynamometer. The tracing is observed for 10 to 20 minutes for baseline rate, long-term variability, and the possible occurrence of spontaneous contractions. The two methods of CST are the nipple-stimulated contraction test and the oxytocin-stimulated contraction test.

Nipple-stimulated contraction test. Several methods of nipple stimulation have been described. In one approach the woman applies warm, moist washcloths to both breasts for several minutes. The woman is then asked to massage one nipple for 10 minutes. Massaging the nipples causes a release of oxytocin from the posterior pituitary. An alternative approach is for her to massage the nipple for 2 minutes, rest for 5 minutes, and repeat the cycles of massage and rest as necessary to achieve adequate uterine activity. When adequate contractions or hyperstimulation (defined as uterine contractions lasting more than 90 seconds or five or more contractions in 10 minutes) occurs, stimulation should be stopped (Druzin, Gabbe, & Reed, 2002).

Oxytocin-stimulated contraction test. Exogenous oxytocin also can be used to stimulate uterine contractions. An intravenous (IV) infusion is begun with a scalp needle. The oxytocin is diluted in an IV solution (e.g., 10 units in 1000 ml of fluid), infused into the tubing of the main IV device through a piggyback port, and delivered by an infusion pump to ensure accurate dosage. One method of oxytocin infusion is to begin at 0.5 milliunits/min and increase the dose by 0.5 millunits/min at 15- to 30-minute intervals until three uterine contractions of good quality are observed within a 10-minute period. A rate of 10 milliunits/min is usually adequate to elicit uterine contractions (Druzin, Gabbe, & Reed, 2002).

Interpretation

If no late decelerations are observed with the contractions, the findings are considered negative (Fig. 21-9, *A*). Repetitive late decelerations render the test results positive (Fig. 21-9, *B*, and Table 21-6).

After interpretation of the FHR pattern, the oxytocin infusion is halted, and the maintenance IV solution infused until uterine activity has returned to the prestimulation level. If the CST is negative, the IV device is removed, and the fetal monitor disconnected. If the CST is positive, continued monitoring and further evaluation of fetal well-being are indicated.

Nursing Role in Antepartal Assessment for Risk

The nurse's role is that of educator and support person when the woman is undergoing such examinations as ultrasonography, MRI, CVS, PUBS, and amniocentesis. In some instances, the nurse may assist the physician with the procedure. In many settings, nurses perform NSTs, CSTs, and BPPs; conduct an initial assessment; and begin necessary interventions for nonreassuring patterns. These nursing procedures are accomplished after additional education and training, under guidance of established protocols, and in collaboration with obstetrics providers (Menihan, 2000; Stringer et al., 2003). Patient teaching, which is an integral component of this role, involves preparing the woman for the procedure, interpreting the findings, and providing psychosocial support when needed.

Psychologic considerations

All women who undergo antepartal assessments are at risk for real and potential problems and may be in an anxious frame of mind. In most instances, the tests are ordered because of suspected fetal compromise, deterioration of a maternal condition, or both. In the third trimester, pregnant women are most concerned about protecting themselves and their fetuses and consider themselves most vulnerable to outside influences. The label of high risk will increase this sense of vulnerability.

When a woman is diagnosed with a high risk pregnancy, she and her family will likely experience stress related to the diagnosis. The woman may exhibit various psychologic responses including anxiety, low self-esteem, guilt, frustration, and inability to function. The development of a high risk pregnancy also can affect parental attachment, accomplishment of the tasks of pregnancy, and family adaptation to the pregnancy (Ramer & Frank, 2001).

Women with complicated pregnancies perceive their risks as higher than do women with uncomplicated pregnancies

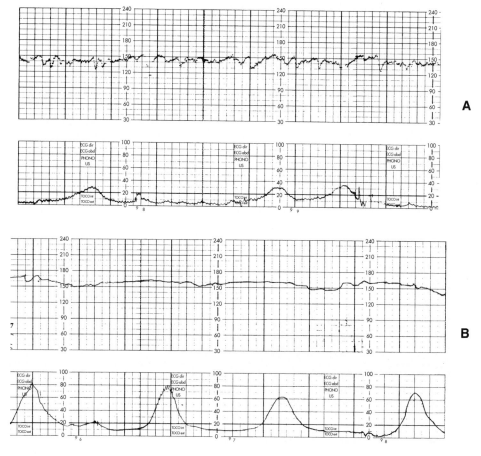

Fig. 21-9 Contraction stress test (CST). **A,** Negative CST. **B,** Positive CST. (From Tucker, S. [2004]. *Pocket guide to fetal monitoring and assessment* [5th ed.]. St. Louis: Mosby.)

(Gupton, Heaman, & Cheung, 2001). If the mother has to be placed on bed rest for pregnancy complications, separation from family, finances, and worry about children and home create further stress (Maloni, Brezinski-Tomasi, & Johnson, 2001).

If the woman is fearful for her own well-being, she may continue to feel ambivalence about the pregnancy or may not accept the reality of the pregnancy. She may not be able to complete preparations for the baby or go to childbirth classes if she is on bed rest or hospitalized. The family may become frustrated because they cannot engage in these activities that prepare them for parenthood.

Antepartal hospitalization is an added stressor for the high risk pregnant woman and her family. The woman may be lonely because she is separated from her home and family. She may feel powerless and unable to make decisions for herself because her care is out of her control. Likewise, preparation for the birth process may be out of control of the woman and her family. Unexpected procedures and care for the woman or fetus may take priority over the usual birth plan and may not allow choices that would have been selected if the pregnancy had been normal.

Attachment to the newborn can be affected if the mother or newborn is ill after the birth. Early contact may not be possible. Time, support, and intervention by the health care

team may be necessary to help the family begin the attachment process.

The nurse can help the woman and her family regain control and balance in their lives by providing support and encouragement, providing information about the pregnancy problem and its management (see Resources list at the end of this chapter), and providing opportunities to make as many choices as possible about the woman's care (Coffman & Ray, 2002).

The impact of the effects of a specific pregnancy complication and its management is discussed in the following chapters in this unit.

COMMUNITY ACTIVITY

Contact the nearest March of Dimes Birth Defects Foundation office to assess the resources available for parents (e.g., pamphlets, websites for high risk pregnancies) and what screening is recommended during pregnancy to identify problems. How can pregnant women get access to the March of Dimes information? What information or resources are available in your community for the problems identified?

Guide for Interpretation of the Contraction Stress Test

INTERPRETATION	CLINICAL SIGNIFICANCE
NEGATIVE No late decelerations, with minimum of three uterine contractions lasting 40 to 60 sec within 10-min period (see Fig. 21-9, *A*)	Reassurance that the fetus is likely to survive labor should it occur within 1 wk; more frequent testing may be indicated by clinical situation
POSITIVE Persistent and consistent late decelerations occurring with more than half of contractions (see Fig. 21-9, *B*)	Management lies between use of other tools of fetal assessment such as BPP and termination of pregnancy (e.g., labor induction, cesarean birth); a positive test result indicates that fetus is at increased risk for perinatal morbidity and mortality; physician may perform expeditious vaginal birth after successful induction or may proceed directly to cesarean birth; decision to intervene is determined by fetal monitoring and presence of FHR reactivity
SUSPICIOUS Late decelerations occurring in less than half of uterine contractions once adequate contraction pattern established	NST and CST should be repeated within 24 hr; if interpretable data cannot be achieved, other methods of fetal assessment must be used*
HYPERSTIMULATION Late decelerations occurring with excessive uterine activity (contractions more often than every 2 min or lasting >90 sec) or persistent increase in uterine tone	
UNSATISFACTORY Inadequate uterine contraction pattern, or tracing too poor to interpret	

Reference: Tucker, S. (2004). *Pocket guide to fetal monitoring and assessment* (5th ed.). St. Louis: Mosby.
BPP, Biophysical profile; *CST,* contraction stress test; *FHR,* fetal heart rate; *NST,* nonstress test.
*Applies to results noted as suspicious, hyperstimulation, or unsatisfactory.

Key Points

- A high risk pregnancy is one in which the life or well-being of the mother or infant is jeopardized by a biophysical or psychosocial disorder coincidental with or unique to pregnancy.
- Biophysical, sociodemographic, psychosocial, and environmental factors place the pregnancy and fetus or neonate at risk.
- Psychosocial perinatal warning indicators include characteristics of the parents, the child, their support systems, and family circumstances.
- Maternal and perinatal mortality rates for Caucasians are considerably lower than for other ethnic groups in the United States.
- Mortality rate decreases when risk is identified early and intensive care is applied.
- Biophysical assessment techniques include fetal movement counts, ultrasonography, and MRI.
- Biochemical monitoring techniques include amniocentesis, PUBS, CVS, and MSAFP.
- Reactive NSTs and negative CSTs suggest fetal well-being.
- Most assessment tests have some degree of risk for the mother and fetus and usually cause some anxiety for the woman and her family.

Answer Guidelines to Critical Thinking Exercise

Down Syndrome

1 Yes, there is sufficient evidence about use of ultrasound in the first trimester to obtain information about the pregnancy other than detecting fetal anomalies.

2 a. There is an increased risk of having a child with Down syndrome with increased maternal age, especially after age 40. For example, the incidence is 1 in 400 at age 35 and 1 in 30 at age 45.

b. Ultrasound is used in the first trimester for determining size and number of fetuses, presence of fetal cardiac and body movements, presence of uterine abnormalities, dating pregnancy, and identifying the presence and location of an intrauterine device (IUD). Fetal anomalies may be detected in the second trimester.

c. The triple-screen test—maternal serum alpha-fetoprotein (MSAFP), unconugated estriol, and beta-human chorionic gonadotropin (β-hCG)—at 16 to 18 weeks may predict up to 60% of cases of Down syndrome, although follow-up diagnostic testing with amniocentesis is needed to confirm the diagnosis. Lower-than-normal MSAFP and unconjugated estriol levels and elevated β-hCG levels in the second trimester are associated with Down syndrome.

3 The priority is to teach Patty what information the ultrasound examination at 8 weeks will provide. Information about other options (e.g., chorionic villus sampling [CVS]) to identify Down syndrome in the first trimester and the screening tests available in the second trimester may also be appropriate.

4 Yes, there is sufficient evidence to support this conclusion.

5 After hearing the choices, Patty and David may decide to have a CVS done or may wait until the second trimester for screening tests and then have amniocentesis if the screening tests warrant follow-up. They may also wait for a second-trimester ultrasound examination.

Resources

Healthy Mothers, Healthy Babies Coalition
409 12th St., SW
Washington, DC 20024
202-863-2458

March of Dimes Birth Defects Foundation
National Foundation/March of Dimes
1275 Mamaroneck Ave.
White Plains, NY 10605
914-428-7100
888-663-4637 (MODIMES)
www.modimes.org

National Clearinghouse for Human Genetic Disease (provides information about inherited diseases)
National Center for Education in Maternal and Child Health
38th and R Sts., NW
Washington, DC 20057

National Institute of Child Health and Human Development (NICHD)
National Institutes of Health
9000 Rockville Pike
Bldg. 31, Room 2A32
Bethesda, MD 20892
301-496-4000
www.nih.gov

Parenthood after Thirty
451 Vermont
Berkeley, CA 94707
415-524-6635

Spina Bifida Association of America
4590 McArthur Blvd., NW, Suite 250
Washington, DC 20007-4226
800-621-3141

References

Alfirevic, Z., Sundberg, K., & Brigham, S. (2003). Amniocentesis and chorionic villi sampling for prenatal diagnosis. (Cochrane Review). In *The Cochrane Library*, Issue 4, 2005. Chichester, UK: John Wiley & Sons.

American Academy of Pediatrics (AAP) & American College of Obstetricians and Gynecologists (ACOG). (2002). *Guidelines for perinatal care* (5th ed.). Elk Grove Village, IL: AAP & ACOG.

American College of Obstetricians and Gynecologists (ACOG). (2004). *ACOG issues position on first-trimester screening methods.* News release. Internet document available at www.acog.org/from_home/publications/press_releases/nr06-30-04.cfm (accessed January 6, 2005).

Arias, E., MacDorman, M., Strobino, D., & Guyer, B. (2003). Annual summary of vital statistics—2003. *Pediatrics, 112*(6 Pt 1), 1215-1230.

Association of Women's Health, Obstetric and Neonatal Nurses (AWHONN). (1998). *Nursing practice competencies and educational guidelines for limited ultrasound examination in obstetric and gynecology/infertility settings* (2nd ed.). Washington, DC: AWHONN.

Athey, P., & Hadlock, F. (1985). *Ultrasound in obstetrics and gynecology* (2nd ed.). St. Louis: Mosby.

Benn, P., Egan, J., Fang, M., & Smith-Bindman, R. (2004). Changes in utilization of prenatal diagnosis. *Obstetrics & Gynecology, 103*(6), 1255-1260.

Chervenak, F., & Gabbe, S. (2002). Obstetric ultrasound: Assessment of fetal growth and anatomy. In S. Gabbe, J. Niebyl, & J. Simpson (Eds.), *Obstetrics: Normal and problem pregnancies* (4th ed.). New York: Churchill Livingstone.

Coffman, S., & Ray, M. (2002). African American women describe support processes during high-risk pregnancy and postpartum. *Journal of Obstetric, Gynecologic, and Neonatal Nursing, 31*(5), 536-544.

Druzin, M., Gabbe, S., & Reed, K. (2002). Antepartum fetal evaluation. In S. Gabbe, J. Niebyl, & J. Simpson (Eds.), *Obstetrics: Normal and problem pregnancies* (4th ed.). New York: Churchill Livingstone.

Enkin, M., Keirse, M., Neilson, J., Crowther, C., Duley, L., Hodnett, E., & Hofmeyr, G. (2001). Effective care in pregnancy and childbirth: A synopsis. *Birth, 28*(1), 41-51.

Fanaroff, A., Martin, J., & Rodriguez, R. (2004). Identification and management of problems in the high-risk neonate. In R. Creasy, R. Resnik, & J. Iams (Eds.), *Maternal-fetal medicine: Principles and practice* (5th ed.). Philadelphia: Saunders.

Garcia, J., Bricker, L., Henderson, J., Martin, M., Mugford, M., Neilson, J., & Roberts, T. (2002). Women's views of pregnancy ultrasound: A systematic review. *Birth, 29*(4), 225-247.

Gilbert, E., & Harmon, J. (2003). *Manual of high risk pregnancy and delivery* (3rd ed.). St. Louis: Mosby.

Gillem-Goldstein, J. et al. (2003). Methods of assessment for pregnancy at risk. In A. DeCherney, & L. Nathan (Eds.), *Current obstetric and gynecologic diagnosis and treatment* (9th ed.). New York: Lange Medical Books/McGraw-Hill.

Glantz, J., & Woods, J. (2004). Significance of amniotic fluid meconium. In R. Creasy, R. Resnik, & J. Iams (Eds.), *Maternal-fetal medicine: Principles and practice* (5th ed.). Philadelphia: Saunders.

Gordon, M. (2002). *Manual of nursing diagnosis* (10th ed.). St. Louis: Mosby.

Gupton, A., Heaman, M., & Cheung, L. (2001). Complicated and uncomplicated pregnancies: Women's perception of risk. *Journal of Obstetric, Gynecologic, and Neonatal Nursing, 30*(2), 192-201.

Harman, C. (2004). Assessment of fetal health. In R. Creasy, R. Resnik, & J. Iams (Eds.), *Maternal-fetal medicine: Principles and practice* (5th ed.). Philadelphia: Saunders.

Jenkins, T., & Wapner, R. (2004). Prenatal diagnosis of congenital disorders. In R. Creasy, R. Resnik, & J. Iams (Eds.), *Maternal-fetal medicine: Principles and practice* (5th ed.). Philadelphia: Saunders.

Kochanek, K., Murphy, S., Anderson, R., & Scott, C. (2004). Deaths: Final data for 2002. *National Vital Statistics Reports, 53*(5), 1-115.

Maloni, J., Brezinski-Tomasi, J., & Johnson, L. (2001). Antepartum bed rest: Effect upon the family. *Journal of Obstetric, Gynecologic, and Neonatal Nursing, 30*(2), 67-77.

Manning, F. (2004). General principles and applications of ultrasound. In R. Creasy, R. Resnik, & J. Iams (Eds.), *Maternal-fetal medicine: Principles and practice* (5th ed.). Philadelphia: Saunders.

Menihan, C. (2000). Limited ultrasound in nursing practice. *Journal of Obstetric, Gynecologic, and Neonatal Nursing, 29*(3), 325-330.

Parer, J., & Nageotte, M. (2004). Intrapartum fetal surveillance. In R. Creasy, R. Resnik, & J. Iams (Eds.), *Maternal-fetal medicine: Principles and practice* (5th ed.). Philadelphia: Saunders.

Ramer, L., & Frank, B. (2001). *Pregnancy: Psychosocial perspectives* (3rd ed.). White Plains, NY: March of Dimes Birth Defects Foundation.

Silbergeld, E. & Patrick, T. (2005). Environmental exposures, toxicologic mechanisms, and adverse pregnancy outcomes. *American Journal of Obstetrics and Gynecology, 192*(5), S11-121.

Simpson, J. (2002). Genetic counseling and prenatal diagnosis. In S. Gabbe, J. Niebyl, & J. Simpson (Eds.), *Obstetrics: Normal and problem pregnancies* (4th ed.). New York: Churchill Livingstone.

Stringer, M., Miesnik, S., Brown, L., Menei, L., & Macones, G. (2003). Limited obstetric ultrasound examinations: Competency and cost. *Journal of Obstetric, Gynecologic, and Neonatal Nursing, 32*(3), 307-312.

Tan, K., & Sabapathy, A. (2001). Maternal glucose administration for facilitating tests of fetal wellbeing (Cochrane Review). In *The Cochrane Library*, Issue 4, 2005. Chichester, UK: John Wiley & Sons.

Tan, K., & Smyth, R. (2001). Fetal vibroacoustic stimulation for facilitation of tests of fetal wellbeing (Cochrane Review). In *The Cochrane Library*, Issue 4, 2005. Chichester, UK: John Wiley & Sons.

Tucker, S. (2004). *Pocket guide to fetal monitoring and assessment* (5th ed.). St. Louis: Mosby.

United States Department of Health and Human Services (USDHHS). (2000). *Healthy People 2010.* (Conference Edition) (Vol. 1-2). Washington, DC: U.S. Government Printing Office.

Wilson, R. (2000). Amniocentesis and chorionic villus sampling. *Current Opinion in Obstetrics and Gynecology, 12*(2), 81-86.

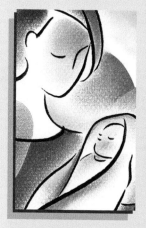

Pregnancy at Risk: Preexisting Conditions

ROBIN WEBB CORBETT

LEARNING OBJECTIVES

- *Differentiate the types of diabetes mellitus and their respective risk factors in pregnancy.*
- *Compare insulin requirements during pregnancy, postpartum, and with lactation.*
- *Identify maternal and fetal risks or complications associated with diabetes in pregnancy.*
- *Develop a plan of care for the pregnant woman with pregestational or gestational diabetes.*
- *Explain the effects of thyroid disorders on pregnancy.*
- *Differentiate the management for pregnant women with class I to class IV cardiac disease.*
- *Describe the different types of anemia and their effects during pregnancy.*

- *Explain the care of pregnant women with pulmonary disorders.*
- *Discuss the effects of gastrointestinal disorders on pregnancy.*
- *Describe the effects of neurologic disorders on pregnancy.*
- *Outline the care of women whose pregnancies are complicated by autoimmune disorders.*
- *Explain effects on and management of pregnant women who have human immunodeficiency virus (HIV) infection.*
- *Discuss the care of pregnant women who use, abuse, or are dependent on alcohol or illicit or prescription drugs.*

KEY TERMS AND DEFINITIONS

autoimmune disorders Group of diseases that disrupt the function of the immune system, causing the body to produce antibodies against itself, resulting in tissue damage

cardiac decompensation Condition of heart failure in which the heart is unable to maintain a sufficient cardiac output

euglycemia Pertaining to a normal blood glucose level; also called *normoglycemia*

gestational diabetes mellitus (GDM) Glucose intolerance first recognized during pregnancy

glycosylated hemoglobin A$_{1c}$ Glycohemoglobin, a minor hemoglobin with glucose attached; the glycosylated hemoglobin concentration represents the average blood glucose level over the previous several weeks and is a measurement of glycemic control in diabetic therapy

hydramnios (polyhydramnios) Amniotic fluid in excess of 2000 ml

hyperglycemia Excess glucose in the blood, usually caused by inadequate secretion of insulin by the islet cells of the pancreas or inadequate control of diabetes mellitus

hyperthyroidism Excessive functional activity of the thyroid gland

hypoglycemia Less than normal amount of glucose in the blood; usually caused by administration of too much insulin, excessive secretion of insulin by the islet cells of the pancreas, or dietary deficiency

hypothyroidism Deficiency of thyroid gland activity with underproduction of thyroxine

ketoacidosis The accumulation of ketone bodies in the blood as a consequence of hyperglycemia; leads to metabolic acidosis

macrosomia Large body size as seen in neonates of mothers with pregestational or gestational diabetes

peripartum cardiomyopathy Inability of the heart to maintain an adequate cardiac output; congestive heart failure occurring during the peripartum

pregestational diabetes mellitus Diabetes mellitus type 1 or type 2 that exists before pregnancy

reflex bradycardia Slowing of the heart in response to a particular stimulus

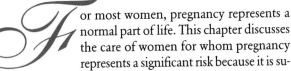

For most women, pregnancy represents a normal part of life. This chapter discusses the care of women for whom pregnancy represents a significant risk because it is superimposed on a preexisting condition. However, with the active participation of well-motivated women in the treatment plan and careful management from a multidisciplinary health care team, positive pregnancy outcomes are often possible.

Providing safe and effective care for women experiencing high risk pregnancy and their fetuses is a challenge. Although there are unique needs related to the preexisting conditions, these high risk women also experience the feelings, needs, and concerns associated with a normal pregnancy. The primary objective of nursing care is to achieve optimal outcomes for both the pregnant woman and the fetus.

This chapter focuses on diabetes mellitus and other metabolic disorders and cardiovascular disorders. Select disorders of the respiratory system, gastrointestinal system, integumentary system, and central nervous system (CNS); substance abuse; and human immunodeficiency virus (HIV) are also discussed.

METABOLIC DISORDERS

Diabetes Mellitus

The perinatal mortality rate for well-managed diabetic pregnancies, excluding major congenital malformations, is approximately the same as for any other pregnancy (Landon, Catalano, & Gabbe, 2002; Moore, 2004). The key to an optimal pregnancy outcome is strict maternal glucose control before conception, as well as throughout the gestational period. Consequently, much emphasis is placed on preconception counseling for women with diabetes.

Pregnancy complicated by diabetes is still considered high risk. It is most successfully managed by a multidisciplinary approach involving the obstetrician, perinatologist, internist or endocrinologist, ophthalmologist, nephrologist, neonatologist, nurse, nutritionist or dietitian, and social worker, as needed. A favorable outcome requires commitment and active participation by the pregnant woman and her family. It is preferable to plan the pregnancy, working with the woman and her family preconceptionally (Slocum et al., 2004).

Pathogenesis

Diabetes mellitus refers to a group of metabolic diseases characterized by hyperglycemia resulting from defects in in-

sulin secretion, insulin action, or both (Expert Committee on the Diagnosis and Classification of Diabetes Mellitus, 2003). Insulin, produced by the beta cells in the islets of Langerhans in the pancreas, regulates blood glucose levels by enabling glucose to enter adipose and muscle cells, where it is used for energy. When insulin is insufficient or ineffective in promoting glucose uptake by the muscle and adipose cells, glucose accumulates in the bloodstream, and hyperglycemia results. Hyperglycemia causes hyperosmolarity of the blood, which attracts intracellular fluid into the vascular system, resulting in cellular dehydration and expanded blood volume. Consequently, the kidneys function to excrete large volumes of urine (polyuria) in an attempt to regulate excess vascular volume and to excrete the unusable glucose (glycosuria). Polyuria, along with cellular dehydration, causes excessive thirst (polydipsia).

The body compensates for its inability to convert carbohydrate (glucose) into energy by burning proteins (muscle) and fats. However, the end products of this metabolism are ketones and fatty acids, which, in excess quantities, produce ketoacidosis and acetonuria. Weight loss occurs as a result of the breakdown of fat and muscle tissue. This tissue breakdown causes a state of starvation that compels the individual to eat excessive amounts of food (polyphagia).

Over time, diabetes causes significant changes in both the microvascular and macrovascular circulations. These structural changes affect a variety of organ systems, particularly the heart, eyes, kidneys, and nerves. Complications resulting from diabetes include premature atherosclerosis, retinopathy, nephropathy, and neuropathy.

Diabetes may be caused by either impaired insulin secretion, when the beta cells of the pancreas are destroyed by an autoimmune process, or by inadequate insulin action in target tissues at one or more points along the metabolic pathway. Both of these conditions are commonly present in the same person, and it is unclear which, if either, abnormality is the primary cause of the disease (Expert Committee on the Diagnosis and Classification of Diabetes Mellitus, 2003).

Classification

The current classification system for diabetes includes four groups: type 1 diabetes, type 2 diabetes, other specific types (e.g., diabetes caused by infection or induced by drugs), and gestational diabetes mellitus (GDM) (Expert Committee on the Diagnosis and Classification of Diabetes Mellitus, 2003). Approximately 8.7% of women greater than 20 years of age have diabetes mellitus (Bernasko, 2004), with approximately 4% to 7% of those women developing gestational diabetes or diabetes in pregnancy (ADA, 2004a; ADA, 2004b). Of the women with pregestational diabetes, the majority (65%) have type 2 diabetes (Chan & Johnson, 2006).

Type 1 diabetes includes those cases that are primarily caused by pancreatic islet beta cell destruction and that are prone to ketoacidosis. People with type 1 diabetes usually have an absolute insulin deficiency. Type 1 diabetes includes cases currently thought to be caused by an autoimmune process, as well as those for which the cause is unknown (Expert Committee on the Diagnosis and Classification of Diabetes Mellitus, 2003).

Type 2 diabetes is the most prevalent form of the disease and includes individuals who have insulin resistance and usually relative (rather than absolute) insulin deficiency. Specific causes of type 2 diabetes are unknown at this time. Type 2 diabetes often goes undiagnosed for years because hyperglycemia develops gradually and often is not severe enough for the patient to recognize the classic signs of polyuria, polydipsia, and polyphagia. Many people who develop type 2 diabetes are obese or have an increased amount of body fat distributed primarily in the abdominal area. Other risk factors for the development of type 2 diabetes include aging, a sedentary lifestyle, hypertension, and prior gestational diabetes. Type 2 diabetes often has a strong genetic predisposition (Expert Committee on the Diagnosis and Classification of Diabetes Mellitus, 2003).

Pregestational diabetes mellitus is the label sometimes given to type 1 or type 2 diabetes that existed before pregnancy. **Gestational diabetes mellitus** is any degree of glucose intolerance with the onset or first recognition occurring during pregnancy. This definition is appropriate whether or not insulin is used for treatment or the diabetes persists after pregnancy. It does not exclude the possibility that the glucose intolerance preceded the pregnancy. Women experiencing gestational diabetes should be reclassified 6 weeks or more after the pregnancy ends (Expert Committee on the Diagnosis and Classification of Diabetes Mellitus, 2003).

Metabolic changes associated with pregnancy

Normal pregnancy is characterized by complex alterations in maternal glucose metabolism, insulin production, and metabolic homeostasis. During normal pregnancy, adjustments in maternal metabolism allow for adequate nutrition for both the mother and the developing fetus. Glucose, the primary fuel used by the fetus, is transported across the placenta through the process of carrier-mediated facilitated diffusion. This means that the glucose levels in the fetus are directly proportional to maternal levels. Although glucose crosses the placenta, insulin does not. Around the tenth week of gestation the fetus begins to secrete its own insulin at levels adequate to use the glucose obtained from the mother. Therefore, as maternal glucose levels rise, fetal glucose levels are increased, resulting in increased fetal insulin secretion.

During the first trimester of pregnancy the pregnant woman's metabolic status is significantly influenced by the rising levels of estrogen and progesterone. These hormones stimulate the beta cells in the pancreas to increase insulin production, which promotes increased peripheral use of glucose and decreased blood glucose, with fasting levels being reduced by approximately 10% (Fig. 22-1, *A*). A concomitant increase in tissue glycogen stores and a decrease in hepatic glucose production occur, which further encourage lower fasting glucose levels. As a result of these normal metabolic changes of pregnancy, women with insulin-dependent diabetes are prone to hypoglycemia during the first trimester.

During the second and third trimesters, pregnancy exerts a "diabetogenic" effect on the maternal metabolic status. Because of the major hormonal changes, there is decreased tolerance to glucose, increased insulin resistance, decreased hepatic glycogen stores, and increased hepatic production of glucose. Increasing levels of human chorionic somatomammotropin, estrogen, progesterone, prolactin, cortisol, and insulinase increase insulin resistance through their actions as insulin antagonists. Insulin resistance is a glucose-sparing mechanism that ensures an abundant supply of glucose for the fetus. Maternal insulin requirements gradually increase from about 18 to 24 weeks of gestation to about 36 weeks of gestation. Maternal insulin requirements may double or quadruple by the end of the pregnancy (Fig. 22-1, *B* and *C*).

At birth, expulsion of the placenta prompts an abrupt drop in levels of circulating placental hormones, cortisol, and insulinase (Fig. 22-1, *D*). Maternal tissues quickly regain their prepregnancy sensitivity to insulin. For the nonbreastfeeding mother the prepregnancy insulin-carbohydrate balance usually returns in approximately 7 to 10 days (Fig. 22-1, *E*). Lactation uses maternal glucose; therefore the breastfeeding mother's insulin requirements will remain low during lactation. On completion of weaning, the mother's prepregnancy insulin requirement is reestablished (Fig. 22-1, *F*).

Pregestational Diabetes Mellitus

Approximately two per 1000 pregnancies are complicated by preexisting diabetes. Women who have pregestational diabetes may have either type 1 or type 2 diabetes, which may or may not be complicated by vascular disease, retinopathy, nephropathy, or other diabetic sequelae. Type 1 diabetes is the more common diagnosis, but as the incidence of type 2 diabetes increases in the general population it may become the more prevalent diagnosis. Almost all women with pregestational diabetes are insulin dependent during pregnancy.

The diabetogenic state of pregnancy imposed on the compromised metabolic system of the woman with pregestational diabetes has significant implications. The normal hormonal adaptations of pregnancy affect glycemic control, and pregnancy may accelerate the progress of vascular complications.

During the first trimester, when maternal blood glucose levels are normally reduced and the insulin response to

Evolve/CD: Case Study—Pregestational Diabetes

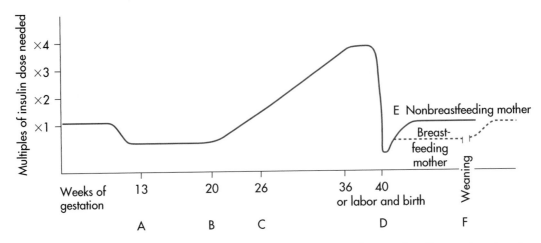

Fig. 22-1   Changing insulin needs during pregnancy. **A,** First trimester: Insulin need is reduced because of increased production by pancreas and increased peripheral sensitivity to insulin; nausea, vomiting, and decreased food intake by mother and glucose transfer to embryo or fetus contribute to hypoglycemia. **B,** Second trimester: Insulin needs begin to increase as placental hormones, cortisol, and insulinase act as insulin antagonists, decreasing insulin's effectiveness. **C,** Third trimester: Insulin needs may double or even quadruple but usually level off after 36 weeks of gestation. **D,** Day of birth: Maternal insulin requirements drop drastically to approach prepregnancy levels. **E,** Breastfeeding mother maintains lower insulin requirements, as much as 25% less than prepregnancy; insulin needs of nonbreastfeeding mother return to prepregnancy levels in 7 to 10 days. **F,** Weaning of breastfeeding infant causes mother's insulin needs to return to prepregnancy levels.

glucose is enhanced, glycemic control is improved. The insulin dosage for the woman with well-controlled diabetes may need to be reduced to avoid hypoglycemia. Nausea, vomiting, and cravings typical of early pregnancy result in dietary fluctuations that influence maternal glucose levels and may also necessitate a reduction in insulin dosage.

Because insulin requirements steadily increase after the first trimester, insulin dosage must be adjusted accordingly to prevent hyperglycemia. Insulin resistance begins as early as 14 to 16 weeks and continues to rise until it stabilizes during the last few weeks of pregnancy.

Diabetic nephropathy has more impact on perinatal outcome than any other vascular complication. Increased risks of preeclampsia, preterm labor, intrauterine growth restriction (IUGR), fetal distress, stillbirth, and neonatal death are associated with this condition (Moore, 2004).

Preconception counseling

Preconception counseling is recommended for all women of reproductive age who have diabetes because it is associated with an improved pregnancy outcome (Moore, 2004). Under ideal circumstances, women with pregestational diabetes are counseled before the time of conception to plan the optimal time for pregnancy, establish glycemic control before conception, and diagnose any vascular complications of diabetes. However, it has been estimated that fewer than 20% of women with diabetes in the United States participate in preconception counseling (Landon, Catalano, & Gabbe, 2002).

The woman's partner should be included in the counseling to assess the couple's level of understanding related to the effects of pregnancy on the diabetic condition and of the potential complications of pregnancy as a result of diabetes. The couple should also be informed of the anticipated alterations in management of diabetes during pregnancy and the need for a multidisciplinary team approach to health care. Financial implications of diabetic pregnancy and other demands related to frequent maternal and fetal surveillance should be discussed. Contraception is another important aspect of preconception counseling to assist the couple in planning effectively for pregnancy.

Maternal risks and complications

Although maternal morbidity and mortality rates have improved significantly, the pregnant woman with diabetes remains at risk for the development of complications during pregnancy. In women who have diabetes, poor glycemic control around the time of conception and in the early weeks of pregnancy is associated with an increased incidence of miscarriage. Women with good glycemic control before conception and in the first trimester are no more likely to miscarry than women who do not have diabetes (Moore, 2004).

Poor glycemic control later in pregnancy, particularly in women without vascular disease, increases the rate of fetal macrosomia. Macrosomia occurs in 20% to 25% of diabetic pregnancies. Macrosomic infants tend to have a disproportionate increase in shoulder and trunk size. Because of this, the risk of shoulder dystocia is greater in these babies than in other macrosomic infants. Women with diabetes therefore face an increased likelihood of cesarean birth because

Critical Thinking Exercise

Diabetes Mellitus

Maria is a 28-year-old pregnant woman, G7P4-2-0-4 who is 30 weeks of gestation. She is 64 inches tall and weighs 277 lbs. Her fasting blood sugar (FBS) is 173 and her HgbA$_{1c}$ is 10.6. She had previously been on glucophage 500 mg bid and took it prior to pregnancy. This is her first visit. The provider prescribes Lantus insulin 37 units and regular insulin 5 units with meals. At her next prenatal visit, she is 32 weeks gestation and reports she is not taking her insulin, "because I can't do that." Her provider prescribes an oral hypoglycemic, glyburide. She asks if she can take this medicine while she is pregnant.

1 Is there sufficient evidence to draw conclusions about her diagnosis and preferred treatment?

2 What assumptions can be made about the following items?
   a. Possible diagnoses.
   b. Physical assessment, laboratory tests, and diagnostic procedures that will be done to make a diagnosis.
   c. Factors contributing to her elevated blood sugar.
   d. Factors contributing to the provider's prescription of an oral hypoglycemic.

3 What implications and priorities for nursing care can be drawn at this time?

4 Does the evidence objectively support your conclusion?

5 Are there alternative perspectives to your conclusion?

---

of failure of fetal descent or labor progress, or of operative vaginal birth (birth involving the use of episiotomy, forceps, or vacuum extractor) (Moore, 2004).

The hypertensive disorder, preeclampsia or eclampsia, occurs more frequently during diabetic pregnancies (Moore, 2004). The highest incidence occurs in women with preexisting vascular changes related to diabetes (Moore, 2004).

Hydramnios (polyhydramnios) occurs approximately 10 times more often in diabetic than in nondiabetic pregnancies. Hydramnios (amniotic fluid in excess of 2000 ml) is associated with premature rupture of membranes (PROM), onset of preterm labor, and postpartum hemorrhage (Cunningham et al., 2005).

Infections are more common and more serious in pregnant women with diabetes. Disorders of carbohydrate metabolism alter the body's normal resistance to infection. The inflammatory response, leukocyte function, and vaginal pH are all affected. Vaginal infections, particularly monilial vaginitis, are more common. Urinary tract infections (UTIs) are also more prevalent. Infection is serious because it causes increased insulin resistance and may result in ketoacidosis. Postpartum infection is more common among women who are insulin dependent.

Ketoacidosis occurs most often during the second and third trimesters, when the diabetogenic effect of pregnancy is the greatest. When the maternal metabolism is stressed by illness or infection, the woman is at increased risk for diabetic ketoacidosis (DKA). The use of tocolytic drugs such as terbutaline to arrest preterm labor may also contribute to the risk for hyperglycemia and subsequent DKA (Cunningham et al., 2005; Iams & Creasy, 2004). DKA may also occur because of the woman's failure to take insulin appropriately. The onset of previously undiagnosed diabetes during pregnancy is another cause. DKA may occur with blood glucose levels barely exceeding 200 mg/dl, compared with 300 to 350 mg/dl in the nonpregnant state. In response to stress factors such as infection or illness, hyperglycemia occurs as a result of increased hepatic glucose production and decreased peripheral glucose use. Stress hormones, which act to impair insulin action and further contribute to insulin deficiency, are released. Fatty acids are mobilized from fat stores to enter into the circulation. As they are oxidized, ketone bodies are released into the peripheral circulation. The woman's buffering system is unable to compensate, and metabolic acidosis develops. The excessive blood glucose and ketone bodies result in osmotic diuresis with subsequent loss of fluid and electrolytes, volume depletion, and cellular dehydration. Prompt treatment of DKA is necessary to avoid maternal coma or death. Ketoacidosis occurring at any time during pregnancy can lead to intrauterine fetal death. It is also a cause of preterm labor. Fetal demise is approximately 10% with maternal ketoacidosis (Moore, 2004) (Table 22-1).

The risk of hypoglycemia is also increased. Early in pregnancy, when hepatic production of glucose is diminished and peripheral use of glucose is enhanced, hypoglycemia occurs frequently, often during sleep. Later in pregnancy hypoglycemia may also result as insulin doses are adjusted to maintain normoglycemia. Women with a prepregnancy history of severe hypoglycemia are at increased risk for severe hypoglycemia during gestation. Mild to moderate hypoglycemic episodes do not appear to have significant deleterious effects on fetal well-being. (see Table 22-1).

Fetal and neonatal risks and complications

From the moment of conception, the infant of a woman with diabetes faces an increased risk of complications that may occur during the antepartum, intrapartum, or neonatal periods. Infant morbidity and mortality rates associated with diabetic pregnancy are significantly reduced with strict control of maternal glucose levels before and during pregnancy.

Despite the improvements in care of pregnant women with diabetes, sudden and unexplained stillbirth is still a major concern. Typically, this is observed in pregnancies after 36 weeks in women with vascular disease or poor glycemic control. It may also be associated with DKA, preeclampsia, hydramnios, or macrosomia. Although the exact cause of stillbirth is unknown, it may be related to chronic intrauterine hypoxia.

The most important cause of perinatal loss in diabetic pregnancy is congenital malformations, accounting for up to 40% of all perinatal deaths. The incidence of congenital

TABLE 22-1

Differentiation of Hypoglycemia (Insulin Shock) and Hyperglycemia (Diabetic Ketoacidosis)

CAUSES	ONSET	SYMPTOMS	INTERVENTIONS
HYPOGLYCEMIA (INSULIN SHOCK)			
Excess insulin	Rapid (regular insulin)	Irritability	Check blood glucose level when symptoms first appear
Insufficient food (delayed or missed meals)	Gradual (modified insulin or oral hypoglycemic agents)	Hunger	Eat or drink 10 to 15 grams simple carbohydrate immediately
Excessive exercise or work		Sweating	Recheck blood glucose level in 15 min and eat or drink another 10 to 15 grams simple carbohydrate if glucose remains low
Indigestion, diarrhea, vomiting		Nervousness	
		Personality change	Recheck blood glucose level in 15 min
		Weakness	
		Fatigue	Notify primary health care provider if no change in glucose level
		Blurred or double vision	
		Dizziness	If woman is unconscious, administer 50% dextrose IV push, 5% to 10% dextrose in water IV drip, or glucagon
		Headache	
		Pallor; clammy skin	
		Shallow respirations	
		Rapid pulse	Obtain blood and urine specimens for laboratory testing
		Laboratory values	
		Urine: negative for sugar and acetone	
		Blood glucose: ≤60 mg/dl	
HYPERGLYCEMIA (DKA)			
Insufficient insulin	Slow (hours to days)	Thirst	Notify primary health care provider
Excess or wrong kind of food		Nausea or vomiting	Administer insulin in accordance with blood glucose levels
Infection, injuries, illness		Abdominal pain	
Emotional stress		Constipation	Give IV fluids such as normal saline solution or one half normal saline solution; potassium when urinary output is adequate; bicarbonate for pH <7
Insufficient exercise		Drowsiness	
		Dim vision	
		Increased urination	
		Headache	Monitor laboratory testing of blood and urine
		Flushed, dry skin	
		Rapid breathing	
		Weak, rapid pulse	
		Acetone (fruity) breath odor	
		Laboratory value	
		Urine: positive for sugar and acetone	
		Blood glucose: ≥200 mg/dl	

DKA, Diabetic ketoacidosis; *IV,* intravenous.

malformations is related to the severity and duration of the diabetes. Anomalies commonly seen in infants primarily affect the cardiovascular system, CNS, and skeletal system (Cunningham et al., 2004; Moore, 2004) (see Chapter 27).

The fetal pancreas begins to secrete insulin at 10 to 14 weeks of gestation. The fetus responds to maternal hyperglycemia by secreting large amounts of insulin (hyperinsulinism). Insulin acts as a growth hormone, causing the fetus to produce excess stores of glycogen, protein, and adipose tissue, leading to increased fetal size, or macrosomia. Macrosomia is often defined as a weight of greater than 4500 g (American College of Obstetricians and Gynecologists [ACOG], 2000a). During birth the macrosomic infant is at risk for a fractured

clavicle, liver or spleen laceration, brachial plexus injury, facial palsy, phrenic nerve injury, or subdural hemorrhage (Moore, 2004) (for further discussion, see Chapter 27).

CARE MANAGEMENT

Assessment and Nursing Diagnoses

Interview

When a pregnant woman with diabetes initiates prenatal care, a thorough evaluation of her health status is completed. In addition to the routine prenatal assessment, a detailed history regarding the onset and course of the diabetes and its management and the degree of glycemic control before pregnancy is obtained. Effective management of the diabetic pregnancy depends on the woman's adherence to a plan of care. At the initial prenatal visit the woman's knowledge regarding diabetes and pregnancy, potential maternal and fetal complications, and the plan of care are also assessed. With subsequent visits, follow-up assessments are completed. Data from these assessments are used to identify the woman's specific learning needs.

The woman's emotional status is assessed to determine how she is coping with pregnancy superimposed on preexisting diabetes. Although normal pregnancy typically evokes some degree of stress and anxiety, pregnancy designated as *high risk* serves to compound anxiety and stress levels. Fear of maternal and fetal complications is a major concern. Strict adherence to the plan of care may necessitate alterations in patterns of daily living and may be an additional source of stress.

The woman's support system is assessed to identify those people significant to her and their roles in her life. It is important to assess reactions of the family or significant other to the pregnancy and to the strict management plan, and their involvement in the treatment regimen.

Physical examination

At the initial visit a thorough physical examination is performed to assess the woman's current health status. In addition to the routine prenatal examination, specific efforts are made to assess the effects of the diabetes, specifically diabetic retinopathy, nephropathy, autonomic neuropathy, and coronary artery disease (ADA, 2003). A baseline electrocardiogram (ECG) may be done to assess cardiovascular status. Evaluation for retinopathy is done, with follow-up by an ophthalmologist each trimester and more frequently if retinopathy is diagnosed. Blood pressure is monitored carefully throughout pregnancy because of the increased risk for preeclampsia. The woman's weight gain is also monitored at each visit. Fundal height is measured, with note made of any abnormal increase in size for dates, which may indicate hydramnios or fetal macrosomia.

Laboratory tests

Routine prenatal laboratory examinations are performed. In addition, baseline renal function may be assessed with a 24-hour urine collection for total protein excretion and creatinine clearance. Urinalysis and culture are performed on the initial prenatal visit and as needed throughout the pregnancy to assess for the presence of UTI, which is common in diabetic pregnancy. At each visit urine is tested for the presence of glucose and ketones. Because of the risk of coexisting thyroid disease, thyroid function tests may also be performed (see later discussion of thyroid disorders).

For the woman with pregestational type 1 or type 2 diabetes, laboratory tests may be done to assess past glycemic control. At the initial prenatal visit, the glycosylated hemoglobin A_{1c} level may be measured. With prolonged hyperglycemia some of the hemoglobin remains saturated with glu-

cose for the life of the red blood cell (RBC). Therefore a test for glycosylated hemoglobin provides a measure of glycemic control over time, specifically over the previous 4 to 6 weeks. Regular measurements of glycosylated hemoglobin provide data for altering the treatment plan and lead to improvement of glycemic control. Values for the measurement of hemoglobin A_{1c}, the most commonly used index of glycosylated hemoglobin, are as follows (Pagana & Pagana, 2003):

- Adult or elderly without diabetes: 2.2% to 4.8%
- Good diabetic control: 2.5% to 5.9%
- Fair diabetic control: 6% to 8%
- Poor diabetic control: greater than 8%

Fasting blood glucose or random (1 to 2 hours after eating) glucose levels may be assessed during antepartum visits (Fig. 22-2). Blood glucose self-monitoring records may also be reviewed.

Nursing diagnoses for the woman with pregestational diabetes include the following:

- *Deficient knowledge related to*
  —diabetic pregnancy, management, and potential effects on pregnant woman and fetus
  —insulin administration and its effects
  —hypoglycemia and hyperglycemia
  —diabetic diet
- *Anxiety, fear, dysfunctional grieving, powerlessness, disturbed body image, situational low self-esteem, spiritual distress, ineffective role performance, interrupted family processes related to*
  —stigma of being labeled "diabetic"
  —effects of diabetes and its potential sequelae on the pregnant woman and the fetus
- *Risk for noncompliance related to*
  —lack of understanding of diabetes and pregnancy and requirements of treatment plan
  —lack of financial resources to purchase blood glucose monitoring supplies or insulin and necessary supplies
  —insufficient funds or lack of transportation to grocery store to follow dietary regimen
- *Risk for injury to fetus related to*
  —uteroplacental insufficiency
  —birth trauma
- *Risk for injury to mother related to*
  —improper insulin administration
  —hypoglycemia and hyperglycemia
  —cesarean or operative vaginal birth
  —postpartum infection

Expected Outcomes of Care

Expected outcomes of management for the pregnant woman with pregestational diabetes include that she will do the following:

- Demonstrate or verbalize understanding of diabetic pregnancy, the plan of care, and the importance of glycemic control

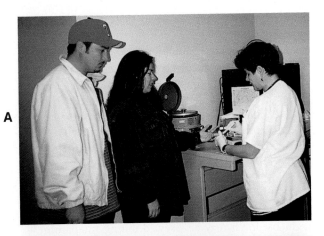

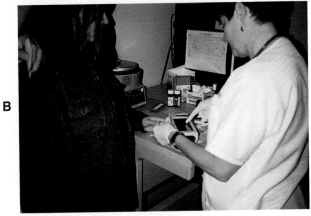

Fig. 22-2 **A,** Clinic nurse collects blood to determine glucose level. **B,** Nurse interprets glucose value displayed by monitor. (Courtesy Dee Lowdermilk, UNC Ambulatory Care Clinics, Chapel Hill, NC.)

- Achieve and maintain glycemic control
- Demonstrate effective coping
- Give birth to a healthy infant at term

Plan of Care and Interventions
Antepartum

Because of her high risk status, a woman with diabetes is monitored much more frequently and thoroughly than are other pregnant women. During the first and second trimesters of pregnancy, her routine prenatal care visits will be scheduled every 1 to 2 weeks. In the last trimester she will likely be seen one or two times each week. In the past, routine hospitalization for management of the diabetes, such as insulin dose changes, was common. With the availability of better home glucose monitoring and the growing reluctance of third-party payers to reimburse for hospitalization, pregnant women with diabetes are now generally managed as outpatients. Some patient and family education and maternal and fetal assessment may be done in the home, depending on the woman's insurance coverage and care provider preference.

Achieving and maintaining constant **euglycemia,** with blood glucose levels in the range of 65 to 105 mg/dl

preprandially (Table 22-2), is the primary goal of medical therapy (ACOG, 2004a; ACOG, 2004b; Moore, 2004). Euglycemia is achieved through a combination of diet, insulin, exercise, and blood glucose determinations. Providing the woman with the knowledge, skill, and motivation she needs to achieve and maintain excellent blood glucose control is the primary nursing goal.

Euglycemia is achieved through a combination of diet, insulin, and exercise. The necessary lifestyle changes for some women and their families can sometimes seem overwhelming. Maintaining tight blood glucose control necessitates that the woman follow a consistent daily schedule. She must get up and go to bed, eat, exercise, and take insulin at the same time each day. Blood glucose measurements are done frequently to determine how well the major components of therapy (diet, insulin, and exercise) are working together to control blood glucose levels. The woman should wear an identification bracelet at all times and carry insulin syringes and "glucose boosters" with her when away from home.

Because the woman is at increased risk for infections, eye problems, and neurologic changes, foot care and general skin care are important. A daily bath that includes good perineal care and foot care is important. For dry skin, lotions, creams, or oils can be applied. Tight clothing should be avoided. Shoes or slippers that fit properly should be worn at all times and are best worn with socks or stockings. Feet should be inspected regularly; toenails should be cut straight across, and professional help should be sought for any foot problems. Extremes of temperature should be avoided.

Diet. The woman with pregestational diabetes has usually had nutritional counseling regarding management of her diabetes. However, pregnancy precipitates special nutritional concerns and needs and the woman must be educated to incorporate these changes into dietary planning. Therefore, for the woman who has "controlled" her diabetes for a number of years, the changes in her insulin and dietary needs mandated by pregnancy may be difficult. Nutritional counseling is usually provided by a registered dietitian.

Dietary management during diabetic pregnancy must be based on blood (not urine) glucose levels. The diet is indi-

TABLE 22-2	
Target Blood Glucose Levels during Pregnancy	
TIME OF DAY	**TARGET PLASMA GLUCOSE LEVEL (MG/DL)**
Premeal/Fasting	>65 but <105
Postmeal (1 hr)	<130–155
Postmeal (2 hr)	<130

From American Diabetes Association (ADA). (2004b). Gestational diabetes mellitus. *Diabetes Care 27* (Suppl 1). S88-S90. Moore, T. (2004). Diabetes in pregnancy. In R. Creasy, R. Resnik, & J. Iams (Eds.). *Maternal-fetal medicine: Principles and practice* (5th ed.). Philadelphia: Saunders.

vidualized to allow for increased fetal and metabolic requirements, with consideration of such factors as prepregnancy weight and dietary habits, overall health, ethnic background, lifestyle, stage of pregnancy, knowledge of nutrition, and insulin therapy. The dietary goals are to provide weight gain consistent with a normal pregnancy, to prevent ketoacidosis, and to minimize wide fluctuation of blood glucose levels.

For nonobese women, dietary counseling based on preconceptional body mass index (BMI) is 30 kcal/kg/day (Cunningham et al., 2005). In contrast, for obese women with a BMI greater than 30, it is recommended that the caloric intake total 25 kcal/kg/day (Moore, 2004). The average diet includes 2200 calories (first trimester) to 2500 calories (second and third trimesters). Total calories may be distributed among three meals and one evening snack or, more commonly, three meals and at least two snacks. Meals should be eaten on time and never skipped. Snacks must be carefully planned in accordance with insulin therapy to avoid fluctuations in blood glucose levels. A large bedtime snack of at least 25 g of carbohydrate with some protein is recommended to help prevent hypoglycemia and starvation ketosis during the night.

The ratio of carbohydrate, protein, and fat or the carbohydrate-to-insulin ratio (C:I ratio) is important to meet the metabolic needs of the woman and the fetus (Bernasko, 2004). Approximately 40% to 50% of the total calories should be carbohydrates, with 30% to 40% fats and proteins providing the remainder of the caloric intake (ADA, 2004d; Bernasko, 2004) (Patient Instructions for Self-Care box below). Simple carbohydrates are limited; complex carbohydrates that are high in fiber content are recommended because the starch and protein in such foods help regulate the blood glucose level by more sustained glucose release. Weight gain for women with a normal BMI (19.8 to 26)

PATIENT INSTRUCTIONS FOR SELF-CARE

Dietary Management of Diabetic Pregnancy

- Follow the prescribed diet plan.
- Eat a well-balanced diet, including daily food requirements for a normal pregnancy.
- Divide daily food intake among three meals and two to four snacks, depending on individual needs.
- Eat a substantial bedtime snack to prevent a severe drop in blood glucose level during the night.
- Limit the intake of fats if weight gain occurs too rapidly.
- Take daily vitamins and iron as prescribed by the health care provider.
- Avoid foods high in refined sugar.
- Eat consistently each day; never skip meals or snacks.
- Reduce the intake of saturated fat and cholesterol.
- Eat foods high in dietary fiber.
- Avoid alcohol, nicotine, and caffeine.

should be approximately 12 kg during the pregnancy (Institute of Medicine [IOM, 1990]).

Exercise. Although it has been shown that exercise enhances the use of glucose and decreases insulin need in women without diabetes, there are limited data regarding exercise in women with pregestational diabetes. Any prescription of exercise during pregnancy for a women with diabetes should be done by the primary health care provider and should be monitored closely to prevent complications, especially for women with vasculopathy. Women with vasculopathy depend completely on exogenous insulin and are at greater risk for wide fluctuations in blood glucose levels and ketoacidosis, which can be made worse by exercise.

Careful instructions are given to the woman. Exercise need not be vigorous to be beneficial: 15 to 30 minutes of walking four to six times a week is satisfactory for most pregnant women. Other exercises that may be recommended are non–weight-bearing activities such as arm exercises or use of a recumbent bicycle. The best time for exercise is after meals, when the blood glucose level is rising. To monitor the effect of insulin on blood glucose levels, the woman can measure blood glucose before, during, and after exercise.

NURSE ALERT *Uterine contractions may occur during exercise; the woman should stop exercising immediately if they are detected.*

Insulin therapy. Adequate insulin is the primary factor in the maintenance of euglycemia during pregnancy, thus ensuring proper glucose metabolism of the woman and fetus. Insulin requirements during pregnancy change dramatically as the pregnancy progresses, necessitating frequent adjustments in insulin dosage. In the first trimester, from 3 to 7 weeks of gestation there is an increase in insulin requirements, followed by a decrease between 7 and 15 weeks of gestation. However, insulin dosage may need to be decreased because of hypoglycemia. The common prescribed insulin dosage is 0.7 units/kg in the first trimester for women with type 1 diabetes (Moore, 2004). During the second and third trimester, because of insulin resistance, dosage must be increased to maintain target glucose levels. As insulin needs rise, women with type 1 diabetes require a dosage increase to 0.8 units/kg during weeks of gestation 18 to 26, 0.9 units/kg during weeks of gestation 27 to 36, and 1 unit/kg from 37 weeks of gestation until labor (ADA, 2004c; Moore, 2004).

For the woman with type 1 pregestational diabetes who has typically been accustomed to one injection per day of intermediate-acting insulin, multiple daily injections of mixed insulin are a new experience. The woman with type 2 diabetes previously treated with oral hypoglycemics is faced with the task of learning to self-administer injections of insulin. The nurse is instrumental in education and support of pregestational diabetic women with regard to insulin administration and adjustment of insulin dosage to maintain euglycemia (Patient Instructions for Self-Care box on p. 682).

Many types of biosynthetic human insulin preparations (Humulin or Novolin) are available, including regular, NPH,

PATIENT INSTRUCTIONS FOR SELF-CARE
Self-Administration of Insulin

PROCEDURE FOR MIXING NPH (INTERMEDIATE-ACTING) AND REGULAR (SHORT-ACTING) INSULIN

- Wash hands thoroughly and gather supplies. Be sure the insulin syringe corresponds to the concentration of insulin you are using.
- Check insulin bottle to be certain it is the appropriate type, and check the expiration date.
- Gently rotate (do not shake) the insulin vial to mix the insulin.
- Wipe off rubber stopper of each vial with alcohol.
- Draw into syringe the amount of air equal to total dose.
- Inject air equal to NPH (intermediate-acting) dose into NPH vial. Remove syringe from vial.
- Inject air equal to regular insulin dose into regular insulin vial.
- Invert regular insulin bottle and withdraw regular insulin dose.
- Without adding more air to NPH vial, carefully withdraw NPH dose.

PROCEDURE FOR SELF-INJECTION OF INSULIN

- Select proper injection site (remember to rotate sites).
- Injection site should be clean. No need to use alcohol. If alcohol is used, let it dry before injecting.
- Pinch the skin up to form a subcutaneous pocket and, holding the syringe like a pencil, puncture the skin at a 45- to 90-degree angle. If there is a great deal of fatty tissue at the site, spread the skin taut and inject the syringe at a 90-degree angle.
- Slowly inject the insulin.
- As you withdraw the needle, cover the injection site with sterile gauze and apply gentle pressure to prevent bleeding.
- Record insulin dosage and time of injection.

Lente, Semi-lente, and mixed. These insulins are less likely to cause antibody formation. Lispro (Humalog), a rapid-acting insulin with a shorter duration than regular insulin, is also available. Advantages of lispro include convenience, because it is injected immediately before mealtime; less hyperglycemia after meals; and fewer hypoglycemic episodes in some patients. Because its effects last 6 to 8 hours, most patients require a longer-acting insulin along with lispro to maintain optimal blood glucose levels (Landon, Catalano, & Gabbe, 2002; Moore, 2004; Weiner & Buhimschi, 2004). In addition, Lantus (insulin glargine) is being used more frequently by providers and is a long-acting insulin lasting approximately 16 to 24 hours in women who are pregnant. Lantus is categorized as a pregnancy category C drug by the U.S. Food and Drug Administration (FDA) (Aventis Pharmaceuticals, 2004). Small amounts of Lantus insulin are slowly released with no pronounced peak. This insulin preparation is most often used with women with insulin resistance diabetes (type 2) requiring high doses of long-acting insulin. Lantus is combined with a rapid-acting insulin to prevent hypoglycemia. Major concerns with Lantus include monitoring for nocturnal hypoglycemia (Moore, 2004) (Table 22-3) and not mixing with other insulins or solutions (Aventis Pharmaceuticals, 2004). It provides a more stable basal blood glucose with less risk of nocturnal hypoglycemia than NPH insulin (Cianni et al., 2005).

Most women with insulin-dependent diabetes are managed with two to three injections per day, also known as *multiple injection therapy (MIT)* (Bernasko, 2004). Usually, two thirds of the daily insulin dose, with longer-acting (NPH) and short-acting (regular or lispro) insulin combined in a 2:1 ratio, is given before breakfast. The remaining one third, again a combination of longer- and short-acting insulin, is administered in the evening before dinner. To reduce the risk of hypoglycemia during the night, separate injections often are administered, with short-acting insulin given before dinner, followed by longer-acting insulin at bedtime. An alternative insulin regimen that works well for some women is to administer short-acting insulin before each meal and longer-acting insulin at bedtime (Moore, 2004).

TABLE 22-3

Insulin Administration during Pregnancy: Expected Time of Action

TYPE OF INSULIN	ONSET	PEAK	DURATION
Lispro (short acting)	Within 15 min	30-90 min	6-8 hr
Regular (short acting)	30 min-1 hr	2-4 hr	8-12 hr
Intermediate acting	1-2½ hr	4-15 hr	24 hr
Long acting	4-8 hr	14-24 hr	24-36 hr
Lantus (long acting)*	60-70 min	No pronounced peak	24 hr

*Lantus is categorized as a category C drug. Category C drugs are drugs in animal studies that an adverse fetal effect has been noted but adequate research has not been conducted in humans (Nursing 2006, 2006).
Reference: Facts and Comparisons. (2003). Drug Facts and Comparisons. St. Louis: Wolters Kluwer Co.

NURSE ALERT *When instructing patients to take insulin before dinner, recognize that some people have eating patterns of breakfast, lunch, and dinner while others follow a pattern of breakfast, dinner, and supper. For some people, the biggest meal is at noon while for others, the biggest meal is the evening meal.*

Continuous subcutaneous insulin infusion (CSII) systems are increasingly used during pregnancy. The insulin pump is designed to mimic more closely the function of the pancreas in secreting insulin (Fig. 22-3). This portable, battery-powered device is worn, like a pager, during most daily activities. The pump infuses regular insulin at a set basal rate and has the capacity to deliver up to four different basal rates in 24 hours. A fine-gauge plastic catheter is inserted into subcutaneous tissue, usually in the abdomen, and attached to the pump syringe by connecting tubing. The subcutaneous catheter and connecting tubing are changed every 2 to 3 days. It also delivers bolus doses of insulin before meals to control postmeal blood glucose levels. The infusion tubing from the insulin pump can be left in place for several weeks without local complications. Although the insulin pump is convenient and generally provides good glycemic control, complications such as DKA, infection, or hypoglycemic coma can still develop (Moore, 2004). Use of the insulin pump requires a knowledgeable, motivated patient, skilled health care providers, and an alternative mode of insulin delivery in case of pump failure (Bernasko, 2004; Moore, 2004).

Monitoring blood glucose levels. Blood glucose testing at home with a glucose reflectance meter or biosensor monitor is the commonly accepted method for monitoring blood glucose levels.

To perform blood glucose monitoring, an individual obtains a drop of blood by means of a finger stick and places it on a test strip. After a specified amount of time, the glucose level can be read by the meter (Patient Instructions for Self-Care box). Blood glucose levels are routinely measured

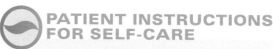

PATIENT INSTRUCTIONS FOR SELF-CARE

Self-Testing of Blood Glucose Level

- Gather supplies, check expiration date, and read instructions on testing materials. Prepare glucose reflectance meter for use according to manufacturer's directions.
- Wash hands in warm water (warmth increases circulation).
- Select site on side of any finger (all fingers should be used in rotation).
- Pierce site with lancet (may use automatic, spring-loaded, puncturing device). Cleaning the site with alcohol is not necessary.
- Drop hand down to side; with other hand gently squeeze finger from hand to fingertip.
- Allow blood to drop onto testing strip. Be sure to cover entire reagent area.
- Determine blood glucose value using the glucose reflectance meter, following manufacturer's instructions.
- Record results.
- Repeat as instructed by health care provider and as needed for signs of hypoglycemia or hyperglycemia.

From American Diabetes Association (ADA). (1995). *Medical management of pregnancy complicated by diabetes* (2nd ed.). Alexandria, VA: ADA.

at various times throughout the day, such as before breakfast, lunch, and dinner; 2 hours after each meal; at bedtime; and in the middle of the night. Hyperglycemia will most likely be identified in 2-hour postprandial values, because blood glucose levels peak approximately 2 hours after a meal. When there is any readjustment in insulin dosage or diet, more frequent measurement of blood glucose is warranted. If nausea, vomiting, or diarrhea occur; or if any infection is present, the woman will be asked to monitor her blood glucose levels more closely.

Target levels of blood glucose during pregnancy are lower than nonpregnant values. Acceptable fasting levels are generally between 65 and 105 mg/dl, and 1-hour postprandial levels should be less than 130 to 155 mg/dl (ADA, 2004b; Moore, 2004). The woman should be told to immediately report episodes of hypoglycemia (less than 60 mg/dl) and hyperglycemia (more than 200 mg/dl) to her health care provider so that adjustments in diet or insulin therapy can be made.

Pregnant women with diabetes are much more likely to develop hypoglycemia than hyperglycemia. Most episodes of mild or moderate hypoglycemia can be treated with oral intake of 10 to 15 grams of simple carbohydrate (Patient Instructions for Self-Care box, Treatment for Hypoglycemia, p. 684). If severe hypoglycemia occurs, in which the woman experiences a decrease in or loss of consciousness or an inability to swallow, she will require a parenteral injection of glucagon or intravenous (IV) glucose. Because hypoglycemia can develop rapidly and because impaired judgment can be associated with even moderate episodes, it is vital that family members, friends, and work colleagues be able to

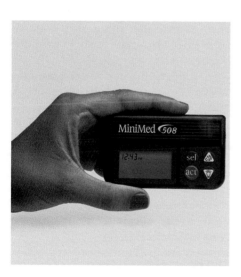

Fig. 22-3 Insulin pump shows basal rate for pregnant women with diabetes. (Courtesy MiniMed, Inc., Sylmar, CA.)

PATIENT INSTRUCTIONS FOR SELF-CARE

Treatment for Hypoglycemia

- Be familiar with signs and symptoms of hypoglycemia (nervousness, headache, shaking, irritability, personality change, hunger, blurred vision, sweaty skin, tingling of mouth or extremities).
- Check blood glucose level immediately when hypoglycemic symptoms occur.
- If blood glucose is <60 mg/dl, immediately eat or drink something that contains 10 to 15 g of simple carbohydrate. Examples are:
  —½ cup (4 ounces) unsweetened fruit juice
  —½ cup (4 ounces) regular (not diet) soda
  —5 to 6 LifeSavers candies
  —1 tablespoon honey or corn (Karo) syrup
  —1 cup (8 ounces) milk
  —2 to 3 glucose tablets
- Rest for 15 minutes, then recheck blood glucose.
- If glucose level is still <60 mg/dl, eat or drink another serving of one of the "glucose boosters" listed above.
- Wait 15 minutes, then recheck blood glucose. If it is still <60 mg/dl, notify health care provider immediately.

From American Diabetes Association (ADA). (1995). *Medical management of pregnancy complicated by diabetes* (2nd ed.). Alexandria, VA: ADA; & Becton Dickinson & Co. (1997). *Controlling low blood sugar reactions.* Franklin Lakes, NJ: Becton Dickinson & Co.

PATIENT INSTRUCTIONS FOR SELF-CARE

What to Do When Illness Occurs

- Be sure to take insulin even though appetite and food intake may be less than normal. (Insulin needs are increased with illness or infection.)
- Call the health care provider and relay the following information:
  —Symptoms of illness (e.g., nausea, vomiting, diarrhea)
  —Fever
  —Most recent blood glucose level
  —Urine ketones
  —Time and amount of last insulin dose
- Increase oral intake of fluids to prevent dehydration.
- Rest as much as possible.
- If unable to reach health care provider and blood glucose exceeds 200 mg/dL with urine ketones present, seek emergency treatment at the nearest health care facility. Do not attempt to self-treat for this.

---

quickly recognize signs and symptoms and initiate proper treatment if necessary.

Hyperglycemia is less likely to occur, but it can rapidly progress to DKA, which is associated with an increased risk of fetal death (Cunningham et al., 2005; Moore, 2004). Maternal hyperglycemia is predictive of macrosomia (ADA, 2004c). Women and family members should be particularly alert for signs and symptoms of hyperglycemia, especially when infections or other illnesses occur (Patient Instructions for Self-Care box, above right).

Urine testing. While urine testing for glucose is not beneficial during pregnancy, urine testing for ketones continues to have a place in diabetic management (ADA, 2004b). Monitoring for urine ketones may detect inadequate caloric or carbohydrate intake (ADA, 2004b).Women may be taught to perform urine testing daily with the first morning urine. Testing may also be done if a meal is missed or delayed, when illness occurs, or when the blood glucose level is greater than 200 mg/dl.

Complications requiring hospitalization. Occasionally, hospitalization is needed to regulate insulin therapy and stabilize glucose levels. Infection, which can lead to hyperglycemia and DKA, is an indication for hospitalization, regardless of gestational age. Hospitalization during the third trimester for closer maternal and fetal observation may be indicated for women whose diabetes is poorly controlled. In addition, women with diabetes are 20% to 30% more likely to also have preexisting hypertension (Moore, 2004), and develop chronic hypertension, preeclampsia, or eclampsia, which may necessitate hospitalization.

Fetal surveillance. Diagnostic techniques for fetal surveillance are often performed to assess fetal growth and well-being. The goals of fetal surveillance are to detect fetal compromise as early as possible and to prevent intrauterine fetal death or unnecessary preterm birth.

Early in pregnancy, the estimated date of birth (EDB) is determined. A baseline sonogram is done during the first trimester to assess gestational age. Follow-up ultrasound examinations are usually performed during the pregnancy (as often as every 4 to 6 weeks) to monitor fetal growth; estimate fetal weight; and detect hydramnios, macrosomia, and congenital anomalies.

Because a fetus in a diabetic pregnancy is at greater risk for neural tube defects (e.g., spina bifida, anencephaly, microcephaly), measurement of maternal serum alpha-fetoprotein is performed between 16 to 20 weeks of gestation (Cunningham et al., 2005). This is often done in conjunction with a detailed ultrasound study to examine the fetus for neural tube defects.

Fetal echocardiography may be performed between 20 and 22 weeks of gestation to detect cardiac anomalies (Moore, 2004). Some practitioners repeat this fetal surveillance test at 34 weeks of gestation. Doppler studies of the umbilical artery may be performed in women with vascular disease to detect placental compromise.

The majority of fetal surveillance measures are concentrated in the third trimester, when the risk of fetal compromise is greatest. Pregnant women should be taught how to do daily fetal movement counts, beginning at 28 weeks of gestation (see Chapter 21) (Moore, 2004).

The nonstress test used to evaluate fetal well-being may be used weekly or more often (twice weekly), typically beginning around 28 weeks of gestation (Moore, 2004). For the woman with vascular disease, testing may begin earlier and continue more frequently. In the presence of a nonreactive nonstress test, a contraction stress test or fetal biophysical profile may be used to evaluate fetal well-being (Landon, Catalano, & Gabbe, 2002; Moore, 2004).

Determination of birth date and mode of birth. Today, most diabetic pregnancies are allowed to progress to 38.5 to 40 weeks of gestation as long as good metabolic control is maintained and all parameters of antepartum fetal surveillance remain within normal limits. Reasons to proceed with birth before term include poor metabolic control, worsening hypertensive disorders, fetal macrosomia, or fetal growth restriction (Cunningham et al., 2005; Moore, 2004).

Many practitioners plan for elective labor induction between 38 and 40 weeks of gestation. To confirm fetal lung maturity before birth, an amniocentesis should be performed in pregnancies between 37 and 38.5 weeks of gestation (Moore, 2004). For the pregnancy complicated by diabetes, fetal lung maturation is better predicted by the amniotic fluid phosphatidylglycerol (>3%) (Moore, 2004) than by the lecithin/sphingomyelin ratio. If the fetal lungs are still immature, birth should be postponed as long as the results of fetal assessment remain reassuring. Amniocentesis may be repeated to monitor lung maturity (Landon, Catalano & Gabbe, 2002). Birth, despite poor fetal lung maturity, may be necessary when testing suggests fetal compromise, worsening maternal renal or visual function, or preeclampsia.

Although vaginal birth is expected for most women with pregestational diabetes, the cesarean rate for these women ranges from 30% to 80% (Cunningham et al., 2005; Moore, 2004). Cesarean birth is often performed when antepartum testing suggests fetal distress or the estimated fetal weight is greater than 4500 grams (Moore, 2004). Also, cesarean birth is necessary when the cervix fails to dilate completely during induction of labor (Moore, 2004).

Intrapartum

During the intrapartum period the woman with pregestational diabetes must be monitored closely to prevent complications related to dehydration, hypoglycemia, and hyperglycemia. Most women use large amounts of energy (calories) to accomplish the work and manage the stress of labor and birth. However, this calorie expenditure varies with the individual. Blood glucose levels and hydration must be carefully controlled during labor. An IV line is inserted for infusion of a maintenance fluid, such as lactated Ringer's solution, 5% dextrose in lactated Ringer's solution, or 10% dextrose (ADA, 2004c). Most commonly, insulin is administered by continuous infusion. Only regular insulin may be administered intravenously. Determinations of blood glucose levels are made every hour, and fluids and insulin are adjusted to maintain blood glucose levels between 80 and 120 mg/dl (ADA, 2004c; Balsells et al., 2000; Bernasko, 2004). It is essential that these target glucose levels be maintained because hyperglycemia during labor can precipitate metabolic problems in the neonate, particularly hypoglycemia.

During labor, continuous fetal heart monitoring is necessary. The woman should assume an upright or side-lying position during bed rest in labor to prevent supine hypotension because of a large fetus or polyhydramnios. Labor is allowed to progress provided normal rates of cervical dilation, fetal descent, and fetal well-being are maintained. Failure to progress may indicate a macrosomic infant and cephalopelvic disproportion, necessitating a cesarean birth. The woman is observed and treated during labor for diabetic complications such as hyperglycemia, ketosis, ketoacidosis, and glycosuria. During second-stage labor, shoulder dystocia may occur with birth of a macrosomic infant (see Chapter 24). A neonatologist, pediatrician, or neonatal nurse practitioner may be present at the birth to initiate assessment and neonatal care.

If a cesarean birth is planned, it should be scheduled in the early morning to facilitate glycemic control. Dependent upon the provider, no morning insulin may be given or the bedtime dose of NPH insulin may be given in the morning and every 8 hours until surgery (Chan & Johnson, 2006). The woman is given nothing by mouth. Epidural anesthesia is recommended because hypoglycemia can be detected earlier if the woman is awake. After surgery, glucose levels should be monitored at least every 2 hours if an IV solution containing 5% dextrose is being infused. Target plasma glucose levels are between 80 and 160 mg/dl (Moore, 2004).

Postpartum

In the immediate 24 hours postpartum, insulin requirements decrease substantially because the major source of insulin resistance, the placenta, has been removed. Women with type 1 diabetes may require only one fourth to one third of the prenatal insulin dose on the first postpartum day, provided that they are eating a full diet (Bernasko, 2004). In women giving birth by cesarean an intravenous infusion of glucose and insulin may be required for the first 2 to 3 days after birth for type 1 diabetics (Moore, 2004). It takes several days after birth to reestablish carbohydrate homeostasis (see Fig. 22-1, *D* and *E*). As insulin needs decrease significantly following birth some women may not require insulin for 24 to 72 hours postpartum (Chan & Johnson, 2006). Blood glucose levels are monitored in the postpartum period, and insulin dosage is adjusted using a sliding scale. The woman who has insulin-dependent diabetes must realize the importance of eating on time even if the baby needs feeding or other pressing demands exist. Women with type 2 diabetes often require only 40% to 50% of their pregnancy insulin dose in the postpartum period and are soon able to maintain euglycemia through diet alone or with oral hypoglycemics (Moore, 2004).

Possible postpartum complications include preeclampsia-eclampsia, hemorrhage, and infection. Hemorrhage is a possibility if the mother's uterus was overdistended (hydramnios, macrosomic fetus) or overstimulated (oxytocin induction). Postpartum infections such as endometritis are more likely to occur in a woman with diabetes.

Mothers are encouraged to breastfeed. In addition to the advantages of maternal satisfaction and pleasure, breast-feeding has an antidiabetogenic effect for the children of women with diabetes and for women with gestational diabetes (Moore, 2004). Insulin requirements may be half of prepregnancy levels because of the carbohydrate used in human milk production. Because glucose levels are lower, breastfeeding women are at increased risk for hypoglycemia, especially in the early postpartum period and after breast-feeding sessions, particularly after late night nursing (Moore, 2004). Breastfeeding mothers with diabetes may be at increased risk for mastitis and yeast infections of the breast. Insulin dosage, which is decreased during lactation, must be recalculated at weaning (Landon, Catalano, & Gabbe, 2002; Lawrence & Lawrence, 2005) (see Fig. 22-1, F).

The mother may have early breastfeeding difficulties. Poor metabolic control may delay lactogenesis and contribute to decreased milk production (Moore, 2004). Initial contact and opportunity to breastfeed the infant may be delayed for mothers who gave birth by cesarean or if infants are placed in neonatal intensive care units or special care nurseries for observation during the first few hours after birth. Support and assistance from nursing staff and lactation specialists can facilitate the mother's early experience with breastfeeding and encourage her to continue.

The new mother needs information about family planning and contraception. Although family planning is important for all women, it is essential for the woman with diabetes to safeguard her own health and to promote optimal outcomes in future pregnancies. The woman and her partner should be informed that the risks associated with pregnancy increase with the duration and severity of the diabetic condition and that pregnancy may contribute to vascular changes associated with diabetes.

The risks and benefits of contraceptive methods should be discussed with the mother and her partner before discharge from the hospital. Barrier methods are often recommended as safe, inexpensive options that have no inherent risks for women with diabetes (Landon, Catalano, & Gabbe, 2002). However, barrier methods such as the diaphragm or condom and spermicide are not as effective as some other forms of contraception, and inconsistent use often leads to unplanned pregnancy (Landon, Catalano, & Gabbe, 2002).

Use of oral contraceptives by diabetic women is controversial because of the risk of thromboembolic and vascular complications and the effect on carbohydrate metabolism. In women without vascular disease or other risk factors, combination low-dose oral contraceptives may be prescribed. Progestin-only oral contraceptives also may be used (Cunningham et al., 2005; Landon, Catalano, & Gabbe, 2002). Close monitoring of blood pressure and lipid levels is necessary to detect complications (Landon, Catalano, & Gabbe, 2002). Some health care providers are reluctant to use intrauterine contraceptive devices (IUDs) in women with diabetes. However, this method has been successfully used with diabetic women though an increased incidence of pelvic infections has been reported in this population (Cunningham et al., 2005).

Opinion is divided about the use of long-acting parenteral progestins, such as Depo-Provera. Some health care providers recommend their use, particularly in women who are non-compliant with daily dosing oral contraceptives. In contrast, other health care providers believe this method may adversely affect diabetic control. Transdermal (patch) and transvaginal (vaginal ring) administration are newer contraceptive methods, particularly effective in women who prefer weekly or every-third-week dosing, respectively. For women weighing more than 90 kg there is a higher contraceptive failure rate with transdermal administration (Cunningham et al., 2005). Therefore, this method would be contraindicated in obese women with diabetes. Limited data are available regarding their use in women with diabetes.

The risks associated with pregnancy increase with duration and severity of diabetes, and vascular changes may worsen. This information needs to be thoroughly discussed with the woman and her partner. Therefore, sterilization should be discussed with the woman who has completed her family, who has poor metabolic control, or who has significant vascular problems.

Evaluation

Evaluation of the care of the pregnant woman with pregestational diabetes is based on the previously stated expected outcomes of care and is closely associated with the degree of maternal metabolic control during pregnancy (Plan of Care).

Gestational Diabetes Mellitus

Gestational diabetes mellitus (GDM) complicates approximately 4% to 7% of all pregnancies in the United States (ADA, 2004a; ADA, 2004b) and accounts for greater than 75% of all cases of diabetic pregnancy (Chan & Johnson, 2006). Prevalence varies (1% - 14%) by racial and ethnic groups (ADA, 2004a). GDM is more likely to occur among Hispanic, Native American, Asian, and African-American populations than in Caucasians (ADA, 2004a; Moore, 2004). GDM is likely to recur in future pregnancies, and there is an increased risk for development of overt diabetes in later life (Moore, 2004). This is especially true of women whose GDM is diagnosed early in pregnancy or who are obese (Landon, Catalano, & Gabbe, 2002). Classic risk factors for GDM include maternal age over 25 years; obesity; family history of type 2 diabetes; and an obstetric history of an infant weighing more than 4500 g, hydramnios, unexplained stillbirth, miscarriage, or an infant with congenital anomalies (Moore, 2004). Women at high risk for GDM are often screened at their initial prenatal visit and then rescreened later (at 24 to 28 weeks of gestation) in pregnancy if the initial screen is negative.

The diagnosis of gestational diabetes is usually made during the second half of pregnancy. As fetal nutrient demands rise during the late second and the third trimesters, mater-

PLAN OF CARE *The Pregnant Woman with Pregestational Diabetes*

NURSING DIAGNOSIS Deficient knowledge related to lack of recall of information as evidenced by woman's questions and concerns

Expected Outcomes *Woman will be able to verbalize important information regarding diabetes, its management, and potential effects on the pregnancy and fetus.*

Nursing Interventions/*Rationales*

- Assess woman's current knowledge base regarding disease process, management, effects on pregnancy and fetus, and potential complications *to provide database for further teaching.*
- Review the pathophysiology of diabetes, effects on pregnancy and fetus, and potential complications *to promote recall of information and compliance with treatment plan.*
- Review procedure for insulin administration, demonstrate procedure for blood glucose monitoring and insulin measurement and administration, and obtain return demonstration *to establish patient comfort and competence with procedures.*
- Discuss diet and exercise as prescribed *to promote self-care.*
- Review signs and symptoms of complications of hypoglycemia and hyperglycemia and appropriate interventions *to promote prompt recognition of complications and self-care.*
- Provide contact numbers for health care team for prompt interventions and answers to questions on an ongoing basis *to promote comfort.*
- Review information on diagnostic tests, schedule of visits to primary health care provider, and expected plan of care *to allay anxiety and enlist cooperation of woman in her care.*

NURSING DIAGNOSIS Risk for fetal injury related to elevated maternal glucose levels

Expected Outcomes *Fetus will remain free of injury and be born at term in a healthy state.*

Nursing Interventions/*Rationales*

- Assess woman's current diabetic control *to identify risk for fetal mortality and congenital anomalies.*
- Monitor fundal height during each prenatal visit *to identify appropriate fetal growth.*
- Monitor for signs and symptoms of gestational hypertension *to identify early manifestations because pregnant women with diabetes are at greater risk.*
- Assess fetal movement and heart rate during each prenatal visit and perform weekly nonstress tests during the last 4 weeks of pregnancy *to assess fetal well-being.*
- Review procedure for blood glucose testing and insulin administration and fetal movement counts *to promote self-care.*

NURSING DIAGNOSIS Anxiety related to threat to maternal and fetal well-being as evidenced by woman verbal expressions of concern

Expected Outcomes *Woman will identify sources of anxiety and report feeling less anxious.*

Nursing Interventions/*Rationales*

- Through therapeutic communication, promote an open relationship with woman *to promote trust.*
- Listen to patient's feelings and concerns *to assess for any misconception or misinformation that may be contributing to anxiety.*
- Review potential dangers by providing factual information *to correct any misconceptions or misinformation.*
- Encourage woman to share concerns with her health care team *to promote collaboration in her care.*

---

nal nutrient ingestion induces greater and more sustained levels of blood glucose. At the same time, maternal insulin resistance is also increasing because of the insulin-antagonistic effects of the placental hormones, cortisol, and insulinase. Consequently, maternal insulin demands rise as much as threefold. Most pregnant women are capable of increasing insulin production to compensate for insulin resistance and to maintain euglycemia. When the pancreas is unable to produce sufficient insulin or the insulin is not used effectively, gestational diabetes can result.

Maternal-fetal risks

Women with GDM have an increased risk (10% to 40%) of developing hypertensive disorders compared with normal pregnant women (ADA, 2004b; Moore, 2004). They also have increased risk for fetal macrosomia, which can lead to increased rates of perineal lacerations, episiotomy, and cesarean birth (ADA, 2004b). In addition, fetal macrosomia may be associated with shoulder dystocia and birth trauma. Diabetes in pregnancy also places the neonate at increased risk for hypoglycemia, hypocalcemia, hyperbilirubinemia, thrombocytopenia, polycythemia, and respiratory distress syndrome (Moore, 2004).

The overall incidence of congenital anomalies among infants of women with gestational diabetes approaches that of the general population because gestational diabetes usually develops after the critical period of organogenesis (first trimester) has passed. However, Anderson and colleagues (2005) found that women who were obese preconceptionally (BMI > 30 kg/m^2) and developed gestational diabetes were at greater risk to give birth to infants with CNS defects.

Screening for gestational diabetes mellitus

ACOG recommends that all pregnant women be screened for GDM, either by history, clinical risk factors, or laboratory screening of blood glucose levels (ACOG, 2001). Based on history and clinical risk factors, some women are at low risk for the development of GDM. Therefore, glucose testing for this low risk population is not cost effective (Expert Committee on the Diagnosis and Classification of Diabetes Mellitus, 2003). This group includes normal weight women younger than 25 years of age who have no family history of diabetes, are not members of an ethnic or a racial group known to have a high prevalence of the disease, and have no previous history of abnormal glucose tolerance or adverse obstetric outcomes usually associated with GDM (ADA, 2004a; ADA 2004b; ACOG, 2001; Expert Committee on the Diagnosis and Classification of Diabetes Mellitus, 2003). Women at high risk for developing GDM should be screened the first prenatal visit and again at 24 to 28 weeks of gestation (ADA, 2004a; ADA, 2004b) The screening test (Glucola screening) most often used consists of a 50-gram oral glucose load, followed by a plasma glucose determination 1 hour later. It is not necessary that the woman be fasting. A glucose value of 135 to 140 mg/dl is considered a positive screen and should be followed by a 2-hour (75-gram) or 3-hour (100-gram) oral glucose tolerance test (OGTT) (ADA, 2004a; ADA, 2004b; Cunningham et al., 2005; Moore, 2004). The OGTT is administered after an overnight fast and at least 3 days of unrestricted diet (at least 150 gram of carbohydrate) and physical activity. The woman is instructed to avoid caffeine because it will increase glucose levels and to abstain from smoking for 12 hours before the test. The 3-hour OGTT, the gold standard test, requires a fasting blood glucose level, which is drawn before giving a 100-gram glucose load. Blood glucose levels are then drawn 1, 2, and 3 hours later. The woman is diagnosed with gestational diabetes if two or more values are met or exceeded (ADA, 2004a; ADA, 2004b; Moore, 2004) (Fig. 22-4).

Nursing diagnoses and expected outcomes of care for women with GDM are basically the same as those for women with pregestational diabetes except that the time frame for planning may be shortened with GDM because the diagnosis is usually made later in pregnancy.

Antepartum care

When the diagnosis of gestational diabetes is made, treatment begins immediately, allowing little or no time for the woman and her family to adjust to the diagnosis before they are expected to participate in the treatment plan. With each step of the treatment plan the nurse and other health care providers should educate the woman and her family, providing detailed and comprehensive explanations to ensure understanding, participation, and adherence to the necessary interventions. Potential complications should be discussed, and the need for maintenance of euglycemia throughout the remainder of the pregnancy is reinforced. It may be reassuring for the woman and her family to know that gestational diabetes typically disappears when the pregnancy is over.

As with pregestational diabetes, the aim of therapy in women with GDM is strict blood glucose control. Fasting blood glucose levels should range from 65 to 105mg/dl, and 1-hour postprandial blood levels should be less than 130 to 155 mg/dl (ADA, 2004b; Moore, 2004).

Diet. Dietary modification is the mainstay of treatment for GDM. The woman with GDM is placed on a standard diabetic diet. The usual prescription is 30 kcal/kg /day based on a normal BMI preconceptional weight. For obese women, the usual prescription is upto 25 kcal/kg/day, which translates into 1500 to 2000 kcal/day for most women (ADA, 2004b; Chan & Johnson, 2006). Carbohydrate intake is restricted to approximately 35% to 40% of caloric intake (ADA, 2004b). Dietary counseling by a nutritionist is recommended.

Exercise. Exercise in women with GDM helps lower blood glucose levels and may be instrumental in decreasing the need for insulin (ADA, 2004b). Women with GDM who already have an active lifestyle should be encouraged to continue an exercise program.

Monitoring blood glucose levels. Blood glucose monitoring is necessary to determine whether euglycemia can be maintained by diet and exercise. Women are encouraged to monitor their blood sugar daily. However,

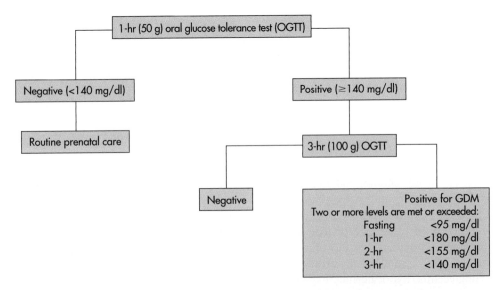

Fig. 22-4 Screening and diagnosis for gestational diabetes. (From American Diabetes Association. [2004b]. Position statement: Gestational diabetes mellitus. *Diabetes Care, 27*[suppl 1], S36-S46.)

fasting and postprandial glucose levels should be monitored minimally at least weekly (ACOG, 2001). The optimal frequency and timing of blood glucose monitoring has not been established (ACOG, 2001). Women with GDM may perform self-monitoring at home, or monitoring may be done at the clinic or office visit.

Insulin therapy. Up to 20% of women with GDM will require insulin during the pregnancy to maintain adequate blood glucose levels, despite compliance with the prescribed diet. In contrast to women with insulin-dependent diabetes, women with gestational diabetes are initially managed with diet and exercise. If fasting glucose levels are greater than 105 mg/dl, then insulin therapy is begun (ADA, 2004b). Either lower or higher thresholds for initiating insulin may be used (Landon, Catalano, & Gabbe, 2002). One oral agent, glyburide, is being used experimentally during pregnancy with women with diabetes. Although limited data exist, minimal placental transfer occurs and maternal and fetal complications were comparable with those of maternal insulin administration (Cianni et al., 2005). Women with diabetes who are unable or unwilling to take insulin by injection or are cognitively impaired may be candidates for glyburide use.

Fetal surveillance. There is no standard recommendation for fetal surveillance in pregnancies complicated by GDM. Women whose blood glucose levels are well controlled by diet are at low risk for fetal complications. Limited antepartum fetal testing is done in women with gestational diabetes as long as their fasting and 2-hour postprandial blood glucose levels remain within normal limits and they have no other risk factors. Daily fetal kick counts are done beginning at 28 weeks of gestation, and nonstress tests may be done twice weekly beginning at 36 weeks of gestation (Moore, 2004). Usually these women progress to term and spontaneous labor without intervention.

Women with GDM whose blood glucose levels are poorly controlled or who require insulin therapy, have hypertension, or have a history of previous stillbirth generally receive more intensive fetal biophysical monitoring. Nonstress tests and biophysical profiles are often performed weekly, beginning at 28 to 36 weeks of gestation (Bernasko, 2004; Moore, 2004).

Intrapartum care

During the labor and birth process, blood glucose levels are monitored at least every 2 hours to maintain levels at 80 to 120 mg/dl (Bernasko, 2004; Moore, 2004). Glucose levels within this range will decrease the incidence of neonatal hypoglycemia. It may be necessary to infuse regular insulin intravenously during labor in order to maintain blood glucose levels within this range. IV fluids containing glucose are not commonly given during labor. Although gestational diabetes is not an indication for cesarean birth, it may be necessary in the presence of preeclampsia or macrosomia. Women with gestational diabetes are encouraged to breast-feed.

Postpartum care

Most women with GDM will return to normal glucose levels after childbirth. However, GDM is likely to recur in future pregnancies, and women with GDM are at significant risk for developing glucose intolerance later in life, so they should be screened with a 75 g oral glucose tolerance test at 6 to 12 weeks postpartum or after breastfeeding has stopped (ADA, 2004b). Obesity is a major risk factor for the later development of diabetes. Therefore women with a history of GDM, particularly those who are overweight, should be encouraged to make lifestyle changes that include weight loss and exercise to reduce this risk (ADA, 2004b). The risk of developing GDM in subsequent pregnancies is 50% or higher. Because infants born to women with GDM are at risk for developing obesity and diabetes in childhood or adolescence, regular health care for these children is essential (Moore, 2004).

Thyroid Disorders
Hyperthyroidism

Hyperthyroidism occurs in approximately 1 or 2 of every 1000 pregnancies. (Cunningham et al., 2005; Nader, 2004b) Graves' disease is the most common cause of hyperthyroidism in 90% to 95% of pregnant women (Nader, 2004b). Clinical manifestations of hyperthyroidism include tachycardia, fatigue, heat intolerance, emotional lability, weight loss, and severe nausea and vomiting. Exophthalmos and enlargement of the thyroid gland (goiter) may also occur. Many of these symptoms also occur with pregnancy, so the disorder can be difficult to diagnose. Laboratory findings include elevated free thyroxine (T_4) and triiodothyronine (T_3) levels and suppressed thyroid-stimulating hormone (TSH) levels (Cunningham et al., 2005; Nader, 2004b). Moderate and severe hyperthyroidism must be treated during pregnancy; untreated or inadequately treated women have an increased risk of preterm birth, stillborns, fetal goiter, and fetal hypothyroidism or hyperthyroidism (Cunningham et al., 2005). Women with hyperthyroidism are also at increased risk to develop severe preeclampsia (Nader, 2004b). Women with hyperemesis gravidarum often present with elevated thyroid hormone levels because of high levels of chorionic gonadotropin (Cunningham et al., 2005).

The primary treatment of hyperthyroidism during pregnancy is drug therapy; the medication of choice is propylthiouracil (PTU). The usual starting dose is 100 to 150 mg every 8 hours, with higher doses required for some women (Nader, 2004b). Women generally show clinical improvement within 2 weeks of beginning therapy, but the medication requires 6 to 8 weeks to reach full effectiveness. During therapy the woman's free T_4 levels are measured monthly, and the results are used to taper the drug to the smallest effective dosage to prevent unnecessary fetal hypothyroidism (Nader, 2004b). PTU is well tolerated by most women. Maternal side effects include pruritus, skin rash, fever, a metallic taste, nausea, bronchospasm, oral ulcerations, hepatitis, and a lupus-like syndrome (Nader, 2004b;

Weiner & Buhimschi, 2004). The most severe side effect is agranulocytosis, which is more common in women over 40 years of age and in those taking high doses of PTU (Nader, 2004b). Symptoms of agranulocytosis are fever and sore throat; these symptoms should be reported immediately to the health care provider, and the woman should stop taking the PTU. Leukopenia of a transient and benign nature may occur as a result of PTU therapy. PTU readily crosses to the placenta and may induce fetal hypothyroidism and goiter (Mestman, 2002; Nader, 2004b).

Beta-adrenergic blockers such as propranolol may be used in severe hyperthyroidism. Long-term use is not recommended because of the potential for IUGR and altered response to anoxic stress, postnatal bradycardia, and hypoglycemia.

Radioactive iodine must not be used in diagnosis or treatment of hyperthyroidism in pregnancy because it may compromise the fetal thyroid. Mothers choosing to breastfeed who are also taking hyperthyroid medication need to be instructed that small amounts are excreted in the breast milk, but PTU has not been found to adversely affect the neonate's thyroid function (Weiner & Buhimschi, 2004).

In severe cases surgical treatment of hyperthyroidism, subtotal thyroidectomy, may be performed during the second or third trimester. Because of the increased risk of miscarriage and preterm labor associated with major surgery, this treatment is usually reserved for women with severe disease, those for whom drug therapy proves toxic, and those who are unable to adhere to the prescribed medical regimen.

NURSE ALERT *A serious but uncommon complication of undiagnosed or partially treated hyperthyroidism is thyroid storm, which may occur in response to stress such as infection, birth, or surgery. A woman with this emergency disorder may have fever, restlessness, tachycardia, vomiting, hypotension, or stupor. Prompt treatment is essential; IV fluids and oxygen are administered, along with high doses of PTU. After administration of PTU, iodide is given. Other medications include antipyretics, dexamethasone, and beta-blockers (Cunningham et al., 2005; Nader, 2004b).*

Hypothyroidism

Hypothyroidism during pregnancy is less common (1.3 per 1000) than hyperthyroidism and is often associated with menstrual and fertility problems and an increased risk of miscarriage (Cunningham et al., 2005). Hypothyroidism is usually caused by glandular destruction by autoantibodies, most commonly because of Hashimoto's thyroiditis. Characteristic symptoms of hypothyroidism include weight gain; fatigue; cold intolerance; constipation; cool, dry skin; coarsened hair; and muscle weakness. Laboratory values in pregnancy include low or low-normal T_3 and T_4 levels and elevated levels of TSH (Cunningham et al., 2005; Nader, 2004b).

Pregnant women with untreated hypothyroidism are at increased risk for preeclampsia, placental abruption, and stillbirth (Cunningham et al., 2005). Infants born to mothers with hypothyroidism may be of low birth weight, but for the most part if such women are treated preconceptionally or early in the pregnancy, the infants are healthy and without evidence of thyroid dysfunction (Nader, 2004b).

Thyroid hormone supplements are used to treat hypothyroidism. Levothyroxine (e.g., l-thyroxine [Synthroid]) is most often prescribed during pregnancy. The usual beginning dosage is 0.1 to 0.15 mg/day with adjustment by 25 to 50 mcg every 4 to 6 weeks as necessary based on the maternal TSH level (Nader, 2004b; Cunningham et al., 2005). The aim of drug therapy is to maintain the woman's level at the lower end of the normal range for pregnant women. In contrast, women on thyroid replacement therapy prior to conception usually will have a dose increase of 25% to 50% during the pregnancy (DiPiro et al., 2005).

NURSE ALERT *If taking iron supplementation, pregnant women should be told to take l-thyroxine 2 hours before or after iron tablets, because ferrous sulfate decreases absorption of T_4 (Spratto & Woods, 2004).*

The fetus depends on maternal thyroid hormones until 12 weeks of gestation, when fetal production begins (Blackburn, 2003). Decreased levels of T_4 in the second trimester have been associated with permanent neonatal neurologic deficits (Cunningham et al., 2005; Nader, 2004b). Careful monitoring of the neonate's thyroid status to detect any abnormalities is important.

Nursing Care

Education of the pregnant woman with thyroid dysfunction is essential to promote compliance with the plan of treatment. It is important to discuss with the woman and her family the disorder and its potential impact on her, her family, and her fetus; the medication regimen and possible side effects; the need for continuing medical supervision; and the importance of compliance. The family is incorporated into the plan of care to foster mutuality and support among the members.

The woman often needs assistance from the nurse in coping with the discomforts and frustrations associated with symptoms of the disorder. For example, the woman with hyperthyroidism who has nervousness and hyperactivity concomitant with weakness and fatigue may benefit from suggestions to channel excess energies into quiet diversional activities such as reading or crafts. Discomfort associated with hypersensitivity to heat (hyperthyroidism) or cold intolerance (hypothyroidism) can be minimized by appropriate clothing and regulation of environmental temperatures, and by avoidance of temperature extremes.

Nutrition counseling with a registered dietitian may provide guidance in selecting a well-balanced diet. The woman with hyperthyroidism who has increased appetite and poor weight gain and the hypothyroid woman who has anorexia and lethargy need counseling to ensure adequate intake of nutritionally sound foods to meet both maternal and fetal needs.

Maternal Phenylketonuria

Phenylketonuria (PKU), a recognized cause of mental retardation, is an inborn error of metabolism caused by an autosomal recessive trait that creates a deficiency in the enzyme phenylalanine hydrolase. Absence of this enzyme impairs the body's ability to metabolize the amino acid phenylalanine, found in all protein foods. Consequently, there is toxic accumulation of phenylalanine in the blood, which interferes with brain development and function. PKU affects 1 in every 15,000 live births in the United States (Cunningham et al., 2005). All newborns are tested soon after birth for this disorder. Prompt diagnosis and therapy with a phenylalanine-restricted diet significantly decrease the incidence of mental retardation. It is recommended that dietary therapy for PKU be continued throughout life (Blackburn, 2003; Brown et al., 2002). Women who discontinue the phenylalanine-restricted diet may demonstrate a decline in intellectual function (Cunningham et al., 2005). Some people discontinue the restricted diet because of the difficulty in adhering to the specially prepared diet (Blackburn, 2003; Brown et al., 2002).

The keys to prevention of fetal anomalies caused by PKU are the identification of women in their reproductive years who have the disorder and dietary compliance for those women diagnosed. Screening for undiagnosed homozygous maternal PKU at the first prenatal visit may be warranted, especially in individuals with a family history of the disorder, with low intelligence of uncertain etiology, or who have given birth to microcephalic infants. Women with PKU should continue the low-protein diet during pregnancy. Nutritional phenylalanine intake and phenylalanine levels must be monitored. It is recommended that maternal phenylalanine levels range between 2 and 6 mg/dl. These levels are associated with a decrease in fetal sequelae (Cunningham et al., 2005). High maternal phenylalanine levels are associated with microcephaly with mental retardation and congenital heart defects (Landon, Catalano, & Gabbe, 2004; Cunningham et al., 2005). Ultrasound examinations are used for fetal surveillance beginning in the first trimester. A spontaneous vaginal birth is anticipated.

Women with PKU may breastfeed but their maternal blood levels are followed closely (Lawrence & Lawrence, 2005; Riordan, 2005) because their milk contains high levels of phenylalanine (Nader, 2004a). Mothers who choose to breastfeed must still supplement the infant's diet with a special milk preparation, phenylalanine (PHE)–free formula that contains little or no phenylalanine (Riordan, 2005).

CARDIOVASCULAR DISORDERS

During a normal pregnancy, the maternal cardiovascular system undergoes many changes that put a physiologic strain on the heart. The major cardiovascular changes that occur during a normal pregnancy and that affect the woman with cardiac disease are increased intravascular volume, decreased systemic vascular resistance, cardiac output changes occurring during labor and birth, and the intravascular volume changes that occur just after childbirth. The strain is present during pregnancy and continues for a few weeks after birth. The normal heart can compensate for the increased workload, so that pregnancy, labor, and birth are generally well tolerated, but the diseased heart is challenged hemodynamically. If the cardiovascular changes are not well tolerated, cardiac failure can develop during pregnancy, labor, or the postpartum period. In addition, if myocardial disease develops, if valvular disease exists, or if a congenital heart defect is present, cardiac decompensation (decreased cardiac output) may occur.

From 1% to 4% of pregnancies are complicated by heart disease (Foley, 2004) the leading cause of nonobstetric maternal death. Rheumatic fever is responsible for about 50% of cardiac complications; congenital diseases and mitral valve disease are the next most common causes. Cardiac disease ranks fourth overall as a cause of maternal death. A maternal mortality rate of up to 50% is anticipated in women with persistent cardiac decompensation. Box 22-1 lists maternal cardiac disease risk groups and their related mortality rates.

The degree of disability experienced by the woman with cardiac disease often is more important in the treatment and prognosis during pregnancy than is the diagnosis of the type of cardiovascular disease. The New York Heart Association's (NYHA's) functional classification of heart disease, a widely accepted standard, is as follows (AHA, 2000):

NYHA Functional Classification of Heart Disease
- Class I: asymptomatic without limitation of physical activity
- Class II: symptomatic with slight limitation of activity

BOX 22-1

Maternal Cardiac Disease Risk Groups

GROUP I (MORTALITY RATE 1%)
- Corrected tetralogy of Fallot
- Pulmonic or tricuspid disease
- Mitral stenosis (classes I and II)
- Patent ductus
- Ventricular septal defect
- Atrial septal defect
- Porcine valve

GROUP II (MORTALITY RATE 5%-15%)
- Mitral stenosis with atrial fibrillation
- Artificial heart valves
- Mitral stenosis (classes III and IV)
- Uncorrected tetralogy
- Aortic coarctation (uncomplicated)
- Aortic stenosis

GROUP III (MORTALITY RATE 25%-50%)
- Aortic coarctation (complicated)
- Myocardial infarction
- Marfan syndrome
- True cardiomyopathy
- Pulmonary hypertension

Source: Gilbert, E., & Harmon, J. (2003). *Manual of high risk pregnancy and delivery* (3rd ed.). St. Louis: Mosby.

Evolve/CD: Case Study—Class III Cardiac Disorder

- Class III: symptomatic with marked limitation of activity
- Class IV: symptomatic with inability to carry on any physical activity without discomfort

No classification of heart disease can be considered rigid or absolute, but the NYHA classification offers a basic practical guide for treatment, assuming that frequent prenatal visits, good patient cooperation, and appropriate obstetric care occur. Medical therapy is conducted as a team approach, including the cardiologist, obstetrician, anesthesiologist, and nurses. The functional classification may change for the pregnant woman because of the hemodynamic changes that occur in the cardiovascular system. There is a 30% to 45% increase in cardiac output compared with nonpregnancy resting values, with the majority of the increase in the first trimester and the peak at 20 to 24 weeks of gestation (Blanchard & Shabetai, 2004). The functional classification of the disease is determined at 3 months and again at 7 or 8 months of gestation. Pregnant women may progress from class I or II to III or IV during pregnancy.

Women with cyanotic congenital heart disease do not fit into the NYHA classification because their exercise-induced symptoms have causes not related to heart failure. An Ability Index was developed for assessment of these patients (Gei & Hankins, 2001).

The incidence of miscarriage is increased, and preterm labor and birth are more prevalent in pregnant women with cardiac problems. In addition, IUGR is common, probably because of low oxygen pressure (Po_2) in the mother. The incidence of congenital heart lesions is increased (2% to 3%) in children of mothers with congenital heart disease (Cunningham et al., 2005). Therefore preconceptional counseling is essential for positive pregnancy outcomes. A diagnosis of cardiac disease depends on the history, physical examination, x-ray findings, and, if indicated, echocardiogram. The differential diagnosis of heart disease also involves ruling out respiratory problems and other potential causes of chest pain. Maternal mortality rates of more than 50% during pregnancy have been associated with pulmonary hypertension. It is important that the woman with cardiac disease be assessed and the diagnosis established as soon as possible (Blanchard & Shabetai, 2004). In addition, the pregnant woman with heart disease must be counseled to avoid tobacco and illicit drugs, such as cocaine—both are lifestyle behaviors that may compromise cardiac functioning.

Peripartum Cardiomyopathy

Peripartum cardiomyopathy is congestive heart failure with cardiomyopathy. Diagnostic criteria include development of cardiac failure in the last month of pregnancy or within the first 5 months postpartum, lack of another cause for heart failure, absence of heart disease before the last month of pregnancy, and a depressed ejection fraction (Blanchard & Shabetai, 2004; Cunningham et al., 2005). The etiology of the disease is unknown. Theories suggest genetic predisposition, autoimmunity, and viral infections. The incidence of

this disease is 1 per 3000 to 4000 live births in the United States (Blanchard & Shabetai, 2004).

Peripartum cardiomyopathy is more common in African-Americans, in twin pregnancies, and in women with preeclampsia (Foley, 2004). The 5-year survival rate for women with peripartum cardiomyopathy is 50% or less, with a worsening prognosis if the cardiomegaly persists after 6 months postpartum (Blanchard & Shabetai, 2004). Symptoms may vary depending on the type of peripartum cardiomyopathy, but all relate to congestive heart failure. Pregnancy is contraindicated for women with persistent cardiomegaly or cardiac dysfunction.

Medical management of cardiomyopathy during pregnancy mimics the regimen used for congestive heart failure. Treatment includes beta-adrenergic blockers, diuretics, digoxin, anticoagulants, and sodium restriction. Angiotensin-converting enzyme (ACE) inhibitors are contraindicated in pregnancy because of their teratogenic potential but may be used postpartally. The nursing care of women with peripartum cardiomyopathy is essentially the same as for women with other cardiac problems.

Rheumatic Heart Disease

Rheumatic fever is increasingly uncommon in the United States but is more common in underdeveloped nations (Blanchard & Shabetai, 2004; Cunningham et al., 2005). When it occurs, it usually develops suddenly, often several symptom-free weeks after an inadequately treated group A β-hemolytic streptococcal throat infection. Episodes of rheumatic fever create an autoimmune reaction in the heart tissue, leading to permanent damage of heart valves (usually the mitral valve) and the chordae tendineae cordis. This damage is referred to as *rheumatic heart disease (RHD)*. RHD may be evident during acute rheumatic fever or discovered years later. Recurrences of rheumatic fever are common, each with the potential to increase the severity of heart damage. If a woman has had rheumatic fever in the past, a recurrence can occur during pregnancy, most likely early in the pregnancy. The American Heart Association recommends lifelong prophylaxis with benzathine G penicillin, even during pregnancy. For those women with penicillin allergies, erythromycin is an acceptable alternative during pregnancy. Heart murmurs resulting from stenosis, valvular insufficiency, or thickening of the walls of the heart characterize RHD. Signs and symptoms include cardiac murmurs, congestive heart failure, and an enlarged heart (Blanchard & Shabetai, 2004; Cunningham et al., 2005). Treatment also includes limited physical activity, diuretics, sodium restriction, and medications such as digoxin, beta-blockers, and calcium channel blockers. It is recommended that affected women give birth vaginally, with use of an epidural anesthetic and strict monitoring of their fluid intake (Cunningham et al., 2005).

Mitral Valve Stenosis

Mitral valve stenosis is a narrowing of the opening of the mitral valve caused by stiffening of valve leaflets, which obstructs blood flow from the atrium to the ventricle and is the characteristic lesion resulting from RHD (Blanchard & Shabetai, 2004). Even though a history of rheumatic fever may be absent, it remains the most likely cause of mitral stenosis. As the mitral valve narrows, dyspnea worsens, occurring first on exertion and eventually at rest. A tight stenosis plus the increase in blood volume and therefore cardiac output of normal pregnancy may cause ventricular failure and pulmonary edema; hemoptysis may occur. About 25% of women with mitral valve stenosis may become symptomatic for the first time during pregnancy (Cunningham et al., 2005).

The care of the woman with mitral stenosis typically is managed by reducing her activity, restricting dietary sodium, and increasing bed rest. The pregnant woman with mitral stenosis should be followed clinically for symptoms and by echocardiograms to monitor the atrial and ventricular size, as well as heart valve function. Prophylaxis for intrapartum endocarditis and pulmonary infections may be provided for women at high risk (Easterling & Otto, 2002).

Mitral Valve Prolapse

Mitral valve prolapse (MVP) is a common, usually benign, condition occurring in 2% to 3% of women of reproductive age (Cunningham, et al., 2005). The mitral valve leaflets prolapse into the left atrium during ventricular systole, allowing some backflow of blood. Midsystolic click and late systolic murmur are hallmarks of this syndrome. Most cases are asymptomatic. A few women have atypical chest pain (sharp and located in the left side of the chest) that occurs at rest and does not respond to nitrates. They may also have anxiety, palpitations, dyspnea on exertion, and syncope. Specific treatment is usually not necessary except for symptomatic tachyarrhythmias and, rarely, heart failure (Cunningham et al., 2005). Patients usually are treated with beta-blockers such as propranolol (Inderal) or beta–adrenergic blockers such as atenolol (Tenormin) (Blanchard & Shabetai, 2004; Cunningham et al., 2005). Pregnancy and its associated hemodynamic changes may change or alleviate the murmur and click of MVP, as well as symptoms. As with RHD, antibiotic prophylaxis may be given before invasive procedures for woman with mitral regurgitation, thickened mitral valves and complicated vaginal births to prevent bacterial endocarditis (Blanchard & Shabetai, 2004; Cunningham et al., 2005).

Infective Endocarditis

Infective endocarditis, or inflammation of the innermost lining (endocardium) of the heart caused by invasion of microorganisms, is an uncommon disorder during pregnancy (Cunningham et al., 2005). It may be seen in women taking street drugs intravenously. Bacterial endocarditis, leading to incompetence of heart valves and thus congestive heart failure and cerebral emboli, can result in death. Treatment is with antibiotics.

Eisenmenger Syndrome

Eisenmenger syndrome is a right-to-left or bidirectional shunting that can be at the atrial or ventricular level and is combined with elevated pulmonary vascular resistance (Blanchard & Shabetai, 2004). The syndrome is associated with a maternal mortality rate of approximately 50%, but this is dependent on the severity of the pulmonary hypertension (Blanchard & Shabetai, 2004). Because of the poor pregnancy outcomes, pregnancy is contraindicated in women with Eisenmenger syndrome (Blanchard & Shabetai, 2004). Maternal morbidity is associated with right ventricular failure and associated cardiogenic shock (Cunningham et al., 2005). If pregnancy occurs, termination may be recommended if the woman has significant pulmonary hypertension.

In women who continue pregnancy, physical activity is strictly limited, and the supine position is avoided in the third trimester. Treatment includes diuretics, vasodilators, oxygen therapy, and skilled intensive nursing care. Maternal hypotension is not tolerated and should be avoided. Intensive monitoring of fluid status and cardiac function is vital (Blanchard & Shabetai, 2004).

Atrial Septal Defect

Atrial septal defect (ASD) is an abnormal opening between the atria. It is one of the causes of a left-to-right shunt and is the most common congenital defect seen during pregnancy. This defect may go undetected because the woman usually is asymptomatic. The pregnant woman with an ASD will most likely have an uncomplicated pregnancy, unless she has pulmonary hypertension (Blanchard & Shabetai, 2004; Cunningham et al., 2005). With complicated ASDs some women may have right-sided heart failure or arrhythmias as the pregnancy progresses, as a result of increased plasma volume.

Tetralogy of Fallot

Tetralogy of Fallot is the most common cyanotic heart disease present during pregnancy (Blanchard & Shabetai, 2004). Other cyanotic congenital heart diseases are rarely seen during pregnancy because women with these conditions rarely survive to adulthood. Components of tetratology of Fallot include a ventricular septal defect (VSD), pulmonary stenosis, overriding aorta, and right ventricular hypertrophy, leading to a right-to-left shunt. Women with a corrected tetralogy of Fallot have a mortality rate of less than 1%; however women with uncorrected tetralogy of Fallot have a 10% to 15% mortality rate (Cunningham et al., 2005; Gie & Hankins, 2001). Medical management for women with uncorrected tetralogy of Fallot includes avoiding hypotensive episodes during labor and monitoring maternal hematocrits, anticoagulant therapy, high concentration oxygen administration, and hemodynamic monitoring during labor and birth. Complications include right-sided heart failure, dysrhythmias, and conduction defects, with the most dangerous time being the late third trimester and early postpartum period (Blanchard & Shabetai, 2004). Women with tetralogy of Fallot are counseled preconceptionally to have surgical repair.

Marfan Syndrome

Marfan syndrome is an autosomal dominant disorder characterized by generalized weakness of the connective tissue, resulting in joint deformities, ocular lens dislocation, and dilation of the aortic root and progressive aortic valve insufficiency (Blackburn, 2003; Blanchard & Shabetai, 2004). Approximately 90% of individuals with this syndrome have MVP. Aortic insufficiency may result, with an increased risk of aortic dissection and rupture during pregnancy, particularly in the third trimester or postpartum. Excruciating chest pain is the most common symptom of aortic dissection, along with dyspnea and an aortic diastolic murmur (Blanchard & Shabetai, 2004). Therapy includes limiting physical activity, preventing hypertensive complications, and administering beta-blockers. Preconception genetic counseling is recommended to make women aware of the risks of pregnancy with this disease, with a 50% risk of inheritance of the syndrome (Blanchard & Shabetai, 2004).

Heart Transplantation

Increasing numbers of heart recipients are successfully completing pregnancies. Before conception, the woman should be assessed for quality of ventricular function and potential rejection of the transplant. The woman should be stabilized on the immunosuppressant regimen with close monitoring of these medications during the pregnancy (Foley, 2004). Conception should be postponed for at least 1 year after transplantation to avoid acute rejection episodes (Blanchard & Shabetai, 2004). Risks to the woman include hypertension, preeclampsia, preterm labor, renal insufficiency, small-for-gestational-age neonate, and infections (Foley, 2004). During labor, beta-blocking agents may be needed to prevent tachycardia resulting from vagal denervation from the transplant surgery. Vaginal birth is desired, but transplant recipients have an increased rate of cesarean births. Management of the intrapartal period requires the coordination of care among all health care providers involved in the care of the woman and her fetus. After birth, the neonate may exhibit immunosuppressive effects during the first week of life. Though information is limited, breastfeeding infants of mothers who are taking cyclosporine absorb undetectable amounts (Weiner & Buhimschi, 2004).

CARE MANAGEMENT

Assessment and Nursing Diagnoses

The presence of cardiac disease makes the decision to become pregnant more difficult. Planned pregnancy requires that the woman understand the peripartum risks. If the pregnancy is unplanned, the nurse needs to explore the woman's desire to continue the pregnancy after examining the risks in relation to the status of her cardiac condition. The woman's partner and family should be included in the discussion. Women with cardiac disease with significant cardiac compromise may choose to terminate the pregnancy.

The pregnant woman with cardiac disease requires detailed assessment to determine the potential for optimal maternal health and a viable fetus throughout the peripartum period. If she chooses to continue the pregnancy, the high risk pregnant woman's condition may be assessed as often as weekly.

Multidisciplinary care will include a cardiologist, obstetrician, anesthesiologist, and nurses skilled in intensive obstetric care.

Interview

The nurse assesses for factors that would increase stress on the heart, such as anemia, infection, and edema, and how the woman is adapting to the physiologic changes of pregnancy. Special attention is given to the review of the cardiovascular and pulmonary systems. The nurse should determine whether the woman has experienced chest pain at rest or on exertion; edema of the face, hands, or feet; hypertension; heart murmurs; palpitations; paroxysmal nocturnal dyspnea; diaphoresis; pallor; or syncope. Pulmonary signs and symptoms such as cough, hemoptysis, shortness of breath, and orthopnea can indicate cardiac disease. Table 22-4 lists normal and abnormal cardiovascular signs and symptoms during pregnancy.

The nurse documents all medication taken by the woman—including over-the-counter (OTC) medications such as supplemental iron—and is alert to their potential side effects and interactions. The woman is also assessed for undue emotional stress that might further compromise her cardiac status. Examples are depression, anxiety about or fear of morbidity or mortality for herself and her fetus, financial concerns related to extended hospitalization, anger because of impaired social interaction, and feelings of inadequacy regarding her inability to meet family and household demands.

The woman's cultural background may affect the amount of support that she is able to receive from significant others. Family size (number of children and extended family members in the home), as well as role expectations within the family, may be dictated by cultural norms. For the woman with cardiac impairment, family expectations may prove to be a cause of major stress if she is unable to bear the expected number of children or if it is unacceptable to receive help with domestic chores.

Physical assessment

Routine assessments continue during the prenatal period, including monitoring the amount and pattern of weight gain, edema, vital signs, and discomforts of pregnancy. In addition, the woman is observed for signs of **cardiac decompensation,** that is, progressive generalized edema, crackles at the base of the lungs, or pulse irregularity (Signs of Potential Complications box). Symptoms of cardiac decompensation may appear abruptly or gradually. Medical intervention must be instituted immediately to maintain optimal cardiac status. Dyspnea, palpitations, syncope, and edema occur commonly in pregnant women and can mask the symptoms of a developing or worsening cardiovascular disorder. A woman's sudden inability to perform activities that she previously was comfortable doing may indicate cardiac decompensation.

Laboratory and diagnostic tests

Routine urinalysis and blood work (complete blood cell count and blood chemistry) are done during the initial visit. The woman with cardiac impairment requires a baseline

TABLE 22-4

Cardiovascular Signs and Symptoms during Pregnancy

NORMAL	ABNORMAL
SIGNS	
Neck vein pulsation	Neck vein distention
Diffuse or displaced apical pulse	Cardiomegaly; heave
Split S_1, accentuated S_2	Loud P_2; wide split of S_2
Third heart sound - loud	Summation gallop
Systolic murmur (1-2/6) (92%- 95%)	Loud systolic murmur (4-6/6)
Venous hum	Diastolic murmur
Sinus dysrhythmia	Sustained dysrhythmia
Peripheral edema, particularly lower extremities	Clubbing or cyanosis
SYMPTOMS	
Fatigue	Symptoms at rest
Chest pain	Exertional chest pain
Dyspnea	Exertional severe dyspnea
Orthopnea	Orthopnea (progressive)
Hyperpnea	Paroxysmal nocturnal dyspnea
Palpitations	Tachycardia (>120 beats/min); dysrhythmia
Syncope (vasovagal)	Exertional syncope

Adapted from Blackburn, S. (2003). *Maternal, fetal, and neonatal physiology: A clinical perspective* (2nd ed.). St. Louis: Saunders.

ECG at the beginning of her pregnancy, if not before pregnancy, which permits vital diagnostic comparisons of subsequent ECGs. Echocardiograms and pulse oximetry studies may be performed as indicated. Chest films may be necessary during late pregnancy, provided the abdomen is carefully shielded. In addition, fetal ultrasound, fetal movement studies, or fetal nonstress tests may be used to determine fetal well-being.

The following nursing diagnoses may be appropriate for the pregnant woman with cardiac disease:

- *Fear related to*
  - increased peripartum risk
- *Risk for ineffective coping related to*
  - the woman's cardiac condition
  - changes in relationships
- *Risk for ineffective tissue perfusion related to*
  - hypotensive syndrome
- *Activity intolerance related to*
  - cardiac condition
- *Deficient knowledge related to*
  - cardiac condition
  - pregnancy and how it affects cardiac condition
  - requirements to alter self-care activities
- *Impaired home maintenance related to*
  - woman's confinement to bed or limited activity level
- *Self-care deficit (bathing, grooming, dressing) related to*
  - fatigue or activity intolerance
  - need for bed rest

Expected Outcomes of Care

The pregnant woman with cardiovascular problems faces significant curtailment of her activities. These restrictions can have physical and emotional implications. The community health nurse, social worker, and physical or occupational therapist are some of the resource people whose services may need to be incorporated into the plan of care. Expected outcomes for the pregnant woman (and family, if appropriate) may include that she (they) will do the following:

- Verbalize understanding of the disorder, management, and probable outcome
- Describe her role in management, including when and how to take medication, adjust diet, and prepare for and participate in treatment

signs of
POTENTIAL COMPLICATIONS

Cardiac Decompensation

PREGNANT WOMAN: SUBJECTIVE SYMPTOMS
- Increasing fatigue or difficulty breathing, or both, with her usual activities
- Feeling of smothering
- Frequent cough
- Palpitations; feeling that her heart is "racing"
- Generalized edema: swelling of face, feet, legs, fingers (e.g., rings do not fit anymore)

NURSE: OBJECTIVE SIGNS
- Irregular, weak, rapid pulse (≥100 beats/min)
- Progressive, generalized edema
- Crackles at base of lungs after two inspirations and exhalations that do not clear after coughing
- Orthopnea; increasing dyspnea
- Rapid respirations (≥25 breaths/min)
- Moist, frequent cough
- Cyanosis of lips and nail beds

- Cope with emotional reactions to the pregnancy and infant at risk
- Adapt to the physiologic stressors of pregnancy, labor, and birth
- Identify and use support systems
- Carry her fetus to the point of viability or to term

Plan of Care and Interventions
Antepartum

Therapy for the pregnant woman with heart disease is focused on minimizing stress on the heart. This stress is greatest between 28 and 32 weeks of pregnancy as the hemodynamic changes reach their maximum. The workload of the cardiovascular system is reduced by appropriate treatment of any coexisting emotional stress, hypertension, anemia, hyperthyroidism, or obesity.

Signs and symptoms of cardiac decompensation are reviewed during the prenatal period. The woman with class I or II heart disease requires 8 to 10 hours of sleep every day and should take 30-minute naps after eating. Her activities are restricted, with housework, shopping, and exercise limited to the amount allowed for the functional classification of her heart disease. Information on how to cope with activity limitations is important in meeting emotional needs of the woman. Referral to a support group may help the woman and her family handle stress.

The pregnant woman with class II cardiac disease should avoid heavy exertion and should stop any activity that causes even minor signs and symptoms of cardiac decompensation. She may be admitted to the hospital near term (earlier if signs of cardiac overload or arrhythmia develop) for evaluation and treatment.

Bed rest for much of each day is necessary for pregnant women with class III cardiac disease. Approximately 30% of these women experience cardiac decompensation during pregnancy. With this possibility the woman may require hospitalization for the remainder of the pregnancy.

Because decompensation occurs even at rest in persons with class IV cardiac disease, a major initial effort must be made to improve the cardiac status of the pregnant woman in this category who chooses to continue her pregnancy (Teaching Guidelines box).

Infections are treated promptly. Women with valvular dysfunction may receive prophylactic antibiotics.

Nutrition counseling is necessary, optimally with the woman's family present. The pregnant woman needs a well-balanced diet, high in iron and folic acid supplementation, with high protein and adequate calories to gain weight. The iron supplements tend to cause constipation. Therefore the pregnant woman should increase her intake of fluids and fiber, and a stool softener may be prescribed. It is important for the pregnant woman with cardiac disease to avoid straining during defecation, thus causing the Valsalva maneuver (forced expiration against a closed airway, which when released causes blood to rush to the heart and overload the cardiac system). The woman's intake of potassium is monitored to prevent hypokalemia, especially if she is taking diuretics. A referral to a registered dietitian is recommended.

Cardiac medications are prescribed as needed for the pregnant woman, with attention to fetal well-being. The hemodynamic changes that occur during pregnancy, such as increased plasma volume and increased renal clearance of drugs, can alter the amount of medication needed to establish and maintain a therapeutic drug level (Blanchard & Shabetai, 2004).

If anticoagulant therapy is required during pregnancy for conditions such as recurrent venous thrombosis, pulmonary embolus, RHD, or prosthetic valves, heparin should be used, because this large-molecule drug does not cross the placenta. The nurse should closely monitor the woman's blood work, specifically the partial thromboplastin time (PTT). The woman may need to learn to self-administer heparin by injection or continuous subcutaneous infusion. She also requires specific nutritional teaching to avoid foods high in

---

TEACHING GUIDELINES
The Pregnant Woman at Risk for Cardiac Decompensation

- Assess lifestyle patterns, emotional status, and environment of woman.
- Arrange for consultations as needed (e.g., dietitian, home care, child care, social work).
- Determine woman's and her family's understanding of her heart disease and how the disease affects her pregnancy.
- Determine stressors in the woman's life. Assist woman in identifying effective coping strategies.
- Instruct woman to report signs of cardiac decompensation or congestive heart failure: generalized edema, distention of neck veins, dyspnea, pulmonary crackles, cough, palpitations, sudden weight gain.
- Instruct woman to be watchful for signs of thromboembolism, such as redness, tenderness, pain, or swelling of

the legs. Instruct woman to seek medical help immediately if such symptoms occur.
- Instruct woman to avoid constipation and consequent straining with bowel movements (Valsalva maneuver) by taking in adequate fluids and fiber. A stool softener may be ordered.
- Explore with woman ways to obtain the needed rest throughout the day. Depending on the level of her cardiac disease, she may need to sleep 10 hours per night and rest 30 minutes after meals (class I or II) or rest for most of the day (class III or IV).
- Help woman make use of community resources, including support groups, as indicated.
- Emphasize the importance of keeping her prenatal visits.

From Gilbert, E. & Harmon, J. (2003). *Manual of high risk pregnancy and delivery* (3rd ed.). St. Louis: Mosby.

vitamin K, such as raw, dark green leafy vegetables, which counteract the effects of the heparin. In addition, she will require a folic acid supplement.

Tests for fetal maturity and well-being, as well as placental sufficiency, may be necessary. Other therapy is directly related to the functional classification of heart disease. The nurse may need to reinforce the need for close medical supervision.

Intrapartum

For all pregnant women and caregivers the intrapartum period is the one that evokes the most apprehension. The woman with impaired cardiac function has additional reasons to be anxious because labor and giving birth place an additional burden on her already compromised cardiovascular system.

Assessments include the routine assessments for all laboring women, as well as assessments for cardiac decompensation. In addition, arterial blood gases (ABGs) may be needed to assess for adequate oxygenation. A Swan-Ganz catheter may be inserted to accurately monitor hemodynamic status during labor and birth. ECG monitoring and continuous monitoring of blood pressure and pulse oximetry are usually instituted for the woman, and the fetus is continuously monitored electronically.

NURSE ALERT *A pulse rate of 100 beats/min or greater or a respiratory rate of 25 breaths/min or greater is a concern. Respiratory status is checked frequently for developing dyspnea, coughing, or crackles at the base of the lungs. The color and temperature of the skin are noted. Pale, cool, clammy skin may indicate cardiac shock.*

Nursing care during labor and birth focuses on the promotion of cardiac function. Anxiety is minimized by maintaining a calm atmosphere in the labor and birth rooms. The nurse provides anticipatory guidance by keeping the woman and her family informed of labor progress and events that will probably occur, as well as answering any questions they have. The woman's childbirth preparation method should be supported to the degree it is feasible for her cardiac condition. Nursing techniques that promote comfort, such as back massage, are used.

Cardiac function is supported by keeping the woman's head and shoulders elevated and body parts resting on pillows. The side-lying position usually facilitates hemodynamics during labor. Discomfort is relieved with medication and supportive care. Epidural regional anesthesia provides better pain relief than narcotics and causes fewer alterations in hemodynamics (Cunningham et al., 2005). Maternal hypotension must be avoided.

The woman may require other types of medication (e.g., anticoagulants, prophylactic antibiotics). If evidence of cardiac decompensation appears, the physician may order deslanoside (Cedilanid-D) for rapid digitalization, furosemide (Lasix) for rapid diuresis, and oxygen by intermittent positive pressure to decrease the development of pulmonary edema.

LEGAL TIP Cardiac and Metabolic Emergencies

The management of emergencies such as maternal cardiopulmonary distress or arrest or maternal metabolic crisis should be documented in policies, procedures, and protocols. Any independent nursing actions appropriate to the emergency should be clearly identified.

Beta-adrenergic agents (e.g., ritodrine and terbutaline) should be not be used for tocolysis in women with cardiac problems. These drugs are associated with various cardiac side effects, including tachycardia and myocardial ischemia. A synthetic oxytocin, Syntocinon, can be used for induction of labor. This drug does not appear to cause significant coronary artery constriction in doses prescribed for labor induction or control of postpartum uterine atony. Cervical ripening agents containing prostaglandin are not contraindicated, but reports of use in pregnant women with cardiac disease are not available.

If there are no obstetric problems, vaginal birth is recommended and may be accomplished with the woman in the side-lying position to facilitate uterine perfusion. If the supine position is used, a pad is positioned under the hip to displace the uterus laterally and minimize the danger of supine hypotension. The knees are flexed, and the feet are flat on the bed. To prevent compression of popliteal veins and an increase in blood volume in the chest and trunk as a result of the effects of gravity, stirrups are not used. Open glottis pushing is recommended, and the Valsalva maneuver must be avoided when pushing because it reduces diastolic ventricular filling and obstructs left ventricular outflow. Mask oxygen is important. Episiotomy and vacuum extraction or outlet forceps may be used because these procedures decrease the length of the second stage of labor and decrease the workload of the heart in second stage labor. Cesarean birth is not routinely recommended for women who have cardiovascular disease because there is risk of dramatic fluid shifts, sustained hemodynamic changes, and increased blood loss.

Penicillin prophylaxis may be ordered for pregnant women with class II or higher cardiac disease to protect against bacterial endocarditis in labor and during the early puerperium. Dilute IV oxytocin immediately after birth may be employed to prevent hemorrhage. Ergot products should not be used because they increase blood pressure. Fluid balance should be maintained, and blood loss replaced. If tubal sterilization is desired, surgery is delayed at least several days to ensure homeostasis.

Postpartum

Monitoring for cardiac decompensation in the postpartum period is essential. The first 24 to 48 hours postpartum are the most hemodynamically difficult for the woman. Hemorrhage or infection, or both, may worsen the cardiac condition. The woman with a cardiac disorder may continue to require a Swan-Ganz catheter and ABG monitoring.

NURSE ALERT *The immediate postbirth period is hazardous for a woman whose heart function is compromised. Cardiac output increases rapidly as extravascular* *fluid is remobilized into the vascular compartment. At the moment of birth intraabdominal pressure is reduced drastically; pressure on veins is removed, the splanchnic vessels engorge, and blood flow to the heart is increased. When blood flow increases to the heart, a reflex bradycardia may result.*

Care in the postpartum period is tailored to the woman's functional capacity. Routine postpartum assessments are done. The head of the bed is elevated, and the woman is encouraged to lie on her side. Bed rest may be ordered, with or without bathroom privileges. Progressive ambulation may be permitted as tolerated. The nurse may need to help the woman meet her grooming and hygiene needs and other activities. Bowel movements without stress or strain for the woman are promoted with stool softeners, diet, and fluids.

The woman may need a family member to help in the care of the infant. Breastfeeding is not contraindicated, but not all women with heart disease will be able to nurse their infants (Lawrence & Lawrence, 2005; Riordan, 2005). The woman who chooses to breastfeed will need the support of her family and the nursing staff to be successful. The woman may need assistance in positioning herself or the infant for feeding. To further conserve the woman's energy, the infant may need to be brought to the mother and taken from her after the feeding. If the woman is unable to breastfeed and her energies do not allow her to bottle-feed the infant, the baby can be kept at the bedside so she can look at and touch her baby to establish an emotional bond with her baby with a low expenditure of energy.

Preparation for discharge is carefully planned with the woman and family. Provision of help for the woman in the home by relatives, friends, and others must be addressed. If necessary, the nurse refers the family to community resources (e.g., homemaking services). Rest and sleep periods, activity, and diet must be planned. The couple may need information about reestablishing sexual relations and contraception or sterilization. Oral contraceptives are often contraindicated because of the risk of thromboembolism. Maternal cardiac output is usually stabilized by 2 weeks postpartum (Easterling & Otto, 2002).

Cardiopulmonary resuscitation of the pregnant woman

Cardiac arrest in a pregnant woman occurs in approximately 1 in 30,000 pregnancies (Hueppchen & Satin, 2004). It is most often related to events at the time of birth such as amniotic fluid embolism, eclampsia, stroke, hemorrhage, and acute respiratory failure. Some modifications of the procedure for cardiopulmonary resuscitation (CPR) (Emergency box) are needed during pregnancy.

Various protocols exist for CPR during pregnancy. The most widely used guide is the American Heart Association (AHA) Advanced Cardiac Life Support Protocol (AHA, 2000). This protocol recommends standard CPR with the uterus displaced laterally, fluid restoration, and defibrillation if indicated. The decision for cesarean birth must be made

---

EMERGENCY

Cardiopulmonary Resuscitation for the Pregnant Woman

CARDIOPULMONARY RESUSCITATION (CPR)

Airway
- Determine unresponsiveness.
- Activate emergency medical system and get the automated external defibrillator (AED) if available.
- Position woman on flat, firm surface with uterus displaced laterally with a wedge (e.g., a rolled towel placed under her hip) or manually, or place her in a lateral position.
- Open airway with head tilt–chin lift maneuver.

Breathing
- Determine breathlessness (look, listen, feel).
- If the woman is not breathing, give two slow breaths.

Circulation
- Determine pulselessness by feeling carotid pulse.
- If there is no pulse, begin chest compressions at rate of 100 per minute. Chest compressions may be performed slightly higher on the sternum if the uterus is enlarged enough to displace the diaphragm into a higher position.
- After four cycles of 15 compressions and two breaths, check her pulse. If pulse is not present, continue CPR.

Defibrillation
- Use an AED according to standard protocol to analyze heart rhythm and deliver shock if indicated.

Relief of foreign-body airway obstruction
- If the pregnant woman is unable to speak or cough, perform chest thrusts. Stand behind the woman and place your arms under her armpits to encircle her chest. Press backward with quick thrusts until the foreign body is expelled (Fig. 22-5). If the woman becomes unresponsive, follow the steps for victims who become unresponsive, but use chest thrusts instead of abdominal thrusts.

Source: American Heart Association (AHA). (2001). Fundamentals of BLS for healthcare providers. Dallas: AHA.

---

within 4 to 5 minutes of the mother's cardiac arrest. The gestational age of the infant and the presence of skilled pediatric support personnel must be considered in the decision.

In the event of cardiac arrest, standard resuscitative efforts with a few modifications are implemented. To prevent supine hypotension, the pregnant woman is placed on a flat, firm surface with the uterus displaced laterally either manually or with a wedge or rolled blanket or towel under her right hip (AHA, 2000). If defibrillation is needed, the paddles need to be placed one rib interspace higher than usual because the heart is displaced slightly by the enlarged uterus. If possible, the fetus should be monitored during the cardiac arrest.

Complications may be associated with CPR of a pregnant woman. These complications may include laceration of the

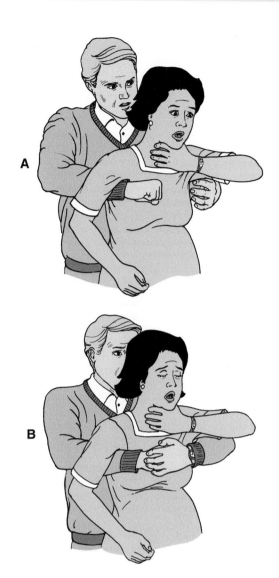

Fig. 22-5 Heimlich maneuver. Clearing airway obstruction in woman in late stages of pregnancy (can also be used in markedly obese victim). **A,** Standing behind victim, place your arms under woman's armpits and across chest. Place thumb side of your clenched fist against middle of sternum, and place other hand over fist. **B,** Perform backward chest thrusts until foreign body is expelled or woman becomes unconscious. If pregnant woman becomes unconscious because of foreign body airway obstruction, place her on her back and kneel close to victim's side. (Be sure uterus is displaced laterally by using, for example, a rolled blanket under her hip.) Open mouth with tongue-jaw lift, perform finger sweep, and attempt rescue breathing. If unable to ventilate, position hands as for chest compression. Deliver five chest thrusts firmly to remove obstruction. Repeat above sequence of Heimlich maneuver, finger sweep, and attempt to ventilate. Continue above sequence until pregnant woman's airway is clear of obstruction or help has arrived to relieve you. If woman is unconscious, give chest compressions as for woman without pulse (AHA, 2001).

liver, rupture of the uterus, fractures of the ribs and sternum, hemothorax, or hemoperitoneum. Fetal complications, including cardiac arrhythmia or asystole related to maternal defibrillation and medications, CNS depression related to

antiarrhythmic drugs and inadequate uteroplacental perfusion, and onset of preterm labor, may also occur (Hueppchen & Satin, 2004).

If resuscitation is successful, the woman and her fetus must receive careful monitoring. The woman remains at increased risk for recurrent pulmonary arrest and arrhythmias (ventricular tachycardia, supraventricular tachycardia, bradycardia). Therefore her cardiovascular, pulmonary, and neurologic status should be assessed continuously. Uterine activity and resting tone must be monitored. Fetal status and gestational age should be determined and used in decision making regarding the continuation of the pregnancy or the timing and route of birth.

Evaluation

The nurse uses the previously stated expected outcomes as criteria to evaluate the care of the woman with cardiac disease (Plan of Care).

ANEMIA

Anemia is the most common medical disorder of pregnancy, affecting from 20% to 60% of pregnant women (Kilpatrick & Laros, 2004). Anemia results in reduction of the oxygen-carrying capacity of the blood. Because the oxygen-carrying capacity of the blood is decreased, the heart tries to compensate by increasing the cardiac output. This effort increases the workload of the heart and stresses ventricular function. Therefore anemia that occurs with any other complication (e.g., preeclampsia) may result in congestive heart failure.

An indirect index of the oxygen-carrying capacity is the packed RBC volume, or hematocrit level. The normal hematocrit range in nonpregnant women is 37% to 47%. However, normal values for pregnant women with adequate iron stores may be as low as 33%. As defined by the CDC, anemia in pregnancy is defined as below 11 g/dl in the first and third trimesters and less than 10.5 g/dl in the second trimester (IOM, 1990). This has been explained by hydremia (dilution of blood), also called the *physiologic anemia of pregnancy.*

At or near sea level, the pregnant woman is anemic when her hemoglobin level is less than 11 g/dl or hematocrit is less than 33%. In areas of high altitude, much higher values indicate anemia; for example, at 1500 m (5000 feet) above sea level, a hemoglobin level less than 14 g/dl indicates anemia (Pagana & Pagana, 2003).

When a woman has anemia during pregnancy, the loss of blood at birth, even if minimal, is not well tolerated. She is at an increased risk for requiring blood transfusions. Women with anemia have a higher incidence of puerperal complications, such as infection, than do pregnant women with normal hematologic values.

Nursing care of the anemic pregnant woman requires that the nurse be able to distinguish between the normal physiologic anemia of pregnancy and the disease states. Approximately 90% of cases of anemia in pregnancy are of the iron

PLAN OF CARE *The Pregnant Woman with Heart Disease*

NURSING DIAGNOSIS Activity intolerance related to effects of pregnancy on the woman with rheumatic heart disease with mitral valve stenosis

Expected Outcome *Woman will verbalize a plan to change lifestyle throughout pregnancy in order to avoid risk of cardiac decompensation.*

Nursing Interventions/*Rationales*

- Assist woman to identify factors that decrease activity tolerance and explore extent of limitations *to establish a baseline for evaluation.*
- Help woman to develop an individualized program of activity and rest, taking into account the living and working environment as well as support of family and friends *to maintain sufficient cardiac output.*
- Teach woman to monitor physiologic response to activity (e.g., pulse rate, respiratory rate) and reduce activity that causes fatigue or pain *to maintain sufficient cardiac output and prevent potential injury to fetus.*
- Enlist family and friends to assist woman in pacing activities and to provide support in performing role functions and self-care activities that are too strenuous *to increase chances of compliance with activity restrictions.*
- Suggest that woman maintain an activity log that records activities, time, duration, intensity, and physiologic response *to evaluate effectiveness of and adherence to activity program.*
- Discuss various quiet diversional activities that could be done by the woman *to decrease the potential for boredom during rest periods.*

NURSING DIAGNOSIS Risk for ineffective therapeutic regimen management related to woman's first pregnancy and perceived sense of wellness

Expected Outcome *Woman will participate in an effective therapeutic regimen for pregnancy complicated by heart disease.*

Nursing Interventions/*Rationales*

- Identify factors, such as insufficient knowledge about the effect of cardiac disease on pregnancy, that could inhibit the woman from participating in a therapeutic regimen *to promote early interventions, such as teaching about the importance of rest.*
- Teach woman and family about factors such as lack of rest or not taking prescribed medications that could adversely affect the pregnancy *to provide information and promote empowerment over the situation.*
- Encourage expression of feelings about the disease and its potential effect on the pregnancy *to promote a sense of trust.*
- Identify resources in the community *to provide a shared sense of common experiences.*
- Encourage woman to verbalize her plan for carrying out the regimen of care *to evaluate the effects of teaching.*

NURSING DIAGNOSIS Decreased cardiac output related to increased circulatory volume secondary to pregnancy and cardiac disease

Expected Outcome *The woman will exhibit signs of adequate cardiac output (i.e., normal pulse and blood pressure, normal heart and breath sounds, normal skin color, tone, and turgor, normal capillary refill, normal urine output, and no evidence of edema).*

Nursing Interventions/*Rationales*

- Reinforce the importance of activity and rest cycles *to prevent cardiac complications.*
- Plan with woman a frequent visit schedule to caregiver *to provide adequate surveillance of high risk pregnancy.*
- Teach woman to lie in lateral position *to increase uteroplacental blood flow* and to elevate legs while sitting *to promote venous return.*
- Monitor intake and output and check for edema *to assess for renal complications or venous return problems.*
- Monitor fetal heart rate and fetal activity, and perform nonstress test as indicated *to assess fetal status and detect uteroplacental insufficiency.*

---

deficiency type. The remaining 10% of cases embrace a considerable variety of acquired and hereditary anemias, including folic acid deficiency, sickle cell anemia, and thalassemia.

Iron Deficiency Anemia

Iron deficiency anemia is the most common anemia of pregnancy (Kilpatrick & Laros, 2004). Because of the increased iron needs necessitated for fetal development and maternal stores, pregnant women who ingest a balanced diet are encouraged to take multivitamins with iron (Blackburn, 2003). Pregnant women with anemia despite iron supplementation need to be questioned regarding the practice of pica, the ingestion of nonfood substances (e.g., clay, cornstarch, freezer frost). If iron deficiency anemia is diagnosed, increased iron dosages are recommended (elemental iron, 60 to 120 mg/day). It is important to teach the pregnant woman the significance of the iron therapy. In addition, the pregnant woman should be instructed about which foods are high in

iron and which are high in ascorbic acid, which facilitates iron absorption from the gastrointestinal tract. In addition, women need to be instructed regarding strategies to decrease the gastrointestinal side effects of iron therapy. Some pregnant women cannot tolerate the prescribed oral iron because of the nausea and vomiting associated with the pregnancy and as a side effect of iron therapy. Therefore, some practitioners may recommend the use of chewable children's vitamins with iron, 2 tablets/day. For women with anemia refractory to oral iron therapy, with a hemoglobin less than 8.5 g/dl, the health care provider may order parenteral iron such as iron dextran (Kilpatrick & Laros, 2004).

Folate Deficiency

Even in well-nourished women, it is common to have a folate deficiency. Poor diet and increased alcohol use may contribute to folate deficiency. Malabsorption may play a part in the development of anemia caused by a lack of folic acid.

Women with megaloblastic anemia caused by folic acid deficiency have the usual presenting symptoms and signs of anemia: pallor, fatigue, and lethargy as well as glossitis and skin roughness, which are associated specifically with megaloblastic anemia (Kilpatrick & Laros, 2004). Folic acid deficiency anemia is common in multiple gestations. Folate deficiency during conception has been associated with increases in the incidence of neural tube defects, cleft lip, and cleft palate. During pregnancy the recommended daily intake is 400 mcg of folic acid per day. Women are instructed to consume foods high in folic acid (fresh, green leafy vegetables and legumes) and encouraged to take a daily prenatal multivitamin.

Sickle Cell Hemoglobinopathy

Sickle cell hemoglobinopathy is a disease caused by the presence of abnormal hemoglobin in the blood. Sickle cell trait (SA hemoglobin pattern) is sickling of the RBCs but with a normal RBC life span. It usually causes only mild clinical symptoms. Sickle cell anemia (sickle cell disease) is a recessive, hereditary, familial hemolytic anemia that affects those of African-American or Mediterranean ancestry (Moore & Martin, 2004). These individuals usually have abnormal hemoglobin types (SS or SC). Beginning in childhood, persons with sickle cell anemia have recurrent attacks (crises) of fever and pain in the abdomen or extremities. These attacks are attributed to vascular occlusion (from abnormal cells), tissue hypoxia, edema, and RBC destruction. Crises are associated with normochromic anemia, jaundice, reticulocytosis, a positive sickle cell test, and the demonstration of abnormal hemoglobin (usually SS or SC).

Almost 10% of African-Americans in North America have the sickle cell trait, but fewer than 1% have sickle cell anemia. The anemia often is complicated by iron and folic acid deficiency.

Women with sickle cell trait usually do well in pregnancy, although they are at increased risk for UTIs and may be deficient in iron (Kilpatrick & Laros, 2004). If the woman has sickle cell anemia, the anemia that occurs in normal pregnancies may aggravate the condition and bring on more crises. Fetal complications include being small for gestational age, IUGR, and skeletal changes. Pregnant women with sickle cell anemia are prone to pyelonephritis, leg ulcers, intense bone pain, strokes, cardiomyopathy, congestive heart failure, acute chest syndrome, and preeclampsia (Cunningham et al., 2005; Moore & Martin, 2004). UTIs and hematuria are common. An aplastic crisis may follow serious infection. Morphine and the adjuvant antihistamines may be given for pain management (Moore & Martin, 2004). Transfusions of the woman have been the usual treatment for symptomatic patients; however, prophylactic red cell transfusions are common as well and significantly reduce the number of painful crises (Cunningham et al., 2005; Kilpatrick & Laros, 2004).

Thalassemia

Thalassemia (Mediterranean or Cooley's anemia) is a relatively common anemia in which there is ineffective erythropoiesis and varying degrees of anemia (Cunningham et al., 2005). Thalassemia is a hereditary disorder that involves the abnormal synthesis of the alpha or beta chains of hemoglobin. Beta thalassemia is the more common variety in the United States and often is diagnosed in persons of Mediterranean, North African, African-American, Middle Eastern, or Asian descent (Kilpatrick & Laros, 2004). The unbalanced synthesis of hemoglobin leads to premature RBC death, resulting in severe anemia. There are two major types, classified according to the missing globin peptide chain (Cunningham et al., 2005). Beta thalassemia major (Cooley's anemia), is the homozygous form of this disorder, and alpha thalassemia minor is the heterozygous form. Thalassemia major is the more severe of the two, and females with beta thalassemia who survive childhood are most often sterile (Cunningham et al., 2005). Couples with the thalassemia trait should seek genetic counseling. Thalassemia must be differentiated from iron deficiency anemia.

Women with thalassemia major have problems conceiving. During pregnancy, women with thalassemia minor may demonstrate a mild persistent anemia, but the RBC level may be normal or even elevated. Supplemental iron and folic acid should be administered (Cunningham et al., 2005).

PULMONARY DISORDERS

As pregnancy advances and the uterus impinges on the thoracic cavity, any pregnant woman may experience increased respiratory difficulty. This difficulty will be compounded by pulmonary disease.

Asthma

Bronchial asthma is an acute respiratory illness characterized by periods of exacerbations and remissions. Exacerbations are triggered by allergens, marked change in ambient temperature, or emotional tension. In many cases the actual cause may be unknown, although a family history of allergy is common. In response to stimuli, there is widespread but reversible narrowing of the hyperreactive airways, making it difficult to breathe. The clinical manifestations are expiratory wheezing, productive cough, thick sputum, and dyspnea.

Prevalence rates for women pregnant with asthma range from 3.7% to 8.4% (Kwon, Belanger, & Bracken, 2004). The physiologic changes associated with pregnancy do not contribute to a worsening of asthma (Whitty & Dombrowski, 2004). The effect of pregnancy on asthma is unpredictable, though women of African-American ethnicity with asthma have an increased morbidity and mortality. Asthma has been associated with IUGR and preterm birth (Whitty & Dombrowski, 2004). Women often experience few symptoms of asthma in the first trimester and in the last weeks of pregnancy. The severity of symptoms usually peaks between 29 and 36 weeks of gestation (Burton & Reyes, 2001).

Therapy for asthma has three objectives: (1) relief of the acute attack, (2) prevention or limitation of later attacks, and (3) adequate maternal and fetal oxygenation (Barth & Stewart, 2004). These goals can be achieved in pregnancy by eliminating environmental triggers (e.g., dust mites, animal dander, pollen), drug therapy (e.g., inhaled beta-agonists, inhaled cromolyn, corticosteroids, antiinflammatory agents), and patient education. Respiratory infections should be treated, and mist or steam inhalation employed to aid expectoration of mucus. Acute episodes may require albuterol, steroids, aminophylline, beta-adrenergic agents, and oxygen. Almost all asthma medications are considered safe in pregnancy (Burton & Reyes, 2001; Gluck & Gluck, 2005).

Asthma attacks can occur in labor; therefore medications for asthma are continued in labor and postpartum. Pulse oximetry should be instituted during labor. Epidural anesthesia reduces oxygen consumption and is recommended for pain relief. Fentanyl, a non–histamine-releasing narcotic may be used also for pain control and is not associated with bronchospasm (Cunningham et al., 2005). During postpartum, women in whom excessive bleeding occurs will receive prostaglandin E_2. The woman usually returns to her prepregnancy asthma status within 3 months after giving birth.

Cystic Fibrosis

Cystic fibrosis is a common autosomal recessive genetic disorder (1 in 3000 live Caucasian births) in which the exocrine glands produce excessive viscous secretions, causing problems with both respiratory and digestive functions (Whitty & Dombrowski, 2004). There is an increase in pulmonary capillary permeability, decrease in lung volume, and shunting, which results in arterial hypoxemia. Respiratory failure and early death (early twenties) may occur. Genetic counseling is encouraged to identify carriers of the disease.

In women with good nutrition, mild obstructive lung disease, and minimal lung impairment, pregnancy is tolerated well (Cunningham et al., 2005; Whitty & Dombrowski, 2004). In those with severe disease, the pregnancy is often complicated by chronic hypoxia and frequent pulmonary infections. Women with cystic fibrosis show a decrease in residual volume during pregnancy, as do normal pregnant women, and are unable to maintain vital capacity. Presumably the pulmonary vasculature cannot accommodate the increased cardiac output of pregnancy. The results are decreased oxygen to the myocardium, decreased cardiac output, and increased hypoxia. A pregnant woman with less than 50% of expected vital capacity usually has a difficult pregnancy. Increased maternal and perinatal mortality is related to severe pulmonary infection.

Maternal weight and symptoms of malabsorption should be monitored at each prenatal visit, and pancreatic enzymes should be adjusted as necessary. A glucose tolerance test should be done at 20 weeks of gestation. Routine respiratory management is continued through the pregnancy. Nonstress tests should be initiated at 32 weeks of ges-

tation. Women with respiratory infections should be hospitalized.

During labor, monitoring for fluid and electrolyte balance is required. Sodium losses through sweat can be significant, and hypovolemia can occur. Cor pulmonale is common, and fluid overload may occur. Oxygen is administered by face mask during labor, and monitoring by pulse oximetry is recommended (Whitty & Dombrowski, 2004). Epidural or local analgesia is the preferred analgesic for birth, with vaginal birth recommended.

Breastfeeding appears to be safe as long as the sodium content of the milk is not abnormal (Lawrence & Lawrence, 2005). Pumping and discarding the milk is done until the sodium content has been determined. Milk samples should be tested periodically for sodium, chloride, and total fat, and the infant's growth pattern should be monitored.

INTEGUMENTARY DISORDERS

The skin surface may exhibit many physiologic and pathologic conditions during pregnancy. Dermatologic disorders induced by pregnancy include melasma (chloasma), herpes gestationis, noninflammatory pruritus of pregnancy, vascular "spiders," palmar erythema, and epulis (tumors on the gingiva). Skin problems generally aggravated by pregnancy are acne vulgaris (acne) (in the first trimester), erythema multiforme, herpetiform dermatitis (fever blisters and genital herpes), granuloma inguinale (Donovan bodies), condylomata acuminata (genital warts), neurofibromatosis (von Recklinghausen disease), and pemphigus. Dermatologic disorders usually improved by pregnancy include acne vulgaris (in the third trimester), seborrheic dermatitis (dandruff), and psoriasis (Cunningham et al., 2005). An unpredictable course during pregnancy may be expected in atopic dermatitis, lupus erythematosus, and herpes simplex.

> **NURSE ALERT** *Isotretinoin (Accutane), commonly prescribed for cystic acne, is highly teratogenic and therefore contraindicated in pregnancy. Fetuses exposed are at increased risk for craniofacial, cardiac, and CNS malformations.*

Explanation, reassurance, and commonsense measures should suffice for normal skin changes. In contrast, disease processes during and soon after pregnancy may be extremely difficult to diagnose and treat.

NEUROLOGIC DISORDERS

The pregnant woman with a neurologic disorder needs to deal with potential teratogenic effects of prescribed medications, changes of mobility during pregnancy, and impaired ability to care for the baby. The nurse should be aware of all drugs the woman is taking and the associated potential for producing congenital anomalies. As the pregnancy progresses, the woman's center of gravity shifts and causes balance and gait changes. The nurse should advise the woman of these expected changes and suggest safety measures as appropriate. Family and community resources may be needed to provide care for the neurologically impaired woman.

Epilepsy

Epilepsy is a disorder of the brain that causes recurrent seizures and is the most common neurologic disorder accompanying pregnancy (Constantino & Varner, 2004). Epilepsy may result from developmental abnormalities or injury, as well as having no known cause. Convulsive seizures may be more frequent or severe during complications of pregnancy, such as edema, alkalosis, fluid-electrolyte imbalance, cerebral hypoxia, hypoglycemia, and hypocalcemia. However, the effects of pregnancy on epilepsy are unpredictable: some women have no change or even a decrease in seizure frequency (Constantino & Varner, 2004).

The differential diagnosis between epilepsy and eclampsia may pose a problem. Epilepsy and eclampsia can coexist. However, a history of seizures and a normal plasma uric acid level, as well as the absence of hypertension, generalized edema, or proteinuria, point to epilepsy.

During pregnancy, the risk of vaginal bleeding is doubled, and there is a threefold risk of abruptio placentae. Abnormal presentations are more common in labor and birth, and there is an increased possibility that the fetus will experience seizures in utero (Aminoff, 2004).

Metabolic changes in pregnancy usually alter pharmacokinetics. In addition, nausea and vomiting may interfere with ingestion and absorption of medication. Failure to take medications is a common factor leading to worsening of seizure activity during pregnancy, particularly during the first trimester (Constantino & Varner, 2004). This is largely because of the message that drugs for epilepsy are harmful to the fetus. Teratogenicity of antiepileptic drugs (AEDs) is well documented. Therefore, polytherapy and the use of the smallest dose possible to control seizures during pregnancy is recommended (Constantino & Varner, 2004; Shehata & Okosun, 2004). Congenital anomalies that can occur with AEDs include cleft lip or palate, congenital heart disease, urogenital defects, and neural tube defects (Weiner & Buhimschi, 2004). AEDs prescribed in pregnancy should also be administered with folic acid. Daily folic acid supplementation is important because of the depletion that occurs when anticonvulsants are taken (Shehata & Okosun, 2004).

The risk of seizures during labor exists; approximately 1% to 2% of women have a tonic-clonic seizure, and another 1% to 2% have a seizure within 24 hours postpartum (Shehata & Okosun, 2004). If the woman cannot take oral AEDs, then phenytoin can be administered intravenously. Serum levels of AEDs should be monitored at 48 hours postpartum and at 1 to 2 weeks postpartum. During the neonatal period, infants can have a hemorrhagic disorder associated with AED-induced vitamin K deficiency. Prophylaxis consists of administering vitamin K during the last month of pregnancy and administering 1 mg intramuscularly to the newborn (Constantino & Varner, 2004).

Multiple Sclerosis

Multiple sclerosis (MS), a patchy demyelinization of the spinal cord and CNS, may be a viral disorder. Women are affected twice as often as men, with the most common onset occurring during the childbearing years between ages 20 to 40 (Shehata & Okosun, 2004). Remissions during pregnancy are common, particularly in the third trimester, and generally MS does not affect the course of the pregnancy (Aminoff, 2004; Shehata & Okosun, 2004). Treatment includes bedrest and steroids for acute exacerbations. Drugs commonly used for MS include beta-interferon and glatiramer acetate but are contraindicated in pregnancy (Shehata & Okosun, 2004). Nursing care of the pregnant women with MS is similar to the care of the normal pregnant women.

Bell's Palsy

The incidence of Bell's palsy (idiopathic facial paralysis) in pregnancy is approximately 57 per 100,000 per year. The incidence usually peaks during the third trimester and the puerperium (Shehata & Okosun, 2004).

The clinical manifestations include the sudden development of a unilateral facial weakness, with maximal weakness within 48 hours after onset (Ahmed, 2005; Cunningham et al., 2005), pain surrounding the ear, difficulty closing the eye on the affected side, and hyperacusis (abnormal acuteness of the sense of hearing) (Aminoff, 2004). In addition, taste on the anterior two thirds of the tongue may be lost, depending on the location of the lesion. There is no relationship between Bell's palsy and maternal and fetal outcomes. The exception is when there is complete nerve conduction block. Antiviral therapy and steroids may be prescribed, although controversy exists regarding whether they hasten recovery. Treatment includes prevention of injury to the exposed cornea, facial muscle massage, careful chewing and manual removal of food from inside the affected cheek, and reassurance that return of normal neurologic function is likely in 85% of affected women (Shehata & Okosun, 2004).

AUTOIMMUNE DISORDERS

Autoimmune disorders make up a large group of diseases that disrupt the function of the immune system of the body. In these types of disorders the body develops antibodies that attack its normally present antigens, causing tissue damage. Autoimmune disorders have a predilection for women in their reproductive years; therefore associations with pregnancy are not uncommon (Nader, 2004a). Pregnancy may affect the disease process. Some disorders adversely affect the course of pregnancy or are detrimental to the fetus. Autoimmune disorders of concern in pregnancy are systemic lupus erythematosus (SLE), myasthenia gravis, and rheumatoid arthritis.

Systemic Lupus Erythematosus

One of the most common serious disorders of childbearing age, systemic lupus erythematosus (SLE) is a chronic, multisystem inflammatory disease characterized by autoimmune antibody production that affects the skin, joints, kidneys, lungs, CNS, liver, and other body organs. The exact cause is unknown, but viral infection and hormonal and genetic factors may be related. SLE affects approximately 1 in 2000 to 3000 births (Hankins & Suarez, 2004). It is three times more common in African-American women.

Early symptoms, such as fatigue, weight loss, skin rashes, and arthralgias, may be overlooked. Anemia and leucopenia are common (Cunningham et al., 2005). Eventually all organs become involved. The condition is characterized by a series of exacerbations and remissions.

If the diagnosis has been established and the woman desires a child, she is advised to wait until she has been in remission for at least 6 months before attempting to get pregnant (Gilbert & Harmon, 2003). An exacerbation of SLE during pregnancy or postpartum occurs in approximately one third of women with SLE. Women are at increased risk for complications such as preeclampsia, renal disease, and preterm birth (Hankins & Suarez, 2004). Because signs and symptoms are similar, it can be difficult to distinguish between a SLE exacerbation and the onset of preeclampsia.

Medical therapy is kept to a minimum in women who are in remission or who have a mild form of SLE. Antiinflammatory drugs such as prednisone and aspirin may be used. It is recommended that aspirin not be used after 24 weeks of gestation, because of an increased risk of premature closure of the fetal ductus arteriosus (Cunningham et al., 2005). Immunosuppressive drugs are not recommended during pregnancy but may be used in some situations when there is greater risk in not treating SLE. Nursing care focuses on early recognition of signs of SLE exacerbation and pregnancy complications, education and support of the woman and her family, and assessment of fetal well-being.

Vaginal birth is preferred, but cesarean birth is common because of maternal and fetal complications. During the postpartum period, the mother should rest as much as possible to prevent an exacerbation of SLE. Adverse perinatal outcomes include preterm births, fetal growth restriction, stillbirth, and neonatal lupus (Cunningham et al., 2005). Breastfeeding is encouraged unless the mother is on immunosuppressive agents. Women with SLE should limit their number of pregnancies because of increased adverse perinatal outcomes, as well as the guarded maternal prognosis (Cunningham et al., 2005). Family planning is important. Oral contraceptives are used with caution secondary to the vascular disease accompanying SLE; however, progestin implants (when available) have been used with no observed negative effects (Cunningham et al., 2005; Hankins & Suarez, 2004).

GASTROINTESTINAL DISORDERS ■

Compromise of GI function during pregnancy is a concern. Obvious physiologic alterations, such as the greatly enlarged uterus, and less apparent changes, such as hormonal differences and hypochlorhydria (deficiency of hydrochloric acid in the stomach's gastric juice), require understanding for proper diagnosis and treatment. Gallbladder disease and inflammatory bowel disease are two GI disorders that may occur during pregnancy.

Cholelithiasis and Cholecystitis

Women are at increased risk to have cholelithiasis (presence of gallstones in the gallbladder), in pregnancy (Blackburn, 2003) with 1 in 1000 pregnant women developing cholecystitis (Cunningham et al., 2005) (Patient Instructions for Self-Care box). Decreased muscle tone allows gallbladder distention and thickening of the bile (biliary sludge) and prolongs emptying time. Increased progesterone levels result in a slight hypercholesterolemia.

Women with acute cholecystitis (inflammation of the gallbladder) usually have colicky abdominal pain in the right upper quadrant and nausea and vomiting, especially after eating a meal high in fat. Fever and an increased leukocyte count may also be present. Ultrasound is often used to detect the presence of stones or for dilation of the common bile duct (Samuels, 2002).

The woman with cholelithiasis or cholecystitis in the first trimester should be treated conservatively with IV fluids, bowel rest, nasogastric suctioning, diet and antibiotics. Meperidine or atropine alleviates ductal spasm and pain. In the past, gallbladder disease has been treated medically but more recently, as women have recurring symptoms cholecystectomies are being performed. Laparoscopic cholecystectomies are performed preferably in the first and second trimesters but if necessary in the third trimester with positive maternal and fetal outcomes (Cunningham et al., 2005;

PATIENT INSTRUCTIONS FOR SELF-CARE

Nutrition for the Pregnant Woman with Cholecystitis or Cholelithiasis

- Assess diet for foods that cause discomfort and flatulence and omit foods that trigger episodes.
- Reduce dietary fat intake
- Choose foods so that most of the calories come from carbohydrates.
- Prepare food without adding fats or oils as much as possible.
- Avoid fried foods.

Landon, 2004). If gallbladder disease is nonacute or nonrecurring then surgery is postponed until the puerperium.

Inflammatory Bowel Disease

The incidence of inflammatory bowel disease, particularly Crohn's disease and ulcerative colitis, is not increased in pregnancy (Cunningham et al., 2005). Active disease at conception may continue during pregnancy and worsen with an increased risk of poor maternal-fetal outcomes (Cunningham et al., Scott & Abu-Hamda, 2004). Treatment of inflammatory bowel disease is the same for the pregnant woman as it is for the nonpregnant woman. Medicines include prednisone and sulfasalazine. Fat soluble vitamin and folic acid supplementation is especially important because of problems with intestinal malabsorption. With complications, such as hemorrhage or if there is no response to medical therapy, surgery may be indicated (Cunningham et al., 2005). Effects of inflammatory bowel disease on pregnancy are usually minimal; however, if the woman is severely debilitated, preterm birth, low birth weight, or fetal death can occur (Scott & Abu-Hamda, 2004). A familial component for inflammatory bowel disease is under investigation but it is unclear whether it is the susceptiblity to the disease or the inflammatory disease itself which is inherited. Presently, with one parent with the disease there is approximately a 10% lifetime risk of developing inflammatory bowel disease with Jewish people disproportionately represented (Scott & Abu-Hamda, 2004).

HIV AND AIDS

Infection with HIV and the resultant acquired immunodeficiency syndrome (AIDS) are increasingly occurring in women. Women, particularly African-American and Hispanic are now the fastest growing population of persons with HIV and AIDS in the United States (CDC, 2001; Minkoff, 2004). Women of color are disproportionately affected; approximately 80% to 85% of HIV-infected women in the United States are African-American or Hispanic (CDC, 2001; Duff, 2002). This section addresses management of the pregnant woman who is HIV positive or has developed full-blown AIDS. See Chapter 5 for more information about the diagnosis and management of nonpregnant women with HIV and Chapter 27 for a discussion of HIV and AIDS in infants.

Preconception Counseling

Pregnancy is not encouraged in HIV-positive women. Preconception counseling is recommended because exposure to the virus has a significant impact on the pregnancy, neonatal feeding method, and neonatal health status. HIV-positive women should be counseled about use of highly active antiretroviral therapy (HAART), the risk of perinatal transmission, and possible obstetric complications. HIV-positive women should be encouraged to seek prenatal care immediately if they suspect pregnancy, to maximize chances for a positive outcome (CDC, 2001).

Pregnancy Risks
Perinatal transmission

Approximately 230 to 370 infants born with AIDS are a result of transmission of the virus from mother to child during the perinatal period (CDC, 2001). Exposure may occur to the fetus through the maternal circulation as early as the first trimester of pregnancy, to the infant during labor and birth by inoculation or ingestion of maternal blood and other infected fluids, or to the infant through breast milk (Lawrence & Lawrence, 2005; Riordan, 2005). Factors that increase the likelihood of perinatal viral transmission are listed in Box 22-2. Women who do not receive prenatal care or who choose not to have earlier HIV testing or are of unknown HIV status may be offered rapid (60-minute turnaround) HIV testing in labor (ACOG, 2004b; CDC, 2004). These women and their infants may receive short-term prophylactic antiretroviral therapy. If a positive HIV test result is confirmed with a second test, then the woman will be counseled regarding long-term care (CDC, 2004). The frequency of perinatal transmission has been reported to vary from a low of 5% to 10% to a high of 50% to 60%.

Treatment of HIV-infected women with the triple drug antiviral drug during pregnancy decreases the mother-to-child transmission to 2% (Stephenson, 2005). Key to preventing vertical transmission is antiretroviral therapy and cesearean birth (ACOG, 2000b; Cunningham et al., 2005). A major concern with monotherapy (predominantly zidovudine) is the development of resistance. Women should be given the option of having a scheduled cesarean birth at 38 weeks to decrease the risk of vertical transmission of HIV to the infant.

Obstetric complications

It is difficult to determine obstetric risk in persons with HIV infection because many confounding variables are often present. Many HIV-positive women also suffer from drug

---

BOX 22-2

Factors That Increase the Risk of Perinatal HIV Transmission

- Previous history of a child with HIV infection
- AIDS
- Preterm birth
- Decreased maternal CD_4 count
- Firstborn twin
- Chorioamnionitis
- Intrapartum blood exposure
- Failure to treat mother and fetus with HAART during the perinatal period
- Breastfeeding

From ACOG, 2004a; Perinatal HIV Guidelines Working Group. (2001). *Public Health Service Task Force recommendations: Use of antiretroviral drugs in pregnant HIV-1-infected women for maternal health and interventions to reduce perinatal HIV-1 transmission in the United States* [Online]. Internet document available at www.hivatis.org (Accessed July 24, 2005) & CDC, 2001.

and alcohol addiction, poor nutrition, limited access to prenatal care, or concurrent sexually transmitted infections (STIs). HIV-positive women are probably at risk for preterm labor and birth, PROM, IUGR, perinatal mortality, and postpartum endometritis (Duff, 2002).

Antepartum care

HIV counseling and testing should be offered to all women at their initial entry into prenatal care, thereby giving them the opportunity to "opt out" (CDC, 2004; Semprini & Fiore, 2004). Universal testing is recommended versus selective testing for maternal HIV, because it results in a greater number of women being screened and treated (CDC, 2004). Identification of HIV-positive pregnant women is especially important, because antepartum and intrapartum HIV antiviral drug therapy (HART) has been shown to improve obstetric outcomes and greatly decrease the risk of viral transmission to the fetus (Tuomala et al., 2005).

HIV-infected women should also be tested for other STIs, such as gonorrhea; syphilis; chlamydial infection; hepatitis B, C, and D; and herpes (CDC, 2002). Cytomegalovirus and toxoplasmosis antibody testing should be done because both infections can cause significant maternal and fetal complications and can be successfully treated with antimicrobial agents. Any history of vaccination and immune status should be documented, and chickenpox (varicella) and rubella titers should be determined. A tuberculin skin test should be performed; a positive test result necessitates the taking of a chest x-ray film to identify active pulmonary disease. A Papanicolaou (Pap) test should be done (Duff, 2002).

All HIV-infected women should be treated with zidovudine or other antiretroviral drug during pregnancy, regardless of their CD_4 counts (Perinatal HIV Guidelines Working Group, 2001). Zidovudine, administered orally, is usually started after the first trimester and continued throughout pregnancy. The major side effect of this drug is bone marrow suppression; periodic hematocrit, white blood cell count, and platelet count assessments should be performed (Duff, 2002). Women with CD_4 counts less than 200 cells/mm^3 should receive prophylactic treatment for *Pneumocystis carinii* pneumonia with daily trimethoprim-sulfamethoxazole (Duff, 2002). Any other opportunistic infections should be treated with medications specific for the infection; often dosages must be higher for women with HIV infection or AIDS.

Women who are HIV positive should also be vaccinated against hepatitis B, pneumococcal infection, *Haemophilus influenzae* type B, and viral influenza. To support any pregnant woman's immune system, appropriate counseling is provided about optimal nutrition, sleep, rest, exercise, and stress reduction. The HIV-infected woman needs nutritional support and counseling about diet choices, food preparation, and food handling. Weight gain or maintenance in pregnancy is a challenge with the HIV-infected patient. The infected patient is counseled regarding "safer sex" practices. Use of condoms is encouraged to minimize further exposure to HIV if her partner is the source. Orogenital sex is discouraged.

Intrapartum care

Several therapy regimens are available. IV zidovudine is administered to the HIV-positive woman during the intrapartum period. A loading dose is initiated on her admission in labor, followed by a continuous maintenance dose throughout labor. Every effort should be made during the birthing process to decrease the neonate's exposure to infected maternal blood and secretions. If feasible, the membranes should be left intact until the birth. Women who give birth within 4 hours following membrane rupture are at twice the risk of vertical transmission (CDC, 2001). The longer the period between the rupture of membranes and birth the greater the risk of maternal-neonatal HIV transmission (Minkoff, 2004) Women who give birth by cesarean with intact membranes and before labor decrease maternal-infant transmission by 50% (Semprini & Fiore, 2004). The best predictor of vertical transmission is maternal plasma viral load (Semprini & Fiore, 2004). Fetal scalp electrode and scalp pH sampling should be avoided, because these procedures may result in inoculation of the virus into the fetus. Likewise, the use of forceps or vacuum extractor should be avoided when possible.

Postpartum and newborn care

Immediately after birth, infants should be wiped free of all body fluids and then bathed as soon as they are in stable condition. All staff members working with the mother or infant must adhere strictly to infection control techniques and observe Standard Precautions for blood and body fluids.

Women who have HIV but who are without symptoms may have an unremarkable postpartum course. Immunosuppressed women with symptoms may be at increased risk for postpartum UTIs, vaginitis, postpartum endometritis, and poor wound healing. Women who are HIV positive but who were not on antiretroviral drugs before pregnancy should be tested in the postpartum period to determine whether therapy that was initiated in pregnancy should be continued (Perinatal HIV Guidelines Working Group, 2001).

After the initial bath, the newborn can be with the mother after birth, but breastfeeding is discouraged because of HIV vertical transmission in breast milk. In planning for discharge, comprehensive care and support services will need to be arranged. After discharge, the woman and her infant are referred to physicians who are experienced in the treatment of AIDS and associated conditions for intensive monitoring and follow-up (Perinatal HIV Guidelines Working Group, 2001).

SUBSTANCE ABUSE

The term *substance abuse* refers to the continued use of substances despite related problems in physical, social, or interpersonal areas (American Psychiatric Association, 2000).

Recurrent abuse results in failure to fulfill major role obligations, and there may be substance-related legal problems and ethical issues (ACOG, 2004a). Any use of alcohol or illicit drugs during pregnancy is considered abuse (American Psychiatric Association, 2000). Chapter 4 discusses the commonly abused illicit and prescription drugs, and Chapter 27 discusses neonatal effects of maternal substance abuse. This discussion focuses on care of the pregnant woman who is a substance abuser. Prevalence rates for substance use during pregnancy range from 0.4% to 27% (Rayburn & Bogenschutz, 2004). Marijuana and cocaine are the illegal drugs most commonly used by pregnant women (Rayburn & Bogenschutz, 2004).

The damaging effects of alcohol and illicit drugs on pregnant women and their unborn babies are well documented (Ludlow, Evans & Hulse, 2004). Alcohol and other drugs easily pass from a mother to her baby through the placenta. Smoking during pregnancy has serious health risks, including bleeding complications, miscarriage, stillbirth, prematurity, low birth weight, and sudden infant death syndrome (Andres, 2004; Savitz, Dole, Terry, Zhou, & Thorp, 2001). Congenital abnormalities have occurred in infants of mothers who have taken drugs. The safest pregnancy is one in which the woman is drug and alcohol free. For pregnant women addicted to heroin, methadone maintenance at the lowest effective dose demonstrates a threefold decrease in drug use (Rayburn & Bogenschutz, 2004).

Pregnant women who abuse substances commonly have little understanding of the ways in which these substances affect them, their pregnancies, and their babies. Often, pregnant mothers who use psychoactive substances receive negative feedback from society, as well as from health care providers, who may not only condemn them for endangering the life of the fetus, but may even withhold support as a result. Stigma, shame, and guilt lead to a high denial of drug problems, alcohol use, or tobacco use both by the woman herself and by family members and friends who conceal the abuse from outsiders to protect the abuser (Windsor, 2003). Traditionally, substance abuse treatment programs have not addressed issues that affect pregnant women, such as concurrent need for obstetric care and child care for other children. Long waiting lists and lack of health insurance present further barriers to treatment.

CARE MANAGEMENT

The care of the substance-dependent pregnant woman is based on historical data, symptoms, physical findings, and laboratory results. Screening questions for alcohol and drug abuse should be included in the overall assessment of the first prenatal visit of all women. Women who are heavily involved in substance abuse often receive no prenatal care or make only a limited number of visits beginning late in pregnancy.

Because women frequently deny or greatly underreport usage when asked directly about drug or alcohol consumption, it is crucial that the nurse display a nonjudgmental and matter-of-fact attitude while taking the history in order to gain the woman's trust and elicit a reasonably accurate estimate. Information about drug use should be obtained by asking first about the woman's intake of OTC and prescribed medications. Next, her usage of "legal" drugs, such as caffeine, nicotine, and alcohol, should be ascertained. Finally, the woman should be questioned about her use of illicit drugs, such as cocaine, heroin, and marijuana.

Screening for alcohol use is commonly done through the use of self-reporting questionnaires. Urine screening is unreliable because alcohol is undetectable within a few hours after ingestion (Russell et al., 1996). Screening questionnaires generally ask about consequences of heavy drinking, alcohol intake, or both. The Michigan Alcoholism Screening Test (MAST) and the CAGE test are two well-known screens that are often used. Two screening tests, the T-ACE (Box 22-3) and the TWEAK, have been developed to screen specifically for alcohol use during pregnancy (Russell et al., 1996).

Urine toxicology testing is often performed to screen for illicit drug use. Drugs may be found in urine, days to weeks after ingestion, depending on how quickly they are metabolized and excreted from the body. Meconium (from the neonate) and hair can also be analyzed to determine past drug use over a longer period of time (Gilbert & Harmon, 2003). In addition to screening for alcohol and drug abuse, the nurse should also screen for physical and sexual abuse and history of psychiatric illness, factors frequently accompanying substance use (Beck et al., 2003).

Because of the risks to the unborn children, pregnant women who abuse substances may face criminal charges under expanded interpretations of child abuse and drug-trafficking statutes. Some states prosecute pregnant women on charges of child abuse because they became pregnant while addicted to drugs. Some policy makers have proposed that pregnant women who abuse substances should be jailed, placed under house arrest, or committed to psychiatric hospitals for the remainder of their pregnancies. Women's health nurses can play a positive role by advocating primary prevention programs for women and counseling and treatment programs for those women already addicted.

LEGAL TIP   Drug Testing during Pregnancy

There is no requirement in the United States for a health care provider to test either the pregnant woman or the newborn for the presence of drugs. However, nurses need to know the practices of the states in which they are working. In some states a woman whose urine drug screen test is positive at the time of labor and birth must be referred to child protective services. If the mother is not in a drug treatment program or is judged unable to provide care, the infant may be placed in foster care. In all states, the U.S. Supreme Court has ruled that it is unlawful to test for drug use without the pregnant woman's permission (Gottlieb, 2001).

Although the ideal long-term outcome is total abstinence, it is not likely that the woman will either desire or be able

BOX 22-3

T-ACE Test

- How many drinks can you hold before getting sleepy or passing out? (TOLERANCE)
- Have people ANNOYED you by criticizing your drinking?
- Have you ever felt you ought to CUT DOWN on your drinking?
- Have you ever had a drink first thing in the morning to steady your nerves or get rid of a hangover? (EYE-OPENER)

Scoring: Two points are given for the TOLERANCE question for the ability to hold at least a six-pack of beer or a bottle of wine. A "yes" answer to any of the other questions receives one point. An overall score of two indicates a high probability that the woman is a risk drinker.

Source: Hankin, J., & Sokol, R. (1995). Identification and care of problems associated with alcohol ingestion in pregnancy. *Seminars in Perinatology*, 19(4), 286-292.

to stop alcohol and drug use suddenly. Indeed, it may be harmful to the fetus for her to do so. A realistic goal may be to decrease substance use, and short-term outcomes will be necessary.

Intervention with the pregnant substance abuser begins with education about specific effects on pregnancy, the fetus, and the newborn for each drug used. Consequences of perinatal drug use should be clearly communicated, and abstinence recommended as the safest course of action. Women are frequently more receptive to making lifestyle changes during pregnancy than at any other time in their lives. The casual, experimental, or recreational drug user is frequently able to achieve and maintain sobriety when she receives education, support, and continued monitoring throughout the remainder of the pregnancy. Periodic screening throughout pregnancy of women who have admitted to drug use may help them to continue abstinence.

Treatment for the substance abuse will be individualized for each woman depending on the type of drug used and the frequency and amount of use. As fetal nicotine levels are greater than maternal serum levels, tobacco use in pregnancy is strongly discouraged (Rayburn & Bogenschutz, 2004). Smoking cessation programs (see Chapter 9) can be successful in decreasing low birth weight, and quitting even in the second and third trimesters can be beneficial to the fetus (Lumley, Oliver, & Waters, 2000; Maloni, 2001). Detoxification, short-term inpatient or outpatient treatment, long-term residential treatment, aftercare services, and self-help support groups are all possible options for alcohol and drug abuse. Women for Sobriety may be a more helpful organization for women than Alcoholics Anonymous or Narcotics Anonymous, which were developed for men who abuse substances. In general, long-term treatment of any sort is becoming increasingly more difficult to obtain, particularly for women who lack insurance coverage. Although some programs allow a woman to keep her children with her at the

treatment facility, far too few of them are available to meet the demand.

Alcohol withdrawal treatment consists of the administration of benzodiazepines, an improvement in the woman's nutritional intake (folic acid and other vitamins), and psychotherapy (Rayburn & Bogenschutz, 2004). The safety of disulfiram (Antabuse) during pregnancy has not been established, so it has limited use for detoxification for pregnant women (Weiner & Buhimschi, 2004).

Methadone treatment for pregnant women dependent on heroin or other narcotics is controversial. If women withdraw from heroin during pregnancy, blood flow to the placenta is impaired. The substitution of methadone for the heroin not only promotes withdrawal from heroin but also does not cause impaired blood flow to the placenta. However, methadone can cause detrimental fetal effects, and withdrawal from it after birth can be worse for the newborn than heroin withdrawal (Weiner & Buhimschi, 2004).

Cocaine use during pregnancy has increased dramatically. Maternal and fetal complications accompany cocaine use, including placental abruption, stillbirth, prematurity, and SGA infants. Pregnant women who use cocaine should be advised to stop using immediately. Such women will need a great deal of assistance, such as an alcohol and drug treatment program, individual or group counseling, and participation in self-help support groups, to successfully accomplish this major lifestyle change.

The increased use of methamphetamine, also known as crystal, meth or its variant, ecstasy, during preganancy is a growing health care concern. Methamphetamine may be snorted, smoked or ingested and is associated with drug dependence. Pregnancy outcomes reported have included maternal mortality, IUGR, and preterm birth (Weiner & Buhimschi, 2004).

Because of the lifestyle often associated with drug use, substance-abusing women are at risk for STIs, including HIV (CDC, 2002). Laboratory assessments will likely include screening for STIs such as gonorrhea and chlamydial infection and antibody determinations for hepatitis B and HIV. A chest x-ray film may be taken to assess for pulmonary problems such as hilar lymphadenopathy, pulmonary edema, bacterial pneumonia, and foreign-body emboli. A skin test to screen for tuberculosis may also be ordered.

Initial and serial ultrasound studies are usually performed to determine gestational age, because the woman may have had amenorrhea as a result of her drug use or may not know when her last menstrual period occurred. Because of concerns about stillbirth, an increased frequency of the birth of infants who are small for gestational age, and the potential for hypoxia, nonstress testing may be done in women who are known substance abusers.

Although substance abusers may be difficult to care for at any time, they are often particularly challenging during the intrapartum and postpartum periods because of manipulative and demanding behavior. Typically, these women display poor control over their behavior and a low

EVIDENCE-BASED PRACTICE
Social Support for Prevention of Low-Birth-Weight Babies

BACKGROUND

- Low-birth-weight (LBW) babies include small-for-gestational-age (SGA) babies, who have not grown adequately during gestation, and preterm babies, who are normal size for gestation but are born too soon (earlier than 37 weeks). These two conditions have different prognoses and treatments. The SGA baby may be at a greater long-term deficit, particularly if brain growth has been compromised. Prematurity is a more acute problem of survival until the lungs mature. One of the major risk factors for LBW babies (less than 2500 g) is chronic poverty, which can lead to malnutrition, unhealthy living conditions, infections, and increased stress. Psychologic stress increases the likelihood of pregnancy and labor complications, fetal growth restriction, preterm birth, and poor health in mother and child. Social support may mitigate this stress somewhat. Accordingly, many countries have attempted to decrease their LBW rates by offering social support programs to women in distress. The programs usually include advice and counseling, tangible assistance, and emotional support. Support is offered by multidisciplinary teams, which may include lay peer counselors. Health care workers have the knowledge and training but may not have experienced social disadvantage, as the lay peer counselor would.

OBJECTIVES

- Reviewers sought to determine the effects of social support for women at high risk for LBW babies, compared with routine care. The authors also planned to compare the effectiveness of health care workers with that of peer counselors. Interventions included some form of emotional support, such as counseling, reassurance, and sympathetic listening, with or without advice about nutrition, rest, stress management, and substance abuse. Tangible assistance included transportation to clinic appointments and household help. Support could start during the first or second trimester and continue at least until birth. Settings could be clinics or home visits, with telephone follow-up. Outcome could include preterm birth, LBW, miscarriage, pregnancy termination, complications of pregnancy or labor, hospitalization, distress, operative birth, perinatal death, length of stay, and postnatal physical or mental health.

METHODS
Search Strategy

- The reviewers searched Cochrane, MEDLINE, 30 journals and conference proceedings, and a current awareness service of 37 journals. Search keywords were not noted.
- Sixteen randomized, controlled trials were selected, representing 13,651 women from Australia, the United Kingdom, France, Latin America, the Netherlands, South Africa, and the United States. The trials were dated 1986 to 2001.

Statistical analyses

- Similar data were pooled. Categoric data were reported by effect size. Continuous data were assigned a weighted mean difference (between intervention and control group).

FINDINGS

- Additional social support did not significantly lower the rate of LBW or preterm births. It did significantly decrease the cesarean birthrate. Women who received additional support were three times more likely to terminate their pregnancy than controls. There was equivocal evidence that the support group required less analgesia than controls. Supported women had improved psychosocial outcomes of significantly less worry and increased satisfaction. No comparison was possible of lay versus professional support.

LIMITATIONS

- The definitions of "high risk for low birth weight" and "social disadvantage" were murky. There was no way to blind the subjects or evaluators to the presence or absence of additional support. Some subjects were lost to follow-up, so long-term data were not available. Various support teams included nurses, doctors, midwives, social workers, psychologists, and trained lay women. Randomization was not consistent.

CONCLUSIONS

- Social support was not able to mitigate the effects on birth weight or prematurity of chronic poverty and the stresses caused by that poverty, or psychologic stress. However, other positive outcomes were seen: a reduction in cesarean birthrate, less worry, and increased satisfaction.

IMPLICATIONS FOR PRACTICE

- The decrease in cesarean birthrate and the improved psychosocial outcomes are reasons to offer support to high risk pregnant women. The additional support may not be powerful enough to overcome the social disadvantage associated with low birth weight and preterm birth. The marked increase in number of pregnancy terminations in the supported group may have been a result of the women's increased awareness of their fragile situations, and feelings of empowerment to change it.

IMPLICATIONS FOR FURTHER RESEARCH

- Researchers have not identified how social disadvantage causes preterm birth and low birth weight. Clear definitions of high risk women may better show any benefits of additional support. The value of lay peer counselors is yet undecided. Lay peer counselors have insight into the lives of the women that professionals may lack, and may offer a cost-effective support system that benefits the community.

Reference: Hodnett, E., & Fredericks, S. (2003). Support during pregnancy for women at increased risk of low birthweight babies (Cochrane Review). In *The Cochrane Library,* Issue 2, 2004. Chichester, UK: John Wiley & Sons.

threshold for pain. Increased dependency needs and poor parenting skills may also be apparent.

Nurses must understand that substance abuse is an illness and that these women deserve to be treated with patience, kindness, consistency, and firmness when necessary. Even women who are actively abusing drugs will experience pain during labor and after giving birth and may need pain medication, as well as nonpharmacologic interventions. It is helpful to develop a standardized plan of care so that patients have limited opportunities to play staff members against one another. Mother-infant attachment should be promoted by identifying the woman's strengths and reinforcing positive maternal feelings and behaviors. Staffing should be sufficient to ensure strict surveillance of visitors and prevent unsupervised drug use.

Advice regarding breastfeeding must be individualized. Although all abused substances appear in breast milk, some in greater amounts than others (Lawrence & Lawrence, 2005), breastfeeding is definitely contraindicated in women who use amphetamines, alcohol, cocaine, heroin, or marijuana. The baby's nutrition and safety needs are of primary importance in this consideration. For some women, a desire to breastfeed may provide strong motivation to achieve and maintain sobriety.

Smoking can interfere with the let-down reflex. Women who smoke in the postpartum period and breastfeed should avoid smoking for 2 hours before a feeding to minimize the nicotine in the milk and improve the let-down reflex. Mothers should also be discouraged from smoking in the same room with the infant because exposure to secondhand smoke can increase the likelihood that the infant will experience behavioral and respiratory health problems (Lawrence & Lawrence, 2005).

Before a known substance abuser is discharged with her baby, the home situation is assessed to determine that the environment is safe and that someone will be available to meet the infant's needs if the mother proves unable to do so. Usually, the hospital's social services department will be involved in interviewing the mother before discharge to ensure that the infant's needs will be met. Sometimes family members or friends will be asked to become actively involved with the mother and infant after discharge. A home care or public health nurse may be asked to make home visits to assess the mother's ability to care for the baby and provide guidance and support. If serious questions about the infant's well-being exist, the case will probably be referred to the state's child protective services agency for further action.

COMMUNITY ACTIVITY

Contact your local health department to assess the resources available for pregnant women who have a substance abuse problem. Assess specific resources for women who report alcohol, tobacco and drug/polydrug use. Ascertain the numbers of women who abuse drugs and alcohol locally and compare with national statistics. Determine the availability of inpatient and outpatient treatment programs for substance abusing women, specifically as covered by private and public monies.

Key Points

- Lack of maternal glycemic control before conception and in the first trimester of pregnancy may be responsible for fetal congenital malformations.

- Maternal insulin requirements increase as the pregnancy progresses and may quadruple by term as a result of insulin resistance created by placental hormones, insulinase, and cortisol.

- Poor glycemic control before and during pregnancy can lead to maternal complications such as miscarriage, infection, and dystocia (difficult labor) caused by fetal macrosomia.

- Careful glucose monitoring, insulin administration when necessary, and dietary counseling are used to create a normal intrauterine environment for fetal growth and development in the pregnancy complicated by diabetes mellitus.

- Because gestational diabetes mellitus (GDM) is asymptomatic in most cases, most women undergo routine screening during pregnancy.

- Thyroid dysfunction during pregnancy requires close monitoring of thyroid hormone levels to regulate therapy and prevent fetal insult.

- The stress of the normal maternal adaptations to pregnancy on a heart whose function is already taxed may cause cardiac decompensation.

- In the case of cardiac arrest in a pregnant woman, the standard resuscitation guidelines should be implemented with the modification of positioning the woman so that the uterus is displaced laterally.

- Maternal morbidity or mortality is a significant risk in a pregnancy complicated by mitral stenosis.

- Anemia, the most common medical disorder of pregnancy, affects at least 20% of pregnant women.

- Autoimmune disorders (e.g., SLE) show a predilection for women in their reproductive years; therefore associations with pregnancy are not uncommon.

- HIV may be transmitted through blood, semen, and perinatal events.

- Perinatal administration of AZT and planned cesarean birth are recommended to decrease transmission of HIV from mother to fetus.

- Because medical history and examination cannot reliably identify all persons with HIV or other blood-borne pathogens, blood and body fluid precautions should be consistently used for everyone.
- Much support from a variety of sources, including family and friends, health care providers, and the recovery community, is needed to help perinatal substance abusers achieve and maintain sobriety.
- It is crucial that health care providers provide compassionate, nonjudgmental care to substance abusers.

Answer Guidelines to Critical Thinking Exercise

Diabetes Mellitus

1 Women who are obese are at greater risk for diabetes mellitus, type 2. Maria's laboratory data, FBS, and HgbA$_{1c}$ are elevated and indicate uncontrolled hyperglycemia. Further assessments are necessary to determine fetal development, such as ultrasound.

2 a. Possible diagnoses for Maria include type 2 diabetes. Less likely diagnoses are type 1 diabetes mellitus and gestational diabetes as determined by her reported use of glucophage.

   b. Physical assessment to include specifically: opthamalogic examination, renal function and cardiovascular status, weekly fasting blood sugars and 2 hour postprandial blood sugars, HgbA$_{1c}$, level 2 ultrasound, fetal heart rate, daily kick counts, and biophysical profile would further ascertain her maternal-fetal status.

   c. Factors contributing to Maria's elevated blood sugar may include excess or wrong kinds of food, insufficient exercise, and obesity. In addition, insulin needs increase during the second and third trimesters.

   d. While oral hypoglycemics are not commonly ordered for pregnant diabetics, they may be the treatment of choice for pregnant diabetics with uncontrolled diabetes who are cognitively impaired or refuse to take insulin.

3 Priorities for nursing care at this time include controlling Maria's blood sugar and monitoring her fetal status. In addition, it is important to answer her questions regarding the safety of the use of oral hypoglycemics during pregnancy. She needs written and verbal information at her level of understanding.

4 Yes, there is initial clinical evidence to support the use of oral hypoglycemics in pregnant diabetics. Adverse maternal and fetal outcomes have not been reported with its use.

5 Some providers may continue to prescribe insulin for pregnant diabetics even when they refuse to comply. This may necessitate teaching family members, or friends how to give insulin injections or having a home health nurse visit to provide injections.

Resources

AIDS Network Hotline
800-342-2437 (AIDS)

AIDS resource list
www.hivnet.org/aidsres.html

American Diabetes Association (ADA)
Diabetes Information Service Center
1660 Duke St.
Alexandria, VA 22314
800-342-2383
www.diabetes.org

American Heart Association
Women's heart information: 1-888-MYHEART (1-888-694-3278)
800-242-8721
www.americanheart.org

Asthma and Allergy Foundation of America
www.aafa.org

Cardiopulmonary resuscitation information
www.cpr-ecc.org

CDC Perinatal HIV Prevention Web Site
http://www.cdc.gov/hiv/projects/perintal/

CDC Rapid Testing Web Site
http://www.cdc.gov/hiv/rapid_testing/

Center for Sickle Cell Disease
2121 Georgia Ave., NW
Washington, DC 20059
202-636-7930

COPE (Coping with the Overall Pregnancy/Parenting Experience)
37 Clarendon St.
Boston, MA 02116
617-357-5588

March of Dimes Birth Defects Foundation
1275 Mamaroneck Ave.
White Plains, NY 10605
914-428-7100
888-663-4637
www.modimes.org

National AIDS Information Clearinghouse
P.O. Box 6003
Rockville, MD 20849-6003
800-458-5231 (English and Spanish)

National Association for Sickle Cell Disease
3345 Wilshire Blvd., Suite 1106
Los Angeles, CA 90010-1880
213-736-5455
800-421-8453

National Bed Rest Support Group
Sidelines
P.O. Box 1808
Laguna Beach, CA 92652
714-497-2265
www.sidelines.org

National Clearinghouse for Alcohol and Drug Abuse Information
P.O. Box 426
Dept DQ
Kensington, MD 20795
800-729-6686
www.health.org

National Multiple Sclerosis Society
733 Third Ave.
New York, NY 10017
800-344-4867
www.nmss.org

National Phenylketonuria Foundation
6301 Tejas Dr.
Pasadena, TX 77503
713-487-4802

National Women's Health Resource Center
120 Albany St., Suite 820
New Brunswick, NJ 08901
877-986-9472
www.healthywomen.org

Pregnancy and Infant Loss
1421 East Wayzata Blvd., Suite 40
Wayzata, MN 55391
614-473-9372

Women for Sobriety, Inc.
POB 618
Quakertown, PA 18951-0618
215-536-8026
215-538-9026 (fax)
www.womenforsobriety.org

References

Ahmed, A. (2005). When is facial paralysis Bell palsy? Current diagnosis and treatment. *Cleveland Clinic Journal of Medicine, 72*(5), 398-405.

American College of Obstetricians and Gynecologists (ACOG). (2004a). *At risk drinking – illicit drug use: Ethical issues in obstetric practice. ACOG committee opinion no. 294.* Washington, DC: ACOG.

American College of Obstetricians and Gynecologists (ACOG). (2000a). *Fetal macrosomia. ACOG practice bulletin no. 22.* Washington, DC: ACOG.

American College of Obstetricians and Gynecologists (ACOG). (2001). *Gestational diabetes. ACOG practice bulletin no. 30.* Washington, DC: ACOG.

American College of Obstetricians and Gynecologists (ACOG). (2004b). *Prenatal and Perinatal human immunodeficiency virus testing; Expanded recommendations. ACOG committee opinion no. 304.* Washington, DC: ACOG.

American College of Obstetricians and Gynecologists (ACOG). (2000b). *Scheduled cesarean delivery and prevention of vertical transmission of HIV infection. ACOG committee opinion no. 234.* Washington, DC: ACOG.

American Diabetes Association (ADA). (2003). Preconception care of women with diabetes. *Diabetes Care, 26*(Suppl 1), S91-S93.

American Diabetes Association (ADA). (2004a). Diagnosis and classification of diabetes mellitus. *Diabetes Care, 27*(Suppl 5-10), 1-19.

American Diabetes Association (ADA). (2004b). Gestational diabetes mellitus. *Diabetes Care, 27*(Suppl 1), S88-S90.

American Diabetes Association (ADA). (2004c). Inpatient diabetes control: Rationale. *Diabetes Care, 27*(8), 2074-2080.

American Diabetes Association (ADA). (1995). *Medical management of pregnancy complicated by diabetes* (2nd ed.). Alexandria, VA: ADA.

American Diabetes Association (ADA). (2004d). Nutrition principles and recommendations in diabetes. *Diabetes Care, 27*(Suppl 1), S36-S46.

American Heart Association Science Advisory. (2000). Assessment of functional capacity in clinical and research applications. *Circulation, 102*(13), 1591-1597.

American Heart Association (AHA). (2001). *Fundamentals of BLS for healthcare providers.* Dallas: American Heart Association.

American Psychiatric Association. (2000). *Diagnostic and statistical manual of mental disorders (DSM-IV-TR)* (4th ed., text revision). Washington, DC: American Psychiatric Association Press.

Aminoff, M. (2004). Neurologic disorders. In R. Creasy, R. Resnik, & J. Iams (Eds.), *Maternal-fetal medicine: Principles and practice* (5th ed.). Philadelphia: Saunders.

Anderson, J., Waller, D., Canfield, M., Shaw G., Watkins, M., & Werler, M. (2005). Maternal obesity, gestational diabetes, and central nervous system birth defects. *Epidemiology, 16*(1), 87-92.

Andres, R. (2004). Effects of therapeutic, diagnositic, and environmental agents and exposure to social and illicit drugs. In R. Creasy, R. Resnik, & J. Iams (Eds.), *Maternal-fetal medicine: Principles and practice* (5th ed.). Philadelphia: Saunders.

Aventis Pharmaceuticals. (2004). *Lantus prescribing information.* Kansas City, MO: Aventis Pharmaceuticals.

Balsells, M., Corcoy, R., Adelantado, J., Garcia-Patterson, A., Altirriba, O., & de Leiva, A. (2000). Gestational diabetes mellitus: Metabolic control during labour. *Diabetes, Nutrition & Metabolism, 13*(5), 257-262.

Barth, W., & Stewart, T. (2004). Cardiac disease. In G. Dildy, M. Belfort, G. Saade, J. Phelan, G. Hankins, & S. Clark (Eds.). *Critical care obstetrics* (4th ed.). Malden, Massachusetts: Blackwell Science.

Beck, L., Johnson, C., Morrow, B., Lipscomb, L., Gaffield, M., Colley Gilbert, B., Rogers, M., & Whitehead, N. (2003). *PRAMS 1999 Surveillance Report.* Atlanta, GA: Division of Reproductive Health, National Center for Chronic Disease Prevention and Health Promotion, Centers for Disease Control and Prevention.

Becton Dickinson & Co. (1997). *Controlling low blood sugar reactions.* Franklin Lakes, NJ: Becton Dickinson & Co.

Bernasko, J. (2004). Contemporary management of type 1 diabetes mellitus in pregnancy. *Obstetrical and Gynecological Survey, 59*(8), 628-636.

Blackburn, S. (2003). *Maternal, fetal, and neonatal physiology: A clinical perspective* (2nd ed.). St. Louis: Saunders.

Blanchard, D., & Shabetai, R. (2004). Cardiac diseases. In R. Creasy, R. Resnik, & J. Iams (Eds.), *Maternal-fetal medicine: Principles and practice* (5th ed.). Philadelphia: Saunders.

Brown, A., Fernhoff, P., Waisbren, S., Frazier, D., Singh, R., Rohr, F., Morris, J., Kenneson, A., MacDonald, P., Gwinn, M., Honein, M., & Rasmussen, S. (2002). Barriers to successful dietary control among pregnant women with phenylketonuria. *Genetics in Medicine, 4*(2) 84-89.

Burton, J., & Reyes, M. (2001). Breathe in, breathe out. Controlling asthma during pregnancy. *AWHONN Lifelines, 5*(1), 24-30.

Centers for Disease Control and Prevention (CDC). (2002). Sexually transmitted diseases treatment guidelines. *Morbidity and Mortality Weekly Report, 51*(RR-6), 1-115.

Centers for Disease Control and Prevention (CDC). (2004). Rapid HIV-1 antibody testing during Labor and delivery for women of unknown HIV status: A practical guide and model protocol. Internet document available at http//www.cdc.gov/hiv/rapid_testing/ Accessed 11/7/05.

Centers for Disease Control and Prevention (CDC). (2001). Revised recommendations for HIV screening of pregnant women: Perinatal counseling and guidelines consultation. *Morbidity and Mortality Weekly Report, 50*(RR19), 59-86.

Chan, P. & Johnson, S. (2006). *Gynecology and obstetrics: Current clinical strategies.* Laguna Hills, CA: CCS Publishing.

Cianni, G., Volpe, L., Lencioni, C., Chatzianagnostou, K. Cuccuru, J., Ghio, A., Benzi, L., & Prato, S. (2005). Use of insulin glargine during the first weeks of pregnancy in five type 1 diabetic women. *Diabetes Care, 28*(4), 982-983.

Constantino, T., & Varner, M. (2004). Seizures and status epilepticus. In G. Dildy, M. Belfort, G. Saade, J. Phelan, G. Hankins & S. Clark (Eds.), *Critical care obstetrics* (4th ed.). Malden, MA: Blackwell Science.

Cunningham, F., Leveno, K., Bloom, S., Hauth, J., Gilstrap, L., & Wenstrom, K. (Eds.). (2005). *Williams obstetrics* (22nd ed.). New York: McGraw-Hill.

DiPiro, J., Talbert, R., Yee, G., Matzke, G., Wells, B., & Posey, L. (2005). *Pharmacotherapy: A pathophysiologic approach* (6th ed.). New York: McGraw-Hill.

Duff, P. (2002). Maternal and perinatal infection. In S. Gabbe, J. Niebyl, & J. Simpson (Eds.), *Obstetrics: Normal and problem pregnancies* (4th ed.). New York: Churchill Livingstone.

Easterling, T., & Otto, C. (2002). Heart disease. In S. Gabbe, J. Niebyl, & J. Simpson (Eds.), *Obstetrics: Normal and problem pregnancies* (4th ed.). New York: Churchill Livingstone.

Expert Committee on the Diagnosis and Classification of Diabetes Mellitus. (2003). Follow-up report on the diagnosis of diabetes mellitus. *Diabetes Care, 26*(11), 3160-3167.

Foley, M. (2004). Cardiac disease. In G. Dildy, M. Belfort, G. Saade, J. Phelan, G. Hankins, & S. Clark (Eds.). *Critical care obstetrics* (4th ed.). Malden, MA: Blackwell Science.

Gei, A., & Hankins, G. (2001). Cardiac disease and pregnancy. *Obstetric and Gynecology Clinics of North America, 28*(3), 465-512.

Gilbert, E., & Harmon, J. (2003). *Manual of high risk pregnancy & delivery* (3rd ed.). St. Louis: Mosby.

Gottlieb, S. (2001). Pregnant women cannot be tested for drugs without consent. *Br Med J, 322*(7289), 753.

Gluck, J., & Gluck, P. (2005). Asthma controller therapy during pregnancy. *American Journal of Obstetrics and Gynecology, 192*(2), 369-380.

Hankin, J., & Sokol, R. (1995). Identification and care of problems associated with alcohol ingestion in pregnancy. *Seminars in Perinatology, 19*(4), 286-292.

Hankins, G.& Suarez, V. (2004). Rheumatologic and connective tissue disorders. In R. Creasy, R. Resnik, & J. Iams (Eds.). *Maternal-fetal medicine: Principles and practice* (5th ed.). Philadelphia: Saunders.

Hodnett, E., & Fredericks, S. (2003). Support during pregnancy for women at increased risk of low birthweight babies (Cochrane Review). In *The Cochrane Library,* Issue 2, 2004. Chichester, UK: John Wiley & Sons.

Hueppchen, N., & Satin, A. (2004). Cardiopulmonary resuscitation. In G. Dildy, M. Belfort, G. Saade, J. Phelan, G. Hankins, & S. Clark (Eds.), *Critical care obstetrics* (4th ed.). Malden, MA: Blackwell Science.

Iams, J., & Creasy, R. (2004). Preterm labor and delivery. In R. Creasy, R. Resnik, & J. Iams (Eds.). *Maternal-fetal medicine: Principles and practice* (5th ed.). Philadelphia: Saunders.

Inzucchi, S., & Burrow, G. (1999). Endocrine disorders in pregnancy. In E. Reece & J. Hobbins (Eds.), *Medicine of the fetus and mother* (2nd ed.). Philadelphia: Lippincott-Raven.

Institute of Medicine (IOM). (1990). *Nutrition during pregnancy, weight gain and nutrient supplements. Report of the subcommittee on nutritional status and weight gain during pregnancy.* Washington, DC: National Academy Press.

Kilpatrick, S., & Laros, R. (2004). Maternal hematologic disorders. In R. Creasy, R. Resnik, & J. Iams. (Eds.), *Maternal-fetal medicine: Principles and practice* (5th ed.). Philadelphia: Saunders.

Kwon, H. Belanger, K., & Bracken, M. (2004). Effect of pregnancy and stage of pregnancy on asthma severity: A systematic review. *American Journal of Obstetrics and Gynecology, 190*(5), 1201-1210.

Landon, M. (2004). Diseases of the liver, biliary system, and pancreas. In R. Creasy, R. Resnik, & J. Iams (Eds.), *Maternal-fetal medicine: Principles and practice* (5th ed.). Philadelphia: Saunders.

Landon, M., Catalano, P., & Gabbe, S. (2002). Diabetes mellitus. In S. Gabbe, J. Niebyl, & J. Simpson (Eds.), *Obstetrics: Normal and problem pregnancies* (4th ed.). New York: Churchill Livingstone.

Lawrence, R., & Lawrence, R. (2005). *Breastfeeding: A guide for the medical profession* (6th ed.). St. Louis: Mosby.

Ludlow, J., Evans, S., & Hulse, G. (2004). Obstetric and perinatal outcomes in pregnancies associated with illicit substance abuse. *Australian and New Zealand Journal of Obstetrics and Gynaecology 44*(4), 302-306.

Lumley, J., Oliver, S., Chamberlain, C., & Oakley, L. (2004). Interventions for promoting smoking cessation during pregnancy (Cochrane Review). In *The Cochrane Library,* Issue 4, 2005. Chichester, UK: John Wiley & Sons.

Maloni, J. (2001). Preventing low birth weight: How smoking cessation counseling can help. *AWHONN Lifelines, 5*(1), 32-35.

Mestman, J. (2002). Endocrine diseases in pregnancy. In S. Gabbe, J. Niebyl, & J. Simpson (Eds.), *Obstetrics: Normal and problem pregnancies* (4th ed.). New York: Churchill Livingstone.

Minkoff, H. (2004). Human immunodeficiency virus. In R. Creasy, R. Resnik, & J. Iams (Eds.), *Maternal-fetal medicine: Principles and practice* (5th ed.). Philadelphia: Saunders.

Moore, T. (2004). Diabetes in pregnancy. In R. Creasy, R. Resnik, & J. Iams (Eds.), *Maternal-fetal medicine: Principles and practice* (5th ed.). Philadelphia: Saunders.

Moore, L., & Martin, J. (2004). Sickle–cell crisis. In G. Dildy, M. Belfort, G. Saade, J. Phelan, G. Hankins, & S. Clark (Eds.). *Critical care obstetrics* (4th ed.). Malden, MA: Blackwell Science.

Nader, S. (2004a). Other endocrine disorders of pregnancy. In R. Creasy, R. Resnik, & J. Iams (Eds.), *Maternal-fetal medicine: Principles and practice* (5th ed.). Philadelphia: Saunders.

Nader, S. (2004b). Thyroid disease and pregnancy. In R. Creasy, R. Resnik, & J. Iams (Eds.), *Maternal-fetal medicine: Principles and practice* (5th ed.). Philadelphia: Saunders.

Nursing 2006. (2006). *Nursing 2006 drug handbook* (26th ed.). Philadelphia: Lippincott Williams & Wilkins.

Pagana, K., & Pagana, T. (2003). *Mosby's diagnostic and laboratory test reference* (6th ed.). St. Louis: Mosby.

Perinatal HIV Guidelines Working Group. (2001). *Public Health Service Task Force recommendations: Use of antiretroviral drugs in pregnant HIV-1-infected women for maternal health and interventions to reduce perinatal HIV-1 transmission in the United States.* Internet document available at www.hivatis.org (accessed July 24, 2005).

Rayburn, W., & Bogenschutz, M. (2004). Pharmacotherapy for pregnant women with addictions. *American Journal of Obstetrics and Gynecology, 191*(6), 1885-1897.

Riordan, J. (2005). *Breastfeeding and human lactation* (3rd ed.). Boston: Jones & Bartlett.

Russell, M., Martier, S., Sokol, R., Mudar, P., Jacobson, S., & Jacobson, J. (1996). Detecting risk drinking during pregnancy: A comparison of four screening questionnaires. *American Journal of Public Health, 86*(10), 1435-1439.

Samuels, P. (2002). Hepatic disease. In S. Gabbe, J. Niebyl, & J. Simpson (Eds.), *Obstetrics: Normal and problem pregnancies* (4th ed.). New York: Churchill Livingstone.

Savitz, D., Dole, N., Terry, J., Zhou, H., & Thorp, J. (2001). Smoking and pregnancy outcome among African-American and white women in central North Carolina. *Epidemiology, 12*(6), 636-642.

Semprini, A., & Fiore, S. (2004). HIV and pregnancy: Is the outlook for mother and baby transformed? *Current Opinion in Obstetrics and Gynecology, 16*(6), 471-475.

Scott, L., & Abu-Hamda, E. (2004). Gastrointestinal disease in pregnancy. In R. Creasy, R. Resnik, & J. Iams (Eds.), *Maternal-fetal medicine: Principles and practice* (5th ed.). Philadelphia: Saunders.

Shehata, H., & Okosun, H. (2004). Neurologic disorders in pregnancy. *Current Opinion in Obstetrics and Gynecology, 16*(2), 117-122.

Slocum, J., Barcio, L., Darany, J., Friedley, K., Homko, C., Mills, J., Roberts, D., & Seifert, H. (2004). Preconception to postpartum: Management of pregnancy complicated by diabetes. *Today's Educator, 30*(5), 740-753.

Spratto, G., & Woods, A. (2004). *PDR: Nurses's drug handbook.* Clifton Park, NY: Delmar.

Stephenson, J. (2005). Reducing HIV vertical transmission scrutinized. *Journal of the American Medical Association 293*(17), 2079-2081.

Tuomala, R., Watts, H., Li, D., Vajarannant, M. Pitt, J., Hammill, H., Landesman, S., Zorrilla, C., & Thompson, B. (2005). Improved obstetric outcomes and few maternal toxicities are associated with antiretroviral therapy, including highly active antiretroviral therapy during pregnancy. *Journal of Acquired Immune Deficiency Syndromes & Human Retrovirology, 38*(4), 449-473.

Weiner, C., & Buhimschi, C. (2004). *Drugs for pregnant and lactating women.* New York: Churchill Livingstone.

Whitty, J., & Dombrowski, M. (2004). Respiratory diseases in pregnancy. In R. Creasy, R. Resnik, & J. Iams (Eds.), *Maternal-fetal medicine: Principles and practice* (5th ed.). Philadelphia: Saunders.

Windsor, R. (2003). Smoking cessation or reduction in pregnancy treatment methods: A meta-evaluation of the impact of dissemination. *The American Journal of Medical Sciences, 326*(4), 216-222.

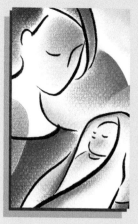

CHAPTER 23

Pregnancy at Risk: Gestational Conditions

ROBIN WEBB CORBETT

LEARNING OBJECTIVES

- *Describe the pathophysiology of preeclampsia and eclampsia.*
- *Differentiate the management of the woman with mild preeclampsia from that of the woman with severe preeclampsia.*
- *Identify the priorities for management of eclamptic seizures.*
- *Describe HELLP syndrome, including appropriate nursing actions.*
- *Explain the effects of hyperemesis gravidarum on maternal and fetal well-being.*
- *Discuss the management of the woman with hyperemesis gravidarum in the hospital and at home.*
- *Differentiate among causes, signs and symptoms, possible complications, and management of miscarriage, ectopic pregnancy, incompetent cervix, and hydatidiform mole.*
- *Compare and contrast placenta previa and abruptio placentae in relation to signs and symptoms, complications, and management.*
- *Discuss the diagnosis and management of disseminated intravascular coagulation.*
- *Differentiate signs and symptoms, effects on pregnancy and the fetus, and management during pregnancy of common sexually transmitted infections and other infections.*
- *Explain the basic principles of care for a pregnant woman undergoing abdominal surgery.*
- *Discuss implications of trauma on the mother and fetus during pregnancy.*
- *Identify priorities in assessment and stabilization measures for the pregnant trauma victim.*

KEY TERMS AND DEFINITIONS

abruptio placentae Partial or complete premature separation of a normally implanted placenta

cerclage Use of nonabsorbable suture to keep a premature dilating cervix closed; usually removed when pregnancy is at term

cervical funneling Effacement of the internal cervical os

chronic hypertension Systolic pressure of 140 mm Hg or higher or diastolic pressure of 90 mm Hg or higher that is present preconceptionally or occurs before 20 weeks of gestation

clonus Spasmodic alternation of muscular contraction and relaxation; counted in beats

Couvelaire uterus Interstitial myometrial hemorrhage after premature separation (abruption) of placenta; purplish-bluish discoloration of the uterus and boardlike rigidity of the uterus are noted

disseminated intravascular coagulation (DIC) Pathologic form of coagulation in which clotting factors are consumed to such an extent that generalized bleeding can occur; associated with abruptio placentae, eclampsia, intrauterine fetal demise, amniotic fluid embolism, and hemorrhage

eclampsia Severe complication of pregnancy of unknown cause and occurring more often in the primigravida; characterized by new onset grand mal seizures in a woman with preeclampsia occurring during pregnancy or shortly after birth

ectopic pregnancy Implantation of the fertilized ovum outside of the uterine cavity; locations include the uterine tubes, ovaries, and abdomen

gestational hypertension The new onset of hypertension without proteinuria after week 20 of pregnancy

HELLP syndrome Condition characterized by hemolysis, elevated liver enzymes, and low platelet count; a complication of severe preeclampsia

hydatidiform mole (molar pregnancy) Gestational trophoblastic neoplasm usually resulting from fertilization of an egg that has no nucleus or an inactivated nucleus

hyperemesis gravidarum Abnormal condition of pregnancy characterized by protracted vomiting, weight loss, and fluid and electrolyte imbalance

miscarriage Loss of pregnancy that occurs naturally without interference or known cause; also called *spontaneous abortion*

Continued

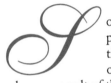 ome women experience significant problems during the months of gestation that can greatly affect pregnancy outcome. Some of these conditions develop as a result of the pregnant state; others are problems that could happen to anyone, at any time of life, but occur in this case during pregnancy. This chapter discusses a variety of disorders that did not exist before pregnancy, all of which have at least one thing in common: their occurrence in pregnancy puts the woman and fetus at risk. Hypertension in pregnancy, hyperemesis gravidarum, hemorrhagic complications of early and late pregnancy, surgery during pregnancy, trauma, and infections are discussed.

HYPERTENSION IN PREGNANCY ■

Significance and Incidence

Hypertension is the most common medical complication of pregnancy (Martin et al., 2005). A significant contributor to maternal and perinatal morbidity and mortality, preeclampsia complicates approximately 9% to 22% of all pregnancies not ending in first-trimester miscarriages (American College of Obstetricians and Gynecologists [ACOG], 2002; Martin et al., 2005). The rate has risen steadily by about 30% to 40%, since 1990, though it has been essentially unchanged since 2000 for all age, racial, and ethnic groups. The current rate is 37.4 per 1000 live births (Martin et al., 2005). In addition, rates for chronic hypertension have increased moderately (8.4 per 1000), whereas the rate for eclampsia has declined to (4.0 per 1000 live births) (Martin et al., 2005). Age distribu-

tion remains U-shaped, with women younger than 20 years of age and older than 40 years of age having the highest rates of occurrence of hypertension. Maternal race also influences the rate of pregnancy-associated hypertension, with the highest rates seen in Native American (49.7 per 1000) and African American (40.2 per 1000) women. Hispanic women have an intermediate rate (25.9 per 1000), and Asian or Pacific Islander women have the lowest rate for hypertension complicating pregnancy (19.6 per 1000) (Martin et al., 2005). In the United States, preeclampsia ranks second only to embolic events as a cause of maternal mortality and accounts for almost 15% of these deaths (National High Blood Pressure Education Program Working Group on High Blood Pressure in Pregnancy [Working Group], 2000). Hypertension (chronic and gestational) complicating pregnancy increases the woman's risk for a cesarean birth.

Preeclampsia predisposes the woman to potentially lethal complications, including eclampsia, abruptio placentae, disseminated intravascular coagulation (DIC), acute renal failure, hepatic failure, adult respiratory distress syndrome, and cerebral hemorrhage (Working Group, 2000). Preeclampsia occurs primarily after the second trimester of pregnancy and contributes significantly to intrauterine fetal death and perinatal mortality (Working Group, 2000). Causes of perinatal death related to preeclampsia are uteroplacental insufficiency and abruptio placentae, which lead to intrauterine death, preterm birth, and low birth weight (Roberts, 2004).

Eclampsia (characterized by seizures) from significant cerebral effects of preeclampsia is the major maternal hazard. As a rule, maternal and perinatal morbidity and mortality rates are highest among cases in which eclampsia is seen early in gestation (before 28 weeks), maternal age is greater than 25 years, the woman is a multigravida, and chronic hypertension or renal disease is present (Mattar & Sibai, 2000). The fetus of the eclamptic woman is at increased risk for hypertension in pregnancy, preterm birth, intrauterine growth restriction (IUGR), and acute hypoxia (Gilbert & Harmon, 2003).

Classification

The hypertensive disorders of pregnancy encompass a variety of conditions featuring an elevation of maternal blood pressure (BP) with a corresponding risk to maternal and fetal well-being. Hypertension is the third leading cause of maternal mortality, accounting for 16% of pregnancy-related deaths (Chang et al., 2003). The classification system most commonly used in the United States today is based on reports from ACOG (2002) and the National High Blood Pressure Education Program Working Group on High Blood Pressure in Pregnancy (2000). This classification system is summarized in Table 23-1.

Gestational hypertension

Gestational hypertension is the onset of hypertension without proteinuria after week 20 of pregnancy (ACOG, 2002; Working Group, 2000). *Gestational hypertension* is a non-specific term that replaces the term *pregnancy-induced hypertension* (PIH). Chronic hypertension and gestational hyper-

tension may occur independently or simultaneously. The diagnosis and differentiation between gestational hypertension and preeclampsia is made in the postpartum period. If the woman has not developed preeclampsia and her BP returns to normal values by 12 weeks after birth, the woman is diagnosed with transient hypertension. If BP values remain elevated, then the diagnosis of chronic hypertension is made (ACOG, 2002; Working Group, 2000).

Preeclampsia

Preeclampsia is a pregnancy-specific condition in which hypertension develops after 20 weeks of gestation in a previously normotensive woman. It is a multisystem, vasospastic disease process characterized by hypertension and proteinuria (ACOG, 2002; Working Group, 2000). Preeclampsia is usually categorized as mild or severe for purposes of management (Table 23-2).

Hypertension is defined as a systolic BP greater than 140 mm Hg or a diastolic BP greater than 90 mm Hg (ACOG, 2002; Working Group, 2000). The diagnosis of a new onset of hypertension during pregnancy is based on at least two measurements at least 4 to 6 hours apart. The Working Group (2000) recommend that the blood pressure, disappearance of sound (Korotkoff phase V) be taken with the woman upright or if hospitalized either upright or in the left lateral recumbent position with the arm at heart level. They further recommend no tobacco or caffeine use within the preceding 30 minutes of blood pressure measurement.

Evolve/CD: Case Study—Preeclampsia

TABLE 23-1

Classification of Hypertensive States of Pregnancy

TYPE	DESCRIPTION
GESTATIONAL HYPERTENSIVE DISORDERS	
Gestational hypertension	Development of mild hypertension during pregnancy in previously normotensive woman without proteinuria or pathologic edema
Gestational proteinuria	Development of proteinuria after 20 weeks of gestation in previously nonproteinuric woman without hypertension
Preeclampsia	Development of hypertension and proteinuria in previously normotensive woman after 20 weeks of gestation or in early postpartum period; in presence of trophoblastic disease it can develop before 20 weeks of gestation
Eclampsia	Development of convulsions or coma in preeclamptic woman
CHRONIC HYPERTENSIVE DISORDERS	
Chronic hypertension	Hypertension and/or proteinuria in pregnant woman with chronic hypertension prior to 20 weeks of gestation and persistent after 12 weeks postpartum
Superimposed preeclampsia or eclampsia	Development of preeclampsia or eclampsia in woman with chronic hypertension prior to 20 weeks of gestation

Modified from Gilbert, E., & Harmon, J. (2003). *Manual of high risk pregnancy and delivery* (3rd ed.). St. Louis: Mosby; Cunningham, F., Leveno, K., Bloom, S., Hauth, J., Gilstrap, L., Wenstrom, K. (2005). *Williams obstetrics* (22nd ed.). New York: McGraw-Hill.

Differentiation between Mild and Severe Preeclampsia

	MILD PREECLAMPSIA	SEVERE PREECLAMPSIA
MATERNAL EFFECTS		
Blood pressure (BP)	BP reading >140/90 mm Hg × 2, 4-6 hr apart	Rise to ≥160/110 mm Hg on two separate occasions 4-6 hr apart with pregnant woman on bed rest
Mean arterial pressure (MAP)	>105 mm Hg	>105 mm Hg
Proteinuria		
—Qualitative dipstick	Proteinuria of ≥300 mg in a 24-hr specimen; ≥1+ on dipstick	Proteinuria of ≥2.0 grams in 24 hr or ≥2+ on dipstick
—Quantitative 24-hr analysis		
Reflexes	May be normal	Hyperreflexia ≥3+, possible ankle clonus
Urine output	Output matching intake, ≥30 ml/hr or <650 ml/24 hr	<20 ml/hr or <400-500 ml/24 hr
Headache	Absent or transient	Persistent or Severe
Visual problems	Absent	Blurred, photophobia, blind spots on funduscopy
Irritability or changes in affect	Transient	Severe
Epigastric pain	Absent	Present
Serum creatinine	Normal	Elevated, >1.2 mg/dl
Thrombocytopenia	Absent	Present, <100,000/mm^3
AST elevation	Normal or minimal	Marked
Pulmonary edema	Absent	Present
FETAL EFFECTS		
Placental perfusion	Reduced	Decreased perfusion expressing as IUGR in fetus; FHR: late decelerations
Premature placental aging	Not apparent	At birth placenta appearing smaller than normal for duration of pregnancy, premature aging apparent with numerous areas of broken syncytia, ischemic necroses (white infarcts) numerous, intervillous fibrin deposition (red infarcts)

AST, Aspartate aminotransferase; *FHR,* fetal heart rate; *IUGR,* intrauterine growth restriction.
Sources: ACOG (2002). *Diagnosis and management of preeclampsia and eclampsia.* AGOG Practice Bulletin number 33, Washington DC: AGOG; Cunningham, F., Leveno, K., Bloom, S., Hauth, J., Gilstrap, L., Wenstrom, K. (2005). *Williams obstetrics* (22nd ed.). New York: McGraw-Hill.

More accurate readings are obtained with use of an appropriate size cuff (1.5 times longer than the upper arm circumference) and with a mercury sphygmomanometer (ACOG, 2002). Women who demonstrate an increase of 30 mm Hg systolic or 15 mm Hg diastolic should be closely monitored if the BP elevation occurs with proteinuria and hyperuricemia (uric acid of 6 mg/dl or more) (ACOG, 2002; Working Group, 2000). See Box 23-1 for instructions for measuring BP.

Proteinuria is defined as a concentration of >30 mg/dl in a random urine or more in at least two random urine specimens collected at least 6 hours apart. In a 24-hour specimen, proteinuria is defined as a concentration of ≥300 mg/24 hours. Due to the discrepancies between a random urine and a 24 hour urine protein, the 24 hour urine is preferred for diagnosis (Working Group, 2000). Pathologic edema is a clinically evident, generalized accumulation of fluid of the face, hands, or abdomen that is not responsive to 12 hours of bed rest. It may also be manifested as a rapid weight gain of more than 2 kg in 1 week. Edema frequently occurs in pregnancy and is no longer considered diagnostic of preeclampsia (ACOG, 2002; Working Group, 2000).

Severe preeclampsia

Severe preeclampsia is the presence of any one of the following in the woman diagnosed with preeclampsia: (1) systolic BP of at least 160 mm Hg or diastolic BP of at least 110 mm Hg; (2) proteinuria of greater than 2 g protein excreted in a 24-hour specimen, or greater than 2+ on two random dipstick measurements taken at least 4 hours apart; (3) oliguria, of less than 500 ml over 24 hours; (4) cerebral or visual disturbances, such as altered level of consciousness (LOC), headache, scotomata, or blurred vision; (5) hepatic involvement, including epigastric pain; (6) thrombocytopenia with a platelet count less than 100,000/mm^3; (7) pul-

BOX 23-1

Blood Pressure Measurement

- Measure blood pressure with the woman seated (ambulatory) or in the left lateral recumbent position with the arm at heart level .
- After positioning, allow the woman at least 10 minutes of quiet rest before blood pressure measurement, to encourage relaxation.
- No tobacco or caffeine use 30 minutes prior to blood pressure measurement.
- Use the same arm each time for blood pressure measurement.
- Hold the arm in a roughly horizontal position at heart level.
- Use the proper-sized cuff (cuff should cover approximately 80% of the upper arm or be 1.5 times the length of the upper arm).
- Maintain a slow, steady deflation rate.
- Take the average of two readings at least 6 hours apart to minimize recorded blood pressure variations across time.
- Use Korotkoff phase V (disappearance of sound) for recording the diastolic value (some sources recommend recording both phase IV [the muffled sound] and phase V).
- Use accurate equipment. The manual sphygmomanometer is the most accurate device.
- If interchanging manual and electronic devices, use caution in interpreting different blood pressure values.

monary edema or cyanosis; or (8) fetal growth restriction (ACOG, 2002; Working Group, 2000).

Eclampsia

Eclampsia is the onset of seizure activity or coma in a patient with preeclampsia, with no history of preexisting pathology that can result in seizure activity (ACOG, 2002; Working Group, 2000). The initial presentation of eclampsia varies; one third of the women develop eclampsia during the pregnancy, one third during labor, and one third within 72 hours postpartum (Emery, 2005).

Chronic hypertension

Chronic hypertension is defined as hypertension present before the pregnancy or diagnosed before the twentieth week of gestation. Hypertension that persists longer than 6 weeks postpartum is also classified as chronic hypertension (Emery, 2005). There is no widely accepted definition of mild hypertension. Severe hypertension is usually defined as a diastolic BP of 110 mm Hg or higher (ACOG, 2002; Working Group, 2000).

Chronic hypertension with superimposed preeclampsia

Superimposed preeclampsia is the development of a new onset proteinuria (300 mg or greater in a 24-hour urine collection), sudden increase in proteinuria, sudden increase in hypertension or the presentation of HELLP syndrome (*he*molysis, *e*levated *liver* enzymes, and *low platelets) in a pregnant woman with hypertension before 20 weeks of gestation (ACOG, 2002; Sibai, 2002).

Etiology

The etiology of high blood pressure in pregnancy is not known. What is known is that with an increased maternal blood pressure, fluid moves from the vascular system to the extravascular spaces. Blood becomes hemoconcentrated with a decreased renal plasma flow and glomerular filtration rate. Pregnant women with chronic high blood pressure have a 20% reduction in sodium excretion. An elevated blood pressure in pregnancy and the subsequent vasoconstriction will reduce uteroplacental perfusion with alterations in fetal growth (Blackburn, 2003).

Preeclampsia is a condition unique to human pregnancy; signs and symptoms usually develop only during pregnancy and disappear quickly after birth of the fetus and passage of the placenta. The cause is unknown. No single patient profile identifies the woman who will have preeclampsia. However, certain high risk factors are associated with the development of preeclampsia: primigravidity, multifetal presentation, preexisting diabetes mellitus, and African-American ethnicity (Box 23-2) (ACOG, 2002; Duckitt & Harrington, 2005).

Current theories regarding the etiology of hypertension in pregnancy include hyperhomocysteinemia (Mignini et al., 2005), antiphospholipid antibodies (Dildy, 2004), increased vascular tone, abnormal vascular response to placentation, abnormal prostaglandin action, endothelial cell dysfunction (Dildy, 2004; Sibai, Dekker & Kupferminc, 2005), coagulation abnormalities, abnormal trophoblast invasion, and dietary factors (ACOG, 2002, Cunningham et al., 2005). Immunologic factors and genetic disposition may also play an important role in the etiology of hypertension in pregnancy (Roberts, 2004).

Pathophysiology

Preeclampsia is characterized by vasospasms, changes in the coagulation system, and disturbances in systems related to volume and BP control. Vasospasms result from an increased sensitivity to circulating pressors, such as angiotensin II, and possibly an imbalance between the prostaglandins prostacyclin and thromboxane A_1 (ACOG, 2002; Working Group, 2000).

Endothelial cell dysfunction, believed to result from decreased placental perfusion, may account for many changes in preeclampsia (Fig. 23-1). Arteriolar vasospasm may cause endothelial damage and contribute to an increased capillary permeability. This increases edema and further decreases intravascular volume, predisposing the woman with preeclampsia to pulmonary edema (ACOG, 2002; Working Group, 2000).

BOX 23-2

Risk Factors Associated with the Development of Preeclampsia

Chronic renal disease
Chronic hypertension
Family history of preeclampsia
Multifetal gestation
Primigravidity or new partner with multiparous woman
Extremes of maternal age <19 years or >40 years
Diabetes
Rh incompatibility
Obesity
African-American ethnicity
Insulin resistance
Limited sperm exposure with same partner
Preeclampsia in a previous pregnancy
Pregnancies after donor insemination, oocyte donation, embryo donation
Maternal infections

Data from: American College of Obstetricians and Gynecologists (ACOG). (2002). *Diagnosis and management of preeclampsia and eclampsia. ACOG Practice Bulletin no. 33.* Washington, DC: ACOG; Gilbert, E., & Harmon, J. (2003). *Manual of high risk pregnancy and delivery* (3rd ed.). St. Louis: Mosby; Sibai, B., Dekker, G., & Kupferminc, M. (2005). Preeclampsia. *Lancet, 365*(9461) 785-799.

Immunologic factors may play an important role in the development of preeclampsia (Roberts, 2004; Sibai, 2002). The presence of a foreign protein, the placenta, or the fetus may be perceived by the mother's immune system as an antigen. This may then trigger an abnormal immunologic response. This theory is supported by the increased incidence of preeclampsia or eclampsia in first-time mothers (first exposure to fetal tissue) or to multiparous women pregnant by a new partner (Cunningham et al., 2005; Li & Wi, 2000). Preeclampsia may be an immune complex disease in which the maternal antibody system is overwhelmed from excessive fetal antigens in the maternal circulation. This theory seems compatible with the high incidence of preeclampsia among women exposed to a large mass of trophoblastic tissue as seen in twin pregnancies or hydatidiform moles.

Genetic predisposition may be another immunologic factor. Dekker (2001) reported a greater frequency of preeclampsia and eclampsia among daughters and granddaughters of women with a history of eclampsia, which suggests an autosomal recessive gene controlling the maternal immune response. Paternal factors are also being examined (Cunningham et al., 2005; Robillard, 2002).

Diets inadequate in nutrients, especially protein, calcium, sodium, magnesium, and vitamins E and C, may be an etiologic factor in preeclampsia. Some practitioners prescribe high-protein diets (90 mg supplemental protein) without caloric restriction and moderate sodium intake in the prevention and treatment of this disorder. However, data are limited regarding the association between diet and preeclampsia.

Preeclampsia progresses along a continuum from mild disease to severe preeclampsia, HELLP syndrome, or eclampsia. The pathophysiology of preeclampsia reflects alterations in the normal adaptations of pregnancy. Normal physiologic adaptations to pregnancy include increased blood plasma volume, vasodilation, decreased systemic vascular resistance, elevated cardiac output, and decreased colloid osmotic pressure (Box 23-3).

Pathologic changes in the endothelial cells of the glomeruli (glomeruloendotheliosis) are uniquely characteristic of preeclampsia, particularly in nulliparous women. The main pathogenic factor is not an increase in BP but poor perfusion as a result of vasospasm. Arteriolar vasospasm diminishes the diameter of blood vessels, which impedes blood flow to all organs and raises BP (Working Group, 2000). Function in organs such as the placenta, kidneys, liver, and brain is decreased by as much as 40% to 60%. The pathophysiologic sequelae are shown in Fig. 23-2.

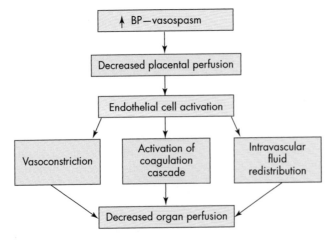

Fig. 23-1 Etiology of preeclampsia: endothelial cell dysfunction.

BOX 23-3

Normal Physiologic Adaptations to Pregnancy

CARDIOVASCULAR

↑ Blood volume; plasma volume expansion greater than red cell mass expansion, leading to physiologic anemia of pregnancy

↓ Total peripheral resistance, decreases in blood pressure readings and mean arterial pressure

↑ Cardiac output resulting from increased blood volume, slight increase in heart rate to compensate for peripheral relaxation

↑ Oxygen consumption

Physiologic edema related to ↓ plasma colloid osmotic pressure and ↑ venous capillary hydrostatic pressure

HEMATOLOGIC

↑ Clotting factors, predisposing to disseminated intravascular coagulation and clotting

↓ Serum albumin resulting in decreases in colloid osmotic pressure, predisposing toward pulmonary edema

RENAL

↑ Renal plasma flow and glomerular filtration rate

ENDOCRINE

↑ Estrogen production resulting in ↑ renin-angiotensin II-aldosterone secretion

↑ Progesterone production blocking aldosterone effect (slight ↓ sodium)

↑ Vasodilator prostaglandins resulting in resistance to angiotensin II (slight ↓ blood pressure)

HELLP syndrome

HELLP syndrome is a laboratory diagnosis for a variant of severe preeclampsia that involves hepatic dysfunction, characterized by hemolysis (H), elevated liver enzymes (EL), and low platelets (LP) (ACOG, 2002; Sibai, 2004). The platelet count must be less than 100,000/mm³, liver enzyme levels (aspartate aminotransferase [AST] and alanine aminotransferase [ALT]) must be elevated, and evidence of intravascular hemolysis (burr cells on peripheral smear or elevated bilirubin [indirect] level) must be present. A unique form of coagulopathy (not DIC) occurs with HELLP syndrome. The platelet count is low, but coagulation factor assays, prothrombin time (PT), partial thromboplastin time (PTT), and bleeding time remain normal. In some instances, hemolysis does not occur and the condition is termed *ELLP* (Sibai, 2004).

A diagnosis of HELLP syndrome is associated with an increased risk for adverse perinatal outcomes, including placental abruption, acute renal failure, subcapsular hepatic hematoma, hepatic rupture, recurrent preeclampsia, preterm birth, and fetal and maternal death (ACOG, 2002; Sibai, 2004). HELLP appears in approximately 20% of women with severe preeclampsia (ACOG, 2002; Emery, 2005). The syn-

drome is associated with an increased risk of maternal death. Perinatal mortality rates range from 7.4% to 20.4% with a maternal mortality of approximately 1% (Sibai, 2004). Preterm labor is greatly increased, 70% with subsequent fetal and neonatal complications associated with preterm delivery such as respiratory distress syndrome and intracerebral hemorrhage (Sibai, 2004).

HELLP syndrome is often nonspecific in clinical presentation. A majority of patients report a history of malaise for several days. Many women (30% to 90%) experience epigastric or right upper quadrant abdominal pain (possibly related to hepatic ischemia), nausea, and vomiting (Sibai, 2004).

NURSE ALERT *It is extremely important to understand that many patients with HELLP syndrome may not have signs or symptoms of severe preeclampsia. For example, many of these women are normotensive or have only slight elevations in BP. Proteinuria also may be absent. As a result, women with HELLP syndrome are often misdiagnosed with a variety of other medical or surgical disorders (Sibai, 2004).*

Recognition of the clinical and laboratory findings associated with HELLP syndrome is important if early, aggressive therapy is to be initiated to prevent maternal and neonatal mortality. Complications reported with HELLP syndrome include renal failure, pulmonary edema, ruptured liver hematoma, DIC, and placental abruption (Sibai, 2004).

CARE MANAGEMENT

Assessment and Nursing Diagnoses

Hypertensive disorders of pregnancy can occur without warning or with the gradual development of symptoms. A key goal is early detection of the disease in order to prevent the catastrophic maternal and fetal sequelae. Therefore each woman is assessed for etiologic factors during the first prenatal visit (see Box 23-2). During each subsequent visit the woman is assessed for signs or symptoms that suggest the onset or presence of preeclampsia.

Interview

The nurse reviews the woman's admission form and prenatal record. The nurse conducts the interview to clarify, expand, or complete the form. The medical history is reviewed, especially the presence of diabetes mellitus, renal disease, and hypertension. Family history is explored for occurrence of preeclamptic or hypertensive conditions, diabetes mellitus, and other chronic conditions. The social and experiential history provides information about the woman's support system, nutritional status, cultural beliefs, activity level, and lifestyle behaviors (e.g., smoking, alcohol and drug use).

A review of systems adds to the database for detecting BP changes from baseline and the presence of proteinuria.

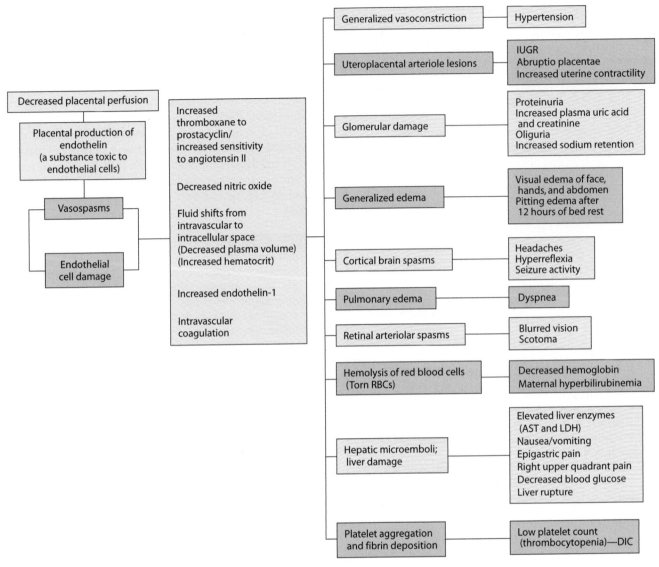

Fig. 23-2   Pathophysiology of preeclampsia. (Modified from Gilbert, E., & Harmon, J. [2003]. *Manual of high risk pregnancy and delivery* [3rd ed.]. St. Louis: Mosby.)

It is important to note whether the woman is having unusual, frequent, or severe headaches; visual disturbances; or epigastric pain. Abnormal amount and pattern of weight gain and increased signs of edema may be present even though they may not be specifically diagnostic signs of preeclampsia.

Physical examination

Personnel caring for pregnant women need to be consistent in taking and recording BP measurements in the standardized manner (see Box 23-1). Electronic BP devices are less accurate in high flow states such as pregnancy or in hypertensive or hypotensive states.

Observation of edema in addition to hypertension warrants additional investigation. Edema is assessed for distribution, degree, and pitting. If periorbital or facial edema is not obvious, the pregnant woman is asked whether it was present when she awoke. Edema may be described as dependent or pitting.

Dependent edema is edema of the lowest or most dependent parts of the body, where hydrostatic pressure is greatest. If a pregnant woman is ambulatory, this edema may first be evident in the feet and ankles. If the pregnant woman is confined to bed, the edema is more likely to occur in the sacral region.

Pitting edema is edema that leaves a small depression or pit after finger pressure is applied to the swollen area. The pit, which is caused by movement of fluid to adjacent tissue away from the point of pressure, normally disappears within 10 to 30 seconds. Although the amount of edema is difficult to quantify, the method shown in Fig. 23-3 may be used to record relative degrees of edema formation.

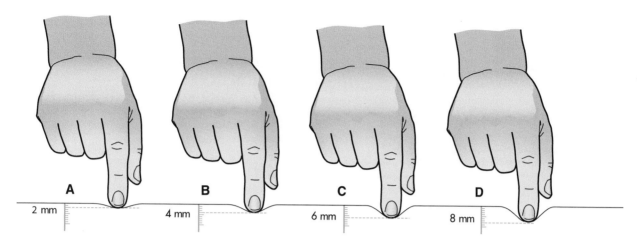

Fig. 23-3 Assessment of pitting edema of lower extremities. **A,** +1; **B,** +2; **C,** +3; **D,** +4.

Symptoms reflecting central nervous system (CNS) and visual system involvement usually accompany facial edema. Although it is not a routine assessment during the prenatal period, evaluation of the fundus of the eye yields valuable data. An initial baseline finding of normal eye grounds assists in differentiating preexisting disease from a new disease process. The woman will also be assessed for epigastric pain and oliguria. Respirations are also assessed for crackles, which may indicate pulmonary edema.

Deep tendon reflexes (DTRs) are evaluated if preeclampsia is suspected. The biceps and patellar reflexes and ankle clonus are assessed, and the findings recorded.

> **NURSE ALERT** *The evaluation of DTRs is especially important if the woman is being treated with magnesium sulfate; absence of DTRs is an early indication of impending magnesium toxicity.*

To elicit the biceps reflex, the examiner strikes a downward blow over the thumb, which is situated over the biceps tendon (Fig. 23-4, *A*). Normal response is flexion of the arm at the elbow, described as a 2+ response (Table 23-3). The patellar reflex is elicited with the woman's legs hanging freely over the end of the examining table or with the woman lying on her left side with the knee slightly flexed. A blow with a percussion hammer is dealt directly to the patellar tendon, inferior to the patella. Normal response is the extension or kicking out of the leg (Fig. 23-4, *B*). To assess for hyperactive reflexes (clonus) at the ankle joint, the examiner supports the leg with the knee flexed (Fig. 23-4, *C*). With one hand, the examiner sharply dorsiflexes the foot, maintains the position for a moment, and then releases the foot. Normal (negative clonus) response is elicited when no rhythmic oscillations (jerks) are felt while the foot is held in dorsiflexion. When the foot is released, no oscillations are seen as the foot drops to the plantar flexed position. Abnormal (positive clonus) response is recognized by rhythmic oscillations of one or more "beats" felt when the foot is in dorsiflexion and seen as the foot drops to the plantar flexed position.

An important assessment is determination of fetal status. Uteroplacental perfusion is decreased in women with preeclampsia, placing the fetus in jeopardy. Daily fetal movement counts are obtained. The fetal heart rate (FHR) is assessed for baseline rate and variability and accelerations, which indicate an intact, oxygenated fetal CNS. Abnormal baseline rate, decreased or absent variability, and late decelerations are indications of fetal intolerance to the intrauterine environment. Biophysical or biochemical monitoring such as nonstress tests (NSTs), contraction stress testing, biophysical profile (BPP), and serial ultrasonography are used to assess fetal status.

Doppler flow velocimetry studies are used for evaluating maternal and fetal well-being (see Chapter 21). Uteroplacental perfusion is assessed by measuring the velocity of blood flow through the uterine artery, umbilical arteries, or both. Abnormal uterine artery Doppler flow is associated with risk of IUGR in women with HELLP syndrome (Bush, O'Brien, & Barton, 2001). Currently, this diagnostic test is not recommended as a general screening test for preeclampsia (Sibai, 2002).

Uterine tonicity is evaluated for signs of labor and abruptio placentae. If labor is suspected, a vaginal examination for

TABLE 23-3

Assessing Deep Tendon Reflexes

GRADE	DEEP TENDON REFLEX RESPONSE
0	No response
1+	Sluggish or diminished
2+	Active or expected response
3+	More brisk than expected, slightly hyperactive
4+	Brisk, hyperactive, with intermittent or transient clonus

From Seidel, H., Ball, J., Dains, J., Benedict, G. (2003). *Mosby's guide to physical examination* (5th ed.). St. Louis: Mosby.

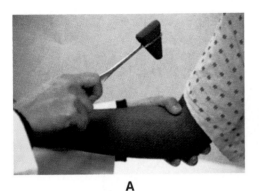
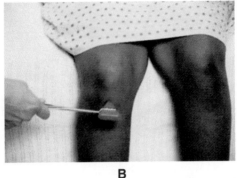
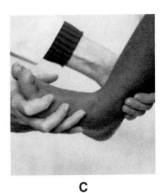

A **B** **C**

Fig. 23-4 **A,** Biceps reflex. **B,** Patellar reflex with patient's legs hanging freely over end of examining table. **C,** Test for ankle clonus. (From Seidel, H., Ball, J., Dains, J., Benedict, G. [2003]. *Mosby's guide to physical examination* [5th ed.]. St. Louis: Mosby.)

cervical changes is indicated (see Table 23-8 for signs of abruptio placentae).

During the physical examination, the pregnant woman is examined for signs of progression of mild preeclampsia to severe preeclampsia or eclampsia. Signs of worsening liver involvement, renal failure, worsening hypertension, cerebral involvement, and developing coagulopathies must be assessed and documented. Respirations are assessed for crackles or diminished breath sounds, which may indicate pulmonary edema. Noninvasive assessment parameters include LOC, BP, hemoglobin oxygen saturation (pulse oximetry), electrocardiographic findings, and urine output. Eclampsia is usually preceded by various premonitory symptoms and signs, including headache, severe epigastric pain, hyperreflexia, and hemoconcentration. However, convulsions can

appear suddenly and without warning in a seemingly stable woman with only minimum BP elevations (Sibai, 2004). Seizures may recur within minutes of the first convulsion, or the woman may never have another. During the seizure, the mother and fetus are not receiving oxygen, so eclamptic seizures produce a metabolic insult to both the mother and fetus.

Laboratory tests

Blood and urine specimens are collected to aid in the diagnosis and treatment of preeclampsia, HELLP syndrome, and chronic hypertension. Baseline laboratory test information is useful in cases of early diagnosis of preeclampsia because it can be compared with later results to evaluate progression and severity of disease (Table 23-4). An

TABLE 23-4

Common Laboratory Changes in Preeclampsia

	NORMAL NONPREGNANT	PREECLAMPSIA	HELLP
Hemoglobin/hematocrit	12 to 16 g/dl/37% to 47%	May ↑	↓
Platelets	150,000 to 400,000/mm³	Unchanged or <100,000/mm³	<100,000/mm³
Prothrombin time (PT)/ partial thromboplastin time (PTT)	12 to 14 sec/60 to 70 sec	Unchanged	Unchanged
Fibrinogen	200 to 400 mg/dl	300 to 600 mg/dl	↓
Fibrin split products (FSP)	Absent	Absent/Present	Present
Blood urea nitrogen (BUN)	10 to 20 mg/dl	↑	↑
Creatinine	0.5 to 1.1 mg/dl	>1.2 mg/dl	↑
Lactate dehydrogenase (LDH) *	45 to 90 units/L	↑	↑ (>600 units/L)
Aspartate aminotransferase (AST)	4 to 20 units/L	Unchanged to minimal ↑	↑ (>70 units/L)
Alanine aminotransferase (ALT)	3 to 21 units/L	Unchanged to minimal ↑	↑
Creatinine clearance	80 to 125 ml/min	130 to 180 ml/min	↓
Burr cells or schistocytes	Absent	Absent	Present
Uric acid	2 to 6.6 mg/dl	>5.9 mg/dl	>10 mg/dl
Bilirubin (total)	0.1 to 1 mg/dl	unchanged or ↑	↑ (>1.2 mg/dl)

Sources: Cunningham, F. et al., (2005). *Williams obstetrics* (22nd ed.). New York: McGraw-Hill.
Dildy, G. (2004) Complications of preeclampsia. In G. Dildy, M. Belfort, G. Saade, J. Phelan, G. Hankins, & S. Clark (Eds.), *Critical care obstetrics* (4th ed.) Malden, MA: Blackwell Science. Roberts, J. (2004). Pregnancy-related chypertension. In R. Creasy, R. Resnik, & J. Iams (Eds.), *Maternal-fetal medicine: Principles and practice* (5th ed.). Philadelphia: Saunders.
*LDH values differ according to the test/assays being done.

initial blood specimen is obtained for the following tests to assess the disease process and its effect on renal and hepatic functioning:

- Complete blood cell count (including a platelet count)
- Clotting studies (including bleeding time, PT, PTT, and fibrinogen)
- Liver enzymes (lactate dehydrogenase [LDH], AST, ALT)
- Chemistry panel (blood urea nitrogen [BUN], creatinine, glucose, uric acid)
- Type and screen, possible crossmatch and antibody screen

The hematocrit, hemoglobin, and platelet levels are monitored closely for changes indicating a worsening of patient status. Because hepatic involvement is a possible complication, serum glucose levels are monitored if liver function tests indicate elevated liver enzymes. Once the platelet count drops below 100,000/mm^3, coagulation profiles are needed to identify developing DIC (Sibai, 2002).

Urine output is assessed for volume of at least 30 ml/hr or 120 ml/4 hr. Proteinuria is determined from dipstick testing of a clean-catch or catheterized urine specimen. A reading of 2+ or 3+ on two or more occasions, at least 6 hours apart, should be followed by a 24-hour urine collection. A 24-hour collection to test for protein and creatinine clearance is more reflective of true renal status. Renal laboratory assessments include monitoring trends in serum creatinine and BUN levels. As renal function becomes compromised, renal excretion of creatinine and other waste products, including magnesium sulfate, decreases. As renal excretion decreases, serum levels of creatinine, BUN, uric acid, and magnesium increase. Proteinuria is usually a late sign in the course of preeclampsia (ACOG, 2002; Working Group, 2000).

Protein readings are designated as follows:

0	negative
Trace	trace
1+	30 mg/dl
2+	100 mg/dl
3+	300 mg/dl
4+	1000 mg (1 g)/dl

Nursing diagnoses for the woman with hypertensive disorders in pregnancy may include the following:

- *Anxiety related to*
  - preeclampsia and its effects on woman and infant
- *Deficient knowledge related to*
  - management (diet, medications, activity restrictions)
- *Ineffective individual or family coping related to*
  - woman's restricted activity and concern over a complicated pregnancy
  - woman's inability to work outside the home and care for her family
  - transfer of woman to tertiary care center for more intensive management

- *Powerlessness related to*
  - inability to prevent or control condition and outcomes
- *Ineffective tissue perfusion related to*
  - hypertension
  - cyclic vasospasms
  - cerebral edema
  - hemorrhage
- *Risk for injury to fetus related to*
  - uteroplacental insufficiency
  - preterm birth
  - abruptio placentae
- *Risk for injury to mother related to*
  - CNS irritability secondary to cerebral edema, vasospasm, decreased renal perfusion
  - magnesium sulfate and antihypertensive therapies
  - abruptio placentae

Expected Outcomes of Care

Expected outcomes for care of women with hypertensive disorders of pregnancy include that the woman will do the following:

- Recognize and immediately report signs and symptoms indicative of worsening condition
- Adhere to the medical regimen to minimize risk to herself and her fetus
- Identify and use available support systems
- Verbalize her fears and concerns to cope with the condition and situation
- Develop no signs of eclampsia and its complications
- Give birth to a healthy infant
- Develop no adverse sequelae from her condition or its management

Plan of Care and Interventions

Nursing actions are derived from medical management, health care provider directives, and nursing diagnoses. The most effective therapy is prevention. Early prenatal care, identification of pregnant women at risk, and recognition and reporting of physical warning signs are essential components for optimizing maternal and perinatal outcomes. The nurse's skills in assessing the woman for factors and symptoms of preeclampsia and educating her about reporting symptoms cannot be overestimated.

The goals of therapy are to ensure maternal safety and to deliver a healthy newborn as close to term as possible. At or near term, the plan of care for a woman with preeclampsia is most likely to be induction of labor, preceded, if necessary, by cervical ripening. When preeclampsia is diagnosed in a woman at less than 37 weeks of gestation, however, immediate birth may not be in the best interest of the fetus. In this situation the initial intervention is usually a thorough evaluation of both the maternal and fetal condition. This evaluation may be done in the high risk clinic or the physician's office. A multidisciplinary plan of care is then developed, based on the assessment findings.

Emotional and psychologic support is essential in assisting the woman and her family to cope. Their perception of the disease process, the reasons for it, and the care received will affect their compliance with and participation in therapy. The family needs to use coping mechanisms and support systems to help them through this crisis. A plan of care specifically designed for the woman with preeclampsia must be superimposed on the nursing care all women need during labor and the birth process.

Mild preeclampsia and home care

If the woman has mild preeclampsia (e.g., BP is stable, urine protein is less than 300 mg in a 24-hour collection, and woman has no subjective complaints), she may be managed expectantly, usually at home. The maternal-fetal condition must be assessed two to three times per week. Many agencies are available to provide this assessment in the home. Arrangements for this service may be made, depending on the woman's insurance coverage. If home nursing care is not an option, the woman may be asked to perform self-assessment daily, including weight, urine dipstick protein determinations, BP measurement, and fetal movement counting. She will be instructed to report the development of any subjective symptoms immediately to her health care provider (Patient Instructions for Self-Care box) and to

return to the physician's office or high risk clinic for assessment as scheduled.

The fetal condition also is closely monitored to allow additional time for fetal growth and maturation. An evaluation of fetal growth by ultrasound should be obtained every 3 weeks. Fetal movement is counted daily. Other fetal assessment tests include an NST once or twice a week and a BPP as needed. Fetal jeopardy as evidenced by inappropriate growth or abnormal test results necessitates immediate interventions for birth (ACOG, 2002; Sibai, 2002; Working Group, 2000).

Activity restriction. Bed rest in the lateral recumbent position is a standard therapy for preeclampsia and may improve uteroplacental blood flow during pregnancy. Bed rest has been shown to be beneficial in decreasing BP and promoting diuresis. However, recommendations for bed rest for all high risk pregnant women is becoming more controversial. Maloni and Kutil (2000) and Maloni (2002) doc-

PATIENT INSTRUCTIONS FOR SELF-CARE

Assessing and Reporting Clinical Signs of Preeclampsia

- Report to your health care provider immediately any *increase in your blood pressure, protein in urine, weight gain greater than 1 lb/wk, or edema.*
- *Take your blood pressure on the same arm in a sitting position* each time for consistent and accurate readings. Support arm on a table in a horizontal position at heart level.
- *Weigh* yourself using the same scale, wearing the same clothes, at the same time each day, after voiding, before breakfast, for reliable daily weights.
- *Dipstick test your clean-catch urine sample* to assess proteinuria; report frequency of or burning on urination.
- *Report to your health care provider* if proteinuria is 2⁺ or more or if you have a decrease in urine output.
- *Assess your baby's activity daily.* Decreased activity (four or fewer movements per hour) may indicate fetal compromise and should be reported.
- *It is important to keep your scheduled prenatal appointments* so that any changes in your or your baby's condition can be detected.
- *Keep a daily log or diary* of your assessments for your home health care nurse, or bring it with you to your next prenatal visit.
- Report to your health care provider immediately any *headache, dizziness, blurring of vision or muscular irritability (seizures)*

⑦ *Critical Thinking Exercise*

Preeclampsia

Demetria is a 16-year-old pregnant African-American, primigravida who is 33 weeks of gestation. Her medical history is positive with type 2 diabetes mellitus and she has a maternal history of hypertension. Her preconceptual weight is 263 and she is 63 inches tall. A baseline BP is not noted. She is admitted from the local health department to the hospital with elevated BPs ranging from 150/92–164/96 while lying on her left side and DTRs of 3+.

Her obstetric provider orders:
V.S. every 4 hours
FHR every shift
Regular diet
Heplock
CBC, chem. 14, liver panel, platelets and uric acid
NST on admission
24-hour urine for total protein and creatinine
Bed rest with bathroom privilege – maintain side lying position
Daily weights
10 mg of hydralazine IV now and recheck BP in 10 minutes with manual cuff
External fetal monitoring
Betamethasone 12 mg IM now, repeat in 24 hours

1 Is there sufficient evidence to draw conclusions about her diagnosis and preferred treatment?
2 What assumptions can be made about the following items:
  a. Possible diagnoses
  b. Physical assessment, laboratory tests, and diagnostic procedures that have been ordered or will be ordered
  c. Factors contributing to her high blood pressure in pregnancy
3 What implications and priorities for nursing care can be drawn at this time?
4 Does the evidence objectively support your conclusion?
5 Are there alternative perspectives to your conclusion?

umented adverse physiologic outcomes related to complete bed rest, including cardiovascular deconditioning; diuresis with accompanying fluid, electrolyte, and weight loss; muscle atrophy; and psychologic stress. These changes begin on the first day of bed rest and continue for the duration of therapy. Sibai (2002) recommends rest at home, rather than strict bed rest, and allows a woman hospitalized with mild preeclampsia to be out of bed.

Women with mild preeclampsia feel reasonably well; boredom from activity restriction is therefore common. Diversionary activities, visits from friends, telephone conversations, and creation of a comfortable and convenient environment are ways to cope with the boredom (Patient Instructions for Self-Care box). Gentle exercise (e.g., range of motion, stretching, Kegel exercises, pelvic tilts) is important in maintaining muscle tone, blood flow, regularity

of bowel function, and a sense of well-being (Maloni & Kutil, 2000; Maloni, 2002). Relaxation techniques can help reduce the stress associated with the high risk condition and prepare the woman for labor and birth.

Diet. Diet and fluid recommendations are much the same as for healthy pregnant women. Diets high in protein and low in salt have been suggested to prevent preeclampsia; however, the efficacy of this has not been proven. Sibai (2004) recommends a regular diet with no restriction of salt. The exception may be the woman with chronic hypertension that was successfully controlled with a low-salt diet before the pregnancy. Adequate fluid intake helps maintain optimum fluid volume and aids in renal perfusion and filtration. The nurse uses assessment data regarding the woman's diet to counsel her in areas of deficiency, as needed (Patient Instructions for Self-Care box).

PATIENT INSTRUCTIONS FOR SELF-CARE
Coping with Bed Rest

QUESTIONS FOR HEALTH CARE PROVIDERS

Clarify with your health care provider: What is bed rest? Question your activity level, positioning, driving, bathroom privileges, working inside the home, child care activities, personal hygiene, mobility, stairs, diet, visitors, and sexual activity.

When should I contact my OB provider?

How often will I need to see my OB provider and what tests will be required and why?

If my pregnancy does not go to term, where will I give birth and who will be my doctor and the baby's doctor?

Will I need to take any medications at home? If so, why?

Will I have any home monitoring equipment or health care providers making home visits?

What symptoms would require me to go to the hospital?

SURVIVING BED REST—TIPS FOR HOME

Stock mini-fridge or cooler with healthy snacks and beverages.

Develop a schedule and follow—pay bills on Monday, make a grocery list on Tuesday.

Contact post office and delivery companies to allow them to leave packages with specific neighbors or ask that signature requirement be waived and package left at door.

Have computer available at bedside or use a laptop. Use for communication with friends, to conduct business, and to shop as necessary. Also use to communicate with Internet support groups and obtain information.

Order supplies, such as stamps, by Internet or phone.

Have a TV and CD with remote, and record programs to watch when bored.

Delegate responsibilities—laundry, pick up groceries, dry cleaning, meet repair people, child care, organize meals.

Have a portable phone bedside—schedule appointments by phone, parent teacher conferences.

Have available:
- Post-it notes
- Cups with lids and flexible straws
- Paper plates
- Plastic forks, spoons, and knives
- Baby monitor or walkie talkies
- Wet wipes
- Big trashbasket
- Notebook to record questions for providers, phone numbers, to-do lists
- Rollable cart or easily moved crate to keep items organized
- Pillows and more pillows (body pillow)
- Eggcrate mattress
- Envelopes and stationery
- Take-out menus
- Telephone answering machine or service
- Reading materials
- Movies/CDs

Plan for family time—visits and interaction, particularly with small children

If possible, hire:
- Housecleaning
- Lawn care
- Child care assistance

Share/trade magazines with friends.

Explore your interest in a new hobby—needlework, new reading content area.

Track your medicine—recording type/times/amount to minimize errors.

Monitor and record a daily fetal movement count.

Question your OB provider regarding the availability of a physical therapist to minimize bed rest complications.

Identify relaxation exercises and activities (music) and implement.

Continued

PATIENT INSTRUCTIONS FOR SELF-CARE
Coping with Bed Rest—cont'd

Drink 6-8 glasses of water a day and eat foods high in fiber. Ask your health care provider if you may have a prenatal vitamin with a stool softener.

SURVIVING BED REST–TIPS FOR HOSPITAL

Clarify with your health care provider: What is bed rest? Question your activity level, positioning, bathroom privileges, children's visits, activities, personal hygiene, mobility, diet, and visitors.

In addition to survival tips for the home, the following may be useful in the hospital setting:

Bring your own pillow, shampoo, and conditioner. Have wheelchair for outside visits or visiting other antepartal patients.

Share/trade magazines with friends and other antepartal patients.

If possible, bring laptop with DVD capabilities to allow you to watch movies.

Ask friends to bring healthy food and snacks when visiting rather than flowers.

Explore your interest in hand-held games.

Explore your interest in a new hobby–needlework, new reading area.

Work with staff regarding scheduling–OB provider exams, vital signs, nursing assessments, etc.

Bring earplugs to block the hospital noise.

Ask for a room with a view.

Have a large calendar and clock for easy viewing. Record significant events on the calendar.

http://fpb.cwru.edu/Bedrest
http://www.momsonbedrest.com
Source: Maloni, J. (2002). Astronauts & pregnancy bed rest: What NASA is teaching us about inactivity. *AWHONN Lifelines, 6*(4), 318-323.
Maloni, J., & Kutil, R. (2000). Antepartum support group for women hospitalized on bed rest. *MCN American Journal of Maternal Child Nursing, 25*(4), 204-210.

PATIENT INSTRUCTIONS FOR SELF-CARE
Nutrition

- Eat a nutritious, balanced diet (60 to 70 g protein, 1200 mg calcium, and adequate zinc, magnesium, and vitamins). Consult with registered dietitian on the diet best suited for you as an individual.
- There is no sodium restriction; however, consider limiting excessively salty foods (luncheon meats, pretzels, potato chips, pickles, sauerkraut).
- Eat foods with roughage (whole grains, raw fruits, and vegetables).
- Drink six to eight 8-oz glasses of water per day.
- Avoid alcohol and tobacco, and limit caffeine intake.

Successful home care requires the woman to be well educated about preeclampsia and motivated to follow the plan of care. She must also be reliable about keeping appointments. The effects of illness, language, age, culture, beliefs, and support systems must be considered. The woman's support systems must be mobilized and involved in planning and implementing her care (Plan of Care).

Severe preeclampsia and HELLP syndrome

If the woman's condition worsens or she already has severe preeclampsia or HELLP syndrome and is critically ill, she should receive appropriate management (usually in a tertiary care center), ranging from immediate birth to conservative management of the pregnancy (ACOG, 2002; Sibai,

2004; Working Group, 2000). Recognition of the clinical and laboratory findings of severe preeclampsia or HELLP syndrome is important if early, aggressive therapy is to be initiated to prevent maternal and perinatal mortality. An unfavorable (uneffaced and undilated) cervix resulting from gestational age, the aggressive nature of this disorder, and the associated perinatal mortality support cesarean birth for these women.

The administration of magnesium sulfate as prophylaxis against seizures and an antihypertensive agent if diastolic BP is higher than 100 mm Hg to 110 mm Hg are important components of management. The woman with severe preeclampsia or HELLP syndrome has multiple problems, and nursing care must focus on both the mother and fetus.

Hospital care. Antepartum care focuses on stabilization and preparation for birth. The woman may be admitted to an antepartum or a labor and birth unit, depending on the hospital. If the woman's condition is severe, she may be placed in a medical intensive care unit for hemody-namic monitoring (ACOG, 2002). Maternal and fetal surveillance, patient education regarding the disease process, and supportive measures directed toward the woman and her family are initiated. Assessments include review of the cardiovascular system, pulmonary system, renal system, hematologic system, and CNS. Monitoring urinary output is critical because magnesium is excreted by the kidneys. Fetal assessments for well-being (e.g., NST, BPP, fetal movement counts) are important because of the potential for hypoxia related to uteroplacental insufficiency. Baseline laboratory assessments include metabolic studies for liver enzyme (AST, ALT, LDH) determination,

PLAN OF CARE *Mild Preeclampsia: Home Care*

NURSING DIAGNOSIS Risk for injury related to signs of preeclampsia

Expected Outcomes *Woman will demonstrate ability to assess self and fetus for signs of worsening preeclampsia; no adverse sequelae will occur as result of preeclamptic condition.*

Nursing Interventions/*Rationales*

- Review warning signs and symptoms of preeclampsia *to ensure adequate knowledge base exists for decision making.*
- Assess home environment, including woman's ability to assume self-care responsibilities, support systems, language, age, culture, beliefs, and effects of illness, *to determine if home care is viable option.*
- Teach woman how to do a self-assessment for clinical signs of preeclampsia (take and record blood pressure, measure urine protein, assess edema formation, assess fetal activity) *to obtain immediate evidence of a worsening condition.*
- Teach woman to report any increases in blood pressure, 2$^+$ proteinuria, presence of edema, and decreased fetal activity to her health care provider immediately *to prevent worsening of preeclamptic condition.*
- Teach woman about use of rest and relaxation as palliative treatment options *to decrease blood pressure and promote diuresis.*

NURSING DIAGNOSIS Fear or anxiety related to preeclampsia and its effect on the fetus

Expected Outcome *Woman's feelings and symptoms of fear or anxiety will decrease or ease.*

Nursing Interventions/*Rationales*

- Provide a calm, soothing atmosphere and teach family *to provide emotional support to facilitate coping.*

- Encourage verbalization of fears *to decrease intensity of emotional response.*
- Involve woman and family in the management of her preeclamptic condition *to promote a greater sense of control.*
- Help woman identify and use appropriate coping strategies and support systems *to reduce fear and anxiety.*
- Explore use of desensitization strategies such as progressive muscle relaxation, visual imagery, or thought stopping *to reduce fear-related emotions and related physical symptoms.*

NURSING DIAGNOSIS Deficient diversional activity related to imposed bed rest

Expected Outcome *Woman will verbalize diminished feelings of boredom.*

Nursing Interventions/*Rationales*

- Assist woman to explore creative personally meaningful activities that can be pursued from the bed *to promote activities that have meaning, purpose, and value to the individual.*
- Maintain emphasis on personal choices of woman *to promote control and minimize imposition of routines by others.*
- Evaluate what support and system resources are available in the environment *to assist in providing diversional activities.*
- Explore ways for woman to remain an active participant in home management and decision making *to promote control.*
- Engage support of family and friends in carrying out chosen activities and making necessary environmental alterations *to ensure success.*
- Teach woman about stress management and relaxation techniques *to help manage tension of confinement.*

CD: Plan of Care—Mild Preeclampsia Home Care

---

complete blood count with platelets, coagulation profile to assess for DIC, and electrolyte studies to establish renal functioning.

Weight is measured on admission and every day thereafter at the same time. An indwelling urinary catheter facilitates monitoring of renal function and effectiveness of therapy but is used only in women with severe preeclampsia, eclampsia, or HELLP syndrome. If appropriate, vaginal examination may be done to check for cervical changes. Abdominal palpation establishes uterine tonicity and fetal size, activity, and position. Electronic monitoring to determine fetal status is initiated at least once a day. The nurse's skill in implementing the techniques described here can be reassuring to the woman and her family. The woman's room must be close to staff and emergency drugs, supplies, and equipment. Noise and external stimuli must be minimized. Seizure precautions are taken (Box 23-4).

Bed rest or restricted activity is commonly ordered, although there is a lack of scientific evidence to support the efficacy of these restrictions (ACOG, 2002; Enkin et al., 2001). The nurse's ingenuity may be called on to help the

woman cope physically and psychologically with the side effects of immobility and an environment limited in stimuli and support. Thromboembolic events, a risk factor during normal pregnancy, pose an even greater risk with preeclampsia (Plan of Care).

Intrapartum nursing care of the woman with severe preeclampsia or HELLP syndrome involves continuous monitoring of maternal and fetal status as labor progresses. The assessment and prevention of tissue hypoxia and hemorrhage, both of which can lead to permanent compromise of vital organs, continue throughout the intrapartum and postpartum periods (Sibai, 2004).

Magnesium sulfate. One of the important goals of care for the woman with severe preeclampsia is prevention or control of convulsions. Magnesium sulfate is the drug of choice in the prevention and treatment of convulsions caused by preeclampsia or eclampsia (ACOG, 2002; Cunningham et al., 2005; Nick, 2004). The routine use of magnesium sulfate is indicated for severe preeclampsia, HELLP syndrome, or eclampsia. However, no data support the routine use of magnesium sulfate for women diagnosed

---

BOX 23-4

Hospital Precautionary Measures

- Environment
  - Quiet
  - Nonstimulating
  - Lighting subdued
- Seizure precautions
  - Suction equipment tested and ready to use
  - Oxygen administration equipment tested and ready to use
- Call button within easy reach
- Emergency medication tray immediately accessible
  - Hydralazine and magnesium sulfate in or adjacent to woman's room
  - Calcium gluconate immediately available
- Emergency birth pack accessible

---

with mild preeclampsia or gestational hypertension (Working Group, 2000).

Magnesium sulfate is administered as a secondary infusion (piggyback) to the main intravenous (IV) line by volumetric infusion pump. An initial loading dose of 4 to 6 g of magnesium sulfate per protocol or physician's order is infused over 15 to 20 minutes. This dose is followed by a maintenance dose of magnesium sulfate that is diluted in an IV solution per physician's order (e.g., 40 g of magnesium sulfate in 1000 ml of lactated Ringer's solution) and administered by infusion pump at 2 g/hr (Cunningham et al., 2005). This dose should maintain a therapeutic serum magnesium level of 4 to 7 mEq/L (Cunningham et al., 2005; Nick, 2004). Levels of magnesium sulfate are often checked daily (Gilbert & Harmon, 2003). After the loading dose, there may be a transient lowering of the arterial BP secondary to relaxation of smooth muscle by the magnesium sulfate. For the initial 24 hours postpartum, magnesium sulfate is usually continued intravenously (Box 23-5).

Intramuscular (IM) magnesium sulfate is rarely used because absorption rate cannot be controlled, injections are painful, and tissue necrosis may occur. However, the IM route may be used with some women who are being transported to a tertiary care center. The IM dose is 4 to 5 g given in each buttock, a total of 10 g (with 1% procaine possibly

---

PLAN OF CARE *Severe Preeclampsia: Hospital Care*

NURSING DIAGNOSIS Risk for injury to woman and fetus related to CNS irritability

Expected Outcome *Woman will show diminished signs of CNS irritability (e.g., DTRs 2+, absence of clonus) and have no convulsions.*

Nursing Interventions/*Rationales*

- Establish baseline data (e.g., DTRs, clonus) *to use as basis for evaluating effectiveness of treatment.*
- Administer IV magnesium sulfate per physician's orders *to decrease hyperreflexia and minimize risk of convulsions.*
- Monitor maternal vital signs, FHR, urine output, DTRs, IV flow rate, and serum levels of magnesium sulfate *to assess for and prevent magnesium sulfate toxicity (e.g., depressed respirations, oliguria, sudden drop in blood pressure, hyporeflexia, fetal distress).*
- Have calcium gluconate at bedside *to be available if needed as antidote for magnesium sulfate toxicity.*
- Maintain a quiet, darkened environment *to avoid stimuli that may precipitate seizure activity.*

NURSING DIAGNOSIS Ineffective tissue perfusion related to preeclampsia secondary to arteriolar vasospasm

Expected Outcome *Woman will exhibit signs of increased vasodilation (i.e., diuresis, decreased edema, weight loss).*

Nursing Interventions/*Rationales*

- Establish baseline data (e.g., weight, degree of edema) *to use as basis for evaluating effectiveness of treatment.*
- Administer intravenous magnesium sulfate per physician order, *which serves to relax vasospasms and increase renal perfusion.*
- Place woman on bed rest in a side-lying position *to maximize uteroplacental blood flow, reduce blood pressure, and promote diuresis.*
- Monitor intake and output, edema, and weight *to assess for evidence of vasodilation and increased tissue perfusion.*

NURSING DIAGNOSIS Risk for

- excess fluid volume related to increased sodium retention secondary to administration of magnesium sulfate
- impaired gas exchange related to pulmonary edema secondary to increased vascular resistance
- decreased cardiac output related to use of antihypertensive drugs
- injury to fetus related to uteroplacental insufficiency secondary to use of antihypertensive medications

Expected Outcomes *Woman will exhibit signs of normal fluid volume (i.e., balanced intake and output, normal serum creatinine levels, normal breath sounds); adequate oxygenation (i.e., normal respirations, full orientation to person, time, and place); normal range of cardiac output (i.e., normal pulse rate and rhythm); and fetal well-being (i.e., adequate fetal movement, normal FHR).*

Nursing Interventions/*Rationales*

- Monitor woman for signs of fluid volume excess (increased edema, decreased urine output, elevated serum creatinine level, weight gain, dyspnea, crackles) *to detect potential complications.*
- Monitor woman for signs of impaired gas exchange (increased respirations, dyspnea, altered blood gases, hypoxemia) *to detect potential complications.*
- Monitor woman for signs of decreased cardiac output (altered pulse rate and rhythm) *to detect potential complications.*
- Monitor fetus for signs of difficulty (decreased fetal activity, decreased FHR) *to prevent complications.*
- Record findings and report signs of increasing problems to physician *to enable timely interventions.*

being added to the solution to reduce injection pain), and can be repeated at 4-hour intervals. Z-track technique should be used for the deep IM injection, followed by gentle massage at the site.

Magnesium sulfate interferes with the release of acetylcholine at the synapses, decreasing neuromuscular irritability, depressing cardiac conduction, and decreasing CNS irritability. Because magnesium circulates in a free state and unbound to protein and is excreted in the urine, accurate recordings of maternal urine output must be obtained and monitored. Diuresis is an excellent prognostic sign; however, if renal function declines, all of the magnesium sulfate will not be excreted and can cause magnesium toxicity.

Because magnesium sulfate is a CNS depressant, the nurse assesses for signs and symptoms of magnesium toxicity. Serum magnesium levels are obtained on the basis of the woman's response and if any signs of toxicity are present. Expected side effects of magnesium sulfate are a feeling of warmth, flushing, and nausea. Symptoms of mild toxicity include lethargy, muscle weakness, decreased DTRs, and slurred speech. Increasing toxicity may be indicated by maternal hypotension, bradycardia, bradypnea, and heart block (Nick, 2004).

NURSE ALERT *Loss of patellar reflexes, respiratory depression, oliguria, and decreased level of consciousness are signs of magnesium toxicity. Actions are needed to prevent respiratory or cardiac arrest. If magnesium toxicity is suspected, the infusion should be discontinued immediately. Calcium gluconate, the antidote for magnesium sulfate, may also be ordered (10 ml of a 10% solution, or 1 g) and given by slow IV push (usually by the physician) over at least 3 minutes to avoid undesirable reactions such as arrhythmias, bradycardia, and ventricular fibrillation (Cunningham et al., 2005; Nick, 2004; Sibai, 2002).*

BOX 23-5

Care of Patient with Preeclampsia Receiving Magnesium Sulfate

PATIENT AND FAMILY TEACHING
Explain technique, rationale, and reactions to expect
- Route and rate
- Purpose of "piggyback"
Reasons for use
- Tailor information to woman's readiness to learn
- Explain that magnesium sulfate is used to prevent disease progression
- Explain that magnesium sulfate is used to prevent seizures
Reactions to expect from medication
- Initially woman will feel flushed, hot, sedated, nauseated, and may experience burning at the IV site, especially during the bolus.
- Sedation will continue
Monitoring to anticipate
- Maternal: blood pressure, pulse, DTRs, level of consciousness, urine output (indwelling catheter), presence of headache, visual disturbances, epigastric pain
- Fetal: FHR and activity

ADMINISTRATION
- Verify physician order
- Position woman in side-lying position
- Prepare solution and administer with an infusion control device (pump)
- Piggyback a solution of 40 g of magnesium sulfate in 1000 ml lactated Ringer's solution with an infusion control device at the ordered rate: loading dose—initial bolus of 4 to 6 g over 15 to 30 min; maintenance dose—1 to 3 g/hr

MATERNAL AND FETAL ASSESSMENTS
- Monitor blood pressure, pulse, respiratory rate, FHR, and contractions every 15 to 30 min, depending on woman's condition

- Monitor intake and output, proteinuria, DTRs, presence of headache, visual disturbances, level of consciousness, and epigastric pain at least hourly
- Restrict hourly fluid intake to a total of 100 to 125 ml/hr; urinary output should be at least 30 ml/hr

REPORTABLE CONDITIONS
- Blood pressure: systolic ≥160 mm Hg, diastolic ≥110 mm Hg, or both
- Respiratory rate: ≤12 breaths/min
- Urinary output <30 ml/hr
- Presence of headache, visual disturbances, or epigastric pain
- Increasing severity or loss of DTRs; increasing edema, proteinuria
- Any abnormal laboratory values (magnesium levels, platelet count, creatinine clearance, levels of uric acid, AST, ALT, prothrombin time, partial thromboplastin time, fibrinogen, fibrin split products)
- Any other significant change in maternal or fetal status

EMERGENCY MEASURES
- Keep emergency drug tray at bedside with calcium gluconate and intubation equipment
- Keep side rails up
- Keep lights dimmed, and maintain a quiet environment

DOCUMENTATION
- All of the above

DTRs, Deep tendon reflexes; *FHR,* fetal heart rate; *AST,* aspirate aminotransferase; *ALT,* alanine aminotransferase.

NURSE ALERT *Because magnesium sulfate is also a tocolytic agent, its use may increase the duration of labor. A preeclamptic woman receiving magnesium sulfate may need augmentation with oxytocin during labor. The amount of oxytocin needed to stimulate labor may be more than that needed for a woman who is not receiving magnesium sulfate.*

Control of blood pressure. For the severely hypertensive preeclamptic woman, antihypertensive medications may be ordered to lower the diastolic BP. Initiation of antihypertensive therapy reduces maternal morbidity and mortality rates associated with left ventricular failure and cerebral hemorrhage. Because a degree of maternal hypertension is necessary to maintain uteroplacental perfusion, antihypertensive therapy must not decrease the arterial pressure too much or too rapidly. The target range for the diastolic pressure is therefore less than 110 mm Hg and the systolic pressure less than 160 mm Hg (ACOG, 2002; Cunningham et al., 2005; Sibai, Dekker, & Kupferminc, 2005).

IV hydralazine remains the antihypertensive agent of choice for the treatment of hypertension in severe preeclampsia (ACOG, 2002; Cunningham et al., 2005). IV labetalol hydrochloride, nifedipine, verapamil, and oral methyldopa are also used (ACOG, 2002; Cunningham et al., 2005). The choice of agent used depends on patient response and physician preference. Table 23-5 compares antihypertensive agents used to treat hypertension in pregnancy.

Magnesium sulfate does not seem to affect FHR in a healthy term fetus. Neonatal serum magnesium levels approximate those levels of the mother (Cunningham et al., 2005). Magnesium sulfate dosage levels adequate to prevent maternal seizures have been determined to be safe for the fetus with neonatal levels nearly equal with maternal levels (Cunningham et al., 2005). Toxic levels in the newborn can cause neonatal depression and occur with "severe" hypermagnesemia at birth (Cunningham et al., 2005). Although rarely needed, calcium and exchange transfusion with mechanical ventilation can be used to treat infants with hypermagnesmia. Long-term effects of magnesium administration on mothers and infants is under study (Magpie Trial Follow-Up Study Management, 2004).

Eclampsia

If eclampsia develops after the initiation of magnesium sulfate therapy, additional magnesium sulfate or another anticonvulsant (e.g., diazepam) may be administered (Roberts, 2004). With adequate blood magnesium levels, the eclamptic woman will rarely continue to have seizures. Approximately 20% of women with eclampsia do not follow the progression from mild disease to convulsion with the abrupt onset of seizures (Sibai, Dekker, & Kupferminc, 2005). However, diazepam is not without fetal and neonatal effects. The FHR loses variability. In the neonate there is depressed sucking ability, hypotonia, and decreased respirations (Weiner & Buhimschi, 2004). The convulsions that occur in eclampsia are frightening to observe. Increased hypertension and tonic contraction of all body muscles (seen as arms flexed, hands clenched, legs inverted) precede the tonic-clonic convulsions (Fig. 23-5). During this stage, muscles alternately relax and contract. Respirations are halted and then begin again with long, deep, stertorous inhalations. Hypotension follows, and coma ensues. Nystagmus and muscular twitching persist for a time. Disorientation and amnesia cloud the immediate recovery. Oliguria and anuria are notable. Seizures may recur within minutes of the first convulsion, or the woman may never have another. Eclamptic seizures can result in tissue damage to the woman during the convulsion, especially if she is in a bed with unpadded side rails. During the convulsion the pregnant woman and fetus are not receiving oxygen, so eclamptic seizures produce a marked metabolic insult to both the woman and the fetus (Cunningham et al., 2005; Sibai, Dekker, & Kupferminc, 2005).

Immediate care. The immediate care during a convulsion is to ensure a patent airway and maintain oxygenation (Emergency box). When convulsions occur, the woman is turned onto her side to prevent aspiration of vomitus and supine hypotension syndrome. After the convulsion ceases, food and fluid are suctioned from the glottis or trachea, and oxygen is administered by face mask. The drug of choice, magnesium sulfate (e.g., 2 to 4 g) is given via IV push and repeated every 15 minutes with a maximum of 6 g. Alternatively another anticonvulsant other than magnesium sulfate such as diazepam may be given (ACOG, 2002; Cunningham et al., 2005; Sibai, Dekker, & Kupferminc, 2005). If an IV is not already infusing then one is begun with at least an 18-gauge needle. Time, duration, and description of convulsions are recorded, and any urinary or fecal incontinence is noted. The fetus is monitored for adverse effects. Transient fetal bradycardia, decreased FHR variability, and compensatory tachycardia are common.

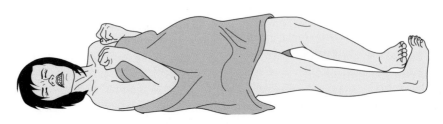

Fig. 23-5 Eclampsia (convulsions or seizures).

TABLE 23-5

Pharmacologic Control of Hypertension in Pregnancy

ACTION	TARGET TISSUE	EFFECTS MATERNAL	FETAL	NURSING ACTIONS
HYDRALAZINE (APRESOLINE, NEOPRESOL)				
Arteriolar vasodilator	Peripheral arterioles: to decrease muscle tone, decrease peripheral resistance; hypothalamus and medullary vasomotor center for minor decrease in sympathetic tone	Headache, flushing, palpitation, tachycardia, some decrease in uteroplacental blood flow, increase in heart rate and cardiac output, increase in oxygen consumption, nausea and vomiting	Tachycardia; late decelerations and bradycardia if maternal diastolic pressure <90 mm Hg	Assess for effects of medications, alert mother (family) to expected effects of medications, assess blood pressure frequently because precipitous drop can lead to shock and perhaps abruptio placentae; assess urinary output; maintain bed rest in a lateral position with side rails up; use with caution in presence of maternal tachycardia
LABETALOL HYDROCHLORIDE (NORMODYNE)				
Beta-blocking agent causing vasodilation without significant change in cardiac output	Peripheral arterioles (see hydralazine)	Minimal: flushing, tremulousness; minimal change in pulse rate	Minimal, if any	See hydralazine; less likely to cause excessive hypotension and tachycardia; less rebound hypertension than hydralazine
METHYLDOPA (ALDOMET)				
Maintenance therapy if needed: 250-500 mg orally every 8 hr (α_2-receptor agonist)	Postganglionic nerve endings: interferes with chemical neurotransmission to reduce peripheral vascular resistance; causes CNS sedation	Sleepiness, postural hypotension, constipation; rare: drug-induced fever in 1% of women and positive Coombs' test result in 20%	After 4 mo maternal therapy, positive Coombs' test result in infant	See hydralazine
NIFEDIPINE (PROCARDIA)				
Calcium channel blocker	Arterioles: to reduce systemic vascular resistance by relaxation of arterial smooth muscle	Headache, flushing; possible potentiation of effects on CNS if administered concurrently with magnesium sulfate; may interfere with labor	Minimal	See hydralazine; use caution if patient also receiving magnesium sulfate

CNS, Central nervous system.

Aspiration is a leading cause of maternal morbidity and mortality after eclamptic seizure. After initial stabilization and airway management, the nurse should anticipate orders for a chest radiograph and possibly arterial blood gases to rule out the possibility of aspiration.

A rapid assessment of uterine activity, cervical status, and fetal status is performed after a convulsion. During the convulsion, membranes may have ruptured; the cervix may have dilated because the uterus becomes hypercontractile and hypertonic; and birth may be imminent. If not, once a woman's seizure activity and BP are controlled, a decision should be made regarding whether birth should take place. The target levels for blood pressure management are a systolic blood pressure between 140 mm Hg and 160 mm Hg and a diastolic between 90 mm Hg and 110 mm Hg. Blood pressure may be managed with hydralazine (10 mg doses) or

EMERGENCY

Eclampsia

TONIC-CLONIC CONVULSION SIGNS

- Stage of invasion: 2 to 3 sec, eyes are fixed, twitching of facial muscles occurs
- Stage of contraction: 15 to 20 sec, eyes protrude and are bloodshot, all body muscles are in tonic contraction
- Stage of convulsion: muscles relax and contract alternately (clonic), respirations are halted and then begin again with long, deep, stertorous inhalation, coma ensues

INTERVENTION

- Keep airway patent: turn head to one side, place pillow under one shoulder or back if possible
- Call for assistance
- Protect with side rails up
- Observe and record convulsion activity

AFTER CONVULSION OR SEIZURE

- Do not leave unattended until fully alert
- Observe for postconvulsion coma, incontinence
- Use suction as needed
- Administer oxygen via face mask at 10 L/min
- Start intravenous fluids, and monitor for potential fluid overload
- Give magnesium sulfate or other anticonvulsant drug as ordered
- Insert indwelling urinary catheter
- Monitor blood pressure
- Monitor fetal and uterine status
- Expedite laboratory work as ordered to monitor kidney function, liver function, coagulation system, and drug levels
- Provide hygiene and a quiet environment
- Support and keep woman and family informed
- Be prepared for assisting with birth when woman is in stable condition

labetalol (20-40 mg intravenously) every 15 minutes (Sibai, 2005). The more serious the condition of the woman, the greater the need to proceed to birth. The route of birth–induction of labor versus cesarean birth–depends on maternal and fetal condition, fetal gestational age, presence of labor and the cervical Bishop score (Sibai, Dekker, & Kupferminc, 2005). In pregnancies of less than 34 weeks of gestation, antenatal corticosteroids may be given to promote fetal lung maturation. If the birth can be delayed for 48 hours, steroids such as betamethasone (12 mg IM 24 hours apart) may be given to the woman (Cunningham et al., 2005; Sibai, Dekker, & Kupferminc, 2005). General anesthesia is generally not recommended as there is an increased risk of aspiration but maternal pain can be controlled with epidural anesthesia or systemic opioids. Regional anesthesia is not recommended for eclamptic women with coagulopathy or a platelet count less than 50,000 (Sibai, Dekker, & Kupferminc, 2005).

The woman may have been incontinent of urine and stool during the convulsion; she will need assistance with hygiene and a change of gown. Oral care with a soft toothbrush may be of comfort.

Immediately after a seizure, the woman may be confused and can be combative, necessitating the temporary use of restraints. It may take several hours for the woman to regain her usual level of mental functioning. The health care provider explains procedures briefly and quietly. The woman is never left alone. The family is also kept informed of management, rationale for treatment, and the woman's progress.

Laboratory tests are ordered to assess for HELLP syndrome and to have blood typed and crossmatched for administration of packed red blood cells as needed. Blood is available for emergency transfusion because abruptio placentae, with accompanying hemorrhage and shock, often occurs in women with eclampsia. Other tests include determination of electrolyte levels, liver function battery, and complete hemogram and clotting profile, including platelet count and fibrin split product levels (to assess for DIC).

If the maternal-fetal dyad's condition deteriorates, a urinary catheter is inserted, and, to monitor fluid status, measurement of central venous pressure (CVP) or pulmonary artery wedge pressure (PAWP) may be required.

Postpartum nursing care

After birth the symptoms of preeclampsia or eclampsia resolve quickly, usually within 48 hours. The hematopoietic and hepatic complications of HELLP syndrome may persist longer. Affected patients often show an abrupt decrease in platelet count, with a concomitant increase in LDH and AST levels, after a trend toward normalization of values has begun. Generally the laboratory abnormalities seen with HELLP syndrome resolve in 72 to 96 hours.

The nursing care of the woman with hypertensive disease differs from that required in the usual postpartum period in a number of respects. The following variations in the nursing process are described.

Careful assessment of the woman with a hypertensive disorder continues throughout the postpartum period. Nursing care will include monitoring of vital signs, increased amounts of intravenous fluids intrapartally and postpartum and subsequent monitoring of intake and outpout and close monitoring of symptoms. BP is measured at least every 4 hours for 48 hours or more frequently as the woman's condition warrants. Even if no convulsions occurred before the birth, they may occur within this period. Magnesium sulfate infusion may be continued 24 hours after the birth. Assessments for effects and side effects continue until the medication is discontinued.

Later postpartum eclampsia is eclampsia occurring after 48 hours but prior to 4 postpartal weeks. These women may present with clinical manifestations of preeclampsia intrapartal or during the immediate postpartum though other women present with the initial symptoms and convulsions after 48 hours postpartum (Sibai, Dekker, & Kupferminc, 2005).

NURSE ALERT *The woman is at risk for a boggy uterus and a large lochia flow as a result of the magnesium sulfate therapy. Uterine tone and lochial flow must be monitored closely.*

The preeclamptic woman is unable to tolerate excessive postpartum blood loss because of hemoconcentration. Oxytocin or prostaglandin products are used to control bleeding. Ergot products (e.g., Ergotrate, Methergine) are contraindicated because they can increase BP. The woman is asked to report symptoms such as headaches and blurred vision. The nurse assesses affect, LOC, BP, pulse, and respiratory status before an analgesic is given for headache. Magnesium sulfate potentiates the action of narcotics, CNS depressants, and calcium channel blockers; these drugs must be administered with caution. The woman may need to continue an antihypertensive medication regimen if her diastolic BP exceeds 100 mm Hg at hospital discharge.

The woman's and family's responses to labor, birth, and the neonate are monitored. Interactions and involvement in the care of the neonate are encouraged to the extent that the woman and her family desire. In addition, the woman and her family need opportunities to discuss their emotional response to complications. The nurse provides information concerning the prognosis. There is a sevenfold increase in the risk of recurrence of preeclampsia and eclampsia in women who developed preeclampsia or eclampsia in their first pregnancy (Duckitt & Harrington, 2005).

Prevention

Early prenatal care for identification of women at risk and early detection of development of preeclampsia is the best prevention because there is no known etiology for preeclampsia. There have been numerous clinical trials studying various methods for prevention. These interventions included the use of low-dose aspirin, antioxidants, calcium, magnesium, zinc, and fish oil dietary supplementation, protein or sodium restriction, heparin or low molecular weight heparin administration and antihypertensive medications in women with chronic hypertension (Sibai, Dekker, & Kupferminc, 2005). Continued research is necessary to identify strategies to reduce the incidence or severity of preeclampsia in healthy pregnant women. Nurses should be aware of what strategies are being studied and use the most reliable evidence about the results so that they can counsel pregnant women about interventions that are evidenced based and likely to be beneficial (Enkin et al., 2001). One excellent resource for evidence-based care is the Cochrane Pregnancy and Childbirth Database (Callister & Hobbins-Garbett, 2000).

Chronic hypertension

Chronic hypertension occurs in up to 5% of pregnant women, with the incidence higher in African-American women and in women older than 40 years of age (Livingston & Sibai, 2001). Chronic hypertension in pregnancy is associated with increased incidence of abruptio placentae, su-

perimposed preeclampsia, and an increased perinatal death rate (threefold to fourfold) (Cunningham et al., 2005). Fetal effects include fetal growth restriction and small-for-gestational-age (SGA) infants (Cunningham et al., 2005; Livingston & Sibai, 2001; Roberts, 2004). Ideally, women with chronic hypertension should be screened preconceptionally. Medications that may be teratogenic, such as angiotensin converting enzyme inhibitors, should be reviewed (Peters & Flack, 2004). Women who are at high risk are usually managed with antihypertensive therapy and frequent assessments of maternal and fetal well-being. Methyldopa (Aldomet) is usually the drug of choice, although beta-blockers and calcium channel blockers are also used (Chan & Johnson, 2006; Cunningham et al., 2005; Working Group, 2000). Women at low risk for complications may be monitored closely, and antihypertensive therapy used as needed. As for any individual with hypertension, lifestyle changes are recommended. These changes include limiting sodium intake, performing exercise as appropriate, ingesting a balanced diet, limiting caffeine intake, and avoiding alcohol and tobacco (Gilbert & Harmon, 2003). Women at low risk may be induced at approximately 40 weeks of gestation. In contrast, women at high risk are followed closely, and method and timing of birth are dependent on maternal and fetal status. Postpartally, women with chronic hypertension are at risk for complications such as renal failure, pulmonary edema, and heart failure. In addition, BP should be closely evaluated at the 6-week postpartal visit to ascertain need for antihypertensive therapy. As all antihypertensive medications are found in breast milk, the drug of choice for women desiring to breastfeed primarily is methyldopa.

Evaluation

Evaluation of the effectiveness of care of the woman with high blood pressure in pregnancy is based on the expected outcomes.

HYPEREMESIS GRAVIDARUM

Nausea and vomiting complicate approximately 70% of all pregnancies beginning typically at 4 to 6 weeks of gestation and are generally confined to the first trimester or the first 16 to 20 weeks of gestation, peaking from 8 to 12 weeks of gestation (Cunningham et al., 2005; Scott & Abu-Hamda, 2004). Although these manifestations are distressing, they are typically benign, with no significant metabolic alterations or risks to the mother or fetus. Theories include increasing levels of estrogens, human chorionic gonadotropin, transient maternal hyperthyroidism, stress and interrelated psychosocial components (Davis, 2004; Meighan & Wood, 2004; Scott & Abu-Hamda, 2004).

When vomiting during pregnancy becomes excessive enough to cause weight loss of at least 5% of prepregnancy weight and is accompanied by dehydration, electrolyte imbalance, ketosis, and acetonuria, the disorder is termed *hyperemesis gravidarum*. The estimated incidence varies from 3.3 to 10 per 1000 births (Scott & Abu-Hamda, 2004). Approximately 1% of women require hospitalization. Hyperemesis gravidarum usually begins during the first 10 weeks of pregnancy. Hyperemesis gravidarum has been associated with women who are nulliparous, have increased body weight, have a history of migraines, are pregnant with twins (Davis, 2004; Scott & Abu-Hamda, 2004), or hydatifiform mole (Berman, Di Saia, & Tewari, 2004). In addition, an interrelated psychologic component has been associated with hyperemesis and must be assessed. (Cunningham et al., 2005; Scott & Abu-Hamda, 2004). The effects of hyperemesis gravidarum on perinatal outcome vary with the severity of the disorder. Women with hyperemesis gravidarum have a decreased risk of miscarriage (Scott & Abu-Hamda, 2004).

Etiology

The etiology of hyperemesis gravidarum remains obscure. Several theories have been proposed as to the cause, although none of them adequately explains the disorder. Hyperemesis gravidarum may be related to high levels of estrogen or human chorionic gonadotropin (hCG) and may be associated with transient hyperthyroidism during pregnancy. Some research has found a woman who has severe nausea and vomiting has a 1.5 increased chance of carrying a female infant, supporting the association between increased estrogen exposure and hyperemesis gravidarum (Cunningham, et al., 2005; Davis, 2004). Esophageal reflux, reduced gastric motility, and decreased secretion of free hydrochloric acid may contribute to the disorder.

Psychosocial factors also may play a part in the development of hyperemesis gravidarum for some women. Ambivalence toward the pregnancy and increased stress may be associated with this condition (Cunningham et al., 2005; Davis, 2004; Scott & Abu-Hamda, 2004). Conflicting feelings regarding prospective motherhood, body changes, and lifestyle alterations may contribute to episodes of vomiting, particularly if these feelings are excessive or unresolved.

Clinical Manifestations

The woman with hyperemesis gravidarum usually has significant weight loss and dehydration. She may have a decreased BP, increased pulse rate, and poor skin turgor (Scott & Abu-Hamda, 2004). She frequently is unable to keep down even clear liquids taken by mouth. Laboratory tests may reveal electrolyte imbalances.

Collaborative Care

Whenever a pregnant woman has nausea and vomiting, the first priority is a thorough assessment to determine the severity of the problem. In most cases the woman should be told to come immediately to the health care provider's office or to the emergency department, because the severity of the illness is often difficult to determine by phone conversation.

The assessment should include frequency, severity, and duration of episodes of nausea and vomiting. If the woman reports vomiting, then the assessment should also include the approximate amount and color of the vomitus. Other symptoms such as diarrhea, indigestion, and abdominal pain or distention are also identified. The woman is asked to report any precipitating factors relating to the onset of her symptoms. Any pharmacologic or nonpharmacologic treatment measures should be recorded. Prepregnancy weight and documented weight gain or loss during pregnancy are important to note.

The woman's weight and vital signs are measured and a complete physical examination is performed, with attention to signs of fluid and electrolyte imbalance and nutritional status. The most important initial laboratory test to be obtained is a dipstick determination of ketonuria. Other laboratory tests that may be ordered are a urinalysis, a complete blood cell count, electrolytes, liver enzymes, and bilirubin levels. These tests help rule out the presence of underlying diseases such as pyelonephritis, pancreatitis, cholecystitis, and hepatitis (Cunningham et al., 2005). Because of the recognized association between hyperemesis gravidarum and hyperthyroidism, thyroid levels may also be measured (Scott & Abu-Hamda, 2004).

Psychosocial assessment includes asking the woman about anxiety, fears, and concerns related to her own health and the effects on pregnancy outcome. Family members should be assessed both for anxiety and with regard to their role in providing support for the woman.

Initial care

Initially, the woman who is unable to keep down clear liquids by mouth will require IV therapy for correction of fluid and electrolyte imbalances. She should be kept on nothing-by-mouth (NPO) status until dehydration has been resolved and for at least 48 hours after vomiting has stopped to prevent rapid recurrence of the problem. In the past, women requiring IV therapy were admitted to the hospital. Today, however, they may be, and often are, successfully managed at home, even if on enteral therapy. Medications may be used if nausea and vomiting are uncontrolled. The most frequently prescribed drugs include pyridoxine (B_6) (25 mg to 75 mg daily) alone or in combination with doxylamine (Unisom) (25 mg), promethazine (Phenergan), and metoclopramide (Reglan) (ACOG, 2004a; Cunningham et al., 2005; Weiner & Buhimschi, 2004). Other less commonly used drugs include meclizine (Antivert), dimenhydrinate (Dramamine), diphenhydramine (Benadryl), prochlorperazine (Compazine), and ondansetron (Zofran) (Cunningham et al., 2005). Corticosteroids (methylprednisolone [Medrol]) may also be used to treat refractory hyperemesis gravidarum (Cunningham et al., 2005). Lastly, enteral or parenteral nutrition may be used for women nonresponsive to other medical therapies (Cunningham et al., 2005). In addition to medical management, some women can also benefit from psychotherapy or stress reduction techniques (Scott & Abu-Hamda, 2004). Once the vomiting has stopped, feedings are started in small amounts at frequent intervals, and the diet is slowly advanced as tolerated until the woman can consume a nutritionally sound diet.

Nursing care of the woman with hyperemesis gravidarum involves implementing the medical plan of care, whether this care be given in the hospital or home setting. Interventions may include initiating and monitoring IV therapy, administering drugs and nutritional supplements, and monitoring the woman's response to interventions. The nurse observes the woman for any signs of complications such as metabolic acidosis (secondary to starvation), jaundice, or hemorrhage and alerts the physician should these occur. Monitoring includes assessment of the woman's nausea, retching without vomiting, and vomiting as the two symptoms while related are separate. A standardized assessment tool such as the PUQE (pregnancy-unique quantification of emesis and nausea) allows quantification of the presence and severity of the nausea and vomiting and promotes accurate monitoring (Davis, 2004).

Accurate measurement of intake and output, including the amount of emesis, is an important aspect of care. Oral hygiene while the woman is receiving nothing by mouth, and after episodes of vomiting, helps allay associated discomforts. Assistance with positioning and providing a quiet, restful environment, free from odors, may increase the woman's comfort. When the woman begins responding to therapy, limited amounts of oral fluids and bland foods such as crackers, toast, or baked chicken are begun. The diet is progressed slowly as tolerated by the woman until she is able to consume a nutritional diet. Because sleep disturbances may accompany hyperemesis gravidarum, promoting adequate rest is important. The nurse can assist in coordinating treatment measures and periods of visitation to provide opportunity for rest periods.

Follow-up Care

Most women are able to take nourishment by mouth after several days of treatment. Women should be encouraged to eat small, frequent meals consisting of low-fat, high-protein foods; to avoid greasy and highly seasoned foods; and to increase dietary intake of potassium and magnesium. Herbal teas such as ginger, chamomile, or raspberry leaf may decrease nausea (Nursing 2006; Jewell & Young, 2003; Smith, Crowther, Willson, Hotham, & McMillian, 2004; Tiran & Mack, 2000). Many pregnant women find exposure to cooking odors nauseating. Having other family members cook may lessen the woman's nausea and vomiting, even if only temporarily. Dietary instructions include ingestion of dry, bland foods, high protein foods, small, frequent meals, cold foods, of a snack before bedtime, drinking liquids from a cup with a lid, and tea or water with lemon slices, and avoidance of high fat or spicy foods (Davis, 2004). The woman is counseled to contact her health care provider if the nausea and vomiting recur. Complications accompanying severe hyperemesis gravidarum include esophageal rupture, and deficiencies of vitamin k and thiamine with resulting Wernicke encephalopathy (central nervous system involvement) (Cunningham et al., 2005).

A few women will continue to experience intractable nausea and vomiting throughout pregnancy. Rarely, it may be necessary to maintain a woman on enteral, parenteral, or total parenteral nutrition to ensure adequate nutrition for the mother and fetus (Cunningham et al., 2005). Many home health agencies are able to provide these services, and arrangements for service may be made depending on the woman's insurance coverage.

The woman with hyperemesis gravidarum needs calm, compassionate, and sympathetic care, with recognition that the manifestations of hyperemesis can be physically and emotionally debilitating to the patient and stressful for the family. Irritability, tearfulness, and mood changes are often consistent with this disorder. Fetal well-being is a primary concern of the woman. The nurse can provide an environment conducive to discussion of concerns and assist the woman and family in identifying and mobilizing sources of support. The family should be included in the plan of care whenever possible. Their participation may help alleviate some of the emotional stress associated with this disorder.

HEMORRHAGIC COMPLICATIONS ■

Bleeding in pregnancy may jeopardize both maternal and fetal well-being and is the second leading cause of pregnancy-related death (Chang et al., 2003). Ectopic pregnancy rupture and abruptio placentae are responsible for most maternal deaths. Maternal blood loss decreases oxygen-carrying capacity, which predisposes the woman to increased risk for hypovolemia, anemia, infection, preterm labor, and preterm birth and adversely affects oxygen delivery to the fetus. Fetal risks from maternal hemorrhage include blood loss or anemia, hypoxemia, hypoxia, anoxia, and preterm birth. Hemorrhagic disorders in pregnancy are medical emergencies. The incidence and type of bleeding vary by trimester. In the first trimester, most bleeding is a result of miscarriage and ectopic pregnancy. Approximately 50% of bleeding in the third trimester is caused by placenta previa and abruptio placentae.

Early Pregnancy Bleeding

Bleeding during early pregnancy is alarming to the woman and of concern to the health care provider and nurse. The common bleeding disorders of early pregnancy include miscarriage, incompetent cervix, ectopic pregnancy, and hydatidiform mole (molar pregnancy).

Miscarriage

Miscarriage is a pregnancy that ends before 20 weeks of gestation. Twenty weeks of gestation is considered the point

EVIDENCE-BASED PRACTICE
Advisability of Routine Bed Rest for Multiple Pregnancy

BACKGROUND

- Since the early 1950s, it has been standard practice to admit all women pregnant with twins to the hospital for bed rest to prolong pregnancy, improve fetal growth, and manage labor. Although multiple pregnancy is associated with perinatal death as a result of preterm birth and intrauterine growth restriction, no controlled trials provided evidence of benefit from hospitalization. Half a century later, it is still widely accepted. Women frequently reported that the hospitalization and bed rest was distressing and disruptive to their families. Hospitalization is costly, and staffing resources are limited.

OBJECTIVES

- The reviewers' goals were to determine the effects of the intervention (routine hospitalization for bed rest of women with multiple pregnancies) on the outcomes of preterm birth, perinatal death, perinatal morbidity, and women's satisfaction with care.

METHODS
Search Strategy

- The reviewers searched the Cochrane database. Search keywords were *hospital, pregnancy, multiple pregnancy, twin pregnancy, triplet pregnancy,* and combinations of these words.
- Six randomized, controlled trials met the selection criteria. The trials represented 600 women and 1400 babies from Zimbabwe, Finland, and Australia and were conducted from 1985 to 1991.

Statistical Analyses

- Similar data were pooled. Reviewers calculated relative risks for dichotomous (categoric) data, and weighted mean differences for continuous data. Results outside the 95% range were accepted as significant differences.

FINDINGS

- Routine hospitalization for bed rest for women with multiple pregnancies did not result in a decrease in preterm birth. There was equivocal evidence of a trend toward decreased low birth weight. There were no differences in very-low-birth-weight (less than 1500 g) infants between groups. The hospitalized group did not have a lower rate of low Apgar score (less than 7), need for admission to the neonatal unit, or a stay of 7 days or more. Some equivocal evidence showed a decreased risk of hypertension in hospitalized women. One trial measured psychosocial outcomes and reported that 6% "appreciated admission," whereas 18% found it "distressing."

- In twin pregnancies, significantly more hospitalized women gave birth very preterm (less than 34 weeks), and there was a nonsignificant trend toward lower gestation ages at birth than controls. No difference was found in perinatal mortality rate.
- In triplet pregnancies, hospitalization showed more beneficial effects and a trend toward decreased very-low-birth-weight births, although the results did not reach significance.
- Twin pregnancies with cervical effacement and dilation before labor showed no differences between the hospitalized group and the controls in any outcomes.

LIMITATIONS

- The small number of studies and small sample sizes limit the power of the study to draw conclusions. Four of the trials took place in Zimbabwe, and all the trials are more than a decade old, further limiting their generalizability. There were some randomization problems. No information about costs was reported.

CONCLUSIONS

- There is no evidence that supports recommending a policy of routine hospitalization for bed rest for women with multiple pregnancies.

IMPLICATIONS FOR PRACTICE

- A policy of routine hospitalization for bed rest for women with multiple pregnancies may, in fact, cause harm by increasing the risk of very preterm births in twins. There was some evidence of beneficial effects for triplets, but it could not be determined if the effects were attributable to chance alone. Some women found the hospitalization distressing. When women are hospitalized because of multiple gestation, nurses can support them and help them deal with the inactivity and boredom that occur. Families can be included. The woman and her family need to be kept informed of the condition of the fetuses.

IMPLICATIONS FOR FURTHER RESEARCH

- Important long-term developmental outcome of the infants remains unknown. Only one trial addressed the psychosocial effects of hospitalization, yet it is very disruptive to the family, leaving other family members to not only care for the woman, but also perform the family duties she cannot perform. Hospitalization frequently puts a financial burden on the family because of medical costs and lost income. Any future research should include these burdens and costs in their outcomes.

Reference: Crowther, C. (2001). Hospitalization and bed rest for multiple pregnancy (Cochrane Review). In *The Cochrane Library,* Issue 2, 2004. Chichester, UK: John Wiley & Sons.

of viability, or when the fetus is able to survive in an extrauterine environment. A fetal weight of less than 500 g may also be used to define miscarriage (Cunningham et al., 2005). A spontaneous abortion results from natural causes. *Miscarriage* is the term frequently used with women and their families, as the term *abortion* may be perceived as an elective, induced abortion despite the definition and may therefore be objectionable to the family. In this text, the term *miscarriage* is used to refer to a natural pregnancy loss, and *abortion* is used when discussing therapeutic or elective, induced abortion (see Chapter 6).

Incidence and etiology.   Approximately 15% of all clinically recognized pregnancies end in miscarriage (Simpson, 2002). The majority—greater than 80% of miscarriages—occur before 12 weeks of gestation (Cunningham et al., 2005). Of all clinically recognized pregnancy losses, 50% to 60% result from chromosomal abnormalities (Cunningham et al., 2005; Hill, 2004; Simpson, 2002). An early miscarriage is defined as pregnancy loss before 8 weeks of gestation. The causes of early miscarriage include endocrine imbalance (as in women who have luteal phase defects or insulin-dependent diabetes mellitus with high blood glucose levels in the first trimester), immunologic factors (such as antiphospholipid antibodies), infections (such as bacteriuria and *Chlamydia trachomatis* infection), systemic disorders (such as lupus erythematosus), and genetic factors (Gilbert & Harmon, 2003; Hill, 2004).

A late miscarriage (pregnancy loss between 12 and 20 weeks of gestation) usually results from maternal causes, such as advancing maternal age and parity, chronic infections, premature dilation of the cervix and other anomalies of the reproductive tract, chronic debilitating diseases, poor nutrition, and recreational drug use (Cunningham et al., 2005). Little can be done to avoid genetically caused pregnancy loss, but correction of maternal disorders, immunization against infectious diseases, adequate early prenatal care, and treatment of pregnancy complications can do much to prevent miscarriage.

Types.   The types of miscarriage include threatened, inevitable, incomplete, complete, and missed. Miscarriages (both early and late) can recur; all but the threatened miscarriage can lead to infection (Fig. 23-6).

Clinical manifestations.   Signs and symptoms of miscarriage depend on the duration of pregnancy. The presence of uterine bleeding, uterine contractions, and uterine pain are ominous signs that must be considered a threatened miscarriage until proven otherwise.

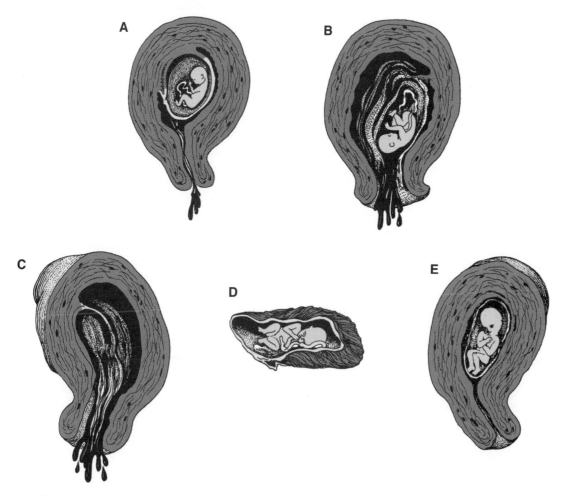

Fig. 23-6   Miscarriage. **A,** Threatened. **B,** Inevitable. **C,** Incomplete. **D,** Complete. **E,** Missed.

If miscarriage occurs before the sixth week of pregnancy, the woman may report a heavy menstrual flow. Miscarriage that occurs between the sixth and twelfth weeks of pregnancy causes moderate discomfort and blood loss. After the twelfth week, miscarriage is typified by more severe pain, similar to that of labor, because the fetus must be expelled. Diagnosis of the type of miscarriage is based on the signs and symptoms present (Table 23-6).

Symptoms of a threatened miscarriage (see Fig. 23-6, *A*) include spotting of blood but with the cervical os closed. Mild uterine cramping may be present.

Inevitable (see Fig. 23-6, *B*) and incomplete (see Fig. 23-6, *C*) miscarriages involve a moderate to heavy amount of bleeding with an open cervical os. Tissue may be present with the bleeding. Mild to severe uterine cramping may be present. An inevitable miscarriage is often accompanied by rupture of membranes (ROM) and cervical dilation; passage of the products of conception will occur. An incomplete miscarriage involves the expulsion of the fetus with retention of the placenta (Cunningham et al., 2005).

In a complete miscarriage (see Fig. 23-6, *D*), all fetal tissue is passed, the cervix is closed, and there may be slight bleeding. Mild uterine cramping may be present.

The term *missed miscarriage* (see Fig. 23-6, *E*) refers to a pregnancy in which the fetus has died but the products of conception are retained in utero for several weeks. It may be diagnosed by ultrasonic examination after the uterus stops increasing in size or even decreases in size. There may be no bleeding or cramping, and the cervical os remains closed.

Recurrent early (habitual) miscarriage is the loss of two or more previable pregnancies, though some providers still define recurrent miscarriage as the loss of three or more pregnancies before 20 weeks of gestation (Cunningham et al., 2005). Recurrent pregnancy loss is associated with the development of placental abruptions and hypertensive disorders (Sheiner, Levy, Katz, & Mazor, 2004).

Miscarriages can become septic, although this is not a common occurrence. Symptoms of a septic miscarriage include fever, abdominal tenderness, and vaginal bleeding, which may be slight to heavy and is malodorous.

Collaborative care. Whenever a woman with vaginal bleeding early in pregnancy seeks treatment, a thorough assessment should be performed (Box 23-6). Information to be obtained includes pain, bleeding, and date of last menstrual period (LMP) to determine approximate gestational age. Pain must be thoroughly assessed; type, location, duration, and precipitating and palliative factors are rated. The initial database should also include vital signs (a temperature higher than 38° C may indicate infection), previous pregnancies, previous pregnancy losses, quantity and nature of the vaginal bleeding, allergies, and emotional status. It is not uncommon for the woman and her family to be anxious and fearful about what may happen to her and to her pregnancy.

Laboratory evaluation of hCG levels, a placental hormone, is used in the diagnosis of pregnancy and pregnancy loss. Low levels of hCG are characteristic of miscarriage.

hCG is produced by the syncytiotrophoblast, and the beta subunit of hCG (β-hCG) can be detected in maternal plasma and urine 7 to 9 days after ovulation if the woman is pregnant. In early pregnancy, the concentration of β-hCG should double every 2 days until about 60 to 70 days of gestation, with peak levels (100,000 milliinternational units/ml) at approximately 8 to 10 weeks of gestation (Cunningham et al., 2005). From 10 to 12 weeks of gestation, hCG levels begin to decrease, with a nadir at approximately 20 weeks of gestation (Cunningham et al., 2005). Before 8 weeks of gestation, if a miscarriage is suspected, two serum quantitative β-hCG levels are drawn 48 hours apart. If a normal pregnancy is present, the β-hCG level doubles within that time.

Ultrasonography can then be used to determine the presence of a viable fetus within a gestational sac. With considerable or persistent blood loss, anemia is likely (hemoglobin level less than 11 g/dl). If infection is present, the white blood cell (WBC) count is greater than 12,000 cells/mm^3.

The following nursing diagnoses are appropriate for the woman experiencing miscarriage:

- *Anxiety or fear related to*
  —unknown outcome and unfamiliarity with medical procedures
- *Deficient fluid volume related to*
  —excessive bleeding secondary to miscarriage
- *Anticipatory grieving related to*
  —unexpected pregnancy outcome
- *Situational low self-esteem related to*
  —inability to successfully carry a pregnancy to term gestation

Medical management. Medical management (see Table 23-6) depends on the classification and on signs and symptoms. Traditionally, threatened miscarriages have been managed with bed rest and supportive care. Though commonly prescribed for women with early vaginal bleeding, bed rest in pregnancy is controversial (Maloni, 2002). Follow-up treatment depends on whether the threatened miscarriage progresses to actual miscarriage or symptoms subside and the pregnancy remains intact. Dilation and curettage (D&C) is a surgical procedure in which the cervix is dilated and a curette is inserted to scrape the uterine walls and remove uterine contents. A D&C is commonly performed to treat inevitable and incomplete miscarriage. The nurse reinforces explanations, answers any questions or concerns, and prepares the woman for surgery.

Dilation and evacuation, performed after 16 weeks of gestation, consists of wide cervical dilation followed by instrumental removal of the uterine contents.

Before either surgical procedure is performed, a full history should be obtained and general and pelvic examinations should be performed. General preoperative and postoperative care is appropriate for the woman requiring surgical intervention for miscarriage. Analgesics or anesthesia appropriate to the procedure are used.

TABLE 23-6

Assessing Miscarriage and the Usual Management

TYPE OF MISCARRIAGE	AMOUNT OF BLEEDING	UTERINE CRAMPING	PASSAGE OF TISSUE	CERVICAL DILATION	MANAGEMENT
Threatened	Slight, spotting	Mild	No	No	Bed rest (controversial), sedation, and avoidance of stress, sexual stimulation, and orgasm usually recommended. Acetaminophen–based analgesics may be given. Further treatment depends on woman's response to treatment.
Inevitable	Moderate	Mild to severe	No	Yes	Bed rest if no pain, fever or bleeding. If pain, rupture of membranes (ROM), bleeding, pain or fever then prompt termination of pregnancy is accomplished, usually by dilation and curettage.
Incomplete	Heavy, profuse	Severe	Yes	Yes, with tissue in cervix	May or may not require additional cervical dilation before curettage. Suction curettage may be done.
Complete	Slight	Mild	Yes	No	No further intervention may be needed if uterine contractions are adequate to prevent hemorrhage and there is no infection. Suction or curettage may be performed to assure no retained fetal or maternal tissue.
Missed	None, spotting	None	No	No	If spontaneous evacuation of the uterus does not occur within 1 month, pregnancy is terminated by method appropriate to duration of pregnancy. Blood clotting factors are monitored until uterus is empty. Disseminated intravascular coagulation (DIC) and incoagulability of blood with uncontrolled hemorrhage may develop in cases of fetal death after the twelfth week, if products of conception are retained for longer than 5 weeks. May be treated with dilation and curettage or 800 micrograms of misoprostol.
Septic	Varies, usually malodorous	Varies	Varies	Yes, usually	Immediate termination of pregnancy by method appropriate to duration of pregnancy. Cervical culture and sensitivity studies are done, and broad-spectrum antibiotic therapy (e.g., ampicillin) is started. Treatment for septic shock is initiated if necessary.
Recurrent (generally defined as 3 or more consecutive abortions)	Varies	Varies	Yes	Yes, usually	Varies, depends on type. Prophylactic cerclage may be done if premature cervical dilation is the cause. Tests of value include: parental cytogenetic analysis and lupus anticoagulant and anticardiolipin antibodies assays.

From Cunningham, F., Leveno, K., Bloom, S., Hauth, J., Gilstrap, L., Wenstrom, K. (2005). *Williams obstetrics* (22nd ed.). New York: McGraw-Hill; Gilbert, E., & Harmon, J. (2003). *Manual of high risk pregnancy and delivery* (3rd ed.). St. Louis: Mosby.

Assessment of Bleeding in Pregnancy

INITIAL DATABASE
- Chief complaint
- Vital signs
- Gravidity, parity
- Date of last menstrual period and estimated date of birth
- Pregnancy history (previous and current)
- Allergies
- Nausea and vomiting
- Pain (onset, quality, precipitating event, and location)
- Bleeding or coagulation problems
- Level of consciousness
- Emotional status

EARLY PREGNANCY
- Confirmation of pregnancy
- Bleeding (bright or dark, intermittent or continuous)
- Pain (type, intensity, persistence)
- Vaginal discharge

LATE PREGNANCY
- Estimated date of birth
- Bleeding (quantity, associated pain)
- Vaginal discharge
- Amniotic membrane status
- Uterine activity
- Abdominal pain
- Fetal status and viability

For late incomplete or inevitable miscarriages and missed miscarriages (16 to 20 weeks of gestation), prostaglandins may be administered into the amniotic sac or by vaginal suppository to induce or augment labor and cause the products of conception to be expelled. IV oxytocin may also be used.

Nursing care. Immediate nursing care focuses on physiologic stabilization. Typical orders to be followed would be initiation of an IV line, request for blood testing of hemoglobin and hematocrit, blood type and Rh, and indirect Coombs' screen. An ultrasound examination is performed for diagnostic confirmation.

Nursing care is similar to the care for any woman whose labor is being induced (see Chapter 24). Special care may be needed for management of side effects of prostaglandin, such as nausea, vomiting, and diarrhea. If the products of conception are not passed in entirety, the woman may be prepared for manual or surgical evacuation of the uterus.

After evacuation of the uterus, 10 to 20 units of oxytocin in 1000 ml of IV fluids may be given to prevent hemorrhage. For excessive bleeding after the miscarriage, ergot products such as ergonovine or a prostaglandin derivative such as carboprost tromethamine may be given to contract the uterus. Three or four doses of ergonovine, 0.2 mg orally or intra-

muscularly every 4 hours, may be given if the woman is normotensive. A 25-mg dose of carboprost may be given intramuscularly every 15 to 90 minutes for a total of as many as eight doses (Cunningham et al., 2005). Side effects associated with the use of carboprost include diarrhea, hypertension, vomiting, fever, and tachycardia (Cunningham et al., 2005). Antibiotics are given as necessary. Analgesics, such as antiprostaglandin agents, may decrease discomfort from cramping. Transfusion therapy may be required for shock or anemia. The woman who is Rh negative and is not isoimmunized is given an IM injection of $Rh_o(D)$ immune globulin within 72 hours of the miscarriage (Cunningham et al., 2005).

Psychosocial aspects of care focus on what the pregnancy loss means to the woman and her family. Women experience feelings of grief and loss after a miscarriage; they may have more intense feelings for a longer time than do men (Abboud & Laimputtong, 2003; Broen, Moum, Bodtkery, & Ekeberg, 2004). Discussions with the family must also be sensitive to the cultural beliefs of the mother and father specific to childbearing and grief. Explanations are provided regarding the nature of the miscarriage, expected procedures, and possible future implications for childbearing.

As with the other fetal or neonatal losses, the woman and her family should be offered the option of seeing the products of conception. They may also want to know what the hospital does with the products of conception or whether they need to make a decision about final disposition of fetal remains. Procedures for disposition of the fetal remains vary by agency and by state. The nurse should be familiar with the agency-specific procedures to minimize misunderstandings and increased discomfort for the family.

Home care. The woman will usually be discharged home postoperatively after a suction D&C when her vital signs are stable, vaginal bleeding is minimal, and she has recovered from anesthesia. Discharge teaching should emphasize the need for rest. If significant blood loss has occurred, iron supplementation may be ordered. Teaching includes information about normal physical findings, such as cramping, type and amount of bleeding, resumption of sexual activity, and family planning. Frequently, the woman and her family want to know when she may become pregnant again. Although this is dependent on the cause of the pregnancy loss, most health care providers suggest waiting approximately 2 to 3 months before becoming pregnant again, dependent upon the provider and the woman. This time allowance facilitates physical and emotional healing. Follow-up care should assess the woman's physical and emotional recovery (Armstrong, 2004). Referrals to local support groups should be provided as needed (Teaching Guidelines box).

Follow-up phone calls after a loss are important. The woman may appreciate a phone call on what would have been her due date. These calls provide opportunities for the woman to ask questions, seek advice, and receive information to help process her grief.

TEACHING GUIDELINES

Discharge Teaching for the Woman after Early Miscarriage

- Advise woman to report any heavy, profuse, or bright red bleeding to health care provider.
- Reassure woman that a scant, dark discharge may persist for 1 to 2 weeks.
- To reduce the risk of infection, remind the woman not to put anything into the vagina until bleeding has stopped (e.g., no tampons, no vaginal intercourse). She should take antibiotics as prescribed.

- Acknowledge that the woman has experienced a loss and that time is required for recovery. She may have mood swings and depression.
- Refer the woman to support groups, clergy, or professional counseling as needed.
- Advise woman that attempts at pregnancy should be postponed for at least 2-3 months to allow body to recover dependent upon health care provider.

Source: Gilbert, E., & Harmon, J. (2003). *Manual of high risk pregnancy and delivery* (3rd ed.). St. Louis: Mosby.

Recurrent premature dilation of the cervix (incompetent cervix)

Passive and painless dilation of the cervical os without labor or contractions of the uterus (incompetent cervix) may occur in the second trimester or early in the third trimester of pregnancy. As a result miscarriage or preterm birth may result. This definition assumes an "all-or-nothing" role for the cervix; it is either "competent" or "incompetent." Current researchers contend that cervical competence is variable and exists as a continuum that is determined in part by cervical length. Other related causative factors include composition of the cervical tissue and the individual circumstances associated with the pregnancy in terms of maternal stress and lifestyle. Iams (2004) refers to this condition as *abnormal or reduced cervical competence*, whereas Freda (1999) refers to this condition as *abnormal or premature dilation of the cervix.*

Etiology. Etiologic factors include a history of previous cervical trauma such as lacerations during childbirth, excessive cervical dilation for curettage or biopsy, or ingestion of diethylstilbestrol (DES) by the woman's mother while pregnant with the woman. Other causes are a congenitally short cervix and cervical or uterine anomalies. Reduced cervical competence is a clinical diagnosis, based on history. Short labors and recurring loss of pregnancy at progressively earlier gestational ages are characteristics of reduced cervical competence. Diagnostic criteria for ultrasound are (1) a short cervix (i.e., less than 20 mm in length) and (2) funneling of the internal os of 30% to 40% of the cervix (Iams, 2004). Effacement of the internal cervical os is sometimes referred to as cervical funneling.

Collaborative care. The nurse assesses the woman's feelings about her pregnancy and her understanding of reduced cervical competence. It is also important to evaluate the woman's support systems. Because the diagnosis of reduced cervical competence is usually not made until the woman has lost one or two pregnancies, she may feel guilty or responsible for this impending loss. It is therefore important to assess for previous reactions to stresses and appropriateness of coping responses. The woman needs the support of her health care providers, as well as that of her family.

Medical management. Conservative management consists of bed rest, hydration, progesterone, antiinflammatory drugs, and antibiotics (Iams, 2004). A cervical cerclage may be performed. During pregnancy, a Shirodkar or a McDonald procedure may be done. With the Shirodkar, maternal fascia lata is threaded submucosally in the cervix anteriorly and posteriorly and tied (Cunningham et al., 2005). In the McDonald cerclage, nonabsorbable ribbon (Mersilene) may be placed around the cervix beneath the mucosa to constrict the internal os of the cervix (Fig. 23-7) (Cunningham et al., 2005). Prophylactic cerclage is placed at 11 to 15 weeks of gestation, after which the woman is told to refrain from intercourse, prolonged (i.e., more than 90 minutes) standing, and heavy lifting (Iams, 2004). She is

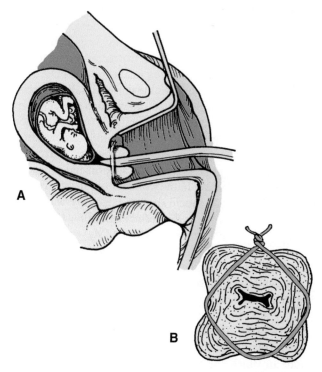

Fig. 23-7 **A,** Cerclage correction of premature dilation of the cervical os. **B,** Cross-sectional view of closed internal os.

monitored during the course of her pregnancy with ultrasound scans to assess for cervical shortening and funneling. The cerclage is electively removed (usually an office or a clinic procedure) when the woman reaches 37 weeks of gestation, or it may be left in place and a cesarean birth performed. If removed, cerclage placement must be repeated with each successive pregnancy. Approximately 80% to 90% of pregnancies treated with cerclage result in live, viable births (Iams, 2004). Recent data suggest that prophylactic cerclage may have no advantage over surveillance by ultrasound (Iams, 2004).

A woman whose reduced cervical competence is diagnosed during the current pregnancy may undergo emergency cerclage placement. Risks of the procedure include premature rupture of membranes (PROM), preterm labor, and chorioamnionitis. Because of these risks, and because bed rest and tocolytic therapy can be used to prolong the pregnancy, cerclage is rarely performed after 25 weeks of gestation (Iams, 2004).

Nursing care. If a cerclage is performed, the nurse monitors the woman postoperatively for contractions, ROM, and signs of infection. Discharge teaching focuses on continued monitoring of these aspects at home. Home uterine monitoring may be indicated with follow-up from a home health agency. The nurse assesses the woman's feelings about her pregnancy and her understanding of reduced cervical competence.

Home care. The woman must understand the importance of activity restriction at home and the need for close observation and supervision. Instruction includes the rationale for bed rest or activity restriction and to report signs of preterm labor, ROM, and infection. Tocolytics may be given to prevent uterine contractions and further dilation of the cervix. The woman must be instructed regarding the importance of taking oral tocolytic medication as prescribed, the expected response, and possible side effects. If home uterine monitoring is implemented, the woman is taught how to apply a uterine contraction monitor and transmit the monitor tracing by telephone to the monitoring center. Nurses at the monitoring center assess the tracing for contractions, answer questions, provide emotional support and education, and report information to the woman's physician or nurse-midwife. The woman should know the signs that would warrant immediate transfer to the hospital, including strong contractions less than 5 minutes apart, ROM, severe perineal pressure, and an urge to push. If management is unsuccessful and the fetus is born before viability, appropriate grief support should be provided. If the fetus is born prematurely, appropriate anticipatory guidance and support are necessary.

Ectopic pregnancy

Incidence and etiology. An ectopic pregnancy is one in which the fertilized ovum is implanted outside the uterine cavity (Fig. 23-8). It accounts for 2% of all pregnancies in the United States (Dialani & Levine, 2004; Sepilian & Wood, 2004). Approximately 95% to 97% of ec-

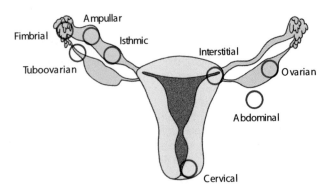

Fig. 23-8 Sites of implantation of ectopic pregnancies. Order of frequency of occurrence is ampulla, isthmus, interstitium, fimbria, tuboovarian ligament, ovary, abdominal cavity, and cervix (external os).

topic pregnancies occur in the uterine (fallopian) tube, with most located in the ampulla (75% to 80%) or largest portion of the tube (Dialani & Levine, 2004). Other sites include the abdominal cavity (3% to 4%) and ovary (0.5%) (Gilbert & Harmon, 2003).

Ectopic pregnancy is the leading pregnancy-related cause of first-trimester maternal deaths and is responsible for 9% of all maternal deaths (Dialani & Levine, 2004; Sepilian & Wood, 2004). Ectopic pregnancy is a leading cause of infertility. Women who have been treated surgically for ectopic pregnancy have a subsequent intrauterine pregnancy rate of 25% to 70%; however, up to 28% of those pregnancies are ectopic. Women treated with methotrexate have an intrauterine pregnancy rate of 64%, and the risk of a recurrent ectopic pregnancy is approximately 11% (Sepilian & Wood, 2004).

The reported incidence of ectopic pregnancy is rising. Some of the increase is due to improved diagnostic techniques, resulting in the identification of more cases. Risk factors for ectopic pregnancy include an increased incidence of sexually transmitted infections (STIs), more effective treatment of pelvic inflammatory disease (PID), increased numbers of tubal sterilizations, use of an intrauterine contraceptive device, diethylstilbestrol exposure in utero, surgical reversal of tubal sterilizations, in vitro fertilization, and previous history of ectopic pregnancy (Dialani & Levine, 2004; Sepilian & Wood, 2004). Ectopic pregnancy is classified according to site of implantation (e.g., tubal, ovarian). The uterus is the only organ capable of containing and sustaining a term pregnancy. However, 5% to 25% of abdominal pregnancies, with birth by laparotomy, may result in a living infant (Fig. 23-9). The risk of deformity is as high as 40% (Gilbert & Harmon, 2003).

Clinical manifestations. Abnormal vaginal bleeding, adnexal fullness, and pain are the classic symptoms of ectopic pregnancy (Dialani & Levine, 2004). Women generally have abdominal pain (97%) as the primary presenting symptom at approximately 5 to 6 weeks of gestation (Dialani & Levine, 2004). The tenderness can progress from a dull

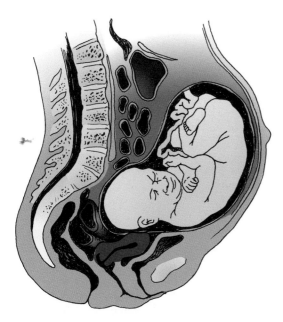

Fig. 23-9 Ectopic pregnancy, abdominal.

pain to a colicky pain when the tube stretches, to sharp, stabbing pain (Cunningham et al., 2005). Pain may be unilateral, bilateral, or diffuse over the abdomen. Dark red or brownish abnormal vaginal bleeding occurs in 50% to 80% of women. If the ectopic pregnancy ruptures, pain increases. This pain may be generalized, unilateral, or acute deep lower quadrant pain caused by blood irritating the peritoneum. Referred shoulder pain can occur as a result of diaphragmatic irritation caused by blood in the peritoneal cavity. The woman may exhibit signs of shock related to the amount of bleeding in the abdominal cavity and not necessarily related to obvious vaginal bleeding. An ecchymotic blueness around the umbilicus (Cullen sign), indicating hematoperitoneum, may develop in an undiagnosed, ruptured intraabdominal ectopic pregnancy. In addition, with abdominal palpation and bimanual examination there is abdominal and adnexal tenderness (Cunninham et al., 2005; Dialani & Levine, 2004). Other presenting symptoms include dizziness and fainting and pregnancy symptoms.

Collaborative care. The differential diagnosis of ectopic pregnancy involves consideration of numerous disorders that share many signs and symptoms. Miscarriage, ruptured corpus luteum cyst, appendicitis, salpingitis, ovarian cysts, torsion of the ovary, and urinary tract infection must be considered (Table 23-7). The key to early detection of ectopic pregnancy is having a high index of suspicion for this condition. Any woman with abdominal pain, vaginal spotting or bleeding, and a positive pregnancy test should undergo screening for ectopic pregnancy. Laboratory screening includes determination of serum progesterone and β-hCG levels. If either of these values is lower than would be expected for a normal pregnancy, the woman is asked to return within 48 hours for serial measurements. For exam-

ple, an intrauterine sac should be visible by ultrasound at 5 to 6 menstrual weeks or 28 days following ovulation or when the β-hCG is 1500 to 2000 milliinternational units/ml (Chan & Johnson, 2006; Cunningham et al., 2005; Dialani & Levine, 2004). As early as 1 week after missed menses the woman will have vaginal sonography to confirm intrauterine or tubal pregnancy. The gestational sac, diagnostic for an ectopic pregnancy, is visible from 4.5–5 weeks of gestation with transvaginal ultrasound and has become the imaging method of choice (Chan & Johnson, 2006; Cunningham et al., 2005).

Hospital care. The woman should be assessed for the presence of active bleeding, associated with tubal rupture. If internal bleeding is present, the woman may report vertigo, shoulder pain, hypotension, and tachycardia. A vaginal examination should be performed only once, and then with great caution. Approximately half of patients with a tubal pregnancy have a palpable mass on examination. It is possible to rupture the mass during a bimanual examination, so care should be taken (Simpson, 2002).

Removal of the ectopic pregnancy by salpingostomy is possible before rupture when the pregnancy is less than 2 cm in length and located in the ampulla (Cunningham et al., 2005). Residual tissue may be dissolved with a dose of methotrexate postoperatively. Methotrexate is an antimetabolite and folic acid antagonist that destroys rapidly dividing cells.

Advanced ectopic abdominal pregnancy requires laparotomy as soon as the woman has been stabilized for surgery. If the placenta of a second- or third-trimester abdominal pregnancy is attached to a vital organ, such as the liver, separation and removal are usually not attempted because of the risk of hemorrhage. The cord is cut flush with the placenta and the abdomen is closed, leaving the placenta in place. Degeneration and absorption of the placenta usually occur without complication, although infection and intestinal obstruction may occur. Methotrexate may be given to dissolve the residual tissue (Cunningham et al., 2005; Gilbert & Harmon, 2003).

If surgery is planned, general preoperative and postoperative care is appropriate for the woman with an ectopic pregnancy. Before surgery, vital signs (pulse, respirations, and BP) are assessed every 15 minutes or as needed, according to severity of the bleeding and the woman's condition. Preoperative laboratory tests include determination of blood type and Rh factor, complete blood cell count, and serum quantitative β-hCG assay. Ultrasonography is used to confirm an extrauterine pregnancy. Blood replacement may be necessary. Postoperatively, the nurse verifies the woman's Rh and antibody status and administers Rh₀(D) immune globulin if appropriate. The woman should be encouraged to verbalize her feelings related to the loss. Referral to community resources may be appropriate.

Hemodynamically stable women with ectopic pregnancies are eligible for methotrexate therapy if the mass is unruptured and measures less than 3.5 cm in diameter by

TABLE 23-7

Differential Diagnosis of Ectopic Pregnancy

	ECTOPIC PREGNANCY	APPENDICITIS	SALPINGITIS	RUPTURED OVARIAN CYST	MISCARRIAGE
Pain	Unilateral cramps and tenderness before rupture May be colicky after rupture Sudden sharp abdominal pelvic pain Abdominal tenderness	Epigastric, peri-umbilical, then right lower quadrant pain, tenderness localizing at McBurney's point, rebound tenderness	Usually in both lower quadrants with or without rebound Mild to severe pelvic pressure	Unilateral, becoming general with progressive bleeding, dull cramping	Mild uterine cramps to severe uterine pain
Nausea and vomiting	Occasionally before, frequently after rupture	Usual, precedes shift of pain to right lower quadrant	Infrequent	Rare	Almost never
Menstruation	Some aberration, missed period, spotting	Unrelated to menses	Hypermenorrhea, metrorrhagia, or both	Period delayed, then bleeding, often with pain	Amenorrhea then spotting, then brisk bleeding
Temperature, pulse, and blood pressure	37.2°-37.8° C, pulse variable, normal before and rapid after rupture, ↓ BP after rupture	37.2°-37.8° C, pulse rapid	37.2°-40° C, pulse elevated in proportion to fever	Not over 37.2° C, pulse normal unless blood loss marked, then rapid	To 37.2° C Signs of shock related to obvious bleeding
Pelvic examination	Unilateral tenderness, especially on movement of cervix, crepitant mass on one side or in cul-de-sac; dark red or brown vaginal discharge	No masses, rectal tenderness high on right side No vaginal discharge	Bilateral tenderness on movement of cervix Purulent discharge	Tenderness over affected ovary, no masses	Cervix open or closed, uterus slightly enlarged, irregularly softened, tender with infection, vaginal bleeding
Laboratory findings	WBC to 15,000/mm³ Pregnancy test result is positive Ultrasound to rule out pregnancy after 6 weeks	WBC 10,000-18,000/mm³ (rarely normal) Pregnancy test result is negative	WBC 15,000-30,000/mm³ Pregnancy test result is negative	WBC normal to 10,000/mm³ Pregnancy test result is negative unless also pregnant Ultrasound will show ovarian cyst	WBC normal Pregnancy test result is positive

Modified from Gilbert, E., & Harmon, J. (2003). *Manual of high risk pregnancy and delivery* (3rd ed.). St. Louis: Mosby.
WBC, White blood cell.

ultrasound (Sepilian & Wood, 2004). Methotrexate therapy avoids surgery and is a safe, effective, and cost-effective way of managing many cases of tubal pregnancy. Management is almost always accomplished on an outpatient basis. The woman is informed of how the medication works, possible side effects, whom to call if she has concerns or if problems develop, and the importance of follow-up care. After receiving the single methotrexate injection, the woman will need to return at least weekly for follow-up laboratory studies and for an average of 2 to 8 weeks or until the β-hCG

level is less than 15 milliinternational units/mL (Kumtepe & Kadanali, 2004; Sepilian & Wood, 2004). A repeat dose of methotrexate may be necessary if β-hCG titers do not drop to 25% by day 7, with approximately 20% of women requiring a second injection. Multiple dose regimens may also be given. During that time, the woman is instructed to put nothing in her vagina (e.g., no tampons or douches, no intercourse) and to avoid sun exposure because the drug may cause photosensitivity (Weiner & Buhimschi, 2004).

NURSE ALERT *The woman on methotrexate therapy who consumes alcohol and takes vitamins containing folic acid (such as prenatal vitamins) increases her risk of experiencing side effects of the drug or exacerbating the ectopic rupture.*

Home care. Future fertility should be discussed. Any woman who has been diagnosed with an ectopic pregnancy should be told to contact her health care provider as soon as she suspects that she might be pregnant, because of the increased risk for recurrent ectopic pregnancy. These women may need referral to grief or infertility support groups. In addition to the loss of the current pregnancy, they are faced with the possibility of future pregnancy losses or infertility.

Hydatidiform mole

Gestational trophoblastic disease (GTD) includes disorders that arise from the placental trophoblast. It includes hydatidiform mole and gestational trophoblastic neoplasia (GTN). A hydatiform mole may be further categorized as a complete or partial mole. GTN refers to persistent trophoblastic tissue that is presumed to be malignant (Berman Di Saia, & Tewari, 2004; Gilbert & Harmon, 2003). Metastatic trophoblastic neoplasia is commonly staged as low risk, intermediate risk and high risk GTN (ACOG, 2004b). Once almost invariably fatal, because of early diagnosis and treatment, GTN is the most curable gynecologic malignancy (Berman, DiSaia, & Tewari, 2004).

Incidence and etiology. Hydatidiform mole occurs in 1 in 1200 pregnancies in the United States and Europe, but a higher incidence has been reported in Asian countries (Berman, DiSaia, & Tewari, 2004). The cause is unknown, although it may be related to an ovular defect or a nutritional deficiency. Women at higher risk for hydatidiform mole formation are those women in their early teens or over 40 years of age and women from the Far East and tropics. The risk of developing a second mole is 1% to 2%.

Types. The complete mole results from fertilization of an egg whose nucleus has been lost or inactivated (Fig. 23-10, *A*). The nucleus of a sperm (23,X) duplicates itself (resulting in the diploid number 46,XX) because the ovum has no genetic material or the material is inactive. The mole resembles a bunch of white grapes (Fig. 23-10, *B*). The hydropic (fluid-filled) vesicles grow rapidly, causing the uterus to be larger than expected for the duration of the pregnancy. Usually the complete mole contains no fetus, placenta, amniotic membranes, or fluid. Maternal blood has no placenta to receive it; therefore, hemorrhage into the uterine cavity and vaginal bleeding occur. In approximately 20% of women with a complete mole, choriocarcinoma or GTN occurs (Cunningham et al., 2005).

A partial mole occurs as a result of two sperm fertilizing an apparently normal ovum. Partial moles often have embryonic or fetal parts and an amniotic sac. Congenital anomalies are usually present (Cunningham et al., 2005). The potential for malignant transformation is 5% to 10% (Cunningham et al., 2005).

Clinical manifestations. In the early stages, the clinical manifestations of a complete hydatidiform mole cannot be distinguished from those of normal pregnancy. Later, vaginal bleeding occurs in almost 95% of cases. The vaginal discharge may be dark brown (resembling prune juice) or bright red and either scant or profuse. It may continue for only a few days or intermittently for weeks. Early in pregnancy the uterus in approximately 50% of affected women is significantly larger than expected from menstrual dates.

Anemia from blood loss, excessive nausea and vomiting (hyperemesis gravidarum), and abdominal cramps caused by uterine distention are relatively common findings. Preeclampsia occurs in approximately 12% of cases, usually between 9 and 12 weeks of gestation, but any symptoms of preeclampsia before 20 weeks of gestation may suggest hydatidiform mole. Hyperthyroidism and pulmonary embolization of trophoblastic elements occur infrequently but are serious complications of hydatidiform mole. Partial

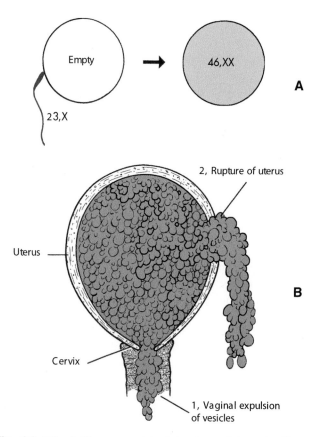

Fig. 23-10 **A,** Chromosomal origin of complete mole. Single sperm (color) fertilizes an "empty" ovum. Reduplication of sperm's 23,X set gives completely homozygous diploid 46,XX. Similar process follows fertilization of empty ovum by two sperm with two independently drawn sets of 23,X or 23,Y; both karyotypes of 46,XX and 46,XY can therefore result. **B,** Uterine rupture with hydatidiform mole. *1,* Evacuation of mole through cervix. *2,* Rupture of uterus and spillage of mole into peritoneal cavity (rare).

moles cause few of these symptoms and may be mistaken for an incomplete or missed miscarriage. Lastly, women may pass vesicles from the uterus which are frequently avascular edematous villi (Berman, DiSaia, & Tewari, 2004)

Collaborative care. Nursing assessments during prenatal visits should include observation for signs of molar pregnancy during the first 24 weeks. If hydatidiform mole is suspected, ultrasonography and serial β-hCG immunoassays are used to confirm the diagnosis. The sonographic pattern of a molar pregnancy is characterized by a diffuse "snowstorm" pattern. The β-hCG titer will remain high or rises above normal peak after the time at which it normally drops (70 to 100 days) (Cunningham et al., 2005).

Although most moles abort spontaneously (around 16 weeks of gestation), suction evacuation (curettage) offers a safe, rapid, and effective method of evacuation of hydatidiform mole if necessary (Cunningham et al., 2005; Gilbert & Harmon, 2003). Induction of labor with oxytocic agents or prostaglandins is not recommended because of the increased risk of embolization of trophoblastic tissue. Administration of Rh$_o$(D) immune globulin to women who are Rh negative is necessary to prevent isoimmunization.

The nurse helps the woman and her family cope with the pregnancy loss and recognize that the pregnancy was abnormal. In addition, the woman and her family are encouraged to verbalize their feelings, and information is provided about support groups or counseling resources as needed. Follow-up management includes frequent physical and pelvic examinations and weekly measurements of β-hCG level until the level drops to normal and remains normal for 2 consecutive weeks. Then β-hCG measurements are taken for every 1 to 2 months for a total of 1 year. A rising titer and an enlarging uterus may indicate choriocarcinoma (malignant GTD). The symptoms (enlarged fundus and rising β-hCG titers) are similar to a normal pregnancy, therefore explanations to the woman and her family must include the need to postpone future pregnancies for at least one year because of the close monitoring required. Any contraceptive method, including oral contraceptives, is appropriate, with the exception of an intrauterine device (IUD). Of particular importance is the necessity of the use of a contraceptive that is reliable and consistently used. Physical examination including pelvic is done monthly until remission and then every 3 months for 1 year. If rising hCG titers are found then chemotherapy is reinitiated (ACOG, 2004b; Berman, Di Saia, & Tewari, 2004).

Late Pregnancy Bleeding

Late pregnancy bleeding disorders include placenta previa, premature separation of placenta (abruptio placentae), and cord insertion and variations in the insertion of the cord and placenta. Expedient assessment for and diagnosis of the cause of bleeding is essential to reduce risk of maternal and perinatal morbidity and mortality (Fig. 23-11).

Placenta Previa

In placenta previa, the placenta is implanted in the lower uterine segment near or over the internal cervical os. Historically, the degree to which the internal cervical os is covered by the placenta has been used to classify four types of placenta previa; total, partial, marginal and low-lying (Fig. 23-12). With a total previa the internal os is entirely covered by the placenta. Partial placenta previa implies incomplete coverage of the internal os. Marginal placenta previa indicates that only an edge of the placenta extends to the margin of the internal os. The term *low-lying placenta* has been used when the placenta is implanted in the lower uterine segment but does not reach the os (Cunningham et al., 2005). Clark (2004) suggests that this classification has become obsolete due in part to better ultrasound diagnosis of placenta previa. Clark offers a more descriptive classification that includes placenta previa (in the third trimester, the placenta covers the internal os) and marginal placenta previa (the distance of the placenta is 2 to 3 cm from the internal os and does not cover it). When the exact relationship of the os to the placenta has not been determined or in the case of apparent placenta previa in the second trimester, the term *low-lying placenta* is used (Clark, 2004).

Incidence and etiology. The incidence of placenta previa is approximately 0.5% of births (Clark, 2004). The most important risk factors are previous placenta previa, previous cesarean birth, and suction curettage for miscarriage or induced abortion, possibly related to endometrial scarring (Ananth, Demissie, Smulian, & Vintzileos, 2001b). The risk also increases with multiple gestation (because of the larger placental area), closely spaced pregnancies, advanced maternal age (older than 35 years), African or Asian ethnicity, male fetal sex, smoking, cocaine use, multiparity, and tobacco use (Clark, 2004; Cunningham et al., 2005).

Clinical manifestations. Approximately 70% of women with placenta previa have painless vaginal bleeding; 20% have vaginal bleeding associated with uterine activity. Previa should be suspected whenever vaginal bleeding occurs after 20 weeks of gestation. This bleeding, bright red in color, is associated with the stretching and thinning of the lower uterine segment that occurs during the third trimester. Placental attachment is gradually disrupted, and bleeding occurs when the uterus is not able to adequately contract and stop blood flow from open vessels (Benedetti, 2002). The initial bleeding is usually a small amount and stops as clots form; however, it can recur at any time (Table 23-8).

Vital signs may be normal, even with heavy blood loss, because a pregnant woman can lose up to 40% of blood volume without showing signs of shock. Clinical presentation and decreasing urinary output may be better indicators of acute blood loss than vital signs alone. The FHR is reassuring unless there is a major detachment of the placenta (Gilbert & Harmon, 2003).

Abdominal examination usually reveals a soft, relaxed, nontender uterus with normal tone. If the fetus is lying

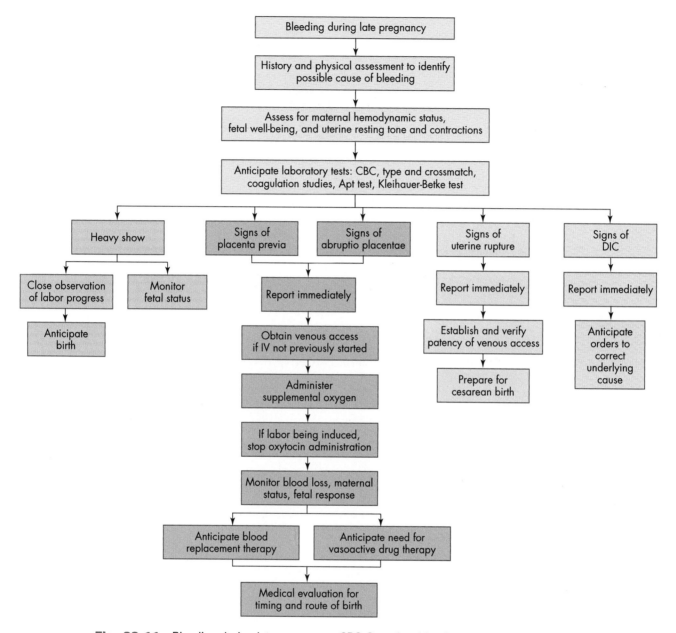

Fig. 23-11 Bleeding during late pregnancy. *CBC,* Complete blood count; *IV,* intravenous.

longitudinally, the fundal height is usually greater than expected for gestational age because the low placenta hinders descent of the presenting fetal part. Leopold's maneuvers may reveal a fetus in an oblique or breech position or lying transverse because of the abnormal site of placental implantation.

Maternal and fetal outcomes. The maternal morbidity rate is approximately 5% and the mortality rate is less than 1% with placenta previa (Clark, 2004). Complications associated with placenta previa include premature ROM, preterm labor and birth, surgery-related trauma to structures adjacent to the uterus, anesthesia complications,

blood transfusion reactions, overinfusion of fluids, abnormal placental attachments, (e.g., placenta accreta), postpartum hemorrhage, thrombophlebitis, anemia, and infection (Ananth et al., 2001b; Crane, Van den Hof, Dodds, Armson, & Liston, 2000).

The greatest risk of fetal death is caused by preterm birth. Other fetal risks include malpresentation and congenital anomalies (Clark, 2004; Gilbert & Harmon, 2003). Infants who are small for gestational age or have IUGR have been associated with placenta previa. This association may be related to poor placental exchange or hypovolemia resulting from maternal blood loss and maternal anemia (Clark, 2004).

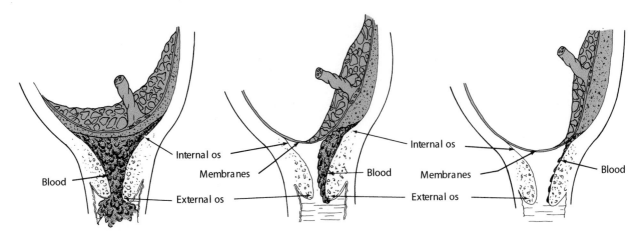

Fig. 23-12 Types of placenta previa after onset of labor. **A,** Complete, or total. **B,** Incomplete, or partial. **C,** Marginal, or low lying.

TABLE 23-8

Summary of Findings: Abruptio Placentae and Placenta Previa

	ABRUPTIO PLACENTAE			
	GRADE 1 MILD SEPARATION (10% TO 20%)	**GRADE 2 MODERATE SEPARATION (20% TO 50%)**	**GRADE 3 SEVERE SEPARATION (>50%)**	**PLACENTA PREVIA**
Bleeding, external, vaginal	Minimal	Absent to moderate	Absent to moderate	Minimal to severe and life-threatening
Total amount of blood loss	<500 ml	1000-1500 ml	>1500 ml	Varies
Color of blood	Dark red	Dark red	Dark red	Bright red
Shock	Rare; none	Mild shock	Common, often sudden, profound	Uncommon
Coagulopathy	Rare, none	Occasional DIC	Frequent DIC	None
Uterine tonicity	Normal	Increased, may be localized to one region or diffuse over uterus, uterus fails to relax between contractions	Tetanic, persistent uterine contraction, boardlike uterus	Normal
Tenderness (pain)	Usually absent	Present	Agonizing, unremitting uterine pain	Absent
ULTRASONOGRAPHIC FINDINGS				
Location of placenta	Normal, upper uterine segment	Normal, upper uterine segment	Normal, upper uterine segment	Abnormal, lower uterine segment
Station of presenting part	Variable to engaged	Variable to engaged	Variable to engaged	High, not engaged
Fetal position	Usual distribution*	Usual distribution*	Usual distribution*	Commonly transverse, breech, or oblique
Gestational or chronic hypertension	Usual distribution*	Commonly present	Commonly present	Usual distribution*
Fetal effects	Normal fetal heart rate pattern	Nonreassuring fetal heart rate pattern	Nonreassuring fetal heart rate pattern, death can occur	Normal fetal heart rate pattern

*Usual distribution refers to the usual variations of incidence seen when there is no concurrent problem.
DIC, Disseminated intravascular coagulation.

CARE MANAGEMENT ■

Assessment and Nursing Diagnoses

A woman with third-trimester vaginal bleeding requires immediate evaluation. Necessary data from the history include gravidity, parity, estimated date of birth (EDB), general status, bleeding (i.e., quantity, quality), precipitating event, and associated pain, vital signs, and fetal status (see Box 23-6). Laboratory studies include a complete blood count, determination of blood type and Rh status, coagulation profile, and possible type and crossmatch.

Placenta previa is diagnosed using transabdominal ultrasound. Transvaginal ultrasounds follow positive transabdominal scans with fewer false-positive results (Cunningham et al., 2005). If ultrasonographic scanning reveals a normally implanted placenta, an examination may be performed to rule out local causes of bleeding (e.g., cervicitis, polyps, or carcinoma of the cervix), and a coagulation profile is obtained to rule out other causes of bleeding. Management of placenta previa depends on the gestational age and condition of the fetus and the amount of bleeding present. It includes expectant management and cesarean birth. Expectant management (observation and bed rest) is implemented if the fetus is not mature. Women may be placed in the hospital on complete bed rest or managed at home. If a woman is bleeding, she is usually placed in the labor and birth unit, where she and the fetus can be closely monitored. If expectant management is to be implemented, a vaginal speculum examination is postponed until fetal viability is reached (preferably after 34 weeks of gestation). If a pelvic examination is needed before that time, anticipate the possibility that an immediate cesarean birth may be required. The woman is taken to a delivery room or an operating room set up for cesarean birth because profound hemorrhage can occur during the examination. This type of vaginal examination, known as the *double-setup procedure*, is rarely performed.

Potential nursing diagnoses for the woman experiencing placenta previa include the following:

- *Decreased cardiac output related to*
  —excessive blood loss secondary to placenta previa
- *Deficient fluid volume related to*
  —excessive blood loss secondary to placenta previa
- *Ineffective peripheral tissue perfusion related to*
  —hypovolemia and shunting of blood to central circulation
- *Anxiety or fear related to*
  —maternal condition and pregnancy outcome
- *Anticipatory grieving related to*
  —actual or perceived threat to self, pregnancy, or infant

Expected Outcomes of Care

Expected outcomes for the woman experiencing placenta previa may include that the woman will do the following:

- Verbalize understanding of her condition and its management
- Identify and use available support systems
- Demonstrate compliance with prescribed activity limitations
- Develop no complications related to bleeding
- Give birth to a healthy term infant

Plan of Care and Interventions
Active management

Once placenta previa has been diagnosed, a management plan is developed based on gestational age, amount of bleeding, and fetal condition. If the woman is at term (longer than or equal to 37 weeks of gestation) and in labor or bleeding persistently, immediate cesarean birth is almost always indicated. In women with placental "migration" or movement of the placenta in relationship to the internal os a vaginal birth may be attempted (Cunningham et al., 2005). Vaginal birth may also be indicated for previable gestations or births involving intrauterine fetal demise (Benedetti, 2002).

Cesarean birth is necessary for the large marjority of women with a placenta previa. The nurse continuously assesses maternal and fetal status while preparing the woman for surgery. Maternal vital signs are assessed frequently for decreasing BP, increasing pulse rate, changes in LOC, and oliguria. Fetal assessment is maintained by continuous electronic fetal monitoring to assess for signs of hypoxia.

Blood loss may not cease with the birth of the infant. The large vascular channels in the lower uterine segment may continue to bleed because of the area's diminished muscle content. The natural mechanism to control bleeding—the interlacing muscle bundles contracting around open vessels (the "living ligature," characteristic of the upper part of the uterus)—is absent in the lower part of the uterus. Postpartum hemorrhage may therefore occur even if the fundus is contracted firmly.

Emotional support for the woman and her family is extremely important. The actively bleeding patient is concerned not only for her own well-being but for the well-being of her fetus. All procedures should be explained, and a support person should be present. The woman should be encouraged to express her concerns and feelings. If the woman and her support person or family desire spiritual support, the nurse can notify the hospital chaplain service or provide information about other supportive resources.

Expectant management.
If the woman is at less than 36 weeks of gestation, she is not in labor, and the bleeding is mild or has stopped, expectant management (i.e., rest and close observation) is generally the treatment of choice to give the fetus time to mature in utero. The woman may remain in the hospital on bed rest with bathroom privileges and limited activity (up in a wheelchair for short periods, [approximately 1 hour daily]). Bleeding is assessed by checking the amount of bleeding on perineal pads, bed pads, and linens. Weighing pads, although not frequently used, is one way to more accurately assess blood loss: 1 g equals 1 ml of blood.

Ultrasonographic examinations may be done every 2 to 3 weeks. Fetal surveillance may include an NST or BPP once or twice weekly. Serial laboratory values are evaluated for decreasing hemoglobin and hematocrit levels and changes in coagulation values. Venous access with an IV infusion or heparin lock may be placed in case blood or blood component therapy is needed. Antepartum steroids (betamethasone) may be ordered to promote fetal lung maturity if gestation is less than 34 weeks. No vaginal or rectal examinations are performed, and the woman is placed on "pelvic rest" (nothing in the vagina). If sonographic findings indicate that the placental edge is located within 2 cm of the internal os then a cesarean birth is necessary (Bhide & Thilaganathan, 2004). Once she reaches 37 weeks of gestation and fetal lung maturity is documented, cesarean birth can be scheduled.

The woman with placenta previa should always be considered a potential emergency because massive blood loss with resulting hypovolemic shock can occur quickly if bleeding resumes. Placenta previa in a preterm gestation may be an indication for transfer to a tertiary perinatal center because a neonatal intensive care unit may be necessary for care of the preterm neonate.

Home care. Criteria for home care management, currently an uncommon practice, vary among primary perinatal providers and are usually determined on a case-by-case basis. To be considered for home care referral, the woman must be in stable condition with no evidence of active bleeding and must have transportation to be able to return to the hospital immediately if active bleeding resumes. She must have close supervision by family or friends in the home. The woman should be taught how to assess fetal and uterine activity and bleeding and told to avoid intercourse, douching, and enemas. She should limit her activities according to the advice of her physician and be advised to keep all appointments for fetal testing, laboratory assessments, and prenatal care. Visits by a perinatal home care nurse may be arranged.

If hospitalization or home care with activity restriction is prolonged, the woman may have concerns about her work- or family-related responsibilities or may become bored with inactivity. She should be encouraged to participate in her own care and decisions about care as much as possible. Provision of diversionary activities or encouragement to participate in activities she enjoys and can do during bed rest is needed (see suggestions for activities in the Self-Care box on p. 727). Participation in support group made up of other women on bed rest while hospitalized, or online if at home may be a helpful coping mechanism (Maloni & Kutil, 2000).

Evaluation

The expected outcomes of care are used to evaluate the care for the woman with placenta previa (Plan of Care).

PLAN OF CARE *Placenta Previa*

NURSING DIAGNOSIS Decreased cardiac output related to bleeding secondary to placenta previa
Expected Outcomes *Woman will exhibit signs of increased blood volume and restoration of cardiac output (i.e., normal pulse and blood pressure; normal heart and breath sounds; normal skin color, tone, and turgor; normal capillary refill).*

Nursing Interventions/*Rationales*

- Palpate uterus for tenderness and tone; assess bleeding rate, amount, color, CBC values, and coagulation profile *to determine severity of situation.* (Do not perform vaginal examination, because it may stimulate further bleeding.)
- Establish baseline data for cardiac output (vital signs; heart and breath sounds; skin color, tone, turgor; capillary refill; level of consciousness; urinary output; pulse oximetry) *to use as basis for evaluating effectiveness of treatment.*
- Initiate intravenous therapy or blood transfusions and medications per physician order *to restore blood volume and prevent organ compromise in mother and fetus.*
- Place woman on bed rest *to decrease oxygen demands.*
- Monitor vital signs, intake and output, hemodynamic status, and laboratory values *to evaluate treatment response.*
- Provide emotional support to woman and her family (i.e., explain procedures and their rationale; explain what is happening and what to expect; keep support person present) *to allay fears and provide the family with some sense of control.*
- After stabilization, teach woman home management, including bed rest, observation for spotting and bleeding, close follow-up with her health care provider, and preparation for immediate return to hospital if needed *to prevent or stem further complications.*

NURSING DIAGNOSIS Risk for injury to the fetus related to decreased uterine or placental perfusion secondary to bleeding
Expected Outcome *Woman will exhibit ongoing signs of fetal well-being (i.e., adequate fetal movement, normal FHR, reactive NST, normal BPP).*

Nursing Interventions/*Rationales*

- Monitor fetus daily for signs of tachycardia, decreased movement, loss of reactivity on NST *to identify and treat changes in fetal status.*
- Obtain BPP per physician order *to assess for signs of chronic asphyxia.*
- Maintain maternal side-lying position *to prevent compression of aorta and vena cava.*

NURSING DIAGNOSIS Risk for infection related to anemia and bleeding secondary to placenta previa
Expected Outcome *Woman will show no signs of intrauterine infection.*

Nursing Interventions/*Rationales*

- Monitor vital signs for elevated temperature, pulse, and blood pressure; monitor laboratory results for elevated WBC count, differential shift; check for uterine tenderness and malodorous vaginal discharge *to detect early signs of infection resulting from exposure of placental tissue.*
- Provide or teach perineal hygiene *to decrease the risk of ascending infection.*

Premature separation of placenta

Premature separation of the placenta, or *abruptio placentae,* is the detachment of part or all of the placenta from its implantation site (Fig. 23-13). Separation occurs in the area of the decidua basalis after 20 weeks of gestation and before the birth of the infant.

Incidence and etiology. Premature separation of the placenta is a serious complication that accounts for significant maternal and fetal morbidity and mortality rates. Approximately 1 in 200 of all pregnancies is complicated by abruptio placentae (Cunningham et al., 2005).

Maternal hypertension is probably the most consistently identified risk factor for abruption (Benedetti, 2002). Cocaine is also a risk factor, believed to be the result of severe hypertension (Andres & Day, 2000). Blunt external abdominal trauma, most often the result of motor vehicle accidents (MVAs) or maternal battering, is an increasingly significant cause of placental abruption (Benedetti, 2002; Clark, 2004). Other risk factors include cigarette smoking, previous abruption (5% to 17%), cocaine use (10%), and preterm rupture of membranes (Clark, 2004; Cunningham et al., 2005). Abruption is more likely to occur in twin gestations (Ananth et al., 2001a). Women who have had two previous abruptions have a recurrence risk of 25% in the next pregnancy (Clark, 2004).

Classification. The most common classification of placental abruption is according to type and severity. This classification system is summarized in Table 23-8.

Clinical manifestations. The separation may be partial or complete, or only the margin of the placenta may be involved. Bleeding from the placental site may dissect (separate) the membranes from the decidua basalis and flow out through the vagina (70% to 80%), it may remain concealed (retroplacental hemorrhage) (10% to 20%), or it may do both (see Fig. 23-13) (Benedetti, 2002). Clinical symptoms vary with degree of separation (see Table 23-8).

Classic symptoms of abruptio placentae include vaginal bleeding, abdominal pain, and uterine tenderness and contractions (Clark, 2004; Cunningham et al., 2005). Although abdominal pain and uterine tenderness are characteristic of abruption, either finding may be absent in the presence of a silent abruption (Clark, 2004). Bleeding may result in maternal hypovolemia (i.e., shock, oliguria, and anuria) and coagulopathy. Mild to severe uterine hypertonicity is present. Pain is mild to severe and localized over one region of the uterus or diffuse over the uterus with a "boardlike" abdomen.

Extensive myometrial bleeding damages the uterine muscle. If blood accumulates between the separated placenta and the uterine wall, it may produce a Couvelaire uterus. The uterus appears purplish and copper colored and is ecchymotic, and contractility is lost. Shock may occur and is out of proportion to blood loss. The Apt test result is positive, hemoglobin and hematocrit levels drop, and coagulation factor levels drop. With the Apt test (blood in the amniotic fluid), vaginal blood is mixed with sodium hydroxide. Maternal blood turns brown while fetal blood remains red. A Kleihauer-Betke (KB) test may be ordered to determine the presence of fetal-to-maternal bleeding (transplacental hemorrhage), although there appears to be no value to this test in the general workup of patients with abruption (Clark, 2004).

Maternal and fetal outcomes. Maternal mortality rate approaches 1% for women with an abruptio placentae (Clark, 2004). This condition remains a leading cause of maternal death. The mother's prognosis depends on the extent of placental detachment, overall blood loss, degree of DIC, and time between placental detachment and birth. Maternal complications are associated with the abruption or its treatment. Hemorrhage, hypovolemic shock, hypofibrinogenemia, and thrombocytopenia are associated with severe abruption. Renal failure and pituitary necrosis may result from ischemia. In rare cases, women who are Rh negative can become sensitized if fetal-to-maternal hemorrhage occurs and the fetal blood type is Rh positive.

Perinatal mortality rates range from 10% to 12% (Cunningham et al., 2005). Death occurs as a result of fetal hypoxia, preterm birth, and SGA status. Risks for neurologic defects are increased (Cunningham et al., 2005). Fetal complications include congenital anomalies (Clark, 2004).

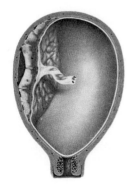
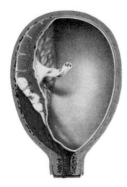
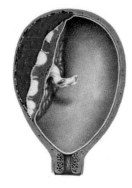

Partial separation
(concealed hemorrhage)

Partial separation
(apparent hemorrhage)

Complete separation
(concealed hemorrhage)

Fig. 23-13 Abruptio placentae. Premature separation of normally implanted placenta.

Collaborative care. Abruptio placentae should be highly suspected in the woman with a sudden onset of intense, usually localized, uterine pain, with or without vaginal bleeding. Initial assessment is much the same as for placenta previa. Physical examination usually reveals abdominal pain, uterine tenderness, and contractions. The fundal height should be measured over time, because an increasing fundal height indicates concealed bleeding. Approximately 60% of live fetuses exhibit nonreassuring signs, such as loss of variability and late decelerations, on the electronic fetal heart monitor; uterine hyperstimulation and increased resting tone may also be noted on the monitor tracing (Benedetti, 2002). Many women demonstrate coagulopathy, as evidenced by abnormal clotting studies (fibrinogen, platelet count, PTT, fibrin split products). Sonographic examination is used to rule out placenta previa; however, it is not always diagnostic for abruption (Cunningham et al., 2005). A retroplacental mass may be detected with ultrasonographic examination, but negative findings do not rule out a life-threatening abruption (Clark, 2004).

Nursing diagnoses and expected outcomes of care are similar to those described for placenta previa.

Treatment depends on the severity of blood loss and fetal maturity and status. Women with abruptio placentae are not usually managed out of the hospital because the placenta can separate further at any time and immediate intervention may be necessary. However, if the abruption is mild and the fetus is less than 36 weeks of gestation and not in distress, expectant management may be implemented. The woman is hospitalized and observed closely for signs of bleeding and labor.

The fetal status is also monitored with intermittent FHR monitoring and NSTs or BPPs until fetal maturity is determined or until the woman's condition deteriorates and immediate birth is indicated. Use of corticosteroids to accelerate fetal lung maturity is appropriately included in the plan of care for expectant management (Cunningham et al., 2005). Women who are Rh negative may be given Rh$_o$(D) immune globulin if fetal-to-maternal hemorrhage occurs.

If the mother is hemodynamically stable, a vaginal birth may be attempted if the fetus is alive and in no acute distress or if the fetus is dead. In the presence of fetal compromise, severe hemorrhage, coagulopathy, poor labor progress, or increasing uterine resting tone, a cesarean birth is performed. At least one large-bore (16 to 18-gauge) IV line should be started. Maternal vital signs are monitored frequently to observe for signs of declining hemodynamic status, such as increasing pulse rate and decreasing BP. Serial laboratory studies include hematocrit or hemoglobin determinations and clotting studies. Continuous electronic fetal monitoring is mandatory. An indwelling Foley catheter is inserted for continuous assessment of urine output, an excellent indirect measure of maternal organ perfusion (Benedetti, 2002).

Blood and fluid volume replacement will most likely be ordered, with a goal of maintaining the urine output at 30 ml/hr or greater and the hematocrit at 30% or greater. If this goal is not reached despite vigorous attempts at replacement, hemodynamic monitoring may be necessary (Benedetti, 2002). Fresh frozen plasma or cryoprecipitate may be given to maintain the fibrinogen level at a minimum of 100 to 150 mg/dl.

Vaginal birth is possible and is especially desirable in cases of fetal demise; however, cesarean birth is common because of fetal or maternal distress.

Nursing care of patients experiencing moderate to severe abruption is demanding because it requires close monitoring of the maternal and fetal condition. All procedures should be explained to the woman and her family. Emotional support is also extremely important. If actively bleeding, the woman is concerned not only for her own well-being but also for the well-being of her fetus.

Cord insertion and placental variations

Velamentous insertion of the cord *(vasa previa)* is a rare placental anomaly associated with placenta previa and multiple gestation. The cord vessels begin to branch at the membranes and then course onto the placenta (Fig. 23-14, *A*). ROM or traction on the cord may tear one or more of the fetal vessels. As a result the fetus may quickly bleed to death.

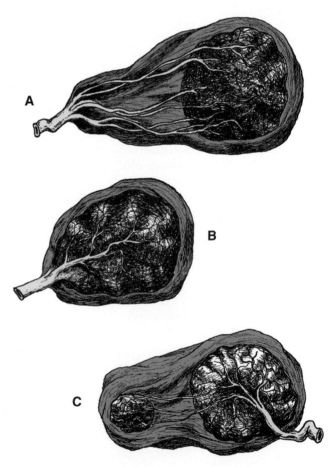

Fig. 23-14 Cord insertion and placental variations. **A,** Velamentous insertion of cord. **B,** Battledore placenta. **C,** Placenta succenturiate.

Battledore (marginal) (Fig. 23-14, *B*) insertion of the cord increases the risk of fetal hemorrhage, especially after marginal separation of the placenta.

Rarely, the placenta may be divided into two or more separate lobes, resulting in *succenturiate* placenta (Fig. 23-14, *C*). Each lobe has a distinct circulation. The vessels collect at the periphery, and the main trunks unite eventually to form the vessels of the cord. Blood vessels joining the lobes may be supported only by the fetal membranes and are therefore in danger of tearing during labor, birth, or expulsion of the placenta. During expulsion of the placenta, one or more of the separate lobes may remain attached to the decidua basalis, preventing uterine contraction and increasing the risk of postpartum hemorrhage.

CLOTTING DISORDERS IN PREGNANCY

Normal Clotting

Normally, there is a delicate balance (homeostasis) between the opposing hemostatic and fibrinolytic systems. The hemostatic system is involved in the lifesaving process. This system stops the flow of blood from injured vessels, in part through the formation of insoluble fibrin, which acts as a hemostatic platelet plug. The coagulation process involves an interaction of the coagulation factors in which each factor sequentially activates the factor next in line, the "cascade effect" sequence. The fibrinolytic system is the process through which the fibrin is split into fibrinolytic degradation products and circulation is restored.

Clotting Problems

A history of abnormal bleeding, inheritance of unusual bleeding tendencies, or a report of significant aberrations of laboratory findings indicate a bleeding or clotting problem. For the pregnant woman, bleeding disorders are suspected if the woman has gestational hypertension, HELLP syndrome, retained dead fetus syndrome, amniotic fluid embolism, sepsis, or hemorrhage. Determination of hemostasis is made by testing the usual mechanisms for the control of bleeding, the function of platelets, and the necessary clotting factors. Most clotting disorders are more a concern in the immediate postpartum period. Recognition in the antepartal period may decrease hemorrhagic problems (see Chapter 25).

Disseminated intravascular coagulation

Disseminated intravascular coagulation (DIC) or consumptive coagulopathy is a pathologic form of clotting that is diffuse and consumes large amounts of clotting factors, causing widespread external bleeding, internal bleeding, or both and clotting (Cunningham et al., 2005). DIC is most often triggered by the release of large amounts of tissue thromboplastin. This occurs in abruptio placentae, retained dead fetus, and amniotic fluid embolus syndrome. Severe preeclampsia, HELLP syndrome, and gram-negative sepsis are

examples of conditions that can trigger DIC because of widespread damage to vascular integrity (Cunningham et al., 2005; Kilpatrick & Laros, 2004). DIC is an overactivation of the clotting cascade and the fibrinolytic system, resulting in depletion of platelets and clotting factors. This results in the formation of multiple fibrin clots throughout the body's vasculature, even in the microcirculation. Blood cells are destroyed as they pass through these fibrin choked vessels. Thus DIC results in a clinical picture of clotting, bleeding, and ischemia (Cunningham et al., 2005; Labelle & Kitchens, 2005). DIC is always a secondary diagnosis. Clinical manifestations and laboratory test results are summarized in Box 23-7.

Collaborative care

Medical management during pregnancy includes correcting the underlying cause and replacement of essential factors and fluid volume. (See Chapter 25 for further discussion.)

The nurse caring for the pregnant woman at risk for DIC must be aware of risk factors. Careful and thorough assessment is required, with particular attention to the signs of bleeding (e.g., petechiae, "oozing" from venous access sites or any break in the skin, and hematuria). Because renal failure is one consequence of DIC, urinary output is carefully monitored (minimum of 30 ml/h) using an indwelling Foley catheter. Vital signs are assessed frequently. Supportive measures include keeping the pregnant woman in a side-lying tilt to maximize

---

BOX 23-7

Antepartal Clinical Manifestations and Laboratory Screening Results for Pregnant Patients with Disseminated Intravascular Coagulation

- Possible Physical Examination Findings
  —Spontaneous bleeding from gums, nose
  —Oozing, excessive bleeding from venipuncture site, intravenous access site, or site of insertion of urinary catheter
  —Petechiae, for example on the arm where blood pressure cuff was placed
  —Other signs of bruising
  —Hematuria
  —Gastrointestinal bleeding
  —Tachycardia
  —Diaphoresis
- Laboratory Coagulation Screening Test Results
  —Platelets–decreased
  —Fibrinogen–decreased
  —Factor V (proaccelerin)–decreased
  —Factor VIII (antihemolytic factor)–decreased
  —Prothrombin time–prolonged
  —Partial prothrombin time–prolonged
  —Fibrin degradation products–increased
  —D-dimer test (specific fibrin degradation fragment)–increased
  —Red blood smear–fragmented red blood cells

Sources: Cunningham et al., 2005; Kilpatrick & Laros, 2004; Labelle & Kitchens, 2005.

blood flow to the uterus. Oxygen may be administered through a tight-fitting rebreathing mask at 8 to 10 L/min, or per hospital protocol or physician order. Blood and blood products must be administered safely. Fetal assessments are done to monitor fetal well-being (Labelle & Kitchens, 2005; Lurie, Feinstein, & Mamet, 2000). DIC usually is "cured" with the birth and as coagulation abnormalites resolve.

INFECTIONS ACQUIRED DURING PREGNANCY

Sexually Transmitted Infections

Sexually transmitted infections (STIs) in pregnancy are responsible for significant morbidity rates. Some consequences of maternal infection, such as infertility and sterility, last a lifetime. Psychosocial sequelae may include altered interpersonal relationships and lowered self-esteem. Congenitally acquired infection may affect the length and quality of a child's life.

Chapter 5 discusses the diagnosis and management of STIs, and Chapter 27 discusses neonatal effects and management. This discussion focuses only on the effects of several common STIs on pregnancy and the fetus (Table 23-9). Effects on pregnancy and the fetus also vary according to whether the infection has been treated at the time of labor and birth.

Collaborative care

The most common STIs in women are *chlamydia*, human papillomavirus, gonorrhea, herpes simplex virus type 2, syphilis, and human immunodeficiency virus (HIV) infection (Centers for Disease Control and Prevention [CDC],

2002). Factors that influence the development and management of STIs during pregnancy include previous history of STI or pelvic inflammatory disease (PID), number of current sexual partners, frequency of intercourse, and anticipated sexual activity during pregnancy. Lifestyle choices also may affect STIs in the perinatal period. Risk factors include use of IV drugs or having a partner who uses IV drugs. Other lifestyle factors that increase susceptibility to STIs (through suppressive effects on the immune system) include smoking, alcohol use, inadequate or poor nutrition, and high levels of fatigue or personal stress (Gibbs, Sweet, & Duff, 2004).

Physical examination and laboratory studies to determine the presence of STIs in the pregnant woman are the same as those done in nonpregnant women (see Chapter 5).

Treatment of specific STIs may be different for the pregnant woman and may even be different at different stages of pregnancy. Table 23-9 describes the maternal, fetal, and neonatal effects. Table 23-10 describes treatment during pregnancy of common STIs. Infected women need instruction regarding how to take prescribed medications, information on whether their partner(s) also need to be evaluated and treated, and a review of preventive measures to avoid reinfection.

TORCH Infections

TORCH infections can affect a pregnant woman and her fetus. Toxoplasmosis, other infections (e.g., hepatitis), rubella virus, cytomegalovirus, and herpes simplex virus, known collectively as *TORCH infections,* are a group of organisms capable of crossing the placenta and adversely affecting the development of the fetus. Generally, all TORCH infections produce influenza-like symptoms in the woman, but fetal

TABLE 23-9

Pregnancy and Fetal Effects of Common Sexually Transmitted Infections

INFECTION	PREGNANCY EFFECTS	FETAL EFFECTS
Chlamydia	Premature rupture of membranes Preterm birth	Preterm labor Conjunctivitis Pneumonia
Gonorrhea	Intraamniotic infection Preterm labor Premature rupture of membranes Postpartum endometritis Miscarriage	Preterm birth Sepsis Conjunctivitis
Group B streptococcus	Preterm labor Premature rupture of membranes Chorioamnionitis Postpartum sepsis Urinary tract infections	Preterm birth Early-onset sepsis
Herpes simplex	Rare—infection	Systemic infection
Human papillomavirus (HPV)	Dystocia from large lesions Excessive bleeding from lesions after birth trauma	Respiratory papillomatosis (rare)
Syphilis	Preterm labor Miscarriage	Preterm birth Stillbirth Congenital infection

Data from Cunningham, F., Leveno, K., Bloom, S., Hauth, J., Gilstrap, L., Wenstrom, K. (2005). *Williams obstetrics* (22nd ed.). New York: McGraw-Hill; & Gilbert, E., & Harmon, J. (2003). *Manual of high risk pregnancy and delivery* (3rd ed.). St. Louis: Mosby.

TABLE 23-10

Treatment of Common Sexually Transmitted Infections in Pregnancy

SEXUALLY TRANSMITTED INFECTION	TREATMENT	NURSING CONSIDERATIONS
Chlamydia	Erythromycin 500 mg PO four times a day × 7 days; or amoxicillin 500 mg PO three times a day × 7 days	Instruct woman to take after meals and with 8 oz water; instruct partner to be tested and treated if needed.
Herpes	Acyclovir is used in pregnancy only if the potential benefit outweighs the potential risk to the fetus; treat symptoms. Analgesics and topical anesthetics may be ordered for severe discomfort.	Instruct woman in comfort measures: keep lesions clean and dry; use compresses on lesions (cold milk, colloidal oatmeal) every 2 to 4 hr, sitz baths; woman should abstain from intercourse while lesions are present; if woman has active lesions at time of labor, a cesarean birth will usually be performed to prevent perinatal transmission.
Gonorrhea	Ceftriaxone 125 mg IM × one dose or Cefixime, 400 mg po X one dose or Spectinomycin, 2 grams IM as single dose plus treatment for chlamydia as listed above	Screening is done at first prenatal visit; repeated in third trimester if high risk. Instruct partner to be tested and treated if needed. Infants are treated within 1 hour of birth with ophthalmic erythromycin or tetracycline ointment.
Group B streptococcus	Penicillin G 5 million units IV initial dose followed by 2.5 million units IV q4 hours during labor or ampicillin 2 grams IV initial dose followed by 1 gram IV q4 hours	Pregnant women should be screened at 36-37 weeks of gestation; if positive or status unknown at time of labor, the woman is treated.
Hepatitis B	For exposure, hepatitis B immune globulin 0.06 mg/kg IM; repeat in 1 mo, followed by hepatitis B vaccine series	Screening should be at first prenatal visit, with rescreening in third trimester for high risk patients; treatment is supportive—bed rest, high-protein, low-fat diet, increased fluid intake; the woman should avoid medications that are metabolized in the liver.
Human papillomavirus	Trichloracetic acid (TCA) or bichloracetic acid (BCA) 80% to 90% applied topically to warts one to three times a week; Xylocaine jelly applied for burning sensations; cryotherapy with liquid nitrogen in second and third trimesters; CO_2 laser ablation therapy	Podophyllum and 5-fluorouracil are possibly teratogenic and should not be used in pregnancy; inform partners to be tested and treated if needed; couples should use condoms for intercourse; inform women that smoking can decrease effects of therapy.
Syphilis	Benzathine penicillin G 2.4 million units IM once; if syphilis of more than one year duration then 2.4 million units IM (one dose per week X 3 weeks) No proven alternatives to penicillin in pregnancy; women who have a history of allergy to penicillin should be desensitized and treated with penicillin	Treatment cures maternal infection and prevents congenital syphilis 98% of the time; routine screening during pregnancy should be at the first prenatal visit and in the third trimester in women at high risk; partners should be tested and treated if needed.
Trichomonas	Metronidazole 2 grams PO once	Inform partners to be treated; women should avoid alcohol and vinegar products to avoid nausea and vomiting, intestinal cramping, and headaches; not recommended during lactation; stop breastfeeding, treat; resume in 48 hours after last dose. Women may use breast pump and discard milk to prevent interruption of milk supply.
Candidiasis	Over-the-counter topical agents; butoconazole, clotrimazole, miconazole, or terconazole; use for 7 days	May be used during lactation.
Bacterial vaginosis	Metronidazole 250 mg PO three times a day × 7 days	See *Trichomonas;* infection may increase risk of preterm labor; women are usually asymptomatic.

IM, Intramuscularly; *IV,* intravenously; *PO,* by mouth;

TABLE 23-11

Maternal Infection: TORCH

INFECTION	MATERNAL EFFECTS	FETAL EFFECTS	COUNSELING: PREVENTION, IDENTIFICATION, AND MANAGEMENT
Toxoplasmosis (protozoa)	Acute infection similar to influenza, lymphadenopathy Woman immune after first episode (except in immuno-compromised patients)	With maternal acute infection, parasitemia Less likely to occur with maternal chronic infection Miscarriage likely with acute infection early in pregnancy	Use good handwashing technique Avoid eating raw meat and exposure to litter used by infected cats; if cats in house, have toxoplasma titer checked If titer is rising during early pregnancy, abortion may be considered an option
OTHER INFECTIONS			
Hepatitis A (infectious hepatitis) (virus)	Miscarriage, cause of liver failure during pregnancy Fever, malaise, nausea, and abdominal discomfort	Exposure during first trimester, fetal anomalies, fetal or neonatal hepatitis, preterm birth, intrauterine fetal death	Usually spread by droplet or hand contact especially by culinary workers; gamma-globulin can be given as prophylaxis for hepatitis A
Hepatitis B (serum hepatitis) (virus)	May be transmitted sexually, symptoms variable—fever, rash, arthralgia, depressed appetite, dyspepsia, abdominal pain, generalized aching, malaise, weakness, jaundice, tender and enlarged liver	Infection occurs during birth Maternal vaccination during pregnancy should present no risk for fetus (however, data are not available)	Generally passed by contaminated needles, syringes, or blood transfusions; also can be transmitted orally or by coitus (but incubation period is longer); hepatitis B immune globulin can be given prophylactically after exposure Hepatitis B vaccine recommended for populations at risk Populations at risk are women from Asia, Pacific islands, Indochina, Haiti, South Africa, Alaska (women of Eskimo descent); other women at risk include health care providers, users of intravenous drugs, those sexually active with multiple partners or single partner with multiple risks

and neonatal effects are more serious. TORCH infections and their maternal and fetal effects are described in Table 23-11. Neonatal effects are discussed in Chapter 27.

SURGICAL EMERGENCIES DURING PREGNANCY

The incidence of surgery requiring anesthesia during pregnancy ranges from 0.2% to 2.2%, affecting an estimated 50,000 to 75,000 pregnant women each year (Kuczkowski, 2004; Ludmir & Stubblefield, 2002). The need for abdominal surgery occurs as frequently among pregnant women as among nonpregnant women of comparable age. However, pregnancy may make diagnosis more difficult. An enlarged uterus and displaced internal organs may make abdominal palpation more difficult, alter the position of an affected organ, or change the usual signs and symptoms associated with a particular disorder. Common conditions necessitating abdominal surgery during pregnancy include cerclage, ovarian cystectomy, and appendectomy (Kuczkowski, 2004). Fetal concerns include teratogenic effects secondary to the anesthetic drugs used, intrauterine fetal death, and premature labor (Kuczkowski, 2004). Regional anesthesia is preferred, with intensive fetal and maternal monitoring. After 24 weeks

TABLE 23-11

Maternal Infection: TORCH–cont'd

INFECTION	MATERNAL EFFECTS	FETAL EFFECTS	COUNSELING: PREVENTION, IDENTIFICATION, AND MANAGEMENT
OTHER INFECTIONS—cont'd			
Rubella (3-day German measles) (virus)	Rash, fever, mild symptoms; suboccipital lymph nodes may be swollen; some photophobia Occasionally arthritis or encephalitis Miscarriage	Incidence of congenital anomalies—first month 50%, second month 25%, third month 10%, fourth month 4% Exposure during first 2 months—malformations of heart, eyes, ears, or brain, abnormal dermatoglyphics Exposure after fourth month—systemic infection, hepatosplenomegaly, intrauterine growth restriction, rash	Vaccination of pregnant women contraindicated; pregnancy should be prevented for 1 month after vaccination; pregnant women nonreactive to hemagglutinin-inhibition antigen can be safely vaccinated after birth
Cytomegalovirus (CMV) (a herpes virus)	Respiratory or sexually transmitted asymptomatic illness or mononucleosis-like syndrome; may have cervical discharge No immunity develops	Fetal death or severe, generalized disease—hemolytic anemia and jaundice, hydrocephaly or microcephaly, pneumonitis, hepatosplenomegaly, deafness	Virus may be reactivated and cause disease in utero or during birth in subsequent pregnancies; fetal infection may occur during passage through infected birth canal; disease is commonly progressive through infancy and childhood
Herpes genitalis (herpes simplex virus, type 2 [HSV-2])	Primary infection with painful blisters, rash, fever, malaise, nausea, headache; pregnancy risks include miscarriage, preterm labor, stillbirths	Transplacental infection is rare; congenital effects include skin lesions and scarring, intrauterine growth restriction, mental retardation, microcephaly	Risk of transmission is greatest during vaginal birth if woman has active lesions Acyclovir not recommended in pregnancy; treat symptomatically (see Table 23-10)

of gestation lateral displacement of the uterus facilitates uteroplacental perfusion (Kuczkowski, 2004).

Appendicitis

Appendicitis occurs in approximately 1 in 2000 pregnancies. This condition occurs with approximately the same frequency during each trimester of pregnancy and the postpartum period (Ludmir & Stubblefield, 2002). The diagnosis of appendicitis is often delayed because the usual signs and symptoms mimic some normal changes of pregnancy such as nausea and vomiting and increased WBC count (Cunningham et al., 2005). As pregnancy progresses, the appendix is pushed upward and to the right of its usual anatomic location (see Fig. 8-13). Because of these changes, rupture of the appendix and the subsequent development of peritonitis occur two to three times more often in pregnant women than in nonpregnant women.

The woman with appendicitis most commonly has right lower quadrant abdominal pain, nausea and vomiting, and loss of appetite. Approximately half of these affected women have muscle guarding. Moving the uterus tends to increase the pain. Temperature may be normal or mildly increased (to 38.3° C). Because of the physiologic increase in WBCs that occurs in pregnancy, elevated WBC counts are not clear indicators of appendicitis (Mourad, Elliott, Erickson, & Lisboa, 2000). Significant increases associated with appendicitis must be monitored either by rising levels on serial samples or by an increasing left shift.

The diagnosis of appendicitis requires a high level of suspicion because the typical signs and symptoms are similar to those found in many other conditions, including pyelonephritis, round ligament pain, placental abruption, torsion of an ovarian cyst, cholecystitis, and preterm labor (Ludmir & Stubblefield, 2002) (see Table 23-7).

Appendectomy before rupture usually does not require either antibiotic or tocolytic therapy. If surgery is delayed until after rupture, multiple antibiotics are ordered. Rupture is likely to result in preterm labor, necessitating the use of tocolytic agents.

Intestinal Obstructions

The second most common nonobstetric abdominal emergency in pregnancy is intestinal obstruction. Any woman with a laparotomy scar is more likely to have an intestinal obstruction (adynamic ileus) during pregnancy. Adhesions as a result of previous surgery or PID, an enlarging uterus, and displacement of the intestines are etiologic factors. Symptoms include constipation; persistent cramplike, abdominal tenderness or pain (continuous or colicky); and vomiting (Cunningham et al., 2005). Auscultatory "rushes" within the abdomen and "laddering" of the intestinal shadows on x-ray films aid in the diagnosis of intestinal obstruction. Immediate surgery is required for release of the obstruction. Pregnancy is rarely affected by the surgery, assuming the absence of complications such as peritonitis.

Gynecologic Problems

Pregnancy predisposes a woman to ovarian problems, especially during the first trimester. Ovarian cysts and twisting (torsion) of ovarian cysts or twisting of adnexal tissues may occur. Other problems include retained or enlarged cystic corpus luteum of pregnancy, and bacterial invasion of reproductive or other intraperitoneal organs. Serial ultrasounds, MRIs and transvaginal color Doppler are used to diagnose most ovarian abnormalities (Cunningham et al., 2005). Ovarian masses generally regress by 16 to 20 weeks of gestation but if not then elective surgery may be done to remove masses. Laparotomy or laparoscopy may be required to discriminate between ovarian problems and early ectopic pregnancy, appendicitis, or an infectious process.

Collaborative Care

The woman and her family are concerned about the effects of the procedure and medication on fetal well-being and the course of pregnancy. An important part of preoperative nursing care is encouraging the woman to express her fears, concerns, and questions. Initial assessment of the pregnant woman requiring surgery focuses on her presenting signs and symptoms. A thorough history is obtained, and a physical examination is performed. Laboratory testing includes, at a minimum, a complete blood count with differential and a urinalysis. FHR, fetal heart activity, and uterine activity

should be monitored; constant vigilance is maintained for symptoms of impending obstetric complications. The extent of preoperative assessment is determined by the immediacy of surgical intervention and the specific condition that necessitates surgery.

Preoperative care for a pregnant woman differs from that for a nonpregnant woman in one significant aspect: the presence of at least one other person, the fetus. Continuous FHR and uterine contraction monitoring should be performed if the fetus is considered viable. Procedures such as preparation of the operative site and time of insertion of IV lines and urinary retention catheters vary with the physician and the facility. Solid foods and liquids are restricted before surgery. If the woman experiences a prolonged NPO status, IV fluids with dextrose should be given. To decrease the risk of vomiting and aspiration, special precautions are taken before anesthetic is administered (e.g., administering an antacid).

Intraoperatively, perinatal nurses may collaborate with the surgical staff to provide for the special needs of pregnant women undergoing surgery. To improve fetal oxygenation, the woman is positioned on the operating table with a lateral tilt to avoid maternal compression of the vena cava. Continuous fetal and uterine monitoring during the procedure is recommended because of the risk for preterm labor. Monitoring may be accomplished using sterile Aquasonic gel and a sterile sleeve for the transducer. During abdominal surgery, uterine contractions may be palpated manually.

In the immediate recovery period, general observations and care pertinent to postoperative recovery are initiated. Frequent assessments are carried out for several hours after surgery. Continuous fetal and uterine monitoring will likely be initiated or resumed because of the increased risk of preterm labor. Tocolysis may be necessary if preterm labor occurs (see Chapter 24).

Plans for the woman's return home and for convalescent care should be completed as early as possible before discharge. Depending on her insurance coverage, nursing care may be provided through a home health agency. If not, the woman and other support persons must be taught necessary skills and procedures, such as wound care. Box 23-8 lists information that should be included in discharge teaching for the postoperative patient. The woman may also need referrals to various community agencies for evaluation of the home situation, child care, home health care, and financial or other assistance.

TRAUMA DURING PREGNANCY ■

Trauma is a common complication during pregnancy because the majority of pregnant women in the United States continue their usual activities. Therefore, pregnant women are at the same risk as other women for vehicular crashes, falls, industrial mishaps, violence, and other injuries in the home and community. Treatment of pregnant trauma victims is complicated because trauma health care providers sel-

Discharge Teaching for Home Care

- Care of incision site
- Diet and elimination related to gastrointestinal function
- Signs and symptoms of developing complications: wound infection, thrombophlebitis, pneumonia
- Equipment needed and technique for assessing temperature
- Recommended schedule for resumption of activities of daily living
- Treatments and medications ordered
- List of resource persons and their telephone numbers
- Schedule of follow-up visits
  If birth has not occurred:
- Assessment of fetal activity (kick counts)
- Signs of preterm labor

dom have the same level of expertise in the care of pregnant women as they do in care of nonpregnant trauma victims (Lutz, 2005).

Significance

Approximately 8% of pregnancies are complicated by physical trauma (Van Hook, 2002). As pregnancy progresses, the risk of trauma seems to increase because more cases of trauma are reported in the third trimester than earlier in gestation.

Acts of violence are a significant health problem in the United States (Beck et al., 2003). The risk of trauma caused by battering and abuse is increased during pregnancy, with estimated rates ranging from 4% to 20% of women abused (Beck et al., 2003; Lutz, 2005). In addition, rates of recurrence are high. Women who are abused during pregnancy have a threefold risk of being murdered compared with nonpregnant abused women (McFarlane, Campbell, Sharps, & Watson, 2002). African-American pregnant women have a threefold higher risk than Caucasian pregnant women (McFarlane et al., 2002). Physical abuse during pregnancy is associated with poor pregnancy outcomes, HIV transmission, and STIs (Beck et al., 2003).

Trauma is the leading nonobstetric cause of maternal death (Ludmir & Stubblefield, 2002). The majority of trauma injuries during pregnancy are minor and have no impact on pregnancy outcomes. However, each case of trauma during pregnancy must be evaluated carefully because pregnancy can mask signs of severe injury.

Trauma increases the incidence of miscarriage, preterm labor, abruptio placentae, and stillbirth (Cunningham et al., 2005). The effect of trauma on pregnancy is influenced by the length of gestation, type and severity of the trauma, and degree of disruption of uterine and fetal physiologic features. Fetal death as a result of trauma is more common than the occurrence of both maternal and fetal death. Careful evaluation of mother and fetus after all types of trauma is imperative. Special considerations for mother and fetus are necessary when

trauma occurs during pregnancy because of the physiologic changes of pregnancy and the presence of the fetus.

Etiology

Blunt abdominal trauma is most commonly the result of motor vehicle accidents but also may be the result of battering or falls (Cunningham et al., 2005). Maternal and fetal mortality and morbidity associated with MVAs are directly correlated with whether the mother remains inside the vehicle or is ejected. Maternal death is usually the result of a head injury or intraabdominal hemorrhage (Van Hook, Gei, & Pacheco, 2004). Fetal death usually correlates with the severity of the maternal injury (Gonik & Foley, 2004; Van Hook, Gei, & Pacheco, 2004). Serious retroperitoneal hemorrhage after lower abdominal and pelvic trauma is reported more frequently during pregnancy. Serious maternal abdominal injuries are usually the result of splenic rupture or liver or renal injury.

Clinical Manifestations

When maternal survival of trauma occurs, fetal death is usually the result of abruptio placentae occurring within 48 hours of the accident (Van Hook, Gei, & Pacheco, 2004).

NURSE ALERT *It is imperative that all pregnant victims be carefully evaluated for signs and symptoms of abruptio placentae after even minor blunt abdominal trauma. Signs and symptoms of abruptio placentae include uterine tenderness or pain, uterine irritability, uterine contractions, vaginal bleeding, leaking of amniotic fluid, and a change in FHR characteristics (e.g., change in baseline rate, loss of accelerations, presence of late decelerations).*

Pelvic fracture may result from severe injury and may produce bladder trauma or retroperitoneal bleeding with the two-point displacement of pelvic bones that usually occurs. One point of displacement is commonly at the symphysis pubis, and the second point is posterior because of the structure of the pelvis. Careful evaluation for clinical signs of internal hemorrhage is indicated (Cunningham et al., 2005).

Direct fetal injury as a complication of trauma during pregnancy most often involves the fetal skull and brain (Gilbert & Harmon, 2003). Most commonly this injury accompanies maternal pelvic fracture in late gestation, after the fetal head becomes engaged. When the force of the impact is great enough to fracture the maternal pelvis, the fetus will often sustain a skull fracture. Evaluation for fetal skull fracture or intracranial hemorrhage is indicated.

Uterine rupture as a result of trauma is rare, occurring in only 0.6% of all reported cases of trauma during pregnancy. Uterine rupture depends on numerous factors, including gestational age, the intensity of the impact, and the presence of a predisposing factor such as a distended uterus caused by polyhydramnios or multiple gestation or the presence of a uterine scar resulting from previous uterine surgery. When uterine rupture occurs, the force responsible is usually a direct, high-energy blow. Fetal death is common with traumatic uterine rupture (Cunningham et al., 2005). However, maternal death occurs less than 10% of the time, and when it occurs it is usually the result of massive injuries sustained from an impact severe enough to rupture the uterus.

Penetrating Abdominal Trauma

Bullet wounds are the most frequent cause of penetrating abdominal injury, followed by stab wounds. In the majority of cases of penetrating abdominal wounds, the woman survives, but the fetus does not (41% to 71%) (Gonik & Foley, 2004). The enlarged uterus may protect other maternal organs, but the fetus is particularly vulnerable (Cunningham et al., 2005). Numerous factors determine the extent and severity of maternal and fetal injury from a bullet wound, including size and velocity of the bullet, anatomic region penetrated, angle of entry, path of the bullet, organs damaged, gestational age, and exit wound. Once the bullet enters the body, it may ricochet several times as it encounters organs or bone, or it may sever a large blood vessel. Gunshot wounds require surgical exploration to determine the extent of injury and repair damage as needed. Stab wounds are limited by the length and width of the penetrating object and are usually confined to the pathway of the weapon. Maternal and fetal injury are less if the stab wound is located in the upper abdomen and if movement of the penetrating object is from above the head downward toward the abdomen rather than from the ground upward toward the lower abdomen. Stab wounds usually require surgical exploration to clean debris, determine extent of injury, and repair damage.

Thoracic Trauma

Thoracic trauma is reported to produce 25% of all trauma deaths (Van Hook, Gei, & Pacheco, 2004). Chest trauma may result in several life threatening injuries which include tension pneumothrorax or open pneumothorax, hemothorax, cardiac tamponade, flail chest, myocardial damage, diaphragmatic rupture, aortic rupture, and pulmonary contusion. Pulmonary contusion results from nearly 75% of blunt thoracic trauma and is a potentially life-threatening condition. Pulmonary contusion can be difficult to recognize, especially if flail chest also is present or if there is no evidence of thoracic injury. Pulmonary contusion should be suspected in cases of thoracic injury, especially after blunt acceleration or deceleration trauma, such as that occurring when a rapidly moving vehicle crashes into an immovable object.

Penetrating wounds into the chest can result in pneumothorax or hemothorax. This type of injury is usually caused by a vehicular crash that results in impalement by the steering column or a loose article in the vehicle that became a projectile with the force of impact. Stab wounds into the chest also may occur as a result of violence.

Collaborative Care

Immediate priorities for stabilization of the pregnant woman after trauma should be identical to those of the nonpregnant trauma patient (Cunningham et al., 2005). Survival of the fetus is dependent on maternal survival and stabilization. The perinatal nurse is often called on to function collaboratively with emergency department or trauma unit staff members in providing care for the pregnant trauma victim. Priorities of care for the pregnant woman after trauma must be to resuscitate the woman and stabilize her condition *first* and then consider fetal needs. Lateral displacement of the uterus may significantly improve maternal cardiac output and therefore fetal oxygenation (Cunningham et al., 2005). On admission after trauma, pregnant women are typed, crossmatched, and screened, with a urinalysis, coagulation panel, ultrasound examination, and assessment of FHR performed as appropriate. A KB test is done for women at greater than 12 weeks of gestation to ascertain fetal red blood cells (fetomaternal hemorrhage) in the maternal circulation regardless of the maternal blood type. $Rh_o(D)$ immunoglobulin administration is indicated for Rh-negative women with fetomaternal bleeding, and tetanus toxoid is administered if indicated (Cunningham et al., 2005).

In cases of minor trauma, the woman is evaluated for vaginal bleeding, uterine irritability, abdominal tenderness, abdominal pain or cramps, and evidence of hypovolemia. A change in or absence of FHR or fetal activity, leakage of amniotic fluid, and presence of fetal cells in the maternal circulation are also included in the assessment.

In cases of major trauma, the systematic evaluation begins with a primary survey and the initial "ABCDEFs" of resuscitation: establishment of and maintaining an *airway*, ensuring adequate *breathing*, maintaining an adequate *circulatory* volume, assessing for *disability* (alert, voice, pain, and unresponsive), *examining* the patient head to toe (Van Hook, Gei, & Pacheco, 2004) and assessing *fetal* status.

Once an airway is established, assessment should focus on adequacy of oxygenation. Rapid placement of two large bore (14- to 16-gauge) IV lines is necessary in the majority of seriously injured women. With maternal blood loss greater than 2,000 ml there is rapid maternal deterioration while the fetus may be compromised with a blood loss less than 2,000 ml (Van Hook, Gei, & Pacheco, 2004). Infusion of IV fluids such as normal saline should use a 3:1 ratio; that is, 3 ml of crystalloid replacement to 1 ml of the estimated blood loss is given over the first 30 to 60 minutes of acute resuscitation. Because of the 50% increase in blood volume during pregnancy, formulas for nonpregnant adults for estimating crystalloid and blood replacement to counter blood loss must be adjusted upward for pregnancy. Replacement of red blood cells and other blood components is anticipated. Vasopressor drugs to restore maternal arterial BP should be avoided, if possible, until volume replacement is administered. Establishing a baseline neurologic status is essential.

After immediate resuscitation and successful stabilization measures, a more detailed secondary survey of the mother and fetus should be accomplished. A complete physical assessment including all body systems is performed. The eval-

TABLE 23-12

Priorities for Perinatal Trauma Management

ACTIVITY	TEAM A (MOTHER)	TEAM B (FETUS)
T = Triage*	Assess ABCs —Airway —Breathing —Circulation	Assess fetus —Cardiac activity —Gestational age Assess placenta for abruption
R = Resuscitation	Perform CPR Infuse crystalloid fluids Administer oxygen at 8-10 L/min by mask Administer blood as indicated (in emergency situation, O-negative blood can be used)	Position mother in lateral tilt
A = Assessment A, B, C, D, E, F	Assess for maternal injuries (similar to that in nonpregnant patient) Assess vital signs; level of consciousness; respiratory status as to depth, irregularity, and breath sounds A–Airway B–Breathing C–Circulatory volume D–Disability (alert, voice, pain, and unresponsive) E–Expose patient for head to toe assessment	F. Assess FHR and uterine contractions with EFM Assess for vaginal bleeding and rupture of membranes; Kleihauer-Betke test may be done to rule out fetal hemorrhage
U = Ultrasound or uterine evaluation	Evaluate uterus for hemorrhage	Evaluate fundal height Palpate for uterine tenderness, contractions, or irritability Ultrasound may be done to determine placental or fetal injury and placental location Amniocentesis may be done to assess fetal lung maturity or intrauterine bleeding
M = Management and monitoring	Decide initial management and needed continual monitoring	Decide to monitor or proceed to cesarean birth depending on status of mother and fetus and risk of prematurity
A = Activate transport or transfer	After stabilization, transport or transfer to critical care, operating suite, or level III perinatal unit	Activate neonatal team for consultation, transfer, or transport as necessary

From Gilbert, E., & Harmon, J. (2003). *Manual of high risk pregnancy and delivery* (3rd ed.). St. Louis: Mosby.
CPR, Cardiopulmonary resuscitation; *EFM,* electronic fetal monitor; *FHR,* fetal heart rate.
*Pregnant woman is first priority, then fetus.

uation and care is usually performed by two teams of care providers. The first team focuses on the mother and the second focuses on the fetus and any pregnancy-related problems. Table 23-12 summarizes posttrauma care for the pregnant woman and fetus.

The greatest clinical concern after vehicular crashes is abruptio placentae, as up to 40% of these women will have an abruption (Van Hook, 2002). Assessments should focus on recognition of this complication, with careful evaluation of fetal monitor tracings, uterine tenderness, labor, or vaginal bleeding. Ultrasound examination may be performed to determine gestational age, viability of the fetus, and placental location.

In addition to assisting with stabilization of the woman, the nurse will likely be providing emotional support for the injured woman and her family. If the trauma is the result of an MVA, other family members may also have been critically injured or killed. The nurse collaborates with staff members in other units of the same hospital, as well as at other hospitals, to make sure that questions are answered and consistent information is given. Grief support may also be necessary.

In the presence of severe, multisystem trauma, perimortem cesarean birth may be indicated. Removal of the fetus early in the process of resuscitation may increase the chance for maternal survival. With maternal death, fetal survival is unlikely if cesarean birth is accomplished more than 20 minutes after maternal demise. Therefore, to facilitate maternal resuscitation, a cesarean birth may be indicated after 4 to 5 minutes of maternal resuscitative efforts are ineffective (Cunningham et al., 2005; Van Hook, Gei, & Pacheco, 2004).

With minor trauma the woman may be discharged home after an adequate period of EFM that demonstrates fetal reassurance and absence of uterine contractions (Cunningham et al., 2005). Her vital signs should be stable, with no evidence of bleeding at the time of discharge. There should be no uterine contractions, and the FHR tracing should be re-assuring before monitoring is discontinued and the woman discharged (Cunningham et al., 2005). Education for the woman and her family is important. She should be instructed to contact her health care provider immediately if changes in fetal movement or signs and symptoms indicative of preterm labor, PROM, or placental abruption develop. If the trauma occurred as a result of a MVA, the woman should be reminded about the importance of wearing a seat belt and given directions for using it correctly during pregnancy (position the lap belt over hips and thighs, rather than across the abdomen) (see Fig. 9-18). If the trauma occurred as a result of domestic violence, the woman may need information about intimate partner violence (see Chapter 4); referral to a crisis center, law enforcement agency, or counseling center; and help in forming a safety plan.

COMMUNITY ACTIVITY

Contact your local hospital, obstetric offices, health department, and mental health counselors to assess resources available for pregnant women and their families who have experienced a pregnancy loss. Assess the availability of written resources reviewing the level of literacy of the resources and support groups. Review the hospital policy and procedure for women experiencing a pregnancy loss to include written materials, parental memorabilia, and disposition of fetus,

Contact your local hospital or obstetric office to identify resources available for women on bed rest due to a high risk pregnancy. Review the hospital policy for these women and their families, i.e., written and electronic materials and support groups. Identify the specific activities allowed, including activity level, home activities, child care, hygiene, ambulation, and sexual activity.

Key Points

- Hypertensive disorders during pregnancy are a leading cause of infant and maternal morbidity and mortality worldwide.
- The cause of preeclampsia is unknown, and there are no known reliable tests for predicting which women are at risk for this condition.
- Preeclampsia is a multisystem disease rather than only an increase in BP.
- HELLP syndrome, which usually becomes apparent during the third trimester, is a variant of severe preeclampsia and is considered life threatening.
- Magnesium sulfate, the anticonvulsive agent of choice for preventing eclampsia, requires careful monitoring of reflexes, respirations, and urinary output; its antidote, calcium gluconate, should be available at the bedside.
- Intent of emergency interventions for eclampsia is to prevent self-injury, ensure adequate oxygenation, reduce aspiration risk, establish seizure control with magnesium sulfate, and correct maternal acidemia.
- The woman with hyperemesis gravidarum may have significant weight loss and dehydration; man-agement focuses on restoring fluid and electrolyte balance and preventing recurrence of nausea and vomiting.
- Some miscarriages occur for unknown reasons, but fetal or placental maldevelopment and maternal factors account for many others.
- The type of miscarriage and signs and symptoms direct care management.
- Recurrent premature dilation of the cervix may be treated with a cervical cerclage; the woman is instructed on activity restriction and recognizing the warning signs of preterm labor, ROM, and infection.
- Ectopic pregnancy is a significant cause of maternal morbidity and mortality.
- There are two categories of gestational trophoblastic disease, hydatiform mole, and or gestational trophoblastic neoplasia (GTN). β-hCG titers are measured to confirm diagnosis and to follow up after treatment.
- Premature separation of the placenta and placenta previa are differentiated by type of bleeding, uterine tonicity, and presence or absence of pain.

Key Points—cont'd

- Clotting disorders are associated with many obstetric complications.
- An enlarged uterus, displaced internal organs, and altered laboratory values may confound differential diagnosis in the pregnant woman when the need for immediate abdominal surgery occurs.
- Preoperative care for a pregnant woman differs from that for a nonpregnant woman in one significant aspect: the presence of at least one other person, the fetus.
- Most traumatic maternal injuries are a result of motor vehicle crashes, followed by falls and direct assaults to the pregnant abdomen.

- Fetal survival depends on maternal survival; after trauma the first priority is resuscitation and stabilization of the pregnant woman before consideration of fetal concerns.
- Minor trauma can be associated with major complications for the pregnancy, including abruptio placentae, fetomaternal hemorrhage, preterm labor and birth, and fetal death.
- Pregnancy confers no immunity against infection, and both mother and fetus must be considered when the pregnant woman contracts an infection.

Answer Guidelines to Critical Thinking Exercise

Preeclampsia

1 Yes. Risk factors for preeclampsia include: obesity, pre-existing diabetes, family history, nulliparity, women at extreme ends of the reproductive continuum and African-American ethnicity.

2 Assumptions:

a. Possible diagnoses for Demetria include: gestational hypertension severe, preeclampsia, HELLP syndrome.

b. Physical assessment will include head to toe baseline physical assessment, V.S., particularly BP with patient on her left side, weight, FHR, fetal movement, deep tendon reflexes, edema (facial, hands, and tibial) and clonus. Nursing assessment will include questioning regarding headache, blurred vision, scotoma, nausea, vomiting, fetal movement, and epigastric discomfort or pain.

Laboratory tests will include CBC, chem. 14 for baseline information and liver panel to assess for elevated liver enzymes. Platelets are ordered to assess for thrombocytopenia which, when coupled with elevated liver enzymes, is indicative of HELLP syndrome, disease severity, and poor pregnancy outcomes. Uric acid is done to assess glomerular filtration rate (GFR). A decrease in uric acid is indicative of a decreasing GFR. An NST is ordered to assess maternal-fetal status and urine dipstick will be done on admission to assess for proteinuria. A 24-hour urine for total protein and creatinine will be started. Increased total protein and creatinine.are indicative of disease severity and contribute to management decisions by the OB provider.

c. Research supports the relationship of obesity to endothelial activation and a systemic inflammatory response. Genetic factors predispose Demetria to preeclampsia. Immunologic maladjustment similar to graft-host rejection is evidenced by microscopic changes at the maternal-placenta bed, as in first pregnancies.

3 Priorities for nursing care at this time include controlling Demetria's blood pressure, facilitating uteroplacental perfusion, and monitoring for neuromuscular irritability and disease status. Hydralazine IV with BP check in 10 minutes and notify obstetric provider if the BP remains elevated. Therefore, nursing care will include: physical assessment every shift, V.S., particularly BP with patient on her left side every 4 hours, daily weights (at the same time of day), FHR every 4 hours, fetal movement every 4 hours, deep tendon reflexes every 4 hours, edema (facial, hands, and tibial) every 4 hours, and clonus every 4 hours. Nursing assessment will include questioning regarding headache, blurred vision, scotoma, nausea, vomiting, fetal movement, and epigastric discomfort or pain. In addition, intake and output (with a minimum urinary output of 30 ml/hour) will be monitored and all urine tested for urinary protein. A heplock is ordered for intravenous access and emergency medications.

4 Yes, there is initial evidence to support the diagnosis of preeclampsia.

5 Further information is necessary to differentiate between gestational hypertension, preeclampsia, superimposed preeclampsia, or chronic hypertension. Her initial prenatal records have been requested from the local health department where she is receiving obstetric care. In addition, results from ordered laboratory and maternal-fetal tests will provide more information for decision making.

Resources

American College of Obstetricians and Gynecologists (ACOG)
409 12th St., SW
Washington, DC 20024
800-762-2264
www.acog.com

American Social Health Association (ASHA)
P.O. Box 13827
Research Triangle Park, NC 27709
1-800-783-9877
www.ashastd.org

Centers for Disease Control and Prevention (CDC)
1600 Clifton Rd., NE
Atlanta, GA 30333
404-329-1819
404-329-3286
www.cdc.gov

Division of Violence Prevention–CDC
Intimate Partner Violence
www.cdc.gov/ncipc

COPE (Coping with the Overall Pregnancy/Parenting Experience)
37 Clarendon St.
Boston, MA 02116
617-357-5588

Family Violence Prevention Fund
383 Rhode Island St., Suite 304
San Francisco, CA 94103
415-252-8900
www.fvpf.org

Left Sidelines Magazine–Bedrest
Sidelines
2805 Park Place
Laguna Beach, CA 92651
949-497-2265
www.sidelines.org

National Domestic Violence and Abuse Hotline
800-799-SAFE

National Institute of Justice
National Criminal Justice Reference Service
P.O. Box 6000
Rockville, MC 20849-6000
800-851-3420
askncjrs@ncjrs.org

National Sexually Transmitted Diseases Hotline
800-227-8922

Moms on Bedrest:
www.momsonbedrest.com

Pregnancy and Infant Loss
1421 East Wayzata Blvd., Suite 40
Wayzata, MN 55391
614-473-9372

Pregnancy Bed Rest
http://fpb.cwru.edu/Bedrest/

Pregnancy Bed Rest
www.pregnancybedrest.com

Rest- Taking to Bed–AmericanBaby
Rest-Coping How to Keep from Going Crazy
http://www.americanbaby

Sexually Transmitted Diseases – CDC
www.cdc.gov/nchstp/dstd/disease_info.htm
www.cdc.gov/std/STDFact-STDs&Pregnancy.htm

Violence Against Women Electronic Network (VAWnet)
www.vawnet.org

References

Abboud, L., & Laimputtong, P. (2003). Pregnancy loss: What it means to women who miscarry and their partners. *Social Work Health Care* 36(3), 37-62.

American College of Obstetricians and Gynecologists (ACOG). (2004b). *Diagnosis and treatment of gestational trophoblastic disease. Practice Bulletin no. 53.* Washington, DC: ACOG.

American College of Obstetricians and Gynecologists (ACOG). (2002). *Diagnosis and management of preclampsia and eclampsia. ACOG Practice Bulletin no. 33.* Washington, DC: ACOG.

American College of Obstetricians and Gynecologists (ACOG). (2004a). *Nausea and vomiting of pregnancy. Practice Bulletin no 52.* Washington, DC: ACOG.

Ananth, C., Smulian, J., Demissie, K., Vintzileos, A., & Knuppel, R. (2001). Placental abruption among singleton and twin births in the United States: Risk factor profiles. *American Journal of Epidemiology, 153*(8), 771-778.

Ananth, C., Demissie, K., Smulian, J., & Vintzileos, A. (2001). Relationship among placenta previa, fetal growth restriction, and preterm delivery: A population-based study. *Obstetrics & Gynecology 98*(2), 299-306.

Andres, R., & Day, M. (2000). Perinatal complications associated with maternal tobacco use. *Seminars in Neonatology, 5*(3), 231-234.

Armstrong, D. (2004). Impact of prior perinatal loss on subsequent pregnancies. *Journal of Obstetric, Gynecologic, and Neonatal Nursing, 33*(6), 765-766.

Beck, L., Johnson, C., Morrow, B., Lipscomb, L., Gaffield, M.,Gilbert, B., Rogers, M., & Whitehead, N. (2003). *PRAMS 1999 Surveillance Report.* Atlanta, GA: Division of Reproductive Health, National Center for Chronic Disease Prevention and Health Promotion, Centers for Disease Control and Prevention.

Benedetti, T. (2002). Obstetric hemorrhage. In S. Gabbe, J. Niebyl, & J. Simpson (Eds.). *Obstetrics: Normal and problem pregnancies* (4th ed.). New York: Churchill Livingstone.

Berman, M., DiSaia, P., & Tewari, K. (2004). Pelvic malignancies, gestational trophoblastic neoplasia, and nonpelvic malignancies. In R. Creasy, R. Resnik, & J. Iams (Eds.). *Maternal-fetal medicine: Principles and practice* (5th ed.). Philadelphia: Saunders.

Bhide, A., & Thilaganathan, B. (2004). Recent advances in the management of placenta previa. *Current Opinion in Obstetrics and Gynecology 16*(6), 447-451.

Blackburn, S. (2003). *Maternal, fetal, and neonatal physiology: A clinical perspective.* (2nd ed.). St. Louis: Saunders.

Broen, A., Moum, T., Bodtker, A., & Ekeberg, O. (2004). Psychological impact on women of miscarriage versus induced abortion: A 2 year follow-up study. *Psychosomatic Medicine, 66*(2), 265-271.

Bush, K., O'Brien, J., & Barton, J. (2001). The utility of umbilical artery Doppler investigatin in women with HELLP (hemolysis, elevated liver enzymes, and low platelets) syndrome. *American Journal of Obstetrics and Gynecology, 184*(6), 1087-1089.

Callister, L., & Hobbins-Garbett, D. (2000). Cochrane pregnancy and childbirth database: Resource for evidence-based practice. *Journal of Obstetric, Gynecologic, and Neonatal Nursing, 29*(2), 123-128.

Centers for Disease Control and Prevention (CDC). (2002). Sexually transmitted diseases treatment guidelines. *Morbidity & Mortality Weekly Report, 51*(RR-6), 1-82.

Chang, J., Elam-Evans, L., Berg, C., Herndon, J., Flowers, L., Seed, K. & Syverson, C. (2003). Pregnancy-related mortality surveillance–United States, 1991-1999. *Morbidity & Mortality Weekly Report Surveillance Summary, 52*(SS-2), 1-8.

Clark, S. (2004). Placenta previa and abruptio placentae. In R. Creasy, R. Resnik, & J. Iams (Eds.). *Maternal-fetal medicine: Principles and practice* (5th ed.). Philadelphia: Saunders.

Crane, J., Van den Hof, M., Dodds, L., Armson, B., & Liston, R. (2000). Maternal complications with placenta previa. *American Journal of Perinatology, 17*(2), 101-105.

Crowther, C. (2001). Hospitalization and bed rest for multiple pregnancy (Cochrane Review). In *The Cochrane Library,* Issue 2, 2004, Chichester, UK: John Wiley & Sons.

Cunningham, F., Leveno, K., Bloom, S., Hauth, J., Gilstrap, L., & Wenstrom, K. (2005). *Williams obstetrics* (22nd ed.). New York: McGraw-Hill.

Davies, B., & Hodnett, E. (2002). Cochrane pregnancy and childbirth database: Resource for evidence-based practice. *Journal of Obstetric, Gynecologic, and Neonatal Nursing, 29*(2), 123-128.

Davis, M. (2004). Nausea and vomiting of pregnancy: An evidence-based review. *Journal of Perinatal and Neonatal Nursing 18*(4), 312-328.

Dekker, G, (2001). Prevention of preclampsia. In B. Sibai (Ed.). *Hypertensive disorders in women.* Philadelphia: Saunders.

Dekker, G., & Sibai, B. (1999). The immunology of preeclampsia. *Seminars in Perinatology, 23*(1), 24-33.

Dialani, V., & Levine, D. (2004). Ectopic pregnancy: A review. *Ultrasound Quarterly, 20*(3), 105-117.

Dildy, G. (2004) Complications of preeclampsia. In G. Dildy, M. Belfort, G. Saade, J. Phelan, G. Hankins, & S. Clark (Eds.). *Critical care obstetrics* (4th ed) Malden, MA: Blackwell Science.

Duckitt, R., & Harrington, D. (2005). Risk factors for pre-eclampsia at antenatal booking: Systematic review of controlled studies. *BMJ 33*(7491), 565.

Emery, S. (2005). Hypertensive disorders of pregnancy: Overdiagnosis is appropriate. *Cleveland Clinic Journal of Medicine, 72*(4), 345-352.

Enkin, M., Keirse, M., Neilson, J., Crowther, C., Duley, L., Hodnett, E., & Hofmeyr, J. (2001). Effective care in pregnancy and childbirth: A synopsis. *Birth, 28*(1), 41-51.

Freda, M. (1999). The power of words. *MCN American Journal of Maternal Child Nursing, 24*(2), 63.

Gibbs, R., Sweet, R., & Duff, P. (2004). Maternal and fetal infectious disorders. In R. Creasy, R. Resnik, & J. Iams (Eds.), *Maternal/fetal medicine: Principles and practice* (5th ed.). Philadelphia: Saunders.

Gilbert, E., & Harmon, J. (2003). *Manual of high risk pregnancy and delivery* (3rd ed.). St. Louis: Mosby.

Gonik, B., & Foley, M. (2004). Intensive care monitoring of the critically ill pregnant patient. In R. Creasy, R. Resnik, & J. Iams (Eds.). *Maternal/fetal medicine: Principles and practice* (5th ed.). Philadelphia: Saunders.

Hill, J. (2004). Recurrent pregnancy loss. In R. Creasy, R. Resnik, & J. Iams (Eds.). *Maternal-fetal medicine: Principles and practice* (5th ed.). Philadelphia: Saunders.

Iams, J. (2004). Abnormal cervical competence. In R. Creasy, R. Resnik, & J. Iams (Eds.). *Maternal-fetal medicine: Principles and practice* (5th ed.). Philadelphia: Saunders.

Jewell, D., & Young, G. (2003). Interventions for nausea and vomiting in early pregnancy. (Cochrane Review). In *The Cochrane Library,* 2004, Issue 2. Chichester, UK: John Wiley & Sons.

Kilpatrick, S., & Laros, R. (2004). Maternal hematologic disorders. In R. Creasy, R. Resnik, & J. Iams (Eds.). *Maternal-fetal medicine: Principles and practice* (5th ed.). Philadelphia: Saunders.

Kuczkowski, K. (2004). Nonobstetric surgery during pregnancy: What are the risks of anesthesia? *Obstetrical and Gynecological Survey, 59*(1), 52-56.

Kumtepe, Y., & Kadanali, I. (2004). Medical treatment of ruptured with hemodynamically stable and unruptured ectopic pregnancy patients. *European Journal of Obstetrics Gynecology and Reproductive Biology 116*(2), 221-225.

Labelle, C., & Kitchens, C. (2005). Disseminated intravascular coagulation: Treat the cause, not the lab values. *Cleveland Clinic Journal of Medicine, 72*(5), 377-397.

Li, D., & Wi, S. (2000). Changing paternity and the risk of preclampsia/eclampsia in the subsequent pregnancy. *American Journal of Epidemiology, 15*(1), 57-62.

Livingston, J., & Sibai, B. (2001). *Chronic hypertension in pregnancy.* Obstetrics and Gynecology Clinics, 28(3), 1-15.

Ludmir, J., & Stubblefield, P. (2002). Surgical procedures in pregnancy. In S. Gabbe, J. Niebyl, & J. Simpson (Eds.). *Obstetrics: Normal and problem pregnancies* (4th ed.). New York: Churchill Livingstone.

Lurie, S., Feinstein, M., & Mamet, Y. (2000). Disseminated intravascular coagulopathy in pregnancy: Thorough comprehension of etiology and management reduces obstetricians' stress. *Archives of Gynecology and Obstetrics, 263*(3), 126-130.

Lutz, K. (2005). Abused pregnant women's interactions with health care providers during the childbearing year. *Journal of Obstetric, Gyencologic, and Neonatal Nursing, 34*(2), 151-162.

Magpie Trial Follow Up Study Management Group. (2004).The Magpie trial follow-up study: Outcome after discharge from hospital for women and children recruited to a trial comparing magnesium sulfate with placebo for pre-eclampsia. *BMC Pregnancy Childbirth, 4*(1), 5.

Maloni, J. (2002). Astronauts & pregnancy bed rest: What NASA is teaching us about inactivity. *AWHONN Lifelines, 6*(4), 318-323.

Maloni J., & Kutil, R. (2000) Antepartum support group for women hospitalized on bed rest. *MCN American Journal of Maternal Child Nursing, 25*(4), 204-10.

Martin, J., Hamilton, B., Sutton, P., Ventura, S., Menacker, F., & Munson, M. (2005). Births: Final data for 2003. *National Vital Statistics Reports, 54*(2), 1-116.

Mattar, F., & Sibai, B. (2000). Eclampsia. VII. Risk factors for maternal morbidity. *American Journal of Obstetrics and Gynecology, 182*(2), 307-312.

McFarlane, J., Campbell, J., Sharps, P., & Watson, K. (2002). Abuse during pregnancy and femicide: Urgent implications for women's health. *Obstetrics and Gynecology 100*(1), 27-36.

Meighan, M., & Wood, A. (2004). The impact of hyperemesis gravidarum on maternal role assumption. *Journal of Obstetric, Gynecologic, and Neonatal Nursing, 34*(2), 172-179.

Mignini, L., Latthe, P., Villar, J., Kilby, M., Carroli, G., & Khalid, S. (2005). Mapping the theories of preeclampsia: The role of homocysteine. *Obstetrics and Gynecology, 105*(2), 411-425.

Mourad, J., Elliott, J., Erickson, L., & Lisboa, L. (2000). Appendicitis in pregnancy: New information that contradicts long-held beliefs. *American Journal of Obstetrics and Gynecology, 182*(5), 1027-1029.

National High Blood Pressure Education Program Working Group on High Blood Pressure in Pregnancy. (2000). Report of the national high blood pressure education program working group on high blood pressure in pregnancy. *American Journal of Obstetrics and Gynecology, 183*(1), S1-S22.

Nick, J. (2004). Deep tendon reflexes, magnesium, and calcium: Assessments and implications. *Journal of Obstetric, Gynecologic, and Neonatal Nursing, 33*(2), 221-230.

Peters, R. & Flack, J. (2004). Hypertensive disorders of pregnancy. *Journal of Obstetric, Gynecologic, and Neonatal Nursing, 33*(2), 209-220.

Roberts, J. (2004). Pregnancy-related hypertension. In R. Creasy, R. Resnik, & J. Iams (Eds.). *Maternal-fetal medicine: Principles and practice* (5th ed.). Philadelphia: Saunders.

Robillard, P. (2002). Interest in preclampsia for researchers in reproduction. *Journal of Reproductive Immunology, 53*(1-2), 279-287.

Scott, L., & Abu-Hamda, E. (2004). Gastrointestinal disease in pregnancy. In R. Creasy, R. Resnik, & J. Iams (Eds.). *Maternal-fetal medicine: Principles and practice* (5th ed.). Philadelphia: Saunders.

Seidel, H., Ball, J., Dains, J., & Benedict, G. (2003). *Mosby's guide to physical examination* (5th ed.). St. Louis: Mosby.

Sepilian, V., & Wood, E. (2004). *Ectopic pregnancy*. Emedicine. Available www.emedicine.com/med/topic3212.htm. (accessed May 2, 2005).

Sheiner, E., Levy, A., Katz, M., & Mazor, M. (2004). Pregnancy outcome following recurrent spontaneous abortions. *European Journal of Obstetrics & Gynecology and Reproductive Biology, 118*(1), 61-65.

Sibai, B. (2004). Diagnosis, controversies, and management of the syndrome of hemolysis, elevated liver enzymes, and low platelet count. *Obstetrics & Gynecology 103*(5 Part 1), 981-991.

Sibai, B. (2002). Hypertension. In S. Gabbe, J. Niebyl, & J. Simpson (Eds.), *Obstetrics: Normal and problem pregnancies* (4th ed.) New York: Churchill Livingstone.

Sibai, B., Dekker, G., Kupferminc, M. (2005). Pre-eclampsia. *Lancet 365*(9461), 785-799.

Simpson, J. (2002). Fetal wastage. In S. Gabbe, J. Niebyl, & J. Simpson (Eds.). *Obstetrics: Normal and problem pregnancies* (4th ed.). New York: Churchill Livingstone.

Smith, C., Crowther, C., Willson, K., Hotham, N., & McMillian, V. (2004). A randomized controlled trial of ginger to treat nausea and vomiting in pregnancy. *Obstetrics & Gynecology, 103*(4), 639-645.

Tiran, D., & Mack, E. (Eds.) (2000). *Complementary therapies for pregnancy and childbirth* (2nd ed.). Edinburgh: Bailliere Tindall.

Van Hook, J. (2002). Trauma in pregnancy. *Clinics in Obstetrics & Gynecology, 45*(2), 414-424.

Van Hook, J., Gei, A., & Pacheco, L. (2004). Trauma in pregnancy. In G. Dildy, M. Belfort, G. Saade, J. Phelan, G. Hankins, & S. Clark (Eds.), *Critical care obstetrics* (4th ed.). Malden, MA: Blackwell Science.

Weiner, C., & Buhimschi, C. (2004). *Drugs for pregnant and lactating women*. New York: Churchill Livingstone.

CHAPTER 24

Labor and Birth at Risk

DEITRA LEONARD LOWDERMILK

LEARNING OBJECTIVES

- Differentiate between preterm birth and low birth weight.
- Identify the risk factors for preterm labor.
- Evaluate current interventions to prevent preterm birth.
- Discuss the use of tocolytics and antenatal glucocorticoids in preterm labor and birth.
- Examine the effects of prescribed bed rest on pregnant women and their families.
- Summarize the nursing care management of women with preterm premature rupture of membranes.

- Demonstrate knowledge of nursing management for a trial of labor, the induction and augmentation of labor, forceps- and vacuum-assisted birth, cesarean birth, and vaginal birth after a cesarean birth.
- Explain the care of a woman with postterm pregnancy.
- Discuss obstetric emergencies and their appropriate management.

KEY TERMS AND DEFINITIONS

amniotic fluid embolism (AFE) Embolism resulting from amniotic fluid entering the maternal bloodstream during labor and birth after rupture of membranes; often fatal to the woman if it is a pulmonary embolism

antenatal glucocorticoids Medications administered to the mother for the purpose of accelerating fetal lung maturity when there is increased risk for preterm birth between 24 and 34 weeks of gestation

augmentation of labor Stimulation of ineffective uterine contractions after labor has started spontaneously but is not progressing satisfactorily

Bishop score Rating system to evaluate inducibility (ripeness) of the cervix; a higher score increases the likelihood of a successful induction of labor

cephalopelvic disproportion (CPD) Condition in which the infant's head is of such a shape, size, or position that it cannot pass through the mother's pelvis or the maternal pelvis is too small, abnormally shaped, or deformed to allow the passage of a fetus of average size

cesarean birth Birth of a fetus by an incision through the abdominal wall and uterus

chorioamnionitis Inflammatory reaction in fetal membranes to bacteria or viruses in the amniotic fluid, which then become infiltrated with polymorphonuclear leukocytes

dysfunctional labor Abnormal uterine contractions that prevent normal progress of cervical dilation, effacement, or descent

dystocia Prolonged, painful, or otherwise difficult labor caused by various conditions associated with the five factors affecting labor (powers, passage, passenger, maternal position, and maternal emotions)

external cephalic version (ECV) Turning of the fetus to a vertex presentation by external exertion of pressure on the fetus through the maternal abdomen

forceps-assisted birth Vaginal birth in which forceps (i.e., curved-bladed instruments) are used to assist in the birth of the fetal head

hypertonic uterine dysfunction Uncoordinated, painful, frequent uterine contractions that do not cause cervical dilation and effacement; primary dysfunctional labor

hypotonic uterine dysfunction Weak, ineffective uterine contractions usually occurring in the active phase of labor; often related to cephalopelvic disproportion or malposition of the fetus; secondary uterine inertia

oxytocin Hormone produced by the posterior pituitary gland that stimulates uterine contractions and the release of milk in the mammary glands (letdown reflex); synthetic oxytocin is a medication that mimics the uterine stimulating action of oxytocin

postterm pregnancy Pregnancy prolonged past 42 weeks of gestation

precipitous labor Rapid or sudden labor lasting less than 3 hours from the onset of uterine contractions to complete birth of the fetus

Continued

KEY TERMS AND DEFINITIONS—cont'd

premature rupture of membranes (PROM) Rupture of the amniotic sac and leakage of amniotic fluid beginning at least 1 hour before the onset of labor at any gestational age

preterm birth Birth occurring before the completion of 37 weeks of gestation

preterm labor Cervical changes and uterine contractions occurring between 20 weeks and 37 weeks of pregnancy

preterm premature rupture of membranes (PPROM) PROM that occurs before 37 weeks of gestation

prolapse of the umbilical cord Protrusion of the umbilical cord in advance of the presenting part

shoulder dystocia Condition in which the head is born but the anterior shoulder cannot pass under the pubic arch

therapeutic rest Administration of analgesics and implementation of comfort or relaxation measures to decrease pain and induce rest for management of hypertonic uterine dysfunction

tocolytics Medications used to suppress uterine activity and relax the uterus in cases of hyperstimulation or preterm labor

trial of labor (TOL) Period of observation to determine whether a laboring woman is likely to be successful in progressing to a vaginal birth

vacuum-assisted birth Birth involving attachment of a vacuum cap to the fetal head (occiput) and application of negative pressure to assist in birth of the fetus

vaginal birth after cesarean (VBAC) Giving birth vaginally after having had a previous cesarean birth

ELECTRONIC RESOURCES

Additional information related to the content in Chapter 24 can be found on

The companion website at **evolve**
http://evolve.elsevier.com/Lowdermilk/Maternity/
- NCLEX Review Questions
- Case Study—Preterm Labor
- Case Study—Postdate Pregnancy
- WebLinks

or on the interactive companion CD
- NCLEX Review Questions
- Case Study—Preterm Labor
- Case Study—Postdate Pregnancy
- Plan of Care—Dysfunctional Labor
- Plan of Care—Preterm Labor

When complications arise during labor and birth, risk of perinatal morbidity and mortality increases. Some complications are anticipated, especially if the mother is identified as high risk during the antepartum period; others are unexpected or unforeseen. The woman, her family, and the obstetric team can feel devastated when things go wrong. Nurses must recognize these feelings if they are to provide effective support. It is crucial for nurses to understand the normal birth process to prevent and detect deviations from normal labor and birth and to implement nursing measures when complications arise. Optimal care of the laboring woman, fetus, and family experiencing complications is possible only when the nurse and other members of the obstetric team use their knowledge and skills in a concerted effort to provide care. This chapter focuses on the problems of preterm labor and birth, dystocia, and postterm pregnancy and obstetric emergencies.

PRETERM LABOR AND BIRTH

Preterm labor is defined as cervical changes and uterine contractions occurring between 20 and 37 weeks of pregnancy. **Preterm birth** is any birth that occurs before the completion of 37 weeks of pregnancy (American College of Obstetricians and Gynecologists [ACOG] & American Academy of Pediatrics [AAP], 2002). Preterm labor and birth are the most serious complications of pregnancy because they lead to about 90% of all neonatal deaths, with more than 75% of these deaths occurring in infants born at fewer than 32 weeks of gestation. Preterm birth is second only to congenital anomalies as a cause of infant mortality. In 2003 the preterm birth rate for all races in the United States was 12.3% (Hamilton, Martin, Sutton, & Centers for Disease Control and Prevention [CDC], National Center for Health Statistics, 2004).

Preterm Birth versus Low Birth Weight

Although they have distinctly different meanings, the terms *preterm birth* or *prematurity* and *low birth weight* are often used interchangeably (Moos, 2004). Preterm birth describes length of gestation (i.e., less than 37 weeks regardless of the weight of the infant), whereas low birth weight describes only weight at the time of birth (i.e., 2500 g or less). Low birth weight is far easier to measure than preterm birth, and therefore in many settings and publications, low birth weight has been used as a substitute term for preterm birth. Preterm birth, however, is a more dangerous health condition for an infant because a decreased length of time in the uterus correlates with immaturity of body systems. Low-birth-weight babies can be, but are not necessarily, preterm; low birth weight can be caused by conditions other than preterm birth, such as intrauterine growth restriction (IUGR), a condition of inadequate fetal growth not necessarily correlated with initiation of labor.

The incidence of preterm birth in the United States is increasing and varies according to race; the 2002 rate for African-Americans (17.7%) was considerably higher than that for American Indians (13.1%), Hispanics (11.6%), Caucasians (11%), and Asians and Pacific Islanders (10.4%) (Martin et al., 2003). The increase in rates is attributed largely to the increase in multiple births. Sociodemographics may play a part in the race-based differences in preterm birth. Preterm birth rates are higher among socially disadvantaged populations, including minorities, women with low levels of education, and women who receive late or no prenatal care (Martin et al., 2003; Maupin et al., 2004). The preterm birth rate is higher among women younger than 15 years of age or older than 45 years (Martin et al., 2003). Multifetal pregnancy from in vitro fertilization also is associated with an increase in preterm births (Moore, 2003).

Predicting Preterm Labor and Birth

The known risk factors for preterm birth are shown in Box 24-1. The risk factors most commonly associated with preterm labor and birth are a history of preterm birth, race (e.g., African-American), and multiple gestation (Martin et al., 2003). Using these risk factors, researchers have tried to determine which women might go into labor prematurely. No risk scoring system has resulted in lowering the preterm birth rate in the United States, however, because at least 50% of all women who ultimately give birth prematurely have no identifiable risk factors (Martin et al., 2003). The March of Dimes has started a 5-year, $75 million campaign to address the problem of prematurity. The Association of Women's Health, Obstetric and Neonatal Nurses (AWHONN) is a partner in this project. AWHONN is helping to increase screening for known risk factors and to teach women the signs and symptoms of preterm labor (Nelson, 2004). It is important that all women be educated about prematurity not only in early pregnancy but also in the preconception period (Freda & Patterson, 2001; Massett et al., 2003).

Biochemical markers

The two most common biochemical markers used in an effort to predict who might experience preterm labor are fetal fibronectin and salivary estriol (Goldenberg et al., 2003).

Fetal fibronectins are glycoproteins found in plasma and produced during fetal life. They appear in the cervical canal early in pregnancy and then again in late pregnancy. Their appearance between 24 and 34 weeks of gestation predicts labor (Bernhardt & Dorman, 2004; Ramsey & Andrews, 2003). The negative predictive value of fetal fibronectin is high (up to 94%). The positive predictive value is lower (46%) (Iams & Creasy, 2004). This means that it may be possible to predict who will *not* go into preterm labor, but not who will (Bernhardt & Dorman, 2004). The test is done during a vaginal examination.

Salivary estriol is a form of estrogen produced by the fetus that is present in plasma at 9 weeks of gestation. Levels of salivary estriol have been shown to increase before

---

BOX 24-1

Risk Factors for Preterm Labor

DEMOGRAPHIC RISKS
- Nonwhite race
- Age (<15 years, >45)
- Low socioeconomic status
- Unmarried
- Less than high school education

BIOPHYSICAL RISKS
- Previous preterm labor or birth
- Second-trimester abortion (more than two spontaneous or therapeutic); stillbirths
- Grand multiparity; short interval between pregnancies, ≤1 year since last birth); fmily history of preterm labor and birth
- Progesterone deficiency
- Uterine anomalies or fibroids; uterine irritability
- Cervical incompetence, trauma, shortened length
- Exposure to DES or other toxic substances
- Medical diseases (e.g., diabetes, hypertension, anemia)
- Small stature (<119 cm in height; <45.5 kg or underweight for height)
- Current pregnancy risks:
  - Multifetal pregnancy
  - Hydramnios
  - Bleeding
  - Placental problems (e.g., placenta previa, abruptio placentae)
  - Infections (e.g., pyelonephritis, recurrent urinary tract infections, asymptomatic bacteriuria, bacterial vaginosis, chorioamnionitis)
  - Gestational hypertension
  - Premature rupture of the membranes
  - Fetal anomalies
  - Inadequate plasma volume expansion; anemia

BEHAVIORAL-PSYCHOSOCIAL RISKS
- Poor nutrition; weight loss or low weight gain
- Smoking (>10 cigarettes a day)
- Substance abuse (e.g., alcohol; illicit drugs, especially cocaine)
- Inadequate prenatal care
- Commutes of more than 1½ hours each way
- Excessive physical activity (heavy physical work, prolonged standing, heavy lifting, care of young child)
- Excessive lifestyle stressors

Sources: Cunningham et al., (2005). *Williams' obstetrics* (22nd ed.). New York: McGraw-Hill; Gilbert, E., & Harmon, J. (2003). *Manual of high risk pregnancy and delivery* (3rd ed.). St. Louis: Mosby; Iams, J. (2002). Preterm birth. In S. Gabbe, J. Niebyl, & J. Simpson (Eds.). *Obstetrics: Normal and problem pregnancies* (4th ed.). New York: Churchill Livingstone; Martin, J. et al. (2003). Births: Final data for 2002. *National Vital Statistics Report, 52*(10), 1-113; & Moore, M. (2003). Preterm labor and birth: What have we learned in the past two decades? *Journal of Obstetric, Gynecologic, and Neonatal Nursing, 32*(5), 638-649.

---

preterm birth. Specimens of salivary estriol are collected by the woman in the home. The testing is done every 2 weeks for about 10 weeks. This marker also has a high negative predictive value (98%) and a lower positive predictive value (7% to 25%) (Bernhardt & Dorman, 2004).

Evolve/CD: Case Study—Preterm Labor

More research is needed before it will be known if these markers offer valuable assistance that is cost effective in the risk assessment for preterm labor.

Endocervical length

Another possible predictor of imminent preterm labor is endocervical length. Some studies have suggested that a shortened cervix precedes preterm labor and can be determined by ultrasound measurement (Bernhardt & Dorman, 2004; Fuchs, Henrich, Osthues, & Dudenhausen, 2004). Women whose cervical length is 35 mm at 24 to 28 weeks of gestation are more likely to have a preterm birth than women whose cervical length exceeds 40 mm. When a woman has a short cervix combined with a positive fetal fibronectin result, her risk for spontaneous preterm birth is substantially higher than that for women positive for only one marker or none at all (Iams & Creasy, 2004).

Causes of preterm labor and birth

The cause of preterm labor is unknown and is assumed to be multifactorial. Infection is thought to be a major etiologic factor in some preterm labors, but trials of antibiotic therapy for all women at risk have not resulted in statistically significant reductions in preterm births (Iams & Creasy, 2004). When cervical, bacterial, or urinary tract infections are present, the risk of preterm birth is increased; therefore early, continuous, and comprehensive prenatal care, which can detect and treat infection, is essential in dealing with this aspect of preterm birth prevention.

Not all preterm births can or even should be prevented. About 25% of all preterm births are iatrogenic, that is, babies are intentionally delivered prematurely because of pregnancy complications that put the life or health of the fetus or mother in danger, not because of preterm labor. Another 25% of all preterm births are preceded by spontaneous rupture of the membranes (preterm premature rupture of the membranes) followed by labor. These preterm births are not known to be preventable. About 50% of preterm births, therefore, are possibly amenable to prevention efforts and are considered idiopathic preterm births (Iams & Creasy, 2004).

Sociodemographic factors such as poverty, low educational level, lack of social support, smoking, little or no prenatal care, domestic violence, and stress are thought to contribute to the 50% of preterm births that may be preventable (Gennaro & Hennessy, 2003; Iams & Creasy, 2004). If prenatal care programs are to be effective in reducing the rate of preterm labor and birth, they must address these sociodemographic factors and develop strategies to attract all women to participate, including those at high risk for preterm labor (Maloni, 2000).

CARE MANAGEMENT

Assessment and Nursing Diagnoses

Because all pregnant women must be considered at risk for preterm labor (as they are for any other pregnancy complication), nursing assessment begins at the time of entry to prenatal care. The onset of preterm labor is often insidious and can be easily mistaken for normal discomforts of pregnancy. It is essential that nurses teach pregnant women how to detect the early symptoms of preterm labor (Box 24-2) (Freda & Patterson, 2001; Witcher, 2002).

The nurse caring for women in a prenatal setting should use known successful modalities for teaching the pregnant woman about early recognition of preterm symptoms and then reassess the woman at each prenatal visit for the symptoms of preterm labor. Pregnant women also must be taught what to do if the symptoms of preterm labor occur. Some women wait hours or days before contacting a health care provider after preterm labor symptoms have begun. Women may ignore the symptoms because of ignorance regarding their significance or a belief that the symptoms are expected during pregnancy. The symptoms may be attributed to other factors such as the flu, incontinence of urine, or working too hard. Some women will become more vigilant, waiting to see

Critical Thinking Exercise

Preterm Labor

You are assigned to Yolanda, who is experiencing preterm labor at 28 weeks of gestation. She has a 2-year-old son at home. This is her third admission for preterm labor during this pregnancy. Her primary health care provider has told her she must remain hospitalized on bed rest until she reaches 37 weeks of gestation or until birth of the baby, whichever comes first. She tearfully asks you why she can't be at home on bed rest, who will help care for her son, and how she will manage to keep from going crazy staying in bed that long. How will you respond to her concerns?

1 Is there sufficient evidence to draw conclusions about the benefits of bed rest to prevent preterm birth?
2 What assumptions can be made about the following issues?
  a. The impact her history might have on the medical and nursing care she receives during this pregnancy
  b. The pros and cons of home management versus hospital management for the prevention of preterm birth for this woman
  c. Ways to reduce the frustration and boredom that are experienced during restriction to bed rest for several weeks
  d. Resources available to assist with care of her 2-year-old son
3 What implications and priorities for nursing care can be drawn at this time?
4 Does the evidence objectively support your conclusion?
5 Are there alternative perspectives to your conclusion?

BOX 24-2

Signs and Symptoms of Preterm Labor

UTERINE ACTIVITY
- Uterine contractions more frequent than every 10 minutes persisting for 1 hour or more
- Uterine contractions may be painful or painless

DISCOMFORT
- Lower abdominal cramping similar to gas pains; may be accompanied by diarrhea
- Dull, intermittent low back pain (below the waist)
- Painful, menstrual-like cramps
- Suprapubic pain or pressure
- Pelvic pressure or heaviness
- Urinary frequency

VAGINAL DISCHARGE
- Change in character and amount of usual discharge: thicker (mucoid) or thinner (watery); bloody, brown, or colorless; increased amount; odor
- Rupture of amniotic membranes

if the symptoms subside, go away, or become worse. Some women may take action by seeking advice about what to do from family or friends, resting more, increasing fluid intake, taking a bath, or rubbing the back or abdomen. Persistence of symptoms and increasing severity finally compel women to seek health care (Weiss, Saks, & Harris, 2002). Waiting too long to see a health care provider could result in inevitable preterm birth without the benefit of the administration of antenatal glucocorticoids (i.e., medication given to accelerate fetal lung maturity). In this event, the neonate is born at higher risk for respiratory distress syndrome and intraventricular hemorrhage.

The nurse must assess the psychosocial and emotional status of women in preterm labor and the impact that treatment (e.g., bed rest, hospitalization) can have on family dynamics. Factors influencing the impact of preterm labor treatment include stability of the support system, financial status, and availability of child support and assistance with household maintenance. Pregnant women who have risk factors for preterm birth are often offered special care with more frequent visits. Although there is no evidence in the literature that this enhanced care results in better outcomes, clinically it makes sense to evaluate at-risk women on a more frequent basis. Freda and Patterson (2001) suggest that the power of nursing care, nursing support, and patient education in the care of women at high risk for preterm birth can affect the occurrence and early detection of preterm labor.

Nursing diagnoses relevant for women at risk for preterm birth include the following:

- *Risk for maternal excess fluid volume related to*
  —administration of tocolytics to suppress preterm labor

- *Interrupted family processes related to*
  —required limitation on maternal activity associated with preterm labor
- *Impaired mobility related to*
  —prescribed bed rest
- *Anticipatory grieving related to*
  —potential for birth of preterm infant
- *Risk for impaired parent-infant attachment related to*
  —care requirements of preterm infant

Expected Outcomes of Care

Expected outcomes include that the woman will do the following:

- Learn the signs and symptoms of preterm labor and be able to assess herself and her need for intervention
- Follow teaching suggestions and call her primary health care provider if symptoms occur
- Not experience preterm symptoms, or, if she does, she will take appropriate action
- Maintain her pregnancy for at least 37 completed weeks
- Give birth to a healthy, full-term infant

Plan of Care and Interventions
Prevention

Prevention strategies that address risk factors associated with preterm labor and birth are less costly in human and financial terms than the high-tech and often lifelong care required by preterm infants and their families. Programs aimed at health promotion and disease prevention that encourage healthy lifestyles for the population in general and women of childbearing age in particular should be developed to prevent preterm labor and birth (Freda, 2003; Heaman, Sprague, & Stewart, 2001; Tiedje, 2003). One of the most important nursing interventions aimed at preventing preterm birth is the education of pregnant women about the early symptoms of preterm labor, so that if symptoms occur the woman can be referred promptly to her care provider for more intensive care (Freda, 2003; Moore, 2003). Box 24-2 identifies the symptoms of preterm labor, and the Guidelines/Guías box identifies what the woman should do if the symptoms appear. Patient education regarding any symptoms of contractions or cramping between 20 and 37 weeks of gestation should be directed toward telling the woman that these symptoms are not normal discomforts of pregnancy, and that contractions or cramping that do not go away should prompt the woman to contact her primary health care provider. Because no one can discriminate between Braxton Hicks contractions and the contractions of early preterm labor, Freda and Patterson (2001) suggest that the term *Braxton Hicks contractions* be eliminated from teaching about pregnancy expectations (Fig. 24-1).

Early recognition and diagnosis

Early recognition of preterm labor is essential to successfully implement interventions such as tocolytic therapy and

GUIDELINES/GUÍAS

What to Do if Symptoms of Preterm Labor Occur

- Empty your bladder.
- *Vacíese la vejiga.*

- Drink two to three glasses of water or juice.
- *Tome dos a tres vasos de agua o jugo.*

- Lie down on your left side for 1 hour.
- *Acuéstese del lado izquierdo por una hora.*

- Palpate for contractions like this.
- *Palpe por contracciones así.*

- If symptoms continue, call your health care provider or go to the hospital.
- *Si continúan los síntomas, llame a su proveedor de los servicios de salud/médico o vaya al hospital.*

- If symptoms abate, resume light activity, but not what you were doing when the symptoms began.
- *Si se alivian los síntomas, resuma sus actividades livianas, pero no haga lo que estaba haciendo cuando empezaron los síntomas.*

- If symptoms return, call your health care provider or go to the hospital.
- *Si se presentan de nuevo los síntomas, llame a su proveedor de los servicios de salud/médico o vaya al hospital.*

- If any of the following symptoms occur, call your health care provider immediately:
- *Si le sucede cualquier de los siguientes síntomas, llame inmediatamente a su proveedor de los servicios de salud/médico:*

  —Uterine contractions every 10 minutes or less for 1 hour or more
  —*Contracciones uterinas cada diez minutos o menos que duran por una hora o más*

  —Vaginal bleeding
  —*Hemorragia vaginal*

  —Odorous vaginal discharge
  —*Flujo vaginal con mal olor*

  —Fluid leaking from the vagina
  —*Flujo que le sale de la vagina*

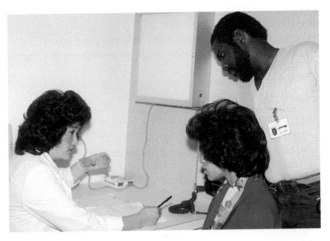

Fig. 24-1 Nurse teaching woman signs and symptoms of preterm labor. (Courtesy Marjorie Pyle, RNC, Lifecircle, Costa Mesa, CA.)

of pharmacologic agents that can be dangerous to the health of the woman, the fetus, or both (Abrahams & Katz, 2002; ACOG/AAP, 2002).

Lifestyle modifications

Nurses caring for women with symptoms of preterm labor should question the woman about whether she has symptoms when engaged in any of the following activities:

- Sexual activity
- Riding long distances in automobiles, trains, or buses
- Carrying heavy loads such as laundry, groceries, or a small child
- Standing more than 50% of the time
- Heavy housework
- Climbing stairs
- Hard physical work
- Being unable to stop and rest when tired

If symptoms occur when the woman is engaged in any of these activities, the woman should consider stopping those activities until 37 weeks of pregnancy when preterm birth is no longer a risk. Counseling about lifestyle modification should be individualized; only women who have symptoms of preterm labor when they are engaged in certain activities need to alter their lifestyles. No specific rules describe which activities are safe for pregnant women and which are not. Each pregnant woman must understand which lifestyle factors might be contributing to her symptoms and be taught to modify only those factors. Sexual activity, for instance, is not contraindicated during pregnancy. If, however, symptoms of preterm labor occur after sexual activity, then that activity may need to be curtailed until 37 weeks of gestation.

Bed rest

Bed rest is a commonly used intervention for the prevention of preterm birth. Although frequently prescribed, bed rest is not a benign intervention, and there is no evi-

administration of antenatal glucocorticoids. The diagnosis of preterm labor is based on three major diagnostic criteria:

- Gestational age between 20 and 37 weeks
- Uterine activity (e.g., contractions)
- Progressive cervical change (e.g., effacement of 80%, or cervical dilation of 2 cm or greater)

If the presence of fetal fibronectin is used as another diagnostic criterion, a sample of cervical mucus for testing should be obtained before an examination for cervical changes, because the lubricant used to examine the cervix can reduce the accuracy of the test for fetal fibronectin.

The pregnant woman at 30 weeks with an irritable uterus but no documented cervical change is not in preterm labor. Misdiagnosis of preterm labor can lead to inappropriate use

dence in the literature to support the efficacy of this intervention in reducing preterm birth rates. It is a form of care of unknown effectiveness (Enkin et al., 2000; Sosa, Athalbe, Belzian, & Bergel, 2004). Maloni and colleagues (1993) described deleterious effects of bed rest on women: after 3 days there is decreased muscle tone, weight loss, calcium loss, and glucose intolerance. Weeks of bed rest lead to bone demineralization, constipation, fatigue, isolation, anxiety, and depression (Box 24-3). Symptoms often are not resolved by 6 weeks postpartum (Maloni & Park, 2005). Bed rest is costly for society; the estimated economic costs are based on lost wages, household help and child care expenses, and hospital costs (Maloni, Brezinski-Tomasi, & Johnson, 2001). Prolongation of pregnancy does not necessarily occur despite the increased costs incurred. Women on bed rest need support and encouragement whether they are at home or are hospitalized. Nurses can create support groups of hospitalized women on bed rest. Internet resources including chat rooms for women on bed rest at home, as well as family and friends, can be important sources of support for the women and reduce the sense of isolation they may feel. Interacting with other women experiencing preterm labor and bed rest has been found to be highly therapeutic (Adler & Zarchin, 2002; Maloni & Kutil, 2000).

Home care

Women who are at high risk for preterm birth commonly are told that it would be best if they were at home on bed rest for weeks or months. The home care of the woman at risk for preterm birth is a challenge for the nurse, who must assist the woman and her family in dealing with the many difficulties faced by families in which one member is incapacitated. The scope of care given to women in their homes ranges from occasional visits to monitor the maternal and fetal condition, to daily telephone consultation and reading of uterine monitoring strips.

Regardless of the frequency of the visits, nursing care for the woman and family in the home demands organization and a sense of just how this family's life has been disrupted by the loss of activity of this essential family member. Families, who are often anxious regarding the health status of the mother and baby, may need help in learning how to organize time and space or to restructure family routines so that the pregnant woman can remain a part of family activity while still maintaining bed rest. It also is important for the nurse to work toward assisting all the family members to explore their feelings regarding the anxieties of preterm labor and help them to share their feelings with one another (Maloni, Brezinski-Tomasi & Johnson, 2001). Box 24-4 and the Patient Instructions for Self-Care Box list activities for women on bed rest and for their children.

The woman's environment can be modified for convenience by using tables and storage units around her bed to keep essential items within reach (e.g., telephone, television, radio, tape or compact disc player, computer with Internet access, snacks, books, magazines, and newspapers, items for hobbies) (Fig. 24-2). Ensuring that the bed or couch is near a window and the bathroom is also helpful. Covering the bed with an egg crate mattress can relieve discomfort. Women often find that a daily schedule of meals, activities, and hygiene and grooming (e.g., shower, dressing in street clothes, applying make-up) that they create reduces boredom and helps them maintain control and normalcy.

BOX 24-3

Adverse Effects of Bed Rest

MATERNAL EFFECTS (PHYSICAL)
- Weight loss
- Muscle wasting, weakness
- Bone demineralization and calcium loss
- Decreased plasma volume and cardiac output
- Increased clotting tendency; risk for thrombophlebitis
- Alteration in bowel function
- Sleep disturbance, fatigue
- Prolonged postpartum recovery

MATERNAL EFFECTS (PSYCHOSOCIAL)
- Loss of control associated with role reversals
- Dysphoria-anxiety, depression, hostility, and anger
- Guilt associated with difficulty complying with activity restriction and inability to meet role responsibilities
- Boredom, loneliness
- Emotional lability (mood swings)

EFFECTS ON SUPPORT SYSTEM
- Stress associated with role reversals, increased responsibilities, and disruption of family routines
- Financial strain associated with loss of maternal income and cost of treatment
- Fear and anxiety regarding the well-being of the mother and fetus

---

BOX 24-4

Activities for Children of Women on Bed Rest

- Schedule brief play periods throughout the day.
- Keep a few favorite toys in a box or basket close to the bed or couch.
- Read to the child(ren).
- Put puzzles together.
- Watch videos, play video games (remote control for TV is ideal).
- Play cards or board games.
- Color in coloring books.
- Cut out pictures from magazines and paste on cardboard.
- Play bed basketball with a soft (sponge) ball or rolled up sock and a trash can or empty laundry basket.

References: McCann, M. (2003). *Days in waiting: A guide to surviving bedrest.* St. Paul, MN: deRuyter-Nelson Publications; &Tracy, A. (2001). *The pregnancy bed rest book: A survival guide for expectant mothers and their families.* New York: Berkley Publishing Group.

PATIENT INSTRUCTIONS FOR SELF-CARE

Suggested Activities for Women on Bed Rest

- Set a routine for daily activities (e.g., getting dressed, moving from the bedroom to a "day bed-rest place," having social time, eating meals, self-monitoring fetal and uterine activity).
- Do passive exercises as allowed.
- Review childbirth education information or have a childbirth class at home, if this can be arranged.
- Plan menus and make up grocery shopping lists.
- Shop by phone.
- Read books about high risk pregnancy or other topics.
- Keep a journal of the pregnancy.
- Keep a calendar of your progress.
- Reorganize files, recipes, household budget.
- Update address book.
- Do mending, sewing.
- Listen to audiotapes, watch videos or television.
- Do crossword puzzles, jigsaw puzzles, etc.
- Do craft projects; make something for the baby.
- Put pictures in photo albums.
- Call a friend, family member, or support person each day or use email.
- Treat yourself to a facial, manicure, neck massage, or other special treat when you need a lift.

Sources: Gilbert, E., & Harmon, J. (2003). *Manual of high risk pregnancy and delivery* (3rd ed.). St. Louis: Mosby; McCann, M. (2003). *Days in waiting: A guide to surviving bedrest.* St. Paul, MN: deRuyter-Nelson Publications; Moondragon Birthing Services. (2005). *Moondragon's pregnancy information: Coping with bedrest during pregnancy.* Internet document available at www.moondragon.org/pregnancy/bedrestcope.html (accessed May 1, 2005); & Tracy, A. (2001). *The pregnancy bed rest book: A survival guide for expectant mothers and their families.* New York: Berkley Publishing Group.

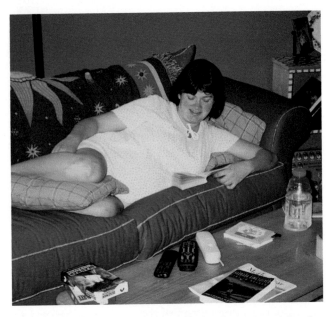

Fig. 24-2 Woman at home on restricted activity for preterm labor prevention. Note how she has arranged her daytime resting area so that needed items are close at hand. (Courtesy Amy Turner, Cary, NC.)

Limiting naps, eating smaller but more frequent meals, and performing gentle range-of-motion exercises can help to reduce some of the detrimental effects of bed rest. It is essential that women and their families recognize that postpartum recovery will be slower as she works to regain strength and stamina (Maloni, 2002).

Home uterine activity monitoring

Home uterine monitoring systems were developed to provide home uterine monitoring services for women diagnosed with preterm labor. Nurses are usually an integral part of the home uterine activity monitoring (HUAM) systems to educate and provide care to the women. The use and effectiveness of HUAM continues to be controversial. Enkin and colleagues (2000) found HUAM a form of care unlikely to be beneficial in preventing preterm birth. However, a comprehensive evidence-based review of clinical data suggests that if used correctly (e.g., twice daily monitoring of uterine activity and daily nursing care) in women at risk for preterm birth, HUAM increases the incidence of early diagnosis of preterm labor, prolongation of pregnancy with fewer preterm births, and reduced neonatal morbidity when study groups are compared with control groups of women receiving standard prenatal care in the United States (Morrison &

Chauhan, 2003). Research should be continued in this area to determine what place HUAM has in preterm labor care.

Suppression of uterine activity

Tocolytics. Should preterm labor occur, women are usually admitted to the hospital for assessment; fetal monitoring; cervical or vaginal cultures; assessment of cervical status, amniotic fluid leakage, and elevated maternal temperature (an early sign of chorioamnionitis). The initiation of tocolytic therapy might be considered at this time. Once the pregnancy has progressed beyond 34 weeks of gestation, the benefits of prolonging the pregnancy do not justify the maternal risk of tocolytic therapy (Witcher, 2002). The use of tocolytics (medications that suppress uterine activity) in an attempt to prevent preterm birth has been the subject of research since the late 1970s. At first, it was thought that use of tocolytic therapy could prolong a threatened pregnancy indefinitely; research has demonstrated only a small improvement in prolonging pregnancy to a term birth. Once uterine contractions are suppressed, maintenance therapy may be implemented in an attempt to continue the suppression, or tocolytic treatment can be discontinued and resumed only if uterine contractions begin again. Research findings suggest that there appears to be no significant difference when tocolytic treatment approaches are compared and that continued maintenance tocolytic therapy has no more than minimal value (Berkman et al., 2003).

It is now thought that the best reason to use tocolytics is that they afford the opportunity to begin administering antenatal glucocorticoids to accelerate fetal lung maturity and reduce the severity of sequelae in infants born preterm ✳

(Anotayanonth, Subhedar, Garner, Neilson, & Harigopal, 2004). Medications used for this purpose include ritodrine (Yutopar), terbutaline (Brethine), magnesium sulfate, indomethacin (Indocin), and nifedipine (Procardia). Ritodrine is the only medication approved by the U.S. Food and Drug Administration (FDA) specifically for the purpose of cessation of uterine contractions; however, magnesium sulfate, terbutaline, and nifedipine are most commonly used in U.S. hospitals (Rideout, 2005). These drugs are used on an "off-label" basis (i.e., drugs known to be effective for a specific purpose, although not specifically developed and tested for this purpose). Important contraindications exist to the use of all tocolytics (Box 24-5). Because these medications have the potential for serious adverse reactions for mother and fetus, close nursing supervision during treatment is critical (Lehne, 2001) (Box 24-6 and Medication Guide).

Magnesium sulfate is the most commonly used tocolytic agent, because maternal and fetal or neonatal adverse reactions are less common than with other tocolytic agents, especially the beta-adrenergic agonists. Although its exact mechanism of action on uterine muscle is unclear, magnesium sulfate does promote relaxation of smooth muscles (Iams, 2002; Witcher, 2002). At the onset of preterm labor, magnesium sulfate is administered via an intravenous infusion. Terbutaline, 0.25 mg, may be injected subcutaneously before the initiation of the magnesium sulfate infusion and then administered again by subcutaneous pump as the infusion is discontinued and the woman prepared for discharge to home care (see Medication Guide).

Ritodrine and terbutaline, beta-adrenergic agonist medications for tocolysis, work by relaxing uterine smooth muscle as a result of stimulation of beta$_2$ receptors on uterine smooth muscle. Although seldom used, ritodrine is usually administered intravenously as one of the first steps in suppressing preterm labor. Terbutaline is most commonly administered by a subcutaneous injection of 0.25 mg to suppress uterine hyperactivity or by a subcutaneous pump. Effectiveness of pump therapy in prolonging gestation is controversial. Terbutaline also may be administered orally. Oral and pump therapy are similar in terms of effectiveness and adverse reactions (Witcher, 2002).

Beta$_2$-adrenergic agonists have many maternal and fetal cardiopulmonary and metabolic adverse reactions in part related to beta$_1$ stimulation and must always be used with extreme caution and careful, conscientious nursing care. Fewer neonatal adverse reactions occur if the administration of the beta-adrenergic agonist is discontinued at least 4 hours before birth (Witcher, 2002). Medication administration and nursing care are aimed at maintaining a therapeutic level of medication and avoiding the most serious side effects while maintaining optimal health of the fetus (see Medication Guide).

NURSE ALERT *Caution must be used when administering intravenous fluids to women in preterm labor because this practice can increase the risk for tocolytic-induced pulmonary edema, especially when a beta-adrenergic agonist or magnesium sulfate is used. It is recommended that the total oral and intravenous fluid intake in 24 hours be restricted to 1500 to 2400 ml. Strict intake and output measurement, daily weight determination, and assessment of pulmonary function should be instituted (Gilbert & Harmon, 2003; Witcher, 2002).*

Nifedipine, a calcium channel blocker, is another tocolytic agent that can suppress contractions. It works by inhibiting calcium from entering smooth muscle cells, thus reducing uterine contractions (Lehne, 2001). Mild maternal side effects and ease of administration have increased its use. When the tocolytic effects and maternal tolerance of nifedipine and beta-adrenergic agonists were compared, no significant

---

BOX 24-6

Nursing Care for Women Receiving Tocolytic Therapy

- Explain the purpose and side effects of tocolytic therapy to woman and her family.
- Position woman on her side to enhance placental perfusion and reduce pressure on the cervix.
- Monitor maternal vital signs, fetal heart rate, and labor status according to hospital protocol and professional standards.
- Assess mother and fetus for signs of adverse reactions related to the tocolytic being administered.
- Determine maternal fluid balance by measuring daily weight and intake and output (I&O).
- Limit fluid intake to 2500 to 3000 ml/day, especially if a beta-adrenergic agonist is being administered.
- Provide psychosocial support and opportunities for women and family to express feelings and concerns.
- Offer comfort measures as required.
- Encourage diversional activities and relaxation techniques.

BOX 24-5

Contraindications to Tocolysis

MATERNAL
- Severe preeclampsia or eclampsia
- Active vaginal bleeding
- Intrauterine infection
- Cardiac disease
- Medical or obstetric condition that contraindicates continuation of pregnancy

FETAL
- Estimated gestational age over 37 weeks
- Dilation over 4 cm
- Fetal demise
- Lethal fetal anomaly
- Chorioamnionitis
- Acute fetal distress
- Chronic intrauterine growth restriction

Medication Guide

Tocolytic Therapy for Preterm Labor

MEDICATION AND ACTION	DOSAGE AND ROUTE	ADVERSE REACTIONS	NURSING CONSIDERATIONS
Magnesium sulfate* CNS depressant; relaxes smooth muscles including uterus	Mix 40 g in 1000 ml intravenous solution, piggyback to primary infusion, and administer loading dose or bolus of 4-6 g using controller pump over 15 to 20 min Continue maintenance infusion at 1 g/hr, increasing to a maximum 3 g/hr until contractions stop or intolerable adverse reactions develop	During loading dose: ● Hot flushes, sweating, nausea and vomiting, drowsiness, and blurred vision; usually subside when loading dose is completed Intolerable adverse reactions: ● Respiratory rate less than 12 breaths/min ● Absent DTRs ● Severe hypotension ● Extreme muscle weakness ● Urine output less than 25-30 ml/hr ● Serum magnesium level of 10 mEq/L or greater	Assess woman and fetus before and after each rate increase and following frequency of agency protocol Monitor serum magnesium levels; therapeutic level should range between 4 and 7.5 mEq/L Discontinue infusion and notify physician if intolerable adverse reactions occur Ensure that calcium gluconate is available for emergency administration to reverse magnesium sulfate toxicity Limit IV fluid intake to 125 ml/hr
Terbutaline* (Brethine) Beta-adrenergic agonist relaxes smooth muscles, inhibiting uterine activity and causing bronchodilation	Subcutaneous injection: ● 0.25 mg q30min for 2 hr ● Maximum dose: 0.5 mg q4-6h Subcutaneous pump: ● Maintenance dose 0.05-0.1 mg/hr ● Bolus: 0.25 mg q4-6h according to contraction pattern ● 3 mg/24 hr maximum dose	Similar to ritodrine	Teach woman and family: ● Assessment measures: pulse, BP, respiratory effort, insertion site for infection, signs of PTL, and adverse reactions of terbutaline ● Whom to call if problems or concerns arise ● Site care and pump maintenance ● Activity restrictions Arrange for follow-up and home care
Nifedipine* (Procardia; Adalat) Calcium channel blocker; relaxes smooth muscles including the uterus by blocking calcium entry	Initial dose: 10-20 mg PO Maintenance dose: 10 to 20 mg q4-6h PO	Transient tachycardia, palpitations Hypotension Dizziness, headache, nervousness Peripheral edema Fatigue Nausea Facial flushing	Do not use with magnesium sulfate Assess woman and fetus according to agency protocol being alert for adverse reactions Do not use sublingual route

differences in length of delay of birth were found, but significantly fewer maternal side effects occurred with nifedipine. Maternal side effects relate primarily to hypotension that occurs with administration. Concerns regarding adverse fetal effects have been reduced. Safety is achieved by following recommended dosages and maintaining maternal blood pressure, thereby preserving effective uteroplacental perfusion (Iams & Creasy, 2004; Witcher, 2002) (see Medication Guide).

Indomethacin, a nonsteroidal antiinflammatory drug (NSAID), has been shown in some trials to suppress preterm labor by blocking the production of prostaglandins. Two prostaglandins are affected, prostacyclin and thromboxane. The decrease in prostacyclin suppresses uterine contractions,

Medication Guide—cont'd

Tocolytic Therapy for Preterm Labor

MEDICATION AND ACTION	DOSAGE AND ROUTE	ADVERSE REACTIONS	NURSING CONSIDERATIONS
Ritodrine (Yutopar) Beta-adrenergic agonist; relaxes smooth muscles, inhibiting uterine activity and causing bronchodilation	Mix 150 mg in 500 ml isotonic intravenous solution Attach to controller pump and piggyback to primary infusion Begin infusion at 0.05-0.1 mg/min Increase rate by 0.05 mg q10min until contractions stop, intolerable adverse reactions develop, or a maximum dose of 0.35 mg/min is reached Maintain effective dose for 12-24 hr	Intravenous adverse reactions: • Shortness of breath, coughing, tachypnea, pulmonary edema • Tachycardia, palpitations, skipped beats • Chest pains • Hypotension • Tremors, dizziness, nervousness • Muscle cramps and weakness • Headache • Hyperglycemia; hypokalemia • Nausea and vomiting • Fetal tachycardia Oral administration adverse reactions: • GI distress • Significant adverse effects are rare	Women should be screened with ECG before therapy begins; maternal heart disease and hypertension are contraindications Use cautiously if woman has type 1 diabetes or hyperthyroidism Validate that woman is in PTL and that pregnancy is over 20 weeks of gestation Assess woman and fetus before and after each rate increase and following frequency of agency protocol Discontinue infusion and notify physician if • Maternal heart rate greater than 120 to 140 beats/min; dysrhythmias, chest pain • BP is less than 90/60 mm Hg • Fetal heart rate greater than 180 beats/min Ensure that propranolol (Inderal) is available to reverse adverse effects related to cardiovascular function
Indomethacin* Prostaglandin inhibitor; relaxes uterine smooth muscle	Initial dose: 50 mg (orally or rectally) Maintenance dose: 25-50 mg, q4-6h for 24-48 hr (PO)	Maternal: Nausea and vomiting, dyspepsia, dizziness, oligohydramnios Fetal: Premature closure of ductus arteriosus Neonate: Bronchopulmonary dysplasia, respiratory distress syndrome, intracranial hemorrhage, necrotizing enterocolitis, hyperbilirubinemia	Used when other methods fail; not recommended after 32 weeks of gestation Do not use in women with bleeding potential Fetal assessment: amniotic fluid level; function of ductus arteriosus

*Caution: Not FDA approved for PTL (off-label use).
BP, Blood pressure; *CNS,* central nervous system; *DTRs,* deep tendon reflexes; *ECG,* electrocardiogram; *GI,* gastrointestinal; *IV,* intravenous; *PO,* by mouth; *PTL,* preterm labor.

and the decrease in thromboxane suppresses platelet aggregation. However, both of these actions increase the risk for postpartum hemorrhage. The severity of fetal side effects associated with the use of indomethacin for tocolysis makes it less common than other classes of tocolytic drugs. Risk for premature closure of the ductus arteriosus increases if treatment goes beyond 48 hours or if the fetus is aged 32 or more weeks of gestation. Therefore, limiting the use of indomethacin to a short duration of treatment (e.g., 48 hours) or to women with less than 32 weeks of gestation is recommended (Iams & Creasy, 2004; Witcher, 2002) (see Medication Guide).

Promotion of fetal lung maturity

Antenatal glucocorticoids. Antenatal glucocorticoids given as intramuscular injections to the mother accelerate fetal lung maturity. Such therapy is viewed as a form of care likely to be beneficial (Enkin et al., 2000). The National Institutes of Health consensus panel recommended that all women at 24 to 34 weeks of gestation should be given antenatal glucocorticoids when preterm birth is threatened, unless there is a medical indication for immediate birth such as cord prolapse, chorioamnionitis, or abruptio placentae (National Institutes of Health, 2000). The regimen for administration of antenatal glucocorticoids is given in the Medication Guide.

NURSE ALERT *Nurses need to know that when any woman is admitted to the hospital and is 24 to 34 weeks pregnant, she should receive antenatal glucocorticoids unless she has chorioamnionitis. These drugs require a 24-hour period to become effective, so timely administration is essential.*

Management of inevitable preterm birth

Labor that has progressed to a cervical dilation of 4 cm is likely to lead to inevitable preterm birth. Preterm births in tertiary care centers lead to better neonatal and maternal outcomes. Women considered at risk for inevitable preterm birth should be transferred quickly to such a facility to ensure the best possible outcome. The first dose of antenatal glucocorticoids should be given before transfer.

Although maternal transport helps to ensure a better health outcome for the mother and the baby, it may have complications. A woman may be transported to a tertiary center far from home, making visits by the family difficult and increasing the anxiety levels of the woman and her family. Attention to the needs of the woman and her family before, during, and after the transport is essential to comprehensive nursing care for these families.

Evaluation

Evaluation of the nursing care provided for a woman at risk for preterm birth is based on achievement of the expected outcomes of care (Plan of Care).

PRETERM PREMATURE RUPTURE OF MEMBRANES

Premature rupture of membranes (PROM) is the rupture of the amniotic sac and leakage of amniotic fluid beginning at least 1 hour before the onset of labor at any gestational age. **Preterm premature rupture of membranes (PPROM)** (i.e., membranes rupture before 37 weeks of gestation) occurs in up to 25% of all cases of preterm labor. Infection often precedes PPROM, but the cause of PPROM remains unknown. PPROM is diagnosed after the woman reports of

---

Medication Guide

Antenatal Glucocorticoid Therapy with Betamethasone, Dexamethasone

ACTION
- Stimulates fetal lung maturation by promoting release of enzymes that induce production or release of lung surfactant. NOTE: The FDA has not approved these medications for this use (i.e., this is an off-label use for obstetrics).

INDICATION
- To prevent or reduce the severity of respiratory distress syndrome in preterm infants between 24 and 34 weeks of gestation.

DOSAGE AND ROUTE
- Betamethasone: 12 mg IM × two doses 12 hr apart
- Dexamethasone: 6 mg IM × two doses 12 hr apart
- May be repeated in 7 days if birth has not occurred.

ADVERSE REACTIONS
- Possible maternal infection, pulmonary edema (if given with beta-adrenergic medications), may worsen maternal condition (diabetes, hypertension).

NURSING CONSIDERATIONS
- Give deep intramuscular injection in gluteal muscle. Teach signs of pulmonary edema. Assess blood glucose levels and lung sounds. Do not give if woman has infection. Use in women with preterm premature rupture of membranes (PPROM) not universally recommended.

IM, Intramuscularly.

either a sudden gush of fluid or a slow leak of fluid from the vagina.

Infection is the serious side effect of PPROM that makes it a major complication of pregnancy. **Chorioamnionitis** is an intraamniotic infection of the chorion and amnion that is potentially life threatening for the fetus and the woman. Most cases of intrauterine infection respond well to antibiotics, yet sepsis can occur and can lead to maternal death. Fetal complications from chorioamnionitis include congenital pneumonia, sepsis, and meningitis (Garite, 2004). Even in the absence of infection, PPROM can precipitate cord prolapse or cause oligohydramnios, leading to cord compression, potentially life-threatening complications for the fetus.

Collaborative Care

Whenever PPROM is suspected, strict sterile technique should be used in any vaginal examination to avoid introduction of infection. A nitrazine or fern test is used to determine if the discharge is amniotic fluid or urine (see Chapter 14: Procedure box: Tests for Rupture of Membranes). A

PLAN OF CARE *Preterm Labor*

NURSING DIAGNOSIS Deficient knowledge related to recognition of preterm labor
Expected Outcome *Woman and significant other delineate the signs and symptoms of preterm labor.*

Nursing Interventions/*Rationales*

- Assess what the partners know about abnormal signs and symptoms during pregnancy *to identify areas of deficit.*
- Discuss signs and symptoms that serve as warning signs of preterm labor *so that the woman or her partner has adequate information to identify problems early.*
- Provide written supplemental materials that include a list of warning signs and instructions regarding what to do if any of the listed signs occur *so that the couple can reinforce and review learning and act swiftly and appropriately should a sign occur.*
- Discuss and demonstrate how to assess and time the contractions *to provide needed skills to assess the signs of labor.*

NURSING DIAGNOSIS Risk for maternal or fetal injury related to recurrence of preterm labor
Expected Outcome *Woman demonstrates ability to assess self and fetus for signs of recurring labor; maternal-fetal well-being is maintained.*

Nursing Interventions/*Rationales*

- Teach woman and partner how to monitor fetal and uterine contraction activity daily *to provide immediate evidence of a worsening condition.*
- Have woman or partner report rupture of membranes, vaginal bleeding, cramping, pelvic pressure, or low backache to appropriate health care resource immediately *because such symptoms are signs of labor.*
- If home uterine activity monitoring is to be used, teach woman and partner how to use the monitoring device and how to transmit the data to the health care provider via telephone *to enhance correct use of monitoring device and increase the accuracy of detection of early labor.*
- Have woman monitor her weight, diet, fluid intake, and vital signs on a daily basis *to evaluate for potential problems.*
- Limit activities to bed rest with bathroom privileges *to decrease the likelihood of onset of labor.*
- Use a side-lying position *to enhance placental perfusion.*
- Abstain from sexual intercourse and nipple stimulation *because such activities may stimulate uterine contractions.*
- Practice relaxation techniques *to decrease uterine tone and decrease anxiety and stress.*
- Take tocolytic or other medications per physician's orders *to inhibit uterine contractions.*
- Teach woman and partner about and have them report any medication side effects immediately *to prevent medication-induced complications.*

- Have family arrange for alternative strategies for carrying out the woman's usual roles and functions *to decrease stress and limit temptations to increase activity.*
- If small children are part of the household, encourage family to make alternative arrangements for child care *to enhance woman's adherence to bed rest protocol.*

NURSING DIAGNOSIS Anxiety related to preterm labor and potentially premature neonate
Expected Outcome *Feelings and symptoms of fear or anxiety abate.*

Nursing Interventions/*Rationales*

- Provide a calm, soothing atmosphere and teach family to provide emotional support *to facilitate coping.*
- Encourage verbalization of fears *to decrease intensity of emotional response.*
- Involve woman and family in the home management of her condition *to promote a greater sense of control.*
- Help the woman identify and use appropriate coping strategies and support systems *to reduce fear and anxiety.*
- Explore the use of desensitization strategies such as progressive muscle relaxation, visual imagery, or thought stopping *to reduce fear-related emotions and related physical symptoms.*
- Provide information about online support groups *to reduce fear and anxiety.*

NURSING DIAGNOSIS Deficient diversional activity related to imposed bed rest
Expected Outcome *Verbalization of diminished feelings of boredom.*

Nursing Interventions/*Rationales*

- Assist woman to creatively explore personally meaningful activities that can be pursued from the bed *to ensure activities that have meaning, purpose, and value to the individual.*
- Maintain emphasis on personal choices of the woman *because doing so promotes control and minimizes imposition of routines by others.*
- Evaluate what support and system resources are available in the environment *to assist in providing diversional activities.*
- Explore ways for the woman to remain an active participant in home management and decision making *to promote control.*
- Engage support of family and friends in carrying out chosen activities and making necessary environmental alterations *to ensure success.*
- Teach woman about stress management and relaxation techniques *to help manage tension of confinement.*

---

woman with this diagnosis can be cared for at home, with more frequent visits to her primary health care provider (Patient Instructions for Self-Care box). Expectant management will continue as long as there are no signs of infection or fetal distress. Nursing support of the woman and her family is critical at this time. She is often anxious about the health of her baby and may fear that she was responsible in some

way for the membrane rupture. The nurse should encourage expression of feelings and concerns, provide information, and make referrals as needed (Weitz, 2001).

Frequent biophysical profiles (BPPs) are performed to determine fetal health status and estimate amniotic fluid volume (AFV). The woman with PPROM also should be taught how to count fetal movements daily, because a slowing of

PATIENT INSTRUCTIONS FOR SELF-CARE

The Woman with Preterm Premature Rupture of Membranes

- Take your temperature and assess pulse every 4 hours when awake.
- Report temperature of more than 38° C.
- Remain on modified bed rest.
- Insert nothing in the vagina.
- Do not engage in sexual activity.
- Assess for uterine contractions.
- Do fetal movement counts daily.
- Do not take tub baths.
- Watch for foul-smelling vaginal discharge.
- Wipe front to back after urinating or having a bowel movement.
- Take antibiotics if prescribed.
- See primary health care provider as scheduled.

PATIENT INSTRUCTIONS FOR SELF-CARE

Counting Fetal Movements (Kick Counts)

- Choose a time of day when you can sit or lie on your side quietly.
- Choices for counting strategies:
  - Starting at 9 AM, count the baby's movements until you have counted 10. If you have not counted 10 movements in 12 hours, notify your primary health care provider.
  - Count four movements, three times a day after meals. Most people count four movements in 1 hour. If you don't, then count for 1 more hour. If at the end of 2 hours you still haven't felt four movements, call your primary health care provider.

fetal movement has been shown to be a precursor to severe fetal compromise. Several methods are commonly used to count fetal movements; two methods are described in the Patient Instructions for Self-Care box. Antenatal glucocorticoids may be administered if chorioamnionitis is absent (Weitz, 2001).

Vigilance for signs of infection is a major part of the nursing care and patient education after PPROM. The woman must be taught how to keep her genital area clean and that nothing should be introduced into her vagina. Signs of infection (e.g., fever, foul-smelling vaginal discharge, rapid pulse) should be reported to the primary health care provider immediately. Prophylactic antibiotic therapy may be ordered in an effort to improve perinatal outcome by preventing infection (Garite, 2004). However, use of prophylactic antibiotics for PROM before labor at term or preterm ✳ is a form of care of unknown effectiveness (Enkin et al., 2000).

DYSTOCIA

Dystocia is defined as long, difficult, or abnormal labor; it is caused by various conditions associated with the five factors affecting labor. It is estimated that dystocia occurs in approximately 8% to 11% of all births and is the primary cause for cesarean births (Gregory, 2000). Dystocia can be caused by any of the following:

- Dysfunctional labor, resulting in ineffective uterine contractions or maternal bearing-down efforts (the powers). This is the most common cause of dystocia (Cunningham et al., 2005).
- Alterations in the pelvic structure (the passage).
- Fetal causes, including abnormal presentation or position, anomalies, excessive size, and number of fetuses (the passenger).
- Maternal position during labor and birth.
- Psychologic responses of the mother to labor related to past experiences, preparation, culture and heritage, and support system.

These five factors are interdependent. In assessing the woman for an abnormal labor pattern, the nurse must consider the way in which these factors interact and influence labor progress. Dystocia is suspected when there is an alteration in the characteristics of uterine contractions, a lack of progress in the rate of cervical dilation, or a lack of progress in fetal descent and expulsion.

Dysfunctional Labor

Dysfunctional labor is described as abnormal uterine contractions that prevent the normal progress of cervical dilation, effacement (primary powers), or descent (secondary powers). Gilbert and Harmon (2003) cited several factors that seem to increase a woman's risk for uterine dystocia including the following:

- Body build (e.g., 30 pounds or more overweight, short stature)
- Uterine abnormalities (e.g., congenital malformations; overdistention, as with multiple gestation; or hydramnios)
- Malpresentations and positions of the fetus
- Cephalopelvic disproportion (CPD) (see p. 785)
- Overstimulation with oxytocin
- Maternal fatigue, dehydration and electrolyte imbalance, and fear
- Inappropriate timing of analgesic or anesthetic administration

Dysfunction of uterine contractions can be further described as being *hypertonic* or *hypotonic*.

Hypertonic uterine dysfunction

The woman experiencing **hypertonic uterine dysfunction**, or primary dysfunctional labor, often is an anxious first-time mother who is having painful and frequent contractions that are ineffective in causing cervical dilation or effacement to progress. These contractions usually occur in the latent stage (cervical dilation of less than 4 cm) and are usually unco-ordinated (Fig. 24-3). The force of the contractions may be in the midsection of the uterus rather than in the fundus, and the uterus is therefore unable to apply downward pressure to push the presenting part against the cervix. The uterus may not relax completely between contractions (Gilbert & Harmon, 2003).

Women with hypertonic uterine dysfunction may be exhausted and express concern about loss of control because of the intense pain they are experiencing and the lack of progress. Therapeutic rest, which is achieved with a warm bath or shower and the administration of analgesics such as morphine, meperidine (Demerol), or nalbuphine (Nubain) to inhibit uterine contractions, reduce pain, and encourage sleep, is usually prescribed for the management of hypertonic uterine dysfunction. After a 4- to 6-hour rest, affected women are likely to awaken in active labor with a normal uterine contraction pattern (Gilbert & Harmon, 2003).

Hypotonic uterine dysfunction

The second and more common type of uterine dysfunction is hypotonic uterine dysfunction, or secondary uterine inertia. The woman initially makes normal progress into the active stage of labor; then the contractions become weak and inefficient or stop altogether (see Fig. 24-3). The uterus is easily indented, even at the peak of contractions. Intrauterine pressure (IUP) during the contraction (usually less than 25 mm Hg) is insufficient for progress of cervical effacement and dilation (Gilbert & Harmon, 2003). CPD and malpositions are common causes of this type of uterine dysfunction.

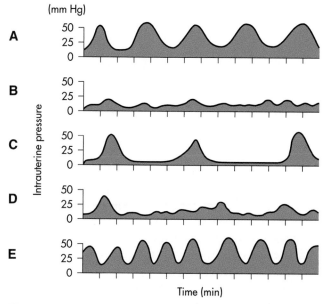

Fig. 24-3 Uterine contractility patterns in labor. **A,** Typical normal labor. **B,** Subnormal intensity, with frequency greater than needed for optimum performance. **C,** Normal contractions but too infrequent for efficient labor. **D,** Incoordinate activity. **E,** Hypercontractility.

A woman with hypotonic uterine dysfunction may become exhausted and be at increased risk for infection. Management usually consists of performing an ultrasound or radiographic examination to rule out CPD and assessing the fetal heart rate (FHR) and pattern, characteristics of amniotic fluid if membranes are ruptured, and maternal well-being. If findings are normal, then measures such as ambulation, hydrotherapy, enema, stripping or rupture of membranes, nipple stimulation, and oxytocin infusion can be used to augment labor.

Secondary powers

Secondary powers, or bearing-down efforts, are compromised when large amounts of analgesia are given. Anesthesia may also block the bearing-down reflex and, as a result, alter the effectiveness of voluntary efforts. Exhaustion resulting from lack of sleep or long labor and fatigue resulting from inadequate hydration and food intake reduce the effectiveness of the woman's voluntary efforts. Maternal position can work against the forces of gravity and decrease the strength and efficiency of the contractions. Table 24-1 summarizes the characteristics of dysfunctional labor.

Abnormal labor patterns

In 2002, prolonged labor patterns occurred at the rate of 7.0 per 1000 live births, with the incidence highest among women under 20 years of age (8.1 per 1000) (Martin et al., 2003).

Six abnormal labor patterns were identified and classified by Friedman (1989) according to the nature of the cervical dilation and fetal descent. The labor patterns seen in normal and abnormal labor are described in Table 24-2.

These patterns may result from a variety of causes, including ineffective uterine contractions, pelvic contractures, CPD, abnormal fetal presentation or position, early use of analgesics, nerve block analgesia or anesthesia, and anxiety and stress. Progress in either the first or second stage of labor can be protracted (prolonged) or arrested (stopped). Abnormal progress can be identified by plotting cervical dilation and fetal descent on a labor graph (partogram) at various intervals after the onset of labor and comparing the resulting curve with the expected labor curve for a nulliparous or multiparous labor (see Fig. 14-8, p. 415).

However, health care providers must be careful when diagnosing a labor pattern as prolonged and when intervening based on this diagnosis. Cesario (2004) found that although the average length of labor today is similar to that found by Friedman, a wider range of normal labor occurs. Parameters to determine if labor is progressing satisfactorily may need to be expanded.

A long and difficult labor can have an adverse psychologic effect on the mother, father, and family. Maternal morbidity and death may occur as a result of uterine rupture, infection, severe dehydration, and postpartum hemorrhage. The fetus is at increased risk for hypoxia.

TABLE 24-1

Dysfunctional Labor: Primary and Secondary Powers

HYPERTONIC UTERINE DYSFUNCTION	HYPOTONIC UTERINE DYSFUNCTION	INADEQUATE VOLUNTARY EXPULSIVE FORCES
DESCRIPTION		
Usually occurs before 4 cm dilation; cause unknown, may be related to fear and tension (primary powers)	Cause may be pelvic contracture and fetal malposition, overdistention of uterus (e.g., twins), or unknown (primary powers)	Involves abdominal and levator ani muscles Occurs in second stage of labor; cause may be related to nerve block anesthetic, analgesia, exhaustion
CHANGE IN PATTERN OF PROGRESS		
Pain out of proportion to intensity of contraction Pain out of proportion to effectiveness of contraction in effacing and dilating the cervix Contractions increase in frequency Contractions uncoordinated Uterus is contracted between contractions, cannot be indented	Contractions decrease in frequency and intensity Uterus easily indentable even at peak of contraction Uterus relaxed between contractions (normal)	No voluntary urge to push or bear down or inadequate or ineffective pushing
POTENTIAL MATERNAL EFFECTS		
Loss of control related to intensity of pain and lack of progress Exhaustion	Infection Exhaustion Psychologic trauma	Spontaneous vaginal birth prevented; assisted birth likely
POTENTIAL FETAL EFFECTS		
Fetal asphyxia with meconium aspiration	Fetal infection Fetal and neonatal death	Fetal asphyxia
CARE MANAGEMENT		
Initiate therapeutic rest measures • Administer analgesic (e.g., morphine, nalbuphine, meperidine) if membranes not ruptured or cephalopelvic disproportion not present • Relieve pain to permit mother to rest • Assist with measures to enhance rest and relaxation (e.g., hydrotherapy)	Rule out cephalopelvic disproportion Stimulate labor with oxytocin (augmentation) Perform amniotomy Assist with measures to enhance the progress of labor (e.g., position changes, ambulation, hydrotherapy)	Coach mother in bearing down with contractions; assist with relaxation between contractions Position mother in favorable position for pushing Reduce epidural infusion rate Assist with low forceps or vacuum-assisted birth Prepare for cesarean birth if nonreassuring fetal status occurs

Precipitous labor. Precipitous labor is defined as labor that lasts less than 3 hours from the onset of contractions to the time of birth. This abnormal labor pattern occurred at a rate of 18.1 per 1000 live births in 2002. Precipitous labor occurred at the highest rate (21.9) among women age 35 to 39 and at the lowest rate (11.7) among women younger than 20 years old (Martin et al., 2003).

Precipitous labor may result from hypertonic uterine contractions that are tetanic in intensity. Maternal and fetal complications can occur as a result. Maternal complications include uterine rupture, lacerations of the birth canal, amniotic fluid embolism (AFE) (p. 813), and postpartum hemorrhage. Fetal complications include hypoxia, caused by decreased periods of uterine relaxation between contractions, and in rare instances, intracranial trauma related to rapid birth (Cunningham et al., 2005).

Women who have experienced precipitous labor often describe feelings of disbelief that their labor began so quickly, alarm that their labor progressed so rapidly, panic about the possibility they would not make it to the hospital in time to give birth, and finally relief when they arrived at the hospital. In addition, women have expressed frustration when nurses did not believe them when they reported their readiness to push.

TABLE 24-2

Labor Patterns in Normal and Abnormal Labor

NORMAL LABOR
1. Dilation: continues
   a. Latent phase: <4 cm and low slope
   b. Active phase: >5 cm or high slope
   c. Deceleration phase: ≥9 cm
2. Descent: active at ≥9 cm dilation

ABNORMAL LABOR

PATTERN	NULLIPARAS	MULTIPARAS
Prolonged latent phase	>20 hr	>14 hr
Protracted active phase dilation	<1.2 cm/hr	<1.5 cm/hr
Secondary arrest: no change	≥2 hr	≥2 hr
Protracted descent	<1 cm/hr	<2 cm/hr
Arrest of descent	≥1 hr	≥½ hr
Failure of descent	No change during deceleration phase and second stage	
Precipitous labor	>5 cm/hr	10 cm/hr

Alterations in Pelvic Structure
Pelvic dystocia

Pelvic dystocia can occur whenever there are contractures of the pelvic diameters that reduce the capacity of the bony pelvis, including the inlet, midpelvis, outlet, or any combination of these planes.

Disproportion of the pelvis is the least common cause of dystocia (Cunningham et al., 2005). Pelvic contractures may be caused by congenital abnormalities, maternal malnutrition, neoplasms, or lower spinal disorders. An immature pelvic size predisposes some adolescent mothers to pelvic dystocia. Pelvic deformities also may be the result of automobile or other accidents or trauma.

An inlet contracture is diagnosed whenever the diagonal conjugate is less than 11.5 cm. The incidence of face and shoulder presentation is increased. Because these presentations interfere with engagement and fetal descent, the risk of prolapse of the umbilical cord is increased. Inlet contracture is associated with maternal rickets and a flat pelvis. Weak uterine contractions may be noted during the first stage of labor in affected women.

Midplane contracture, the most common cause of pelvic dystocia, is diagnosed whenever the sum of the interischial spinous and posterior sagittal diameters of the midpelvis is 13.5 cm or less. Fetal descent is arrested (transverse arrest of the fetal head) in such births because the head cannot rotate internally. These infants are usually born by cesarean, but vacuum-assisted birth has been used safely when the cervix is fully dilated. Midforceps-assisted birth usually is not done

because of the increased perinatal morbidity associated with this intervention.

Outlet contracture exists when the interischial diameter is 8 cm or less. It rarely occurs in the absence of midplane contracture. Women with outlet contracture have a long, narrow pubic arch and an android pelvis, and this causes fetal descent to be arrested. Maternal complications include extensive perineal lacerations during vaginal birth because the fetal head is pushed posteriorly.

Soft-tissue dystocia

Soft-tissue dystocia results from obstruction of the birth passage by an anatomic abnormality other than that involving the bony pelvis. The obstruction may result from placenta previa (low-lying placenta) that partially or completely obstructs the internal os of the cervix. Other causes, such as leiomyomas (uterine fibroids) in the lower uterine segment, ovarian tumors, and a full bladder or rectum, may prevent the fetus from entering the pelvis. Occasionally cervical edema occurs during labor when the cervix is caught between the presenting part and the symphysis pubis or when the woman begins bearing-down efforts prematurely, thereby inhibiting complete dilation. Sexually transmitted infections (e.g., human papillomavirus) can alter cervical tissue integrity and thus interfere with adequate effacement and dilation.

Bandl ring, a pathologic retraction ring that forms between the upper and lower uterine segments (see Fig. 11-10), is associated with prolonged rupture of membranes, protracted labor, and increased risk for uterine rupture (Cunningham et al., 2005).

Fetal Causes

Dystocia of fetal origin may be caused by anomalies, excessive fetal size and malpresentation, malposition, or multifetal pregnancy. Complications associated with dystocia of fetal origin include neonatal asphyxia, fetal injuries or fractures, and maternal vaginal lacerations. Although spontaneous vaginal birth is possible in these instances, a low forceps-assisted, vacuum-assisted, or cesarean birth often is necessary.

Anomalies

Gross ascites, large tumors, and open neural tube defects (e.g., myelomeningocele, hydrocephalus) are fetal anomalies that can cause dystocia. The anomalies affect the relation of the fetal anatomy to the maternal pelvic capacity, with the result that the fetus is unable to descend through the birth canal.

Cephalopelvic disproportion

Cephalopelvic disproportion (CPD), also called *fetopelvic disproportion (FPD)*, is often related to excessive fetal size (i.e., 4000 g or more). When CPD is present, the fetus cannot fit through the maternal pelvis to be born vaginally. Excessive fetal size, or macrosomia, is associated with maternal diabetes mellitus, obesity, multiparity, or the large size of one or both parents. If the maternal pelvis is too small, abnormally shaped, or deformed, CPD may be of maternal origin. In this case, the fetus may be of average size or even smaller.

Malposition

The most common fetal malposition is persistent occipitoposterior position (i.e., right occipitoposterior [ROP] or left occipitoposterior [LOP]; see Chapter 11), occurring in about 25% of all labors. Labor, especially the second stage, is prolonged; the woman typically complains of severe back pain from the pressure of the fetal head (occiput) pressing against her sacrum. Box 24-7 identifies suggested measures to relieve back pain and facilitate rotation of the fetal occiput

---

BOX 24-7

Back Labor—Occiput Posterior Position

MEASURES TO RELIEVE BACK PAIN AND FACILITATE ROTATION OF FETAL HEAD

Measures to reduce back pain during a contraction
- *Counterpressure:* apply fist or heel of hand to sacral area
- *Heat or cold applications:* apply to sacral area
- *Double hip squeeze:*
  - Woman assumes a position with hip joints flexed, such as knee-chest
  - Partner, nurse, or doula places hands over gluteal muscles and presses with palms of hands up and inward toward the center of the pelvis
- *Knee press:*
  - Woman assumes a sitting position with knees a few inches apart and feet flat on the floor or on a stool
  - Partner, nurse, or doula cups a knee in each hand with heels of hands on top of tibia then presses the knees straight back toward the woman's hips while leaning forward toward the woman

Measures to facilitate the rotation of the fetal head (may also relieve back pain)
- *Lateral abdominal stroking:* stroke the abdomen in direction that the fetal head should rotate
- *Hands-and-knees position* (all-fours): can also be accomplished by kneeling while leaning forward over a birth ball, padded chair seat, bed, or over-the-bed table
- *Squatting*
- *Pelvic rocking*
- *Stair climbing*
- *Lateral position:* lie on side toward which the fetus should turn
- *Lunges:* widens pelvis on side toward which woman lunges
  - Woman stands, facing forward, next to or alongside a chair so that she can lunge toward the side the fetal back is on or in the direction of the fetal occiput
  - Places foot on seat of chair with toes pointed toward the back of the chair, then lunges
  - Alternative position for lunge: kneeling

---

to an anterior position, which will facilitate birth (Gilbert & Harmon, 2003; Simkin & Ancheta, 2000).

Malpresentation

Malpresentation is the third most commonly reported complication of labor and birth. Breech presentation is the most common form of malpresentation. The four main types of breech presentation are frank breech (thighs flexed, knees extended), complete breech (thighs and knees flexed), and two types of incomplete breech, one in which the knee extends below the buttocks and the other in which the foot extends below the buttocks (Fig. 24-4). Breech presentations are associated with multifetal gestation, preterm birth, fetal and maternal anomalies, hydramnios, and oligohydramnios. Diagnosis is made by abdominal palpation (e.g., Leopold maneuvers) and vaginal examination and usually is confirmed by ultrasound scan (Lanni & Seeds, 2002).

During labor, the descent of the fetus in a breech presentation may be slow because the breech is not so good a dilating wedge as is the fetal head; the labor itself usually is not prolonged. There is risk of prolapse of the cord if the membranes rupture in early labor. The presence of meconium in amniotic fluid is not necessarily a sign of fetal distress because it results from pressure on the fetal abdominal wall as it traverses the birth canal. Assessment of FHR and pattern should be used to determine whether the passage of meconium is an expected finding associated with breech presentation or is a nonreassuring sign associated with fetal hypoxia. The fetal heart tones of infants in a breech position are best heard at or above the umbilicus.

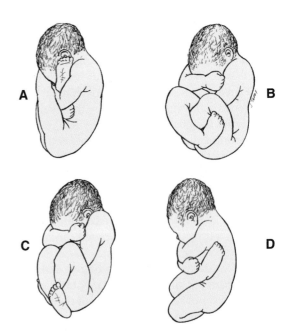

Fig. 24-4   Types of breech presentation. **A,** Frank breech: thighs are flexed on hips; knees are extended. **B,** Complete breech: thighs and knees are flexed. **C,** Incomplete breech: foot extends below the buttocks. **D,** Incomplete breech: knee extends below the buttocks.

EVIDENCE-BASED PRACTICE
Planned Caesarean Birth versus Vaginal Birth for Term Breech Presentation

BACKGROUND

- Breech presentation at birth has been associated with nulliparity, previous breech, uterine or pelvic anomaly, placental malplacement, too much or too little amniotic fluid, extended fetal legs, multiple pregnancy, preterm birth, shortened umbilical cord, decreased fetal activity, intrauterine growth restriction (IUGR), fetal anomaly, and stillbirth. Commonly, breech presentation is an indication for a cesarean birth. Some researchers speculate that the breech position itself is an indicator of poor outcome. For example, the rate of childhood handicaps among breech babies is high, no matter what method of birth is employed. In addition, cesarean birth exposes the mother and baby to all the risks of operative procedures: anesthesia problems, infection, pain, delayed recovery, immobility, ileus, uterine rupture in future pregnancies, and neonatal respiratory problems. Length of stay and cost also rise considerably.

OBJECTIVES

- The reviewers sought to compare the maternal and perinatal outcomes of routine cesarean birth for term breech presentation, compared with term breech presentations delivered vaginally. The perinatal outcomes are death (excluding fatal anomalies), serious neonatal morbidity (Apgar score less than 7, cord blood pH less than 7.0, neonatal intensive care admission, birth asphyxia, birth trauma), and disability in childhood. Maternal outcomes include death, pain, incontinence, instrumental delivery, hemorrhage, infection, depression, self-esteem, relationship with infant and family, problems with future pregnancies and deliveries, satisfaction, and costs. All women should be considered suitable for vaginal birth.

METHODS

Search Strategy

- The authors searched the Cochrane database, MEDLINE, 30 journals and conference proceedings, and a weekly current awareness service of 37 journals. Search keyword was *breech*.
- Three randomized, controlled trials met the criteria, representing 2396 women. Two trials, dated 1980 and 1983, were from the United States. The other trial, dated 2000, was a large, international multicenter trial whose countries were not noted in the review.

Statistical Analyses

- Similar data were pooled. Reviewers calculated relative risks for dichotomous data, and weighted mean differences for continuous data. Countries with low (20 per 1000 or less) and high (more than 20 per 1000) perinatal mortality rates were subgrouped for comparison.

FINDINGS

- Of the women with term breech presentation allocated to vaginal birth, 45% gave birth by cesarean. Those scheduled for cesarean births experienced significantly fewer perinatal deaths (excluding fatal anomalies), decreased short-term neonatal morbidity, fewer low Apgar (less than 7) or very low Apgar (less than 4) scores, less acidotic cord blood, and less cord base excess (15 or more) than did the planned vaginal birth group. The reduction in risk of perinatal mortality and morbidity was less in countries with high perinatal mortality rates. No difference in infant birth trauma was noted between groups. A small but significant increase in short-term maternal morbidity was found in the planned cesarean group. At 3 months postpartum the planned cesarean group experienced less urinary incontinence and perineal pain, and more abdominal pain, than the planned vaginal birth group.

LIMITATIONS

- The two smaller U.S. studies from 1980 and 1983 did not specify the method of randomization. One of those studies had a large discrepancy in numbers between groups. The large multicenter trial used a wide variety of clinical settings and had good follow-up rates, which were strengths.

CONCLUSIONS

- There is evidence that planned caesarean birth in term breech presentations is associated with decreased perinatal death and morbidity rates and an increase in short-term maternal morbidity.

IMPLICATIONS FOR PRACTICE

- Planned caesarean birth is not always desirable or feasible in all settings. External cephalic version, or the ultrasound-guided process of manually changing the fetal presentation from outside the abdomen, is one alternative. Promising results have been noted in other alternative practices, such as using various positions and moxibustion. (Moxibustion is a method of producing analgesia by holding slow-burning moxa or another substance near the skin without causing pain or burning; sometimes used in conjunction with acupuncture.) Even cesarean birth does not totally eliminate the problems associated with breech presentation. Diagnosis of the presentation before labor is desirable.

IMPLICATIONS FOR FURTHER RESEARCH

- Much more evidence is needed on the effects of cesarean births, for breech presentation or other indication, on long-term outcomes, such as reproductive function of women and child development. Researchers need to assess the psychologic impact of cesarean birth on women and their adaptation to parenting. Cost was not addressed in these trials but remains a primary factor in policy making and decision making.

Reference: Hofmeyr, G., & Hannah, M. (2003). Planned caesarean section for term breech delivery (Cochrane Review). In *The Cochrane Library*, Issue 3, 2005. Chichester, UK: John Wiley & Sons.

Vaginal birth is accomplished by mechanisms of labor that manipulate the buttocks and lower extremities as they emerge from the birth canal (Fig. 24-5). Piper forceps sometimes are used to deliver the head. External cephalic version (ECV) (see later discussion) may be tried to turn the fetus to a vertex presentation (Fig. 24-6). Cesarean birth may be necessary (Bowes & Thorp, 2004).

Although opinions vary, a cesarean birth is commonly performed when the fetus is estimated to be larger than 3800 g or smaller than 1500 g, if this is a first pregnancy, if labor is ineffective, or if complications occur. Although cesarean birth reduces the risks to the fetus, the maternal risks are increased. ECV also poses risks and is not always successful. Women whose breech presentation occurs late in pregnancy need to be informed of the options for birth, as well as the risks associated with each option.

Face and brow presentations are uncommon and are associated with fetal anomalies, pelvic contractures, and CPD. Vaginal birth is possible if the fetus flexes to a vertex presentation, although forceps often are used. Cesarean birth is indicated if the presentation persists, if there is fetal distress, or if labor stops progressing.

Cesarean birth is usually necessary for a fetus in a shoulder presentation (i.e., the fetus is in a transverse lie), although ECV may be attempted after 38 weeks of gestation (Bowes & Thorp, 2004).

Multifetal pregnancy

Multifetal pregnancy is the gestation of twins, triplets, quadruplets, or more infants. The twin birth rate was 31.1 per 1000 live births in 2002. The higher-order multiple birth rate (i.e., triplet and more) was 184 per 100,000 live births in 2002 (Martin et al., 2003). The incidence of multiple births has been increasing since 1980. It is likely that this trend is related to the use of fertility-enhancing medications and procedures and the older age of childbearing women. When compared with younger women, women age 35 years and older are naturally more likely to have a multifetal pregnancy.

Multiple births are associated with more complications (e.g., dysfunctional labor) than are single births. The higher incidence of fetal and newborn complications and higher risk of perinatal mortality primarily stem from the birth of low-birth-weight infants resulting from preterm birth and/or IUGR in part related to placental dysfunction and twin-to-twin transfusion. Fetuses may experience distress and asphyxia during the birth process as a result of cord prolapse and the onset of placental separation with the birth of the first fetus. As a result, the risk for long-term problems such as cerebral palsy is higher among infants who were part of a multiple birth.

In addition, fetal complications such as congenital anomalies and abnormal presentations can result in dystocia and an increased incidence of cesarean birth. For example, in only half of all twin pregnancies do both fetuses present in the vertex position, the most favorable for vaginal birth; in one third of the pregnancies, one twin may present in the vertex position and one in the breech (Cunningham et al., 2005).

The health status of the mother may be compromised by an increased risk for hypertension, anemia, and hemorrhage

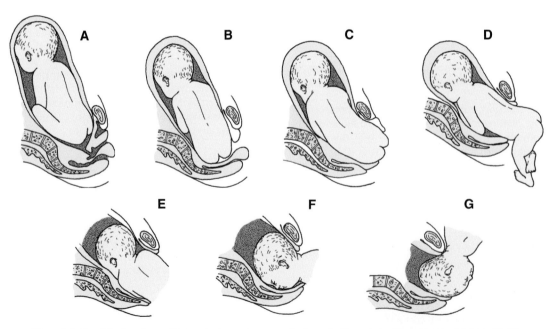

Fig. 24-5 Mechanism of labor in breech presentation. **A,** Breech before onset of labor. **B,** Engagement and internal rotation. **C,** Lateral flexion. **D,** External rotation or restitution. **E,** Internal rotation of shoulders and head. **F,** Face rotates to sacrum when occiput is anterior. **G,** Head is born by gradual flexion during elevation of fetal body.

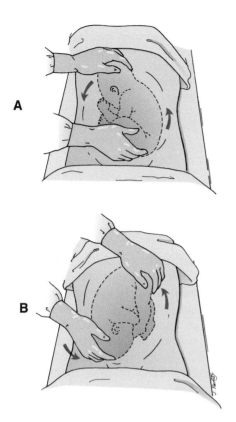

Fig. 24-6 External version of fetus from breech to vertex presentation. This must be achieved without force. **A,** Breech is pushed up out of pelvic inlet while head is pulled toward inlet. **B,** Head is pushed toward inlet while breech is pulled upward.

associated with uterine atony, abruptio placentae, and multiple or adherent placentas. Duration of the phases and stages of labor may vary from the duration experienced with singleton births.

Teamwork and planning are essential components of the management of childbirth in multiple pregnancies, especially those of the higher-order multiples. The nurse plays a key role in coordinating the activities of many highly skilled health care professionals. Early detection and care of the maternal, fetal, and newborn complications associated with multiple births are essential to achieve a positive outcome for mother and babies. Maternal positioning and active support are used to enhance labor progress and placental perfusion. Stimulation of labor with oxytocin, epidural anesthesia, forceps and vacuum assistance, and internal or external version may be used to accomplish the vaginal birth of twins. Cesarean birth is most likely with higher-order multiple births. Each infant may have its own team of health care providers present at the birth. Emotional support that includes expression of feelings and full explanations of events as they occur and of the status of the mother and the fetuses and newborns is important to reduce the anxiety and stress that the mother and her family experience.

Position of the Woman

The functional relationship among the uterine contractions, the fetus, and the mother's pelvis are altered by the maternal position. In addition, the position can provide either a mechanical advantage or disadvantage to the mechanisms of labor by altering the effects of gravity and the body-part relations important to the progress of labor. For example, the hands-and-knees position facilitates rotation from a posterior occiput position more effectively than does the lateral position. Upright positions such as sitting and squatting facilitate fetal descent during pushing and shorten the second stage of labor (Mayberry et al., 2000; Simkin & Ancheta, 2000). Discouraging maternal movement or restricting labor to the recumbent or lithotomy position may compromise progress. The incidence of dystocia in women confined to these positions is increased, resulting in increased need for augmentation of labor or forceps-assisted, vacuum-assisted, or cesarean birth.

Psychologic Responses

Hormones and neurotransmitters released in response to stress (e.g., catecholamines) can cause dystocia. Sources of stress vary for each woman, but pain and the absence of a support person are two recognized factors. Confinement to bed and restriction of maternal movement can be a source of psychologic stress that compounds the physiologic stress caused by immobility in the unmedicated laboring woman. When anxiety is excessive, it can inhibit cervical dilation and result in prolonged labor and increased pain perception. Anxiety also causes increased levels of stress-related hormones (e.g., beta-endorphin, adrenocorticotropic hormone, cortisol, and epinephrine). These hormones act on the smooth muscles of the uterus; increased levels can cause dystocia by reducing uterine contractility.

CARE MANAGEMENT

Assessment and Nursing Diagnoses

Risk assessment is a continuous process in the laboring woman. Review of the findings obtained during the initial interview conducted at the woman's admission to the labor unit and ongoing observations of her psychologic response to labor may reveal factors that can be a source of dysfunctional labor. These factors may include anxiety or fear, a complication of pregnancy, or previous labor complications. The initial physical assessment and ongoing assessments provide information about maternal well-being; status of labor in terms of the characteristics of uterine contractions and progress of cervical effacement and dilation; fetal well-being in terms of FHR and pattern, presentation, station, and position; and status of the amniotic membranes. Ultrasound scanning can identify potential dysfunctional labor problems related to the fetus or maternal pelvis. All these assessments contribute to accurate identification of potential and actual nursing diagnoses related to dystocia and maternal-fetal compromise.

Nursing diagnoses that might be identified in women experiencing dystocia include the following:

> - *Risk for maternal or fetal injury related to*
>   —interventions implemented for dystocia
> - *Powerlessness related to:*
>   —loss of control
> - *Risk for infection related to:*
>   —PPROM
>   —operative procedures
> - *Ineffective individual coping related to*
>   —inadequate support system.
>   —exhaustion
>   —pain

Expected Outcomes of Care

Expected outcomes for the woman with dystocia include the following. The woman will:

- Understand the causes and treatment of dysfunctional labor
- Use measures recommended by the health care team to enhance the progress of labor and birth
- Express relief of pain
- Experience labor and birth with minimal or no complications, such as infection, injury, or hemorrhage
- Give birth to a healthy infant who has experienced no fetal distress or birth injury

Plan of Care and Interventions

Nurses assume many caregiving roles when labor is complicated. They also work collaboratively with other health care providers in providing care. Interventions that the nurse may implement or assist with include ECV, trial of labor, cervical ripening with prostaglandins, induction or augmentation with oxytocin, amniotomy, and operative procedures (e.g., forceps- or vacuum-assisted birth). The nursing role is identified with each of the procedures described.

LEGAL TIP Standard of Care—Labor and Birth Complications

- *Document all assessment findings, interventions, and patient responses on patient record and monitor strips according to unit protocols, procedures, and policies and professional standards.*
- *Assess whether the woman (and her family, if appropriate) is fully informed about procedures for which she is consenting.*
- *Provide full explanations regarding what is happening and what needs to be done to help her and her baby (see Guidelines/Guías boxes: Induction of Labor, p. 791, and Cesarean Birth, p. 802).*
- *Maintain safety by administering medications and treatments correctly.*
- *Have verbal orders signed as soon as possible.*
- *Provide care at the acceptable standard (e.g., according to hospital protocols and professional standards).*

- *If short staffing occurs in the unit and the nurse is assigned additional patients, the nurse should document that rejecting this additional assignment would have placed these patients in danger as a result of abandonment.*
- *Maternal and fetal monitoring continues until birth according to the policies, procedures, and protocols of the birthing facility, even when a decision to carry out cesarean birth is made.*

Version

Version is the turning of the fetus from one presentation to another and may be done either externally or internally by the physician.

External cephalic version. External cephalic version (ECV) is used to attempt to turn the fetus from a breech or shoulder presentation to a vertex presentation for birth. It may be attempted in a labor and birth setting after 37 weeks of gestation. ECV is accomplished by the exertion of gentle, constant pressure on the abdomen (see Fig. 24-6). Before ECV is attempted, ultrasound scanning is done to determine the fetal position; locate the umbilical cord; rule out placenta previa; evaluate the adequacy of the maternal pelvis; and assess the amount of amniotic fluid, the fetal age, and the presence of any anomalies. A nonstress test (NST) is performed to confirm fetal well-being, or the FHR pattern is monitored for a period of time (e.g., 10 to 20 minutes). Informed consent is obtained. A tocolytic agent such as magnesium sulfate or terbutaline often is given to relax the uterus and to facilitate the maneuver (Bowes & Thorp, 2004). Factors that are associated with unsuccessful version include maternal obesity, oligohydramnios, deep engagement of the buttocks, and posterior position of the fetal back. ECV is controversial in women who have had a previous cesarean birth (Cunningham et al., 2005; Lanni & Seeds, 2002). ECV performed at term to avoid breech birth is a beneficial form of care (Enkin et al., 2000). ✳

During an attempted ECV, the nurse continuously monitors the FHR and pattern, especially for bradycardia and variable decelerations; checks the maternal vital signs; and assesses the woman's level of comfort because the procedure may cause discomfort. After the procedure is completed, the nurse continues to monitor maternal vital signs, uterine activity, and FHR and pattern and to assess for vaginal bleeding until the woman's condition is stable. Women who are Rh negative should receive Rh immune globulin because the manipulation can cause fetomaternal bleeding (Bowes & Thorp, 2004).

Internal version. With internal version, the fetus is turned by the physician, who inserts a hand into the uterus and changes the presentation to cephalic (head) or podalic (foot). Internal version may be used in multifetal pregnancies to deliver the second fetus. The safety of this procedure has not been documented; maternal and fetal injury is possible. Cesarean birth is the usual method for managing malpresentation in multifetal pregnancies. The nurse's role is to monitor the status of the fetus and to provide support to the woman.

Trial of labor

A trial of labor (TOL) is the observance of a woman and her fetus for a reasonable period (e.g., 4 to 6 hours) of spontaneous active labor to assess safety of vaginal birth for the mother and infant. It may be initiated if the mother's pelvis is of questionable size or shape, if the fetus is in an abnormal presentation, or if the woman wishes to have a vaginal birth after a previous cesarean birth. It is a form of care likely to be beneficial when implemented after a previous low-segment cesarean birth (Enkin et al., 2000). Fetal sonography, maternal pelvimetry, or both may be done before a TOL to rule out CPD. The cervix must be ripe (e.g., soft, dilatable). During a TOL, the woman is evaluated for the occurrence of active labor, including adequate contractions, engagement and descent of the presenting part, and effacement and dilation of the cervix.

The nurse assesses maternal vital signs and FHR and pattern and is alert for signs of potential complications. If complications develop, the nurse is responsible for initiating appropriate actions, including notifying the primary health care provider, and for evaluating and documenting the maternal and fetal responses to the interventions. Nurses must recognize that the woman and her partner are often anxious about her health and well-being and that of their baby. Supporting and encouraging the woman and her partner and providing information regarding progress can reduce stress, enhance the labor process, and facilitate a successful outcome.

Induction of labor

Induction of labor is the chemical or mechanical initiation of uterine contractions before their spontaneous onset for the purpose of bringing about the birth (Guidelines/Guías: Induction of Labor). Induction may be indicated for a variety of medical and obstetric reasons. These include preeclampsia, diabetes mellitus, chorioamnionitis, and other medical problems, PROM, postterm pregnancy, suspected fetal jeopardy (e.g., IUGR), logistic factors such as history of previous rapid birth or distance of the woman's home from the hospital, and fetal death. Under such conditions the risk to the mother or fetus is less than the risk of continuing the pregnancy (Bowes & Thorp, 2004). Two thirds of the inductions in the United States are elective (i.e., for the convenience of the woman or the health care practitioner) (Ramsey, Ramin, & Ramin, 2000).

Both chemical and mechanical methods are used to induce labor. Intravenous oxytocin and amniotomy are the most common methods used in the United States. Prostaglandins are increasingly used for inducing labor. The most effective protocol (e.g., dose, frequency) to follow when using prostaglandins continues to be investigated (Simpson, 2002; Simpson & Atterbury, 2003).

Less commonly used methods include stripping of membranes, nipple stimulation (manual or with a breast pump), and acupuncture (Bowes & Thorp, 2004). The ingestion of a laxative (e.g., castor oil), herbal preparations (e.g., green, chamomile, or raspberry tea; blue or black cohosh), or spicy food and administration of a soapsuds enema are other methods (Simpson, 2002). Many folk beliefs exist regarding methods to induce labor. These methods include activity (e.g., walking, exercise, strenuous work, intercourse), fasting, and increasing stress (e.g., frightening the woman). It is important for the nurse to know the practices a woman may believe in and follow, because some of these methods can be harmful (e.g., strenuous activity) (Schaffir, 2002).

Success rates for induction of labor are higher when the condition of the cervix is favorable, or inducible. A rating system such as the Bishop score (Table 24-3) can be used to evaluate inducibility. For example, a score of 9 or more on this 13-point scale indicates that the cervix is soft, anterior, 50% or more effaced, and dilated 2 cm or more; and that the presenting part is engaged. Induction of labor is likely to be more successful if the score is 9 or more for nulliparas and 5 or more for multiparas (Gilbert & Harmon, 2003).

Cervical ripening methods

Chemical agents. A prostaglandin E_2 gel (a cervical ripening agent) was approved by the FDA in 1993. Preparations of prostaglandin E_1 and prostaglandin E_2 can be used before induction to "ripen" (soften and thin) the cervix (Medication Guides). This treatment usually results in a

---

GUIDELINES/GUÍAS

Induction of Labor

- Your labor is not progressing.
- *Su trabajo de parto no está progresando.*
- We need to stimulate the contractions.
- *Necesitamos provocar las contracciones.*
- I'm going to give you some medication to make your contractions stronger.
- *Le voy a dar una medicina para hacer más fuertes las contracciones.*
- I'm going to give you Pitocin through your intravenous line.
- *Le voy a dar pitufina por medio del suero.*

TABLE 24-3

Bishop Score

	SCORE			
	0	1	2	3
Dilation (cm)	0	1-2	3-4	≥5
Effacement (%)	0-30	40-50	60-70	≥80
Station (cm)	-3	-2	-1	+1,+2
Cervical consistency	Firm	Medium	Soft	Soft
Cervix position	Posterior	Mid-position	Anterior	Anterior

Medication Guide

Cervical Ripening Using Prostaglandin E₁ (PGE₁): Misoprostol (Cytotec)

ACTION

- PGE₁ ripens the cervix, making it softer and causing it to begin to dilate and efface; stimulates uterine contractions.

INDICATIONS

- PGE₁ is used for preinduction cervical ripening (ripening of cervix before oxytocin induction of labor when the Bishop score is 4 or less) and to induce labor or abortion (abortifacient agent).

DOSAGE

- Insert 25 to 50 mcg (¼ to ½ of a 100-mcg tablet) intravaginally into the posterior fornix using the tips of index and middle fingers without the use of a lubricant. Repeat every 3 to 6 hours as needed to a maximum of 300 to 400 mcg in a 24-hour period or until an effective contraction pattern is established (three or more uterine contractions in 10 minutes), the cervix ripens (Bishop score of 8 or greater), or significant adverse reactions occur.
- Administer 50-100 mcg, PO q4-6h (GI effects increased; may be less effective; data insufficient to recommend giving orally).

ADVERSE REACTIONS

- Higher dosages are more likely to result in adverse reactions such as nausea and vomiting, diarrhea, fever, tachysystole (12 or more uterine contractions in 20 minutes without alteration of FHR pattern), hyperstimulation of the uterus (tachysystole with nonreassuring FHR patterns), or fetal passage of meconium.

NURSING CONSIDERATIONS

- Explain procedure to woman and her family. Ensure that an informed consent has been obtained as per agency policy.
- Assess maternal-fetal unit, before each insertion and during treatment, following agency protocol for frequency. Assess maternal vital signs and health status, FHR pattern, and status of pregnancy, including indications for cervical ripening or induction of labor, signs of labor or impending labor, and the Bishop score. Recognize that a nonreassuring FHR pattern; maternal fever, infection, vaginal bleeding, or hypersensitivity; and regular, progressive uterine contractions contraindicate the use of misoprostol.
- Use caution if the woman has a history of asthma, glaucoma, or renal, hepatic, or cardiovascular disorders.
- Have woman void before procedure.
- Assist woman to maintain a supine position with lateral tilt or a side-lying position for 30 to 40 minutes after insertion.
- Prepare to swab vagina to remove unabsorbed medication using a saline-soaked gauze wrapped around fingers and to administer terbutaline 0.25 mg subcutaneously or intravenously if significant adverse reactions occur.
- Initiate oxytocin for induction of labor no sooner than 4 hours after last dose of misoprostol was administered, following agency protocol, if ripening has occurred and labor has not begun.
- Document all assessment findings and administration procedures.
- Not recommended for use if woman has had previous cesarean birth or if she has a uterine scar.
- Misoprostol (Cytotec) has not yet been approved by the FDA for cervical ripening or labor induction.

FHR, Fetal heart rate; *GI,* gastrointestinal; *PO,* by mouth.

---

higher success rate for the induction of labor, the need for lower dosages of oxytocin during the induction, and shorter induction times. The use of prostaglandins to increase cervical readiness for induction of labor is a beneficial form of care (Enkin et al., 2000). In some cases, women will go into labor after the administration of prostaglandin, thereby eliminating the need to administer oxytocin to induce labor (Gilbert & Harmon, 2003; Simpson, 2002). Prostaglandin E₁, although less expensive and more effective than oxytocin or prostaglandin E₂ for inducing labor and birth, is associated with a higher risk for hyperstimulation of the uterus and nonreassuring changes in FHR and pattern (Goldberg, Greenberg, & Darney, 2001).

Mechanical methods. Mechanical dilators ripen the cervix by stimulating the release of endogenous prostaglandins. Their use is a form of care with a trade-off between beneficial and adverse effects (Enkin et al., 2000). Balloon catheters (e.g., Foley catheter) can be inserted into the intracervical canal to ripen and dilate the cervix. Hydroscopic dilators (substances that absorb fluid from surrounding tis-

sues and then enlarge) also can be used for cervical ripening. Laminaria tents (natural cervical dilators made from desiccated seaweed) and synthetic dilators containing magnesium sulfate (Lamicel) are inserted into the endocervix without rupturing the membranes. As they absorb fluid, they expand and cause cervical dilation. These dilators are left in place for 6 to 12 hours before being removed to assess cervical dilation. Fresh dilators are inserted if further cervical dilation is necessary. Synthetic dilators swell faster than natural dilators and become larger with less discomfort (Simpson, 2002). Amniotomy and membrane stripping also can be used to ripen the cervix (Norwitz, Robinson, & Repke, 2002).

Amniotomy. Amniotomy (i.e., artificial rupture of membranes [AROM]) can be used to induce labor when the condition of the cervix is favorable (ripe) or to augment labor if progress begins to slow. Labor usually begins within 12 hours of the rupture. However, if amniotomy does not stimulate labor, the resulting prolonged rupture may lead to infection. Other potential risks include umbilical cord pro-

Medication Guide

Cervical Ripening Using Prostaglandin E₂ (PGE₂): Dinoprostone (Cervidil Insert; Prepidil Gel)

ACTION

- PGE₂ ripens the cervix, making it softer and causing it to begin to dilate and efface; stimulates uterine contractions.

INDICATIONS

- PGE₂ is used for preinduction cervical ripening (ripening of cervix before oxytocin induction of labor when the Bishop score is 4 or less) and for inducement of labor or abortion (abortifacient agent).

DOSAGE

Cervidil Insert:

- Dosage is 10 mg of dinoprostone designed to be released gradually (approximately 0.3 mg /hr) over 12 hr. Insert is placed transversely into the posterior fornix of vagina. The insert is removed at the onset of active labor or after 12 hours.

Prepidil Gel:

- Dosage is 0.5 mg dinoprostone in 2.5-ml syringe. Gel is administered through a catheter attached to the syringe into the cervical canal just below internal cervical os. Dose may be repeated every 6 hr as needed for cervical ripening up to a maximum of 1.5 mg in a 24-hr period.

ADVERSE REACTIONS

- Potential adverse reactions include headache, nausea and vomiting, diarrhea, fever, hypotension, tachysystole (12 or more uterine contractions in 20 minutes without alteration of fetal heart rate [FHR] pattern), hyperstimulation of the uterus (tachysystole with nonreassuring FHR patterns), or fetal passage of meconium.

NURSING CONSIDERATIONS

- Explain procedure to woman and her family. Ensure that an informed consent has been obtained as per agency policy.
- Assess maternal-fetal unit before each insertion and during treatment following agency protocol for frequency. Assess maternal vital signs and health status, FHR pattern, and status of pregnancy, including indications for cervical ripening or induction of labor, signs of labor or impending labor, and the Bishop score. Recognize that a nonreassuring FHR pattern; maternal fever, infection, vaginal bleeding, or hypersensitivity; and regular, progressive uterine contractions contraindicate the use of dinoprostone.
- Use caution if the woman has a history of asthma; glaucoma; or renal, hepatic, or cardiovascular disorders.
- Bring gel to room temperature before administration. Do not force warming process by using a warm water bath or other source of external heat (e.g., microwave).
- Keep insert frozen until immediately before use; no need to warm.
- Have woman void before insertion.
- Assist woman to maintain a supine position with lateral tilt or a side-lying position for 15 to 30 min after insertion of gel or for 2 hr after placement of insert.
- Prepare to swab vagina to remove remaining gel using a saline-soaked gauze, or pull string to remove insert and to administer terbutaline 0.25 mg subcutaneously or intravenously if significant adverse reactions occur.
- Initiate oxytocin for induction of labor within 6 to 12 hr after last instillation of gel or within 30 min after removal of the insert or follow agency protocol for induction if ripening has occurred and labor has not begun.
- Document all assessment findings and administration procedures.
- Not recommended for use if woman has had previous cesarean birth or if she has a uterine scar.
- Dinoprostone is the only FDA-approved medication for cervical ripening or labor induction.

---

lapse and fetal injury. Once an amniotomy is performed, the woman is committed to labor with an unknown outcome for how and when she will give birth.

Before the procedure, the woman should be told what to expect; she also should be assured that the actual rupture of the membranes is painless for her and the fetus, although she may experience some discomfort when the Amnihook or other sharp instrument is inserted through the vagina and cervix (Procedure box).

The presenting part of the fetus should be engaged and well applied to the cervix to prevent cord prolapse. The woman should be free of active infection of the genital tract (e.g., herpes) and human immunodeficiency virus (HIV) infection (Norwitz, Robinson, & Repke, 2002). The membranes are ruptured with an Amnihook or other sharp instrument, and the amniotic fluid is allowed to drain slowly. The color, odor, and consistency of the fluid is assessed (i.e.,

for the presence or absence of meconium or blood). The time of rupture is recorded.

NURSE ALERT *The FHR is assessed before and immediately after the amniotomy to detect any changes (e.g., transient tachycardia is common, but bradycardia and variable decelerations are not) that may indicate cord compression or prolapse.*

The woman's temperature should be checked at least every 2 hours to rule out possible infection. If her temperature is 38° C or higher, the primary health care provider should be notified. The nurse assesses for other signs and symptoms of infection, such as maternal chills, uterine tenderness on palpation, foul-smelling vaginal drainage, and fetal tachycardia (Simpson, 2002). Comfort measures, such as frequently changing the woman's underpads and perineal cleansing, are implemented.

Oxytocin. Oxytocin is a hormone normally produced by the posterior pituitary gland; it stimulates uterine contractions. Synthetic oxytocin may be used either to induce labor or to augment a labor that is progressing slowly because of inadequate uterine contractions.

The indications for oxytocin induction or augmentation of labor may include, but are not limited to, the following:
- Suspected fetal jeopardy (e.g., IUGR)
- Inadequate uterine contractions; dystocia
- PROM
- Postterm pregnancy
- Chorioamnionitis
- Maternal medical problems (e.g., woman with severe Rh isoimmunization, inadequately controlled diabetes mellitus, chronic renal disease, or chronic pulmonary disease)
- Severe preeclampsia
- Fetal death
- Multiparous women with a history of precipitous labor or who live far from the hospital

The management of stimulation of labor is the same regardless of the indication. Because of the potential dangers associated with the injection of oxytocin in the prenatal and intrapartal periods, the FDA has issued certain restrictions to its use.

Contraindications to oxytocin stimulation of labor include, but are not limited to, the following:
- CPD, prolapsed cord, transverse lie
- Nonreassuring fetal status
- Placenta previa or vasa previa
- Prior classic uterine incision or uterine surgery
- Active genital herpes infection

Certain maternal and fetal conditions, although not contraindications to the use of oxytocin to stimulate labor, do require special caution during its administration. These conditions include the following:
- Multifetal presentation
- Breech presentation
- Presenting part above the pelvic inlet
- Abnormal fetal heart pattern not requiring emergency birth
- Polyhydramnios
- Grand multiparity
- Maternal cardiac disease; hypertension

Oxytocin use can present hazards to the mother and fetus. These hazards are primarily dose related, with most problems caused by high doses that are given rapidly. Maternal hazards include water intoxication and tumultuous labor with tetanic contractions, which may cause premature separation of the placenta, rupture of the uterus, lacerations of the cervix, or postpartum hemorrhage. These complications can lead to infection, disseminated intravascular coagulation, or amniotic fluid embolism. Women may become anxious or fearful if the induction is not successful because they may then have concerns about the method of birth.

Uterine hyperstimulation reduces the blood flow through the placenta and results in FHR decelerations (bradycardia, diminished variability, late decelerations), fetal asphyxia, and neonatal hypoxia. If the estimated date of birth is inaccurate, physical injury, neonatal hyperbilirubinemia, and prematurity are other hazards.

The primary health care provider orders induction or augmentation of labor with oxytocin. The nurse implements the order by initiating the primary intravenous infusion and administering the oxytocin solution through a secondary line. The nurse's actions related to assessment and care of a woman whose labor is being induced are guided by hos-

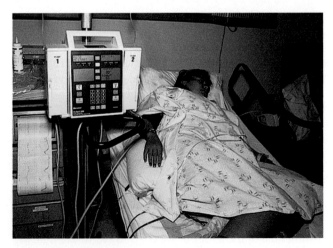

Fig. 24-7 Woman in side-lying position receiving oxytocin. (Courtesy Michael S. Clement, MD, Mesa, AZ.)

pital protocol and professional standards (Fig. 24-7; Box 24-8).

A commonly recommended initial dosage is 0.5 to 1 milliunits/min with increments of 1 or 2 milliunits/min every 30 to 60 minutes because 30 to 40 minutes is required for a steady state of oxytocin to be reached and for the full effect of a dosage increment to be reflected in more intense, frequent, and longer contractions (Simpson & Atterbury, 2003). Such an approach reduces the amount of oxytocin required to achieve a spontaneous vaginal birth and decreases the risk for uterine hyperstimulation, dysfunctional labor, fetal distress, and other adverse reactions such as water intoxication (Norwitz, Robinson, & Repke, 2002; Simpson, 2002).

Nursing considerations. An evidence-based written protocol for the preparation and administration of oxytocin should be established by the obstetric department (physicians, nurses) in each institution (see Box 24-8).

NURSE ALERT *Oxytocin is discontinued immediately and the primary health care provider notified if uterine hyperstimulation, nonreassuring FHR and pattern, or both occur.*

Other nursing interventions, such as administering oxygen by face mask, positioning the woman on her side, and infusing more intravenous fluids are implemented immediately (Emergency box). Based on the status of the

---

BOX 24-8

Protocol: Induction of Labor with Oxytocin

PATIENT AND FAMILY TEACHING

Explain technique, rationale, and reactions to expect:

- Route and rate for administration of medication
- What "piggyback" (Secondary intravenous line inserted into primary intravenous line) is for
- Reasons for use:
  - Induce labor, improve labor
- Reactions to expect concerning the nature of contractions: the intensity of contraction increases more rapidly, holds the peak longer, and ends more quickly; contractions will come regularly and more often
- Monitoring to anticipate:
  - Maternal: blood pressure, pulse, uterine contractions, uterine tone
  - Fetal: heart rate, activity
- Success to expect: a favorable outcome will depend on inducibility of the cervix (e.g., Bishop score of 9 for a primipara)
- Keep woman and support person informed of progress

ADMINISTRATION

Position woman in side-lying or upright position
Assess status of maternal fetal unit
Prepare solutions and administer with pump delivery system according to prescribed orders:

- Infusion pump and solution are set up (e.g., 10 units/1000 ml isotonic electrolyte solution)
- Piggyback solution is connected to IV line at proximal port (port nearest point of venous insertion)
- Solution with oxytocin is flagged with a medication label
- Begin induction at 0.5 to 2 milliunits/min
- Increase dose 1 to 2 milliunits/min at intervals of 15 to 60 minutes until a dose of up to 20 to 40 milliunits/min is reached

MAINTAIN DOSE IF

- Intensity of contractions results in intrauterine pressures of 40 to 90 mm Hg (shown by internal monitor)
- Duration of contractions is 40 to 90 seconds
- Frequency of contractions is 2- to 3-minute intervals
- Cervical dilation of 1 cm/hr occurs in the active phase

MATERNAL AND FETAL ASSESSMENTS

- Monitor blood pressure, pulse, and respirations every 30 to 60 minutes and with every increment in dose
- Monitor contraction pattern and uterine resting tone every 15 minutes and with every increment in dose
- Assess intake and output; limit IV intake to 1000 ml/8 hr; output should be 120 ml or more every 4 hours
- Perform vaginal examination as indicated
- Monitor for nausea, vomiting, headache, hypotension
- Assess fetal status using electronic fetal monitoring; evaluate tracing every 15 minutes and with every increment in dose
- Observe emotional responses of woman and her partner

REPORTABLE CONDITIONS

- Uterine hyperstimulation
- Nonreassuring FHR pattern
- Suspected uterine rupture
- Inadequate uterine response at 20 milliunits/min

EMERGENCY MEASURES

Discontinue use of oxytocin per hospital protocol:

- Turn woman on her side
- Increase primary IV rate up to 200 ml/hr, unless patient has water intoxication, in which case, the rate is decreased to one that keeps the vein open
- Give woman oxygen by face mask at 8 to 10 L/min or per protocol or physician's or nurse-midwife's order

DOCUMENTATION

- Medication: kind, amount, time of beginning, increasing dose, maintaining dose, and discontinuing medication in patient record and on monitor strip
- Reactions of mother and fetus
  - Pattern of labor
  - Progress of labor
  - FHR and pattern
  - Maternal vital signs
  - Nursing interventions and woman's response
- Notification of physician or nurse-midwife

From Ruchata, P., Metheby, N., Essenpreis, H., & Borcherding, K. (2002). Current practices in oxytocin dilution land fluid administration for induction of labor. *Journal of Obstetric, Gynecologic, and Neonatal Nursing, 31*(5), 545-550; Simpson, K. (2002). *Cervical ripening and induction and augmentation of labor* (2nd ed.). Washington, DC: AWHONN.
FHR, Fetal heart rate; *IV,* intravenous.

EMERGENCY

Uterine Hyperstimulation with Oxytocin

SIGNS
- Uterine contractions lasting more than 90 seconds and occurring more frequently than every 2 minutes
- Uterine resting tone greater than 20 mm Hg
- Nonreassuring FHR:
  - —Abnormal baseline ($<$110 or $>$160 beats/min)
  - —Absent variability
  - —Repeated late decelerations or prolonged decelerations

INTERVENTIONS
- Maintain woman in side-lying position.
- Turn off oxytocin infusion; keep maintenance IV line open; increase rate.
- Start administering oxygen by face mask, per protocol or physician's order.
- Notify primary health care provider.
- Prepare to administer terbutaline (Brethine) 0.25 mg subcutaneously if ordered to decrease uterine activity.
- Continue monitoring FHR and uterine activity.
- Document responses to actions.

FHR, Fetal heart rate; *IV,* intravenous.

maternal-fetal unit, the primary health care provider may order that the infusion be restarted once the FHR and uterine activity return to acceptable levels. Depending on the length of time the infusion was discontinued, the induction may be restarted at half the rate that resulted in hyperstimulation (e.g., discontinued for 10 to 20 minutes) or at the same rate as the initial rate (e.g., discontinued for more than 30 to 40 minutes) (Simpson, 2002) (Plan of Care: Dysfunctional Labor).

Augmentation of labor

Augmentation of labor is the stimulation of uterine contractions after labor has started spontaneously but progress is unsatisfactory. Augmentation is usually implemented for the management of hypotonic uterine dysfunction, resulting in a slowing of the labor process (protracted active phase). Common augmentation methods include oxytocin infusion, amniotomy, and nipple stimulation. Noninvasive methods such as emptying the bladder, ambulation and position changes, relaxation measures, nourishment and hydration, and hydrotherapy should be attempted before invasive interventions are initiated. The administration procedure and nursing assessment and care measures for augmentation of labor with oxytocin are similar to those used for induction of labor with oxytocin; protocols for dosage and frequency of increments may vary (e.g., lower dosages may be needed to achieve spontaneous vaginal birth (Gilbert & Harmon, 2003; Simpson, 2002).

Some physicians advocate *active management of labor,* that is, the augmentation of labor to establish efficient labor with the aggressive use of oxytocin so that the woman gives birth within 12 hours of admission to the labor unit. Advocates of active management believe that intervening early (as soon as a nulliparous labor is not progressing at least 1 cm/hr) with use of higher pharmacologic oxytocin doses administered at frequent increment intervals (e.g., a starting dose of 6 milliunits/min with increases of 6 milliunits/min every 15 minutes to a maximum dose of 40 milliunits/min) shortens labor and is associated with a lower incidence of cesarean birth (Norwitz, Robinson, & Repke, 2002; Simpson, 2002).

Additional components of the active management of labor include strict criteria to diagnose that the woman is in active labor with 100% effacement, amniotomy within 1 hour of admission of a woman in labor if spontaneous rupture of the membranes has not occurred, and continuous presence of a personal nurse who provides one-on-one care for the woman while she is in labor. When all components are fully implemented, active management of labor is associated with a lower incidence of cesarean birth. Active management of labor continues to be under study in the United States to determine effectiveness and impact on perinatal morbidity and mortality. Thus far, results have been disappointing, especially in terms of reducing the rate of cesarean births. The disappointing results have been attributed in part to a greater than one-to-one nurse-patient ratio and the high rate of epidural anesthesia. It is considered to be a form of care of unknown effectiveness (Enkin et al., 2000; Gilbert & Harmon, 2003).

Forceps-assisted birth

A **forceps-assisted birth** is one in which an instrument with two curved blades is used to assist in the birth of the fetal head. The cephalic-like curve of the forceps commonly used is similar to the shape of the fetal head, with a pelvic curve to the blades conforming to the curve of the pelvic axis. The blades are joined by a pin, screw, or groove arrangement. These locks prevent the forceps from compressing the fetal skull. Maternal indications for forceps-assisted birth include the need to shorten the second stage of labor in the event of dystocia or to compensate for the woman's deficient expulsive efforts (e.g., if she is tired or has been given spinal or epidural anesthesia), or to reverse a dangerous condition (e.g., cardiac decompensation).

Fetal indications include birth of a fetus in distress or in certain abnormal presentations; arrest of rotation; or delivery of the head in a breech presentation. The use of forceps during childbirth has been decreasing. In 2002, forceps or vacuum were used to assist 5.9% of births (Martin et al., 2003).

Certain conditions are required for a forceps-assisted birth to be successful. The woman's cervix must be fully dilated to avert lacerations and hemorrhage. The bladder should be empty. The presenting part must be engaged, and a vertex presentation is desired. Membranes must be ruptured so that the position of the fetal head can be determined and the forceps can firmly grasp the head during birth (Fig. 24-8). In addition, CPD should not be present.

Nursing considerations. When a forceps-assisted birth is deemed necessary, the nurse obtains the type

PLAN OF CARE *Dysfunctional Labor: Hypotonic Uterine Dysfunction with Protracted Active Phase*

NURSING DIAGNOSIS Risk for injury to mother and/or fetus related to oxytocin augmentation secondary to dysfunctional labor
Expected Outcomes *Maternal-fetal well-being is maintained; labor progresses and birth occurs.*
Nursing Interventions/*Rationales*

- Explain oxytocin protocol to woman and her labor partner *to allay apprehension and enhance participation.*
- Encourage woman to void before beginning protocol *to prevent discomfort and remove a barrier to labor progress.*
- Apply the electronic fetal monitor per hospital protocol and obtain a 15- to 20-min baseline strip *to ensure adequate assessment of FHR and contractions.*
- Position woman in a side-lying position and administer the oxytocin per physician order using an IV infusion pump *to stimulate uterine activity and provide adequate control of the flow rate.*
- Regulate the oxytocin per protocol (e.g., advancing the dose in increments of 1 to 2 milliunits/min every 30 to 60 min) *to allow adequate evaluation of the woman's response to stimulation and to prevent hyperstimulation and fetal hypoxia.*
- Maintain oxytocin dose and rate when contractions occur every 2 to 3 min with a duration of 40 to 90 sec and intrauterine pressures of 60 to 90 mm Hg (if internal monitoring is used) *to produce effective uterine stimulation without risk of hyperstimulation.*
- Monitor maternal vital signs every 30 to 60 min *to assess for oxytocin-induced hypertension.*
- Monitor contractility pattern and FHR and pattern every 15 min *to assess uterine activity for possible hypertonicity or ineffective uterine response to oxytocin and to detect evidence of fetal distress.*
- Monitor intake, output, and specific gravity (limit intake to 1000 ml/8 hr; output should be at least 120 ml/4 hr) *to assess for urinary retention and prevent water intoxication.*
- Monitor cervical dilation, effacement, and station *to assess progress of labor.*
- If hypertonicity or signs of fetal distress are detected, discontinue oxytocin immediately *to arrest the progress of hypertonicity;* turn woman on her side *to increase placental blood flow;* increase primary IV rate to 200 ml/hr (unless signs of water toxicity are present); administer oxygen via face mask *to enhance placental perfusion;* notify primary health care provider; and continuously monitor maternal vital signs and FHR *to provide ongoing assessment of maternal and fetal status.*

- Maintain Standard Precautions and use scrupulous handwashing techniques when providing care *to prevent the spread of infection.*

NURSING DIAGNOSIS Acute pain related to increasing frequency, regularity, intensity, and prolonged peak of contractions
Expected Outcome *The woman exhibits signs of decreased discomfort.*
Nursing Interventions/*Rationales*

- Prepare woman and labor partner for the change in the nature of the contractions once the oxytocin drip is initiated *to prepare them and allow for more effective coping.*
- Review the use of specific techniques such as conscious relaxation, focused breathing, effleurage, massage, and application of sacral pressure *to increase relaxation, decrease intensity of pain of contractions, and promote use of controlled thought and direction of energy.*
- Provide comfort measures such as frequent mouth care *to prevent dry mouth,* application of damp cloth to forehead and changing of damp gown or bed covers *to relieve discomfort of diaphoresis,* and changing of position *to reduce stiffness.*
- Encourage conscious relaxation between contractions *to prevent fatigue, which contributes to increased pain perceptions.*
- Remind woman and labor partner that analgesics are available for use during labor *to provide knowledge to help them make decisions about pain control.*

NURSING DIAGNOSIS Anxiety related to prolonged labor, increased pain, and fatigue
Expected Outcomes *Woman's anxiety is reduced; woman actively participates in the labor process.*
Nursing Interventions/*Rationales*

- Provide ongoing feedback to woman and partner *to allay anxiety and enhance participation.*
- Present care options when possible *to increase feelings of control.*
- Continue to provide comfort measures *to maintain a posture of support and caring and to aid woman in focusing on the labor process.*
- Encourage woman and partner to continue to use those mechanisms that promote effective labor (e.g., breathing, activity, positioning) *to keep woman and partner actively involved in process.*

FHR, Fetal heart rate; *IV,* intravenous.

of forceps requested by the primary health care provider. The nurse may explain to the mother that the forceps blades fit like two tablespoons around an egg, with the blades placed in front of the baby's ears. The nurse usually coaches the woman not to push during contractions unless the primary health care provider instructs the woman to push as traction is being applied during contractions.

NURSE ALERT *Because compression of the cord between the fetal head and the forceps will cause a decrease in FHR, the FHR and pattern are assessed, re-* *ported, and recorded before and after application of the forceps.*

If a decrease in FHR occurs, the primary health care provider removes and reapplies the forceps. After birth the mother is assessed for vaginal and cervical lacerations (e.g., bleeding that occurs even with a contracted uterus); urine retention, which may result from bladder or urethral injuries; and hematoma formation in the pelvic soft tissues, which may result from blood vessel damage. The infant should be assessed for bruising or abrasions at the site of the blade applications, facial palsy resulting from pressure of the blades

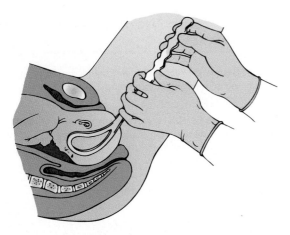

Fig. 24-8 Outlet forceps-assisted extraction of the head.

on the facial nerve (cranial nerve VII), and subdural hematoma. Newborn and postpartum caregivers should be told that a forceps-assisted birth was performed.

Vacuum-assisted birth

Vacuum-assisted birth, or vacuum extraction, is a birth method involving the attachment of a vacuum cup to the fetal head, using negative pressure to assist in the birth of the head. Indications and prerequisites for its use are similar to those for outlet forceps. It is usually not used to assist birth before 34 weeks of gestation (Cunningham et al., 2005). When an operative vaginal birth is required, vacuum ✳ assistance is preferred as a beneficial form of care when compared with forceps assistance (Enkin et al., 2000).

When the birth is to be vacuum assisted, the woman is prepared for a vaginal birth in the lithotomy position to allow sufficient traction. The cup is applied to the fetal head, and a caput develops inside the cup as the pressure is initiated (Fig. 24-9). Traction is applied to facilitate descent of the fetal head, and the woman is encouraged to push as suction is applied. As the head crowns, an episiotomy is performed if necessary. The vacuum cup is released and re-

moved after birth of the head. If vacuum extraction is not successful, a or cesarean birth is usually performed.

Risks to the newborn include cephalhematoma, scalp lacerations, and subdural hematoma. Fetal complications can be reduced by strict adherence to the manufacturer's recommendations for method of application, degree of suction, and duration of application. Maternal complications are uncommon but can include perineal, vaginal, or cervical lacerations and soft-tissue hematomas.

Nursing considerations. The nurse's role for the woman who has a vacuum-assisted birth is one of support person and educator. The nurse can prepare the woman for birth and encourage her to remain active in the birth process by pushing during contractions. The FHR should be assessed frequently during the procedure. After birth, the newborn should be observed for signs of trauma and infection at the application site and for cerebral irritation (e.g., poor sucking or listlessness). The newborn may be at risk for neonatal jaundice as bruising resolves. The parents may need to be reassured that the caput succedaneum will begin to disappear in a few hours. Neonatal caregivers should be told that the birth was vacuum assisted.

Cesarean birth

Cesarean birth is the birth of a fetus through a transabdominal incision in the uterus. Whether cesarean birth is planned (scheduled) or unplanned (emergency), the loss of the experience of giving birth to a child in the traditional manner may have a negative effect on a woman's self-concept. An effort is therefore made to maintain the focus on the birth of a child rather than on the operative procedure.

The purpose of cesarean birth is to preserve the life or health of the mother and her fetus; it may be the best choice for birth when there is evidence of maternal or fetal complications. Since the advent of modern surgical methods and care and the use of antibiotics, maternal and fetal morbidity and mortality have decreased. In addition, incisions are made in the lower uterine segment rather than in the muscular body of the uterus and thus more effective healing

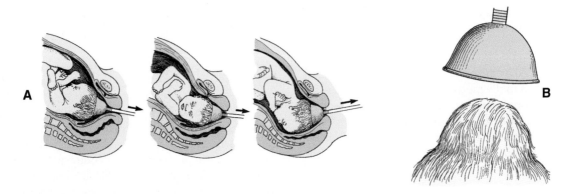

Fig. 24-9 Use of vacuum extraction to rotate fetal head and assist with descent. **A,** Arrow indicates direction of traction on the vacuum cup. **B,** Caput succedaneum formed by the vacuum cup.

is promoted. However, despite these advances, cesarean birth still poses threats to the health of the mother and infant.

The incidence of cesarean births increased to 27.6% in 2003, the highest rate ever reported in the United States, with the primary cesarean birth rate at 19.1% (Hamilton et al., 2004). In Canada the rate was 22.1% in 2001 (Liu et al., 2004). Factors cited in this increase include use of electronic fetal monitoring and epidural anesthesia; an increase in the number of first-time pregnancies, as well as the number of pregnancies at an older age; and the decline in the rate of vaginal birth after cesarean (VBAC) (10.6% in 2003 in the United States; 28.5% in 2001 in Canada) (Hamilton et al., 2004; Liu et al., 2004). Women 35 to 39 years of age have a cesarean birth rate of 35%, and those 40 to 54 years of age have a rate of 40.7%, over twice the rate for teenage women (18%) (Martin et al., 2003).

Women who have private insurance, who are of a higher socioeconomic status, or who give birth in a private hospital are more likely to experience cesarean birth than are women who are poor, who have no insurance, who are receiving public assistance (e.g., Medicaid), or who give birth in a public hospital (Gilbert & Harmon, 2003; Moore, 2003).

Approaches for the management of labor and birth to reduce the rate of cesarean births while increasing the rate of VBAC are presented in Box 24-9. However, the rate of VBAC is decreasing. This decline may be a result of reports of risks of VBAC, legal pressures, conservative practice guidelines, and debate regarding the relative benefits and risks of the cesarean versus the vaginal route for births (Martin et al., 2003).

The type of nursing care given also may influence the rate of cesarean births. A labor management approach that uses one-to-one support and emphasizes ambulation, maternal position changes, relaxation measures, oral fluids and nutrition, hydrotherapy, and nonpharmacologic pain relief facilitates the progress of labor and reduces the incidence of dystocia (AWHONN, 2000; Hodnett, 2002; Miltner, 2002).

The labor management approach that most consistently reduced cesarean birth rates was one-to-one support of the laboring woman by another woman such as a nurse, nurse-midwife, or doula (Hodnett, Gates, Hofmeyr, & Sakala, 2003; Hodnett et al., 2002).

Indications. Few absolute indications exist for cesarean birth. Today most are performed primarily for the benefit of the fetus. The most common indications for cesarean birth are related to labor and birth complications. The complications most closely associated with cesarean birth include CPD, malpresentations such as breech and shoulder, placental abnormalities (e.g., previa, abruptio), dysfunctional

---

BOX 24-9

Selected Measures to Reduce Cesarean Birth Rate and Increase Rate of Vaginal Birth after Cesarean

EDUCATE WOMEN REGARDING
- Advantages and safety of the home environment for early or latent labor
- Indicators for hospital admission
- Management techniques to use during labor to enhance progress
- Nonpharmacologic measures to reduce pain and discomfort and enhance relaxation
- Safety and effectiveness of TOL and VBAC

ESTABLISH ADMISSION CRITERIA FOR WOMEN IN LABOR
- Distinguish clinical manifestations for false labor, latent or early labor, and active labor
- Conduct admission assessments in a separate admissions area
- Send women in false or early or latent labor home or keep them in the admissions area
- Admit women in active labor to the labor and birth unit

USE APPROPRIATE ASSESSMENT TECHNIQUES TO
- Determine status of the maternal-fetal unit
- Establish an individualized rationale for initiating labor interventions such as epidural anesthesia, induction or augmentation, amniotomy, cesarean birth

INITIATE A DOULA PROGRAM THAT
- Provides one-to-one support for women in labor

DEVELOP A PHILOSOPHY OF LABOR MANAGEMENT THAT
- Schedules admission during active labor
- Avoids automatic interventions such as routine induction for spontaneous rupture of membranes at term or post-term pregnancy and cesarean birth for breech presentation, twin gestation, genital herpes, or failure to progress
- Relies on assessment findings reflective of the status of the maternal-fetal unit rather than strict adherence to set ranges for the duration of the stages and phases of labor
- Employs intermittent rather than continuous electronic fetal monitoring of low risk pregnant women
- Focuses on measures that are known to enhance the progress of labor such as upright positions, frequent position changes, ambulation, oral nutrition and hydration, relaxation techniques, hydrotherapy
- Emphasizes nonpharmacologic measures to relieve pain
- Uses nonpharmacologic measures in a manner that reduces their labor-inhibiting effects
- Establishes criteria for elective cesarean birth and TOL
- Encourages women who have had a previous cesarean birth to participate in TOL to attempt a vaginal birth

TOL, Trial of labor; *VBAC*, vaginal birth after cesarean.

labor pattern, umbilical cord prolapse, fetal distress, and multiple gestation (see Evidence-Based Practice Box) on p. 787. Medical risk factors most closely associated with cesarean birth include hypertensive disorders, active genital herpes, positive HIV status, and diabetes (Martin et al., 2003).

Elective cesarean birth. Women are requesting cesarean births for reasons other than medical, obstetric, or fetal indications. These reasons include the belief that the surgery will prevent future problems with pelvic support or sexual dysfunction and the convenience of planning a date or having control and choice about when to give birth (Williams, 2005). Some multiparous women may request a cesarean after a previous traumatic vaginal birth or psychologic trauma (Gardner, 2003). In a committee opinion ACOG notes that the right of patients to refuse surgery is well known (ACOG, 2003). It is less clear if they have the right to ask for surgery. The Society of Obstetricians and Gynaecologists of Canada (SOGC) promotes natural childbirth, does not promote elective cesarean birth but believes that the final decision as to the safest route for childbirth rests with the woman and her health care provider (SOGC, 2004). It is essential that women are fully informed about the risks and benefits of cesarean birth when they consider the request for elective cesarean (McFarlin, 2004).

Forced cesarean birth. A woman's refusal to undergo cesarean birth when indicated for fetal reasons is often described as a *maternal-fetal conflict.* Health care providers are ethically obliged to protect the well-being of both the mother and the fetus; a decision for one affects the other. If a woman refuses a cesarean birth that is recommended because of fetal jeopardy, health care providers must make every effort to find out why she is refusing and provide information that may persuade her to change her mind. If the woman continues to refuse surgery, then health care providers must decide if it is ethical to get a court order for the surgery; however, every effort should be made to avoid this legal step.

Surgical techniques. The two main types of cesarean operation are the classic and the lower-segment cesarean incisions. Classic cesarean birth is rarely performed today, although it may be used when rapid birth is necessary and in some cases of shoulder presentation and placenta previa. The incision is made vertically into the upper body of the uterus (Fig. 24-10, *A*). Because the procedure is associated with a higher incidence of blood loss, infection, and uterine rupture in subsequent pregnancies than is lower-segment cesarean birth, vaginal birth after a classic cesarean birth is contraindicated.

Lower-segment cesarean birth can be achieved through a vertical or transverse incision into the uterus (Fig. 24-10, *B* and *C*). The transverse incision is more popular, however, because it is easier to perform, is associated with less blood loss and fewer postoperative infections, and is less likely to rupture in subsequent pregnancies (Bowes & Thorp, 2004).

Complications and risks. Maternal complications of cesarean births include aspiration, pulmonary

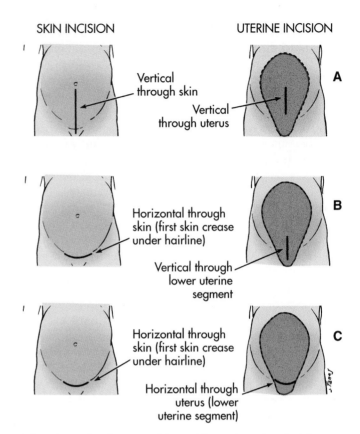

SKIN INCISION   UTERINE INCISION

Vertical through skin
Vertical through uterus   **A**

Horizontal through skin (first skin crease under hairline)
Vertical through lower uterine segment   **B**

Horizontal through skin (first skin crease under hairline)
Horizontal through uterus (lower uterine segment)   **C**

Fig. 24-10 Cesarean birth; skin and uterine incisions. **A,** Classic: vertical incisions of skin and uterus. **B,** Low cervical: horizontal incision of skin; vertical incision of uterus. **C,** Low cervical: horizontal incisions of skin and uterus.

embolism, wound infection, wound dehiscence, thrombophlebitis, hemorrhage, urinary tract infection, injuries to the bladder or bowel, and complications related to anesthesia. The fetus may be born prematurely if the gestational age has not been accurately determined; fetal injuries can occur during the surgery (Bowes & Thorp, 2004). Besides these risks, the woman is at economic risk because the cost of cesarean birth is higher than that of vaginal birth, and a longer recovery period may require additional expenditures.

Many women who have a cesarean birth speak of having feelings that interfere with their maintaining an adequate self-concept. These feelings include fear, disappointment, frustration at losing control, anger (the "why me" syndrome), and loss of self-esteem related to a change in body image and perceived inability to give birth as they had expected and hoped. Often women experience a delay in their ability to interact with their newborns after birth. These women are less likely to breastfeed and may even have some difficulty expressing positive feelings about their newborns for some time after birth. They are often less satisfied with their childbirth experience and report more fatigue and poor physical functioning during the first few weeks after discharge. Success at mothering and in the recovery process can do much to restore the self-esteem of these women. Some women see the scar as mutilating, and worries concerning sexual attractiveness may surface. Some men are fearful of resuming intercourse because of the fear of hurting their partners. Parents may wonder if a cesarean birth was absolutely necessary, and such feelings may surface even years later. They should therefore be given opportunities to discuss the experience to try to understand and resolve concerns after the birth.

Anesthesia. Spinal, epidural, and general anesthetics are used for cesarean births. Epidural blocks are popular because women want to be awake for and aware of the birth experience. However, the choice of anesthetic depends on several factors. The mother's medical history or present condition, such as a spinal injury, hemorrhage, or coagulopathy, may rule out the use of regional anesthesia. Time is another factor, especially if there is an emergency and the life of the mother or infant is at stake. In such a case, general anesthesia will most likely be used unless the woman already has an epidural block in effect. The woman herself is a factor. Either she may not know all the options or may have fears about having "a needle in her back" or about being awake and feeling pain. She needs to be fully informed about the risks and benefits of the different types of anesthesia so that she can participate in the decision whenever there is a choice.

Scheduled cesarean birth. Cesarean birth is scheduled or planned if labor and vaginal birth are contraindicated (e.g., complete placenta previa, active genital herpes, positive HIV status), if birth is necessary but labor is not inducible (e.g., hypertensive states that cause a poor intrauterine environment that threatens the fetus), or if this has been decided on by the primary health care provider and the woman (e.g., a repeat cesarean birth).

Women who are scheduled to have a cesarean birth have time to prepare for it psychologically. However, the psychologic responses of these women may differ. Those having a repeat cesarean birth may have disturbing memories of the conditions preceding the initial surgical birth (primary cesarean birth) and of their experiences in the postoperative recovery period. They may be concerned about the added burdens of caring for an infant and perhaps other children while recovering from a surgical operation. Others may feel glad that they have been relieved of the uncertainty about the date and time of the birth and are free of the pain of labor.

Unplanned cesarean birth. The psychosocial outcomes of unplanned or emergency cesarean birth are usually more pronounced and negative when compared with the outcomes associated with a scheduled or planned cesarean birth. Women and their families experience abrupt changes in their expectations for birth, postbirth care, and the care of the new baby at home. This may be an extremely traumatic experience for all.

The woman usually approaches the procedure tired and discouraged after an ineffective and difficult labor. Fear predominates as she worries about her own safety and well-being and that of her fetus. She may be dehydrated, with low

glycogen reserves. Because preoperative procedures must be done quickly and competently, the time for explanation of the procedures and operation is often short. Because maternal and family anxiety levels are high at this time, much of what is said may be forgotten or misunderstood. The woman may experience feelings of anger or guilt in the postpartum period. Fatigue is often noticeable in these women, and they need much supportive care.

After surgery, counseling strategies that have been implemented by nurses include providing women with opportunities to talk about their birth experience, express their feelings about what happened, have their questions answered, address gaps in knowledge or understanding of events, connect the event with emotions and behavior, and talk about future pregnancies. More research is needed to determine how effective these strategies are for these women in influencing their views about the unplanned cesarean birth experience or about future pregnancies (Gamble & Creedy, 2004).

Prenatal preparation. Concerned professional and lay groups in the community have established councils for cesarean birth to meet the needs of these women and their families. Such groups advocate that a discussion of cesarean birth be included in all parenthood preparation classes. No woman can be guaranteed a vaginal birth, even if she is in good health and there is no indication of danger to the fetus before the onset of labor. For this reason, every woman needs to be aware of and prepared for this eventuality.

Childbirth educators stress the importance of emphasizing the similarities and differences between a cesarean and a vaginal birth. In support of the philosophy of family-centered birth, many hospitals have instituted policies that permit fathers and other partners and family members to share in these births as they do in vaginal ones. Women who have undergone cesarean birth agree that the continued presence and support of their partners helped them respond positively to the entire experience. In addition to preparing women for the possibility of cesarean birth, childbirth educators should empower women to believe in their ability to give birth vaginally and to seek care measures during labor that will enhance the progress of their labors and reduce their risk for cesarean birth.

Preoperative care. Family-centered care is the goal for the woman who is to undergo cesarean birth and for her family. The preparation of the woman for cesarean birth is the same as that done for other elective or emergency surgery. The primary health care provider discusses, with the woman and her family, the need for the cesarean birth and the prognosis for the mother and infant. The anesthesiologist assesses the woman's cardiopulmonary system and describes the options for anesthesia. Informed consent is obtained for the procedure (Guidelines/Guías: Cesarean Birth).

Blood and urine tests are usually done a day or two before a planned cesarean birth or on admission to the labor and birth unit. Laboratory tests, most commonly ordered to establish baseline data, include a complete blood cell count and

GUIDELINES/GUÍAS

Cesarean Birth—Informed Consent

- You need a cesarean.
- *Necesita una operación cesárea.*

- Has your doctor discussed with you the reason for needing a cesarean?
- *¿Ha hablado el doctor con usted sobre la necesidad de tener una operación cesárea?*

- Do you understand why you need a cesarean?
- *¿Entiende usted por qué necesita una operación cesárea?*

- Your signature on this form will allow us to proceed with the surgery.
- *Su firma en este formulario nos permitirá seguir adelante con la operación.*

- Please sign this consent form.
- *Por favor, firme este formulario de autorización.*

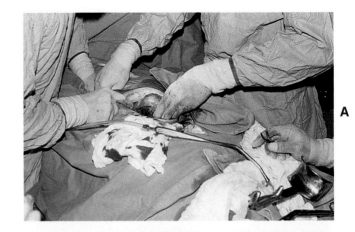

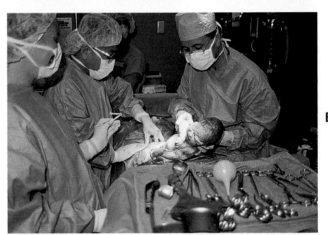

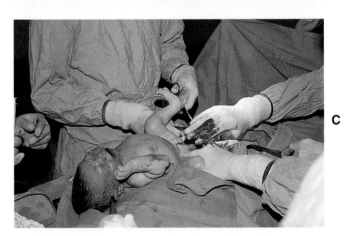

chemistry, blood typing and crossmatching, and urinalysis. Maternal vital signs and blood pressure and FHR and pattern continue to be assessed per the hospital routine until the operation begins. Physical preoperative preparation usually includes inserting a retention catheter to keep the bladder empty and administering prescribed preoperative medications. An abdominal-mons shave or a clipping of pubic hair may be ordered by the primary health care provider. In the event that general anesthesia will be used, an antacid, administered orally to neutralize gastric secretions in case of aspiration, is a beneficial form of care (Enkin et al., 2000). Intravenous fluids are started to maintain hydration and to provide an open line for the administration of blood or medications if needed.

Removal of dentures, nail polish, and jewelry may be optional, depending on hospital policies and type of anesthesia used. If the woman wears glasses and is going to be awake, the nurse should make sure her glasses accompany her to the operating room so she can see her infant. If the woman wears contact lenses, the nurse can find out whether they can be worn for the birth.

During the preoperative preparation, the support person is encouraged to remain with the woman as much as possible to provide continuing emotional support (if this action is culturally acceptable to the woman and support person). The nurse provides essential information about the preoperative procedures during this time. Although the nursing actions may be carried out quickly if a cesarean birth is unplanned, verbal communication, particularly explanation, is important. Silence can be frightening to the woman and her support person. The nurse's use of touch can communicate feelings of care and concern for the woman. The nurse can assess the woman's and her partner's perceptions about cesarean birth (e.g., the woman feels that she is a failure because she did not have a vaginal birth). As the woman expresses her feelings, the nurse may identify a potential for

Fig. 24-11 Cesarean birth. **A,** "Bikini" incision has been made, the muscle layer is separated, the abdomen is entered, and the uterus has been exposed and incised; suctioning of amniotic fluid continues as head is brought up through the incision. Note small amount of bleeding. **B,** The neonate's birth through the uterine incision is nearly complete. **C,** A quick assessment is performed; note extreme molding of head resulting from cephalopelvic disproportion. (Courtesy Marjorie Pyle, RNC, Lifecircle, Costa Mesa, CA.)

a disturbance in self-concept during the postpartum period that may need to be addressed. If there is time before the birth, the nurse can teach the woman about postoperative expectations and about pain relief, turning, coughing, and deep-breathing measures.

Intraoperative care. Cesarean births occur in operating rooms in the surgical suite or in the labor and birth unit. Once the woman has been taken to the operating room, her care becomes the responsibility of the obstetric team, surgeon, anesthesiologist, pediatrician, and surgical nursing staff (Fig. 24-11). If possible, the partner, who is dressed appropriately for the operating room, accompanies the mother to the operating room and remains close to her so that continued support and comfort can be provided.

The nurse who is circulating may assist with positioning the woman on the birth (surgical) table. It is important to position her so that the uterus is displaced laterally to prevent compression of the inferior vena cava, which causes decreased placental perfusion. This is usually accomplished by placing a wedge under the hip. A Foley catheter is inserted into the bladder at this time if one is not already in place.

If the partner is not allowed or chooses not to be present, the nurse can stay in communication with him or her and give progress reports whenever possible. If the woman is awake during the birth, the nurse, anesthesiologist, or both can tell her what is happening and provide support. She may be anxious about the sensations she is experiencing, such as the coldness of solutions used to prepare the abdomen and pressure or pulling during the actual birth of the infant. She also may be apprehensive because of the bright lights or the presence of unfamiliar equipment and masked and gowned personnel in the room. Explanations by the nurse can help to decrease the woman's anxiety.

Care of the infant usually is delegated to a pediatrician or a nurse team skilled in neonatal resuscitation, because these infants are considered to be at risk until there is evidence of physiologic stability after the birth.

A crib with resuscitation equipment is readied before surgery. Those responsible for care are expert not only in resuscitative techniques but also in their ability to detect normal and abnormal infant responses. After birth, if the infant's condition permits and the mother is awake, the baby may be placed skin-to-skin on the mother or can be given to the woman's partner to hold (Fig. 24-12). The infant whose condition is compromised is transported after initial stabilization to the nursery for observation and the implementation of appropriate interventions. In some institutions, the partner may accompany the infant; if not, personnel keep the family informed of the infant's progress, and parent-infant contacts are initiated as soon as possible.

If the family cannot accompany the woman during surgery, the family is directed to the surgical or obstetric waiting room. The physician then reports on the condition of the mother and child to the family members after the birth is completed. Family members may accompany the infant as she or he is transferred to the nursery, giving them an opportunity to see and admire the new baby.

> **LEGAL TIP** **Discosure of Patient Information**
>
> *Some mothers or fathers want the privilege of informing family and friends of the sex of the infant (if it was not known before birth) or other information about the birth. Before responding to requests for such information from people waiting outside the birthing area, the nurse should check to see if the mother has given consent for such information to be released.*

Immediate postoperative care. Once surgery is completed, the mother is transferred to a recovery room or back to her labor room. After a cesarean birth, women have both postoperative and postpartum needs that must be

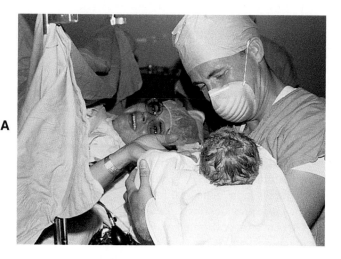
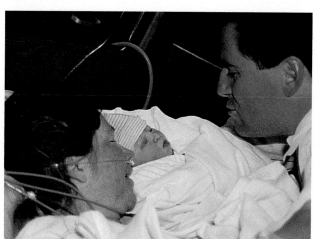

Fig. 24-12 **A,** Parents and their newborn. The physician manually removes the placenta, suctions the remaining amniotic fluid and blood from the uterine cavity, and closes the uterine incision, peritoneum, muscle layer, fatty tissue, and finally the skin, while the new family shares some time together. **B,** Parents become better acquainted with their newborn while mother rests after surgery. (Courtesy Marjorie Pyle, RNC, Lifecircle, Costa Mesa, CA.)

addressed. They are surgical patients as well as new mothers. Nursing assessments in this immediate postbirth period follow agency protocol and include degree of recovery from the effects of anesthesia, postoperative and postbirth status, and degree of pain. A patent airway is maintained, and the woman is positioned to prevent possible aspiration. Vital signs are taken every 15 minutes for 1 to 2 hours or until stable. The condition of the incisional dressing, the fundus, and the amount of lochia are assessed, as well as the intravenous intake and the urine output through the Foley catheter. The woman is helped to turn and do coughing, deep-breathing, and leg exercises. Medications to relieve pain may be administered.

If the baby is present, the mother and her partner are given some time alone with him or her to facilitate bonding and attachment. Breastfeeding can be initiated if the mother feels like trying. If the woman is in a recovery area or in her labor room, she usually is transferred to the postpartum unit after 1 to 2 hours or once her condition is stable and the effects of anesthesia have worn off (i.e., she is alert, oriented, and able to feel and move extremities) (Care Path).

Postoperative or postpartum care. The attitude of the nurse and other health team members can influence the woman's perception of herself after a cesarean birth. The caregivers should stress that the woman is a new mother first and a surgical patient second. This attitude helps the woman perceive herself as having the same problems and needs as other new mothers, while requiring supportive postoperative care.

The women's physiologic concerns for the first few days may be dominated by pain at the incision site and pain resulting from intestinal gas, and hence the need for pain relief. If epidural anesthesia was used for the surgery, epidural opioids can be given in the immediate postoperative period to provide pain relief for approximately 24 hours. Otherwise, pain medications usually are given every 3 to 4 hours, or patient-controlled analgesia may be ordered instead. Other comfort measures such as position changes, splinting of the incision with pillows, and relaxation and breathing techniques (e.g., those learned in childbirth classes) may be implemented. Women are often the best judges of what their bodies need and can tolerate, including the postoperative ingestion of foods and fluids. If desired by the woman, the early introduction of solid food is safe. Women who eat early have been found to require less analgesia, and gastrointestinal problems do not occur (Abrams, Minassian, & Pickett, 2004). Ambulation and rocking in a rocking chair may relieve gas pains, and avoiding the consumption of gas-forming foods and carbonated beverages may help minimize them.

Nurses must be alert to a woman's physiologic needs, managing care to ensure adequate rest and pain relief. Mother-baby care (couplet care) for a cesarean birth mother may need to be modified according to her physiologic limitations as a surgical patient.

Daily care includes perineal care, breast care, and routine hygienic care, including showering after the dressing has been removed (if showering is acceptable according to the women's cultural beliefs and practices). The nurse assesses the woman's vital signs, incision, fundus, and lochia according to hospital policies, procedures, or protocols. Breath sounds, bowel sounds, circulatory status of lower extremities, and urinary and bowel elimination also are assessed. It is important to note maternal emotional status.

During the postpartum period, the nurse also can provide care that meets the psychologic and teaching needs of mothers who have had cesarean births. The nurse can explain postpartum procedures to help the woman participate in her recovery from surgery. The nurse can help the woman plan care and visits from family and friends that will allow adequate rest periods. Information on and assistance with infant care can facilitate adjustment to her role as a mother. The woman is supported as she breastfeeds her baby by receiving individualized assistance to comfortably hold and position the baby at her breast. The side-lying position and the use of pillows to support the newborn can enhance comfort and facilitate successful breastfeeding. The partner can be included in infant teaching sessions, and in explanations about the woman's recovery. The couple also should be encouraged to express their feelings about the birth experience. Some parents are angry, frustrated, or disappointed that a vaginal birth was not possible. Some women express feelings of low self-esteem or a negative self-image. Others express relief and gratitude that the baby is healthy and safely born. It may be helpful for them to have the nurse who was present during the birth visit and help fill in "gaps" about the experience. Other psychologic and lifestyle concerns that have been reported include depression, feeling limited in activities, and changes in family interactions (Gamble & Creedy, 2004).

Discharge after cesarean birth is usually by the third postoperative day. The time is often determined by criteria established by the woman's insurance carrier or the federal government (e.g., diagnosis-related groups).

The Newborn's and Mother's Health Protection Act of 1996 provides for a length of stay of up to 96 hours for cesarean births. These criteria may not coincide with the woman's physical or psychosocial readiness for discharge. Some states have added home care provisions for mothers who meet appropriate criteria for discharge and choose to leave sooner than the allowed length of stay. This policy recognizes that home care is less costly than hospital care and in most cases is more beneficial for recovery.

The nurse provides discharge teaching to prepare women for self-care and newborn care in a limited time, while trying to ensure that the woman is comfortable and able to rest. Discharge teaching and planning should include information about nutrition; measures to relieve pain and discomfort; exercise and specific activity restrictions; time management that includes periods of uninterrupted rest and sleep; hygiene, breast, and incision care; timing for resumption of

CARE PATH	*Cesarean Birth without Complications: Expected Length of Stay—48 to 72 Hours*				
	IMMEDIATE POSTOP CESAREAN	**BY FOURTH HOUR AFTER ADMISSION TO PP UNIT**	**5 TO 24 HOURS**	**25 TO 48 HOURS**	**BY DISCHARGE**
ASSESSMENTS	Recovery room or PACU admission assessment complete	PP admission assessment and care plan completed			
Vital Signs	q15min × 1 hr; q30min × 4 hr, WNL	q1h × 3, WNL	q4-8h, WNL	q8h, WNL	q8h, WNL
Postpartum Assessment	q15min × 1 hr, WNL	q1h × 3, WNL	q4-8h, WNL	q8-12h, WNL	q8-12h, WNL
Abdominal Incision	Dressing dry and intact	Dressing dry and intact	Dressing dry and intact	Dressing off or changed, incision intact	Incision intact; staples may be removed and Steri-Strips in place, incision WNL
Genitourinary	Retention catheter output >30 ml/hr	Retention catheter output >30 ml/hr	Retention catheter output >30 ml/hr; usually discontinued by 24 hours	Catheter discontinued, output >100 ml/void or 240 ml/8 hr	Urine output >240 ml/8 hr
Gastrointestinal		Absent or hypoactive BS	Hypoactive to active BS	Active BS + flatus	Active BS + flatus; may or may not have BM
Musculoskeletal	Alert or easily aroused, can move legs	Alert and oriented, moving all extremities	Ambulating with help	Ambulating unassisted	Ambulating ad lib
Bonding	Evidence of parent-infant bonding; first breastfeeding if desired		Parent-infant bonding continues	Parent-infant bonding progressing	
Laboratory Tests			Intrapartal CBC results on chart or computer; determine Rh status and need for anti-Rh globulin; check for rubella immunity	PP HCT WNL, give anti-Rh globulin if indicated	Give rubella vaccine if indicated

BS, bowel sounds; *BM,* bowel movement; *CBC,* complete blood count; *HCT,* hematocrit; *PACU,* postanesthesia care unit; *Postop,* postoperative; *PP,* postpartum; *WNL,* within normal limits

Continued

CARE PATH — Cesarean Birth without Complications: Expected Length of Stay—48 to 72 Hours—cont'd

	IMMEDIATE POSTOP CESAREAN	BY FOURTH HOUR AFTER ADMISSION TO PP UNIT	5 TO 24 HOURS	25 TO 48 HOURS	BY DISCHARGE
INTERVENTIONS					
IV	IV continues	IV continues	IV continues	IV may be discontinued	
Diet	NPO	Ice chips, sips of clear liquids	Clear liquids	Regular diet or as tolerated	Regular diet
Perineal		Pericare by nurse	Pericare with help	Self-pericare	
Activity	Bed rest	Bed rest	OOB × 3 with help, ADLs assisted, assisted to comfortable position to hold and feed baby	Holds baby comfortably, ambulates without assistance, ADLs unassisted	Activity ad lib
Pulmonary Care	Patent airway; O₂ discontinued	TCDB q2h with splinting, incentive spirometry q1h if ordered, lungs clear	TCDB q2h, continue incentive spriometry if ordered while awake; lungs clear	TCDB as needed; lungs clear	
Medications	Oxytocin added to IV. Pain control: analgesics, IV, or epidural narcotic as ordered	Oxytocin continued. Pain control: analgesics—PCA, IM, PO, or epidural narcotic as ordered	Oxytocin may be discontinued. Pain control: IM, PO, PCA narcotics or analgesics as needed	Oxytocin discontinued. Pain control: PO analgesics, NSAIDs as needed; PCA discontinued; stool softener, PNV as ordered	Rx filled or given to take home

ADLs, activities of daily living; *IM,* intramuscularly; *IV,* intravenous; *NPO,* nothing by mouth; *NSAIDs,* nonsteroidal antiinflammatory drugs; *OOB,* out of bed; *PCA,* patient-controlled analgesia; *PNV,* prenatal vitamins; *PO,* nothing by mouth; *Rx,* prescription; *TCDB,* turn, cough, deep breathe

sexual activity and contraception; signs of complications (see Teaching Guidelines: Patient Instructions for Self-Care: on p. 808) and infant care. The nurse assesses the woman's need for continued support or counseling to facilitate her emotional recovery from the birth. The woman's family and friends should be educated regarding her needs during the recovery process, and their assistance should be coordinated before discharge. Referral to support groups or to community agencies may be indicated to promote the recovery process further. A postdischarge program of telephone follow-up and home visits can facilitate the woman's full recovery after cesarean birth.

Vaginal birth after cesarean

Indications for primary cesarean birth, such as dystocia, breech presentation, or fetal distress, often are nonrecurring. Therefore a woman who has had a cesarean birth may subsequently become pregnant and not have any contraindications to labor and vaginal birth in that pregnancy and may attempt a vaginal birth after cesarean (VBAC).

ACOG (2004a) encourages a TOL and VBAC attempt in women who have had one previous cesarean birth by low transverse incision. Vaginal birth is relatively safe, but there is risk for uterine rupture through a lower uterine segment scar. Increased reports of uterine rupture in the United States

CARE PATH	*Cesarean Birth without Complications: Expected Length of Stay—48 to 72 Hours—cont'd*				
	IMMEDIATE POSTOP CESAREAN	**BY FOURTH HOUR AFTER ADMISSION TO PP UNIT**	**5 TO 24 HOURS**	**25 TO 48 HOURS**	**BY DISCHARGE**
Teaching, Discharge Plan	Breastfeeding, positioning, leg exercises	Verbalize understanding and unit routines, how to achieve rest, TCDB, involution, pain control	*Self:* comfort measures and care; reinforce TCDB and positioning; introduce teaching videos, lactation promotion or suppression *Infant:* Handwashing, infant safety, positioning for feeding and burping; if breastfeeding, then positioning baby, latching on, timing, removing from breast	*Self:* diet; activity and rest; bowel and bladder function; perineal care *Infant:* bonding; parent concerns; feeding; infant bath, cord care; need for car seat; newborn characteristics; circumcision care if procedure performed; answer questions	*Self:* home care, signs of complications (infections, bleeding), normal psychologic adjustments, normal ADLs; resumption of sexual activities; contraception; identification of support system at home; self-concept issues related to cesarean birth. Inform whom to call if problems; review need to keep follow-up appointment; provide information about community resources; provide copy of home care instructions *Infant:* parents to demonstrate infant care; reinforce use of booklets for infant care, whom to call if problems; discuss immunization needs; review need to keep follow-up appointments

and Canada in the 1990s have raised concerns about the safety of VBAC. Labor and vaginal birth are not recommended if there are contraindications, such as a previous fundal classic cesarean scar, a scar from uterine surgery, or evidence of CPD. Women are strongly advised against attempting VBACs in birth centers because the health risks are too great (Bowes & Thorp, 2004; Lieberman, Ernst, Rooks, Stapleton, & Flamm, 2004).

Women are most often the primary decision makers with regard to choice of birth method. During the antepartal period, the woman should be given information about VBAC and encouraged to choose it as an alternative to repeat cesarean birth, as long as no contraindications exist (Ridley,

Davis, Bright, & Sinclair, 2002). VBAC support groups and prenatal classes can help prepare the woman psychologically for labor and vaginal birth.

This labor should occur in a hospital facility that has the equipment and personnel available to begin the surgery within 30 minutes from the time a decision is made to perform cesarean birth (ACOG, 2004a). Ideally the woman is admitted to the labor and birth unit at the onset of spontaneous labor. In the latent phase of labor, the nurse encourages her to engage in normal activities such as ambulation. In the active phase of labor, FHR and pattern and uterine activity usually are monitored electronically, and intravenous access such as a saline lock may be established. The

TEACHING GUIDELINES

Postpartum Pain Relief after Cesarean Birth

INCISIONAL
- Splint incision with a pillow when moving or coughing.
- Use relaxation techniques such as music, breathing, and dim lights.
- Apply a heating pad to the abdomen.

GAS
- Walk as often as you can.
- Do not eat or drink gas-forming foods, carbonated beverages, or whole milk.
- Do not use straws for drinking fluids.
- Take antiflatulence medication if prescribed.
- Lie on your left side to expel gas.
- Rock in a rocking chair.

PATIENT INSTRUCTIONS FOR SELF-CARE

Signs of Postoperative Complications after Discharge

Report the following signs to your health care provider:
- Temperature exceeding 38° C
- Painful urination
- Lochia heavier than a normal period
- Wound separation
- Redness or oozing at the incision site
- Severe abdominal pain

physician or nurse-midwife should be immediately available during active labor.

There is no evidence that administering oxytocin to induce or augment labor or the use of epidural anesthesia is contraindicated, although caution and close monitoring of the laboring woman are urged if these are used (Bowes & Thorp, 2004). However, use of prostaglandins, especially misoprostol (prostaglandin E$_1$), to ripen the cervix or induce labor is not recommended because they have been associated with an increased risk for uterine rupture (ACOG, 2004a).

Attention should be paid to the woman's psychologic, as well as physical, needs during the TOL. Anxiety increases the release of catecholamines and can inhibit the release of oxytocin, thus delaying the progress of labor and possibly leading to a repeat cesarean birth. To alleviate such anxiety, the nurse can encourage the woman to use breathing and relaxation techniques and to change positions to promote labor progress. The woman's partner can be encouraged to provide comfort measures and emotional support. Collaboration among the woman in labor, her partner, the nurse, and other health care providers often results in a successful VBAC. If a TOL does not proceed to vaginal birth, the woman will need support and encouragement to express her

feelings about having another cesarean birth. It is very important that this outcome not be labeled a failed VBAC.

Evaluation

To evaluate the effectiveness of nursing care for a woman experiencing dystocia, the nurse reviews the expected outcomes of care that were met and assesses the woman's and the family's level of satisfaction with the care received.

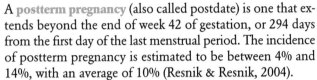

POSTTERM PREGNANCY, LABOR, AND BIRTH

A **postterm pregnancy** (also called postdate) is one that extends beyond the end of week 42 of gestation, or 294 days from the first day of the last menstrual period. The incidence of postterm pregnancy is estimated to be between 4% and 14%, with an average of 10% (Resnik & Resnik, 2004).

Many pregnancies are misdiagnosed as prolonged. This can occur because the pregnancy is inaccurately dated because the woman has an irregular menstrual cycle pattern, an accurate date of the last menstrual period is unknown, or entry into prenatal care was delayed or did not occur.

Although the exact cause of postterm pregnancy is still unknown, a possible cause may be deficiency of placental estrogen and continued secretion of progesterone. Low levels of estrogen may result in a decrease in prostaglandin precursors and reduced formation of oxytocin receptors in the myometrium (Gilbert & Harmon, 2003). A woman who experiences one postterm pregnancy is more likely to experience it again in subsequent pregnancies (Divon, 2002).

Clinical manifestations of postterm pregnancy include maternal weight loss (more than 1.4 kg/wk) and decreased uterine size (related to decreased amniotic fluid), meconium in the amniotic fluid, and advanced bone maturation of the fetal skeleton with an exceptionally hard fetal skull (Gilbert & Harmon, 2003).

Maternal and Fetal Risks

Maternal risks are often related to the birth of an excessively large infant. The woman is at increased risk for dysfunctional labor; birth canal trauma, including perineal lacerations and extension of episiotomy during vaginal birth; postpartum hemorrhage; and infection. Interventions such as induction of labor with prostaglandins or oxytocin, forceps- or vacuum-assisted birth, and cesarean birth are more likely to be necessary. The woman also may experience fatigue and psychologic reactions such as depression, frustration, and feelings of inadequacy as she passes her estimated date of birth (ACOG, 2000; Gilbert & Harmon, 2003).

Fetal risks appear to be twofold. The first is the possibility of prolonged labor, shoulder dystocia, birth trauma, and asphyxia from macrosomia. Macrosomia occurs when the placenta continues to provide adequate nutrients to support fetal growth after 40 weeks of gestation. It is estimated to occur in approximately 25% of prolonged pregnancies (Divon, 2002). The second risk is the compromising effects on the

Critical Thinking Exercise

Postterm Pregnancy

Shelly is 36 years old, G2, P1001, at 41 weeks of gestation. She was sent to the perinatal unit at the antepartal clinic for a biophysical profile. She asks why she just can't be admitted to the Labor and Birth Unit and have a cesarean birth. How will you respond to her question?

1 Is there sufficient evidence to draw conclusions about the benefits of cesarean birth for postterm pregnancy?
2 What assumptions can be made about the following issues?
   a. Elective cesarean for postterm pregnancy
   b. Timing of induction of labor for postterm pregnancy.
   c. Antepartal testing for postterm pregnancy
3 What implications and priorities for nursing care can be drawn at this time?
4 Does the evidence objectively support your conclusion?
5 Are there alternative perspectives to your conclusion?

fetus of an "aging" placenta. Placental function gradually decreases after 37 weeks of gestation. Amniotic fluid volume declines to approximately 800 ml by 40 weeks of gestation and to about 400 ml by 42 weeks of gestation. The resulting oligohydramnios can lead to fetal hypoxia related to cord compression. If placental insufficiency is present, there is a high likelihood of signs of non-reassuring fetal status occurring during labor. Neonatal problems may include asphyxia, meconium aspiration syndrome, dysmaturity syndrome, hypoglycemia, polycythemia, and respiratory distress (Gilbert & Harmon, 2003). Whether an infant born after a postterm pregnancy has neurologic, behavioral, intellectual, or developmental problems must be further investigated.

Collaborative Care

The management of postterm pregnancy is still controversial. The induction of labor at 41 to 42 weeks is suggested by some authorities as a means of reducing the rate of cesarean birth and stillbirth or neonatal death (ACOG, 2004b; Resnik & Resnik, 2004). Others follow a more individualized approach, allowing the pregnancy to proceed to 43 weeks of gestation as long as assessment of fetal well-being with a combination of tests is performed and the results of the tests are normal. Tests are usually performed on a weekly or twice-weekly basis (ACOG, 2004b; Divon, 2002; Myers et al., 2002).

Antepartum assessments for postterm pregnancy may include daily fetal movement counts, NSTs, AFV assessments, contraction stress tests (CSTs), BPPs, and Doppler flow measurements. The BPP may be the best way of gauging fetal well-being because it combines nonstress testing with real-time ultrasound scanning to assess fetal movements, fetal breathing movements, and the AFV. Determining the AFV is critical in women with postterm pregnancies because

a decreased AFV (i.e., oligohydramnios) has been associated with fetal stress. The woman and her family should be fully informed regarding the tests, including why they are performed and the meaning of the results obtained in terms of the health of the mother and fetus.

Cervical checks usually are performed weekly after 40 weeks of gestation to determine whether the condition of the cervix is favorable for induction (5 or greater on the Bishop score for multiparas and 9 or more for nulliparas) (see Table 24-3). Vaginal secretions may be assessed for the amount of fetal fibronectin; a low concentration may predict increased risk for prolonged pregnancy, but results of studies have thus far been inconclusive (Divon, 2002; Gilbert & Harmon, 2003).

During the postterm period, the woman is encouraged to assess fetal activity daily, assess for signs of labor, and keep appointments with her primary health care provider (Patient Instructions for Self-Care). The woman and her family should be encouraged to express their feelings (e.g., frustration, anger, impatience, fear) about the prolonged pregnancy and should be helped to realize that these feelings are normal. At times the emotional and physical strain of a postterm pregnancy may seem insurmountable. Referral to a support group or another supportive resource may be needed.

If the woman's cervix is favorable, labor is usually induced with oxytocin. If not, continued fetal surveillance or a cervical ripening agent (e.g., prostaglandin insert or gel) may be administered, followed by oxytocin induction (ACOG, 2004b; Gilbert & Harmon, 2003; Resnik & Resnik, 2004).

The fetus of a woman with a postterm pregnancy should be monitored electronically for a more accurate assessment of the FHR and pattern. Fetal scalp pH sampling or fetal oxygen saturation monitoring may be done to determine whether acidosis is occurring. Inadequate fluid volume leads to compression of the cord, which results in fetal hypoxia that is reflected in variable or prolonged deceleration patterns and passage of meconium. If oligohydramnios is present, an amnioinfusion may be performed to restore amniotic fluid volume to maintain a cushioning of the cord. The use of amnioinfusion to treat fetal distress associated with oligohydramnios in labor is a form of care likely to be beneficial ❋ (Enkin et al., 2000).

PATIENT INSTRUCTIONS FOR SELF-CARE

Postterm Pregnancy

- Perform daily fetal movement counts.
- Assess for signs of labor.
- Call your primary health care provider if your membranes rupture or if you perceive a decrease in or no fetal movement.
- Keep appointments for fetal assessment tests or cervical checks.
- Come to the hospital soon after labor begins.

Emotional support is essential for the woman with a post-term pregnancy and her family. A vaginal birth is anticipated, but the couple should be prepared for a forceps-assisted, vacuum-assisted, or cesarean birth if complications arise.

Expected outcomes of care include that the woman and her family use appropriate coping mechanisms to deal with the emotional aspects of her postterm pregnancy and that the woman and her newborn experience no injury during the birth.

OBSTETRIC EMERGENCIES

Shoulder Dystocia

Shoulder dystocia is an uncommon obstetric emergency that increases the risk for fetal and maternal morbidity and mortality during the attempt to deliver the fetus vaginally. It is a condition in which the head is born, but the anterior shoulder cannot pass under the pubic arch. FPD related to excessive fetal size (greater than 4000 g) or maternal pelvic abnormalities may be a cause of shoulder dystocia, although shoulder dystocia can occur in the absence of any known risk factors. The nurse should be observant for signs that could indicate the presence of shoulder dystocia, including slowing of the progress of labor and formation of a caput succedaneum that increases in size. When the head emerges, it retracts against the perineum (turtle sign), and external rotation does not occur (Bowes & Thorp, 2004).

The fetus is more likely to experience birth injuries related to asphyxia, brachial plexus damage, and fracture, especially of the humerus or clavicle. The mother's primary risk stems from excessive blood loss as a result of uterine atony or rupture, lacerations, extension of the episiotomy, or endometritis. It is estimated that 0.24% to 2% of all vaginal births are complicated by shoulder dystocia (Bowes & Thorp, 2004).

Collaborative care

Many maneuvers such as suprapubic pressure and maternal position changes have been suggested and tried to free the anterior shoulder, although no one particular maneuver has been found to be most effective (Bowes & Thorp, 2004). Suprapubic pressure can be applied to the anterior shoulder by using the Mazzanti or Rubin technique (Fig. 24-13) in an attempt to push the shoulder under the symphysis pubis (Baskett, 2002).

In the McRoberts maneuver (Fig. 24-14), the woman's legs are flexed apart, with her knees on her abdomen (Baskett, 2002; Baxley & Gobbo, 2004). This maneuver causes the sacrum to straighten, and the symphysis pubis rotates toward the mother's head; the angle of pelvic inclination is decreased, freeing the shoulder. Suprapubic pressure can be applied at this time. The McRoberts maneuver is the preferred method when a woman is receiving epidural anesthesia.

Having the woman move to the hands-and-knees position (the Gaskin maneuver), squatting position, or lateral recumbent position also has been used to resolve cases of shoulder dystocia (Baskett, 2002; Bowes & Thorp, 2004).

Fundal pressure is usually not advised as a method of relieving shoulder dystocia (Nocon, 2000; Simpson & Knox, 2001).

When shoulder dystocia is diagnosed, the nurse helps the woman to assume the position(s) that may facilitate birth of the shoulders, assists the primary health care provider with these maneuvers and techniques during birth, and documents the maneuvers. The nurse also provides encouragement and support to reduce anxiety and fear.

Newborn assessment should include examination for fracture of the clavicle or humerus as well as brachial plexus injuries and asphyxia (Bowes & Thorp, 2004). Maternal assessment should focus on early detection of hemorrhage and trauma to the soft tissue of the birth canal.

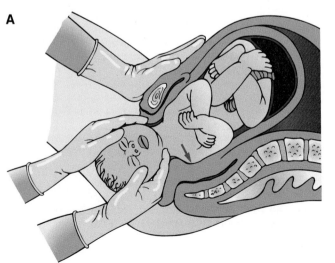

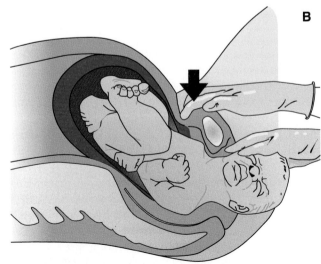

Fig. 24-13 Application of suprapubic pressure. **A,** Mazzanti technique. Pressure is applied directly posteriorly and laterally above the symphysis pubis. **B,** Rubin technique. Pressure is applied obliquely posteriorly against the anterior shoulder.

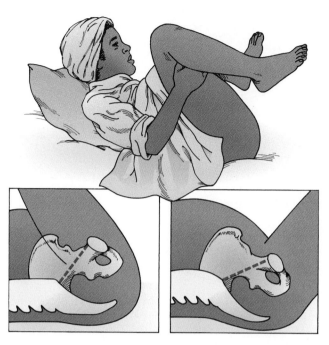

Fig. 24-14 McRoberts maneuver. (Modified from Lanni, S., & Seeds, J. [2002]. Malpresentations. In S. Gabbe, J. Niebyl, & J. Simpson (Eds.), *Obstetrics: Normal and problem pregnancies* [4th ed.]. New York: Churchill Livingstone.)

Prolapsed Umbilical Cord

Prolapse of the umbilical cord occurs when the cord lies below the presenting part of the fetus. Umbilical cord prolapse may be occult (hidden, not visible) at any time during labor whether or not the membranes are ruptured (Fig. 24-15, *A* and *B*). It is most common to see frank (visible) prolapse directly after rupture of membranes, when gravity washes the cord in front of the presenting part (Fig. 24-15, *C* and *D*). Contributing factors include a long cord (longer than 100 cm), malpresentation (breech), transverse lie, or unengaged presenting part.

If the presenting part does not fit snugly into the lower uterine segment (e.g., as in hydramnios), when the membranes rupture, a sudden gush of amniotic fluid may cause the cord to be displaced downward. Similarly the cord may prolapse during amniotomy if the presenting part is high. A small fetus may not fit snugly into the lower uterine segment; as a result, cord prolapse is more likely to occur.

Collaborative care

Prompt recognition of a prolapsed umbilical cord is important because fetal hypoxia resulting from prolonged cord compression (i.e., occlusion of blood flow to and from the fetus for more than 5 minutes) usually results in central nervous system damage or death of the fetus. Pressure on the cord may be relieved by the examiner putting a sterile gloved hand into the vagina and holding the presenting part off of the umbilical cord (Fig. 24-16, *A* and *B*). The woman is assisted into a position such as a modified Sims (Fig. 24-16, *C*), Trendelenburg, or knee-chest (Fig. 24-16, *D*) position, in which gravity keeps the pressure of the presenting part off the cord. If the cervix is fully dilated, a forceps- or vacuum-assisted birth can be performed for the fetus in a cephalic presentation; otherwise, a cesarean birth is likely to be performed. Nonreassuring FHR patterns, inadequate uterine relaxation, and bleeding also can occur as a result of a prolapsed umbilical cord. Indications for immediate interventions are presented in the Emergency box on p. 813. Ongoing assessment of the woman and her fetus is critical to determine the effectiveness of each action taken. The woman and her family are often aware of the seriousness of the situation; therefore the nurse must provide support by giving explanations for the interventions being implemented and their effect on the status of the fetus.

Rupture of the Uterus

Rupture of the uterus is a rare but very serious obstetric injury that occurs in 1 in 1500 to 2000 births. The most

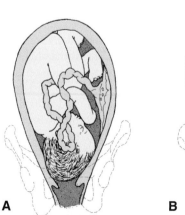
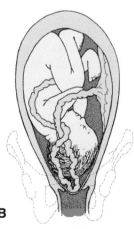
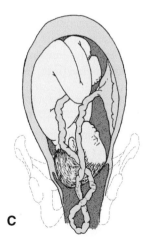
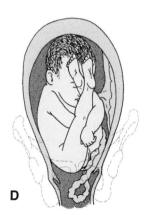

A **B** **C** **D**

Fig. 24-15 Prolapse of umbilical cord. Note pressure of presenting part on umbilical cord, which endangers fetal circulation. **A,** Occult (hidden) prolapse of cord. **B,** Complete prolapse of cord. Note that membranes are intact. **C,** Cord presenting in front of the fetal head may be seen in vagina. **D,** Frank breech presentation with prolapsed cord.

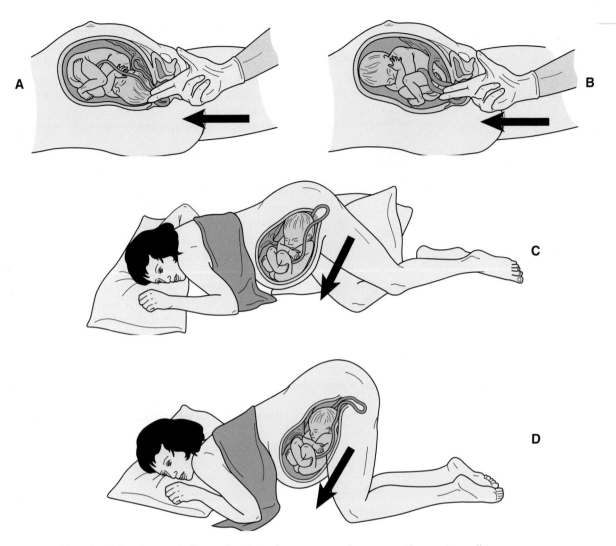

Fig. 24-16 *Arrows* indicate direction of pressure against presenting part to relieve compression of prolapsed umbilical cord. Pressure exerted by examiner's fingers in **A**, vertex presentation, and **B**, breech presentation. **C**, Gravity relieves pressure when woman is in modified Sims position with hips elevated as high as possible with pillows. **D**, Knee-chest position.

frequent causes of uterine rupture during pregnancy are separation of the scar of a previous classic cesarean birth, uterine trauma (e.g., accidents, surgery), and a congenital uterine anomaly. During labor and birth, uterine rupture may be caused by intense spontaneous uterine contractions, labor stimulation (e.g., oxytocin, prostaglandin), an overdistended uterus (e.g., multifetal gestation), malpresentation, external or internal version, or a difficult forceps-assisted birth. It occurs more commonly in multigravidas than in primigravidas.

A uterine rupture is classified as either complete or incomplete. A complete rupture extends through the entire uterine wall into the peritoneal cavity or broad ligament. An incomplete rupture extends into the peritoneum but not into the peritoneal cavity or broad ligament. Bleeding is usually internal. An incomplete rupture also may be a partial separation at an old cesarean scar and may go unnoticed unless the woman undergoes a subsequent cesarean birth or other uterine surgery.

Signs and symptoms vary with the extent of the rupture and may be silent or dramatic. In an incomplete rupture, pain may not be present. The fetus may or may not have late decelerations, decreased variability, an increased or decreased heart rate, or other nonreassuring signs. The woman may experience vomiting, faintness, increased abdominal tenderness, hypotonic uterine contractions, and lack of progress. Eventually, bleeding and the effects of blood loss will be noted. Fetal heart tones may be lost. In a complete rupture, the woman may complain of sudden, sharp shooting abdominal pain and may state that "something gave way." If she is in labor, her contractions will cease, and pain is relieved. She may exhibit signs of hypovolemic shock caused by hemorrhage (i.e., hypotension, tachypnea, pallor, and cool, clammy skin). If the placenta separates, the FHR will be absent. Fetal parts may be palpable through the abdomen. The nurse should suspect pulmonary embolism if the woman complains of chest pain.

EMERGENCY

Prolapsed Cord

SIGNS

- Fetal bradycardia with variable deceleration during uterine contraction.
- Woman reports feeling the cord after membranes rupture.
- Cord is seen or felt in or protruding from the vagina.

INTERVENTIONS

- Call for assistance.
- Notify primary health care provider immediately.
- Glove the examining hand quickly and insert two fingers into the vagina to the cervix. With one finger on either side of the cord or both fingers to one side, exert upward pressure against the presenting part to relieve compression of the cord (Fig. 24-16, *A* and *B*). Place a rolled towel under the woman's right or left hip.
- Place woman into the extreme Trendelenburg or a modified Sims position (Fig. 24-16, *C*), or a knee-chest position (Fig. 24-16, *D*).
- If cord is protruding from vagina, wrap loosely in a sterile towel saturated with warm sterile normal saline solution.
- Administer oxygen to the woman by mask at 8 to 10 L/min until birth is accomplished.
- Start IV fluids or increase existing drip rate.
- Continue to monitor FHR by internal fetal scalp electrode, if possible.
- Explain to woman and support person what is happening and the way it is being managed.
- Prepare for immediate vaginal birth if cervix is fully dilated or cesarean birth if it is not.

Collaborative care

Prevention is the best treatment. Women who have had a previous classic cesarean birth are advised not to attempt vaginal birth in subsequent pregnancies. Women at risk for uterine rupture are assessed closely during labor. Women whose labor is induced with oxytocin or prostaglandin (especially if their previous birth was cesarean) are monitored for signs of uterine hyperstimulation, because this can precipitate uterine rupture. If hyperstimulation occurs, the oxytocin infusion is discontinued or decreased, and a tocolytic medication may be given to decrease the intensity of the uterine contractions. After giving birth, women are assessed for excessive bleeding, especially if the fundus is firm and signs of hemorrhagic shock are present.

If rupture occurs, the type of medical management depends on the severity. A small rupture may be managed with a laparotomy and birth of the infant, repair of the laceration, and blood transfusions, if needed. For a complete rupture, hysterectomy and blood replacement is the usual treatment.

The nurse's role may include starting intravenous fluids, transfusing blood products, administering oxygen, and assisting with the preparation for immediate surgery. Supporting the woman's family and providing information

about the treatment is important during this emergency. The associated fetal mortality rate is high (50% to 75%), and the maternal mortality rate may be high if the woman is not treated immediately (Cunningham et al., 2005). Providing information about spiritual support services or suggesting that the family contact their own support system may be warranted.

Amniotic Fluid Embolism

Amniotic fluid embolism (AFE) occurs when amniotic fluid containing particles of debris (e.g., vernix, hair, skin cells, or meconium) enters the maternal circulation and obstructs pulmonary vessels, causing respiratory distress and circulatory collapse. This can occur because fluid can enter the maternal circulation any time there is an opening in the amniotic sac or maternal uterine veins. Although rare, this complication is estimated to be the cause of 10% of maternal deaths in the United States. The fetal mortality rate is estimated to be as high as 30%, and 50% of the surviving infants will have neurologic damage (Cunningham et al., 2005)

Amniotic fluid is more damaging if it contains meconium and other particulate matter such as mucus, fat globules, lanugo, bacterial products, or debris from a dead fetus because emboli can then form more readily. Maternal death occurs most often when thick meconium is present in the amniotic fluid, because this clogs the pulmonary veins more completely than other debris. Even if death does not occur immediately, serious coagulation problems such as disseminated intravascular coagulopathy (see Chapter 26) usually occur (Cunningham et al., 2005).

Collaborative care

The immediate interventions for AFE are summarized in the Emergency box on p. 814. Such medical management must be instituted immediately. Cardiopulmonary resuscitation is often necessary. The woman is usually placed on mechanical ventilation, and blood replacement is initiated; coagulation defects are treated. Although the incidence of possible complications is small, their immediate recognition and prompt initiation of treatment are important.

NURSE ALERT *Automatic blood pressure devices, FHR monitors, and pulse oximeters may be inadequate and inaccurate during extreme clinical conditions. Assessment by a competent nurse is often more accurate than that provided by any one piece of equipment (Curran, 2003).*

The nurse's immediate responsibility is to assist with the resuscitation efforts. If the woman survives, she is usually moved to a critical care unit, where hemodynamic monitoring, blood replacement, and coagulopathy treatment are implemented. If cardiopulmonary arrest occurs, for optimal fetal survival, a perimortem cesarean birth should occur within 5 minutes (Curran, 2003).

Support of the woman's partner and family is needed; they will be anxious and distressed. Brief explanations of what is happening are important during the emergency and can be reinforced after the immediate crisis is over. If the woman dies, emotional support and involvement of the perinatal loss support team or other resource for grief counseling is needed. Referral to grief and loss support groups would be appropriate (see Chapter 28). The nursing staff also may need help in coping with feelings and emotions that result from a maternal death.

EMERGENCY

Amniotic Fluid Embolism

SIGNS

Respiratory Distress
- Restlessness
- Dyspnea
- Cyanosis
- Pulmonary edema
- Respiratory arrest

Circulatory Collapse
- Hypotension
- Tachycardia
- Shock
- Cardiac arrest

Hemorrhage
- Coagulation failure: bleeding from incisions, venipuncture sites, trauma (lacerations); petechiae, ecchymoses, purpura
- Uterine atony

INTERVENTIONS

Oxygenate
- Administer oxygen by face mask (8 to 10 L/min) or resuscitation bag delivering 100% oxygen.
- Prepare for intubation and mechanical ventilation.
- Initiate or assist with cardiopulmonary resuscitation. Tilt pregnant woman 30 degrees to side to displace uterus.

Maintain cardiac output and replace fluid losses
- Position woman on her side.
- Administer intravenous fluids.
- Administer blood: packed cells, fresh frozen plasma.
- Insert indwelling catheter, and measure hourly urine output.

Correct coagulation failure

Monitor fetal and maternal status

Prepare for emergency birth once woman's condition is stabilized

Provide emotional support to woman, her partner, and family

COMMUNITY ACTIVITY

Meet with different childbirth educators in the community (e.g., at the health department, at the hospital clinic or birth center, or private practice educator) whose class participants plan to give birth at your hospital. Evaluate what information pregnant couples are given about measures they can use to enhance the woman's progress in labor and reduce the possibility of unwanted interventions such as labor augmentation or cesarean birth. Offer suggestions to the educators based on evidence-based practice if needed.

Key Points

- Preterm labor is cervical change and uterine contractions occurring between 20 weeks and 37 weeks of pregnancy; preterm birth is any birth that occurs before the completion of 37 weeks of pregnancy.
- The cause of preterm labor is unknown and is assumed to be multifactorial; therefore it is not possible to predict with certainty which women will experience preterm labor and birth.
- Because the onset of preterm labor is often insidious and can be mistaken for normal discomforts of pregnancy, nurses should teach all pregnant women how to detect the early symptoms of preterm labor and to call their primary health care provider when symptoms occur.

- Bed rest, a commonly prescribed intervention for preterm labor, has many deleterious side effects and has never been shown to decrease preterm birth rates.
- Research has demonstrated that a gain of 48 hours to several days is the best outcome that can be expected with the use of tocolytics. The best reason to use tocolytic therapy is to achieve sufficient time to administer glucocorticoids in an effort to accelerate fetal lung maturity and reduce the severity of respiratory complications in infants born preterm.
- Vigilance for signs of infection is a major part of the care for women with PPROM.

Key Points—cont'd

- Dystocia results from differences in the normal relations among any of the five factors affecting labor and is characterized by differences in the pattern of progress in labor.
- Dysfunctional labor occurs as a result of hypertonic uterine dysfunction, hypotonic uterine dysfunction, or inadequate voluntary expulsive forces.
- The functional relations among the uterine contractions, the fetus, and the mother's pelvis are altered by maternal positioning.
- Uterine contractility is increased by the effects of oxytocin and prostaglandin and is decreased by tocolytic agents.
- Cervical ripening using chemical or mechanical measures can increase the success of labor induction.
- Expectant parents benefit from learning about operative obstetrics (e.g., forceps-assisted, vacuum-

assisted, or cesarean birth) during the prenatal period.
- The basic purpose of cesarean birth is to preserve the life or health of the mother and her fetus.
- Unless contraindicated, vaginal birth is possible after a previous cesarean birth.
- Labor management that emphasizes one-to-one support of the laboring woman by another woman (e.g., doula, nurse, nurse-midwife) can reduce the rate of cesarean birth and increase the rate of VBACs.
- A postterm pregnancy poses a risk to both the mother and the fetus.
- Obstetric emergencies (e.g., shoulder dystocia, prolapsed cord, rupture of the uterus, and amniotic fluid embolism) occur rarely but require immediate intervention to preserve the health or life of the mother and fetus.

Answer Guidelines to Critical Thinking Exercises

Preterm Labor

1 There is no evidence in the literature to support the efficacy of bed rest in reducing preterm birth rates; it is a form of care with unknown effectiveness (Enkin et al., 2000; Maloni, 1998). Deleterious effects of bed rest on women include decreased muscle tone, weight loss, calcium loss, and glucose intolerance. Weeks of bed rest lead to bone demineralization, constipation, fatigue, isolation, anxiety, and depression.

2 a. Because this is Yolanda's third hospitalization for preterm labor, her risks of giving birth prematurely are increased. Her primary health care provider could choose to have her remain hospitalized until birth to increase the chances of a good outcome for the baby.
   b. Bed rest is often ordered as an intervention to prevent preterm birth even though it is of unknown effectiveness. Hospitalization at a facility that can handle high risk or preterm infants increases the chances of a good outcome. Although the home is an ideal location for a pregnant woman, the primary health care provider may have knowledge that Yolanda would be unlikely to remain on bed rest at home because of the need to care for her husband and child.
   c. The nurse can coach Yolanda and her family in ways to reduce the frustration and boredom that accompany restriction to bed rest for several weeks. The environment can be modified for convenience, and essential items placed within reach (e.g., telephone, television, radio, tape or compact disc player, computer with Internet access, snacks, books, magazines, newspapers, and items for hobbies). Families, who are often anxious regarding the health status of the mother and baby, may need help in learning how to organize time and space or to restructure family routines so that the pregnant woman can remain a part of family activity while still maintaining bed rest.
   d. The nurse can explore resources available in the community to assist with care of Yolanda's 2-year-old son. Referral to a social worker can be made. Family members can be asked to help; church and social groups can be helpful.

3 The priority for nursing care is to work with Yolanda to prevent preterm birth. Assisting Yolanda to maintain bed rest as ordered, providing diversions, reducing anxiety, and coaching her in ex-

ercises she can perform in bed to maintain muscle tone and prevent bone loss are actions to take. Providing explanations and keeping the family informed are essential. The fetus and uterine contractions are monitored as required by protocol or the primary health care provider's orders.

4 Although bed rest has not been shown to be effective in preventing preterm birth, it is a common intervention. Therefore the nurse can implement actions to mitigate or prevent the deleterious effects of bed rest. She can work with the family to ensure emotional support and with the social worker to ensure child care for the 2-year-old.

5 Alternatively and importantly, the nurse can also work to ensure that an evidence base exists for care provided. The nurse can work with other health care providers to identify and use the best available evidence on which to base practice. The nurse can provide evidence about the deleterious effects of bed rest and seek to change practice.

Postterm Pregnancy

1 There is no evidence in the literature to support elective cesarean for prolonged pregnancy when there is no maternal or fetal compromise.

2 a. Elective cesarean for any pregnant woman, whether or not she is postterm, may carry iatrogenic risks, such as increased rates of infection, hemorrhage, or other complications.
   b. There is insufficient evidence to recommend one specific time for labor induction. The common practices are to induce labor at 41 or 42 weeks in the presence of a favorable (inducible) cervix. If the cervix is not favorable, management alternatives include use of cervical ripening agents followed by induction or expectant management with antenatal fetal monitoring twice a week.
   c. There is no direct, unbiased evidence that antepartal testing reduces perinatal morbidity and mortality in prolonged gestation. Although the risk of antepartal stillbirth increases with increasing gestational age, there is no evidence that allows determination of the optimal time to initiate antepartal testing. However, common practice is to initiate the BPP or some part of it such as the NST and AFV assessment to assess

fetal condition and to identify oligohydramnios at 41 or 42 weeks of gestation. Testing is usually done twice weekly.

3 Nursing priorities are to encourage the woman to express her feelings about having a prolonged pregnancy, to provide support, to teach her how to assess daily fetal movement (kick counts), and to recognize signs of labor. She should also be encouraged to keep all appointments for fetal assessment tests and cervical checks and to come to the labor and birth unit as soon as her membranes rupture or labor begins.

4 Yes, the evidence objectively supports these conclusions, as there is no one way to manage postterm pregnancy.

5 Yes. Alternative ways to stimulate labor have been studied (e.g., caster oil, stripping membranes, nipple stimulation, sexual intercourse). In general, there is a tradeoff between the effectiveness of induction agents in terms of achieving the labor and risks of uterine tachysystole, hyperstimulation, and potential fetal compromise.

References: ACOG, 2004b; Bowes & Thorp, 2004; Gilbert & Harmon, 2003; Myers et al., 2002; Resnik & Resnik, 2004; Simpson, 2002.

Resources

American College of Obstetricians and Gynecologists (ACOG)
409 12th St., SW
P.O. Box 96920
Washington, DC 20090-6920
800-762-2264
www.acog.org

Birthrites: Healing after Cesarean, Inc.
www.birthrites.org

C/SEC, Inc. (Cesarean/Support Education and Concern)
22 Forest Rd.
Framingham, MA 01701
508-877-8266

A Free Home for Moms on Bedrest
www.momsonbedrest.com

International Cesarean Awareness Network (ICAN)
1304 Kingsdale Ave.
Redondo Beach, CA 90278
310-542-6400
www.ican-online.org

Mothers of Supertwins (MOST)
P.O. Box 951
Brentwood, NY 11717
631-859-1110
www.mostonline.org

National Organization of Mothers of Twins Clubs, Inc. (NOMOTC)
P.O. Box 438
Thompsons Station, TN 37179-0438
615-595-0936
www.nomotc.org

National Perinatal Association
3500 East Fletcher Ave., Suite 205
Tampa, FL 33613-4712
813-971-1008
www.nationalperinatal.org

Pregnancy Bedrest: A Reading Room to Help You Survive and Thrive during Your Days of Waiting
Amy E. Tracy
445C E. Cheyenne Mtn. Blvd., #194
Colorado Springs, CO 80906
www.pregnancybedrest.com

Sidelines: High Risk Pregnancy Support Group
P.O. Box 1808
Laguna Beach, CA 92652
888-447-4754
www.sidelines.org

The Triplet Connection
P.O. Box 99571
Stockton, CA 95209
209-474-0885
www.tripletconnection.org

VBAC.com—A Woman-Centered Evidence Based Resource
Nicette Jukelevics
Center for Family
24050 Madison St., Suite 200
Torrance, CA 90505
310-375-3141
www.vbac.com

References

Abrahams, C., & Katz, M. (2002). A perspective on the diagnosis of preterm labor. *Journal of Perinatal and Neonatal Nursing, 16*(1), 1-11.

Abrams., B., Minassian, D., & Pickett K. (2004). Maternal nutrition. In R. Creasy, R. Resnik, & J. Iams (Eds.). *Maternal-fetal medicine: Principles and practice* (5th ed.). Philadelphia: Saunders.

Adler, C., & Zarchin, Y. (2002). The "Virtual Focus Group": Using the internet to reach pregnant women on home bed rest. *Journal of Obstetric, Gynecologic, and Neonatal Nursing, 31*(4), 418-427.

American College of Obstetricians and Gynecologists (ACOG). (2000). *Fetal macrosomia. ACOG Practice Bulletin no. 22.* Washington, DC: ACOG.

American College of Obstetricians and Gynecologists. (2003). *New ACOG opinion addresses elective cesarean controversy.* News release, October 31, 2003. Washington, DC: ACOG.

American College of Obstetricians and Gynecologists (ACOG). (2004a). *Vaginal birth after a previous cesarean delivery. ACOG Practice Bulletin no. 54.* Washington, DC: ACOG.

American College of Obstetricians and Gynecologists. (ACOG). (2004b). *Management of postterm pregnancy. ACOG Practice Bulletin no. 55.* Washington, DC: ACOG.

American College of Obstetricians and Gynecologists (ACOG) & American Academy of Pediatrics (AAP). (2002). *Guidelines for perinatal care* (5th ed.). Washington, DC: ACOG.

Anotayanonth, S., Subhedar, N., Garner, P., Neilson, J., & Harigopal, S. (2004). Betamimetics for inhibiting preterm labour. *Cochrane Database Systematic Reviews*, Issue 3, Article CD004352.

Association of Women's Health, Obstetric and Neonatal Nurses (AWHONN). (2000). *Issue: Professional nursing support of laboring women.* Washington, DC: AWHONN.

Baskett, T. (2002). Shoulder dystocia. *Best Practices Research in Clinical Obstetrics and Gynaecology, 16*(10), 57-68.

Baxley, E., & Gobbo, R. (2004). Shoulder dystocia. *American Family Physician, 69*(7), 1610, 1612-1613.

Berkman, N. et al. (2003). Tocolytic treatment for the management of preterm labor: A review of the evidence. *American Journal of Obstetrics and Gynecology, 188*(6), 1648-1659.

Bernhardt, J., & Dorman, K. (2004). Pre-term birth risk assessment tools. Exploring fetal fibronectin and cervical length for validating risk. *AWHONN Lifelines, 8*(1), 38-44.

Bowes, W., & Thorp, J. (2004) Clinical aspects of normal and abnormal labor. In R. Creasy, R. Resnik, & J. Iams (Eds.) *Maternal-fetal medicine: Principles and practice* (5th ed.). Philadelphia: Saunders.

Cesario, S. (2004). Reevaluation of Friedman's labor curve: A pilot study. *Journal of Obstetric, Gynecologic, and Neonatal Nursing, 33*(6), 713-722.

Cunningham, F., Leveno, K., Bloom, S., Hauth, J., Gilstrap, L., & Wenstrom, K. (2005). *Williams' obstetrics* (22nd ed.). New York: McGraw-Hill.

Curran, C. (2003). Intrapartum emergencies, *Journal of Obstetric, Gynecologic, and Neonatal Nursing, 32*(6), 802-813.

Divon, M. (2002). Prolonged pregnancy. In S. Gabbe, J. Niebyl, & J. Simpson (Eds.). *Obstetrics: Normal and problem pregnancies* (4th ed.). New York: Churchill Livingstone.

Enkin, M. et al. (2000). *A guide to effective care in pregnancy and childbirth* (3rd ed.). Oxford, NY: Oxford University Press.

Freda, M. (2003). Nursing's contribution to the literature on preterm labor and birth. *Journal of Obstetric, Gynecologic, and Neonatal Nursing, 32*(5), 659-667.

Freda, M., & Patterson, E. (2001). *Preterm birth: Prevention and nursing management* (2nd ed.). March of Dimes Nursing Module Series. White Plains, NY: March of Dimes Birth Defects Foundation.

Friedman, E. (1989). Normal and dysfunctional labor. In W. Cohen et al. (Eds.), *Management of labor* (2nd ed.). Rockville, MD: Aspen.

Fuchs, I., Henrich, W., Osthues, K., & Dudenhausen, J. (2004). Sonographic cervical length in singleton pregnancies with intact membranes presenting in threatened preterm labor. *Ultrasound in Obstetrics and Gynecology, 24*(5), 554-557.

Gamble, J., & Creedy, D. (2004). Content and processes of postpartum counseling after a distressing birth experience: A review. *Birth, 31*(3), 213-218.

Gardner, P. (2003). Previous traumatic birth: An impetus for requested cesarean birth. *Journal of Perinatal and Neonatal Education, 12*(1), 1-5.

Garite, T. (2004). Premature rupture of membranes. In R. Creasy, R. Resnik, & J. Iams (Eds.), *Maternal-fetal medicine: Principles and practice* (5th ed.). Philadelphia: Saunders.

Gennaro, S., & Hennessy, M. (2003). Physiological and psychological stress: Impact on preterm birth. *Journal of Obstetric, Gynecologic, and Neonatal Nursing, 32*(5), 669-675.

Gilbert, E., & Harmon, J. (2003). *Manual of high risk pregnancy and delivery* (3rd ed.). St. Louis: Mosby.

Goldberg, A., Greenberg, M., & Darney, P. (2001). Drug therapy: Misoprostol and pregnancy. *New England Journal of Medicine, 344*(1), 38-47.

Goldenberg, R., Iams, J., Mercer, B., Meis, P., Moawad, A., Das, A., Copper, R., Johnson, F., & National Institute of Child Health and Human Development Maternal-Fetal Medicine Units Network. (2003). What we have learned about the predictors of preterm birth. *Seminars in Perinatology, 27*(3), 636-643.

Gregory, K. (2000). Monitoring risk adjustment and strategies to decrease cesarean rates. *Current Opinion in Obstetrics and Gynecology, 12*(6), 481-486.

Hamilton, B., Martin, J., Sutton, P., & Centers for Disease Control and Prevention, National Center for Health Statistics. (2004). Births: Preliminary data for 2003. *National Vital Statistics Report, 23*(9), 1-17.

Heaman, M., Sprague, A., & Stewart, P. (2001). Reducing the preterm birth rate: A population health strategy. *Journal of Obstetric, Gynecologic, and Neonatal Nursing, 30*(1), 20-29.

Hodnett, E. (2002). Caregiver support for women during childbirth. *Cochrane Database Systematic Reviews,* Issue 1, Article CD000199.

Hodnett, E., Gates, S., Hofmeyr, G., & Sakala, C. (2003). Continuous support for women during childbirth. *Cochrane Database Systematic Reviews,* Issue 3, Article CD003766.

Hodnett, E., Lowe, N., Hannah, M., Willan, A., Stevens, B., & Weston, J. (2002). Effectiveness of nurses as providers of birth support in North American hospitals. *Journal of the American Medical Association, 288*(11), 1373-1381.

Hofmeyr, G., & Hannah, M. (2003). Planned caesarean section for term breech delivery (Cochrane Review). In *The Cochrane Library,* Issue 3, 2005. Chichester, UK: John Wiley & Sons.

Iams, J. (2002). Preterm birth. In S. Gabbe, J. Niebyl, & J. Simpson (Eds.), *Obstetrics: Normal and problem pregnancies* (4th ed.). New York: Churchill Livingstone.

Iams, J., & Creasy, R. (2004). Preterm labor and delivery. In R. Creasy, R. Resnik, & J. Iams (Eds.). *Maternal-fetal medicine: Principles and practice* (5th ed.). Philadelphia: Saunders.

Lanni, S., & Seeds, J. (2002). Malpresentations. In S. Gabbe, J. Niebyl, & J. Simpson (Eds.), *Obstetrics: Normal and problem pregnancies* (4th ed.). New York: Churchill Livingstone.

Lehne, R. (2001). *Pharmacology for nursing care.* Philadelphia: Saunders.

Lieberman, E., Ernst, E., Rooks, J., Stapleton, S., & Flamm, B. (2004). Results of the national study of vaginal birth after cesarean in birth centers. *Obstetrics & Gynecology, 104*(5 Pt 1), 933-942.

Liu, S. et al. (2004). Recent trends in caesarean delivery rates and indications for caesarean delivery in Canada. *Journal of Obstetrics and Gynaecology of Canada, 26*(8), 735-742.

Maloni, J. (1998). *Antepartum bedrest: Case studies, research, and nursing care.* Washington, DC: AWHONN.

Maloni, J. (2000). *The prevention of preterm birth: Research-based practice, nursing interventions, and practice scenarios.* Washington, DC: AWHONN.

Maloni, J. (2002). Astronauts & pregnancy bed rest: What NASA is teaching us about inactivity. *AWHONN Lifelines, 6*(4), 318-323.

Maloni, J., & Kutil, R. (2000). Antepartum support group for women hospitalized on bedrest. *MCN American Journal of Maternal/Child Nursing, 25*(4), 204-210.

Maloni, J., & Park, S. (2005). Postpartum symptoms after antepartum bedrest. *Journal of Obstetric, Gynecologic, and Neonatal Nursing, 34*(2), 163-171.

Maloni, J., Brezinski-Tomasi, J., & Johnson, L. (2001). Antepartum bedrest: Effect upon the family. *Journal of Obstetric, Gynecologic, and Neonatal Nursing, 30*(2), 165-173.

Maloni, J. et al. (1993). Physical and psychosocial side effects of antepartum bed rest. *Nursing Research, 42*(4), 197-203.

Martin, J. et al. (2003). Births: Final data for 2002. *National Vital Statistics Report, 52*(10), 1-113.

Massett, H., Greenup, M., Ryan, C., Staples, D., Green, N., & Maibach, E. (2003). Public perceptions about prematurity: A national survey. *American Journal of Preventive Medicine, 24*(2), 120-127.

Maupin R., Lyman, R., Fatsis, J, Prystowiski, E., Nguyen, A., Wright, C., Kissinger, P., & Miller, J. (2004). Characteristics of women who deliver with no prenatal care. *Journal of Maternal Fetal Neonatal Medicine, 16*(1), 45-50.

Mayberry, L., Wood, S., Strange, L., Lee, L., Heisler, D., Nielsen-Smith, K.. (2000). *Second stage labor management: Promotion of evidence-based practice and a collaborative approach to patient care.* Washington, DC: AWHONN.

McCann, M. (2003). *Days in waiting: A guide to surviving bedrest.* St. Paul, MN: deRuyter-Nelson Publications.

McFarlin, B. (2004). Elective cesarean birth: Issues and ethics of informed choice. *Journal of Midwifery and Women's Health, 49*(5), 421-429.

Miltner, R. (2002). More than support: Nursing interventions provided to women in labor. *Journal of Obstetric, Gynecologic, and Neonatal Nursing, 31*(6), 753-761.

Moondragon Birthing Services. (2005). *Moondragon's pregnancy information: Coping with bedrest during pregnancy.* Internet document available at www.moondragon.org/pregnancy/bedrestcope.html (accessed May 1, 2005).

Moore, M. (2003). Preterm labor and birth: What have we learned in the past two decades? *Journal of Obstetric, Gynecologic, and Neonatal Nursing, 32*(5), 638-649.

Moos, M. (2004). Understanding prematurity: Sorting fact from fiction. *AWHONN Lifelines, 8*(1), 32-37.

Morrison, J., & Chauhan, S. (2003). Current status of home uterine activity monitoring. *Clinics in Perinatology, 30*(4), 757-801.

Myers, E. et al. (2002). *Management of prolonged pregnancy. Evidence Report/Technology Assessment no. 53.* AHRQ Publication 02-E018. Rockville, MD: Agency for Healthcare Research and Quality.

National Institutes of Health. (2000). *Antenatal corticosteroids revisited. Consensus Development Conference Statement.* Maryland: NIH. Internet document available at http://consensus.nih.gov. (Accessed 9/6/05).

Nelson, R. (2004). Premature births on the rise. *American Journal of Nursing, 104*(6), 23-24.

Nocon, J. (2000). Shoulder dystocia and macrosomia. In L. Kean, P. Baker, & D. Edlestone (Eds.), *Best practice in labor ward management.* Philadelphia: Saunders.

Norwitz, E., Robinson, J., & Repke, J. (2002). Labor and delivery. In S. Gabbe, J. Niebyl, & J. Simpson (Eds.), *Obstetrics: Normal and problem pregnancies* (4th ed.). New York: Churchill Livingstone.

Ramsey, P., & Andrews, W. (2003). Biochemical predictors of preterm labor: Fetal fibronectin and salivary estriol. *Clinics in Perinatology, 30*(4), 701-733.

Ramsey, P., Ramin, K., & Ramin, S. (2000). Labor induction. *Current Opinion Obstetrics and Gynecology, 12*(6), 463-473.

Resnik, J., & Resnik, R. (2004). Post-term pregnancy. In R. Creasy, R. Resnik, & J. Iams (Eds.), *Maternal-fetal medicine: Principles and practice,* (5th ed.), Philadelphia: Saunders.

Rideout, S. (2005). Tocolytics of pre-term labor: What nurses need to know. *AWHONN Lifelines, 9*(1), 56-61.

Ridley, R., Davis, P., Bright, J., & Sinclair, D. (2002). What influences a woman to choose vaginal birth after cesarean? *Journal of Obstetric, Gynecologic, and Neonatal Nursing, 31*(6), 665-672.

Ruchata, P., Metheby, N., Essenpreis, H., & Borcherding, K. (2002). Current practices in oxytocin dilution and fluid administration for induction of labor. *Journal of Obstetric, Gynecologic, and Neonatal Nursing, 31*(5), 545-550.

Schaffir, J. (2002). Survey of folk beliefs about induction of labor. *Birth, 29*(1), 47-51.

Simkin, P., & Ancheta, R. (2000). *The labor progress handbook.* Malden, MA: Blackwell Science.

Simpson, K. (2002). *Cervical ripening and induction and augmentation of labor* (2nd ed.). Washington, DC: AWHONN.

Simpson, K., & Atterbury, J. (2003). Trends and issues in labor induction in the United States: Implications for clinical practice. *Journal of Obstetric, Gynecologic, and Neonatal Nursing, 32*(6), 767-779.

Simpson, K., & Knox, G. (2001). Fundal pressure during second stage of labor. *MCN American Journal of Maternal Child Nursing, 26*(6), 64-70.

Society of Obstetricians and Gynaecologists of Canada (SOGC). (2004). News. C-sections on demand–SOGC's position. *Birth, 31*(2),154.

Sosa, C., Athalbe, F., Belzian, J., & Bergel, E. (2004). Bed rest in singleton pregnancies for preventing preterm birth. *Cochrane Database of Systematic Reviews,* Issue 1, Article CD003581.

Tiedje, L. (2003). Psychosocial pathways to prematurity: Changing our thinking toward a lifecourse and community approach. *Journal of Obstetric, Gynecologic, and Neonatal Nursing, 32*(5), 650-658.

Tracy, A. (2001). *The pregnancy bed rest book: A survival guide for expectant mothers and their families.* New York: Berkley Publishing Group.

Weiss, M., Saks, N., & Harris, S. (2002). Resolving the uncertainty of preterm symptoms: Women's experiences with the onset of preterm labor. *Journal of Obstetric, Gynecologic, and Neonatal Nursing, 31*(1), 66-76.

Weitz, B. (2001). Premature rupture of the fetal membranes: An update for advanced practice nurses. *MCN American Journal of Maternal Child Nursing, 26*(2), 86-92.

Williams, D. (2005). The top 10 reasons elective cesarean section should be on the decline. *AWHONN Lifelines, 9*(1), 23-24.

Witcher, P. (2002). Treatment of preterm labor. *Journal of Perinatal and Neonatal Nursing, 16*(1), 25-46.

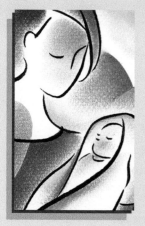

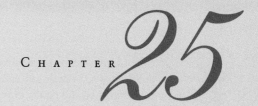

CHAPTER 25

Postpartum Complications

DEITRA LEONARD LOWDERMILK

LEARNING OBJECTIVES

- Identify causes, signs and symptoms, possible complications, and medical and nursing management of postpartum hemorrhage.
- Differentiate the causes of postpartum infection.
- Summarize assessment and care of women with postpartum infection.
- Describe thromboembolic disorders, including incidence, etiology, signs and symptoms, and management.
- Describe sequelae of childbirth trauma.
- Discuss postpartum emotional complications, including incidence, risk factors, signs and symptoms, and management.
- Summarize the role of the nurse in the home setting in assessing potential problems and managing care of women with postpartum complications.

KEY TERMS AND DEFINITIONS

endometritis Postpartum uterine infection, often beginning at the site of the placental implantation

hemorrhagic (hypovolemic) shock Clinical condition in which the peripheral blood flow is inadequate to return sufficient blood to the heart for normal function, particularly oxygen transport to the organs or tissue

inversion of the uterus Condition in which the uterus is turned inside out so that the fundus intrudes into the cervix or vagina

mastitis Infection in a breast, usually confined to a milk duct, characterized by influenza-like symptoms and redness and tenderness in the affected breast

mood disorders Disorders that have a disturbance in the prevailing emotional state as the dominant feature; cause is unknown

pelvic relaxation Refers to the lengthening and weakening of the fascial supports of pelvic structures

postpartum depression (PPD) Depression occurring within 4 weeks of childbirth, lasting longer than postpartum blues and characterized by a variety of symptoms that interfere with activities of daily living and care of the baby

postpartum hemorrhage (PPH) Excessive bleeding after childbirth; traditionally defined as a loss of 500 ml or more after a vaginal birth and 1000 ml after a cesarean birth

puerperal infection Infection of the pelvic organs during the postbirth period; also called *postpartum infection*

subinvolution Failure of a part (e.g., the uterus) to reduce to its normal size and condition after enlargement from functional activity (e.g., pregnancy)

thrombophlebitis inflammation of a vein with secondary clot formation

urinary incontinence (UI) Uncontrollable leakage of urine

uterine atony Relaxation of uterus; leads to postpartum hemorrhage

ELECTRONIC RESOURCES

Additional information related to the content in Chapter 25 can be found on

the companion website at **evolve**
http://evolve.elsevier.com/Lowdermilk/Maternity/
- NCLEX Review Questions
- WebLinks

or on the interactive companion CD
- NCLEX Review Questions
- Plan of Care—Postpartum Hemorrhage
- Plan of Care—Postpartum Depression

*C*ollaborative efforts of the health care team are needed to provide safe and effective care to the woman and family experiencing postpartum complications. This chapter focuses on hemorrhage, infection, sequelae of childbirth trauma, and psychologic complications.

POSTPARTUM HEMORRHAGE

Definition and Incidence

Postpartum hemorrhage (PPH) continues to be a leading cause of maternal morbidity and mortality in the United States (Papp, 2003) and worldwide. It is a life-threatening event that can occur with little warning and is often unrecognized until the mother has profound symptoms. PPH has been traditionally defined as the loss of more than 500 ml of blood after vaginal birth and 1000 ml after cesarean birth. A 10% change in hematocrit between admission for labor and postpartum or the need for erythrocyte transfusion also has been used to define PPH (American College of Obstetricians and Gynecologists [ACOG], 1998). However, defining PPH is not a clear-cut issue. ACOG states that hemorrhage is difficult to define clinically. Diagnosis is often based on subjective observations, with blood loss often being underestimated by as much as 50% (ACOG, 1998).

Traditionally, PPH has been classified as early or late with respect to the birth. Early, acute, or primary PPH occurs within 24 hours of the birth. Late or secondary PPH occurs more than 24 hours but less than 6 weeks postpartum (ACOG, 1998). Today's health care environment encourages shortened stays after birth, thereby increasing the potential for acute episodes of PPH to occur outside the traditional hospital or birth center setting.

Etiology and Risk Factors

It is helpful to consider the problem of excessive bleeding with reference to the stages of labor. From birth of the infant until separation of the placenta, the character and quantity of blood passed may suggest excessive bleeding. For example, dark blood is probably of venous origin, perhaps from varices or superficial lacerations of the birth canal. Bright blood is arterial and may indicate deep lacerations of the cervix. Spurts of blood with clots may indicate partial placental separation. Failure of blood to clot or remain clotted indicates a pathologic condition or coagulopathy such as disseminated intravascular coagulation (DIC) (ACOG, 1998).

Excessive bleeding may occur during the period from the separation of the placenta to its expulsion or removal. Commonly such excessive bleeding is the result of incomplete placental separation, undue manipulation of the fundus, or excessive traction on the cord. After the placenta has been expelled or removed, persistent or excessive blood loss usually is the result of atony of the uterus or inversion of the uterus into the vagina. Late PPH may be the result of subinvolution of the uterus, endometritis, or retained placental fragments (ACOG, 1998). Risk factors for PPH are listed in Box 25-1.

Uterine Atony

Uterine atony is marked hypotonia of the uterus. Normally, placental separation and expulsion are facilitated by contraction of the uterus, which also prevents hemorrhage from the placental site. The corpus is in essence a basket-weave of strong, interlacing smooth muscle bundles through which many large maternal blood vessels pass (see Fig. 4-3). If the uterus is flaccid after detachment of all or part of the placenta, brisk venous bleeding occurs, and normal coagulation of the open vasculature is impaired and continues until the uterine muscle is contracted.

Uterine atony is the leading cause of PPH, complicating approximately one in 20 births (Shevell & Malone, 2003). It is associated with high parity, hydramnios, a macrosomic fetus, and multifetal gestation. In such conditions, the uterus is "overstretched" and contracts poorly after the birth. Other causes of atony include traumatic birth, use of halogenated anesthesia (e.g., halothane) or magnesium sulfate, rapid or prolonged labor, chorioamnionitis, and use of oxytocin for labor induction or augmentation (Shevell & Malone, 2003).

BOX 25-1

Risk Factors for Postpartum Hemorrhage

Uterine atony
- Overdistended uterus
  - Large fetus
  - Multiple fetuses
  - Hydramnios
  - Distention with clots
- Anesthesia and analgesia
  - Conduction anesthesia
- Previous history of uterine atony
- High parity
- Prolonged labor, oxytocin-induced labor
- Trauma during labor and birth
  - Forceps-assisted birth
  - Vacuum-assisted birth
  - Cesarean birth

Lacerations of the birth canal
Retained placental fragments
Ruptured uterus
Inversion of the uterus
Placenta accreta
Coagulation disorders
Placental abruption
Placenta previa
Manual removal of a retained placenta
Magnesium sulfate administration during labor or postpartum period
Endometritis
Uterine subinvolution

Lacerations of the Genital Tract

Lacerations of the cervix, vagina, and perineum also are causes of PPH. Hemorrhage related to lacerations should be suspected if bleeding continues despite a firm, contracted uterine fundus. This bleeding can be a slow trickle, an oozing, or frank hemorrhage. Factors that influence the causes and incidence of obstetric lacerations of the lower genital tract include operative birth, precipitate birth, congenital abnormalities of the maternal soft parts, and contracted pelvis. Size, abnormal presentation, and position of the fetus; relative size of the presenting part and the birth canal; previous scarring from infection, injury, or operation; and vulvar, perineal, and vaginal varicosities also can cause lacerations.

Extreme vascularity in the labial and periclitoral areas often results in profuse bleeding if laceration occurs. Hematomas also may be present.

Lacerations of the perineum are the most common of all injuries in the lower portion of the genital tract. These are classified as first, second, third, and fourth degree (see Chapter 14). An episiotomy may extend to become either third- or fourth-degree laceration.

Prolonged pressure of the fetal head on the vaginal mucosa ultimately interferes with the circulation and may produce ischemic or pressure necrosis. The state of the tissues in combination with the type of birth may result in deep vaginal lacerations, with consequent predisposition to vaginal hematomas.

Pelvic hematomas may be vulvar, vaginal, or retroperitoneal in origin. Vulvar hematomas are the most common. Pain is the most common symptom, and most vulvar hematomas are visible. Vaginal hematomas occur more commonly in association with a forceps-assisted birth, an episiotomy, or primigravidity (Benedetti, 2002). During the postpartum period, if the woman reports a persistent perineal or rectal pain or a feeling of pressure in the vagina, a careful examination is made. However, a retroperitoneal hematoma may cause minimal pain, and the initial symptoms may be signs of shock (Benedetti, 2002).

Cervical lacerations usually occur at the lateral angles of the external os. Most are shallow, and bleeding is minimal. More extensive lacerations may extend into the vaginal vault or into the lower uterine segment.

Retained Placenta
Nonadherent retained placenta

Retained placenta may result from partial separation of a normal placenta, entrapment of the partially or completely separated placenta by an hourglass constriction ring of the uterus, mismanagement of the third stage of labor, or abnormal adherence of the entire placenta or a portion of the placenta to the uterine wall. Placental retention because of poor separation is common in very preterm births (20 to 24 weeks of gestation).

Management of nonadherent retained placenta is by manual separation and removal by the primary health care provider. Supplementary anesthesia is not usually needed for women who have had regional anesthesia for birth. For other women, administration of light nitrous oxide and oxygen inhalation anesthesia or intravenous (IV) thiopental facilitates uterine exploration and placental removal. After this removal, the woman is at continued risk for PPH and for infection.

Adherent retained placenta

Abnormal adherence of the placenta occurs for reasons unknown, but it is thought to result from zygotic implantation in an area of defective endometrium so that there is no zone of separation between the placenta and the decidua. Attempts to remove the placenta in the usual manner are unsuccessful, and laceration or perforation of the uterine wall may result, putting the woman at great risk for severe PPH and infection (Cunningham et al., 2005).

Unusual placental adherence may be partial or complete. The following degrees of attachment are recognized:

- *Placenta accreta*—slight penetration of myometrium by placental trophoblast
- *Placenta increta*—deep penetration of myometrium by placenta
- *Placenta percreta*—perforation of uterus by placenta

Bleeding with complete or total placenta accreta may not occur unless separation of the placenta is attempted. With more extensive involvement, bleeding will become profuse when removal of the placenta is attempted. Treatment includes blood component replacement therapy, and hysterectomy may be indicated (Clark, 2004).

Inversion of the Uterus

Inversion of the uterus after birth is a potentially life-threatening but rare complication. The incidence of uterine inversion is approximately 1 in 2000 to 2500 births (ACOG, 1998), and the condition may recur with a subsequent birth. Uterine inversion may be partial or complete. Complete inversion of the uterus is obvious; a large, red, rounded mass (perhaps with the placenta attached) protrudes 20 to 30 cm outside the introitus. Incomplete inversion cannot be seen but must be felt; a smooth mass will be palpated through the dilated cervix. Contributing factors to uterine inversion include fundal implantation of the placenta, vigorous fundal pressure, excessive traction applied to the cord, uterine atony, leiomyomas, and abnormally adherent placental tissue (Bowes & Thorp, 2004). Uterine inversion occurs most often in multiparous women and with placenta accreta or increta. The primary presenting signs of uterine inversion are hemorrhage, shock, and pain.

Prevention—always the easiest, cheapest, and most effective therapy—is especially appropriate for uterine inversion. The umbilical cord should not be pulled on strongly unless the placenta has definitely separated.

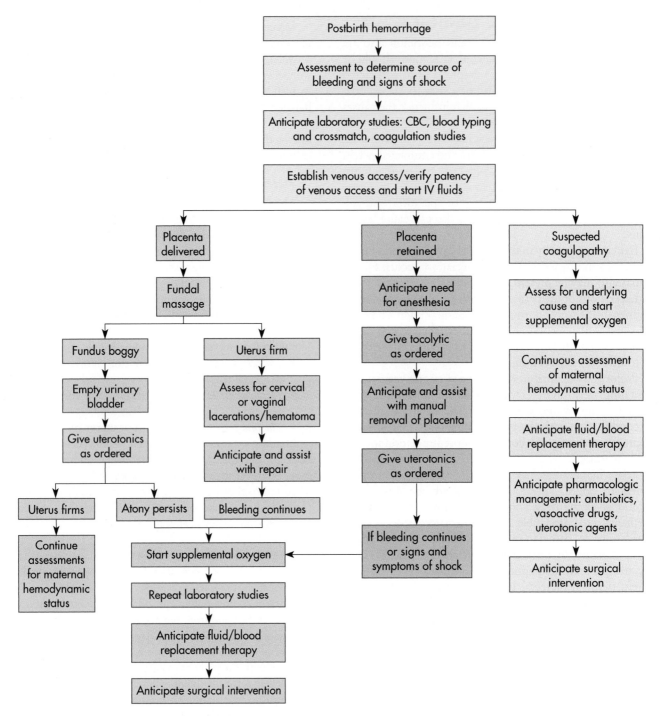

Fig. 25-1 Nursing assessments for postpartum bleeding. *CBC,* Complete blood count; *IV,* intravenous; *s/s,* signs and symptoms; *uterotonics,* medications to contract the uterus.

Subinvolution of the Uterus

Late postpartum bleeding may occur as a result of subinvolution of the uterus. Recognized causes of subinvolution include retained placental fragments and pelvic infection.

Signs and symptoms include prolonged lochial discharge, irregular or excessive bleeding, and sometimes hemorrhage. A pelvic examination usually reveals a uterus that is larger than normal and that may be boggy.

CARE MANAGEMENT

Assessment and Nursing Diagnoses

PPH may be sudden and even exsanguinating. The nurse must therefore be alert to the symptoms of hemorrhage and hypovolemic shock and be prepared to act quickly to minimize blood loss (Fig. 25-1 and Box 25-2).

Noninvasive Assessments of Cardiac Output in Postpartum Patients Who Are Bleeding

- Palpation of pulses (rate, quality, equality)
  - Arterial
  - Blood pressure
- Auscultation
  - Heart sounds and murmurs
  - Breath sounds
- Inspection
  - Skin color, temperature, turgor
  - Level of consciousness
  - Capillary refill
  - Urinary output
  - Neck veins
  - Pulse oximetry
  - Mucous membranes
- Observation
  - Presence or absence of anxiety, apprehension, restlessness, disorientation

The woman's history should be reviewed for factors that cause predisposition to PPH (see Box 25-1). The fundus is assessed to determine whether it is firmly contracted at or near the level of the umbilicus. Bleeding should be assessed for color and amount. The perineum is inspected for signs of lacerations or hematomas to determine the possible source of bleeding.

Vital signs may not be reliable indicators of shock immediately postpartum because of the physiologic adaptations of this period. However, frequent vital sign measurements during the first 2 hours after birth may identify trends related to blood loss (e.g., tachycardia, tachypnea, decreasing blood pressure).

Assessment for bladder distention is important because a distended bladder can displace the uterus and prevent contraction. The skin is assessed for warmth and dryness; nail beds are checked for color and promptness of capillary refill. Laboratory studies include evaluation of hemoglobin and hematocrit levels.

Late PPH develops at least 24 hours after the birth or later in the postpartum period. The woman may be at home when the symptoms occur. Discharge teaching should emphasize the signs of normal involution, as well as potential complications. Nursing diagnoses for women experiencing PPH include the following:

- *Deficient fluid volume related to*
  - excessive blood loss secondary to uterine atony, lacerations, or uterine inversion
- *Risk for imbalanced fluid volume related to*
  - blood and fluid volume replacement therapy
- *Risk for infection related to*
  - excessive blood loss or exposed placental attachment site

- *Risk for injury related to*
  - attempted manual removal of retained placenta
  - administration of blood products
  - operative procedures
- *Fear or anxiety related to*
  - threat to self
  - deficient knowledge regarding procedures and operative management
- *Risk for impaired parenting related to*
  - separation from infant secondary to treatment regimen
- *Ineffective (peripheral) tissue perfusion related to*
  - excessive blood loss and shunting of blood to central circulation

Expected Outcomes of Care

Expected outcomes of care for the woman experiencing PPH may include that the woman will do the following:
- Maintain normal vital signs and laboratory values
- Develop no complications related to excessive bleeding
- Express understanding of her condition, its management, and discharge instructions
- Identify and use available support systems

Plan of Care and Interventions
Medical management

Early recognition and acknowledgment of the diagnosis of PPH are critical to care management. The first step is to evaluate the contractility of the uterus. If the uterus is hypotonic, management is directed toward increasing contractility and minimizing blood loss.

The initial management of excessive postpartum bleeding is firm massage of the uterine fundus, expression of any clots in the uterus, elimination of any bladder distention, and continuous IV infusion of 10 to 40 units of oxytocin added to 1000 ml of lactated Ringer's or normal saline solution. If the uterus fails to respond to oxytocin, a 0.2-mg dose of ergonovine (Ergotrate) or methylergonovine (Methergine) may be given intramuscularly to produce sustained uterine contractions. However, it is more common to administer a 0.25-mg dose of a derivative of prostaglandin $F_{2\alpha}$ (carboprost tromethamine) intramuscularly. It also can be given intramyometrially at cesarean birth or intraabdominally after vaginal birth. Oral (400 mcg) and rectal (1000 mcg) administration of misoprostol also is used, but there is no consensus about efficacy (Berg & Smith, 2002). See Table 25-1 for a comparison of drugs used to manage PPH. In addition to the medications used to contract the uterus, rapid administration of crystalloid solutions and/or blood or blood products will be needed to restore the woman's intravascular volume (Mousa & Walkinshaw, 2001).

NURSE ALERT *Use of ergonovine or methylergonovine is contraindicated in the presence of hypertension or cardiovascular disease. Prostaglandin $F_{2\alpha}$ should be*

TABLE 25-1

Drugs Used to Manage Postpartum Hemorrhage

	OXYTOCIN (PITOCIN)	METHYLERGONOVINE (METHERGINE)*	PROSTAGLANDIN F$_{2\alpha}$ (PROSTIN/15M; HEMABATE)
Action	Contraction of uterus; decreases bleeding	Contraction of uterus	Contraction of uterus
Side effects	Infrequent; water intoxication; nausea and vomiting	Hypertension, nausea, vomiting, headache	Headache, nausea, vomiting, fever
Contraindications	None for PPH	Hypertension, cardiac disease	Asthma, hypersensitivity
Dosage and route	10-40 units/L diluted in lactated Ringer's solution or normal saline at 125 to 200 milliunits/min IV or 10 to 20 units IM	0.2 mg IM q2-4h up to five doses; 0.2 mg IV only for emergency	0.25 mg IM or intramyometrially every 15 to 90 min up to eight doses
Nursing considerations	Continue to monitor vaginal bleeding and uterine tone	Check blood pressure before giving and do not give if >140/90 mm Hg; continue monitoring vaginal bleeding and uterine tone	Continue to monitor vaginal bleeding and uterine tone

IM, Intramuscularly; *IV,* intravenously.
*Information about methylergonovine may also be used to describe ergonovine (Ergotrate).

used cautiously in women with cardiovascular disease or asthma (Bowes & Thorp, 2004).

Hypotonic uterus. Oxygen can be given to enhance oxygen delivery to the cells. A urinary catheter is usually inserted to monitor urine output as a measure of intravascular volume. Laboratory studies usually include a complete blood count with platelet count, fibrinogen, fibrin split products, prothrombin time, and partial thromboplastin time. Blood type and antibody screen are done if not previously performed (ACOG, 1998).

If bleeding persists, bimanual compression may be considered by the obstetrician or nurse-midwife. This procedure involves inserting a fist into the vagina and pressing the knuckles against the anterior side of the uterus, and then placing the other hand on the abdomen and massaging the posterior uterus with it. If the uterus still does not become firm, manual exploration of the uterine cavity for retained placental fragments is implemented. If the preceding procedures are ineffective, surgical management may be the only alternative. Surgical management options include vessel ligation (uteroovarian, uterine, hypogastric), selective arterial embolization, and hysterectomy (Shevell & Malone, 2003).

Bleeding with a contracted uterus. If the uterus is firmly contracted and bleeding continues, the source of bleeding still must be identified and treated. Assessment may include visual or manual inspection of the perineum, vagina, uterus, cervix, or rectum and laboratory studies (e.g., hemoglobin, hematocrit, coagulation studies, platelet count). Treatment depends on the source of the bleeding. Lacerations are usually sutured. Hematomas may be managed with observation, cold therapy, ligation of the bleeding vessel, or evacuation. Fluids and or blood replacement may be needed (Benedetti, 2002).

Uterine inversion. Uterine inversion is an emergency situation requiring immediate recognition, replacement of the uterus within the pelvic cavity, and correction of associated clinical conditions. Tocolytics (e.g., magnesium sulfate, terbutaline) or halogenated anesthetics may be given to relax the uterus before attempting replacement (Hostetler & Bosworth, 2000). Medical management of this condition includes repositioning the uterus, giving oxytocin after the uterus is repositioned, treating shock, and initiating broad-spectrum antibiotics (Benedetti, 2002; Bowes & Thorp, 2004).

Subinvolution. Treatment of subinvolution depends on the cause. Ergonovine, 0.2 mg every 4 hours for 2 or 3 days, and antibiotic therapy are the most common medications used (Cunningham et al., 2005). Dilation and curettage (D&C) may be needed to remove retained placental fragments or to debride the placental site.

Herbal remedies

Herbal remedies have been used with some success to control PPH after the initial management and control of bleeding, particularly outside the United States. Some herbs have homeostatic actions, whereas others work as oxytocic agents to contract the uterus (Tiran & Mack, 2000). Box 25-3 lists herbs that have been used and their actions. However, published evidence of the safety and efficacy of herbal therapy is lacking. Evidence from well-controlled studies is needed before recommendation for practice should be made (Brucker, 2001).

BOX 25-3

Herbal Remedies for Postpartum Hemorrhage

HERB	ACTION
Witch hazel	Homeostatic
Lady's mantle	Homeostatic
Blue cohosh	Oxytocic
Cotton root bark	Oxytocic
Motherwort	Promotes uterine contraction; vasoconstrictive
Shepherd's purse	Promotes uterine contraction
Alfalfa leaf	Increases availability of vitamin K; increases hemoglobin
Nettle	Increases availability of vitamin K; increases hemoglobin
Raspberry leaf	Homeostatic; promotes uterine contraction

Source: Beal, M. (1998). Use of complementary and alternative therapies in reproductive medicine. *Journal of Nurse-Midwifery, 43*(3), 224-233; Schirmer, G. (1998). *Herbal medicine.* Bedford TX: MED2000; Skidmore-Roth, L. (2004). *Mosby's handbook of herbs and natural supplements* (2nd ed.). St. Louis: Mosby; & Tiran, D., & Mack, S. (Eds.). (2000). *Complementary therapies for pregnancy and childbirth* (2nd ed.). Edinburgh: BaillièreTindall.

Nursing interventions

Immediate nursing care of the woman with PPH includes assessment of vital signs, uterine consistency, bleeding, and administration of oxytocin or other drugs to stimulate uterine contraction according to standing orders or protocols. Venous access is established if not already in place. The primary health care provider is notified if not present.

The woman and her family will be anxious about her condition. The nurse can intervene by calmly providing explanations about interventions being performed and the need to act quickly.

After the bleeding has been controlled, the care of the woman with lacerations of the perineum is similar to that of women with episiotomies (analgesia as needed for pain and hot or cold applications as necessary). The need for increased roughage in the diet and increased intake of fluids is emphasized. Stool softeners may be used to assist the woman in reestablishing bowel habits without straining and putting stress on the suture lines.

NURSE ALERT *To avoid injury to the suture line, a woman with third- or fourth-degree lacerations is not given rectal suppositories or enemas or digital rectal examinations.*

The care of the woman who has experienced an inversion of the uterus focuses on immediate stabilization of hemodynamic status. This requires close observation of her response to treatment to prevent shock or fluid overload. If the uterus has been repositioned manually, care must be taken to avoid aggressive fundal massage.

Discharge instructions for the woman who has had PPH are similar to those for any postpartum woman. In addition, she should be told that she will probably feel fatigue, even exhaustion, and will need to limit her physical activities to conserve her strength. She may need instructions in increasing her dietary iron and protein intake and iron supplementation to rebuild lost red blood cell (RBC) volume. She may need assistance with infant care and household activities until she has regained strength. Some women have problems with delayed or insufficient lactation and postpartum depression (PPD). Referrals for home care follow-up or to community resources may be needed (see Resources at the end of this chapter).

Evaluation

The nurse can be reasonably assured that care was effective to the extent that the expected outcomes were achieved (Plan of Care).

HEMORRHAGIC (HYPOVOLEMIC) SHOCK ◼

Hemorrhage may result in hemorrhagic (hypovolemic) shock. Shock is an emergency situation in which the perfusion of body organs may become severely compromised and death may occur. Physiologic compensatory mechanisms are activated in response to hemorrhage. The adrenal glands release catecholamines, causing arterioles and venules in the skin, lungs, gastrointestinal tract, liver, and kidneys to constrict. The available blood flow is diverted to the brain and heart and away from other organs, including the uterus. If shock is prolonged, the continued reduction in cellular oxygenation results in an accumulation of lactic acid and acidosis (from anaerobic glucose metabolism). Acidosis (reduced serum pH) causes arteriolar vasodilation; venule vasoconstriction persists. A circular pattern is established; that is, decreased perfusion, increased tissue anoxia and acidosis, edema formation, and pooling of blood further decrease the perfusion. Cellular death occurs. See the Emergency box for assessments and interventions for hemorrhagic shock.

Medical Management

Vigorous treatment is necessary to prevent adverse sequelae. Medical management of hypovolemic shock involves restoring circulating blood volume and treating the cause of the hemorrhage (e.g., lacerations, uterine atony, or inversion). To restore circulating blood volume, a rapid IV infusion of crystalloid solution is given at a rate of 3 ml infused for every 1 ml of estimated blood loss (e.g., 3000 ml infused for 1000 ml of blood loss). Packed RBCs are usually infused if the woman is still actively bleeding and no improvement in her condition is noted after the initial crystalloid infusion. Infusion of fresh-frozen plasma may be needed if clotting factors and platelet counts are below normal values (Cunningham et al., 2005).

Nursing Interventions

Hemorrhagic shock can occur rapidly, but the classic signs of shock may not appear until the postpartum woman has

PLAN OF CARE *Postpartum Hemorrhage*

NURSING DIAGNOSIS Deficient fluid volume related to postpartum hemorrhage

Expected Outcome *Woman will demonstrate fluid balance as evidenced by stable vital signs, prompt capillary refill time, and balanced intake and output.*

Nursing Interventions/*Rationales*

- Monitor vital signs, oxygen saturation, urine specific gravity, and capillary refill *to provide baseline data.*
- Measure and record amount and type of bleeding by weighing and counting saturated pads. If woman is at home, teach her to count pads and save any clots or tissue. If woman is admitted to hospital, save any clots and tissue for further examination *to estimate type and amount of blood loss for fluid replacement.*
- Provide quiet environment *to promote rest and decrease metabolic demands.*
- Give explanation of all procedures *to reduce anxiety.*
- Begin IV access with 18-gauge or larger needle for infusion of isotonic solution as ordered *to provide fluid or blood replacement.*
- Administer medications as ordered, such as oxytocin, methylergonovine, or prostaglandin $F_{2\alpha}$, *to increase contractility of the uterus.*
- Insert indwelling urinary catheter *to provide most accurate assessment of renal function and hypovolemia.*
- Prepare for surgical intervention as needed *to stop the source of bleeding.*

NURSING DIAGNOSIS Ineffective tissue perfusion related to hypovolemia

Expected Outcome *Woman will have stable vital signs, oxygen saturation, arterial blood gases, and adequate hematocrit and hemoglobin.*

Nursing Interventions/*Rationales*

- Monitor vital signs, oxygen saturation, arterial blood gases, and hematocrit and hemoglobin *to assess for hypovolemic shock and decreased tissue perfusion.*
- Assess for any changes in level of consciousness *to assess for evidence of hypoxia.*
- Assess capillary refill, mucous membranes, and skin temperature *to note indicators of vasoconstriction.*
- Give supplementary oxygen as ordered *to provide additional oxygenation to tissues.*
- Suction as needed, insert oral airway, *to maintain clear, open airway for oxygenation.*
- Monitor arterial blood gases *to provide information about acidosis or hypoxia.*
- Administer sodium bicarbonate if ordered *to reverse metabolic acidosis.*

NURSING DIAGNOSIS Anxiety related to sudden change in health status

Expected Outcome *Woman will verbalize that anxious feelings are diminished.*

Nursing Interventions/*Rationales*

- Using therapeutic communication, evaluate woman's understanding of events *to provide clarification of any misconceptions.*
- Provide calm, competent attitude and environment *to aid in decreasing anxiety.*
- Explain all procedures *to decrease anxiety about the unknown.*
- Allow woman to verbalize feelings *to permit clarification of information and promote trust.*
- Continue to assess vital signs or other clinical indicators of hypovolemic shock *to evaluate if psychologic response of anxiety intensifies physiologic indicators.*

NURSING DIAGNOSIS Risk for infection related to blood loss and invasive procedures as a result of postpartum hemorrhage

Expected Outcomes *Woman will verbalize understanding of risk factors. Woman will demonstrate no signs of infection.*

Nursing Interventions/*Rationales*

- Maintain Standard Precautions and use good handwashing technique when providing care *to prevent introduction of or spread of infection.*
- Teach woman to maintain good handwashing technique (particularly before handling her newborn) and to maintain scrupulous perineal care with frequent change and careful disposal of perineal pads *to avoid spread of microorganisms.*
- Monitor vital signs *to detect signs of systemic infection.*
- Monitor level of fatigue and lethargy, evidence of chills, loss of appetite, nausea and vomiting, and abdominal pain, *which are indicative of extent of infection and serve as indicators of status of infection.*
- Monitor lochia for foul smell and profusion *as indicators of infection state.*
- Assist with collection of intrauterine cultures or other specimens for laboratory analysis *to identify specific causative organism.*
- Monitor laboratory values (i.e., white blood cell [WBC] count, cultures) *for indicators of type and status of infection.*
- Ensure adequate fluid and nutritional intake *to fight infection.*
- Administer and monitor broad-spectrum antibiotics if ordered *to prevent infection.*
- Administer antipyretics as ordered and necessary to reduce elevated temperature.

lost 30% to 40% of blood volume. The nurse must continue to reassess the woman's condition, as evidenced by the degree of measurable and anticipated blood loss, and mobilize appropriate resources.

Most interventions are instituted to improve or monitor tissue perfusion. The nurse continues to monitor the woman's pulse and blood pressure. If invasive hemodynamic monitoring is ordered, the nurse may assist with the placement of the central venous pressure (CVP) or pulmonary artery (Swan-Ganz) catheter and monitor CVP, pulmonary artery pressure, or pulmonary artery wedge pressure as ordered (Poole & White, 2003).

Additional assessments to be made include evaluation of skin temperature, color, and turgor, as well as assessment of the woman's mucous membranes. Breath sounds should be auscultated before fluid volume replacement, if possible, to provide a baseline for future assessment. Inspection for oozing at the sites of incisions or injections and assessment of the presence of petechiae or ecchymosis in areas not associated with surgery or trauma are critical in the evaluation for DIC.

EMERGENCY

Hemorrhagic Shock

ASSESSMENTS
- Respirations
- Pulse
- Blood pressure
- Skin
- Urinary output
- Level of consciousness
- Mental status
- Central venous pressure

CHARACTERISTICS
- Rapid and shallow
- Rapid, weak, irregular
- Decreasing (late sign)
- Cool, pale, clammy
- Decreasing
- Lethargy → coma
- Anxiety → coma
- Decreased

INTERVENTION
- Summon assistance and equipment.
- Start intravenous infusion per standing orders.
- Ensure patent airway; administer oxygen.
- Continue to monitor status.

Oxygen is administered, preferably by nonrebreathing face mask, at 10 to 12 L/min to maintain oxygen saturation. Oxygen saturation should be monitored with a pulse oximeter, although measurements may not always be accurate in a woman with hypovolemia or decreased perfusion. Level of consciousness is assessed frequently and provides additional indications of blood volume and oxygen saturation. In early stages of decreased blood flow the woman may report "seeing stars" or feeling dizzy or nauseated. She may become restless and orthopneic. As cerebral hypoxia increases, she may become confused and react slowly or not at all to stimuli. Some women complain of headaches (Curran, 2003). An improved sensorium is an indicator of improved perfusion.

Continuous electrocardiographic monitoring may be indicated for the woman who is hypotensive or tachycardic, continues to bleed profusely, or is in shock. A Foley catheter with a urometer is inserted to allow hourly assessment of urinary output. The most objective and least invasive assessment of adequate organ perfusion and oxygenation is urinary output of at least 30 ml/hr (Benedetti, 2002). Blood may be drawn and sent to the laboratory for studies that include hemoglobin and hematocrit levels, platelet count, and coagulation profile.

Fluid or Blood Replacement Therapy

Critical to successful management of the woman with a hemorrhagic complication is establishment of venous access, preferably with a large-bore IV catheter. The establishment of two IV lines facilitates fluid resuscitation. Vigorous fluid resuscitation includes the administration of crystalloids (lactated Ringer's, normal saline solutions), colloids (albumin), blood, and blood components (Benedetti, 2002). Fluid resuscitation must be carefully monitored because fluid overload may occur. Intravascular fluid overload occurs more frequently with colloid therapy. Transfusion reactions may follow administration of blood or blood components,

including cryoprecipitates. Even in an emergency, each unit must be checked per hospital protocol. Complications of fluid or blood replacement therapy include hemolytic reactions, febrile reactions, allergic reactions, circulatory overload, and air embolism.

> **LEGAL TIP** Standard of Care for Bleeding Emergencies
>
> *The standard of care for obstetric emergency situations such as PPH or hypovolemic shock is that provision should be made for the nurse to implement actions independently. Policies, procedures, standing orders or protocols, and clinical guidelines should be established by each health care facility in which births occur and should be agreed on by health care providers involved in the care of obstetric patients.*

COAGULOPATHIES

When bleeding is continuous and there is no identifiable source, a coagulopathy may be the cause. The woman's coagulation status must be assessed quickly and continuously. The nurse may draw and send blood to the laboratory for studies. Abnormal results depend on the cause and may include increased prothrombin time, increased partial thromboplastin time, decreased platelets, decreased fibrinogen level, increased fibrin degradation products, and prolonged bleeding time. Causes of coagulopathies may be pregnancy complications such as idiopathic thrombocytopenic purpura (ITP), or von Willebrand disease and DIC.

Idiopathic Thrombocytopenic Purpura

ITP is an autoimmune disorder in which antiplatelet antibodies decrease the life span of the platelets. Thrombocytopenia, capillary fragility, and increased bleeding time are diagnostic findings. ITP may cause severe hemorrhage after cesarean birth or from cervical or vaginal lacerations. The incidence of postpartum uterine bleeding and vaginal hematomas also is increased. Neonatal thrombocytopenia, a result of the maternal disease process, occurs in about 50% of cases and is associated with high mortality (Kilpatrick & Laros, 2004).

Medical management focuses on control of platelet stability. If ITP was diagnosed during pregnancy, the woman likely was treated with corticosteroids or IV immunoglobulin. Platelet transfusions are usually given when there is significant bleeding. A splenectomy may be needed if the ITP does not respond to medical management.

von Willebrand Disease

von Willebrand disease, a type of hemophilia, is probably the most common of all hereditary bleeding disorders (Strozewski, 2000). Although von Willebrand disease is rare, it is among the most common congenital clotting defects in U.S. women of childbearing age. It results from a factor VIII deficiency and platelet dysfunction that is transmitted as an incomplete autosomal dominant trait to both sexes. Symptoms include a familial bleeding tendency, previous bleeding episodes, prolonged bleeding time (the most important test), factor VIII deficiency (mild to moderate), and bleeding from mucous membranes. Although factor VIII increases during pregnancy, there is still a risk for PPH as levels of von Willebrand factor begin to decrease (Roque, Funai, & Lockwood, 2000).

The woman may be at risk for bleeding for up to 4 weeks postpartum. Treatment of von Willebrand disease may include replacement of factor VIII and administration of desmopressin or antifibrinolytics (Strozewski, 2000).

NURSE ALERT *Cryoprecipitate is no longer recommended by the Medical and Scientific Advisory Council of the National Hemophilia Association as a treatment for von Willebrand disease because it may contain donor viruses (Strozewski, 2000).*

Disseminated Intravascular Coagulation

DIC is a pathologic form of clotting that is diffuse and consumes large amounts of clotting factors, including platelets, fibrinogen, prothrombin, and factors V and VII. Widespread external bleeding, internal bleeding, or both can result. DIC also causes vascular occlusion of small vessels resulting from small clots forming in the microcirculation. In the obstetric population, DIC may occur as a result of abruptio placentae, amniotic fluid embolism, dead fetus syndrome (fetus has died but is retained in utero for at least 6 weeks), severe preeclampsia, septicemia, cardiopulmonary arrest, and hemorrhage.

The diagnosis of DIC is made according to clinical findings and laboratory markers. Physical examination reveals unusual bleeding; spontaneous bleeding from the woman's gums or nose may be noted. Petechiae may appear around a blood pressure cuff placed on the woman's arm. Excessive bleeding may occur from the site of a slight trauma (e.g., venipuncture sites, intramuscular or subcutaneous injection sites, nicks from shaving of perineum or abdomen, and injury from insertion of a urinary catheter). Symptoms also may include tachycardia and diaphoresis. Laboratory tests reveal decreased levels of platelets, fibrinogen, proaccelerin, antihemophiliac factor, and prothrombin (the factors consumed during coagulation). Fibrinolysis is increased at first but is later severely depressed. Degradation of fibrin leads to the accumulation of fibrin split products in the blood; these have anticoagulant properties and prolong the prothrombin time. Bleeding time is normal, coagulation time shows no clot, clot-retraction time shows no clot, and partial thromboplastin time is increased. DIC must be distinguished from other clotting disorders before therapy is initiated.

Primary medical management in all cases of DIC involves correction of the underlying cause (e.g., removal of the dead fetus, treatment of existing infection or of preeclampsia or

eclampsia, or removal of a placental abruption). Volume replacement, blood component therapy, optimization of oxygenation and perfusion status, and continued reassessment of laboratory parameters are the usual forms of treatment. Plasma levels usually return to normal within 24 hours after birth. Platelet counts usually return to normal within 7 days (Kilpatrick & Laros, 2004).

Nursing interventions include assessment for signs of bleeding and signs of complications from the administration of blood and blood products, administering fluid or blood replacement as ordered, and protecting the woman from injury. Because renal failure is one consequence of DIC, urinary output is monitored, usually by insertion of an indwelling urinary catheter. Urinary output must be maintained at more than 30 ml/hr.

The woman and her family will be anxious or concerned about her condition and prognosis. The nurse offers explanations about care and provides emotional support to the woman and her family through this critical time.

THROMBOEMBOLIC DISEASE ■

A thrombosis results from the formation of a blood clot or clots inside a blood vessel and is caused by inflammation (**thrombophlebitis**) or partial obstruction of the vessel. Three thromboembolic conditions are of concern in the postpartum period:

- *Superficial venous thrombosis*: Involvement of the superficial saphenous venous system
- *Deep venous thrombosis*: Involvement varies but can extend from the foot to the iliofemoral region
- *Pulmonary embolism*: Complication of deep venous thrombosis occurring when part of a blood clot dislodges and is carried to the pulmonary artery, where it occludes the vessel and obstructs blood flow to the lungs

Incidence and Etiology

The incidence of thromboembolic disease in the postpartum period varies from about 0.5 to 3 per 1000 women (Laros, 2004). The incidence has declined in the last 20 years because early ambulation after childbirth has become the standard practice. The major causes of thromboembolic disease are venous stasis and hypercoagulation, both of which are present in pregnancy and continue into the postpartum period. Other risk factors include cesarean birth, history of venous thrombosis or varicosities, obesity, maternal age older than 35 years, multiparity, and smoking (Weiss & Bernstein, 2000).

Clinical Manifestations

Superficial venous thrombosis is the most frequent form of postpartum thrombophlebitis. It is characterized by pain and tenderness in the lower extremity. Physical examination may reveal warmth, redness, and an enlarged, hardened vein over the site of the thrombosis. Deep vein thrombosis is more common in pregnancy and is characterized by unilateral leg pain, calf tenderness, and swelling (Fig. 25-2). Physical examination may reveal redness and warmth, but women also may have a large amount of clot and have few symptoms (Stenchever, Droegemueller, Herbst, & Mishell, 2001). A positive Homans sign may be present, but further evaluation is needed because the calf pain may be attributed to other causes such as a strained muscle resulting from the birthing position. Pulmonary embolism is characterized by dyspnea and tachypnea. Other signs and symptoms frequently seen include apprehension, cough, tachycardia, hemoptysis, elevated temperature, and pleuritic chest pain (Laros, 2004).

Physical examination is not a sensitive diagnostic indicator for thrombosis. Venography is the most accurate method for diagnosing deep venous thrombosis; however, it is an invasive procedure that exposes the woman and fetus to ionizing radiation and is associated with serious complications. Noninvasive diagnostic methods are more commonly used; these include real-time and color Doppler ultrasound. Cardiac auscultation may reveal murmurs with pulmonary embolism. Electrocardiograms are usually normal. Arterial P_{O_2} may be lower than normal. A ventilation/perfusion scan, Doppler ultrasound, and pulmonary arteriogram may be used for diagnosis (Laros, 2004).

Medical Management

Superficial venous thrombosis is treated with analgesia (nonsteroidal antiinflammatory agents), rest with elevation of the affected leg, and elastic stockings (Laros, 2004). Local application of heat also may be used. Deep venous thrombosis is initially treated with anticoagulant (usually continuous IV heparin) therapy, bed rest with the affected leg elevated, and analgesia. After the symptoms have decreased, the woman may be fitted with elastic stockings to use when she is allowed to ambulate. IV heparin therapy continues for 3 to 5 days or until symptoms resolve. Oral anticoagulant therapy (warfarin) is started during this time and will be continued for about 3 months. Continuous IV heparin therapy is used for pulmonary embolism until symptoms have resolved. Intermittent subcutaneous heparin or oral anticoagulant therapy is usually continued for 6 months.

Nursing Interventions

In the hospital setting, nursing care of the woman with a thrombosis consists of continued assessments: inspection and palpation of the affected area; palpation of peripheral pulses; checking Homans sign; measurement and comparison of leg circumferences; inspection for signs of bleeding; monitoring for signs of pulmonary embolism including chest pain, coughing, dyspnea, and tachypnea; and respiratory status for presence of crackles. Laboratory reports are monitored for prothrombin or partial thromboplastin times. The woman and her family are assessed for their level of understanding about the diagnosis and their ability to cope during the unexpected extended period of recovery.

Interventions include explanations and education about the diagnosis and the treatment. The woman will need assistance with personal care as long as she is on bed rest; the family should be encouraged to participate in the care if that is what she and they wish. While the woman is on bed rest, she should be encouraged to change positions frequently but not to place the knees in a sharply flexed position that could cause pooling of blood in the lower extremities. She also should be cautioned not to rub the affected area, as this action could cause the clot to dislodge. Once the woman is allowed to ambulate, she is taught how to prevent venous congestion by putting on the elastic stockings before getting out of bed.

Heparin and warfarin are administered as ordered, and the physician is notified if clotting times are outside the therapeutic level. If the woman is breastfeeding, she is assured that neither heparin nor warfarin is excreted in significant quantities in breast milk. If the infant has been discharged, the family is encouraged to bring the infant for feedings as

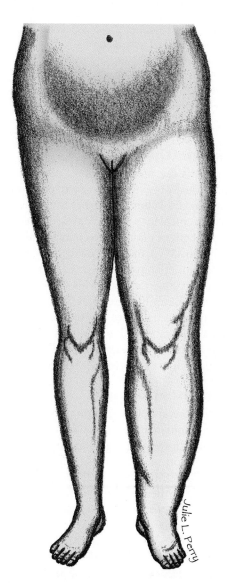

Fig. 25-2 Deep vein thrombophlebitis.

permitted by hospital policy; the mother also can express milk to be sent home.

Pain can be managed with a variety of measures. Position changes, elevating the leg, and application of moist warm heat may decrease discomfort. Administration of analgesics and antiinflammatory medications may be needed.

NURSE ALERT *Medications containing aspirin are not given to women receiving anticoagulant therapy because aspirin inhibits synthesis of clotting factors and can lead to prolonged clotting time and increased risk of bleeding.*

The woman is usually discharged home with oral anticoagulants and will need explanations about the treatment schedule and possible side effects. If subcutaneous injections are to be given, the woman and family are taught how to administer the medication and about site rotation. The woman and her family also should be given information about safe care practices to prevent bleeding and injury while she is receiving anticoagulant therapy, such as using a soft toothbrush and using an electric razor. She also will need information about follow-up with her health care provider to monitor clotting times and to make sure the correct dose of anticoagulant therapy is maintained. The woman also should use a reliable method of contraception if taking warfarin, because this medication is considered teratogenic (Gilbert & Harmon, 2003).

POSTPARTUM INFECTIONS

Postpartum or *puerperal infection* is any clinical infection of the genital canal that occurs within 28 days after miscarriage, induced abortion, or childbirth. The definition used in the United States continues to be the presence of a fever of 38° C or more on 2 successive days of the first 10 postpartum days (not counting the first 24 hours after birth) (Cunningham et al., 2005). Puerperal infection is probably the major cause of maternal morbidity and mortality throughout the world; however, it occurs after about 6% of births in the United States (5 to 10 times higher after cesarean births than after vaginal births) (Gibbs, Sweet, & Duff, 2004). Common postpartum infections include endometritis, wound infections, mastitis, urinary tract infections (UTIs), and respiratory tract infections.

The most common infecting organisms are the numerous streptococcal and anaerobic organisms. *Staphylococcus aureus*, gonococci, coliform bacteria, and clostridia are less common but serious pathogenic organisms that also cause puerperal infection. Postpartum infections are more common in women who have concurrent medical or immunosuppressive conditions or who had a cesarean or other operative birth. Intrapartal factors such as prolonged rupture of membranes, prolonged labor, and internal maternal or fetal monitoring also increase the risk of infection (Gibbs, Sweet, & Duff, 2004). Factors that predispose the woman to postpartum infection are listed in Box 25-4.

BOX 25-4

Predisposing Factors for Postpartum Infection

PRECONCEPTION OR ANTEPARTAL FACTORS
- History of previous venous thrombosis, urinary tract infection, mastitis, pneumonia
- Diabetes mellitus
- Alcoholism
- Drug abuse
- Immunosuppression
- Anemia
- Malnutrition

INTRAPARTAL FACTORS
- Cesarean birth
- Prolonged rupture of membranes
- Chorioamnionitis
- Prolonged labor
- Bladder catheterization
- Internal fetal or uterine pressure monitoring
- Multiple vaginal examinations after rupture of membranes
- Epidural anesthesia
- Retained placental fragments
- Postpartum hemorrhage
- Episiotomy or lacerations
- Hematomas

Endometritis

Endometritis is the most common cause of postpartum infection. It usually begins as a localized infection at the placental site (Fig. 25-3) but can spread to involve the entire endometrium. Incidence is higher after cesarean birth. Assessment for signs of endometritis may reveal a fever (usually greater than 38° C); increased pulse; chills; anorexia; nausea; fatigue and lethargy; pelvic pain; uterine tenderness; and/or foul-smelling, profuse lochia (Duff, 2002). Leukocytosis and a markedly increased RBC sedimentation rate are typical laboratory findings of postpartum infections. Anemia also may be present. Blood cultures or intracervical or intrauterine bacterial cultures (aerobic and anaerobic) should reveal the offending pathogens within 36 to 48 hours.

Wound Infections

Wound infections also are common postpartum infections but often develop after the woman is at home. Sites of infection include the cesarean incision and the episiotomy or repaired laceration site. Predisposing factors are similar to those for endometritis (see Box 25-4). Signs of wound infection include erythema, edema, warmth, tenderness, seropurulent drainage, and wound separation. Fever and pain also may be present.

Urinary Tract Infections

Urinary tract infections (UTIs) occur in 2% to 4% of postpartum women. Risk factors include urinary catheterization,

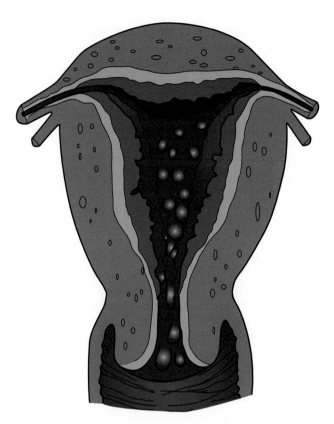

Fig. 25-3 Postpartum infection—endometritis.

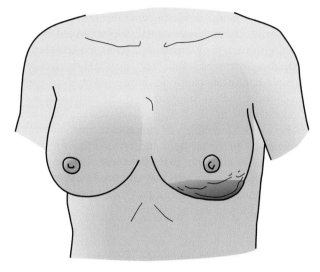

Fig. 25-4 Mastitis.

frequent pelvic examinations, epidural anesthesia, genital tract injury, history of UTI, and cesarean birth. Signs and symptoms include dysuria, frequency and urgency, low-grade fever, urinary retention, hematuria, and pyuria. Costovertebral angle (CVA) tenderness or flank pain may indicate upper UTI. Urinalysis results may reveal *Escherichia coli*, although other gram-negative aerobic bacilli also may cause UTIs.

Mastitis

Mastitis affects about 1% of women soon after childbirth, most of whom are first-time mothers who are breastfeeding. Mastitis almost always is unilateral and develops well after the flow of milk has been established (Fig. 25-4). The infecting organism generally is the hemolytic *S. aureus*. An infected nipple fissure usually is the initial lesion, but the ductal system is involved next. Inflammatory edema and engorgement of the breast soon obstruct the flow of milk in a lobe; regional, then generalized, mastitis follows. If treatment is not prompt, mastitis may progress to a breast abscess.

Symptoms rarely appear before the end of the first postpartum week and are more common in the second to fourth weeks. Chills, fever, malaise, and local breast tenderness are noted first. Localized breast tenderness, pain, swelling, redness, and axillary adenopathy also may occur. Antibiotics are prescribed. Lactation can be maintained by emptying the breasts every 2 to 4 hours by breastfeeding, manual expression, or breast pump.

CARE MANAGEMENT

Signs and symptoms associated with postpartum infection were discussed with each infection. Laboratory tests usually performed include a complete blood count, venous blood cultures, and uterine tissue cultures. Nursing diagnoses for women experiencing postpartum infection include the following:

- *Deficient knowledge related to*
  -cause, management, course of infection
  -transmission and prevention of infection
- *Impaired tissue integrity related to*
  -effects of infection process
- *Acute pain related to*
  -mastitis
  -puerperal infection
  -UTI
- *Interrupted family processes related to*
  -unexpected complication to expected postpartum recovery
  -possible separation from newborn
  -interruption in process of realigning relationships after the addition of the new family member
- *Risk for impaired parenting related to*
  -fear of spread of infection to newborn

The most effective and least expensive treatment of postpartum infection is prevention. Preventive measures include good prenatal nutrition to control anemia and intrapartal hemorrhage. Good maternal perineal hygiene with thorough handwashing is emphasized. Strict adherence by all health care personnel to aseptic techniques during childbirth and the postpartum period is very important.

Management of endometritis consists of IV broad-spectrum antibiotic therapy (cephalosporins, penicillins, or clindamycin and gentamicin) and supportive care, including hydration, rest, and pain relief (French & Smaill, 2002). Antibiotic therapy is usually discontinued 24 hours after the woman is asymptomatic (Gibbs, Sweet, & Duff, 2004). Assessments of lochia, vital signs, and changes in the woman's condition continue during treatment. Comfort measures depend on the symptoms and may include cool compresses, warm blankets, perineal care, and sitz baths. Teaching should include side effects of therapy, prevention of spread of infection, signs and symptoms of worsening condition, and adherence to the treatment plan and the need for follow-up care. Women may need to be encouraged or assisted to maintain mother-infant interactions and breastfeeding (if allowed during treatment).

Postpartum women are usually discharged to home by 48 hours after birth. This is often before signs of infection are evident. Nurses in birth centers and hospital settings must be able to identify women at risk for postpartum infection and to provide anticipatory teaching and counseling before discharge. After discharge, telephone follow-up, hot lines, support groups, lactation counselors, home visits by nurses, and teaching materials (videos, written materials) are all interventions that can be implemented to prevent or increase recognition of postpartum infections. Home care nurses must be able to recognize signs and symptoms of postpartum infection so that the woman can contact her primary health care provider. These nurses also must be able to provide the appropriate nursing care for women who need follow-up home care.

Treatment of wound infections may combine antibiotic therapy with wound debridement. Wounds may be opened and drained. Nursing care includes frequent wound and vital sign assessments and wound care. Comfort measures include sitz baths, warm compresses, and perineal care. Teaching includes good hygiene techniques (e.g., changing perineal pads front to back, handwashing before and after perineal care), self-care measures, and signs of worsening conditions to report to the health care provider. The woman is usually discharged to home for self-care or home nursing care after treatment is initiated in the inpatient setting.

Medical management for UTIs consists of antibiotic therapy, analgesia, and hydration. Postpartum women are usually treated on an outpatient basis; therefore teaching should include instructions on how to monitor temperature, bladder function, and appearance of urine. The woman also should be taught about signs of potential complications and the importance of taking all antibiotics as prescribed. Other suggestions for prevention of UTIs include using proper perineal care, wiping from front to back after urinating or having a bowel movement, and increasing fluid intake.

Because mastitis rarely occurs before the postpartum woman who is breastfeeding is discharged, teaching should include warning signs of mastitis and counseling about prevention of cracked nipples. Management includes intensive antibiotic therapy (e.g., cephalosporins and vancomycin, which are particularly useful in staphylococcal infections), support of breasts, local heat (or cold), adequate hydration, and analgesics.

Almost all instances of acute mastitis can be avoided by using proper breastfeeding technique to prevent cracked nipples. Missed feedings, waiting too long between feedings, and abrupt weaning may lead to clogged nipples and mastitis. Cleanliness practiced by all who have contact with the newborn and new mother also reduces the incidence of mastitis. See Chapter 20 for further information.

SEQUELAE OF CHILDBIRTH TRAUMA

Women are at risk for problems related to the reproductive system from the age of menarche through menopause and the older years. These problems include structural disorders of the uterus and vagina related to pelvic relaxation and **urinary incontinence (UI)**. They can be a delayed result of childbearing. For example, the structures and soft tissues of the vagina and bladder may be injured during a prolonged labor, during a precipitous birth, or when cephalopelvic disproportion occurs. Defects can also occur in women who have never been pregnant.

Uterine Displacement and Prolapse

Normally, the round ligaments hold the uterus in anteversion, and the uterosacral ligaments pull the cervix backward and upward (see Fig. 4-2). Uterine displacement is a variation of this normal placement. The most common type of displacement is posterior displacement, or retroversion, in which the uterus is tilted posteriorly and the cervix rotates anteriorly. Other variations include retroflexion and anteflexion (Fig. 25-5).

By 2 months postpartum the ligaments should return to normal length, but in approximately one third of women the uterus remains retroverted. This condition is rarely symptomatic, but conception may be difficult because the cervix points toward the anterior vaginal wall and away from the posterior fornix, where seminal fluid pools after coitus. If symptoms occur, they may include pelvic and low back pain, dyspareunia, and exaggeration of premenstrual symptoms.

Uterine prolapse is a more serious type of displacement. The degree of prolapse can vary from mild to complete. In complete prolapse, the cervix and body of the uterus protrude through the vagina and the vagina is inverted (Fig. 25-6).

Uterine displacement and prolapse can be caused by congenital or acquired weakness of the pelvic support structures (often referred to as **pelvic relaxation**). In many cases problems can be related to a delayed but direct result of childbearing. Although extensive damage may be noted and repaired shortly after birth, symptoms related to pelvic relaxation most often appear during the perimenopausal period, when the effects of ovarian hormones on pelvic tissues are lost and atrophic changes begin. Pelvic trauma, stress and strain, and the aging process are also contributing causes. Other causes of pelvic relaxation include reproductive surgery and pelvic radiation.

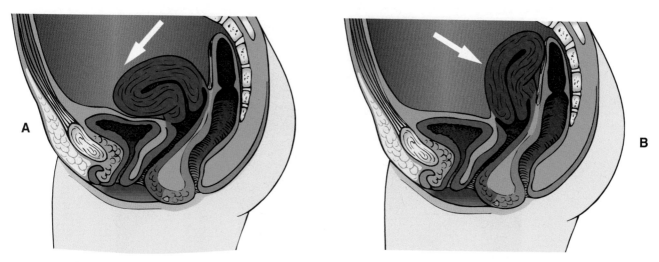

Fig. 25-5 Types of uterine displacement. **A,** Anterior displacement. **B,** Retroversion (backward displacement of uterus).

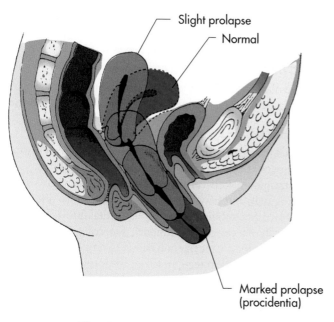

Slight prolapse

Normal

Marked prolapse (procidentia)

Fig. 25-6 Prolapse of uterus.

Clinical manifestations

Generally, symptoms of pelvic relaxation relate to the structure involved: urethra, bladder, uterus, vagina, cul-de-sac, or rectum. The most common complaints are pulling and dragging sensations, pressure, protrusions, fatigue, and low backache. Symptoms may be worse after prolonged standing or deep penile penetration during intercourse. Urinary incontinence may be present.

Cystocele and Rectocele

Cystocele and rectocele almost always accompany uterine prolapse, causing the uterus to sag even further backward and downward into the vagina. *Cystocele* (Fig. 25-7, *A*) is the protrusion of the bladder downward into the vagina that develops when supporting structures in the vesicovaginal septum are injured. Anterior wall relaxation gradually develops over time as a result of congenital defects of supports, childbearing, obesity, or advanced age. When the woman stands, the weakened anterior vaginal wall cannot support the weight of the urine in the bladder; the vesicovaginal septum is forced downward, the bladder is stretched, and its capacity is increased. With time the cystocele enlarges until it protrudes into the vagina. Complete emptying of the bladder is difficult because the cystocele sags below the bladder neck. *Rectocele* is the herniation of the anterior rectal wall through the relaxed or ruptured vaginal fascia and rectovaginal septum; it appears as a large bulge that may be seen through the relaxed introitus (Fig. 25-7, *B*).

Clinical manifestations

Cystoceles and rectoceles often are asymptomatic. If symptoms of cystocele are present, they may include complaints of a bearing-down sensation or that "something is in my vagina." Other symptoms include urinary frequency, retention, incontinence, and possible recurrent cystitis and UTIs. Pelvic examination will reveal a bulging of the anterior wall of the vagina when the woman is asked to bear down. Unless the bladder neck and urethra are damaged, urinary continence is unaffected. Women with large cystoceles complain of having to push upward on the sagging anterior vaginal wall to be able to void.

Rectoceles may be small and produce few symptoms, but some are so large that they protrude outside of the vagina when the woman stands. Symptoms are absent when the woman is lying down. A rectocele causes a disturbance in bowel function, the sensation of "bearing down," or the sensation that the pelvic organs are falling out. With a very large rectocele, it may be difficult to have a bowel movement. Each time the woman strains during bowel

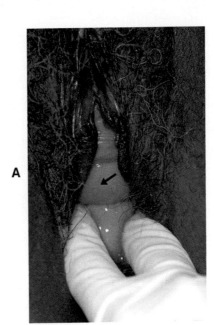
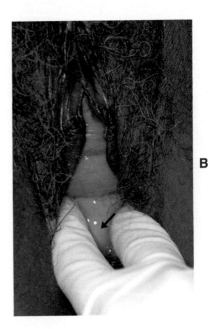

Fig. 25-7 **A,** Cystocele. **B,** Rectocele. (From Seidel, H., Ball, J., Dains, J., & Benedict, G. [2003]. *Mosby's guide to physical examination* [5th ed.]. St. Louis: Mosby.)

evacuation, the feces are forced against the thinned rectovaginal wall, stretching it more. Some women facilitate evacuation by applying digital pressure vaginally to hold up the rectal pouch.

Urinary Incontinence

Urinary incontinence (UI) affects young and middle-aged women, with the prevalence increasing as the woman ages (Sampselle, 2003). Although nulliparous women can have UI, the incidence is higher in women who have given birth and also increases with parity (Sampselle, 2003). Conditions that disturb urinary control include stress incontinence, because of sudden increases in intraabdominal pressure (such as from sneezing or coughing); urge incontinence, caused by disorders of the bladder and urethra, such as urethritis and urethral stricture, trigonitis, and cystitis; neuropathies, such as multiple sclerosis, diabetic neuritis, and pathologic conditions of the spinal cord; and congenital and acquired urinary tract abnormalities.

Stress incontinence may follow injury to bladder neck structures. A sphincter mechanism at the bladder neck compresses the upper urethra, pulls it upward behind the symphysis, and forms an acute angle at the junction of the posterior urethral wall and the base of the bladder (Fig. 25-8). To empty the bladder, the sphincter complex relaxes and the trigone contracts to open the internal urethral orifice and pull the contracting bladder wall upward, forcing urine out. The angle between the urethra and the base of the bladder is lost or increased if the supporting pubococcygeus muscle is injured; this change, coupled with urethrocele, causes incontinence. Urine spurts out when the woman is asked to bear down or cough in the lithotomy position.

Clinical manifestations

Involuntary leaking of urine is the main sign. Episodes of leaking are common during coughing, laughing, and exercise.

Genital Fistulas

Genital fistulas are perforations between genital tract organs. Most occur between the bladder and the genital tract (e.g., vesicovaginal); between the urethra and the vagina (urethrovaginal); and between the rectum or sigmoid colon and the vagina (rectovaginal) (Fig. 25-9). Genital fistulas may also be a result of a congenital anomaly, gynecologic surgery, obstetric trauma, cancer, radiation therapy, gynecologic trauma, or infection (e.g., in the episiotomy).

Clinical manifestations

Signs and symptoms of vaginal fistulas depend on the site but may include presence of urine, flatus, or feces in the vagina; odors of urine or feces in the vagina; and irritation of vaginal tissues.

CARE MANAGEMENT ■

Assessment for problems related to structural disorders of the uterus and vagina focuses primarily on the genitourinary tract, the reproductive organs, bowel elimination, and psychosocial and sexual factors. A complete health history, physical examination, and laboratory tests are done to support the appropriate medical diagnosis. The nurse needs to assess the woman's knowledge of the disorder, its management, and the possible prognosis.

The health care team works together to treat the disorders related to alterations in pelvic support and to assist the

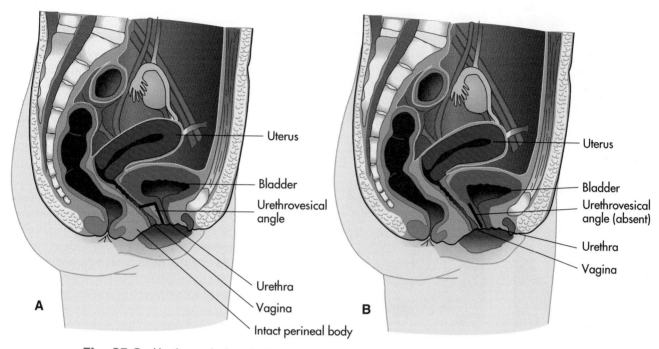

Fig. 25-8 Urethrovesical angle. **A,** Normal angle. **B,** Widening (absence) of angle.

woman in management of her symptoms. In general, nurses working with these women can provide information and self-care education to prevent problems before they occur, to manage or reduce symptoms and promote comfort and hygiene if symptoms are already present, and to recognize when further intervention is needed. This information can be part of all postpartum discharge teaching or can be provided at

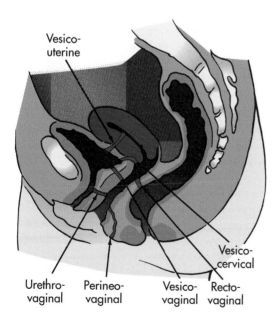

Fig. 25-9 Types of fistulas that may develop in vagina, uterus, and rectum. (From Phipps, W., Sands, J., & Marek, J. [2003]. *Medical-surgical nursing: Health and illness perspectives* [7th ed.]. St. Louis: Mosby.)

postpartum follow-up visits in clinics or physician or nurse-midwife offices or during postpartum home visits.

Interventions for specific problems depend on the problem and the severity of the symptoms. If discomfort related to uterine displacement is a problem, several interventions can be implemented to treat uterine displacement. Kegel exercises (see p. 93) can be performed several times daily to increase muscle strength. A knee-chest position performed for a few minutes several times a day can correct a mildly retroverted uterus. A fitted pessary device may be inserted in the vagina to support the uterus and hold it in the correct position (Fig. 25-10). Usually a pessary is used only for a short time because it can lead to pressure necrosis and vaginitis. Good hygiene is important; some women may be taught to remove the pessary at night, cleanse it, and replace it in the morning. If the pessary is always left in place, regular douching with commercially prepared solutions or weak vinegar solutions (1 tablespoon to 1 quart of water) to remove increased secretions and keep the vaginal pH at 4 to 4.5 are suggested. After a period of treatment, most women are free of symptoms and do not require the pessary. Surgical correction is rarely indicated.

Treatment for uterine prolapse depends on the degree of prolapse. Pessaries may be useful in mild prolapse to support the uterus in the correct position. Estrogen therapy also may be used in the older woman to improve tissue tone. If these conservative treatments do not correct the problem, or if there is a significant degree of prolapse, abdominal or vaginal hysterectomy is usually recommended.

Treatment for a cystocele includes use of a vaginal pessary or surgical repair. Pessaries may not be effective.

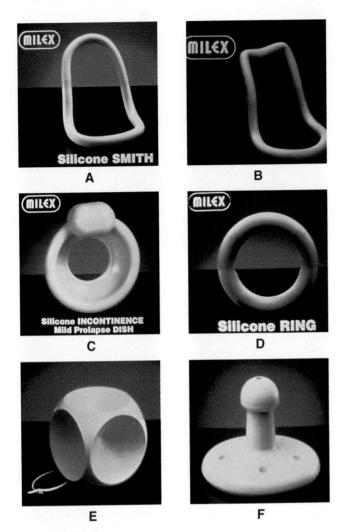

Fig. 25-10 Examples of pessaries. **A,** Smith. **B,** Hodge without support. **C,** Incontinence dish without support. **D,** Ring without support. **E,** Cube. **F,** Gellhorn. (Courtesy Milex Products, Inc., a division of CooperSurgical, Trumbull, CT.)

Anterior repair (colporrhaphy) is the usual surgical procedure and is usually done for large, symptomatic cystoceles. This involves a surgical shortening of pelvic muscles to provide better support for the bladder. An anterior repair is often combined with a vaginal hysterectomy.

Small rectoceles may not need treatment. The woman with mild symptoms may get relief from a high-fiber diet and adequate fluid intake, stool softeners, or mild laxatives. Vaginal pessaries usually are not effective. Large rectoceles that are causing significant symptoms are usually repaired surgically. A posterior repair (colporrhaphy) is the usual procedure. This surgery is performed vaginally and involves shortening the pelvic muscles to provide better support for the rectum. Anterior and posterior repairs may be performed at the same time and with a vaginal hysterectomy.

Mild to moderate UI can be significantly decreased or relieved in many women by bladder training and pelvic muscle (Kegel) exercises (Sampselle, 2003). Other management strategies include pelvic flow support devices (i.e., pessaries),

estrogen therapy, insertion of an artificial urethral sphincter, and surgery (e.g., anterior repair) (Stenchever et al., 2001).

Nursing care of the woman with a cystocele, rectocele, or fistula requires great sensitivity, because the woman's reactions are often intense. She may become withdrawn or hostile because of embarrassment caused by odors and soiling of her clothing that are beyond her control. She may have concerns about engaging in sexual activities because her partner is repelled by these problems. The nurse may tactfully suggest hygiene practices that reduce odor. Commercial deodorizing douches are available, or noncommercial solutions, such as chlorine solution (1 teaspoon of chlorine household bleach to 1 quart of water) may be used. The chlorine solution is also useful for external perineal irrigation. Sitz baths and thorough washing of the genitals with unscented, mild soap and warm water help. Sparse dusting with deodorizing powders can be useful. If a rectovaginal fistula is present, enemas given before leaving the house may provide temporary relief from oozing of fecal material until corrective surgery is performed. Irritated skin and tissues may benefit from use of a heat lamp or application of an emollient ointment. Hygienic care is time consuming and may need to be repeated frequently throughout the day; protective pads or pants may need to be worn. All of these activities can be demoralizing to the woman and frustrating to her and her family.

POSTPARTUM PSYCHOLOGIC COMPLICATIONS

Mental health disorders have implications for the mother, the newborn, and the entire family. Such conditions can interfere with attachment to the newborn and family integration, and some may threaten the safety and well-being of the mother, newborn, and other children.

Mood Disorders

Mood disorders are the predominant mental health disorder in the postpartum period, typically occurring within 4 weeks of childbirth (American Psychiatric Association [APA], 2000). Many women experience a mild depression, or "baby blues," after the birth of a child. Others can have more serious depressions that can eventually incapacitate them to the point of being unable to care for themselves or their babies. Nurses are strategically positioned to offer anticipatory guidance, to assess the mental health of new mothers, to offer therapeutic interventions, and to refer when necessary. Failure to do so may result in tragic consequences.

The Diagnostic and Statistical Manual of Mental Disorders contains the official guidelines for the assessment and diagnosis of psychiatric illness (APA, 2000). However, specific criteria for postpartum depression (PPD) are not listed. Instead, postpartum onset can be specified for any mood disorder either without psychotic features (i.e., PPD) or with psychotic features (i.e., postpartum psychosis) if the onset occurs within 4 weeks of childbirth (APA, 2000).

Etiology and risk factors

The cause of PPD may be biologic, psychologic, situational, or multifactorial. A personal history or a family history of mood disorder, mood and anxiety symptoms in the antepartal period, as well as postpartum blues increases the risk for PPD (APA, 2000). In a metaanalysis of 84 studies published in the 1990s, Beck (2001) found 13 risk factors for PPD, four of which had not been identified previously as predictors. The effect sizes of the risk factors identified in an updated metaanalysis revealed that 10 predictors have a medium relation with PPD, and three predictors have a small relation (Beck, 2002). A revised version of the Postpartum Depression Predictors Inventory (PDPI) has been published (Beck, 2002). Box 25-5 lists all 13 risk factors for PPD, with those having the greater effect size listed first.

In addition, research has found that fatigue is an important predictor of PPD (Bozoky & Corwin, 2002). As early as 7 postpartum days, fatigue is predictive of depression at postpartum day 28.

Postpartum depression without psychotic features

PPD is an intense and pervasive sadness with severe and labile mood swings and is more serious and persistent than postpartum blues. Intense fears, anger, anxiety, and despondency that persist past the baby's first few weeks are not a normal part of postpartum blues. Occurring in approximately 10% to 15% of new mothers, these symptoms rarely disappear without outside help. The majority of these mothers do not seek help from any source, and only about 20% consult a health professional. The occurrence of PPD among teenage mothers was more than 2.5 times that for older mothers (Herrick, 2002). African-American mothers were twice as likely as Caucasian mothers to experience PPD. Younger mothers (younger than 20 years) and those with less than a high school education were significantly less likely to

seek help and had higher rates of PPD (Herrick, 2002). Mothers who had no one to talk to about their problems after giving birth had a high rate of PPD and a low rate of help seeking.

The symptoms of postpartum major depression do not differ from the symptoms of nonpostpartum mood disorders except that the mother's ruminations of guilt and inadequacy feed her worries about being an incompetent and inadequate parent. In PPD, there may be odd food cravings (often sweet desserts) and binges with abnormal appetite and weight gain. New mothers report an increased yearning for sleep, sleeping heavily but awakening instantly with any infant noise, and an inability to go back to sleep after infant feedings.

A distinguishing feature of PPD is irritability. These episodes of irritability may flare up with little provocation, and they may sometimes escalate to violent outbursts or dissolve into uncontrollable sobbing. Many of these outbursts are directed against significant others ("He never helps me") or the baby ("She cries all the time and I feel like hitting her"). Women with postpartum major depressive episodes often have severe anxiety, panic attacks, and spontaneous crying long after the usual duration of baby blues.

Many women feel especially guilty about having depressive feelings at a time when they believe they should be happy. They may be reluctant to discuss their symptoms or their negative feelings toward the child. A prominent feature of PPD is rejection of the infant, often caused by abnormal jealousy (APA, 2000). The mother may be obsessed by the

---

BOX 25-5

Risk Factors for Postpartum Depression

- Prenatal depression
- Low self-esteem
- Stress of child care
- Prenatal anxiety
- Life stress
- Lack of social support
- Marital relationship problems
- History of depression
- "Difficult" infant temperament
- Postpartum blues
- Single status
- Low socioeconomic status
- Unplanned or unwanted pregnancy

Source: Beck, C. (2001). Predictors of postpartum depression: An update. *Nursing Research, 50*(5), 275-282; & Beck, C. (2002). Revision of the Postpartum Depression Predictors Inventory. *Journal of Obstetric, Gynecologic, and Neonatal Nursing, 31*(4), 394-402.

Critical Thinking Exercise

Postpartum Depression

The nurses on the postpartum unit are revising their discharge teaching plan. Sara would like to include a section on postpartum depression (PPD). Joan thinks this information is not needed as she believes most of the mothers are happy and there is so much else to teach. They ask you, the nurse educator on the unit, for advice on making a decision about including information about postpartum depression. What advice will you give?

1 Evidence—Is there sufficient evidence to draw conclusions about advice to give about the inclusion of postpartum depression information in discharge teaching?
2 Assumptions—Describe underlying assumptions about each of following issues:
   a. Anticipatory guidance as a nursing intervention for PPD
   b. Women and risks of depression, including PPD
   c. Effects of PPD on parenting
3 What implications and priorities are needed in developing a discharge teaching plan?
4 Does the evidence objectively support your conclusion?
5 Are there alternative perspectives to your conclusion?

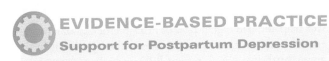

EVIDENCE-BASED PRACTICE
Support for Postpartum Depression

BACKGROUND

- Clinicians use various definitions of postpartum depression, with ranges of incidence varying from 7% to 30%. Although many define any depression lasting longer than 6 months as chronic, there is no consensus regarding duration. Symptoms can be disabling to the woman, including excessive fatigue, insomnia, inability to cope, suicidal ideation, and lack of maternal feelings for the baby. It is distinguished from postpartum psychosis, a psychiatric emergency that may include hallucinations, delusions, and disorganized thoughts and behaviors. Postpartum depression can disrupt relationships, especially with her partner, and her infant can experience attachment disorders and cognitive delays. Causes of postpartum depression are unknown. Hormones may challenge some threshold after birth in the psychologically vulnerable woman. Some factors associated with postpartum depression include age, parity, anxiety, social class, obstetric complications, past psychiatric history, psychosocial and marital stressors, and unplanned pregnancy. Isolation seems to exacerbate the symptoms, and support seems to relieve them. Support has been found to be beneficial to pregnant and laboring women (see "Continuous Labor Support," Evidence-Based Practice box for Chapter 14). A meaningful relationship with a supportive caregiver reinforces the concept that the woman matters to someone, increasing feelings of well-being, control, and positive affect. Although medications are sometimes useful in postpartum depression, researchers have found compliance to be low.

OBJECTIVES

- The authors sought evidence of the effectiveness of professional and/or social support for women who have been diagnosed with postpartum depression. The interventions were emotional support, counseling, or tangible assistance (child care, household assistance) via phone, home or clinic visits, individually or in groups, to women with postpartum depression. The controls were women with postpartum depression receiving "usual care" in that setting.
- Outcome measures could include unbiased indicators of maternal or family morbidity, duration and resolution of depression, and social functioning.

METHODS
Search Strategy

- The reviewers searched Cochrane, MEDLINE, and 38 relevant journals via Zetoc, an electronic current awareness service. Search keywords were not noted.
- Two randomized, controlled trials met the criteria, representing 137 women from the United Kingdom. In the 1989 trial, the intervention began at 12 weeks postpartum

and was provided by health visitors trained in nondirective counseling who made eight half-hour home visits. The 1997 trial also began at 12 weeks and involved six sessions with a psychologist trained in cognitive-behavior therapy.

Statistical Analyses

- Both trials used the Edinburgh Postnatal Depression Scale, which not only has good evidence of reliability and validity but also allowed pooling of the data. The odds ratio and 95% confidence intervals were calculated for the categoric data.

FINDINGS

- At 25 weeks postpartum, the mothers who had received the intervention were significantly less depressed than the controls.

LIMITATIONS

- Postpartum depression was confirmed by a clinical interview, but the reliability and validity of that was not addressed. The participants were not blinded to the treatment allocation, but the health assessors and outcome assessors were blinded to group. One study had a 30% dropout rate, which may have introduced bias. Both the number of studies (i.e., both are from one country) and samples are small, limiting generalizability.

CONCLUSIONS

- Supportive intervention in the postpartum period may be effective in relieving postpartum depression.

IMPLICATIONS FOR PRACTICE

- Isolation may contribute to postpartum depression. Social or professional support may, in theory, help alleviate depression in the vulnerable postpartum woman, but the evidence is too scanty to make policy recommendations.

IMPLICATIONS FOR FURTHER RESEARCH

- Larger studies of the benefits suggested by this small review for improving postpartum depression with increased support are needed. Of urgent interest is the optimum timing and duration of such intervention, especially as a preventive measure. The type and training of effective support caregivers, the type of intervention, and the setting are important to determine. Perhaps the family can become involved in the support intervention. Cost is a primary driving factor in mental health services, which need evidence of cost-effectiveness. Long-term follow-up may provide insight into the benefits derived for the mother and the infant and family by alleviating postpartum depression.

Reference: Ray, K., & Hodnett, E. (2001). Caregiver support for postpartum depression (Cochrane Review), In *The Cochrane Library*, Issue 2, 2004. Chichester, UK: John Wiley & Sons.

notion that the offspring may take her place in her partner's affections. Attitudes toward the infant may include disinterest, annoyance with care demands, and blaming because of her lack of maternal feeling. When observed, she may appear awkward in her responses to the baby. Obsessive thoughts about harming the child are very frightening to her. Often she does not share these thoughts because of embarrassment, but when she does, other family members become very frightened.

Medical management. The natural course is one of gradual improvement over the 6 months after birth. Support treatment alone is not efficacious for major postpartum depression. Pharmacologic intervention is needed in most instances. Treatment options include antidepressants, anxiolytic agents, and electroconvulsive therapy (ECT). Psychotherapy focuses on the mother's fears and concerns regarding her new responsibilities and roles, as well as monitoring for suicidal or homicidal thoughts. For some women, hospitalization is necessary.

Postpartum depression with psychotic features

Postpartum psychosis is a syndrome most often characterized by depression (as described previously), delusions, and thoughts by the mother of harming either the infant or herself (Sadock & Sadock, 2000). A postpartum mood disorder with psychotic features occurs in 1 to 2 per 1000 births and may occur more often in primiparas (Sadock & Sadock, 2000). Once a woman has had one postpartum episode with psychotic features, there is a 30% to 50% likelihood of recurrence with each subsequent birth (APA, 2000).

Symptoms often begin within days after the birth, although the mean time to onset is 2 to 3 weeks and almost always within 8 weeks of birth (Sadock & Sadock, 2000). Characteristically, the woman begins to complain of fatigue, insomnia, and restlessness and may have episodes of tearfulness and emotional lability. Complaints regarding the inability to move, stand, or work are also common. Later, suspiciousness, confusion, incoherence, irrational statements, and obsessive concerns about the baby's health and welfare may be present (Sadock & Sadock, 2000). Delusions may be present in 50% of all women, and hallucinations in approximately 25%. Auditory hallucinations that command the mother to kill the infant can also occur in severe cases. When delusions are present, they are often related to the infant. The mother may think the infant is possessed by the devil, has special powers, or is destined for a terrible fate (APA, 2000). Grossly disorganized behavior may be manifested as a disinterest in the infant or an inability to provide care. Some will insist that something is wrong with the baby or accuse nurses or family members of hurting or poisoning him or her. Nurses are advised to be alert for mothers who are agitated, overactive, confused, complaining, or suspicious.

A specific illness included in depression with psychotic features is bipolar disorder. This mood disorder is preceded or accompanied by manic episodes, characterized by elevated, expansive, or irritable moods. Clinical manifestations of a manic episode include at least three of the following symptoms that have been significantly present for at least 1 week: grandiosity, decreased need for sleep, pressured speech, flight of ideas, distractibility, psychomotor agitation, and excessive involvement in pleasurable activities without regard for negative consequences (APA, 2000). Because these women are hyperactive, they may not take the time to eat or sleep, which leads to inadequate nutrition, dehydration, and sleep deprivation. While in a manic state, mothers will need constant supervision when caring for their infants. Mostly they will be too preoccupied to provide child care.

Medical management. A favorable outcome is associated with a good premorbid adjustment (before the onset of the disorder) and a supportive family network (Sadock & Sadock, 2000). Because mood disorders are usually episodic, women may experience another episode of symptoms within a year or two of the birth. Postpartum psychosis is a psychiatric emergency, and the mother will probably need psychiatric hospitalization. Antipsychotics and mood stabilizers such as lithium are the treatments of choice. If the mother is breastfeeding, some sources recommend that no pharmacologic agents should be prescribed (Sadock & Sadock, 2000), but other sources advise caution while prescribing some agents (Stowe, Strader, & Nemeroff, 2001). Antipsychotics and lithium should be avoided in breastfeeding mothers, but other mood stabilizers may be compatible with breastfeeding (see later discussion). It is usually advantageous for the mother to have contact with her baby if she so desires, but visits must be closely supervised. Psychotherapy is indicated after the period of acute psychosis is past.

CARE MANAGEMENT

Even though the prevalence of PPD is fairly well established, women are unlikely to seek help from a mental health care provider. Primary health care providers can usually recognize severe PPD or postpartum psychosis but may miss milder forms; even if the disorder is recognized, the woman may be treated inappropriately or subtherapeutically (Gold, 2002). In as many as 50% of women with PPD, the disorder will go undetected (Beck & Gable, 2001).

Assessment and Nursing Diagnoses

To recognize symptoms of PPD as early as possible, the nurse should be an active listener and demonstrate a caring attitude. Nurses cannot depend on women volunteering unsolicited information about their depression or asking for help. The nurse should observe for signs of depression and ask appropriate questions to determine moods, appetite, sleep, energy and fatigue levels, and ability to concentrate. Examples of ways to initiate conversation include the following: "Now that you have had your baby, how are things going for you? Have you had to change many things in your life since having the baby?" and "How much time do you spend crying?" If the nurse assesses that the new mother is depressed, she or he must ask if the mother has thought about hurting herself or the baby. The woman may be more willing to answer honestly if the nurse says, "Lots of women feel depressed after having a baby, and some feel so badly that they think about hurting themselves or the baby. Have you had these thoughts?"

Nurses can use screening tools in assessing whether the depressive symptoms have progressed from postpartum blues to PPD. Examples are the Edinburgh Postnatal Depression Scale (EPDS) (Cox, Holden, & Sagovsky, 1987) and the PDPI (Beck, 2002).

The EPDS is a self-report assessment designed specifically to identify women experiencing PPD. It has been used and validated in studies in numerous cultures (Eberhard-Gran, Eskild, Tambs, Opjordsmoen, & Samuelsen, 2001) and has even been used to measure depression and anxiety in fathers (partners) (Matthey, Barnett, Kavanagh, & Howie, 2001). The assessment tool asks the woman to respond to 10 statements about the common symptoms of depression. The woman is asked to choose the response that is closest to describing how she has felt for the past week.

Through focused research over at least a decade, Beck has developed and continues to refine the Postpartum Depression Checklist (PDC) and the Postpartum Depression Screening Scale (PDSS) (Beck & Gable, 2000; Beck & Gable, 2001). The latest revision (PDPI) is a checklist of 13 symptoms of PPD. The published tool is designed to be used by nurses and other health care providers to elicit information from the woman during an interview during pregnancy and continuing in the postpartum period to assess risk (Beck, 2002). Areas assessed include the predictors of depression as listed in Box 25-5.

If the initial interaction reveals some question that the woman might be depressed, a formal screening is helpful in determining the urgency of the referral and the type of provider. Also important is the need to assess the woman's family members because they may be able to offer valuable information, as well as have a need to express how they have been affected by the woman's emotional disorder (Maley, 2002).

Planning is focused on meeting the individualized needs of the family to ensure safety, especially for the mother and infant and any other children, and to facilitate functional family coping. Nursing diagnoses may include the following:

- *Risk for self-directed (mother) or other-directed (children) violence related to*
  —postpartum depression
- *Situational low self-esteem in the mother related to*
  —stresses associated with role changes
- *Disabled family coping related to*
  —increased care needs of mother and infant
- *Risk for impaired parenting related to*
  —inability of depressed mother to attach to infant

- *Risk for injury to newborn related to*
  —mother's depression (inattention to infant's needs for hygiene, nutrition, safety) and psychotropic medications via breast milk

Expected Outcomes of Care

Specific measurable criteria can be developed based on the following general outcomes:
- The mother will no longer be depressed.
- The mother's and infant's physical well-being will be maintained.
- The family will cope effectively.
- Family members will demonstrate continued healthy growth and development.
- The infant will be fully integrated into the family.

Plan of Care and Interventions
On the postpartum unit

The postpartum nurse must observe the new mother carefully for any signs of tearfulness and conduct further assessments as necessary. PPD must be discussed by nurses to prepare new parents for potential problems in the postpartum period (Patient Instructions for Self-Care box and Chapter 17). The family must be able to recognize the symptoms and know where to go for help. Written materials that explain what the woman can do to prevent depression could be used as part of discharge planning.

Mothers are often discharged from the hospital before the blues or depression occurs. If the postpartum nurse is concerned about the mother, a mental health consultation should be requested before the mother leaves the hospital. Routine instructions regarding PPD should be given to the person who comes to take the woman home; for example, "If you notice that your wife (or daughter) is upset or crying a lot, please call the postpartum care provider immediately—don't wait for the routine postpartum appointment."

NURSE ALERT *Because the newborn may be scheduled for a checkup before the mother's 6-week checkup, nurses in well-baby clinics or pediatrician offices should be alert for signs of PPD in new mothers and be knowledgeable about community referral resources.*

In the home and community

Postpartum home visits can reduce the incidence of or complications from depression. A brief home visit or phone call at least once a week until the new mother returns for her postpartum visit may save the life of a mother and her infant; however, these contacts may not be feasible or available. Supervision of the mother with emotional complications may become a prime concern. Because depression can greatly interfere with her mothering functions, family and friends may need to participate in the infant's care. This is a time for the extended family and friends to determine what they can do to help, and the nurse can work with them to

PATIENT INSTRUCTIONS FOR SELF-CARE

Activities to Prevent Postpartum Depression

- Share knowledge about postpartum emotional problems with close family and friends.
- Take care of yourself: eat a balanced diet, exercise on a regular basis, and get enough sleep. Ask someone to take care of the baby so that you can get a full night's sleep.
- Share your feelings with someone close to you; don't isolate yourself at home.
- Don't overcommit yourself or feel like you need to be a superwoman.
- Don't place unrealistic expectations on yourself.
- Don't be ashamed of having emotional problems after your baby is born—it happens to approximately 15% of women.

ensure adequate supervision of the woman and their understanding of the woman's mental illness.

When the woman has PPD, a partner often reacts with confusion, shock, denial, and anger and feels neglected and blamed. The nurse can talk with the woman about how her condition is hard for him, too, and that he is probably very worried about her. Men often withdraw or criticize when they are deeply worried about their significant others. The nurse can provide nonjudgmental opportunities for the partner to verbalize feelings and concerns, help the partner identify positive coping strategies, and be a source of encouragement for the partner to continue supporting the woman. Both the woman and her partner need an opportunity to express their needs, fears, thoughts, and feelings in a nonjudgmental environment.

Even if the mother is severely depressed, hospitalization can be avoided if adequate resources can be mobilized to ensure safety for both mother and infant. The nurse in home health care will need to make frequent phone calls or home visits to do assessment and counseling. Community resources that may be helpful are temporary child care or foster care, homemaker service, Meals on Wheels, parenting guidance centers, mother's-day-out programs, and telephone support groups or other support programs (Wroblewski & Tallon, 2004) (see Resources at end of chapter).

Referral. Women with moderate to severe PPD should be referred to a mental health therapist, such as an advanced practice psychiatric nurse, for evaluation and therapy to avoid the effects that PPD can have on the woman and on her relationships with her partner, baby, and other children (Brown, 2001). Inpatient psychiatric hospitalization may be necessary. This decision is made when the safety needs of the mother or children are threatened.

Providing safety. When depression is suspected, the nurse asks, "Have you thought about hurting yourself?" If delusional thinking about the baby is suspected, the nurse asks, "Have you thought about hurting your baby?" There

are four criteria to measure in assessing the seriousness of a suicidal plan: method, availability, specificity, and lethality. Has the woman specified a method? Is the method of choice available? How specific is the plan? If the method is concrete and detailed, with access to it right at hand, the suicide risk increases. How lethal is the method? The most lethal method is shooting, with hanging a close second. The least lethal is slashing one's wrists. Medication overdose can also be used to cause death.

NURSE ALERT *Suicidal thoughts or attempts are one of the most serious symptoms of PPD and require immediate assessment and intervention (Levy, Sanders, & Sabraw, 2002).*

Psychiatric hospitalization. Women with postpartum psychosis are a psychiatric emergency and must be referred immediately to a psychiatrist who is experienced in working with women with PPD, who can prescribe medication and other forms of therapy and assess the need for hospitalization.

LEGAL TIP **Legal Commitment**

If a woman with PPD is experiencing active suicidal ideation or harmful delusions about the baby and is unwilling to seek treatment, legal intervention may be necessary to commit the woman to an inpatient setting for treatment.

Within the hospital setting, the reintroduction of the baby to the mother can occur at the mother's own pace. A schedule is set for increasing the number of hours the mother cares for the baby over several days, culminating in the infant staying overnight in the mother's room. This allows the mother to experience meeting the infant's needs and giving up sleep for the baby, a situation difficult for new mothers even under ideal conditions. The mother's readiness for discharge and caring for the baby is assessed. Her interactions with her baby are also carefully supervised and guided.

Nurses should also observe the mother for signs of bonding with the baby. Attachment behaviors are defined as eye-to-eye contact; physical contact that involves holding, touching, cuddling, and talking to the baby and calling the baby by name; and the initiation of appropriate care. A staff member is assigned to keep the baby in sight at all times. Indirect teaching, praise, and encouragement are designed to bolster the mother's self-esteem and self-confidence.

Psychotropic medications. PPD is usually treated with antidepressant medications. If the woman with PPD is not breastfeeding, antidepressants can be prescribed without special precautions. The commonly used antidepressant drugs are often divided into four groups: selective serotonin reuptake inhibitors (SSRIs), heterocyclics (including the tricyclic antidepressants [TCAs]), monoamine oxidase inhibitors (MAOIs), and other antidepressant agents not in the above classifications (Keltner & Folks, 2001) (Box 25-6).

BOX 25-6

Antidepressant Medications

SELECTIVE SEROTONIN REUPTAKE INHIBITORS
Citalopram (Celexa)
Fluoxetine (Prozac)
Fluvoxamine (Luvox)
Paroxetine (Paxil)
Sertraline (Zoloft)

TRICYCLICS
Amitriptyline (Elavil)
Amoxapine (Asendin)
Clomipramine (Anafranil)
Desipramine (Norpramin)
Doxepin (Sinequan)
Imipramine (Tofranil)
Nortriptyline (Pamelor)
Protriptyline (Vivactil)

QUADRICYCLICS
Maprotiline (Ludiomil)
Mirtazapine (Remeron)

MONOAMINE OXIDASE INHIBITORS
Phenelzine (Nardil)
Tranylcypromine (Parnate)

OTHER AGENTS
Bupropion (Wellbutrin) IR and SR
Nefazodone (Serzone)
Trazodone (Desyrel)
Venlafaxine (Effexor)

The SSRIs are prescribed more frequently today than other groups of antidepressant medications. They are relatively safe and carry fewer side effects than the TCAs. The most frequent side effects with the SSRIs are gastrointestinal disturbances (nausea, diarrhea), headache, and insomnia. In approximately one third of patients the SSRIs reduce libido, arousal, or orgasmic function.

The TCAs cause many central nervous system (CNS) and peripheral nervous system (PNS) side effects. A common CNS effect is sedation, and this could easily interfere with mothers caring for their babies. A mother could fall asleep while holding the baby and drop him or her, or she could have trouble getting fully awake during the night to care for the baby. Other side effects include weight gain, tremors, grand mal seizures, nightmares, agitation or mania, and extrapyramidal side effects. Anticholinergic side effects include dry mouth, blurred vision (usually temporary), difficulty voiding, constipation, sweating, and orgasm difficulty (Keltner & Folks, 2001).

Hypertensive crisis is the main reason that MAOIs are not prescribed more frequently. The woman should be taught to watch for signs of hypertensive crisis—throbbing, occipital headache, stiff neck, chills, nausea, flushing, retroorbital pain, apprehension, pallor, sweating, chest pain, and palpi-

tations (Keltner & Folks, 2001). This crisis is brought on by the woman eating foods that contain tyramine, a sympathomimetic pressor amine, which normally is broken down by the enzyme monoamine oxidase. The nurse must do extensive teaching about avoidance of foods that contain tyramine such as aged cheeses, nuts, soy sauce, preserved meats, and tap beers (National Headache Foundation, 2005).

The woman taking mood stabilizers (Box 25-7) must be taught about the many side effects, and especially, for those on lithium, the need to have serum lithium levels assessed every 6 months. Women with severe psychiatric syndromes such as schizophrenia, bipolar disorder, or psychotic depression will probably require antipsychotic medications (Box 25-8). Most of these antipsychotic medications can cause sedation and orthostatic hypotension—both of which could interfere with the mother being able to safely care for her baby. They can also cause PNS effects such as constipation, dry mouth, blurred vision, tachycardia, urinary retention, weight gain, and agranulocytosis. CNS effects may include akathisia, dystonias, parkinsonism-like symptoms, tardive dyskinesia (irreversible), and neuroleptic malignant syndrome (potentially fatal).

Psychotropic medications and lactation. A major clinical dilemma is the psychopharmacologic treatment of women with PPD who want to breastfeed their infants. In the past, women were told to discontinue lactation.

BOX 25-7

Mood Stabilizers

- Carbamazepine (Tegretol XR)
- Clonazepam (Klonopin)
- Divalproex (Depakote)
- Lithium carbonate (Eskalith)

BOX 25-8

Commonly Used Antipsychotic Medications

PHENOTHIAZINES
- Chlorpromazine (Thorazine)
- Fluphenazine (Prolixin)
- Perphenazine (Trilafon)
- Thioridazine (Mellaril)
- Trifluoperazine (Stelazine)

OTHER
- Clozapine (Clozaril)
- Haloperidol (Haldol)
- Loxapine (Loxitane)
- Olanzapine (Zyprexa)
- Pimozide (Orap)
- Quetiapine (Seroquel)
- Risperidone (Risperdal)
- Thiothixene (Navane)
- Ziprasidone (Geodon)

Today, we know that 5% to 17% of all nursing mothers take a prescription medication (Stowe, Strader, & Nemeroff, 2001). The FDA has not approved any psychotropic medication for use during lactation. However, the American Academy of Pediatrics (AAP) has published reports on excretion of medications into human breast milk since 1983. Almost all of the psychotropic medications listed in the 2001 report are drugs for which the effects on the breastfeeding newborn are "unknown but still may be of concern" (AAP, 2001). The reason for the concern is that although the medications appear to be in low concentrations in breast milk (commonly a milk-to-serum ratio of 0.5 to 1), many drugs have a long half-life, and levels may build up in plasma and tissue of nursing infants. Long-term effects on the newborn are unknown (AAP, 2001). Because all psychotropic medications pass through breast milk to the infant, the risks associated with the use of such medication must be weighed against the risks associated with maternal agitation and potentially self-destructive behavior.

Breast milk-excretion studies have demonstrated that antidepressants are present in breast milk, with a milk-to-serum ratio that is typically greater than 1:1 (Stowe, Strader, & Nemeroff, 2001) and often in higher concentrations in the fatty hind milk (Newport, Wilcox, & Stowe, 2001). Most TCAs appear to be safe during breastfeeding. Minimal data are available concerning the SSRIs, so earlier reviews recommended using the secondary amine TCAs. In light of the increasing data on SSRIs, and the lack of adverse reports, these recommendations are likely to be revised (Stowe, Strader, & Nemeroff, 2001). MAOIs are usually avoided; no human data have been published on the newer antidepressants.

The elapsed time between maternal dosing and infant feeding has been shown to affect the amount of antidepressant medication to which the infant is exposed. Adjusting both the schedule of dosing of the antidepressant and the infant's feeding schedule may considerably reduce the concentration of the drug to which the infant is exposed. In addition, eliminating the one daily feeding with the highest concentration may be necessary (Stowe, Strader, & Nemeroff, 2001). Most of the drugs listed in Boxes 25-6 and 25-7 are classified as drugs whose effects on infants are unknown but may be of concern.

Antipsychotic medications are excreted into breast milk. None of these medications has been proven safe during lactation; the AAP does not rate any of the antipsychotic medications as compatible with breastfeeding.

Mood-stabilizing and antimanic medications are present in breast milk. Lithium is contraindicated in breastfeeding. The benefits of breastfeeding and the potential risks must be carefully considered before use of other mood stabilizers (AAP, 2001).

In summary, all psychotropic medications studied to date are excreted in breast milk. The information about adverse effects of psychotropic agents on infants are limited to case reports. The nursing infant's daily dose of psychotropic agents is less than the maternal daily dose. Psychotropic medications are excreted into breast milk with a specific individual time course, allowing the minimization of infant exposure with continuation of breastfeeding. The long-term neurobehavioral effects of infant exposure to psychotropic medications through breastfeeding are unknown. Psychotropic medications for breastfeeding women should be selected if they have greater documentation of prior use, lower FDA risk category, few or no metabolites, and fewer side effects (Stowe, Strader, & Nemeroff, 2001).

Nursing implications. When breastfeeding women have emotional complications and need psychotropic medications, referral to a psychiatrist who specializes in postpartum disorders is preferred. The nurse should reinforce the need to take antidepressants as ordered. Because they do not exert any effect for approximately 2 weeks and usually do not reach full effect for 4 to 6 weeks, many women discontinue taking the medication on their own. Patient and family teaching should reinforce the schedule for taking medications in conjunction with the infant's feeding schedule.

Other treatments for PPD. Other treatments for PPD include complementary or alternative therapies such as those listed in Box 25-9, ECT, and psychotherapy. Alternative therapies may be used alone but often are used with other treatments for PPD. Safety and efficacy studies of these alternative therapies are needed to ensure that care and advice is based on evidence (Tiran & Mack, 2000).

NURSE ALERT *St. John's wort is often used to treat depression. It has not been proven safe for women who are breastfeeding.*

ECT may be used for women with PPD who have not improved with antidepressant therapy. Psychotherapy in the form of group therapy or individual (interpersonal) therapy also has been used with positive results alone and in

---

BOX 25-9

Possible Alternative or Complementary Therapies for Postpartum Depression

- Acupuncture
- Acupressure
- Aromatherapy
- Jasmine
- Ylang-ylang
- Rose
- Herbal remedies
- Lavender tea
- Healing touch or therapeutic touch
- Massage
- Relaxation techniques
- Reflexology
- Yoga

Source: Skidmore-Roth, L. (2004). *Mosby's handbook of herbs and natural supplements* (2nd ed.). St. Louis: Mosby; & Tiran, D., & Mack, S. (Eds.). (2000). *Complementary therapies for pregnancy and childbirth* (2nd ed.). Edinburgh: Baillière Tindall.

conjunction with antidepressant therapy; however, more studies are needed to determine what types of professional support are most effective (Ray & Hodnett, 2001).

Evaluation

The nurse can be assured that care has been effective if the physical well-being of the mother and infant is maintained, the mother and family are able to cope effectively, and each family member continues to show a healthy adaptation to the presence of the new member of the family (Plan of Care).

Postpartum Onset of Panic Disorder

Approximately 3% to 5% of women develop panic disorder or obsessive-compulsive disorder in the postpartum period. Panic attacks are discrete periods in which there is the sudden onset of intense apprehension, fearfulness, or terror

(APA, 2000). During these attacks, symptoms such as shortness of breath, palpitations, chest pain, choking, smothering sensations, and fear of losing control are present. They have intrusive thoughts about terrible injury done to the infant, such as stabbing or burns, sometimes by themselves. Rarely do they harm the baby. Nurses need only to listen to hear symptoms of panic disorder. Usually these women are so distraught that they will share with whomever will listen. Oftentimes the family has tried to tell them that what they are experiencing is normal, but they know differently.

Medical management

Treatment is usually a combination of medications, education, psychotherapy, and cognitive behavioral interventions, along with an attempt to identify any medical or physiologic contributors. Antidepressants such as SSRIs may be prescribed (Brown, 2001), and sertraline (Zoloft) and

---

CD: Plan of Care—Postpartum Depression

✍ PLAN OF CARE *Postpartum Depression*

NURSING DIAGNOSIS Risk for injury to the woman and/or newborn related to woman's emotional state and/or treatment

Expected Outcomes *The mother and newborn will remain free of injury. The woman's family will verbalize understanding of the need for maternal and infant supervision and have a plan to provide that supervision.*

Nursing Interventions/*Rationales*

- Assess the postpartum woman for risk factors for depression (before discharge) *to determine if she is at risk and in need of prompt interventions or referral.*
- Provide information about signs of PPD to woman and family *to promote prompt recognition of problems.*
- Observe maternal-infant interactions before discharge *to determine appropriateness.*
- Maintain frequent contact with woman by telephone calls and home visits *to determine if further interventions are necessary, because most postpartum mothers are discharged early from the inpatient setting.*
- Counsel woman and family to telephone health care provider if behaviors indicating depression, such as crying, increase *to provide prompt care and referral if necessary and avoid injury to newborn and mother.*
- Provide opportunities for woman and family to verbalize feelings and concerns in a nonjudgmental setting *to promote a trusting relationship.*
- Assess woman for any suicidal thoughts or plans *to provide for safety of woman and infant.*
- Assist family to develop a plan for maternal and infant supervision *to provide for safety of woman and infant.*
- Provide information about community resources for assistance *to ensure care if woman is unable to care for herself or infant.*
- Reinforce teaching or refer breastfeeding mother to lactation consultant *to obtain information regarding effects of antidepressant and antipsychotic medications.*

NURSING DIAGNOSIS Disabled family coping related to postpartum maternal depression as evidenced by family members' denial of woman's illness

Expected Outcomes *Family will identify positive coping mechanisms and initiate a plan to cope with the woman's depression.*

Nursing Interventions/*Rationales*

- Provide opportunity for family and significant others to verbalize feelings and concerns *to establish a trusting relationship.*
- Give information to the family regarding postpartum depression *to clarify any misconceptions or misinformation.*
- Assist family to identify positive coping mechanisms that have been effective during past crises *to promote active participation in care.*
- Assist family to identify community sources of support *to provide additional resources as needed.*
- Refer family to mental health counselor as needed *to provide further expertise from a mental health professional.*

NURSING DIAGNOSIS Risk for impaired parenting related to inability of mother to attach to infant

Expected Outcomes *Woman demonstrates appropriate attachment behaviors in infant interactions. Woman expresses satisfaction with infant.*

Nursing Interventions/*Rationales*

- Observe maternal-infant interactions *to assess quality of interactions and to determine need for interventions.*
- Encourage woman to express her anxiety, fears, or other feelings *to allow woman to ventilate her concerns and have them accepted.*
- Encourage the woman to have as much contact with infant as possible *to minimize separation and to promote attachment.*
- Demonstrate infant care and explain infant behaviors *to enhance mother's care abilities and understanding of infant's abilities.*
- Make referrals as needed to community resources *to assist the woman in developing parenting skills or promoting confidence in infant care.*

paroxetine (Paxil) are approved in the United States for the treatment of panic disorder; fluvoxamine (Luvox) may be especially helpful with obsessions (Keltner & Folks, 2001).

Nursing considerations

The following nursing interventions are suggested:

- Education is a crucial nursing intervention. New mothers should be provided with anticipatory guidance concerning the possibility of panic attacks during the postpartum period. Preparing for the attacks may help decrease their unexpected, terrifying nature (Beck, 1998).
- Women can be reassured that it is common to feel a sense of impending doom and fear of insanity during panic attacks. These fears are temporary and disappear once the panic attack is over (Beck, 1998).
- Nurses can help women identify panic triggers that are particular to their own lives. Keeping a diary can help identify the triggers (Beck, 1998).
- Family and social supports are helpful. The new mother is encouraged to put usual chores on hold and to ask for and accept help.

- Support groups allow these mothers to experience comfort in seeing others like themselves.
- Sensory interventions such as music therapy and aromatherapy are nonintrusive and inexpensive.
- Behavioral interventions such as breathing exercises and progressive muscle relaxation can be helpful (Fishel, 1998).
- Cognitive interventions such as positive self-talk training, reframing and redefining, and reassurance can alter the negative thinking (Fishel, 1998).

COMMUNITY ACTIVITY

Identify resources in your community for women with postpartum depression. Develop criteria to evaluate these resources (e.g., accessibility, costs), and compare the resources according to the results of your analysis including the strengths and weaknesses (or pros and cons) of each resource.

Key Points

- PPH is the most common and most serious type of excessive obstetric blood loss.
- Hemorrhagic (hypovolemic) shock is an emergency situation in which the perfusion of body organs may become severely compromised, leading to significant risk of morbidity or death for the mother.
- The potential hazards of the therapeutic interventions may further compromise the woman with a hemorrhagic disorder.
- Clotting disorders are associated with many obstetric complications.
- The first symptom of postpartum infection is usually fever greater than 38° C on 2 consecutive days in the first 10 postpartum days (after the first 24 hours).
- Prevention is the most effective and inexpensive treatment of postpartum infection.

- Structural disorders of the uterus and vagina related to pelvic relaxation and UI may be a delayed result of childbearing.
- Bladder training and pelvic muscle exercises can significantly decrease or relieve mild to moderate UI.
- Mood disorders account for most mental health disorders in the postpartum period.
- Identification of women at greatest risk for postpartum depression can be facilitated by use of various screening tools.
- Suicidal thoughts or attempts are one of the most serious symptoms of postpartum depression.
- Antidepressant medications are the usual treatment for postpartum depression; however, specific precautions are needed for breastfeeding women.

Answer Guidelines to Critical Thinking Exercise

Postpartum Depression

1 Yes, there is evidence to draw conclusions about including information on postpartum depression in discharge teaching.

2 a. Nurses have a major opportunity and responsibility to help women understand risk factors and to motivate them to adopt healthy lifestyles that prevent disease. Women need to be prepared for potential problems in the postpartum period such as PPD and to be counseled to engage in self care practices for their own health promotion and illness prevention. Teaching activities include taking care of oneself by eating a balanced diet, getting exercise, and getting adequate sleep; sharing feelings; not overcommitting or setting unrealistic expectations for oneself; and making sure family and friends also have knowledge about PPD.

b. Women experience depression twice as often as men. It occurs in approximately 10% to 15% of postpartum women. Assessment tools can be used to identify women at risk for PPD to see whether the woman has progressed from postpartum blues to PPD. These screening tools elicit information from the woman about the common symptoms of depression. The tool developed by Beck (2002) includes predictors of depression that include prenatal depression, low self-esteem, stress of child care, prenatal anxiety, life stress, lack of social support, marital relationship problems, history of depression, "difficult" infant temperament, postpartum blues, single status, low socioeconomic status, and unplanned or unwanted pregnancy.

c. Impaired parenting is a major risk of PPD. A prominent feature of PPD is rejection of the infant. The woman may be obsessed that the infant is taking her place in her partner's affections. She may show disinterest, annoyance with care demands, blaming self because of her lack of maternal feeling. She may appear awkward in her responses to the baby and may not be able to provide care for the baby. She may have thoughts of harming the baby or accuse others of trying to harm the baby. Friends and family may need to provide infant care, or temporary foster care may be needed if there is no support system.

3 The plan should be developed to include what screening methods will be used on the postpartum unit, what written materials will be provided, whether classes or individual sessions will be included, who will be included in the teaching session, what follow-up will be provided (e.g., phone calls, home visits), and what resources are available in the community for referral or support.

4 Yes. Depression is treatable if identified early and adequate treatment is given. It will not go away by itself. Women who are not informed may not seek help.

5 An alternative argument is to develop prenatal assessments and information about the risks of PPD and to assess throughout pregnancy for signs of problems. Classes and written materials can be provided during pregnancy as well by childbirth educators or health care providers (see Wroblewski & Tallon, 2004).

Resources

AHCPR website
www.hcfa.gov/medicaid/siq/siqipg/htm

Depression after Delivery (DAD)
P.O. Box 1282
Morrisville, PA 19067
908-575-9121
www.depressionafterdelivery.com

National Association for Continence
1-800-252-3337
www.nafc.org

National Depressive and Manic-Depressive Association
730 N. Franklin St., Suite 501
Chicago, IL 60610
800-826-3632
www.ndmda.org

National Headache Foundation
1-888-NHF-5552
www.headaches.org/consumer/topicsheets/tyramine.html

Postpartum Support International
927 North Kellog Ave.
Santa Barbara, CA 93111
805-967-7636
www.chss.iup.edu/postpartum

References

American Academy of Pediatrics (AAP) Committee on Drugs. (2001). The transfer of drugs and other chemicals into human milk. *Pediatrics, 108*(3), 776-789.

American College of Obstetricians and Gynecologists (ACOG). (1998). *Postpartum hemorrhage. ACOG Education Bulletin no. 243.* Washington, DC: ACOG.

American Psychiatric Association (APA). (2000). *Diagnostic and statistical manual of mental disorders* (4th ed., text revision). Washington, DC: American Psychiatric Association Press.

Beal, M. (1998). Use of complementary and alternative therapies in reproductive medicine. *Journal of Nurse-Midwifery, 43*(3), 224-233.

Beck, C. (1998). Postpartum onset of panic disorder. *Journal of Nursing Scholarship, 30*(2), 131-135.

Beck, C. (2001). Predictors of postpartum depression: An update. *Nursing Research, 50*(5), 275-282.

Beck, C. (2002). Revision of the Postpartum Depression Predictors Inventory. *Journal of Obstetric, Gynecologic, and Neonatal Nursing, 31*(4), 394-402.

Beck, C., & Gable, R. (2000). Postpartum Depression Screening Scale: Development and psychometric testing. *Nursing Research, 49*(5), 272-282.

Beck, C., & Gable, R. (2001). Further validation of the Postpartum Depression Screening Scale. *Nursing Research, 50*(3), 155-164.

Benedetti, T. (2002). Obstetric hemorrhage. In S. Gabbe, J. Niebyl, & J. Simpson (Eds.), *Obstetrics: Normal and problem pregnancies* (4th ed.), New York: Churchill Livingstone.

Berg, T., & Smith, C. (2002). Pharmacologic therapy for peripartum emergencies. *Clinical Obstetrics and Gynecology, 45*(1), 125-135.

Bowes, W., & Thorp, J. (2004). Clinical aspects of normal and abnormal labor. In R. Creasy, R. Resnik, & J. Iams (Eds.), *Maternal-fetal medicine: Principles and practice* (5th ed.). Philadelphia: Saunders.

Bozoky, I., & Corwin, E. (2002). Fatigue as a predictor of postpartum depression. *Journal of Obstetric, Gynecologic, and Neonatal Nursing, 31*(4), 436-443.

Brown, C. (2001). Depression and anxiety disorders. *Obstetrics and Gynecology Clinics of North America, 28*(2), 241-268.

Brucker, M. (2001). Management of the third stage of labor: An evidence-based approach. *Journal of Midwifery & Women's Health, 46*(6), 381-392.

Clark, S. (2004). Placenta previa and abruptio placentae. In R. Creasy, R. Resnik, & J. Iams (Eds.), *Maternal-fetal medicine: Principles and practice* (5th ed.). Philadelphia: Saunders.

Cox, J., Holden, J., & Sagovsky, R. (1987). Detection of postnatal depression. Development of the 10-item Edinburgh Postnatal Depression Scale. *British Journal of Psychiatry, 150,* 782-786.

Cunningham, F. G., Leveno, K., Bloom, S., Hauth, J., Gilstrap, L., & Wenstrom, K. (2005). *Williams obstetrics* (22nd ed.). New York: McGraw-Hill.

Curran, C. (2003). Intrapartum emergencies. *Journal of Obstetric, Gynecologic, and Neonatal Nursing, 32*(6), 802-813.

Duff, P. (2002). Maternal and perinatal infection. In S. Gabbe, J. Niebyl, & J. Simpson (Eds.), *Obstetrics: Normal and problem pregnancies* (4th ed.). New York: Churchill Livingstone.

Eberhard-Gran, M., Eskild, A., Tambs, K., Opjordsmoen, S., & Samuelsen, S. (2001). Review of validation studies of the Edinburgh Postnatal Depression Scale. *Acta Psychiatrica Scandinavica, 104*(4), 243-249.

Fishel, A. (1998). Nursing management of anxiety and panic. *Nursing Clinics of North America, 33*(1), 135-151.

French, L., & Smaill, F. (2002). Antibiotic regimens for endometritis after delivery (Cochrane Review). In *The Cochrane Library*, Issue 2. Oxford: Update Software.

Gibbs, R., Sweet, R., & Duff, P. (2004). Maternal and fetal infectious disorders. In R. Creasy, R. Resnik, & J. Iams (Eds.), *Maternal-fetal medicine: Principles and practice* (5th ed.). Philadelphia: Saunders.

Gilbert, E., & Harmon, J. (2003). *Manual of high risk pregnancy and delivery* (3rd ed.). St. Louis: Mosby.

Gold, L. (2002). Postpartum disorders in primary care: Diagnosis and treatment. *Primary Care, 29*(1), 27-41.

Herrick, H. (2002). *Postpartum depression: Who gets help? Statistical Brief no. 24.* Raleigh, NC: Department of Health and Human Services.

Hostetler, D., & Bosworth, M. (2000). Uterine inversion: A life-threatening obstetric emergency. *Journal of the American Board of Family Practice, 13*(2), 120-123.

Keltner, N., & Folks, D. (2001). *Psychotropic drugs* (3rd ed.). St. Louis: Mosby.

Kilpatrick, S., & Laros, R. (2004). Maternal hematologic disorders. In R. Creasy, R. Resnik, & J. Iams (Eds.), *Maternal-fetal medicine: Principles and practice* (5th ed.). Philadelphia: Saunders.

Laros, R. (2004). Thromboembolic disease. In R. Creasy, R. Resnik, & J. Iams (Eds.), *Maternal-fetal medicine: Principles and practice* (5th ed.). Philadelphia: Saunders.

Levy, M., Sanders, D., & Sabraw, S. (2002). Moms who kill, when depression turns deadly. *Psychology Today, November-December 2002*, 13-17.

Maley, B. (2002). Creating a postpartum depression support group. *AWHONN Lifelines, 6*(1), 62-65.

Matthey, S., Barnett, B., Kavanagh, D., & Howie, P. (2001). Validation of the Edinburgh Postnatal Depression Scale for men, and comparison of item endorsement with their partner. *Journal of Affective Disorders, 64*(2-3), 175-184.

Mousa, H., & Walkinshaw, S. (2001). Major postpartum haemorrhage. *Current Opinions in Obstetrics and Gynecology, 13*(6), 595-603.

Newport, D., Wilcox, M., & Stowe, Z. (2001). Antidepressants during pregnancy and lactation: Defining exposure and treatment issues. *Seminars in Perinatology, 25*(3), 177-190.

Papp, Z. (2003). Massive obstetric hemorrhage. *Journal of Perinatal Medicine, 31*(5), 408-414.

Phipps, W., Sands, J., & Marek, J. (2003). *Medical-surgical nursing: Health and illness perspectives* (7th ed.). St. Louis: Mosby.

Poole, J., & White D. (Eds.). (2003). *Obstetrical emergencies for the perinatal nurse.* White Plains, NY: March of Dimes Birth Defects Foundation.

Ray, K., & Hodnett, E. (2001). Caregiver support for postpartum depression (Cochrane Review). In *The Cochrane Library*, Issue 2, 2004. Chichester, UK: John Wiley & Sons.

Roque, H., Funai, R., & Lockwood, C. (2000). von Willebrand disease and pregnancy. *Journal of Maternal and Fetal Medicine, 9*(5), 257-266.

Sadock, H., & Sadock, B. (2000). *Kaplan and Sadock's comprehensive textbook of psychiatry* (7th ed.). Philadelphia: Lippincott Williams & Wilkins.

Sampselle, C. (2003). Behavior interventions in young and middle-aged women: Simple interventions to combat a complex problem. *American Journal of Nursing, 103*(suppl, March 2003), 9-19.

Schirmer, G. (1998). *Herbal medicine.* Bedford, TX: MED2000.

Seidel, H., Ball., J., Dains, J., & Benedict, G. (2003). *Mosby's guide to physical examination* (5th ed.). St. Louis: Mosby.

Shevell, T., & Malone, F. (2003). Management of obstetric hemorrhage. *Seminars in Perinatology, 27*(1), 86-104.

Skidmore-Roth, L. (2004). *Mosby's handbook of herbs and natural supplements* (2nd ed.). St. Louis: Mosby.

Stenchever, M., Droegemueller, W., Herbst, A., & Mishell, D. (2001). *Comprehensive gynecology* (4th ed.). St. Louis: Mosby.

Stowe, J., Strader, J., & Nemeroff, C. (2001). Psychopharmacology during pregnancy and lactation. In A. Schartzberg & C. Nemeroff (Eds.), *Essentials of clinical psychopharmacology.* Washington, DC: American Psychiatric Publishing.

Strozewski, S. (2000). Von Willebrand's disease: What you need to know about this inherited bleeding disorder. *American Journal of Nursing, 100*(2), 24AA-24DD.

Tiran, D., & Mack, S. (Eds.). (2000). *Complementary therapies for pregnancy and childbirth* (2nd ed.). Edinburgh: Baillière Tindall.

Weiss, N., & Bernstein, P. (2000). Risk factor scoring for predicting venous thromboembolism in obstetric patients. *American Journal of Obstetrics and Gynecology, 182*(5), 1073-1075.

Wroblewski, M., & Tallon, D. (2004). Implementing a comprehensive postpartum depression support program. *AWHONN Lifelines, 8*(3), 248-252.

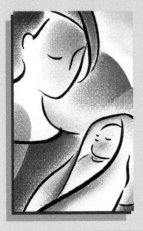

The Newborn at Risk: Problems Related to Gestational Age

SHANNON E. PERRY

LEARNING OBJECTIVES

- *Compare and contrast the characteristics of preterm, term, postterm, and postmature neonates.*
- *Discuss respiratory distress syndrome and the approach to treatment.*
- *Compare methods of oxygen therapy for the sick infant.*
- *Describe nursing interventions for nutritional care of the preterm infant.*
- *Discuss the pathophysiology of retinopathy of prematurity and chronic lung disease (bron-*

- *chopulmonary dysplasia), and identify risk factors that predispose preterm infants to these problems.*
- *Describe the treatment of the infant with meconium aspiration.*
- *Describe risk factors associated with the birth and transition of an infant of a diabetic mother.*
- *Plan developmentally appropriate care for high risk infants.*
- *Develop a plan to meet the needs of parents of high risk infants.*

KEY TERMS AND DEFINITIONS

barotrauma Physical injury resulting from changing air pressure; often associated with ventilatory assistance in preterm infants

chronic lung disease (bronchopulmonary dysplasia [BPD]) Pulmonary condition affecting preterm infants who have experienced respiratory failure and have been oxygen dependent for more than 28 days

continuous positive airway pressure (CPAP) Means of infusing oxygen or air under a preset pressure via nasal prongs, a face mask, or an endotracheal tube

corrected age Taking into account the gestational age and the postnatal age of a preterm infant when determining expectations for development

developmentally appropriate care Care that takes into consideration the gestational age and condition of the infant and promotes the development of the infant

extracorporeal membrane oxygenation (ECMO) Oxygenation of blood external to body using cardiopulmonary bypass and a membrane oxygenator; used primarily for newborns with refractory respiratory failure or meconium aspiration syndrome

insensible water loss Evaporative water loss that occurs mainly through the skin and respiratory tract

kangaroo care Skin-to-skin infant care, especially for preterm infants, that provides warmth to infant; infant is placed naked or diapered against

mother's or father's bare chest and is covered with parent's shirt or a warm blanket

mechanical ventilation Technique used to provide predetermined amount of oxygen; requires intubation

meconium aspiration syndrome (MAS) Function of fetal hypoxia; with hypoxia, the anal sphincter relaxes and meconium is released; reflex gasping movements draw meconium and other particulate matter in the amniotic fluid into the infant's bronchial tree, obstructing the airflow after birth

necrotizing enterocolitis (NEC) Acute inflammatory bowel disorder that occurs primarily in preterm or low-birth-weight neonates; characterized by ischemic necrosis (death) of the gastrointestinal mucosa, which may lead to perforation and peritonitis; formula-fed infants are at higher risk for this disease

neutral thermal environment (NTE) Environment that enables the neonate to maintain a normal body temperature with minimum use of oxygen and energy

nonnutritive sucking Use of a pacifier by infants

patent ductus arteriosus (PDA) Failure of the fetal ductus arteriosus to close after birth

periventricular-intraventricular hemorrhage (PV-IVH) Hemorrhage into the ventricles of the brain; a common type of brain injury in preterm infants; prognosis depends on the severity of hemorrhage

respiratory distress syndrome (RDS) Condition resulting from decreased pulmonary gas exchange,

KEY TERMS AND DEFINITIONS—cont'd

leading to retention of carbon dioxide (increase in arterial Pco_2); most common neonatal causes are prematurity, perinatal asphyxia, and maternal diabetes mellitus; also called *hyaline membrane disease*

retinopathy of prematurity (ROP) Complex, multicausal disorder that affects the developing reti-

nal vessels of premature infants resulting in capillary hemorrhages, fibrotic resolution, and possible retinal detachment; visual impairment may be mild or severe: formerly known as retrolental fibroplasia (RLF)

trophic feedings Very small feedings given to stimulate maturation of the gut

ELECTRONIC RESOURCES

Additional information related to the content in Chapter 26 can be found on

the companion website at **evolve**
http://evolve.elsevier.com/Lowdermilk/Maternity/
• NCLEX Review Questions
• WebLinks

or on the interactive companion CD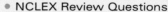
• NCLEX Review Questions
• Critical Thinking Exercise—Patent Ductus Arteriosus
• Plan of Care—The High Risk Preterm Newborn
• Plan of Care—The Infant of Mother with Diabetes Mellitus

*M*odern technology and expert nursing care have made important contributions to improving the health and overall survival of high risk infants. However, infants who are born considerably before term and survive are particularly susceptible to the development of sequelae related to their preterm birth. These conditions include necrotizing enterocolitis, chronic lung disease (bronchopulmonary dysplasia), intraventricular and periventricular hemorrhage, and retinopathy of prematurity. The focus of this chapter is on care of the preterm infant, but care of other high risk infants with gestational age–related problems is also discussed. Discussion of infants born of mothers with diabetes are included because these infants may experience problems that place them at risk for proper function and development.

High risk infants are most often classified according to birth weight, gestational age, and predominant pathophysiologic problems (Box 26-1). Intrauterine growth rates are not the same for all infants, and other factors (e.g., heredity, placental insufficiency, and maternal disease) influence intrauterine growth and birth weight. The classification system in the box encompasses birth weight and gestational age.

THE PRETERM INFANT

Preterm infants, those born before 37 weeks of gestation, are at risk because their organ systems are immature and they lack adequate physiologic reserves to function in an extrauterine environment. The range of birth weight and physiologic problems varies widely among preterm infants as a result of increased survivability among those who weigh less than 1000 g. However, one general concept is that the lower the weight and the gestational age, the fewer chances of survival exist among infants born preterm. Preterm birth is

responsible for almost two thirds of infant deaths. The cause of preterm birth is largely unknown; however, the incidence of preterm birth is highest among low socioeconomic groups. This is likely a result of the lack of comprehensive prenatal health care. Other factors found to be associated with preterm birth include gestational hypertension; maternal infection; multifetal pregnancy; HELLP syndrome (hemolysis, elevated liver enzymes, and low platelet count occurring in association with preeclampsia); premature dilation of the cervix; and placental or umbilical cord conditions that affect the fetus' receipt of nutrients.

There are varying opinions about the practical and ethical dimensions of resuscitation of extremely low-birth-weight (ELBW) infants (those infants whose birth weight is 1000 g or less). Ethical issues associated with resuscitation of these infants include whether to resuscitate, who should make that decision, whether the cost of resuscitation is justified, and whether the benefits of technology outweigh the burdens on the infant, family, and society in relation to quality of life.

The potential problems and care needs of the preterm infant weighing 2000 g differ from those of the term, postterm, or postmature infant of equal weight. The presence of physiologic disorders and anomalies affects the infant's response to treatment. In general, the closer infants are to term, the easier their adjustment to the external environment.

CARE MANAGEMENT

Assessment and Nursing Diagnoses

For the high risk infant, an accurate assessment of gestational age (see Chapter 19) is critical in helping the nurse identify the potential problems the newborn is likely to experience. Assessment of the infant's behavior using a tool such as the

Classification of High Risk Infants

CLASSIFICATION ACCORDING TO SIZE

- *Low-birth-weight (LBW) infant*—An infant whose birth weight is less than 2500 g, regardless of gestational age
- *Very low-birth-weight (VLBW) infant*—An infant whose birth weight is less than 1500 g
- *Extremely low-birth-weight (ELBW) infant*—An infant whose birth weight is less than 1000 g
- *Appropriate-for-gestational-age (AGA) infant*—An infant whose birth weight falls between the 10th and 90th percentiles on intrauterine growth curves
- *Small-for-date (SFD) or small-for-gestational-age (SGA) infant*—An infant whose rate of intrauterine growth was restricted and whose birth weight falls below the 10th percentile on intrauterine growth curves
- *Large-for-gestational-age (LGA) infant*—An infant whose birth weight falls above the 90th percentile on intrauterine growth charts
- *Intrauterine growth restriction (IUGR)*—Found in infants whose intrauterine growth is restricted (sometimes used as a more descriptive term for the SGA infant)
  - *Symmetric IUGR*—Growth restriction in which the weight, length, and head circumference are all affected
  - *Asymmetric IUGR*—Growth restriction in which the head circumference remains within normal parameters while the birth weight falls below the 10th percentile

CLASSIFICATION ACCORDING TO GESTATIONAL AGE

- *Premature (preterm) infant*—An infant born before completion of 37 weeks of gestation, regardless of birth weight
- *Full-term infant*—An infant born between the beginning of 38 weeks and the completion of 42 weeks of gestation, regardless of birth weight
- *Postmature (postterm) infant*—An infant born after 42 weeks of gestation, regardless of birth weight

CLASSIFICATION ACCORDING TO MORTALITY

- *Live birth*—Birth in which the neonate manifests any heart beat, breathes, or displays voluntary movement, regardless of gestational age
- *Fetal death*—Death of the fetus after 20 weeks of gestation and before birth, with absence of any signs of life after birth
- *Neonatal death*—Death that occurs in the first 27 days of life; early neonatal death occurs in the first week of life; late neonatal death occurs at 7 to 27 days
- *Perinatal mortality*—Total number of fetal and early neonatal deaths per 1000 live births

Assessment of Preterm Infants' Behavior (APIB) assists the caregiver in determining infant competence and readiness for behavioral intervention and individualizing supportive care (Als, Butler, Kosta, & McAnulty, 2005) (Box 26-2).

The response of the preterm or postterm infant to extrauterine life is different from that of the term infant. By understanding the physiologic basis of these differences, the nurse can assess these infants, determine the response of the preterm or postterm infant, and discern which of the potential problems are more likely to occur.

Respiratory function

Pink color, adequate tissue perfusion, and respiratory patterns are quickly established in nonstressed newborns, and they are soon vigorous and show appropriate muscle tone. However, infants with a potential for respiratory depression at birth because of asphyxia, maternal analgesia or illness, immaturity, prematurity, or congenital malformations may exhibit cyanosis, decreased tissue perfusion, retractions, nasal flaring, tachypnea, or a combination of these problems.

The preterm infant is likely to have difficulty making the pulmonary transition from intrauterine to extrauterine life. Numerous problems may affect the respiratory system of preterm infants and may include the following:

- Decreased number of functional alveoli
- Deficient surfactant levels
- Smaller lumen in the respiratory system
- Greater collapsibility or obstruction of respiratory passages
- Insufficient calcification of the bony thorax
- Circulating hormones that may affect cardiovascular function
- Immature and fragile capillaries in the lungs
- Greater distance between functional alveoli and capillary bed

In combination, these deficits severely hinder the infant's respiratory efforts and can produce respiratory distress or apnea. Early signs of respiratory distress include flaring of the nares and expiratory grunting. Depending on the severity of respiratory distress and cause, retractions may begin as subcostal, intercostal, or suprasternal. Increasing respiratory effort (e.g., paradoxic breathing patterns, retractions, nasal flaring, expiratory grunting, tachypnea, or apnea) indicates increasing distress. Initially a compromised infant's color may be cyanotic centrally or pale. Acrocyanosis is a normal finding in the neonate, but central cyanosis indicates the existence of an underlying problem.

Periodic breathing is a respiratory pattern commonly seen in premature infants. Such infants exhibit 5- to 10-second respiratory pauses followed by 10 to 15 seconds of compensatory rapid respirations. Such periodic breathing should not be confused with apnea, which is a cessation of respirations of 20 seconds or more. The nurse must be prepared to provide oxygen and artificial ventilation as

BOX 26-2

Assessment of the Preterm Infants' Behavior (APIB)

The APIB is a neurobehavioral assessment that is appropriate for use with preterm, at-risk, and full-term infants. It can be used from birth until 1 month after the expected date of birth. The focus of the APIB is on assessment of mutually interacting behavioral subsystems that are simultaneously interacting with the environment. The subsystems that are assessed include the following:

- Autonomic: respiration, digestion, color
- Motor: tone, movement, postures
- State organization: range, robustness, transition patterns
- Attention: robustness, transitions
- Self-regulation: effort, success.

The degree of facilitation which is required to support reorganization and balance of the subsystem is also assessed.

The environment is assessed through challenging distal, proximal, tactile, and vestibular items that are derived from the Brazelton Neonatal Behavioral Assessment Scale (BNBAS).

The APIB requires training before use. It has good interrater reliability and concurrent and construct validity. It is relevant clinically for behavioral intervention and for determining appropriate and supportive care.

Adapted from Als, H., Butler, S., Kosta, S., & McAnulty, G. (2005). The Assessment of Preterm Infants' Behavior (APIB): Furthering the understanding and measurement of neurodevelopmental competence in preterm and full-term infants. *Mental Retardation and Developmental Disabilities Research Review, 11*(1), 94-102.

necessary when the newborn demonstrates an inability to initiate or maintain adequate respiratory function.

Cardiovascular function

Evaluation of heart rate and rhythm, color, blood pressure (BP), perfusion, pulses, oxygen saturation, and acid-base status provides information on cardiovascular status. The nurse must be prepared to intervene if symptoms of hypovolemia, shock, or both are found. These symptoms include hypotension, prolonged capillary refill (>3 seconds), tachycardia initially then bradycardia, and continued respiratory distress despite the provision of oxygen and ventilation.

BP is monitored routinely in the sick neonate by either internal or external means. Direct recording with arterial catheters is often used but carries the risks inherent in any procedure in which a catheter is introduced into an artery. An umbilical venous catheter may also be used to monitor the neonate's central venous pressure. Oscillometry (Dinamap) and Doppler transcutaneous apparatus are simple, effective means for detecting alterations in systemic BP (hypotension or hypertension).

Maintaining body temperature

Preterm infants are susceptible to temperature instability as a result of numerous factors. Preterm infants are at high risk for heat loss because of the large surface area in relation to body weight. Other factors that place preterm infants at risk for temperature instability include the following:

- Minimal insulating subcutaneous fat
- Limited stores of brown fat (an internal source for the generation of heat present in normal term infants)
- Decreased or absent reflex control of skin capillaries (vasoconstriction)
- Inadequate muscle mass activity (therefore the preterm infant is unable to produce its own heat)
- Poor muscle tone, resulting in more body surface area being exposed to the cooling effects of the environment
- An immature temperature regulation center in the brain
- Increased insensible water loss
- Decreased ability to increase oxygen consumption
- Decreased caloric intake

The goal of thermoregulation is a **neutral thermal environment (NTE),** which is the environmental temperature at which oxygen consumption and metabolic rate are minimal but adequate to maintain the body temperature (Horns, 2002). The NTE for preterm infants weighing less than 1000 g is very narrow, and the prediction of the NTE for each infant is impossible. With knowledge of the four mechanisms of heat transfer (i.e., convection, conduction, radiation, and evaporation), the nurse can create an environment for the preterm infant that prevents temperature instability (see Chapter 19). The infant is kept in a radiant warmer or incubator with control settings at a temperature to maintain the NTE. Because overheating produces an increase in oxygen and calorie consumption, the infant is also jeopardized if he or she becomes hyperthermic (apnea and flushed color may indicate hyperthermia). Unlike older children, the preterm infant is not able to sweat and thus dissipate heat.

Skin-to-skin (kangaroo) contact between the stable preterm infant and parent is also a viable option for interaction because of the maintenance of appropriate body temperature by the infant.

Central nervous system function

The preterm infant's central nervous system (CNS) is susceptible to injury as a result of the following problems:

- Birth trauma with damage to immature structures
- Bleeding from fragile capillaries
- Impaired coagulation process, including prolonged prothrombin time
- Recurrent anoxic and hyperoxic episodes
- Predisposition to hypoglycemia
- Fluctuating systemic BP with concomitant variation in cerebral flow and pressure

In the preterm neonate neurologic function is dependent on gestational age, associated illness factors, and predisposing factors such as intrauterine asphyxia, which may have caused neurologic damage. Clinical signs of neurologic dysfunction may be subtle, nonspecific, or specific; however, five categories of clinical manifestations should be carefully evaluated in the preterm infant. These clinical signs include seizure activity, hyperirritability, CNS depression, elevated intracranial pressure, and abnormal movements such as decorticate posturing. Primary and tendon reflexes are generally present in preterm infants by 28 weeks of gestation and should be part of the neurologic examination. Ongoing assessment and documentation of these neurologic signs are needed both for the purposes of discharge teaching and making follow-up recommendations, as well as for their predictive value.

Maintaining adequate nutrition

The initial goal of neonatal nutrition in the preterm infant is to prevent catabolism and excess fluid losses. Once the infant's respiratory and cardiac function have been stabilized, the goal of nutrition is to promote normal growth and development. However, the maintenance of adequate nutrition in the preterm infant is complicated by problems with intake and metabolism of nutrients sufficient to promote physical and brain growth. The preterm infant has the following disadvantages with regard to intake: weak or absent suck, swallow, and gag reflexes; a small stomach capacity; and immature digestive enzymes. The preterm infant's metabolic functions are compromised by a limited store of nutrients, a decreased ability to digest proteins and absorb nutrients, and immature enzyme systems.

The nurse must continuously assess the infant's nutritional status. Some preterm infants, because of gestational age and birth weight and existing illness factors such as respiratory distress, require gavage or intravenous (IV) feedings instead of oral feedings.

Maintaining renal function

The preterm infant's immature renal system is unable to (1) adequately excrete metabolites and drugs; (2) concentrate urine; or (3) maintain acid-base, fluid, or electrolyte balance. Therefore intake and output, as well as specific gravity, must be assessed. Laboratory tests must be performed to assess acid-base and electrolyte balance. Medication levels are also monitored in preterm infants because metabolism by renal and hepatic routes is often hindered. Because of great variability in drug metabolism, serum levels are obtained to ensure adequate therapeutic range for treatment and to prevent toxicity.

Maintaining hematologic status

The preterm infant is predisposed to hematologic problems because of the following conditions:
- Increased capillary fragility
- Increased tendency to bleed (prolonged prothrombin time and partial thromboplastin time)
- Decreased production of red blood cells (RBCs) resulting from physiologic rapid decrease in erythropoiesis after birth
- Large amount of fetal hemoglobin
- Loss of blood attributable to frequent blood sampling for laboratory tests

- Decreased RBC survival related to the relatively larger size of the RBC and its increased permeability to sodium and potassium
- Decreased levels of circulating albumin

The nurse assesses such infants for any evidence of bleeding from puncture sites and the gastrointestinal (GI) tract. Infants are also examined for signs of anemia (e.g., decreased hemoglobin and hematocrit levels, pale skin, increased apnea, lethargy, tachycardia, and poor weight gain). The amount of blood withdrawn for laboratory testing is monitored.

Resisting infection

Preterm infants are at increased risk for infection because they have a shortage of stored maternal immunoglobulins, an impaired ability to make antibodies, and a compromised integumentary system (i.e., thin skin). Preterm and term infants exhibit various nonspecific signs and symptoms of infection (Box 26-3). Early identification and treatment of sepsis is essential. Stoll and co-workers (2004) found that compared with uninfected infants, ELBW survivors were more likely to have adverse neurodevelopmental outcomes and impaired head growth (Box 26-4).

Protection from infection

Protection from infection is an integral part of all newborn care, but preterm and sick infants are particularly susceptible to infectious organisms. As with all aspects of care, strict handwashing is the single most important measure to prevent nosocomial infections. Personnel with known infectious disorders are barred from the unit until they are no longer infectious. Standard Precautions are instituted in all nursery areas as a method of infection control to protect the infants and staff.

Skin care

The skin of preterm infants is characteristically immature relative to that of full-term infants. Because of its increased sensitivity and fragility, the use of alkaline-based soap that might destroy the acid mantle of the skin is avoided. The increased permeability of the skin facilitates absorption of ingredients that may become toxic. All skin products (e.g., alcohol, povidone-iodine) are used with caution, and the skin is rinsed with water afterward because these substances may cause severe irritation and chemical burns in preterm infants. Adhesives used after heel sticks or to secure monitoring equipment or IV infusions may excoriate the skin or adhere to the skin surface so firmly that the epidermis can be separated from understructures and pulled away with the tape. The use of pectin barriers and hydrocolloid adhesives may be useful because these products mold well to skin contours and adhere in moist conditions. Recommendations for protecting the integrity of premature skin include using minimal adhesive tape, backing the tape with cotton, and delaying adhesive and pectin barrier removal until adherence is reduced (Lund & Kuller, 2003). An emollient such as

BOX 26-3

Signs of Neonatal Infection

Many signs are subtle and nonspecific.
- Temperature instability
- Hypothermia—most common
- Hyperthermia—rare

CENTRAL NERVOUS SYSTEM CHANGES
- Lethargy
- Irritability
- Altered level of consciousness (LOC)

CHANGES IN COLOR
- Cyanosis, pallor
- Mottling (marbling)
- Jaundice

CARDIOVASCULAR INSTABILITY
- Poor perfusion
- Hypotension
- Bradycardia or tachycardia
- Prolonged capillary refill (>3 seconds)

RESPIRATORY DISTRESS
- Tachypnea or bradypnea
- Apnea
- Retractions, nasal flaring, grunting

GASTROINTESTINAL PROBLEMS
- Feeding intolerance, increased residuals
- Vomiting
- Diarrhea
- Bloody stools (frank or occult positive)
- Abdominal distention

METABOLIC INSTABILITY
- Glucose instability
- Metabolic acidosis

OTHER
- Electrolyte imbalance
- Decreased urinary output

BOX 26-4

Ethical Considerations of Negative Sequelae of Increased Survival Rates for Extremely Low-Birth-Weight Infants

Advances in perinatal and neonatal care have resulted in improved survival rates (67%) for extremely low-birth-weight infants (those weighing less than 1000 g). Although the survival rates for those without impairment has increased, the improved survival rate has been accompanied by an increase in the rate of infants with morbidity and neurodevelopment impairment. Neonatal morbidity includes sepsis (51%), periventricular leukomalacia (nerve fibers along the ventricles of the brain are damaged and replaced with fluid) (7%), and chronic lung disease (43%). Impairment includes cerebral palsy (25%), deafness (7%), major neurosensory abnormality, and Bayley Mental Developmental Index score of <70 (36%) (Wilson-Costello, Friedman, Minich, Fanaroff, & Hack, 2005). Head ultrasound may be normal, but the infant may have an adverse outcome (Laptook, O'Shea, Shankaran, Bhaskar, & NICHD Neonatal Network, 2005).

At the birth of a very preterm infant, health care providers and parents must make the decision about whether to try to resuscitate the infant. If parents know the substantial risk of having a child with significant impairment, would they still choose vigorous resuscitation? Who should make the decision about whether or not to resuscitate? How much information should parents be given about possible sequelae to a preterm birth? What factors should enter into the decision to resuscitate? Should ability to pay or insurance status of the parents be considered? Should gravity and parity be a factor in the decision?

Eucerin or Aquaphor may also be used to promote skin integrity and prevent dry, cracking, and peeling skin in infants at risk for skin breakdown (Horii & Lane, 2001; Lund & Kuller, 2003). Solvents used to remove tape are avoided because they tend to dry and burn the delicate skin. Guidelines for skin care are listed in the Teaching Guidelines box.

Growth and Development Potential

Although it is impossible to predict with complete accuracy the growth and development potential of each preterm newborn, some findings support an anticipated favorable outcome in the absence of ongoing medical sequelae that can affect growth, such as chronic lung disease (CLD) (formerly called *bronchopulmonary dysplasia*), necrotizing enterocolitis

(NEC), and CNS problems. The lower the birth weight, the greater the likelihood of negative sequelae. The growth and development milestones (e.g., motor milestones, vocalization, and growth) are corrected for gestational age until the child is approximately 2½ years of age.

The age of a preterm newborn is corrected by adding the gestational age and the postnatal age. For example, an infant born at 32 weeks of gestation 4 weeks ago would now be considered 36 weeks of age. The infant's corrected age 6 months after the birth date is then 4 months, and the infant's responses are evaluated against the norm expected for a 4-month-old infant.

Certain measurable factors predict normal growth and development. The preterm infant experiences catch-up body growth during the first 2 to 3 years of life, with maximum growth occurring between 36 and 40 weeks of postconceptional age. The head is the first to experience catch-up growth, followed by a gain in weight and height. An effective discharge plan should include frequent outpatient follow-up with a primary care provider and developmental specialist for monitoring growth and achievement of developmental milestones.

TEACHING GUIDELINES
Neonatal Skin Care

GENERAL SKIN CARE

Assessment

- Assess skin every day or once a shift for redness, dryness, flaking, scaling, rashes, lesions, excoriation, or breakdown.
- Evaluate and report abnormal skin findings and analyze for possible causation.
- Intervene according to interpretation of findings or physician order.

BATHING

Initial Bath

- Assess for stable temperature a minimum of 2 to 4 hours before first bath.
- Use cleansing agents with neutral pH or minimal dyes or perfume in water.
- Do not completely remove vernix.
- Bathe preterm infant (<32 weeks) in sterile water only.

Routine

- Decrease frequency of baths to every second or third day by daily cleansing of eye, oral, and diaper areas and pressure points.
- Use cleanser or soaps no more than two or three times a week.
- Avoid rubbing skin during bathing or drying.
- Immerse stable infants fully (except head) in an appropriately sized tub.
- Use swaddled immersion bathing technique: slow unwrapping after gently lowering into water for sensitive, but stable, infants needing assistance with motor system reactivity.

EMOLLIENTS

- Follow hospital protocol or consider the following:
  - Apply petroleum-based ointment without preservative sparingly to body (avoid face, head) every 6 to 12 hours during the first 2 to 4 weeks for infants <32 weeks (except when neonate is in radiant heat source).
  - Apply emollient as needed to infants >32 weeks for dry, flaking skin.

ADHESIVES

- Decrease use as much as possible.

- Use transparent adhesive dressings to secure IVs, catheters, and central lines.
- Use hydrogel or limb electrodes.
- Consider pectin barriers (Hollihesive*, Duoderm†) beneath adhesives to protect skin.
- Secure pulse oximeter probe or electrodes with elasticized dressing material (carefully avoid restricting blood flow). Change pulse oximeter site at least every 8 hours or more often, especially with compromised circulation.
- Do not use adhesive remover, solvents, and bonding agents.
- Avoid removing adhesives for at least 24 hours after application.
- Adhesive removal can be facilitated using water, mineral oil, or petrolatum.
- Remove adhesives or skin barriers slowly, supporting the skin underneath with one hand and gently peeling away the product from the skin with the other hand.‡

ANTISEPTIC AGENTS

- Apply before invasive procedures.
- Apply povidone-iodine two times, air dry for 30 seconds; remove completely with sterile water or sterile saline solution after procedure.
- Avoid use of alcohol.

TRANSEPIDERMAL WATER LOSS

- Minimize transepidermal water loss and heat loss in small premature infants <30 weeks by:
  - Measuring ambient humidity during first weeks of life.
  - Considering an increase in humidity to >70% by using one or more of the following options or hospital guidelines:
    - Transparent dressings
    - Emollient application every 6 to 8 hours or according to hospital protocol
    - Servo-controlled humidifying incubator

SKIN BREAKDOWN

Prevention

- Decrease pressure from externally applied forces using water, air, or gel mattresses, sheepskin, or cotton bedding.

---

*Hollister, Libertyville, IL.
†ConvaTec/Bristol-Myers Squibb Co., Princeton, NJ.
‡Caution: Scissors are not to be used for tape or dressing removal because of hazard of cutting skin or amputating tiny digits.

Parental Adaptation to Preterm Infant

Parents who experience the preterm birth of their infant have an experience that is much different from that of parents giving birth to a full-term infant. Because of this difference, parental attachment and adaptation to the parental role may differ as well.

Parental tasks

Parents must accomplish a number of psychologic tasks before effective relationships and parenting patterns can evolve. These tasks include the following:

- Experiencing anticipatory grief over the potential loss of an infant. The parent grieves in preparation for the infant's possible death, although the parent clings to

TEACHING GUIDELINES—cont'd

Neonatal Skin Care

- Provide adequate nutrition, including protein, fat, and zinc.
- Apply transparent adhesive dressings to protect arms, elbows, and knees from friction injury.
- Use tracheostomy and gastrostomy dressings for drainage and relief of pressure from tracheostomy or G tube (Hydrasorb or Lyofoam).[†]
- Use emollient in the diaper area (groin and thighs) to reduce urine irritation.

Treatment

- Irrigate wound every 4 to 8 hours with warm half-strength normal saline (NS) using a 30-ml or larger syringe and 20-gauge Teflon catheter.
- Culture wound and treat if signs of infection (excessive redness, swelling, pain on touch, heat, or resistance to healing) are present.
- Use transparent adhesive dressing for uninfected wounds.
- Apply hydrogel with or without antibacterial or antifungal ointments (as ordered) for infected wounds (may need to moisten before removal).
- Use hydrocolloid for deep, uninfected wounds (leave in place for 5 to 7 days) or as an ostomy barrier and to improve appliance adhesion; warm barrier in hand for several minutes to soften before applying to skin.
- Avoid use of antiseptic solutions for wound cleansing (use for intact skin only).

Treating Diaper Dermatitis

- Maintain clean, dry skin; use absorbent diapers; and change often.
- If mild irritation occurs, use petrolatum barrier.
- For developing dermatitis, apply a generous quantity of zinc-oxide barrier.
- For severe dermatitis, identify cause (frequent stooling from spina bifida, severe opiate withdrawal, or malabsorption syndrome) and treat.
- Treat *Candida albicans* with antifungal ointment or cream.
- Avoid powders and antibiotic ointments (not recommended). (See Cord and Circumcision Care, Chapter 19.)

OTHER SKIN CARE CONCERNS

Use of Substances on Skin

- Evaluate all substances that come in contact with infant's skin.

- Before using any topical agent, analyze components of preparation and:
  - Use sparingly and only when necessary.
  - Confine use to smallest possible area.
  - Whenever possible and appropriate, wash off with water.
  - Monitor infant carefully for signs of toxicity and systemic effects.

Use of Thermal Devices

- Avoid heat lamps because of increased potential for burns. If needed, measure actual temperature of exposed skin every 15 minutes.
- When using heating pads (Aqua-K pads):
  - Change infant's position every 15 minutes initially and then every 1 to 2 hours.
  - Preset temperature of heating pads to <40° C.
- When using preheated transcutaneous electrodes:
  - Avoid use on infants weighing less than 1000 g.
  - Set at lowest possible temperature (<44° C) and secure with plastic wrap.
  - Use pulse oximetry rather than transcutaneous monitoring whenever possible.
- When prewarming heels before phlebotomy, avoid temperatures >40° C.
- Warm ambient humidity, direct away from infant; use aerosolized sterile water, and maintain ambient temperature so as not to exceed 40° C.
- Document use of all heating devices.

Use of Fluid Therapy/Hemodynamic Monitoring

- Be certain fingers or toes are visible whenever extremity is used for intravenous (IV) or arterial line.
- Assess extremity distal to insertion site hourly for signs of poor circulation, edema, or inadequate perfusion.
- Secure catheter or needle with transparent dressing or tape to promote easy visualization of site.
- Assess site hourly for signs of ischemia, infiltration, and inadequate perfusion (check capillary refill).
- Avoid use of restraints (e.g., arm boards); if used, check that they are secured safely and not restricting circulation or movement (check for pressure areas).
- Use commercial IV protector (i.e., I.V. House) with minimal tape.

Modified from Kuller, J. (2001). Skin breakdown: Risk factors, prevention, and treatment. *Newborn and Infant Nursing Reviews, 1*(1), 33-42; Johnson, F., & Maikler, V. (2001). Nurses' adoption of the AWHONN/NANN Neonatal Skin Care Project. *Newborn and Infant Nursing Reviews, 1*(1), 59-67; Lund, C., Kuller, J., & Lott, J. (2001). Neonatal skin care: Clinical outcomes of the AWHONN/NANN evidence-based clinical practice guideline. *Journal of Obstetric, Gynecologic, and Neonatal Nursing, 30*(1), 41-51; & Taquino, L. (2000). Promoting wound healing in the neonatal setting: Process versus protocol. *Journal of Perinatal and Neonatal Nursing, 14*(1), 108-118.

Critical Thinking Exercise

Preterm Infant

After having two full-term pregnancies, Charlotte gave birth to her third baby at 28 weeks of gestation. The infant was transported to a tertiary center that could provide the care the infant needed. Charlotte lives 60 miles from the city in which the tertiary center is located, and she is to be discharged tomorrow. It is anticipated that the infant will require a stay in the NICU for at least 8 more weeks. You have been caring for Charlotte and are preparing her for discharge. You have spoken to the nurse caring for the baby. The infant is stable at present, receiving a small amount of oxygen, and has started gavage feeding. The IV is to be discontinued when the infant can tolerate adequate amounts of milk. The nursery has asked for breast milk from Charlotte to feed the baby.

1 Evidence—Is there sufficient evidence to draw conclusions about what to tell Charlotte about her own recovery and the expected progress of the baby?
2 Assumption—What assumptions can be made about the following?
  a. Charlotte's postpartum recovery
  b. The infant's expected progress
  c. The possibility of Charlotte furnishing breast milk for the baby
  d. The long-term outcome for the baby
3 What implications and priorities for nursing care can be drawn at this time?
4 Does the evidence objectively support your conclusion?
5 Are there alternative perspectives to your conclusion?

the hope that the infant will survive. This begins during labor and lasts until the infant dies or shows evidence of surviving.

- Acceptance by the mother of her failure to give birth to a healthy, full-term infant. Grief and depression typify this phase, which persists until the infant is out of danger and is expected to survive.
- Resuming the process of relating to the infant. As the infant's condition begins to improve and the infant gains weight, feeds by nipple, and is weaned from the incubator, the parent can begin the process of developing an attachment to the infant that was interrupted by the infant's critical condition at birth.
- Learning how this infant differs in special needs and growth patterns, caregiving needs, and growth and development expectations.
- Adjusting the home environment to the needs of the new infant. Visitors may be limited to reduce the risk of exposure to pathogens, and the environmental temperature may be altered to optimize conditions for the infant.

Grandparents and siblings also react to the birth of the preterm infant. Parents must deal with the grief of grandparents and the bewilderment and anger of the infant's siblings at the apparent disproportionate amount of parental time spent with the newborn.

Parental responses

Parents progress through stages as they interact with their infants, from maintaining an en face position and stroking and touching their infant (Fig. 26-1) to assuming some child care activities such as feeding, bathing, and diapering the infant.

Parenting disorders

The incidence of physical and emotional abuse is greater in infants who, because of preterm birth or illness, are separated from their parents for a time after birth. Physical abuse includes varying degrees of poor nutrition, poor hygiene, and bodily harm. Emotional abuse ranges from subtle disinterest to outright dislike of the infant. Appropriate resources should be made available to assess the parent's feelings regarding the preterm infant's birth. In addition, proper guidance and counseling are made available, including posthospital discharge, to help families adjust to and care for the preterm infant. The ultimate goal is for the family to incorporate the infant as a regular family member.

Factors surrounding the birth may predispose parents to subconsciously or overtly reject the infant. These factors might include parental pain and anxiety, a heavy financial burden because of the cost of the infant's care, unresolved anticipatory grief, threat to self-esteem, or the fact that the infant was the product of an unwanted pregnancy. The goal of health professionals is early identification of inadequate coping skills and potentially dysfunctional parenting so that further problems can be prevented and early intervention accessed.

Potential nursing diagnoses for high risk infants and their parents include the following:

- *Ineffective breathing pattern related to*
  —decreased number of functional alveoli
  —surfactant deficiency
  —immature respiratory control
  —increased pulmonary vascular resistance (PVR)
- *Ineffective thermoregulation related to*
  —immature CNS thermoregulation
  —increased heat loss to environment and inability to produce heat
  —greater body surface exposed to environment
  —decreased brown fat reserves to produce body heat
- *Risk for infection related to*
  —invasive procedures
  —decreased immune response
  —ineffective skin barrier
- *Parental anxiety related to*
  —lack of knowledge about infant's condition
  —lack of knowledge regarding infant's prognosis (uncertain outcome)
  —inability to perform expected caregiving activities
  —neonatal intensive care unit (NICU) environment, noise, and high-tech care

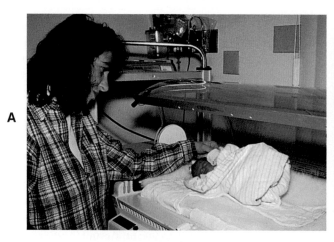 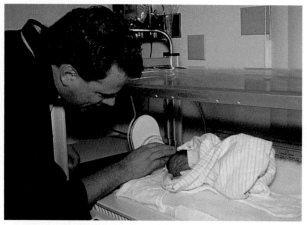

Fig. 26-1 **A,** Mother interacts with her preterm infant by touch. **B,** Father interacts with his newborn by stroking and touching infant with fingertips. (Courtesy Michael S. Clement, MD, Mesa, AZ.)

Expected Outcomes of Care

The nursing plan of care for the preterm infant is dictated by the physiologic needs of the infant's immature systems and often involves emergency treatments and procedures. Nursing care is a critical element in the infant's chances for survival. In addition to meeting the infant's physical needs, nursing care is planned in conjunction with parents to promote parent-infant attachment and interaction. Expected outcomes are presented in patient-centered terms and include that the infant will do the following:

- Maintain adequate physiologic functioning (airway, breathing, circulation)
- Receive adequate nutrition
- Maintain body temperature
- Remain free of infection
- Experience appropriate parent-infant interactions

Expected outcomes for the parents include that they will do the following:

- Perceive the infant as potentially normal (if this is medically substantiated)
- Provide care comfortably
- Experience pride and satisfaction in the care of the infant
- Organize their time and energies to meet the love, attention, and care needs of the other members of the family as well as their own needs

Plan of Care and Interventions

The best environment for fetal growth and development is in the uterus of a healthy, well-nourished woman. The goal of care for the preterm infant is to provide an extrauterine environment that approximates a healthy intrauterine environment in order to promote normal growth and development. Nursing and medical personnel, respiratory therapists, occupational and physical therapists, dietitians, social workers, and pharmacists work as a team to provide the intensive care needed.

The admission of a preterm newborn to the intensive care nursery is usually an emergency situation. Resuscitation is started in the birthing unit, and warmth and oxygen are provided during transport to the nursery. A rapid initial assessment is done to determine the infant's need for lifesaving treatment.

The nurse uses many technologic support systems to monitor body responses and maintain body functions in the infant. Technical skill needs to be combined with a gentle touch and concern about the traumatic effects of harsh lighting and the volume of machinery noise. The NICU environment may be a major contributing factor to learning and behavioral problems in preterm infants (Gardner & Goldson, 2002).

Physical care

The preterm infant's environmental support typically consists of the following equipment and procedures:

- Incubator or radiant warmer to control body temperature (NTE)
- Oxygen administration, depending on infant's pulmonary and circulatory status
- Electronic monitors as needed for observation of respiratory and cardiac functions
- Assistive devices for positioning the infant
- Clustering of care and minimization of stimulation

Various metabolic support measures that may be instituted consist of the following:

- Parenteral fluids to support nutrition and hydration
- IV access to facilitate antibiotic therapy if sepsis is a concern
- Blood work to monitor arterial blood gases (ABGs), blood glucose level, and electrolytes and for other diagnostic studies (C-reactive protein, white blood cell count with differential, hemoglobin and hematocrit) as indicated.

Maintaining body temperature

The high risk infant is susceptible to heat loss and its complications (see Fig. 18-3). In addition, LBW infants may be unable to increase their metabolic rate because of impaired gas exchange, caloric intake restrictions in relation to high expenditure, or poor thermoregulation. Transepidermal water loss is greater because of skin immaturity in ELBW and very low-birth-weight (VLBW) infants (i.e., those weighing less than 1000 g and 1500 g, respectively) and can contribute to temperature instability.

High risk infants are cared for in the thermoneutral environment created by use of an external heat source. A probe applied to the infant is attached to an external heat source supplied by a radiant warmer or a servocontrolled incubator. Studies indicate that optimum thermoneutrality cannot be predicted for every high risk infant's needs. Guidelines for providing an optimum thermal environment for the VLBW infant suggest maintaining the infant's core temperature at rest within a range of 36.3° to 36.9° C, with core and mean temperatures changing less than 0.2° and 0.3° C an hour. Standard guidelines for maintaining an NTE in the LBW infant are published (Blake & Murray, 2002). Further research is needed to define an NTE for the ELBW infant.

Warming the hypothermic infant. Rapid changes in body temperature may cause apnea and acidosis in the neonate. Therefore the warming of a hypothermic infant should occur over a period of hours; rapid rewarming may cause apnea, and rewarming too slowly increases metabolic distress and oxygen consumption. Rewarming must therefore be individualized for each infant according to illness and ability to produce heat. To accomplish this, the infant is placed either under a radiant warmer or in an incubator with a servocontrol mechanism. It has been suggested that rewarming proceed at a rate of 1° to 2° C per hour. Another approach is to gradually increase the environmental temperature of the incubator and increase the humidity (above 70%) (Blackburn, 2003). Appropriate guidelines for rewarming the hypothermic infant should be consulted for further information.

Weaning the infant from the incubator. To wean the infant from the incubator, the incubator heat is decreased slowly over at least several hours. On average, infants who are medically stable, gaining weight, and tolerating enteral feedings and weigh 1300 to 1500 g may be weaned (depending on institution protocol). The following general guidelines may be followed to wean the infant from the incubator:

- Dress the infant in a diaper, shirt, and cap.
- Disconnect the servocontrol probe (if still in use).
- Lower the incubator temperature by no more than 0.5° C per each 2-hour period.
- Record the temperature of both the infant and incubator.
- Assess the infant's responses to the changes every hour until four stable readings are obtained.
- Monitor the infant's temperature and other vital signs.

This procedure is repeated until the incubator temperature is the same as the room temperature, and the infant's body temperature consistently remains in the range of 36° to 37° C. The infant is placed in an open bassinet when the body temperature is stable, after which it is reassessed in conjunction with the delivery of routine care. If necessary, the infant may be returned to the incubator and weaning repeated once the infant is able to regulate his or her temperature.

Oxygen therapy

The goals of oxygen therapy are to provide adequate oxygen to the tissues, prevent lactic acid accumulation resulting from hypoxia, and at the same time avoid the potentially negative effects of oxygen barotraumas (injury resulting from changing air pressure associated with ventilation). Numerous methods have been devised to improve oxygenation. All require that the gas be warmed and humidified before entering the respiratory tract. If the infant does not require mechanical ventilation, oxygen can be connected to a plastic hood placed over the infant's head to supply variable concentrations of humidified oxygen. Because oxygen therapy is not without inherent hazards, each infant must be carefully monitored to prevent hyperoxemia and hypoxemia.

Infants who require oxygen should have their respiratory status assessed accurately every 1 to 2 hours; this includes a continuous pulse oximetry reading and, as warranted, ABG measurement. Vital signs including heart rate and BP are assessed to monitor adequate respiratory function and adequate circulation and perfusion of tissues. The interventions implemented range from hood oxygen administration to ventilator therapy.

Interest in the resuscitation of asphyxiated newborns with 21% oxygen (room air) rather than 100% oxygen has increased; preliminary studies demonstrate no significant neurologic morbidities at 18 to 24 months in newborns resuscitated with 21% oxygen (Saugstad, 2005). Proponents of room air resuscitation suggest fewer complications are associated with oxidative stress and hyperoxemia when room air is administered (Saugstad, 2005). Large multicenter studies are currently in progress to determine the optimum concentration of oxygen for resuscitation.

Oxygen hood. Oxygen in a specified concentration can be administered by hood to infants who do not require mechanical pressure support. The hood is a clear plastic cover that is sized to fit over the head and neck of the infant (Fig. 26-2, *A*). The oxygen level is checked every 1 to 2 hours and the concentration adjusted in response to the infant's condition.

Nasal cannula. Low-flow amounts of oxygen can be administered by nasal cannula (Fig. 26-2, *B*). Nasal cannulas are used for infants who are out of the acute phase of illness and recuperating but still require supplemental oxygen; they are the preferred method for home oxygen administration. The infant receives an adequate, continuous flow of oxygen while allowing optimal vision, positioning, and

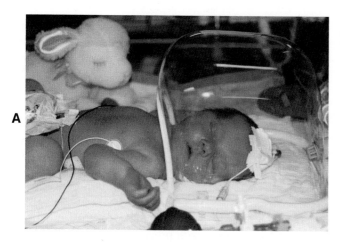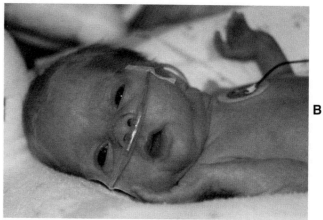

Fig. 26-2 **A,** Infant under hood. **B,** Infant with nasal cannula. (Courtesy Victoria Langer, RNC, MSN, NNP; from Dickason, E., Silverman, B., & Kaplan, J. [1998]. *Maternal-infant nursing care* [3rd ed.]. St. Louis: Mosby.)

parental holding. Infants can also breastfeed while receiving oxygen by this method. The nasal prongs must be inspected often to ensure that they are not partially obstructed by milk or secretions.

Continuous distending pressure. Infants who are unable to maintain an adequate PaO$_2$ despite the administration of oxygen by hood or nasal cannula may require the delivery of oxygen using continuous distending airway pressure via continuous positive airway pressure (CPAP) or continuous negative pressure. CPAP delivers oxygen at a preset pressure (Fig. 26-3, *A*) by means of nasal prongs, nasal pharyngeal tubes, endotracheal tube, or face mask. Nasal prongs are the most common method of CPAP delivery. An orogastric tube may be necessary for decompression of the stomach during use of nasal prongs. CPAP increases the functional residual capacity; improves the diffusion time of pulmonary gases, including oxygen; and can decrease PVR

and intrapulmonary shunting. If implemented early enough, CPAP may preclude the need for mechanical ventilation. CPAP is the preferred mode for infants who require minor distending pressure without the trauma associated with endotracheal intubation and its inherent complications (Hagedorn, Gardner, & Abman, 2002).

Mechanical ventilation. Mechanical ventilation must be implemented if other methods of therapy cannot correct abnormalities in oxygenation (Fig. 26-3, *B*). Its use is indicated whenever blood gas values reveal the existence of severe hypoxemia or severe hypercapnia. The condition of the infant experiencing apnea with bradycardia, ineffective respiratory effort, shock, asphyxia, infection, meconium aspiration syndrome (MAS), respiratory distress syndrome (RDS), or congenital defects that affect ventilation may also deteriorate and require intubation to reverse the process.

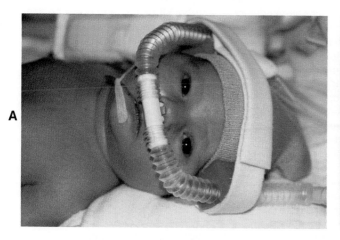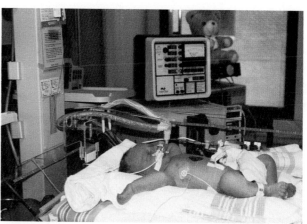

Fig. 26-3 **A,** Infant receiving ventilatory assistance with nasal continuous positive airway pressure (CPAP). **B,** Infant intubated and on ventilator. (Courtesy Victoria Langer, RNC, MSN, NNP; from Dickason, E., Silverman, B., & Kaplan, J. [1998]. *Maternal-infant nursing care* [3rd ed.]. St. Louis: Mosby.)

Ventilator settings are determined by the infant's particular needs. The ventilator is set to provide a predetermined amount of oxygen to the infant during spontaneous respirations and also to provide mechanical ventilation in the absence of spontaneous respirations. Newer technologies in ventilation allow oxygen to be delivered at lower pressures and in assist modes, thereby preventing the overriding of the infant's spontaneous breathing and providing distending pressures within a physiologic range, decreasing barotrauma and associated complications such as pneumothorax (accumulation of air in the pleural space) and pulmonary interstitial emphysema (PIE) (free air that accumulates in interstitial tissue). See Table 26-1 for an explanation of types of mechanical ventilation used in newborns.

Surfactant replacement therapy. Surfactant is a surface-active phospholipid secreted by the alveolar epithelium. Acting much like a detergent, this substance reduces the surface tension of fluids that line the alveoli and respiratory passages, resulting in uniform expansion and maintenance of lung expansion at low intraalveolar pressure. Immature development of these functions produces consequences that seriously compromise respiratory efficiency. Deficient surfactant production causes unequal inflation of alveoli on inspiration and the collapse of alveoli on end expiration. Without surfactant, infants are unable to keep their lungs inflated and therefore exert a great deal of effort to reexpand the alveoli with each breath. With increasing exhaustion, infants are able to open fewer and fewer alveoli. This inability to maintain lung expansion produces widespread atelectasis.

In the absence of alveolar stability (normal functional residual capacity) and with progressive atelectasis, PVR increases, whereas with normal lung expansion PVR decreases. Consequently, there is hypoperfusion to the lung tissue, with a decrease in effective pulmonary blood flow. The increase in PVR causes partial reversion to the fetal circulation, with

TABLE 26-1

*Common Methods for Assisted Ventilation in Neonatal Respiratory Distress**

METHOD	DESCRIPTION	HOW PROVIDED
Continuous distending pressure—continuous positive airway pressure (CPAP)	Provides constant distending pressure to airway in spontaneously breathing infant	Nasal prongs Endotracheal tube Face mask Nasal cannula or nasopharyngeal tubes Bubble CPAP uses water resistance
Intermittent mandatory ventilation (IMV)	Allows infant to breathe spontaneously at own rate but provides mechanical cycled respirations and pressure at regular preset intervals; infant may maintain asynchronous ventilation efforts, which diminishes effective gas exchange, air leaks, and air trapping; uses positive end-expiratory pressure (PEEP)	Endotracheal intubation
Synchronized intermittent mandatory ventilation (SIMV)	Mechanically delivered breaths are synchronized to the onset of spontaneous patient breaths; assist or control mode facilitates full inspiratory synchrony; involves signal detection of onset of spontaneous respiration from abdominal movement, thoracic impedance, and airway pressure or flow changes; pressure support ventilation provides an inspiratory pressure assist when spontaneous breathing is detected to decrease infant's work of breathing	Patient-triggered infant ventilator with signal detector and assist or control (A/C) mode; endotracheal tube; SIMV, A/C, and pressure support are also referred to as *patient-triggered ventilation*
Volume guarantee ventilation	Delivers a predetermined volume of gas using an inspiratory pressure that varies according to the infant's lung compliance (often used in conjunction with SIMV)	Volume guarantee ventilator with flow sensor; endotracheal tube
High-frequency oscillation (HFO)	Application of high-frequency, low-volume, sine-wave flow oscillations to airway at rates between 480 and 1200 breaths/min	Variable-speed piston pump (or loudspeaker, fluidic oscillator); endotracheal tube
High-frequency jet ventilation (HFJV)	Uses a separate, parallel, low-compliant circuit and injector port to deliver small pulses or jets of fresh gas deep into airway at rates between 250 and 900 breaths/min	May be used alone or with low-rate IMV; endotracheal tube

*This is not a comprehensive list of available ventilation modes. For more information, consult specific references on mechanical ventilation such as Donn, S., & Sinha, S. (2003). Invasive and noninvasive neonatal mechanical ventilation. *Respiratory Care, 48*(4), 426-441.

a right-to-left shunting of blood through the persisting fetal communications—the ductus arteriosus and foramen ovale. Inadequate pulmonary perfusion and ventilation produce hypoxemia and hypercapnia. Pulmonary arterioles, with their thick muscular layer, are markedly reactive to diminished oxygen concentration. Therefore a decrease in oxygen tension causes vasoconstriction in the pulmonary arterioles that is further enhanced by a decrease in blood pH. This vasoconstriction contributes to a significant increase in PVR. In normal ventilation with increased oxygen concentration, the ductus arteriosus constricts, and the pulmonary vessels dilate to decrease PVR.

Surfactant can be administered as an adjunct to oxygen and ventilation therapy. Generally, infants born before 32 weeks of gestation do not have adequate amounts of pulmonary surfactant to survive extrauterine life. In many centers the use of prophylactic surfactant is reserved for infants younger than 29 weeks who will likely have RDS (Hagedorn, Gardner, & Abman, 2002). Exogenous surfactant is manufactured artificially or extracted from bovine, porcine, or calf lung extract and is given as one or more doses through an endotracheal tube. The infant must be monitored for the occurrence of potential side effects such as patent ductus arteriosus (PDA) and pulmonary hemorrhage.

Although use of this medication has been associated with a significantly reduced length of time on mechanical ventilation and oxygen therapy and an increased survival rate in premature infants, it has not significantly decreased the incidence of CLD, intraventricular hemorrhage, or PDA. The administration of antenatal steroids to the mother and surfactant replacement have decreased the incidence of RDS and concomitant morbidities.

Inhaled nitric oxide, extracorporeal membrane oxygenation, liquid ventilation. Inhaled nitric oxide (INO), extracorporeal membrane oxygenation (ECMO), and liquid ventilation (LV) are additional therapies used in the treatment of respiratory distress and respiratory failure in neonates. INO is used in term and near-term infants with conditions such as persistent pulmonary hypertension, MAS, pneumonia, sepsis, and congenital diaphragmatic hernia to decrease or reverse pulmonary hypertension, pulmonary vasoconstriction, acidosis, and hypoxemia. Nitric oxide is a colorless, highly diffusible gas that can be administered through the ventilator circuit blended with oxygen. INO therapy may be used in conjunction with surfactant replacement therapy, high-frequency ventilation, or ECMO. Clinical trials have demonstrated that use of INO in infants with severe and moderate persistent pulmonary hypertension improved ventilatory status, decreased requirements for ventilatory support, and decreased the need for ECMO (Sadiq, Mantych, Bemawra, Devaslar, & Hocker, 2003). INO has not proved to be effective in decreasing RDS or in improved survival rates in preterm infants, although clinical trials are still ongoing (Kinsella & Abman, 2000; Sadiq et al., 2003).

Extracorporeal membrane oxygenation (ECMO) may be used in the management of term infants with acute

severe respiratory failure for the same conditions as those mentioned for INO. This therapy involves a modified heart-lung machine, although in ECMO, the heart is not stopped, and blood does not entirely bypass the lungs. Blood is shunted from a catheter in the right atrium or right internal jugular vein by gravity to a servo-regulated roller pump, pumped through a membrane lung where it is oxygenated, through a small heat exchanger where it is warmed, and then returned to the systemic circulation through a major artery such as the carotid artery to the aortic arch. ECMO provides oxygen to the circulation, allowing the lungs to "rest," and decreases pulmonary hypertension and hypoxemia in such conditions as persistent pulmonary hypertension of the newborn (PPHN), congenital diaphragmatic hernia, sepsis, meconium aspiration, and severe pneumonia. ECMO is not used in preterm infants younger than 34 weeks of gestation because of the anticoagulant therapy required in the pump and circuits; this may increase the potential for intraventricular hemorrhage in such infants. In some centers the success of high frequency ventilation and INO has greatly decreased the demand for and use of ECMO.

Liquid ventilation has been used experimentally in various neonatal clinical trials to increase pulmonary compliance, decrease lung surface tension, and decrease inflating pressures and subsequent barotrauma in newborn respiratory failure. This therapy involves the use of perfluorocarbons, which are inert liquids derived by replacing all the carbon-bound hydrogen atoms in organic compounds with fluorine. Oxygen delivery in the compromised neonate is significantly improved with perfluorocarbons; antibiotics and surfactant may be administered directly into the lungs with LV, and removal of debris such as meconium is facilitated.

The use of permissive hypercapnia to decrease lung damage and the incidence of CLD in neonates has had varying results, and trial studies to date have not demonstrated decreased mortality, lung tissue damage, or pulmonary and neurodevelopmental morbidity (Thome & Carlo, 2002; Woodgate & Davies, 2001). In permissive hypercapnia, the $PaCO_2$ is allowed to reach levels in the range of 45 to 55 mm Hg, whereas the previous goal was to maintain the $PaCO_2$ in the range of 35 to 45 mm Hg. Hypercapnia has been linked with an increased incidence of intraventricular hemorrhage.

High-frequency ventilation. Other modes of ventilator therapy include high-frequency oscillator ventilation and jet ventilation (see Table 26-1). These methods of high-frequency ventilation work by providing smaller volumes of oxygen at a significantly more rapid rate (more than 300 breaths/min) than traditional mechanical ventilators. As a result, the intrathoracic pressure and the risk of barotrauma are decreased.

Weaning from respiratory assistance

The infant is ready to be weaned from respiratory assistance when the ABG and oxygen saturation levels are maintained within normal limits (WNL) and the infant is able to establish spontaneous ventilation sufficient to maintain acid-base balance. A spontaneous, adequate respiratory effort must be present, and the infant must show improved muscle tone during increased activity. Weaning is done in a stepwise and gradual manner. This may consist of the infant being extubated, placed on nasal CPAP, and then weaned to oxygen by means of a hood or nasal cannula. Throughout the weaning process the infant's oxygen levels are monitored by pulse oximetry, tcPo₂ monitoring, and blood gas levels.

Some infants are not able to be weaned from all oxygen support by the time of discharge from the hospital and may require home oxygen therapy for several months. CLD (bronchopulmonary dysplasia), or congenital anomalies such as repaired congenital diaphragmatic hernia or tracheoesophageal fistula, or a neurologic insult with resultant dysfunction may prevent weaning.

The parents need to be given consistent information and be reassured about the infant's respiratory progress. Decisions regarding the nature of continued interventions should be included in a multidisciplinary plan of care, and the therapy should be explained frequently to the family.

Nutritional care

Optimum nutrition is critical in the management of LBW and preterm infants, but there are difficulties in providing for their nutritional needs. The various mechanisms for ingestion and digestion of foods are not fully developed; the more immature the infant, the greater the problem. In addition, the nutritional requirements for this group of infants are not known with certainty. It is known that all preterm infants are at risk because of poor nutritional stores and several physical and developmental characteristics.

An infant's need for rapid growth and daily maintenance must be met in the presence of several anatomic and physiologic disabilities. Although some sucking and swallowing activities are demonstrated before birth and in premature infants, coordination of these mechanisms does not occur until approximately 32 to 34 weeks of gestation, and they are not fully synchronized until 36 to 37 weeks. Initial sucking is not accompanied by swallowing, and esophageal contractions are uncoordinated. The gag reflex may not be developed until 36 weeks of gestation. Consequently, infants are highly prone to aspiration and its attendant problems. As infants mature, the suck-swallow pattern develops but is slow and ineffectual, and these reflexes may also become easily exhausted.

The amount and method of feeding are determined by the size and condition of the infant. Nutrition can be provided by either the parenteral or enteral route or by a combination of the two. Infants who are ELBW, VLBW, or critically ill are often fed exclusively by the parenteral route because of their inability to digest and absorb enteral nutrition. Illness factors resulting in hypoxia and major organ immaturity further preclude the use of enteral feeding until the infant's condition has stabilized; NEC has previously

been associated with enteral feedings in acutely ill or distressed infants (see Necrotizing Enterocolitis, p. 874). Total parenteral nutrition (TPN) support of acutely ill infants may be accomplished quite successfully with commercially available IV solutions specifically designed to meet the infant's nutritional needs, including protein, amino acids, trace minerals, vitamins, carbohydrates (dextrose), and fat (lipid emulsion).

Studies have shown that the early introduction of small amounts of enteral feedings in metabolically stable preterm infants is beneficial. These minimal enteral or **trophic feedings** have been shown to stimulate the infant's GI tract, preventing mucosal atrophy and subsequent enteral feeding difficulties. Minimal enteral feedings with as little as 0.1 to 4 ml of preterm formula or breast milk per kilogram may be given by gavage as early as the second or third postnatal day. Parenteral hydration and nutrition are continued until the infant is able to tolerate an amount of enteral feeding sufficient to sustain growth. An increased incidence of NEC in those VLBW infants fed enterally has not been substantiated (Evans & Thureen, 2001). In fact, minimal enteral feedings increase mineral absorption, increase serum calcium and alkaline phosphatase activity, and substantially decrease the incidence of bilious gastric residuals and feeding intolerance in preterm infants (Schanler, Shulman, Lau, Smith, & Heitkemper, 1999). Minimal enteral feedings have been recommended as the standard of care for feeding VLBW infants (Denne et al., 2002).

Type of nourishment. The types of formulas used, the mode and volume of feeding, and the infant's feeding schedule are based on the findings yielded by assessment of the following variables:

- Weight of the infant
- Pattern of weight gain or loss (infants weighing less than 1500 g require more energy for growth and thermoregulation)
- Presence or absence of suck and swallow reflexes
- Behavioral readiness to take oral feedings
- Physical condition, including presence or absence of bowel sounds, abdominal distention, or bloody stools, as well as presence and degree of respiratory distress or apneic episodes
- Residual from previous feeding, if being gavage fed
- Malformations (especially GI defects)
- Renal function, including urinary output and laboratory values (e.g., nitrogen balance, electrolyte balance, and glucose level)

Sufficient evidence now indicates that human milk is the best source of nutrition for term and preterm infants. Preterm infants may be able to successfully breastfeed earlier than previously believed (28 to 36 weeks). Even small preterm infants are able to breastfeed, if they have adequate sucking and swallowing reflexes and no other contraindications, such as respiratory complications or concurrent illness, are present (Morton, 2002). Preterm infants who are breastfed rather than bottle-fed demonstrate fewer oxygen desaturations, absence of bradycardia, warmer skin temperature, and better coordination of breathing, sucking, and swallowing (Gardner, Snell, & Lawrence, 2002).

Mothers who wish to breastfeed their preterm infants are encouraged to pump their breasts until their infants are sufficiently stable to tolerate breastfeeding. Appropriate guidelines for the storage of expressed mother's milk (EMM) should be followed to decrease the risk of milk contamination and destruction of its beneficial properties.

Commercially available preterm formulas are cow's milk based and whey predominant and have a higher concentration of protein, calcium, and phosphorus than term formulas to meet the unique needs of the preterm infant (American Academy of Pediatrics [AAP], 2004). Most preterm formulas are either 22 cal/oz or 24 cal/oz (breast milk and formula for term infants contain 20 cal/oz).

NURSE ALERT *Contamination of powdered infant formula in hospitals by* Enterobacter sakazakii *has been associated with serious neonatal infections, NEC, and mortality (Centers for Disease Control and Prevention [CDC], 2002; van Acker et al., 2001). The preparation of powdered formula in preterm infants should be carefully performed under strict aseptic technique, preferably in a pharmacy, and the formula properly refrigerated to prevent infection (AAP, 2004). When possible, alternatives to powdered formula should be chosen. Continuous infusion of powdered formula should not exceed 4 hours (CDC, 2002).*

Hydration. High risk infants often receive supplemental parenteral fluids to supply additional calories, electrolytes, or water. Adequate hydration is particularly important in preterm infants because their extracellular water content is higher (70% in full-term infants and up to 90% in preterm infants), their body surface is larger, and the capacity for osmotic diuresis is limited in preterm infants' underdeveloped kidneys. Therefore these infants are highly vulnerable to fluid depletion.

Infants who are ELBW, tachypneic, receiving phototherapy, or in a radiant warmer have increased insensible water loss (loss that occurs mainly through the skin and respiratory tract) that requires appropriate fluid adjustments. Nurses must monitor fluid status by daily (or more frequent) weights and accurate intake and output of all fluids, including medications and blood products. Urine-specific gravity and dipstick measurements are monitored per unit protocol, and serum electrolytes are obtained as warranted by the infant's condition. ELBW infants often require more frequent monitoring of these parameters because of their excessive fluid loss through the skin, immature renal function, and propensity to dehydration or overhydration. Intolerance of even dextrose 5% is not uncommon in the ELBW infant, with subsequent glycosuria and osmotic diuresis. Alterations in behavior, alertness, or activity level in these infants re-

ceiving IV fluids may signal an electrolyte imbalance, hypoglycemia, or hyperglycemia. The nurse must be observant for tremors or seizures in the VLBW or ELBW infant, because these may be a sign of hyponatremia or hypernatremia. Weight gain from fluid overload in the sick preterm infant may occur as a result of fluid retention (renal failure), inappropriate fluid administration (parenteral), or congestive heart failure. A fluid gain may result in the opening of a previously closed PDA, thus exacerbating associated illness. Growing preterm infants, especially those with CLD, receiving oral electrolyte supplements should be carefully monitored for rapid weight gain that may result in pulmonary congestion, PDA, and electrolyte imbalance. See Box 26-5 for calculation of a weight loss or gain.

Elimination patterns. Frequency of urination, as well as the amount, color, pH, and specific gravity of the urine is assessed. The assessment of bowel movements includes frequency of stooling and character of the stool, as well as whether there is constipation, diarrhea, or loss of fats (steatorrhea). Infants with unexplained abdominal distention are assessed carefully to rule out the presence of necrotizing enterocolitis or obstruction of the GI tract.

Oral feeding. Nourishment by the oral route is preferred for the infant who has adequate strength and GI function. Breast milk may be fed by breast, bottle, or gavage. Formula may be fed by bottle or gavage.

Many high risk infants cannot suck well enough to breastfeed or bottle-feed until they have recovered from their initial illness or matured physically. Infants may be put to breast for practice feeds as soon as medically stable.

Gavage feeding. Gavage feeding is a method of providing breast milk or formula through a nasogastric or orogastric tube (Fig. 26-4). Gavage feeding can be accomplished either with a tube inserted at each feeding (bolus) or continuously through an indwelling feeding tube. Breast milk or formula can be supplied intermittently using a syringe

---

BOX 26-5

Calculation of a Weight Loss or Gain

EXAMPLE 1

Day 1	1,750 g (birth weight)	$\dfrac{70}{1,750} = \dfrac{X\%}{100\%}$
Day 3	1,680 g	
	70 g loss	$1750X = 7,000$

$$1,750\overline{)7,000.0}$$

X = 4.0% weight loss

EXAMPLE 2

Day 3	1680 g	$\dfrac{40}{1,680} = \dfrac{X\%}{100\%}$
Day 4	1720 g	
	40 g gain	$1,680X = 4,000$

$$1,680\overline{)4,000.00}$$

X= 2.4% weight gain

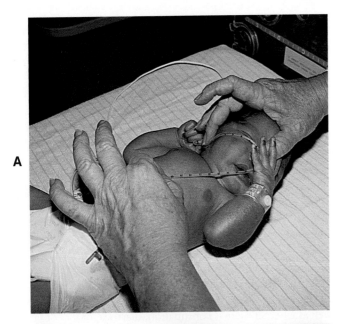

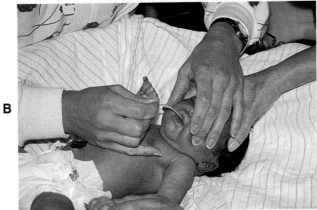

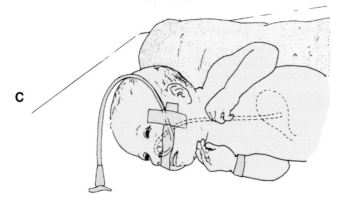

Fig. 26-4 Gavage feeding. **A,** Measurement of gavage feeding tube from tip of nose to earlobe and to midpoint between end of xiphoid process and umbilicus. Tape may be used to mark correct length on tube. **B,** Insertion of gavage tube using orogastric route. **C,** Indwelling gavage tube, nasogastric route. After feeding by orogastric or nasogastric tube, infant is propped on right side or placed prone (preterm infant) for 1 hour to facilitate emptying of stomach into small intestine. Note rolled towel for support. (**A** and **B,** Courtesy Marjorie Pyle, RNC, Lifecircle, Costa Mesa, CA.)

with gravity-controlled flow or can be given continuously using an infusion pump. The type of fluid instilled is recorded with every syringe change. The volume of the continuous feedings is recorded hourly, and the residual gastric aspirate is measured before each feeding. Residuals of less than a quarter of a feeding can be refed to the infant, depending largely on unit protocol. Feeding may be stopped if the residual is greater than 2 to 4 ml/kg or greater than the volume to be infused in 1 hour and is not resumed until the infant can be assessed for a possible feeding intolerance (Anderson, Johnson, Townsend, & Hay, 2002).

The orogastric route of gavage feedings is preferred because most infants are preferential nose breathers. However, some infants do not tolerate oral tube placement. The procedure for inserting a gavage feeding tube is described in the Procedure box.

Procedure

Inserting a Gavage Feeding Tube

1 Measure the length of the gavage tube from the tip of the nose to the lobe of the ear to the midpoint between the xiphoid process and the umbilicus (Fig. 26-4, *A*). Mark the tube with a piece of tape.

2 Lubricate the tip of the tube with sterile water, and insert gently through the nose or mouth (Fig. 26-4, *B*) until the predetermined mark is reached. Placement of the tube in the trachea will cause the infant to gag, cough, or become cyanotic.

3 Check correct placement of the tube by:
  a. Pulling back on the plunger to aspirate stomach contents. Lack of stomach aspirate or fluid is not necessarily evidence of improper placement. Aspiration of respiratory secretions may be mistaken for stomach contents; however, the pH of the stomach contents is much lower (more acidic) than the pH of respiratory secretions.
  b. Injecting a small amount of air (1 to 3 ml) into the tube while listening for gurgling by using a stethoscope placed over the stomach. Ensure that the tube is inserted to the mark; it is possible to hear air entering the stomach even if the tube is positioned above the gastroesophageal (cardiac) sphincter.

4 Tape the tube in place and also tape it to the cheek to prevent accidental dislodgement and incorrect positioning (Fig. 26-4, *C*).
  a. Assess the infant's skin integrity before taping the tube.
  b. Edematous or very preterm infants should have a pectin barrier placed under the tape to prevent abrasions, or use a zinc oxide base tape to prevent epidermal stripping.*

5 Tube placement *must* be assessed before each feeding.

*Lund, C., & Durand, D. (2002). Skin and skin care. In G. Merenstein & S. Gardner (Eds.), *Handbook of neonatal intensive care* (5th ed.). St. Louis: Mosby.

EVIDENCE-BASED PRACTICE
Early Discharge of Gavage-Fed Preterm Infants

BACKGROUND

- Preterm babies (<37 weeks of gestation) typically remain hospitalized until full oral feeding is established. Stable preterm infants could be discharged 1 to 2 weeks earlier, if the transition from gavage feeding to oral feeding could happen at home. The benefits of such a policy include uniting the family sooner, decreased nosocomial (hospital-acquired) infections, and considerable cost savings. Possible adverse outcomes include extra care burden for the family and complications such as aspiration pneumonia or growth failure. Health care support offered to families of preterm infants discharged while still on gavage feeding has included outpatient clinic visits, professional home visits, phone contact, and emergency room visits. Several studies of early discharge with home gavage infants show no evidence of inadequate weight gain or increase of readmissions.

OBJECTIVES

- To establish safety, the reviewers compared the effects of early discharge of stable, gavage-fed preterm infants to the usual practice of hospitalizing preterm infants until full oral feeding is established. Also of interest was any difference in outcomes dependent on the type of support (home versus clinic). The infants could not have intravenous supplementation. Outcomes could include number of days to transition to full sucking, breastfeeding prevalence, weight gain, length of hospitalization, neurodevelopment, readmission, milk aspiration, infection, death, satisfaction, cost, and health service use.

METHODS
Search Strategy

- The authors searched MEDLINE, Cochrane, CINAHL, and EMBASE for trials relating to early discharge. Search keywords included *early discharge, hospital in the home, gavage, tube, feed, low birth weight, preterm, premature infant, premature infant diseases, patient discharge, length of stay,* and *enteral nutrition.* Only one quasi-randomized trial met the criteria for the review. It was a 1999 Swedish trial of 88 infants from 75 families. The intervention group (n = 45) received early discharge with home visits by a registered nurse. The control group (n = 43) stayed in the hospital until full oral feeding was established.

Statistical Analyses

- Reviewers calculated relative risks for dichotomous (categoric) data and mean differences for continuous data. Results outside the 95% confidence intervals were accepted as significantly different.

FINDINGS

- The early discharge group had mean reductions in lengths of stay of 9.3 days. During that time, the inter-

vention group had significantly fewer infections than the hospitalized controls. While the controls were still hospitalized, eight of the 45 intervention group infants were readmitted during the home gavage program (two for jaundice, two for blood transfusions, one for inguinal herniorrhaphy and cryotherapy for retinopathy, one for removal of apnea monitor, one for skin condition and maternal anxiety, and one for respiratory syncytial virus). No differences were found in duration or exclusivity of breastfeeding, weight gain, readmission, health care use, maternal anxiety, or maternal confidence. Intervention mothers did score higher on feeling prepared to care for their infant, but the difference did not meet the level of significance. Cost was not measured directly, but the reviewers estimated the hospitalization costs of the control group exceeded the cost of health care support used by the intervention group. One infant in the control group died of sudden infant death syndrome (SIDS).

LIMITATIONS

- The trial was quasi-randomized and small, limiting generalizability. The paucity of trials led to this single study being included, even though nine of the 45 infants in the intervention (20%) never actually received home gavage feedings but were hospitalized until full oral feedings were established. Their data were included in the intervention group statistics, which follows the usual statistical guidelines of keeping subjects in "intention-to-treat" grouping. Nevertheless, one out of five in the intervention group actually received the control protocol.

CONCLUSIONS

- Although the early discharge group had mean reductions in lengths of stay of 9.3 days and the intervention group had significantly fewer infections than the hospitalized controls, no conclusions can be drawn because of the inclusion of only one study.

IMPLICATIONS FOR PRACTICE

- Policy changes for early versus usual discharge for stable preterm gavage-fed infants cannot be made on the basis of one small, quasi-randomized trial.

IMPLICATIONS FOR FURTHER RESEARCH

- Large randomized, controlled trials are needed to be able to suggest safety and efficacy of early discharge of stable gavage-fed preterm infants. Outcomes need to include growth, infection rates, costs, family impact, complications, and long-term outcomes. Of great interest to community health nurses are the types of support most effective to families with special-needs infants.

Reference: Collins, C., Makrides, M., & McPhee, A. (2003). Early discharge with home support of gavage feeding for stable preterm infants who have not established full oral feeds (Cochrane Review). In *The Cochrane Library*, Issue 2, 2004. Chichester, UK: John Wiley & Sons.

To begin the feeding, the nurse connects the barrel of a syringe to the gavage tube. While crimping the feeding tube, the nurse pours the specified amount of breast milk or formula into the syringe. The crimp in the tube is then released and the feeding allowed to flow by gravity at a rate that approximates that of an oral feeding (about 1 ml/min). The infant can be held or swaddled to help the infant associate the feeding with positive interactions.

Once the prescribed volume has been delivered, the tube is crimped or pinched and the syringe removed. The gavage tube is capped (or the nurse continues to pinch it) while removing it in one steady motion. Capping or pinching the tube prevents breast milk or formula from leaking from the tube and being aspirated during removal of the tube.

After the feeding, the infant is positioned to prevent aspiration. The documentation of the procedure includes the size of the feeding tube, the amount and quality of the residual from the previous feeding, the type and quantity of fluid instilled, and the infant's response to the procedure.

Gastrostomy feeding. Gastrostomy feeding involves the surgical placement of a tube through the skin of the abdomen into the stomach. With percutaneous gastrostomy insertion, feedings are often started within hours of insertion. Feedings by gravity are done slowly over 20 to 30 minutes. Special care must be taken to prevent rapid bolusing of the fluid because this may lead to abdominal distention, GI reflux into the esophagus, diarrhea with malabsorption, or respiratory compromise. Meticulous skin care at the tube insertion site is necessary to prevent skin breakdown or infection. Intake and output is carefully monitored to ensure adequate fluid and calorie intake and adequate renal function.

Advancing infant feedings. Feedings are advanced from passive (parenteral and gavage) to active (nipple and breastfeeding) as assessment data and the infant's ability to tolerate feedings warrant. The infant's sucking patterns and demonstration of a quiet alert state can also be used to determine readiness to nipple feed.

The infant receiving nutrition parenterally is gradually weaned off this type of nutrition. The nourishment given by gavage feedings is increased as parenteral fluids are decreased, depending on the infant's tolerance of enteral feeding. Feedings are advanced slowly and cautiously; if feedings are advanced too rapidly, vomiting, diarrhea, abdominal distention, and apneic episodes may result.

The infant receiving gavage feedings progresses to bottle-feeding or breast milk feedings. Gavage feedings are decreased as the infant's ability to suckle breast milk or formula improves. Often the infant is fed by both nipple and gavage feeding during this transition; this ensures intake of the prescribed volumes of both fluid and nutrients. The parents should be encouraged to interact by talking and making eye contact with the infant during feedings.

Because preterm infants are often discharged at weights equal to 1500 g, the need to continue nutritional intake and growth to match intrauterine growth remains. A concern in recent years has been the delayed growth of preterm infants

discharged home after neonatal intensive care. To address these growth needs, it is now recommended that formerly infants born prematurely receive either human breast milk with a preterm human milk fortifier or a 22 cal/oz formula until the postnatal age of 9 months.

Nonnutritive sucking. For the infant who requires gavage or parenteral feedings, nonnutritive sucking on a pacifier during the gavage procedure may improve oxygenation and facilitate earlier transition to nipple feeding (Fig. 26-5). Such nonnutritive sucking may lead to decreased energy expenditure with less restlessness.

Mothers of premature infants should be encouraged to let their infants start sucking at the breast during kangaroo care; some infant's suck and swallow reflexes may be coordinated by as early as 32 weeks of gestation.

Environmental concerns

Infants in NICUs are exposed to high levels of auditory input from the various machine alarms, and this can have adverse effects (Fig. 26-6). Although the AAP recommends that noise levels be lower than 45 decibels (db), continuous noise levels of 38 to 90 db are common in NICUs. An incubator produces a constant noise level of 50 to 75 db (Gardner & Goldson, 2002), and each new piece of life-support equipment used adds another 20 db to the background noise. The infant's hearing may be damaged if he or she is exposed to a constant decibel level of 90 db or frequent decibel swings higher than 110 db.

The infant's vision may be altered by the overhead lights or a phototherapy mask, making it difficult for the infant to interact with caregivers and family members. The infant may be unable to establish diurnal and nocturnal rhythms because of the continuous exposure to overhead lighting. In addition, sedation or pain medications affect the way in which the infant perceives the environment.

Effects of environmental hazards can be potentiated by some drugs used for infant therapy. Diuretics (especially

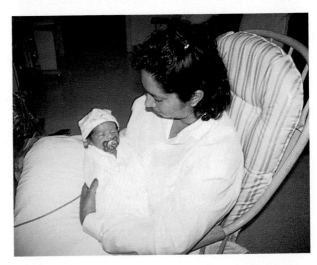

Fig. 26-5 Nonnutritive sucking by infant. (Courtesy Marjorie Pyle, RNC, Lifecircle, Costa Mesa, CA.)

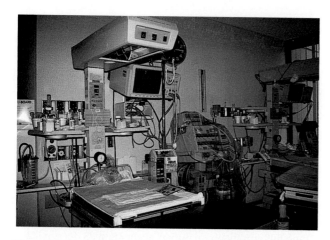

Fig. 26-6 NICU equipment, which, although necessary, may contribute to significant environmental stimulation. Note bed, wall oxygen attachments, monitor, ventilator, incubator, and pumps, all of which have alarm systems. (Courtesy Marjorie Pyle, RNC, Lifecircle, Costa Mesa, CA.)

furosemide [Lasix]), antibiotics (gentamicin), and antimalarial agents can potentiate noise-induced hearing loss. Routine hearing screening should be performed on all infants before discharge (see Fig. 19-9).

Nurses can modify the environment to provide a developmentally supportive milieu. In that way, the infant's neurobehavioral and physiologic needs can be better met, the infant's developing organization can be supported, and growth and development can be fostered (Byers, 2003; Martucci, 2004).

In one study, preterm infants with less than 32 weeks of gestation grew faster than similar cohorts when cycled lighting was provided instead of continuous near darkness (Brandon, Holditch-Davis, & Belyea, 2002). Other studies have found varying results regarding the provision of near darkness by dimming NICU lights and the incidence of retinopathy of prematurity in NICUs.

Developmental care

The goal of developmentally appropriate care is to support each infant's efforts to become as well-organized, competent, and stable as possible. Developmental care includes all care procedures and the physical and social aspects of care in the NICU (Byers, 2003; Johnson, Abraham, & Parrish, 2004; Martucci, 2004). The caregiver uses the infant's own behavior and physiologic functioning as the basis for planning care and providing interventions. Through caregiver observation, the infant's strengths, thresholds for disorganization, and areas in which the infant is vulnerable can be identified (Byers, 2003). The family is included in developmental care as the primary co-regulators (Als et al., 2003; Whitfield, 2003). Working together, the family and other caregivers provide opportunities to enhance the strengths of the family and the infant and to reduce the stress associated with the birth and care of high risk infants.

Lowering light and noise levels by instituting "quiet hours" during each 8-hour shift and positioning are just two of the ways in which nurses can support infants in their development. Sleep interruptions are minimized, and positioning and bundling the infant help promote self-regulation and prevent disorganization.

Positioning. The motor development of preterm infants permits less flexion than their full-term counterparts have. Caregivers can provide a variety of positions for infants; side-lying and prone are preferred to supine while in the intensive care setting. Body containment with use of blanket rolls, swaddling, holding the infant's arms in a crossed position, and secure holding provide boundaries and promote self-regulation during feeding, procedures, and other stressful interventions (Gardner & Goldson, 2002). The prone position encourages flexion of the extremities; a sling or hip roll assists in maintenance of flexion. Holding the limbs close to the body (containment) when the infant is moved decreases stimulation that produces jerky, uncoordinated movements. Proper body alignment is necessary to prevent developmental problems that may affect the ability to walk as the child matures.

Reducing inappropriate stimuli. Staff can reduce unnecessary noise by closing doors or portholes on incubators quietly, by not placing objects on top of incubators, avoiding radios, speaking quietly, and handling equipment noiselessly.

Nursing care affects sleep-wake behaviors in preterm infants. Infants can be protected from light by dimming the lights during the night or placing a blanket over the incubator (Fig. 26-7). Sleep-wake cycles can be induced with such measures. Infants need periods when they are completely undisturbed. Signs placed on incubators can remind staff and parents of quiet time.

Infant communication. Infants communicate their needs and ability to tolerate sensory stimulation through physiologic responses. The nurses and parents of

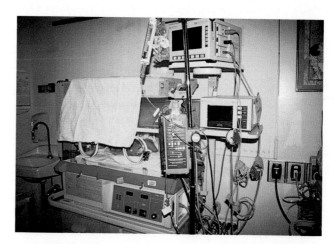

Fig. 26-7 Infant in double-walled incubator with a blanket for a light shield. (Courtesy Marjorie Pyle, RNC, Lifecircle, Costa Mesa, CA.)

high risk infants must therefore be alert to such cues. Although full-term infants may thrive on stimulation, this same stimulation in high risk infants can instead provoke physical symptoms of stress and anxiety (Gardner & Goldson, 2002).

Problems with noxious stimuli and barriers to normal contact may cause anxiety and tension. Clues to overstimulation include gaze aversion, hiccupping, gagging, or regurgitating food. Term infants exhibit a startle reflex, and premature infants move all of their limbs in an uncoordinated fashion in response to noxious stimuli. An irregular respiratory rate or an increased heart rate may develop in severely distressed infants, who may then be unable to regain a calm state.

A relaxed infant state is indicated by stabilization of vital signs, closed eyes, and a relaxed posture. Nonintubated infants may make soothing verbal sounds when they are relaxed. Infants requiring artificial ventilation cannot cry audibly and often show their distress through posturing; they then relax once their needs are met. As high risk infants heal and mature, they increasingly respond to stimuli in a self-regulated manner rather than with a dissociated response. Infants who do not demonstrate ability for self-regulation should be further evaluated for potential neurologic problems.

Infant stimulation. A Neonatal Individualized Development Care and Assessment Program (NIDCAP) routinely integrates aspects of neurodevelopmental theory with caregivers' observations, environmental interventions, and parental support (Byers, 2003; Gardner & Goldson, 2002). Routine reassessment is built into the program's design. Developmental stimuli may consist of such simple measures as placing a waterbed on top of the infant's mattress, or kangaroo (skin-to-skin) holding by the parents. The care of the infant is organized to allow extended periods of undisturbed rest and sleep. Pain medications or sedatives should be administered consistently per the unit's protocol.

Infants acquire a sense of trust as they learn the feel, sound, and smell of their parents (Gardner & Goldson, 2002). High risk infants must also learn to trust their caregivers to obtain comfort. However, caregivers in the nursery may inflict pain as part of the care they must give. For this reason, it is important for both the parents and the caregivers to employ comforting interventions such as removing painful stimuli, stopping hunger, and changing wet or soiled clothing to foster trust (Box 26-6). The simplest calming technique is to contain the infant's extremities close to the body using both hands.

When the infant is ready for interaction, the nurse has many options. All infants can tolerate being held, even if only for short periods. Additional ways for the nurse or parents to stimulate infants include cuddling, rocking, singing, and talking to the infant (Fig. 26-8). These activities are beneficial, increase weight gain, and decrease time to discharge. Stroking the infant's skin during medical therapy can provide tactile stimulation. The caregiver responds to the infant's cues by offering reassurance, providing for nonnutritive

BOX 26-6

Neonatal Health Psychology—
An Emerging Field

Health psychology was established as a discipline in 1994 and is defined as "the scientific study of the psychological processes and behavior in health, illness and health care." Neonatology is a subdiscipline of medicine that includes care for infants at risk for developmental disabilities. Psychology can make a contribution to the theory and care of the preterm infant, who is viewed as a "unique, emergent, coactional and hierarchical human being." Neonatal health psychology (NNHP) is defined as "the scientific study of biopyschosocial and behavioral processes in health, illness, and health care of the preterm (and fullterm) neonate during his/her first 28 days of life, and the relationship of such processes with later outcome." NNHP has significant interdisciplinary connotations reflecting the diverse ways in which information is derived from nonverbal neonates.

From Adamson-Macedo, E. (2004). Neonatal health psychology (NNHP): Theories and practice. *Neuro Endocrinology Letters, 25*(Suppl 1), 9-34.

sucking, stroking the infant's back, and talking to the infant. Music during endotracheal suctioning improves oxygen saturation (Chou, Wang, Chen, & Pai, 2003).

Mobiles and decals that can be changed frequently may also be placed within the infant's visual range to stimulate the infant visually. Wind-up musical toys provide rhythmic distractions as long as they are not too loud. If the infant is receiving phototherapy, the protective eye patches are removed periodically (e.g., during feeding) so that the infant can see the caregiver's face for short, comforting sessions. Although much beneficial infant interaction with caregivers

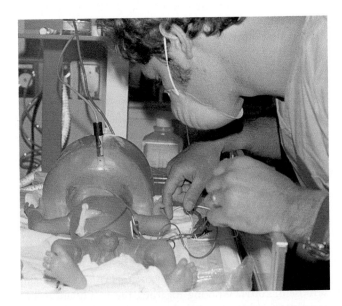

Fig. 26-8 A father caresses his tiny preterm infant receiving oxygen by hood in the NICU. (Courtesy Marjorie Pyle, RNC, Lifecircle, Costa Mesa, CA.)

may be desired, it is important to continually assess the infant's response to interactions designed to improve neurodevelopment. The caregivers cannot assume that the infant likes the mobile because the arms are extended and fingers splayed; this is actually a "time out" signal indicating stress. It is particularly important to help parents understand the infant's neurodevelopmental cues as not being a rejection of their caretaking abilities; at times preterm infants who are still disorganized need a time out from parental interaction in order to fully recover. The nurse can promote feelings of parental involvement by jointly developing an individualized plan of care for the infant. This may involve a written sign at the bedside with a brief message such as "Hello, Mom. This is Josh. I just had blood drawn at 1:00 PM so I need a 1-hour nap. I will see you at 2:00 PM. Love, Josh." Individualized care can influence brain development and behavioral function assessed at 9 months corrected age (Als et al., 2004).

Kangaroo care.   Kangaroo care (skin-to-skin holding) helps infants to directly interact with their parents (Brown, 2004). In this technique the infant, dressed only in a diaper, is placed directly on the parent's bare chest and then covered with the parent's clothing, a warmed blanket, or an overhead warmer lamp (Fig. 26-9). In this way, the parent's body temperature also functions as an external heat source that enhances the infant's temperature regulation. Even ventilator-dependent infants weighing less than 1000 g have been found to benefit from this measure, although they usually tolerate it for 30 minutes or less at a time.

Preterm infants experiencing kangaroo care recover rapidly from birth-related fatigue. Infants and parents who participate in kangaroo care have been observed to have dramatically better outcomes. The mothers report increased breast milk output and fewer feelings of helplessness related to their experiences in the NICU. Infants have been found to maintain their temperatures and oxygenation levels better and to experience fewer episodes of crying, apnea, and periodic respirations (Neu, Browne, & Vojir, 2000). They have also been observed to be alert and quiet longer and to have slightly higher heart rates. Kangaroo care also meets developmental needs by fostering neurobehavioral development.

Parental support

The nurse as support person and teacher shapes the environment and makes caregiving more responsive to the needs of parents and infant. Nurses are instrumental in helping parents learn who their infant is and recognize behavioral cues in his or her development.

If a high risk birth is anticipated, the family can be given a tour of the NICU or shown a video to prepare them for the sights and activities of the unit. After the birth, the parents can be given a booklet, be shown a video, or have someone describe what they will see when they go to the unit to see their infant. As soon as possible, the parents should see and touch their infant so that they can begin to acknowledge

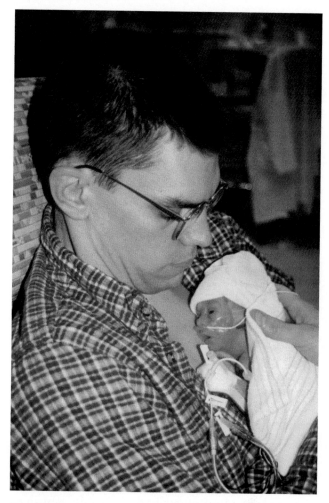

Fig. 26-9   Father providing kangaroo care. (Courtesy Judy Meyr, St. Louis, MO.)

the reality of the birth and the infant's true appearance and condition. They will need encouragement to begin to accomplish the psychologic tasks imposed by the preterm birth. A nurse and primary health care provider should be present during the parent's first visit to see the infant for the following reasons:

- To help them "see" the infant rather than focus on equipment. The significance and function of the apparatus that surrounds the infant should be explained.
- To explain the characteristics normal for an infant of their baby's gestational age. In this way, parents do not compare their infant with a full-term healthy baby.
- To encourage the parent to express feelings about the pregnancy, labor, and birth and the experience of having a preterm infant.
- To assess the parent's perceptions of the infant and determine the appropriate time for them to become actively involved in care.

As soon after the birth as possible, the parents are given the opportunity to meet the infant in the en face position, to touch the infant, and to see his or her favorable characteristics. Both parents, but especially the mother, encouraged to visit the nursery as desired and help with the infant's care. When the family cannot be present physically, for example, when the infant has been transported from another hospital, staff members can devise appropriate methods to keep the family in frequent touch with the newborn, such as daily phone calls, notes written as if from the infant, and video or photographs of the baby.

Many hospitals have support groups for parents of infants in intensive care nurseries. These groups encourage parents experiencing anxiety and grief to share their feelings. A parent with NICU experience often makes contact with a new member and provides additional support. These parents provide support for the new NICU parent through hospital visits, phone contact, and home visits.

In one testimonial, parents of infants in an NICU identified the following four central themes for NICU staff to consider when caring for the NICU family: (1) nurturing the parents; (2) providing accurate and consistent information; (3) clarifying NICU policies for neonatal treatment and family interaction; and (4) helping parents of NICU neonates connect with other parents in the NICU and graduates of NICU care (Woodwell, 2002).

Ward (2001) developed a 20-item NICU Family Needs Inventory to help identify the particular needs of parents with an infant in the NICU. Perceived needs identified in the initial study included providing information about the infant's condition and treatment plan, answering parents' questions honestly, actively listening to parents' fears and concerns, assisting parents in understanding the infant's responses, and providing assurance.

Some high risk infants can be discharged earlier than expected. Criteria for early discharge require the infant to be physiologically stable, receiving adequate nutrition and gaining weight daily, and to have a stable body temperature in an open bassinet. The parents or other caregivers must exhibit physical, emotional, and educational readiness to assume care of the infant. Ideally, the home environment is adequate for meeting the needs of the infant. The parents need to show that they know the way to take the infant's temperature and what signs and symptoms to report, and that they understand the dietary needs of the infant. Inadequate postnatal nutrition can be a serious problem and result in continued growth failure. After discharge, nutrient-enriched formula should be continued for about 9 months postterm for both breast and bottlefed infants (Dusick, Poindexter, Ehrenkranz, & Lemons, 2003).

Parent education

Cardiopulmonary resuscitation.   Sudden infant death syndrome (SIDS) is more likely to occur in preterm infants than in term infants; infants discharged from an NICU are about twice as likely to die unexpectedly during the first year of life as infants in the general population. Instruction in cardiopulmonary resuscitation (CPR) is essential for parents of all infants but especially for parents of infants at risk for life-threatening events. Risk factors include prematurity,

apneic and/or bradycardic spells, and the tendency to choke. All parents should be encouraged to obtain instruction in CPR at the hospital, local Red Cross, or other community agency. It should be emphasized that CPR knowledge does not preclude or substitute for proper positioning of the infant in the crib (i.e., supine) when put to sleep, unless otherwise directed by the primary care physician. In addition, the bed should have a firm mattress and be free of extra blankets, stuffed animals, or toys, which may cause the infant to become entangled and subsequently smothered.

Evaluation

The nurse uses the previously stated outcomes of care to evaluate the effectiveness of the physical and psychosocial aspects of care (Plan of Care).

COMPLICATIONS ASSOCIATED WITH PREMATURITY ■

Respiratory Distress Syndrome

Respiratory distress syndrome (RDS) is a lung disorder affecting mostly preterm infants, although a small percentage of term or near-term infants may also be affected. Maternal and fetal conditions associated with a decreased incidence and severity of RDS include female infant; African-American race; maternal steroid (betamethasone) therapy; and stressors such as maternal gestational hypertension, maternal drug abuse, chronic retroplacental abruption, prolonged rupture of membranes, and intrauterine growth restriction (IUGR) (Hagedorn, Gardner, & Abman, 2002). The incidence and severity of RDS increase with a decrease in gestational age. Perinatal asphyxia, hypovolemia, male infant, Caucasian race, maternal diabetes, second-born twin, familial predisposition, maternal hypotension, cesarean birth without labor, hydrops fetalis, and third-trimester bleeding are all factors that place an infant at increased risk for RDS (Hagedorn, Gardner, & Abman, 2002).

RDS is caused by a lack of pulmonary surfactant, which leads to progressive atelectasis, loss of functional residual capacity, and ventilation-perfusion imbalance with an uneven distribution of ventilation. Surfactant deficiency may be caused by insufficient surfactant production, abnormal composition and function, disruption of surfactant production, or a combination of these factors. The sequence of events that occurs is further compromised by weak respiratory muscles and an overly compliant chest wall, which are common to premature infants. Lung capacity is compromised by the presence of proteinaceous material and epithelial debris in the airways. The resulting decreased oxygenation, cyanosis, and metabolic or respiratory acidosis can increase PVR. This increased PVR can lead to right-to-left shunting and a reopening of the ductus arteriosus and foramen ovale (Hagedorn, Gardner, & Abman, 2002).

Clinical symptoms of RDS include tachypnea, grunting, nasal flaring, intercostal or subcostal retractions, hypercapnia, respiratory or mixed acidosis, hypotension, and shock.

These respiratory symptoms usually present immediately after birth or within 6 hours of birth. Physical examination reveals crackles, poor air exchange, pallor, use of accessory muscles (retractions), and occasionally apnea. Radiographic findings include uniform reticulogranular appearance and air bronchograms. The infant's clinical course is variable. There is usually an increased oxygen requirement and increased respiratory effort as atelectasis, loss of functional residual capacity, and ventilation-perfusion imbalance worsen.

Severe RDS is often associated with a shocklike state, as manifested by diminished cardiac inflow and low arterial BP. The ELBW or VLBW infant, as a result of extreme pulmonary immaturity, decreased glycogen stores, and lack of accessory muscles, may have severe RDS at birth.

RDS is a self-limiting disease with respiratory symptoms abating after 72 hours. The disappearance of respiratory symptoms coincides with the production of surfactant in type II cells of the alveoli.

The treatment for RDS is supportive. Adequate ventilation and oxygenation must be established and maintained in an attempt to prevent ventilation-perfusion mismatch and atelectasis. Exogenous surfactant, which alters the typical course of RDS, may be administered at or shortly after birth. Positive-pressure ventilation, CPAP, and oxygen therapy may be needed during the respiratory illness. Prevention of complications associated with mechanical ventilation is critical. These complications include pulmonary interstitial emphysema, pneumothorax, pneumomediastinum (accumulation of air in the mediastinum), and pneumopericardium (accumulation of air in the space surrounding the heart).

Acid-base balance is evaluated by monitoring ABG values (Table 26-2). Frequent blood sampling requires arterial access either by umbilical artery catheter (UAC) or by a peripheral arterial line. Pulse oximetry and transcutaneous carbon dioxide and oxygen monitors document trends in ventilation and oxygenation. Capillary blood gas values may be used to evaluate pH and Pco_2 in infants whose condition is more stable.

TABLE 26-2

Normal Arterial Blood Gas Values for Neonates

VALUE	RANGE
pH	7.35-7.45
Arterial oxygen pressure (Pao$_2$)	60-80 mm Hg
Carbon dioxide pressure (Paco$_2$)	35-45 mm Hg
Bicarbonate (Hco$_3$)	22-26 mEq/L
Base excess	(−4) to (+4)
Oxygen saturation	92%-94%

From Parry, W., & Zimmer, J. (2002). Acid-base homeostasis and oxygenation. In G. Merenstein & S. Gardner (Eds.), *Handbook of neonatal intensive care* (5th ed.). St. Louis: Mosby.

The maintenance of an NTE continues to be of critical importance in infants with RDS; infants with hypoxemia are unable to increase their metabolic rate when cold stressed.

The clinical and radiographic presentation of neonatal pneumonia may be similar to that of RDS. Therefore sepsis evaluation, including blood culture, complete blood count (CBC) with differential, and occasionally a lumbar puncture, is done in infants with RDS to rule out systemic infection. Laboratory and radiographic tests rarely confirm the diagnosis of neonatal pneumonia; rather, it is the clinical history and presenting clinical signs that provide a basis for the diagnosis and treatment (Stoll & Gotoff, 2004). Broad-spectrum antibiotics are begun while the results of cultures are awaited.

Fluid and nutrition must be maintained for the infant critically ill with RDS. Parenteral nutrition can provide protein and fat to promote a positive nitrogen balance. Daily monitoring of electrolytes, urine output, specific gravity, and weight assists in the evaluation of hydration status.

Respiratory distress of a nonpulmonary origin in neonates may also be caused by sepsis, cardiac defects (structural or functional), exposure to cold, airway obstruction (atresia), intraventricular hemorrhage, hypoglycemia, metabolic acidosis, acute blood loss, and drugs. Pneumonia in the neonatal period may present as respiratory distress caused by bacterial or viral agents and may occur alone or as a complication of RDS.

Patent Ductus Arteriosus

The ductus arteriosus is a muscular contractile structure in the fetus connecting the left pulmonary artery and the dorsal aorta. The ductus constricts after birth as oxygenation, the levels of circulating prostaglandins, and the muscle mass increase. Other factors that promote ductal closure include catecholamines, low pH, bradykinin, and acetylcholine. When the fetal ductus arteriosus fails to close after birth, **patent ductus arteriosus (PDA)** occurs. Ductal closure usually occurs within hours or days in the term infant but may be delayed in preterm infants as a result of oxygenation and circulating hormones (prostaglandins).

The clinical presentation in an infant with a PDA includes systolic murmur, active precordium, bounding peripheral pulses, tachycardia, tachypnea, crackles, and hepatomegaly. The systolic murmur is heard best at the second or third intercostal space at the upper left sternal border. An active precordium is caused by an increased left ventricular stroke volume. A widened pulse pressure may result in an increase in peripheral pulses.

Radiographic studies of infants with a large shunting PDA typically show cardiac enlargement and pulmonary edema; with a smaller PDA the radiograph may appear normal for the infant's age (Montoya & Washington, 2002). ABG findings reveal hypercarbia and metabolic acidosis. A color flow Doppler echocardiogram can demonstrate a PDA, identify the direction of the shunting (left-to-right, right-to-left, or both), and quantitate the amount of blood shunting across the PDA.

CD: Critical Thinking Exercise—Patent Ductus Arteriosus

NURSING DIAGNOSIS Ineffective breathing pattern related to pulmonary, cardiovascular, and neuromuscular immaturity, decreased energy reserves as evidenced by assessment findings (e.g., nasal flaring, tachypnea, grunting)

Expected Outcomes *Infant exhibits adequate oxygenation (i.e., arterial blood gas [ABG] levels and acid-base balance within normal limits [WNL] for age; oxygen saturations 92% or greater; respiratory rate and pattern WNL for age; breath sounds clear; absence of grunting and nasal flaring; minimal retractions; skin color appropriate).*

Nursing Interventions/*Rationales*

- Position neonate prone or supine, avoiding neck hyperextension *to promote optimum air exchange.* Use a side-lying position after feeding or in cases of excessive mucous production *to avoid aspiration.* Avoid Trendelenburg position *because it can cause increased intracranial pressure and reduce lung capacity.*
- Suction nasopharynx, trachea, and endotracheal tube only as necessary *to remove mucus and secretions.* Avoid oversuctioning *because it can cause bronchospasm, bradycardia, and hypoxia and predispose neonate to intraventricular hemorrhage.*
- Administer percussion, vibration, and postural drainage only as necessary *to facilitate drainage of secretions.*
- Administer oxygen and monitor neonatal response *to maintain oxygen saturation.*
- Maintain a neutral thermal environment *to conserve oxygen and glucose.*
- Monitor ABG levels, acid-base balance, oxygen saturation, respiratory rate and pattern, breath sounds, and airway patency; observe for grunting, nasal flaring, retractions, and cyanosis *to detect signs of respiratory distress.*

NURSING DIAGNOSIS Ineffective thermoregulation related to immature central nervous system [CNS] temperature regulation, decreased brown fat, inability to produce body heat, and minimal subcutaneous fat stores as evidenced by assessment findings (e.g., absent or decreased subcutaneous tissue, body temperature less than 36.5° C)

Expected Outcome *Infant exhibits maintenance of stable body temperature within normal range for postconceptional age (36.5° to 37.2° C).*

Nursing Interventions/*Rationales*

- Place neonate in a prewarmed radiant warmer *to maintain stable temperature.*
- Place temperature probe over tissue (not bone) such as abdomen *to control heat levels delivered by radiant warmer.*
- Take axillary temperature periodically *to monitor temperature and cross-check functioning of warmer unit.*
- Avoid exposing infant to cool air and drafts, cold scales, cold stethoscopes, cold examination tables, and prolonged bathing, *which predispose the infant to heat loss.*
- Use additional shield or cover in warmer (plastic wrap) *to prevent further heat loss from exposure to drafts and air currents and to minimize insensible water loss.*
- Monitor probe function and status frequently *because detachment can cause overheating or warmer-induced hyperthermia.*
- Transfer infant to a servocontrolled open warmer bed or incubator *when temperature has stabilized.*

NURSING DIAGNOSIS Risk for infection related to immature immune system, exposure to multiple sources of infection (invasive procedures, maternal infection) as evidenced by assessment findings (e.g., feeding intolerance, apnea, temperature instability)

Expected Outcome *Infant exhibits no evidence of infection.*

Nursing Interventions/*Rationales*

- Institute scrupulous handwashing techniques before and after handling neonate; ensure all supplies and/or equipment are clean before use; and ensure strict aseptic technique with invasive procedures *to minimize exposure to infective organisms.*
- Prevent contact with persons who have communicable infections and instruct parents in infection control procedures *to minimize infection risk.*
- Continuously monitor vital signs for stability *because instability, hypothermia, or prolonged temperature elevations are indicators of infection.*
- Administer prescribed antibiotics *to provide coverage for infection during sepsis workup.*

NURSING DIAGNOSIS Risk for imbalanced nutrition: less than body requirements related to inability to ingest adequate nutrients for growth secondary to gastrointestinal (GI) immaturity, decreased stomach capacity, and associated illness factors as evidenced by inadequate weight gain

Expected Outcomes *Infant receives adequate amount of nutrients with sufficient caloric intake to maintain positive nitrogen balance; demonstrates steady weight gain (as appropriate to acuity).*

Nursing Interventions/*Rationales*

- Administer parenteral fluid or total parenteral nutrition (TPN) as prescribed *to provide adequate nutrition and fluid intake.*
- Monitor for signs of intolerance to TPN, *which can interfere with effective replenishment of nutrients.*
- Periodically assess readiness to orally feed (i.e., strong suck, swallow, and gag reflexes) *to provide appropriate transition from TPN to oral feeding as soon as neonate is ready.*
- Advance volume and concentration of formula when orally feeding per unit protocol *to avoid overfeeding and feeding intolerance.*
- Provide expressed breast milk (including colostrum) when infant's condition is stable *to enhance GI development, promote natural immunity, and achieve other benefits of human milk (digestive enzymes).*
- If mother desires to breastfeed when neonate's condition is stable, demonstrate how to express milk *to establish and maintain lactation until infant can breastfeed.*

NURSING DIAGNOSIS Risk for imbalanced (specify if deficient or excess) fluid volume related to large extracellular fluid (ECF) volume, decreased ability to regulate fluid shifts, renal immaturity, permeable skin, and insensible and transepidermal water losses as evidenced by excessive weight gain or loss

Expected Outcome *Infant exhibits evidence of fluid homeostasis.*

Nursing Interventions/*Rationales*

- Administer parenteral fluids as prescribed and regulate carefully *to maintain fluid balance.* Avoid hypertonic fluids such

PLAN OF CARE   *The High Risk Preterm Newborn—cont'd*

as undiluted medications and concentrated glucose *because they can cause excess solute load on immature kidneys.*

- Implement strategies (e.g., use of plastic covers and increase of ambient humidity) *that minimize insensible water loss.*
- Monitor hydration status (i.e., skin turgor, blood pressure, edema, weight, mucous membranes, fontanels, urine specific gravity, and electrolytes) and intake and output *to evaluate for evidence of dehydration or overhydration.*

NURSING DIAGNOSIS **Risk for impaired skin integrity related to immature skin structure, poor perfusion, immobility, and invasive procedures as evidenced by epidermal stripping with adhesive removal or placement and translucent skin, erythema, and abrasions**

Expected Outcome *Infant's skin remains intact with no evidence of irritation or injury.*

Nursing Interventions/*Rationales*

- Cleanse skin as needed with plain warm water and apply moisturizing agents to skin *to prevent dryness and reduce friction across skin surface.*
- When performing procedures, minimize use of tape and apply a skin barrier between tape and skin; use transparent elastic film for securing central and peripheral lines; use limb electrodes for monitoring or attach with hydrogel and rotate electrodes often; remove adhesives with soap and water rather than alcohol or acetone-based adhesive removers *to minimize skin damage.*
- Carefully monitor use of thermal devices such as pulse oximeter probes, BiliBlankets, or thermal heating pads *to prevent burns.*
- Monitor skin closely for evidence of redness, rash, irritation, bruising, breakdown, ischemia, and infiltration *to detect and treat potential complications early.*

NURSING DIAGNOSIS **Risk for injury of the CNS related to fluctuating systemic and intracranial pressures, immature vascular bed, immature state regulatory ability, environmental stimuli, and episodes of hyperoxia and hypoxia as evidenced by episodes of hypoxia associated with handling, and fluctuating blood pressure readings.**

Expected Outcome *Infant will exhibit normal intracranial pressure (ICP) with no evidence of intraventricular hemorrhage.*

Nursing Interventions/*Rationales*

- Institute minimum stimulation protocol (i.e., minimizing handling, clustering care techniques, avoiding sudden head movements to one side, ensuring undisturbed sleep periods, using light variations to simulate day and night, limiting personnel and equipment noise in environment) *to decrease stress responses, which can increase ICP.*
- Institute ordered pharmacologic and nonpharmacologic pain control methods *to manage pain and reduce physical stress.*

- Avoid hypertonic solutions and medications *because they increase cerebral blood flow.*
- Elevate head of bed 15 to 20 degrees *to decrease ICP.*
- Monitor vital signs *for evidence of ICP.*
- Recognize signs of overstimulation (e.g., flaccidity, yawning, irritability, crying, staring, and active averting) *so stimulation can be stopped to allow rest.*

NURSING DIAGNOSIS **Risk for impaired parenting related to separation and interruption of parent-infant attachment secondary to premature birth, severity of infant's illness, high-tech neonatal intensive care unit (NICU) environment; and anticipatory grieving over loss of perfect newborn as evidenced by physical separation from parents, verbalization of shock and disbelief at appearance of infant, lack of contact between infant and parent**

Expected Outcomes *Parents establish contact with neonate; demonstrate competent parenting skills and willingness to care for neonate.*

Nursing Interventions/*Rationales*

- Before parents' first visit to the NICU, prepare them by explaining what the neonate will look like, what the equipment will look like, and what the equipment does, *to diminish fear and decrease sense of shock.*
- Keep parents informed about infant's condition (e.g., improvements and setbacks) and important aspects of infant's care; encourage and answer parental questions; actively listen to parent concerns *to establish trust, open communication, and caring atmosphere to aid in coping.*
- Encourage parents to contact NICU staff any time, day or night, for concerns regarding the infant's condition *to maintain open channels of communication regarding infant's status and decrease parents' fear of unknown.*
- Encourage parents to visit the NICU often; to name infant; to touch, hold, or caress infant as physical condition permits; to be actively involved in infant's care; to bring personal items (e.g., clothing, stuffed animals, or pictures of family) *to allow formation of emotional bond.*
- Reinforce parent involvement and praise care endeavors *to increase self-confidence in their contribution.*
- Encourage parents to bring other siblings to visit preterm infant as age-appropriate; explain to siblings what they are seeing; encourage siblings to draw pictures or write letters for infant and place in or near infant's crib *to promote family involvement, help ease sibling fears, and let them contribute to infant's care.*
- Refer parents to social services as needed *to ensure comprehensive care.*
- Provide consistent and frequent information regarding infant's condition through multidisciplinary conferences *to promote parent trust in caregivers and provide consistent information.*
- Encourage parental involvement in a support group *to share feelings and decrease anxiety.*

The PDA can be managed medically or surgically. Medical management consists of ventilatory support, fluid restriction, and the administration of diuretics and indomethacin. Indomethacin is a prostaglandin synthetase inhibitor that blocks the effect of the arachidonic acid products on the ductus and causes the PDA to constrict. Ventilatory support is adjusted based on ABG levels. Fluid restriction is implemented to decrease cardiovascular volume overload in association with the diuretic therapy. Surgical ligation is performed when PDA is clinically significant and medical management has failed. The nonsteroidal antiinflammatory drug (NSAID), ibuprofen, has been used with some success in the medical closure of PDA in preterm infants. This drug has fewer side effects than indomethacin and acts by inhibiting prostaglandin formation (Flores, 2003).

Nursing care of the infant with PDA focuses on supportive care. The infant needs an NTE, adequate oxygenation, meticulous fluid balance, and parental support.

Periventricular-Intraventricular Hemorrhage

Periventricular-intraventricular hemorrhage (PV-IVH) is one of the most common types of brain injury that occurs in neonates and is among the most severe in both short-term and long-term outcomes. The true incidence of PV-IVH is unknown, but the general estimate is 15% in infants at less than 32 weeks of gestation or weighing under 1501 g (Volpe, 2001). PV-IVH occurs in approximately 3.5% to 5% of term infants, with 50% of those cases caused by asphyxia or trauma. In term infants the symptoms appear within 48 hours of birth (Paige & Carney, 2002).

The pathogenesis of PV-IVH includes intravascular factors (e.g., fluctuating or increasing cerebral blood flow, increases in cerebral venous pressure, and coagulopathy), vascular factors, extravascular factors (hypoglycemia, acidosis), and routine nursery care (rapid volume expansion, blood transfusion). PV-IVH events typically occur within the first week of life. PV-IVH is classified according to severity, which determines long-term neurodevelopmental outcomes.

Nursing care focuses on recognition of factors that increase the risk of PV-IVH, interventions to decrease the risk of bleeding, and supportive care to infants who have bleeding episodes. The infant is positioned with the head in midline and the head of the bed elevated slightly to prevent or minimize fluctuations in intracranial BP. An NTE is maintained, as well as oxygenation. Rapid infusions of fluids should be avoided. BP is monitored closely for fluctuations. The infant is monitored for signs of pneumothorax because it often precedes PV-IVH.

Necrotizing Enterocolitis

Necrotizing enterocolitis (NEC) is an acute inflammatory disease of the GI mucosa, commonly complicated by perforation. This often fatal disease occurs in about 2% to 5% of newborns in NICUs. Three factors appear to play an important role in the development of NEC: intestinal ischemia, colonization by pathogenic bacteria, and substrate (formula feeding) in the intestinal lumen. The precise cause of NEC is still uncertain, but it appears to occur in infants whose GI tract has suffered vascular compromise. Intestinal ischemia of unknown etiology, immature GI host defenses, bacterial proliferation, and feeding substrate are now believed to have a multifactorial role in the etiology of NEC. Prematurity remains the most prominent risk factor in the development of NEC.

The onset of NEC in the full-term infant usually occurs between 4 and 10 days after birth. In the preterm infant the onset may be delayed for up to 30 days. Signs of developing NEC are nonspecific, which is characteristic of many neonatal disease processes. Some generalized signs include decreased activity, hypotonia, pallor, recurrent apnea and bradycardia, decreased oxygen saturation, respiratory distress, metabolic acidosis, oliguria, hypotension, decreased perfusion, temperature instability, and cyanosis. GI symptoms include abdominal distention, increasing or bile-stained residual gastric aspirates, vomiting (bile or blood), grossly bloody stools, abdominal tenderness, and erythema of the abdominal wall (Bensard, Calkins, Partrick, & Price, 2002).

Diagnosis of NEC is confirmed by radiographic examination that reveals bowel loop distention, pneumatosis intestinalis, pneumoperitoneum, portal air, or a combination of these findings. The abnormal radiographic findings are caused by the bacterial colonization of the GI tract associated with NEC, resulting in an ileus. Pneumatosis intestinalis, pneumoperitoneum, and portal air are caused by gas produced by the bacteria that invade the wall of the intestines and escape into the peritoneum and portal system when perforation occurs. Laboratory evaluation includes a complete blood cell count with differential, coagulation studies, ABG analysis, serum electrolyte levels, and blood culture. The white blood cell (WBC) count may be either increased or decreased. The platelet count and coagulation studies may be abnormal, with thrombocytopenia and disseminated intravascular coagulation (DIC). Electrolyte levels may be abnormal, with leaking capillary beds and fluid shifts with the infection.

Treatment of infants with NEC is supportive and preventive for bowel perforation. Oral or tube feedings are discontinued to rest the GI tract. A nasogastric tube is inserted and placed to low suction to provide gastric decompression. Parenteral therapy (often by TPN) is begun. NEC is an infectious disease; control of infection is imperative, with an emphasis on careful handwashing before and after infant contact. Systemic antibiotic therapy is instituted, and surgical resection is performed if perforation or clinical deterioration occurs.

With early recognition and treatment, medical management is increasingly successful. If there is progressive deterioration under medical management or evidence of perforation, surgical resection and anastomosis are performed. Extensive involvement may necessitate surgical intervention and establishment of an ileostomy, jejunostomy, or colostomy. Sequelae in surviving infants include short-gut syndrome, colonic stricture with obstruction, fat malabsorption, and failure to thrive secondary to intestinal dysfunction. Various surgical interventions for NEC are available and depend on the extent of bowel necrosis, associated illness factors, and infant stability. Intestinal transplantation has been successful in some preterm infants with NEC-associated short-gut syndrome who had already developed life-threatening TPN-related complications. Transplantation may be a lifesaving option for infants who previously faced high morbidity and mortality (Vennarecci et al., 2000). Therapy may be prolonged and recovery may be delayed by adhesions, complications of bowel resection, short-gut syndrome (especially if the ileocecal valve is removed), and intolerance of oral feedings.

NURSE ALERT *Observe for indications of early development of NEC by checking the appearance of the abdomen for distention (measuring abdominal girth, measuring residual gastric contents before feedings, and listening for the presence of bowel sounds) and performing all routine assessments for high risk neonates.*

Minimal enteral feedings (trophic feeding, GI priming) have gained acceptance with no evidence of increased incidence of NEC. Early experience indicates such feedings may in fact be protective against NEC in nonasphyxiated preterm infants in addition to exerting other potential benefits. There is evidence that human milk may have a protective effect against the development of NEC (Diehl-Jones & Askin, 2004).

Complications of Oxygen Therapy

Retinopathy of prematurity

Retinopathy of prematurity (ROP) is a complex, multicausal disorder that affects the developing retinal vessels of premature infants. The normal retinal vessels begin to form in utero at approximately 16 weeks of gestation in response to an unknown stimulus. The retinal vessels continue to develop until they reach maturity at approximately 42 to 43 weeks after conception. Once the retina is completely vascularized, the retinal vessels are not susceptible to ROP. The mechanism of injury in ROP is unclear. Oxygen tensions that are too high for the level of retinal maturity initially result in vasoconstriction. After oxygen therapy is discontinued, neovascularization occurs in the retina and vitreous, with capillary hemorrhages, fibrotic resolution, and possible retinal detachment. Scar tissue formation and consequent visual impairment may be mild or severe. The entire disease process in severe cases may take as long as 5 months to evolve. Examination by an ophthalmologist before discharge and a schedule for repeat examinations thereafter are recommended for the parents' guidance.

The key to management of ROP is prevention and early detection of premature birth.

Although exposure to bright light has not proven to contribute to ROP, such exposure is nevertheless undesirable from a neurobehavioral developmental perspective. All caregivers should use supplemental oxygen judiciously, monitor oxygen blood levels carefully, attend to saturation monitor alarms promptly, and prevent wide fluctuations in oxygen blood levels (hyperoxemia and hypoxemia).

Circumferential cryopexy, laser photocoagulation, vitamin E therapy, and decreased intensity of ambient light are used in the treatment of ROP with varying results (Box 26-7).

BOX 26-7

Treatments for Retinopathy of Prematurity

- *Circumferential cryopexy*—Use of a freezing probe around the edge of the retina to seal tears
- *Laser photocoagulation*—Use of a light (laser) that can be microscopically focused; used to seal leaky blood vessels or retinal tears
- *Vitamin E*—Fat-soluble vitamin with antioxidant properties that encourages healing and reduces scarring

---

Early screening and detection should be provided for infants born at less than 28 weeks of gestation and whose weight is less than 1500 g and for infants weighing between 1500 g and 2000 g who are believed to be at high risk for development of ROP (AAP, 2001).

Chronic Lung Disease

Chronic lung disease, formerly called bronchopulmonary dysplasia, is a chronic pulmonary iatrogenic condition caused by barotrauma from pressure ventilation and oxygen toxicity (Hagedorn, Gardner, & Abman, 2002). The etiology of CLD is multifactorial and includes pulmonary immaturity, surfactant deficiency, lung injury and stretch, barotrauma, inflammation caused by oxygen exposure, fluid overload, ligation of a PDA, and genetic predisposition (Hagedorn, Gardner, & Abman, 2002). The incidence of CLD in infants weighing less than 1500 g who require mechanical ventilation for RDS ranges from 23% to 80% (Berger, Bachmann, Adams, & Schubiger, 2004; Gracey, Talbot, Lankford, & Dodge, 2002). In some institutions, the overall incidence of CLD has decreased over the past decade (Byrne, Mellen, Lindstrom, & Cotton, 2002).

Clinical signs of CLD include tachypnea, retractions, nasal flaring, increased work of breathing, exercise intolerance (to handling and feeding), and tachycardia (Hagedorn, Gardner, & Abman, 2002). Auscultation of lung fields in affected infants reveals crackles, decreased air movement, and occasionally expiratory wheezing.

Treatment for CLD includes oxygen therapy, nutrition, fluid restriction, and medications (e.g., diuretics, corticosteroids, and bronchodilators). The use of corticosteroids to prevent or treat CLD is controversial because of the side effects and varied results in clinical trials; however, corticosteroids are used in many centers to treat or prevent CLD (AAP, 2002). The key to the management of CLD is prevention by reducing the incidence of prematurity and RDS and by using surfactant and antenatal steroids and minimizing lung trauma from mechanical ventilation and high oxygen concentrations.

The prognosis for infants with CLD depends on the degree of pulmonary dysfunction. Most deaths occur within the first year of life as a result of cardiorespiratory failure, sepsis, or respiratory infection; in some infants the deaths are sudden and unexplained.

THE POSTMATURE INFANT

Postterm infants are those whose gestation is prolonged beyond 42 weeks, regardless of birth weight; the infant is called *postmature*. These infants may be large for gestational age (LGA) or small for gestational age (SGA), but most often their weight is appropriate for gestational age (AGA). It is important to determine whether the pregnancy is actually prolonged and also whether there is any evidence of fetal jeopardy as a result. The cause of prolonged pregnancy is unknown. Postmaturity can be associated with placental insufficiency, resulting in a newborn who has a thin, emaciated appearance (dysmature) at birth because of loss of subcutaneous fat and muscle mass. There may be meconium staining of the fingernails, the hair and nails may be long, and vernix may be absent. The skin may peel off. Not all postmature infants show signs of dysmaturity; some continue to grow in utero and are large at birth.

Perinatal mortality is significantly higher in the postmature fetus and neonate. During labor and birth, increased oxygen demands of the postmature fetus may not be met. Insufficient gas exchange in the postmature placenta increases the likelihood of intrauterine hypoxia, which may result in the passage of meconium in utero, thereby increasing the risk for meconium aspiration syndrome. Of all the deaths of postmature newborns, half occur during labor and birth, about one third occur before the onset of labor, and one sixth occur in the newborn period.

Meconium Aspiration Syndrome

Meconium staining of the amniotic fluid can be indicative of nonreassuring fetal status, especially in a vertex presentation. It appears in from 8% to 20% of all births. Many infants with meconium staining exhibit no signs of depression at birth; however, the presence of meconium in the amniotic fluid necessitates careful supervision of labor and close monitoring of fetal well-being. The presence of a team skilled in neonatal resuscitation is required at the birth of any infant with meconium-stained amniotic fluid. The mouth and nares of the infant are routinely suctioned on the perineum before the infant's first breath. However, Vain and coworkers (2004) in a multicentered randomized, controlled trial found no difference in outcomes between those infant who were suctioned and those who were not. The current practice needs further study.

Meconium in the airway at birth can migrate down to the terminal airways, causing mechanical obstruction leading to meconium aspiration syndrome (MAS). The fetus may have aspirated meconium in utero, which can cause a chemical pneumonitis. These infants may develop persistent pulmonary hypertension of the newborn (PPHN), further complicating their management. Infants with moderate-to-severe MAS may receive surfactant replacement to improve alveolar function.

Persistent Pulmonary Hypertension of the Newborn

Persistent pulmonary hypertension of the newborn is a term applied to the combined findings of pulmonary hypertension, right-to-left shunting, and a structurally normal heart. PPHN may occur either as a single entity or as the main component of MAS, congenital diaphragmatic hernia, RDS, hyperviscosity syndrome, or neonatal pneumonia or sepsis. PPHN is also called *persistent fetal circulation (PFC)* because the syndrome includes reversion to fetal pathways for blood flow.

A brief review of fetal blood flow can help in the visualization of the problems with PPHN (see Fig. 7-12). In utero, oxygen-rich blood leaves the placenta through the umbilical vein, goes through the ductus venosus, and enters the inferior vena cava. From there, it empties into the right atrium and is mostly shunted across the foramen ovale to the left atrium, effectively bypassing the lungs. This blood enters the left ventricle, leaves through the aorta, and preferentially perfuses the carotid and coronary arteries. Thus the heart and brain receive the most oxygenated blood. Blood drains from the brain into the superior vena cava, reenters the right atrium, proceeds to the right ventricle, and exits through the main pulmonary artery. The lungs are a high-pressure circuit, needing only enough perfusion for growth and nutrition. The ductus arteriosus (connecting the main pulmonary artery and the aorta) is the path of least resistance for the blood leaving the right side of the fetal heart, shunting most of the cardiac output away from the lungs and toward the systemic system. This right-to-left shunting is the key to fetal circulation.

After birth, both the foramen ovale and the ductus arteriosus close in response to various biochemical processes, pressure changes within the heart, and dilation of the pulmonary vessels. This dilation allows virtually all of the cardiac output to enter the lungs, become oxygenated, and provide oxygen-rich blood to the tissues for normal metabolism. Any process that interferes with this transition from fetal to neonatal circulation may precipitate PPHN. PPHN characteristically proceeds into a downward spiral of exacerbating hypoxia and pulmonary vasoconstriction. Prompt recognition and aggressive intervention are required to reverse this process.

The infant with PPHN is typically born at term or postterm, has tachycardia and cyanosis as presenting signs, and within minutes or hours progresses to severe respiratory compromise with concomitant acidosis, which further compromises pulmonary perfusion and deteriorating oxygenation. Management depends on the underlying cause of the persistent pulmonary hypertension. The use of INO and ECMO (see previous discussion) has improved the chances of survival of these infants.

Another mode of treatment for PPHN and other respiratory disorders of the newborn is high-frequency ventilation, an assisted-ventilation method that delivers small volumes of gas at high frequencies and limits the development of high airway pressure, thus theoretically reducing barotrauma.

OTHER PROBLEMS RELATED TO GESTATION

Small-for-Gestational-Age Infants and Intrauterine Growth Restriction

Infants who are SGA (i.e., weight is below the 10th percentile expected at term) or infants who have IUGR (i.e., rate of growth does not meet expected growth pattern) are considered high risk, with the perimortality rate 10 to 20 times greater than that for the normal term infant (Kliegman & Das, 2002).

Various conditions can affect and impede growth in the developing fetus. Conditions occurring in the first trimester that affect all aspects of fetal growth (e.g., infections, teratogens, and chromosomal abnormalities) or extrinsic conditions early in pregnancy result in symmetric IUGR (i.e., head circumference, length, and weight are all less than the 10th percentile). Conditions causing symmetric growth restriction result in an SGA infant, usually with a smaller head circumference and reduced brain capacity. Growth restriction in later stages of pregnancy, as a result of maternal or placental factors, results in asymmetric growth restriction (with respect to gestational age, weight will be less than the 10th percentile, whereas length and head circumference will be greater than the 10th percentile). Infants with asymmetric IUGR have the potential for normal growth and development. Abnormal fetal size may indicate an adaptive response, with diminished fetal weight-sparing brain growth.

Care of the SGA infant is based on the clinical problems present and is the same given to preterm infants with similar problems. Gas exchange is supported by maintaining a clear airway and preventing cold stress. Hypoglycemia is treated with oral feedings (e.g., breast, formula, or IV dextrose) as the infant's condition warrants. An external heat source (radiant warmer or incubator) is used until the infant is able to maintain an adequate body temperature. Nursing support of parents is the same as that given to parents of preterm infants.

Common problems that affect SGA infants who experienced IUGR are perinatal asphyxia, meconium aspiration (discussed previously), immunodeficiency, hypoglycemia, polycythemia, and temperature instability.

Perinatal asphyxia

Commonly, IUGR infants have been exposed to chronic hypoxia for varying periods before labor and birth. Labor is a stressor to the normal fetus; it is an even greater stressor for the growth-restricted fetus. The chronically hypoxic infant is severely compromised by a normal labor and has difficulty compensating after birth. The alert, wide-eyed appearance of the newborn is attributed to prolonged fetal hypoxia. Appropriate management and resuscitation are essential for the depressed infant.

The birth of the SGA newborn with perinatal asphyxia may be associated with a maternal history of heavy cigarette smoking; gestational hypertension; low socioeconomic status; multifetal gestation; gestational infections such as rubella, cytomegalovirus, and toxoplasmosis; advanced diabetes mellitus; and cardiac problems. Sequelae to perinatal asphyxia include MAS and hypoglycemia.

Hypoglycemia

All high risk infants are at risk for the development of hypoglycemia. Infants who are asphyxiated or have other physiologic stress may experience hypoglycemia as a result of a decreased glycogen supply, inadequate gluconeogenesis, or overuse of glycogen stored during fetal life. The concept of hypoglycemia as being a single cutoff value has received criticism because of the wide variability of glucose values from one newborn to another, expressed along a continuum of falling blood glucose values (Blackburn, 2003). Cornblath and associates (2000) have suggested operational thresholds at which interventions to increase serum blood glucose levels should be implemented to prevent serious effects. The threshold criteria are as follows:

- At-risk infants (neonatal factors: infant of diabetic mother, hypothermia, hyperinsulinism, respiratory distress, congenital abnormalities, SGA, prematurity; maternal factors: gestational hypertension, terbutaline administration for preterm labor) should have glucose values equal to 36 mg/dl within the first few hours of life, with a therapeutic objective of 45 mg/dl. In these infants it is recommended that close observation and blood glucose levels be monitored within 2 to 3 hours of birth. If the newborn has a blood glucose below 36 mg/dl (2 mmol/L), intervention such as breastfeeding or bottle-feeding should be instituted; if levels remain low despite feeding, IV dextrose is warranted.
- Blood glucose levels for infants with severe hyperinsulinism may need to be higher (60 mg/dl; 3.3 mmol/L) to prevent serious effects.
- Hypoglycemia in preterm infants requires further studies, but it has been suggested that values be maintained above 47 mg/dl (2.6 mmol/L) (Cornblath et al., 2000).

Because hypoglycemia is often asymptomatic in newborns, dependence on clinical signs or a single blood glucose value alone is inadequate.

Symptoms of hypoglycemia include poor feeding, hypothermia, and diaphoresis. CNS symptoms can include tremors and jitteriness, weak cry, lethargy, floppy posture, seizures, or coma. Diagnosis is confirmed by laboratory blood glucose determinations or glucose reflectance meter. The use of reagent strips alone is reported to be unreliable, especially at values lower than 40 to 50 mg/dl, and may be affected by the hematocrit (Blackburn, 2003).

Heat loss

SGA infants are particularly susceptible to temperature instability; therefore, close attention must be given to maintain a thermoneutral environment. Nursing considerations focus on maintenance of thermoneutrality to promote recovery from perinatal asphyxia because cold stress jeopardizes such recovery.

Large-for-Gestational-Age Infants

The LGA infant is defined as an infant weighing 4000 g or more at birth. An infant is considered LGA despite gestation when the weight is above the 90th percentile on growth charts or two standard deviations above the mean weight for gestational age. Certain fetal disorders, including transposition of the great vessels and Beckwith-Wiedemann syndrome, can also result in LGA status.

Maternal pelvic diameters have not kept pace with the better maternal health and nutrition that results in larger newborns; therefore fetopelvic disproportion may occur, particularly in obese women, women who gain 16 kg or more during gestation, and women with undiagnosed and/or uncontrolled diabetes who are prone to have large newborns. Birth trauma, especially associated with breech or shoulder presentation, is a serious hazard for the oversized neonate. Asphyxia, CNS injury, or both may occur.

All pregnancies of longer than 42 weeks of gestation must be carefully evaluated. All large fetuses are monitored during a trial of labor, and preparation is made for a cesarean birth if nonreassuring fetal status or poor progress of labor occurs. LGA newborns may be preterm, term, or postdate; they may be infants of diabetic mothers (IDMs); or they may be postmature. Each of these problems carries special concerns. Regardless of coexisting potential problems, the LGA infant is at risk by virtue of size alone.

The nurse assesses the LGA infant for hypoglycemia and trauma resulting from vaginal or cesarean birth. The blood glucose levels of LGA infants are monitored, and hypoglycemia is corrected. Any specific birth injuries are identified and treated appropriately.

Infants of Diabetic Mothers

All infants born to mothers with diabetes are at some risk for complications. The degree of risk is influenced by the severity and duration of maternal disease. Problems seen in infants of diabetic mothers include congenital anomalies, macrosomia, birth trauma and perinatal asphyxia, RDS, hypoglycemia, hypocalcemia and hypomagnesemia, cardiomyopathy, hyperbilirubinemia, and polycythemia. Because some of these problems are also seen in infants with gestational age–related problems, discussion of IDMs is included here.

Pathophysiology

The mechanisms responsible for the problems seen in IDMs are not fully understood. Congenital anomalies are believed to be caused by fluctuations in blood glucose levels and episodes of ketoacidosis in early pregnancy. Later in pregnancy, when the mother's pancreas cannot release sufficient insulin to meet increased demands, maternal hyperglycemia results. The high levels of glucose cross the placenta and stimulate the fetal pancreas to release more insulin. The combination of the increased supply of maternal glucose and other nutrients, the inability of maternal insulin to cross the placenta, and increased fetal insulin results in excessive fetal growth called *macrosomia* (see the discussion that follows).

Hyperinsulinemia accounts for many of the problems the fetus or infant develops. In addition to fluctuating glucose levels, maternal vascular involvement or superimposed maternal infection adversely affects the fetus. Normally, maternal blood has a more alkaline pH than does carbon dioxide–rich fetal blood. This phenomenon encourages the exchange of oxygen and carbon dioxide across the placental membrane. When the maternal blood is more acidotic than the fetal blood, such as during ketoacidosis, little carbon dioxide or oxygen exchange occurs at the level of the placenta. The mortality for the unborn infant resulting from an episode of maternal ketoacidosis may be as high as 50% or more (Kalhan & Parimi, 2002).

There are indications that some neonatal conditions (e.g., macrosomia, hypoglycemia, polyhydramnios, preterm birth, and perhaps fetal lung immaturity) may be eliminated, or the incidence decreased, by maintaining tight control over maternal glucose levels within narrow limits. Tight glucose control is defined as the maintenance of maternal blood glucose levels between 100 and 120 mg/dl.

Congenital anomalies

Congenital anomalies occur in about 7% to 10% of IDMs. Their incidence is two to four times that in infants born to mothers without diabetes. The incidence is greatest among SGA newborns. IUGR leading to SGA status is seen in IDMs with severe vascular disease. The most commonly occurring anomalies involve the cardiac system, musculoskeletal system, and CNS. In most defects associated with diabetic pregnancies the structural abnormality occurs before the eighth week after conception. This reinforces the importance of control of blood glucose both before conception and in the early stages of pregnancy.

The incidence of congenital heart lesions in these infants is five times higher than that in the general population. Coarctation of the aorta, transposition of the great vessels, and atrial or ventricular septal defects are the most common lesions encountered in the IDM. Maternal diabetic control is correlated with the incidence of defects; that is, the better the control, the fewer defects.

CNS anomalies include anencephaly, encephalocele, meningomyelocele, and hydrocephalus. The musculoskeletal system may be affected by caudal regression syndrome (i.e., sacral agenesis, with weakness or deformities of the lower extremities, malformation and fixation of the hip joints, and shortening or deformity of the femurs). Hypertrichosis on the pinnae (excessive hair growth on the external ear) has been added to the list of characteristic clinical features. Other defects noted in this population include GI atresia and urinary tract malformations.

Macrosomia

Despite improvements in the control of maternal blood sugar levels, the incidence of macrosomia in the insulin-dependent diabetic is higher than in infants born of mothers who are not diabetic. At birth the typical LGA infant has a round, cherubic ("tomato" or cushingoid) face, a chubby body, and a plethoric or flushed complexion (Fig. 26-10). The infant has enlarged internal organs (i.e., hepatosplenomegaly, splanchnomegaly, and cardiomegaly) and increased body fat, especially around the shoulders. The placenta and umbilical cord are larger than average. The brain is the only organ that is not enlarged. IDMs may be LGA but physiologically immature.

The macrosomic infant is at risk for hypoglycemia, hypocalcemia, hyperviscosity, and hyperbilirubinemia. The excessive shoulder size in these infants often leads to dystocia, particularly because the head may be smaller in proportion to the shoulders than in a nonmacrosomic infant. Macrosomic infants born vaginally or by cesarean birth after a trial of labor may incur birth trauma.

Birth trauma and perinatal asphyxia

Birth injury (resulting from macrosomia or method of birth) and perinatal asphyxia occur in 20% of infants of gestational diabetic mothers (IGDMs) and 35% of IDMs. Examples of birth trauma include cephalhematoma; paralysis of the facial nerve (seventh cranial nerve) (see Fig. 27-3); fracture of the clavicle (see Fig. 27-1) or humerus; brachial plexus

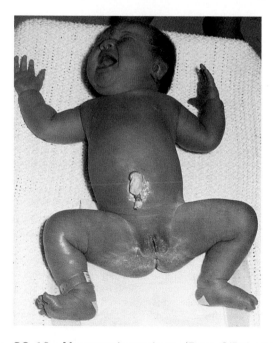

Fig. 26-10 Macrosomic newborn. (From O'Doherty, N. [1986]. *Neonatology: Micro atlas of the newborn.* Nutley, NJ: Hoffmann-La Roche.)

paralysis, usually Erb-Duchenne (right upper arm) palsy (see Fig. 27-2); and phrenic nerve paralysis, invariably associated with diaphragmatic paralysis.

Respiratory distress syndrome

IDMs are four to six times more likely than normal infants to develop RDS. With improved maternal glucose control, this risk is substantially reduced. In the fetus exposed to high levels of maternal glucose, synthesis of surfactant may be delayed because of the high fetal serum level of insulin. Fetal lung maturity, as evidenced by a lecithin/sphingomyelin (L/S) ratio of 2:1, is not reassuring if the mother has pregestational or gestational diabetes mellitus. For the infants of such mothers, an L/S ratio of 3:1 or more or the presence of phosphatidylglycerol in the amniotic fluid is more indicative of adequate lung maturity.

Hypoglycemia

Hypoglycemia affects many IDMs. After constant exposure to high circulating levels of glucose, hyperplasia of the fetal pancreas occurs, resulting in hyperinsulinemia. Disruption of the fetal glucose supply occurs with the clamping of the umbilical cord, and the neonate's blood glucose level falls rapidly in the presence of fetal hyperinsulinism. Hypoglycemia is most common in the macrosomic or SGA infant, but blood glucose levels should be monitored in all infants of known or suspected diabetic mothers.

Asymptomatic or symptomatic hypoglycemia most commonly becomes evident within the first 1 to 3 hours after birth. Signs of hypoglycemia include jitteriness, apnea, tachypnea, and cyanosis. Significant hypoglycemia may result in seizures. Hypoglycemia is worsened by the presence of hypothermia or respiratory distress.

Hypocalcemia and hypomagnesemia

Hypocalcemia occurs in as many as 50% of IDMs. A number of these cases are related to hypoxia or prematurity; however, the overall incidence of hypocalcemia is higher than in nondiabetic pregnancies. Hypomagnesemia is believed to develop because of maternal renal losses that occur in diabetes. Hypocalcemia is associated with preterm birth, birth trauma, and perinatal asphyxia. Signs of hypocalcemia are similar to those of hypoglycemia, but they occur within the first 24 hours of age.

Cardiomyopathy

All IDMs need careful observation for cardiomyopathy because an increased heart size is often found among these infants. Two types of cardiomyopathy can occur. Clinicians must be alert to identify the type of lesion correctly so that appropriate therapy is instituted. Both types of lesions are associated with respiratory symptoms and congestive heart failure.

Hypertrophic cardiomyopathy (HCM) is characterized by a hypercontractile and thickened myocardium. The ventricular walls are thickened, as is the septum, which in severe cases results in outflow tract obstructions. The mitral valve is poorly functioning. In nonhypertrophic cardiomyopathy (non-HCM) the myocardium is poorly contractile and overstretched. The ventricles are increased in size, and there is no outflow obstruction. Most infants are asymptomatic, but severe outflow obstruction may cause left ventricular heart failure. HCM may be treated with a beta-adrenergic blocker (such as propranolol to decrease contractility and heart rate). A cardiotonic agent is used to treat non-HCM (such as digoxin to increase contractility and decrease heart rate). The abnormality usually resolves in 3 to 12 months.

Hyperbilirubinemia and polycythemia

IDMs are at increased risk of developing hyperbilirubinemia (see Chapter 18). Many IDMs are also polycythemic. Polycythemia increases blood viscosity, thereby impairing circulation. In addition, this increased number of RBCs to be hemolyzed increases the potential bilirubin load that the neonate must clear. The excessive RBCs are produced in extramedullary foci (liver and spleen) in addition to the usual sites in bone marrow. Therefore both liver function and bilirubin clearance may be adversely affected. Bruising associated with birth of a macrosomic infant will contribute further to high bilirubin levels.

Nursing care

Ideally, planning for the IDM begins during the antenatal period. Pediatric staff members are present at the birth. Implementation of care depends on the neonate's particular problems. If the maternal blood glucose level was well controlled throughout the pregnancy, the infant may require only monitoring. Because euglycemia is not always possible, the nurse must promptly recognize and treat any consequences of maternal diabetes that arise (Plan of Care).

DISCHARGE PLANNING ■

Discharge planning for the high risk newborn begins early in the hospitalization. Throughout the infant's hospitalization, the nurse gathers information from the health care team members and the family. This information is used to determine the infant's and family's readiness for discharge.

As home care needs of the infant's parents are assessed, steps are taken to eliminate any knowledge deficits. Discharge teaching for the high risk newborn family is extensive, requires time, and cannot be adequately accomplished on the day of discharge. Information is provided about

---

CD: Plan of Care—The Infant of Mother with Diabetes Mellitus

PLAN OF CARE   *The Infant of Mother with Diabetes Mellitus*

NURSING DIAGNOSIS Risk for injury related to hypoglycemia secondary to hyperinsulinemia and maternal diabetes
Expected Outcome *Infant will exhibit serum blood glucose levels that are WNL.*
Nursing Interventions/Rationales
- Monitor blood glucose levels in infants at known risk for hypoglycemia (e.g., SGA, preterm [ELBW, VLBW] infant of diabetic mother) *to assess and detect early onset to prevent complications.*
- Observe for signs of hypoglycemia (e.g., jitteriness, twitching, lethargy, apathy, seizures, cyanosis, sweating, eye rolling, and refusal to eat) *to assess and detect signs of onset to prevent complications.*
- Institute early feeding of breast milk or infant formula *to prevent or treat early hypoglycemia.*
- Reduce adverse environmental factors (e.g., cold stress, hypoxia, and respiratory distress) *that can predispose infant to hypoglycemia.*

NURSING DIAGNOSIS Ineffective breathing pattern related to lung immaturity secondary to maternal diabetes
Expected Outcome *Infant will exhibit breathing pattern adequate to maintain oxygenation (i.e., respiratory rate, rhythm, and amplitude).*
Nursing Interventions/Rationales
- Monitor infant vital signs and patency of airway *to evaluate pulmonary and circulatory status.*

- Avoid activities that may lower body temperature and lead to cold stress, *which can induce respiratory distress.*
- Suction as needed *to keep airway patent and prevent aspiration.*
- Position infant on side initially *to facilitate mucous drainage.*
- Have resuscitation equipment and oxygen available *for quick treatment of respiratory distress.*

NURSING DIAGNOSIS Risk for imbalanced body temperature related to physiologic immaturity
See the Plan of Care for the term newborn in Chapter 19.

NURSING DIAGNOSIS Anxiety; risks for powerlessness, situational low self-esteem, ineffective coping, related to neonate's condition, management, and prognosis
Expected Outcome *Parents demonstrate understanding of prognosis and therapy for infant.*
Nursing Interventions/Rationales
- Explain potential effects of maternal diabetic condition on newborn *to relieve fear of unknown and support ability to cope.*
- Encourage open communication (e.g., inform parents of ongoing condition, procedures, and treatment; answer questions; correct misperceptions; actively listen to parental concerns) *to provide support and help provide sense of control.*
- Encourage parents to interact with infant and to become involved in care routines *to foster emotional connection.*

ELBW, Extremely low birth weight; *SGA,* small for gestational age; *VLBW,* very low birth weight; *WNL,* within normal limits.

infant care, especially as it pertains to the particular infant's home needs (e.g., supplemental oxygen, gastrostomy feedings). Parent education includes having the parents give return demonstrations of their infant care skills to show whether they are becoming increasingly independent in the provision of this care. Parents of infants who have special needs or who were born at less than 34 weeks of gestation should be given the opportunity to spend a night or two in a predischarge room providing care for the infant away from the NICU to become better acquainted with the necessary care and to have a time of transition in which questions may be answered regarding home care. Additional parent teaching should include bathing and skin care; requirements for meeting nutritional needs after discharge; safety in the home, including supine sleep position and prevention of infection (e.g., respiratory syncytial virus); and medication administration.

Preterm infants have a high rate of readmission to acute care centers and visits to the emergency room. It is imperative that the family have a health professional they can contact for questions regarding infant care and behavior once they are home. Parents should obtain an age-appropriate car seat before the discharge of their infant and demonstrate its use with the infant. In many cases, the car seat for the preterm infant will require adjustments. It is recommended that a period of time be used to monitor the infant in the car seat for oxygen desaturations so adjustments can be made. Before discharge all high risk or preterm infants should receive the appropriate immunizations, metabolic screening, hematology assessment (bilirubin risk as appropriate), and evaluation of hearing.

Successful discharge of high risk infants to their homes requires a multidisciplinary approach. Medical, nursing, social services, and other professionals (physical therapy, occupational therapy, nutritionist, developmental follow-up specialist) are crucial to the smooth transition of these infants and their families to the community and home. If the infant is transported back to the community hospital that referred either the mother before birth or the infant after birth, interfacility communication is essential to continuity of care.

Discharge to home for high risk infants does not mean they can be treated like healthy term newborns. Follow-up with a specialized practitioner familiar with the complications common to the high risk newborn is essential. Further follow-up of specific complications by qualified specialists and referral to centers for developmental interventions can help ensure the best outcome possible for these infants.

Referrals for appropriate resources also need to be made. Infants with developmental disabilities, or those infants who may be at risk for further problems (preterm infants), are referred to appropriate community programs. Social service involvement is especially important for young or psychosocially high risk parents (e.g., substance abusers or those with a mental illness).

For the family of the child who is technology dependent, special education needs are discussed before discharge.

TRANSPORT OF HIGH RISK INFANTS

Transport to a Regional Center

If a hospital is not equipped to care for a high risk mother and fetus or a high risk infant, transfer to a specialized perinatal or regional tertiary care center is arranged. Maternal transport ideally occurs with the fetus in utero because this has two distinct advantages: (1) neonatal morbidity and mortality are decreased, and (2) the mother and infant are not separated at birth.

For a variety of reasons, it is not always possible to transport the mother before the birth. Therefore, physicians and nurses in all facilities must have the skills and equipment necessary for making an accurate diagnosis and implementing emergency interventions to stabilize the infant's condition until transport can occur (Pettett, Sewell, & Merenstein, 2002). The goal of these interventions is to maintain the infant's condition within the normal physiologic range. Specific attention is given to vital signs, oxygenation and ventilation, thermoregulation, acid-base balance, fluid and electrolyte status, blood glucose, and developmental interventions.

Arrangements for transport to an intensive care facility are made as soon as the high risk infant is identified. Each hospital where infants are born should be able to provide for appropriate neonatal stabilization and arrange for transport to a tertiary care facility. The infant must be kept warm and adequately oxygenated (including intubation and surfactant replacement as indicated); have vital signs and oxygen saturation monitored; and, when indicated, receive an IV infusion. The infant is transported in a specially designed incubator unit containing a complete life-support system and other emergency equipment that can be carried by ambulance, van, or helicopter (Fig. 26-11).

The transport team may consist of physicians, nurse-practitioners, nurses, and respiratory therapists. Commonly a nurse trained in neonatal intensive care and a respiratory therapist constitute the team. The team must have experience in resuscitation, stabilization, and provision of critical care during the transport. Teams provide information for the parents about the tertiary center (Box 26-8).

There may be instances when transport in a special transport incubator is not possible and alternate means of transport may be identified.

Instead of the usual incubator method of transport, Sontheimer, Fischer, and Buch (2004) transported 31 stable infants to and from a regional center using kangaroo transport. Transports were conducted in helicopter (2) and ambulance (29) by mothers (27), father (1), nurses (2), and physician (1). The infants were monitored, and their conditions remained stable. Parents felt safe and comfortable with this method.

The birth of any high risk infant can cause profound parental stress. Parents can grieve the loss of the ideal infant. They are fearful of the possible eventual outcomes for the infant. They must also deal with the technologic world surrounding their infant. Amid all the equipment, it is some-

BOX 26-8

Information for Parents about the Tertiary Center

- Information about the special care unit—what it is, what it does
- Exact location of the unit—address, map, waiting area for relatives and friends
- Names of individuals likely to be involved in the newborn's care (e.g., primary nurse, neonatologist, clinical manager)
- Visiting hours and hospital rules
- Telephone numbers
- Any particular rules or regulations regarding the special care unit
- Location of parking facilities, nearby lodging, and rules regarding young children (siblings)

From Pettett, G., Sewell, S., & Merenstein, G. (2002). Regionalization and transport in perinatal care. In G. Merenstein & S. Gardner (Eds.), *Handbook of neonatal intensive care* (5th ed.). St. Louis: Mosby.

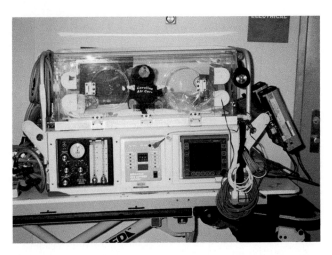

Fig. 26-11 Total life support system for transport of high risk newborns. (Courtesy UNC Hospitals, Carolina Air Care, Chapel Hill, NC.)

times difficult for them to perceive the infant and respond to its needs. Parents of high risk infants who have been transported to regional centers therefore need special support.

Transport from a Regional Center

Infants may need to be transferred back to the referring facility; however, in many cases the infant is discharged home from the tertiary center. Often premature infants who require thermoregulation and gavage feedings can be cared for in community hospitals closer to the parents' home. This allows parents to visit their infant more easily and to work with their personal health care provider on the long-range expected outcomes for the infant. Specialized incubators make these trips possible (see Fig. 26-11). However, parents may express mixed feelings about such return transports and may be reluctant to adapt to a different facility and group of caregivers. To minimize some of these concerns, it is important to give the parents very clear information about return transports during the initial discharge planning.

Although at the time of discharge parents may not recognize the need for information on the various resources available to help them in the care of their infant, they can be given such lists of agencies and telephone numbers for later use. Providing them with a patient-specific directory covering special programs, social support, and community and funding resources can help them make the transition to the home care of their infants. As the nurse continually reinforces the idea that the infant will go home, this prompts the parents to plan for the days ahead and therefore be ready to take their infant home when the time comes.

COMMUNITY ACTIVITY

During a scheduled clinical experience in the NICU, a special care nursery, or community hospital nursery, observe a transport team leaving to pick up an infant from a referring hospital, bringing in an infant to the special care nursery, or arriving at the community hospital to pick up an infant for transport to the special care nursery. Who are the transport team members? What equipment are they using? How was the referral made? What communication links are there between the special care nursery and the community hospitals in the surrounding area? How are parents kept informed of the infant's condition? How much does such a transport cost? Who pays for the transport?

Key Points

- Preterm infants are at risk for problems related to the immaturity of their organ systems.
- RDS, ROP, and CLD (bronchopulmonary dysplasia) are associated with prematurity.
- High risk infants must be observed for respiratory distress and other early signs of physiologic distress.
- Metabolic abnormalities of diabetes mellitus in pregnancy adversely affect embryonic and fetal development.
- Infants born to diabetic mothers are at risk for hypoglycemia and RDS.
- The adaptation of parents to preterm or high risk infants differs from that of parents of full-term infants.
- SGA infants are considered to be at risk because of fetal growth restriction.
- Nonreassuring fetal status among postmature infants is related to the progressive placental insufficiency that can occur in a postterm pregnancy.
- Specially trained nurses may transport high risk infants to and from special care units.
- Parents need special instruction (e.g., CPR, oxygen therapy, suctioning, developmental care) before they take a high risk infant home.

Answer Guidelines to Critical Thinking Exercise

Preterm Infant

1 Yes, there is sufficient evidence. The normal progress in recovery from childbirth is well documented. Because the baby was born preterm, Charlotte was not prepared for the birth at this time nor for the probability of a long-term stay in the NICU for the infant. At 28 weeks, the infant has a good chance for survival. In the absence of problems during the nursery stay, the prognosis is good. If Charlotte chooses to breastfeed, she will have to pump regularly for a considerable amount of time before she can actually nurse the baby. In addition, she has the problem of transporting the milk to the nursery.

2 a. Charlotte's physical recovery should progress easily. However, her emotional and psychologic recovery may be difficult. She is likely to ask herself what she did to cause the preterm birth and may feel guilt, particularly if the infant develops problems. The relationship among her husband and herself and the other two children may be strained by the worry about the baby and the time she spends traveling to see the infant.

   b. Barring complications, the infant can be expected to progress and develop normally. However, the infant's hospitalization and separation from the family will likely put a strain on family members, who will be worried about the infant as long as it is in the NICU and until the baby is home.

   c. Charlotte can be informed that the cause of the majority of preterm births is unknown and that she need not feel guilt for having the baby early. Charlotte can pump and freeze her breast milk and transport it to the hospital in a cooler; however, she will likely not be able to travel that distance to see the infant every day. Obtaining breast milk at 28 weeks takes perseverance and regular pumping. Although this puts a burden on Charlotte, it is important for the infant's well-being.

   d. Infants born at 28 weeks with no concomitant problems can develop normally. However, they are at risk for nosocomial infections, and some infants have developmental delays.

3 Charlotte and her family need information about postpartum recovery, the possibility of postpartum "blues" or depression associated with a preterm birth, and stresses associated with a preterm birth and neonatal transport. They may need assistance in talking to their two older children about the baby and the need for the baby to be in the hospital. They need to be informed about how to contact the NICU and care providers, given information about usual care in that setting, given directions to the hospital, and prepared for back transport to their local hospital when the infant's condition improves such that NICU care is no longer required. They need to be kept informed daily about the progress of the baby.

4 Phases of postpartum recovery and the stresses associated with preterm birth and neonatal transport are well documented. Long-term outcomes for preterm infants, parental responses to preterm birth, and integration of the infant into the family have been studied extensively. The nurse can use those studies and patient education materials to assist the family.

5 The above recommendations assume the infant is progressing normally with no problems. If the infant has or develops problems, additional support for the family will be necessary. Participation in parent groups is helpful. They may be referred to the clergy of their choice for additional support. If the infant does not survive, the bereavement service at the hospital can provide information and support.

Resources

Academy of Neonatal Nursing
2270 Northpoint Pkwy.
Santa Rosa, CA 95407-7398
707-568-2168
707-569-0786 (fax)
www.academyonline.org

Advances in Neonatal Care
Elsevier
360 Park Ave., South
New York, NY 10010

American Academy of Pediatrics (AAP)
141 Northwest Point Blvd.
Elk Grove, IL 60007-1098
847-228-5005
www.aap.org

Journal of Perinatal and Neonatal Nursing
Lippincott Williams & Wilkins
530 Walnut St.
Philadelphia, PA 19106-3621
215-521-8300
215-521-8902 (fax)
www.lww.com

National Association of Neonatal Nurses
4700 W. Lake Ave.
Glenview, IL 60025-1485
800-451-3795
888-477-6266 (fax)
www.nann.org
info@nann.org

Neonatal Network
2270 Northpoint Pkwy.
Santa Rosa, CA 95407-7398
707-569-1415
707-569-0786 (fax)
www.neonatalnetwork.com

Parents of Prematures
13613 NE 26th Pl.
Bellevue, WA 98005
206-283-7466

Recommended Standards for NICU Design
www.nd.edu/~kkolberg/frmain.htm

References

Adamson-Macedo, E. (2004). Neonatal health psychology (NNHP): Theories and practice. *Neuro Endocrinology Letters, 25*(Suppl 1), 9-34.

Als, H. et al. (2003). A three-center, randomized, controlled trial of individualized developmental care for very low birth weight preterm infants: Medical, neurodevelopmental, parenting, and caregiving effects. *Journal of Developmental and Behavioral Pediatrics, 24*(6), 399-408.

Als, H. et al. (2004). Early experience alters brain function and structure. *Pediatrics, 113*(4), 846-857.

Als, H. Butler, S., Kosta, S., & McAnulty, G. (2005). The Assessment of Preterm Infants' Behavior (APIB): Furthering the understanding and measurement of neurodevelopmental competence in preterm and full-term infants. *Mental Retardation and Developmental Disabilities Research Review, 11*(1), 94-102.

American Academy of Pediatrics (AAP), Committee on Fetus and Newborn. (2002). Postnatal corticosteroids to treat or prevent chronic lung disease in preterm infants. *Pediatrics, 109*(2), 330-337.

American Academy of Pediatrics (AAP), Committee on Nutrition. (2004). *Pediatric nutrition handbook* (5th ed.). Elk Grove Village, IL: AAP.

American Academy of Pediatrics (AAP), Section on Ophthalmology. (2001). Screening examination of premature infants for retinopathy of prematurity. *Pediatrics, 108*(3), 809-811.

Anderson, M., Johnson, C., Townsend, S., & Hay, W. (2002). Enteral nutrition. In G. Merenstein & S. Gardner (Eds.), *Handbook of neonatal intensive care* (5th ed.). St. Louis: Mosby.

Bensard, D., Calkins, C., Partrick, D., & Price, F. (2002). Neonatal surgery. In G. Merenstein & S. Gardner (Eds.), *Handbook of neonatal intensive care* (5th ed.). St. Louis: Mosby.

Berger, T., Bachmann, I., Adams, M., & Schubiger, G. (2004). Impact of improved survival of very low-birth-weight infants on incidence and severity of bronchopulmonary dysplasia. *Biology of the Neonate, 86*(2), 124-130.

Blackburn, S. (2003). *Maternal, fetal, and neonatal physiology: A clinical perspective* (2nd ed.). St. Louis: Saunders.

Blake, W., & Murray, J. (2002). Heat balance. In G. Merenstein & S. Gardner (Eds.), *Handbook of neonatal intensive care* (5th ed.). St. Louis: Mosby.

Brandon, D., Holditch-Davis, D., & Belyea, M. (2002). Preterm infants born at less than 31 weeks' gestation have improved growth in cycled light compared with continuous near darkness. *Journal of Pediatrics, 140*(2), 192-199.

Brown, J. (2004). Early relationship environments: Physiology of skin-to-skin contact for parents and their preterm infants. *Clinics in Perinatology, 31*(2), 287-298, vii.

Byers, J. (2003). Components of developmental care and the evidence for their use in the NICU. *MCN American Journal of Maternal Child Nursing, 28*(3), 174-180.

Byrne, B., Mellen, B., Lindstrom, D., & Cotton, R. (2002). Is the BPD epidemic diminishing? *Seminars in Perinatology, 26*(6), 461-466.

Centers for Disease Control and Prevention (CDC). (2002). *Enterobacter sakazakii* infections associated with the use of powdered infant formula—Tennessee, 2001. *Morbidity and Mortality Weekly Report, 51*(14), 297-300.

Chou, L., Wang, R., Chen, S., & Pai, L. (2003). Effects of music therapy on oxygen saturation in premature infants receiving endotracheal suctioning. *Journal of Nursing Research, 11*(3), 209-216.

Collins, C., Makrides, M., & McPhee, A. (2003). Early discharge with home support of gavage feeding for stable preterm infants who have not established full oral feeds (Cochrane Review). In *The Cochrane Library*, Issue 2, 2004. Chichester, UK: John Wiley & Sons.

Cornblath, M., Hawdon, J., Williams, A., Aynsley-Green, A., Ward-Platt, M., Schwartz, R., & Kalhan, S. (2000). Controversies regarding operational definition of neonatal hypoglycemia: Suggested thresholds. *Pediatrics, 105*(5), 1141-1145.

Denne, S., Poindexter, B., Leitch, C., Ernst, J., Lemons, P., & Lemons, J. (2002). Nutrition and metabolism in the high-risk neonate. Part One. Enteral nutrition. In A. Fanaroff & R. Martin (Eds.), *Neonatal-perinatal medicine: Diseases of the fetus and infant* (7th ed.). St. Louis: Mosby.

Dickason, E., Silverman, B., & Kaplan, J. (1998). *Maternal-infant nursing care* (3rd ed.). St. Louis: Mosby.

Diehl-Jones, W., & Askin, D. (2004). Nutritional modulation of neonatal outcomes. *AACN Clinical Issues, 15*(1), 83-96.

Dusick, A., Poindexter, B., Ehrenkranz, R., & Lemons, J. (2003). Growth failure in the preterm infant: Can we catch up? *Seminars in Perinatology, 27*(4), 302-310.

Evans, R., & Thureen, P. (2001). Early feeding strategies in preterm & critically ill neonates. *Neonatal Network, 20*(7), 7-18.

Flores, M. (2003). Ibuprofen: Alternative treatment for patent ductus arteriosus. *Neonatal Network, 22*(2), 26-31.

Gardner, S., & Goldson, E. (2002). The neonate and the environment: Impact on development. In G. Merenstein & S. Gardner (Eds.), *Handbook of neonatal intensive care* (5th ed.). St. Louis: Mosby.

Gardner, S., Snell, B., & Lawrence, R. (2002). Breastfeeding the neonate with special needs. In G. Merenstein & S. Gardner (Eds.), *Handbook of neonatal intensive care* (5th ed.). St. Louis: Mosby.

Gracey, K., Talbot, D., Lankford, R., & Dodge, P. (2002). The changing face of bronchopulmonary dysplasia: Part 1. *Advances in Neonatal Care, 2*(6), 326-338.

Hagedorn, M., Gardner, S., & Abman, H. (2002). Respiratory diseases. In G. Merenstein & S. Gardner (Eds.), *Handbook of neonatal intensive care* (5th ed.). St. Louis: Mosby.

Horii, K., & Lane, A. (2001). Evidence-based use of emollients in neonates. *Newborn and Infant Nursing Reviews, 1*(1), 21-24.

Horns, K. (2002). Comparison of two microenvironments and nurse caregiving on thermal stability of ELBW infants. *Advances in Neonatal Care, 2*(3), 149-160.

Johnson, B., Abraham, M., & Parrish, R. (2004). Designing the neonatal intensive care unit for optimal family involvement. *Clinics in Perinatology, 31*(2), ix, 353-382.

Johnson, F., & Maikler, V. (2001). Nurses' adoption of the AWHONN/NANN Neonatal Skin Care Project. *Newborn and Infant Nursing Reviews, 1*(1), 59-67.

Kalhan, S., & Parimi, P. (2002). Disorders of carbohydrate metabolism. In A. Fanaroff & R. Martin (Eds.), *Neonatal-perinatal medicine: Diseases of the fetus and infant* (7th ed.). St. Louis: Mosby.

Kinsella, J., & Abman, S. (2000). Inhaled nitric oxide: Current and future uses in neonates. *Seminars in Perinatology, 24*(6), 387-395.

Kliegman, R., & Das, U. (2002). Intrauterine growth retardation. In A. Fanaroff & R. Martin (Eds.), *Neonatal-perinatal medicine: Diseases of the fetus and infant* (7th ed.). St. Louis: Mosby.

Kuller, J. (2001). Skin breakdown: Risk factors, prevention, and treatment. *Newborn and Infant Nursing Reviews, 1*(1), 33-42.

Laptook, A., O'Shea, T., Shankaran, S., Bhaskar, B., & NICHD Neonatal Network. (2005). Adverse neurodevelopmental outcomes among extremely low birth weight infants with a normal head ultrasound: Prevalence and antecedents. *Pediatrics, 115*(3), 673-680.

Lund, C., & Durand, D. (2002). Skin and skin care. In G. Merenstein & S. Gardner (Eds.), *Handbook of neonatal intensive care* (5th ed.). St. Louis: Mosby.

Lund, C., & Kuller, J. (2003). Assessment and management of the integumentary system. In C. Kenner & J. Lott (Eds.), *Comprehensive neonatal nursing: A physiologic perspective* (3rd ed.). St. Louis: Saunders.

Lund, C., Kuller, J., & Lott, J. (2001). Neonatal skin care: Clinical outcomes of the AWHONN/NANN evidence-based clinical practice guideline. *Journal of Obstetric, Gynecologic, and Neonatal Nursing, 30*(1), 41-51.

Martucci, M. (2004). Considerations in planning a newborn developmental care program in a community hospital setting. *Advances in Neonatal Care, 4*(2), 59-66.

Montoya, K., & Washington, R. (2002). Cardiovascular disease and surgical interventions. In G. Merenstein & S. Gardner (Eds.), *Handbook of neonatal intensive care* (5th ed.). St. Louis: Mosby.

Morton, J. (2002). Strategies to support extended breastfeeding of the premature infant. *Advances in Neonatal Care, 2*(5), 267-282.

Neu, M., Browne, J., & Vojir, C. (2000). The impact of two transfer techniques used during skin-to-skin care on the physiologic and behavioral responses of preterm infants. *Nursing Research, 49*(4), 215-223.

O'Doherty, N. (1986). *Neonatology: Micro atlas of the newborn.* Nutley, NJ: Hoffmann-La Roche.

Paige, P., & Carney, P. (2002). Neurologic disorders. In G. Merenstein & S. Gardner (Eds.), *Handbook of neonatal intensive care* (5th ed.). St. Louis: Mosby.

Parry, W., & Zimmer, J. (2002). Acid-base homeostasis and oxygenation. In G. Merenstein & S. Gardner (Eds.), *Handbook of neonatal intensive care* (5th ed.). St. Louis: Mosby.

Pettett, G., Sewell, S., & Merenstein, G. (2002). Regionalization and transport in perinatal care. In G. Merenstein & S. Gardner (Eds.), *Handbook of neonatal intensive care* (5th ed.). St. Louis: Mosby.

Sadiq, H., Mantych, G., Bemawra, R., Devaslar, U., & Hocker, J. (2003). Inhaled nitric oxide in the treatment of moderate persistent pulmonary hypertension of the newborn: A randomized controlled, multicenter trial. *Journal of Perinatology, 23*(2), 98-103.

Saugstad, O. (2005). Oxygen for newborns: How much is too much? *Journal of Perinatology, 25*(Suppl 2), S45-S49.

Schanler, R., Shulman, R., Lau, C., Smith, E., & Heitkemper, M. (1999). Feeding strategies for premature infants: Randomized trial of gastrointestinal priming and tube-feeding method. *Pediatrics, 103*(2), 434-439.

Sontheimer, D., Fischer, C., & Buch, K. (2004). Kangaroo transport instead of incubator transport. *Pediatrics, 113*(4), 920-923.

Stoll, B., & Gotoff, S. (2004). Infections in the neonatal infant. In R. Behrman, R. Kliegman, & H. Jenson (Eds), *Nelson textbook of pediatrics* (17th ed.). Philadelphia: Saunders.

Stoll, B., Hansen, N., Adams-Chapman, I., Fanaroff, A., Hintz, S., Vohr, B., Higgins, R., & National Institute of Child Health and Human Development Neonatal Research Network. (2004). Neurodevelopmental and growth impairment among extremely low-birth-weight infants with neonatal infection. *Journal of the American Medical Association, 292*(19), 2357-2365.

Taquino, L. (2000). Promoting wound healing in the neonatal setting: Process versus protocol. *Journal of Perinatal and Neonatal Nursing, 14*(1), 108-118.

Thome, U., & Carlo, W. (2002). Permissive hypercapnia. *Seminars in Neonatology, 7*(5), 409-419.

Vain, N., Szyld, E., Prudent, L., Wiswell, T., Aguilar, A., & Vivas, N. (2004). Oropharyngeal and nasopharyngeal suctioning of meconium-stained neonates before delivery of their shoulders: Multicenter, randomized, controlled trial. *Lancet, 364*(9434), 597-602.

van Acker, J., de Smet, F., Muyldermans, G., Bougatef, A., Naessens, A., & Lauwers, S. (2001). Outbreak of necrotizing enterocolitis associated with *Enterobacter sakazakii* in powdered milk formula. *Journal of Clinical Microbiology, 39*(1), 293-297.

Vennarecci, G., Kato, T., Misiakos, E., Neto, A., Verzaro, R., Pinna, A., Nery, J., Khan, F., Thompson, J., & Tzakis, A. (2000). Intestinal transplantation for short gut syndrome attributable to necrotizing enterocolitis. *Pediatrics, 105*(2), E25.

Volpe, J. (2001). *Neurology of the newborn* (4th ed.). Philadelphia: Saunders.

Ward, K. (2001). Perceived needs of parents of critically ill infants in a neonatal intensive care unit (NICU). *Pediatric Nursing, 27*(3), 281-286.

Whitfield, M. (2003). Psychosocial effects of intensive care on infants and families after discharge. *Seminars in Neonatology, 8*(2), 185-193.

Wilson-Costello, D., Friedman, H., Minich, N., Fanaroff, A., & Hack, M. (2005). Improved survival rates with increased neurodevelopmental disability for extremely low birth weight infants in the 1990s. *Pediatrics, 115*(4), 997-1003.

Woodgate, P., & Davies, M. (2001). Permissive hypercapnia for the prevention of morbidity and mortality in mechanically ventilated newborn infants (Cochrane Review). In *The Cochrane Library*, Issue 2, 2005. Chichester, UK: John Wiley & Sons.

Woodwell, W. (2002). The long road home: Perspectives on parenting in the NICU. *Advances in Neonatal Care, 2*(3), 161-169.

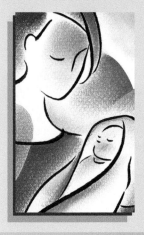

CHAPTER 27

The Newborn at Risk: Acquired and Congenital Problems

SHANNON E. PERRY

LEARNING OBJECTIVES

- *Summarize assessment and care of the new-born with soft-tissue, skeletal, and nervous system injuries caused by birth trauma.*
- *Identify maternal conditions that place the new-born at risk for infection.*
- *Describe methods used to identify infection in the newborn.*
- *Identify clinical signs of infection in the newborn.*
- *Identify the effects of maternal use of alcohol, heroin, methadone, marijuana, methampheta-mine, cocaine, and smoking tobacco on the fetus and newborn.*
- *Outline the assessment of a newborn exposed to recreational drugs in utero.*
- *Compare neonatal Rh and ABO incompatibility.*
- *Describe preoperative and postoperative nursing care of the newborn.*
- *Explain congenital disorders presented in this chapter and identify the priority of nursing care for each.*

KEY TERMS AND DEFINITIONS

ABO incompatibility Hemolytic disease that occurs when the mother's blood type is O and the new-born's is A, B, or AB

alcohol-related birth defects (ARBD) Congenital abnormality or anomaly resulting from excessive maternal alcohol intake during pregnancy; characterized by typical craniofacial and limb defects, cardiovascular defects, intrauterine growth restriction, and developmental delay; newer terminology for *fetal alcohol syndrome (FAS)*

alcohol-related neurodevelopmental disorder (ARND) Disorder in infants affected by prenatal exposure to alcohol but who do not meet the criteria for FAS; previously referred to as *fetal alcohol effects (FAE)*

anencephaly Congenital deformity characterized by the absence of cerebrum, cerebellum, and flat bones of the skull

cleft lip Incomplete closure of the lip; lay term is *harelip*

cleft palate Incomplete closure of the palate or roof of the mouth; a congenital fissure

Coombs' test Indirect: Determination of Rh-positive antibodies in maternal blood; **direct**: determination of maternal Rh-positive antibodies in fetal cord blood; positive test result indicates the presence of antibodies or titer

developmental dysplasia of the hip Abnormal development of the hip joint, resulting in instability of the hip causing one or both of the femoral heads to be displaced from the acetabulum (hip socket)

erythroblastosis fetalis Hemolytic disease of the newborn usually caused by isoimmunization resulting from Rh incompatibility or ABO incompatibility

exchange transfusion Replacement of 75% to 85% of circulating blood by withdrawal of the recipient's blood and injection of a donor's blood in equal amounts, the purposes of which are to prevent an accumulation of bilirubin in the blood above a dangerous level, to prevent the accumulation of other by-products of hemolysis in hemolytic disease, and to correct anemia and acidosis

gastroschisis Abdominal wall defect at the base of the umbilical stalk

hydrocephalus Accumulation of fluid in the subdural or subarachnoid spaces

hydrops fetalis Most severe expression of fetal hemolytic disorder, a possible sequela to maternal Rh isoimmunization; infants exhibit gross edema (anasarca), cardiac decompensation, and profound pallor from anemia and seldom survive

inborn error of metabolism Group of recessive disorders caused by a metabolic defect that results from the absence of or change in a protein, usually an enzyme, and mediated by the action of a certain gene.

microcephaly Abnormal smallness of the head in relation to the rest of the body and underdevelopment of the brain, resulting in some degree of mental retardation

myelomeningocele External sac containing meninges, spinal fluid, and nerves that protrudes through defect in vertebral column

KEY TERMS AND DEFINITIONS—cont'd

neonatal abstinence syndrome Signs and symptoms associated with drug withdrawal in the neonate

omphalocele Congenital defect resulting from failure of closure of the abdominal wall or muscles and leading to herniation of abdominal contents through the navel

thrush Fungal infection of the mouth or throat characterized by the formation of white patches on a red, moist, inflamed mucous membrane; caused by *Candida albicans*

TORCH infections Infections caused by organisms that damage the embryo or fetus; acronym for *tox*oplasmosis, *o*ther (e.g., syphilis), *r*ubella, *c*ytomegalovirus (CMV), and *h*erpes simplex

ELECTRONIC RESOURCES

Additional information related to the content in Chapter 27 can be found on

the companion website at 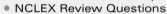 **evolve**
http://evolve.elsevier.com/Lowdermilk/Maternity/
- NCLEX Review Questions
- WebLinks

or on the interactive companion CD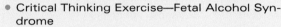
- NCLEX Review Questions
- Critical Thinking Exercise—Fetal Alcohol Syndrome
- Plan of Care—The Drug-Exposed Newborn

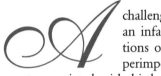challenge for the nurse is the birth of an infant at risk because of conditions or circumstances that are superimposed on the normal course of events associated with birth and the adjustment to extrauterine existence. The infant may be considered high risk because of birth trauma, maternal substance abuse, infection, or congenital anomalies. Birth trauma includes physical injuries a neonate sustains during labor and birth. Congenital anomalies include such conditions as gastrointestinal (GI) malformations, neural tube defects (NTDs), abdominal wall defects, and cardiac defects.

At times the nurse is able to anticipate problems, such as when a woman is admitted in premature labor or a congenital anomaly is diagnosed by ultrasound before birth. At other times the birth of a high risk infant is unanticipated. In either case the personnel and equipment necessary for immediate care of the infant must be available.

BIRTH TRAUMA

Birth trauma (injury) is physical injury sustained by a neonate during labor and birth. It remains an important source of neonatal morbidity.

In theory, most birth injuries may be avoidable, especially if careful assessment of risk factors and appropriate planning of birth occur. The use of fetal ultrasonography allows antepartum diagnosis of many conditions that may be treated in utero or shortly after birth. Elective cesarean birth can be chosen for some pregnancies to prevent significant birth injury. A small percentage of significant birth injuries are unavoidable despite skilled and competent obstetric care, such as in especially difficult or prolonged labor or when the infant is in an abnormal fetal presentation. Some injuries cannot be anticipated until the specific circumstances are encountered during childbirth. Emergency cesarean birth may provide a last-minute salvage, but in these circumstances the injury may be truly unavoidable. The same injury might be caused in several ways; for example, a cephalhematoma could result from an obstetric technique such as forceps birth or vacuum extraction or from pressure of the fetal skull against the maternal pelvis.

Many injuries are minor and resolve readily in the neonatal period without treatment. Other trauma requires some degree of intervention; few are serious enough to be fatal. The nurse's contributions to the welfare of the newborn begin with early observation of the newborn's transition. The prompt reporting of signs that indicate deviations from normal permits early initiation of appropriate therapy. Table 27-1 provides an overview of neurologic birth injuries and the sites in which they occur.

CARE MANAGEMENT

When the infant is born the nurse makes a rapid inspection and physical assessment to determine if there are any life-threatening conditions requiring immediate medical or surgical attention. A comprehensive physical assessment of the newborn is performed after the parents have had the opportunity to interact with the newborn. Because evidence of some birth injuries may not be apparent at the initial examination, assessment continues during each contact with the neonate.

Soft-tissue injuries that commonly occur at birth including caput succedaneum and cephalhematoma are discussed in Chapter 19.

Skeletal Injuries

The newborn's immature, flexible skull can withstand a great degree of deformation (molding) before fracture results. Considerable force is required to fracture the newborn's skull.

TABLE 27-1

Types of Birth Injuries

SITE OF INJURY	TYPE OF INJURY
Scalp	Caput succedaneum
	Subgaleal hemorrhage
	Cephalhematoma
Skull	Linear fracture
	Depressed fracture
	Occipital osteodiastasis
Intracranial	Epidural hematoma
	Subdural hematoma (laceration of falx, tentorium, or superficial veins)
	Subarachnoid hemorrhage
	Cerebral contusion
	Cerebellar contusion
	Intracerebellar hematoma
Spinal cord (cervical)	Vertebral artery injury
	Intraspinal hemorrhage
	Spinal cord transection or injury
Plexus	Erb palsy
	Klumpke paralysis
	Total (mixed) brachial plexus injury
	Horner syndrome
	Diaphragmatic paralysis
	Lumbosacral plexus injury
Cranial and peripheral nerve	Radial nerve palsy
	Medial nerve palsy
	Sciatic nerve palsy
	Laryngeal nerve palsy
	Diaphragmatic paralysis
	Facial nerve palsy

From Paige, P., & Carney, P. (2002). Neurologic disorders. In G. Merenstein & S. Gardner (Eds.). *Handbook of neonatal intensive care* (5th ed.). St. Louis: Mosby.

Two types of skull fractures typically are identified in the newborn: linear fractures and depressed fractures. The location of the fracture and involvement of underlying structures determine its significance.

If an artery lying in a groove on the undersurface of the skull is torn as a result of the fracture, increased intracranial pressure (ICP) will follow. Unless a blood vessel is involved, linear fractures, which account for 70% of all fractures for this age group, heal without special treatment. The soft skull may become indented without laceration of either the skin or the dural membrane. These depressed fractures, or ping-pong ball indentations, may occur during difficult births from pressure of the head on the bony pelvis. They also can occur as a result of injudicious application of forceps. Spontaneous or nonsurgical elevation of the indentation by using a hand breast pump or vacuum extractor has been reported (Mangurten, 2002).

The clavicle is the bone most often fractured during birth. Generally the break is in the middle third of the bone (Fig. 27-1). Dystocia, particularly shoulder impaction, may be the predisposing problem. Limitation of motion of the arm,

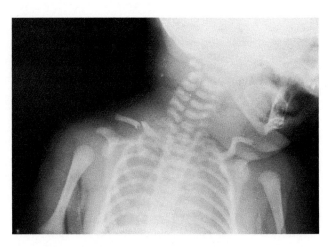

Fig. 27-1 Fractured clavicle after shoulder dystocia. (From O'Doherty, N. [1986]. *Neonatology: Micro atlas of the newborn.* Nutley, NJ: Hoffmann-La Roche.)

crepitus over the bone, and the absence of the Moro reflex on the affected side are diagnostic. Except for use of gentle rather than vigorous handling, no accepted treatment for fractured clavicle in the newborn exists, and the prognosis is good. The humerus and femur are other bones that may be fractured during a difficult birth. Fractures in newborns generally heal rapidly. Immobilization is accomplished with slings, splints, swaddling, and other immobilization devices.

The parents need support in handling these infants because they often are fearful of hurting them. Parents are encouraged to practice handling, changing diapers, and feeding the affected neonate under the guidance of nursery personnel. This increases their confidence and knowledge and facilitates attachment. A plan for follow-up therapy is developed with the parents so that the times and arrangements for therapy are acceptable to them.

Peripheral Nervous System Injuries

Plexus injury results from forces that alter the normal position and relationship of the arm, shoulder, and neck. Erb palsy (Erb-Duchenne paralysis) is caused by damage to the upper plexus and usually results from a stretching or pulling away of the shoulder from the head such as might occur with shoulder dystocia or with a difficult vertex or breech birth. The less common lower plexus palsy, or Klumpke palsy, results from severe stretching of the upper extremity while the trunk is relatively less mobile.

The clinical manifestations of Erb palsy are related to the paralysis of the affected extremity and muscles. The arm hangs limp alongside the body. The shoulder and arm are adducted and internally rotated. The elbow is extended, and the forearm is pronated, with the wrist and fingers flexed; a grasp reflex may be present because finger and wrist movement remain normal (Tappero, 2003) (Fig. 27-2). In lower plexus palsy, the muscles of the hand are paralyzed, with consequent wrist drop and relaxed fingers. In a third and

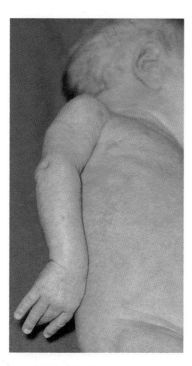

Fig. 27-2 Erb-Duchenne paralysis in newborn infant. Moro reflex is absent in right upper extremity. Recovery was complete. (From O'Doherty, N. [1986]. *Neonatology: Micro atlas of the newborn.* Nutley, NJ: Hoffmann-La Roche.)

more severe form of brachial palsy the entire arm is paralyzed and hangs limp and motionless at the side. The Moro reflex is absent on the affected side for all of the forms of brachial palsy (Dunham, 2003).

Treatment of the affected arm is aimed at preventing contractures of the paralyzed muscles and maintaining correct placement of the humeral head within the glenoid fossa of the scapula. Complete recovery from stretched nerves usually takes 3 to 6 months. However, avulsion of the nerves (complete disconnection of the ganglia from the spinal cord that involves both anterior and posterior roots) results in permanent damage. For those injuries that do not improve spontaneously by 3 months, surgical intervention may be needed to relieve pressure on the nerves or to repair the nerves with grafting (Volpe, 2001). In some cases, injection of botulinum toxin A into the triceps muscle may be effective in reducing muscle contractures after birth-related brachial plexus injuries (Rollnik et al., 2000).

Nursing care of the newborn with brachial palsy is concerned primarily with proper positioning of the affected arm. The affected arm should be gently immobilized on the upper abdomen; passive range-of-motion exercises of the shoulder, wrist, elbow, and fingers are initiated in the latter part of the first week (Volpe, 2001). Wrist flexion contractures may be prevented with the use of supportive splints. In dressing the infant, preference is given to the affected arm. Undressing begins with the unaffected arm, and redressing begins with the affected arm to prevent unnecessary manipulation and stress on the paralyzed muscles. Parents are

taught to use the "football" position when holding the infant and to avoid picking the child up from under the axillae or by pulling on the arms.

Pressure on the facial nerve during birth may result in injury to cranial nerve VII. The primary clinical manifestations are loss of movement on the affected side, such as an inability to completely close the eye, drooping of the corner of the mouth, and absence of wrinkling of the forehead and nasolabial fold (Fig. 27-3). Facial palsy or paralysis is most noticeable when the infant cries. The mouth is drawn to the unaffected side, the wrinkles are deeper on the normal side, and the eye on the involved side remains open. Often the condition is temporary, resolving within hours or days of birth. Permanent paralysis is rare.

Nursing care of the infant with facial nerve paralysis involves aiding the infant in sucking and helping the mother with feeding techniques. The infant may require gavage feeding to prevent aspiration. Breastfeeding is not contraindicated, but the mother will need additional assistance in helping the infant grasp and compress the areolar area.

If the lid of the eye on the affected side does not close completely, artificial tears can be instilled daily to prevent drying of the conjunctiva, sclera, and cornea. The lid is often taped shut to prevent accidental injury. If eye care is needed at home, the parents are taught the procedure for administering eye drops before the infant is discharged from the nursery.

Phrenic nerve paralysis results in diaphragmatic paralysis as demonstrated by ultrasonography, which shows paradoxic chest movement and an elevated diaphragm. Initially, radiography may not demonstrate an elevated diaphragm if the

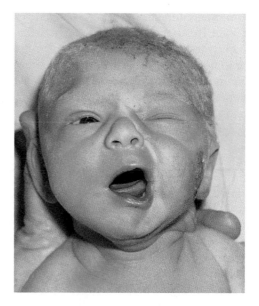

Fig. 27-3 Facial paralysis 15 minutes after forceps birth. Absence of movement on affected side is especially noticeable when infant cries. (From O'Doherty, N. [1986]. *Neonatology: Micro atlas of the newborn.* Nutley, NJ: Hoffmann-La Roche.)

neonate is receiving positive pressure ventilation (Volpe, 2001). The injury sometimes occurs in conjunction with brachial palsy. Respiratory distress is the most common and important sign of injury. Because injury to the phrenic nerve is usually unilateral, the lung on the affected side does not expand, and respiratory efforts are ineffectual. The infant is positioned on the affected side to facilitate maximum expansion of the uninvolved lung. Breathing is primarily thoracic, and cyanosis, tachypnea, or complete respiratory failure may be seen. Pneumonia and atelectasis on the affected side may also occur.

The infant with phrenic nerve paralysis requires the same nursing care as any infant with respiratory distress. As with other birth injuries, the emotional needs of the family are similar to those discussed for soft-tissue injury (see Chapter 19). Follow-up is also essential because of the extended length of recovery.

Central Nervous System Injuries

All types of intracranial hemorrhage (ICH) occur in newborns. ICH as a result of birth trauma is more likely to occur in the full-term, large infant. The frequency and degree of severity of ICH are different in the newborn than in older children or adults. In the newborn, more than one type of hemorrhage can and does commonly occur.

A subdural hematoma, or life-threatening collection of blood in the subdural space, most often is produced by the stretching and tearing of the large veins in the tentorium of the cerebellum, the dural membrane that separates the cerebrum from the cerebellum. When this type of bleeding occurs, the typical history includes a primiparous mother, with the total labor and birth occurring in less than 2 or 3 hours; a difficult birth; or a large-for-gestational-age infant. Subdural hematoma occurs infrequently because of improvements in obstetric care. However, it is especially serious because of its inaccessibility to aspiration by subdural tap.

Subarachnoid hemorrhage, the most common type of ICH, occurs in term infants as a result of trauma and in preterm infants as a result of hypoxia. Small hemorrhages are the most common. Bleeding is of venous origin, and underlying contusion also may occur.

The clinical presentation of hemorrhage in the full-term infant can vary considerably. In many infants, signs are absent, and hemorrhaging is diagnosed only because of abnormal findings on lumbar puncture—for example, red blood cells (RBCs) in the cerebrospinal fluid (CSF) or a hemorrhage is seen on a computed tomography (CT) scan. The initial clinical manifestations of neonatal subarachnoid hemorrhage may be the early onset of alternating central nervous system (CNS) depression and irritability, with refractory seizure. Poor feeding, apnea, and unequal pupils may suggest an intracranial insult. Occasionally the infant appears normal initially then has seizures on the second or third day of life, followed by no apparent sequelae.

In general, nursing care of an infant with ICH is supportive and includes monitoring neurologic signs, intra-

venous (IV) therapy, observation and management of seizures, and prevention of increased ICP.

Spinal cord injuries almost always result from breech births, especially difficult ones in which version and extraction are used. This type of injury is rarely seen today because cesarean birth is often used for breech presentation (Paige & Carney, 2002).

NEONATAL INFECTIONS ■

Sepsis

Sepsis (the presence of microorganisms or their toxins in the blood or other tissues) continues to be one of the most significant causes of neonatal morbidity and mortality. Maternal immunoglobulin M (IgM) does not cross the placenta. Immunoglobulin A (IgA) and IgM require time to reach optimum levels after birth. Phagocytosis (process by which cells engulf and destroy microorganisms and cellular debris) is less efficient. Serum complement levels are inadequate; serum complement (C1 through C6) is involved in immunologic reactions, some of which kill or lyse bacteria and enhance phagocytosis. Dysmaturity seen with intrauterine growth restriction (IUGR) and preterm and postdate birth further compromises the neonate's immune system.

Table 27-2 outlines risk factors for neonatal sepsis. Special precautions for preventing infection, as well as prompt recognition when it occurs, are necessary for optimum newborn care. Neonatal infections may be acquired in utero, during birth or resuscitation, and nosocomially.

TABLE 27-2

Risk Factors for Neonatal Sepsis

SOURCE	RISK FACTORS
Maternal	Low socioeconomic status
	Poor prenatal care
	Poor nutrition
	Substance abuse
Intrapartum	Premature rupture of fetal membranes
	Maternal fever
	Chorioamnionitis
	Prolonged labor
	Rupture of membranes >12 to 18 hr
	Premature labor
	Maternal urinary tract infection
Neonatal	Twin or multiple gestation
	Male
	Birth asphyxia
	Meconium aspiration
	Congenital anomalies of skin or mucous membranes
	Galactosemia
	Absence of spleen
	Low birth weight or prematurity
	Malnourishment
	Prolonged hospitalization

Neonatal bacterial infection is classified into two patterns according to the time of presentation. Early-onset or congenital sepsis usually manifests within 24 to 48 hours of birth, progresses more rapidly than later-onset infection, and carries a mortality rate as high as 50%. Early-onset infection is usually caused by microorganisms from the normal flora of the maternal vaginal tract, including group B streptococci (GBS), *Haemophilus influenzae, Listeria monocytogenes, Escherichia coli,* and *Streptococcus pneumoniae* (Merenstein, Adams, & Weisman, 2002). With the widespread use of intrapartum penicillin for prevention of GBS infection, *E. coli* has been reported to be the most common offending pathogen in early-onset sepsis (Stoll et al., 2002). *Coagulase-negative staphylococcus* has also been reported in some centers as the most common pathogen (Edwards et al., 2003), but this is debatable because some consider it to be a contaminant (Polak, Ringler, & Daugherty, 2004). Early-onset sepsis is associated with a history of obstetric events such as preterm labor, prolonged rupture of membranes (>12–18 hours), maternal fever during labor, and chorioamnionitis (Merenstein, Adams, & Weisman, 2002).

Nosocomial infection (late-onset) is most commonly seen after 2 weeks of age and is slower in progression. Bacteria responsible for late-onset sepsis are varied, may be acquired from the birth canal or from the external environment, and include *Staphylococcus aureus, Staphylococcus epidermidis, Pseudomonas* organisms, and GBS.

Viral infections may cause miscarriage, stillbirth, intrauterine infection, congenital malformations, and acute neonatal disease. These pathogens also may cause chronic infection, with subtle manifestations that may be recognized only after a prolonged period. It is important to recognize these manifestations in the neonatal period to be able to treat the acute infection, to prevent nosocomial infections in other infants, and to anticipate effects on the infant's subsequent growth and development.

Fungal infections are of greatest concern in the immunocompromised or premature infant. Occasionally, fungal infections such as thrush are found in otherwise healthy term infants.

The term *septicemia* refers to a generalized infection in the bloodstream. Pneumonia, the most common form of neonatal infection, is one of the leading causes of perinatal death. Bacterial meningitis affects 1 in 2500 live-born infants. Gastroenteritis is sporadic, depending on epidemic outbreaks. Local infections such as conjunctivitis and omphalitis occur commonly. Infection continues to be a significant factor in fetal and neonatal morbidity and mortality.

CARE MANAGEMENT ■

Assessment and Nursing Diagnoses

The prenatal record is reviewed for risk factors associated with infection and the signs and symptoms suggestive of infection. Maternal vaginal or perineal infection may be transmitted directly to the infant during passage through the birth canal. Psychosocial history and history of sexually transmitted infections (STIs) may indicate possible human immunodeficiency virus (HIV), hepatitis B virus (HBV), herpes (HSV-2), or CMV infection.

Perinatal events also are reviewed. Premature rupture of membranes (PROM) may be caused by maternal or intrauterine infection. Ascending infection may occur after prolonged PROM, prolonged labor, or intrauterine fetal monitoring. In some cases infection may occur with intact membranes or contribute to early rupture. A maternal history of fever during labor or the presence of foul-smelling amniotic fluid may also indicate the presence of infection. Antibiotic therapy initiated during labor should be noted. The neonate's gestational age, maturity, birth weight, and sex all affect the incidence of infection. Sepsis occurs about twice as often and results in a higher mortality in male than in female infants. The neonate is assessed for respiratory distress, skin abscesses, rashes, and other indications of infection.

During the postnatal period, the time of onset of suspicious signs is noted. Onset within the first 48 hours of life is more often associated with prenatal or perinatal predisposing factors. Onset after 2 or 3 days more often reflects disease acquired at or subsequent to birth.

The earliest clinical signs of neonatal sepsis are characterized by a lack of specificity. The nonspecific signs include lethargy, poor feeding, poor weight gain, and irritability. The nurse or parent may simply note that the infant is just not doing as well as before. Differential diagnosis may be difficult because signs of sepsis are similar to signs of noninfectious neonatal problems such as hypoglycemia and stress. Additional clinical and laboratory information and appropriate cultures supplement the findings described. Table 27-3 outlines the clinical signs associated with neonatal sepsis.

Laboratory studies are important. Specimens for cultures include blood, CSF, stool, and urine. Fluids such as urine and CSF may be evaluated by counterimmune electrophoresis (CIE) or latex agglutination (LA) to assist in the identification of the bacteria. A complete blood cell count with differential is performed to determine the presence of bacterial infection or increased or decreased white blood cell (WBC) count (the latter is an ominous sign). The total neutrophil count, immature to total neutrophil (I:T) ratio, absolute neutrophil count (ANC), and C-reactive protein level may be used to determine the presence of sepsis (Table 27-4). Newer technology includes detection of viral DNA or antibodies by polymerase chain reaction (PCR) amplification in fluids (Frenkel, 2005). Detection of antepartal infection can now be successfully treated with a number of antiviral medications to decrease viral replication and fetal transmission of disease; neonates may also be treated with antiviral medications such as ganciclovir. Treatment with antibiotics is initiated after cultures are obtained in neonates. In high risk infants with significant illness, antiviral or antibiotic treatment may begin once cultures are obtained;

TABLE 27-3

*Signs of Sepsis**

SYSTEM	SIGNS
Respiratory	Apnea, bradycardia
	Tachypnea
	Grunting, nasal flaring
	Retractions
	Decreased oxygen saturation
	Metabolic acidosis
Cardiovascular	Decreased cardiac output
	Tachycardia
	Hypotension
	Decreased perfusion
Central nervous	Temperature instability
	Lethargy
	Hypotonia
	Irritability, seizures
Gastrointestinal	Feeding intolerance (decreased suck strength and intake; increasing residuals)
	Abdominal distention
	Vomiting, diarrhea
Integumentary	Jaundice
	Pallor
	Petechiae
	Mottling

Adapted from Askin, D. (1995). Bacterial and fungal sepsis in the neonate. *Journal of Obstetric, Gynecologic, and Neonatal Nursing, 24*(7), 635-643, 1995.
*Laboratory findings include neutropenia, increased bands, hypoglycemia or hyperglycemia, metabolic acidosis, and thrombocytopenia.

when the pathogen is identified, antibiotic therapy may be modified.

Vigilant assessment continues during and after treatment. The newborn continues to be assessed for sequelae to septicemia, which include meningitis, disseminated intravascular coagulation (DIC), necrotizing enterocolitis, pneumonia, and septic shock. Septic shock results from the toxins released into the bloodstream. The most common signs include decreasing oxygen saturations, poor perfusion, tachycardia, respiratory distress, and hypotension.

Various nursing diagnoses are possible, depending on the infant's gestational age and birth weight, the organ systems involved, and the nature of the infection. Examples of nursing diagnoses related to neonatal infections include the following:

Newborn

- *Risk for infection related to*
  - maternal vaginal (or other) infection
  - indwelling umbilical catheters, parenteral fluids (invasive procedures)
  - intrauterine electronic fetal monitoring
  - dysmaturity, IUGR, gestational age
- *Ineffective thermoregulation related to*
  - systemic infection

- *Impaired skin integrity related to*
  - use of multiple supportive invasive measures (e.g., physiologic monitoring, parenteral fluid therapy, inhalation therapy)
- *Acute pain related to*
  - multiple supportive invasive measures

Parents and family

- *Anxiety, fear, or anticipatory grieving related to*
  - uncertainty about infant's prognosis
  - therapy (invasive)
- *Risk for impaired parent-infant attachment related to*
  - separation of parent and newborn
  - feelings of inadequacy in caring for infant
- *Powerlessness or spiritual distress related to*
  - perinatal events or newborn's condition beyond parents' control

Expected Outcomes

Expected outcomes include the following:
- The newborn will remain free of infection.
- The newborn's early signs of sepsis will be recognized, and appropriate therapy will be instituted.
- If therapy is necessary, the newborn will suffer no harmful sequelae.
- Parents will begin interacting and caring for newborn and be involved in his or her care.
- Parents will maintain self-esteem by understanding that their role as parents is important to the infant's well-being.

Plan of Care and Interventions
Prevention

Virtually all controlled clinical trials have demonstrated that effective handwashing is responsible for the prevention of nosocomial infection in nursery units. Nursing is directly or indirectly responsible for minimizing or eliminating environmental sources of infectious agents in the nursery. Measures to be taken include Standard Precautions, careful and thorough cleaning of contaminated equipment, frequent replacement of used equipment (e.g., changing IV and nasogastric tubing per hospital protocol, and cleaning resuscitation and ventilation equipment, IV pumps, and incubators), and disposal of contaminated linens and diapers in an appropriate manner. Overcrowding must be avoided in nurseries. Guidelines for space, visitation, and general infection control in areas where newborns receive care have been established and published (American Academy of Pediatrics [AAP] & American College of Obstetricians and Gynecologists [ACOG], 2002).

Infants cared for in neonatal intensive care units (NICUs) are at high risk for infection. There is center-to-center variability, with infection rates from 11.5% to 34% (Buus-Frank, 2004). Handwashing is the single most effective measure to reduce nosocomial infection. However, the rate of compliance with standards for hand hygiene is only

TABLE 27-4

Suspected Neonatal Sepsis

ASSESSMENTS	1. Potential maternal risk factors and unstable vital signs, especially temperature instability 2. Sepsis screen in first hour (CBC with differential, platelets, and CRP level) if there are significant maternal risk factors (prolonged rupture of membranes, maternal temperature) or if infant demonstrates physiologic signs of sepsis
TREATMENT	1. Start IV administration of antibiotics by peripheral IV 2. Provide other treatments as needed for additional physiologic problems (supplemental oxygen or ventilator for respiratory distress, incubator for temperature instability)
POSSIBLE CONSULTATIONS	1. Neonatologists and advanced practice nurses for care of unstable infants 2. Medical specialists for care of infants with additional problems (congenital deformities) 3. Lactation consultant, interpreter, social worker, and chaplain as needed or requested
ADDITIONAL ASSESSMENTS	1. Weight and measurements 2. Blood culture, chest x-ray examination, urinalysis, and lumbar puncture, if infant is symptomatic or CRP level is positive 3. Repeat determination of CRP level in the morning for 2 days; if negative and infant not symptomatic, stop antibiotic treatment 4. Continuous cardiac and oxygen saturation monitor assessment if infant's condition is unstable
DIRECT INFANT CARE	1. Vital signs every 1 to 2 hr for the first 4 hr, then every 4 hr 2. Advance oral feedings as tolerated (infant on NPO status only if condition is physiologically unstable) 3. Bath and cord care done per unit protocols
TEACHING AND DISCHARGE PLANNING	1. Initiate on admission. Provide parents with written and oral information on suspected sepsis 2. Reinforce information and determine parents' understanding of information before discharge. Include information on well-baby care and community follow-up with the family's primary health care provider

From Lucile Salter Packard Children's Hospital at Stanford, CA.
CBC, complete blood count; *CRP,* C-reactive protein; *IV,* intravenous; *NPO,* nothing by mouth.

22%. The combined use of alcohol, hand hygiene, and gloves is effective in reducing the incidence of systemic infection (Buus-Frank, 2004). It is incumbent on caregivers to strictly adhere to recommended guidelines for hand hygiene.

The skin, its secretions, and normal flora are natural defenses that protect against invading pathogens. Warm water may be used to remove blood and meconium from the neonate's face, head, and body. A mild nonmedicated soap (in single-use container or in the form of a small bar reserved for a single newborn) can be used with careful water rinsing.

NURSE ALERT *Artificial and long natural fingernails worn by nurses and other caregivers have been associated with serious neonatal infection and morbidity from Pseudomonas aeruginosa in the NICU (Moolenaar et al., 2000).*

Breastfeeding or feeding the newborn breast milk from the mother is encouraged. Breast milk provides protective mechanisms. Colostrum contains IgA, which offers protection against infection in the GI tract. Human milk contains iron-binding protein that exerts a bacteriostatic effect on *E. coli.* Human milk also contains macrophages and lymphocytes. The vulnerability of infants to common mucosal pathogens such as respiratory syncytial virus (RSV) may be reduced by passive transfer of maternal immunity in the colostrum and breast milk. Some evidence indicates that early enteral feedings (trophic or minimal enteral feedings) may be beneficial in establishing a natural barrier to infection in extremely low-birth-weight (ELBW) and very low-birth-weight (VLBW) infants; further studies are needed to make general recommendations and establish protocols (Strodtbeck, 2003).

Administering medications, taking precautions when performing treatments, and following isolation procedures are also interventions to be considered in the prevention and treatment of neonatal sepsis.

Monitoring the IV infusion rate and administering antibiotics are nursing responsibilities. It is important to administer the prescribed dose of antibiotic within 1 hour after it is prepared to avoid loss of drug stability. If the IV fluid the infant is receiving contains electrolytes, vitamins, or other medications, the nurse should check with the hospital pharmacy before adding antibiotics. The antibiotic (or other medication) may be deactivated or may form a precipitate when combined with other medications. In that case a piggyback solution of the prescribed fluid is attached with a three-way stopcock at the infusion site.

Care must be taken in suctioning secretions from any newborn's oropharynx or trachea. Routine suctioning is not recommended and may further compromise the infant's immune status as well as cause hypoxia and increase ICP. Isolation procedures are implemented as indicated according to hospital policy. Isolation protocols are changing rapidly, and the nurse is urged to participate in continuing education and in-service programs to remain up to date.

Evaluation

The nurse can be reasonably assured that care was effective if the outcomes established for care are met.

TORCH Infections

The occurrence of certain maternal infections during early pregnancy is known to be associated with various congenital malformations and disorders. The most common and best understood infections are represented by the acronym TORCH (Box 27-1). One of the problems with these viral infections—TORCH infections—is the lack of maternal symptomatology, resulting in lack of treatment and thus often producing an affected newborn at birth. With the advent of newer diagnostic methods these viral infections may be diagnosed in utero and interventions planned based on the availability of intrauterine treatments. HSV may result in a severe, often fatal systemic illness in neonates. Survivors of herpetic infection may have residual CNS damage (encephalitis) and chorioretinitis. The other congenital infections also may result in encephalopathy with various anomalies, including microcephaly, chorioretinitis, intracranial calcifications, microphthalmus, and cataracts. To a certain extent, the varied clinical manifestations of these infections overlap, but a specific diagnosis can be made by the clustering of clinical findings, as well as specific antibody studies.

Toxoplasmosis

Toxoplasmosis is a multisystem disease caused by the protozoan *Toxoplasma gondii*. Cats who hunt infected birds and mice harbor the parasite and excrete the infective oocysts in their feces. Human infection follows hand-to-mouth contact, such as after disposal of cat litter or after handling or ingesting raw meat from cattle or sheep that grazed in contaminated fields. The transplacental transmission rate increases as pregnancy progresses: 20% in the first trimester, 50% in the second trimester, and 65% in the third trimester (Cowles & Gonik, 2002). First trimester exposure to the protozoan is more serious for the fetus than third trimester or perinatal transmission. Intrauterine detection of the condition may occur as early as 18 weeks of gestation using PCR (polymerase chain reaction) of the gene (B1) of the protozoa in amniotic fluid. The detection of intrauterine infection and subsequent maternal treatment with spiramycin may prevent fetal infection (Boyer & Boyer, 2004). More than 70% of affected infants are free of symptoms. The clinical features of toxoplasmosis resemble cytomegalic inclusion disease (CMID) in the infant. Both diseases are responsible for serious perinatal mortality and morbidity: 10% to 15% of affected infants die, 50% have visual problems by age 1 year, and 85% have severe psychomotor problems or mental retardation by age 2 to 4 years.

Severe toxoplasmosis is associated with preterm birth, growth restriction, microcephaly or hydrocephaly, microphthalmos, chorioretinitis, CNS calcification, thrombocytopenia, jaundice, and fever. Petechiae or a maculopapular rash may also be evident. Some clinical manifestations do not develop until later in life. The affected infant may be treated with pyrimethamine, as well as oral sulfadiazine, but folic acid supplementation will be required to prevent anemia.

Gonorrhea

The incidence of gonococcal infection in pregnant women ranges from 2.5% to 7.3%. With this high incidence, it is not surprising that neonatal infection with *Neisseria gonorrhoeae* occurs. After rupture of membranes, ascending infection can result in orogastric contamination of the fetus. The organism also may invade mucosal surfaces such as the conjunctiva (ophthalmia neonatorum), rectal mucosa, and pharynx. Contamination may occur as the infant passes through the birth canal, or it may occur postnatally from an infected adult. Neonatal gonococcal arthritis, septicemia, meningitis, vaginitis, and scalp abscesses can also develop.

Eye prophylaxis (e.g., with 0.5% erythromycin ointment) is administered at or shortly after birth to prevent oph-

---

BOX 27-1

TORCH Infections Affecting Newborns

T	Toxoplasmosis
O	Other: gonorrhea, syphilis, varicella, hepatitis B virus (HBV), human parvovirus B19, human immunodeficiency virus (HIV)
R	Rubella
C	Cytomegalovirus (CMV) infection
H	Herpes simplex virus (HSV) infection

thalmia neonatorum. The infant with a mild infection often recovers completely with appropriate treatment (e.g., single dose of intramuscular [IM] or IV ceftriaxone). Occasionally, infants die of overwhelming infection in the early neonatal period. The newborn with clinical disease should be admitted to a hospital for treatment (AAP & ACOG, 2002).

Syphilis

Congenital and neonatal syphilis have reemerged in recent years as significant health problems. It is estimated that for every 100 women diagnosed with primary or secondary disease, two to five infants will contract congenital syphilis. If syphilis during pregnancy is untreated, 40% to 50% of neonates born to these women will have symptomatic congenital syphilis. Treatment failure can occur, particularly when treatment is given in the third trimester; therefore, infants born to women treated after 20 weeks of gestation should be investigated for congenital syphilis.

Fetal infestation with the spirochete *Treponema pallidum* is blocked by Langhans' layer in the chorion until this layer begins to atrophy at between 16 and 18 weeks of gestation. If spirochetemia is untreated, it will result in fetal death by midtrimester, miscarriage, or stillbirth (in one in four cases). All neonates in whom the infection occurs before 7 months of gestation are affected. Only 60% are affected if the infection occurs late in pregnancy. If maternal infection is treated adequately before the eighteenth week, neonates seldom demonstrate signs of the disease. Although treatment after the eighteenth week may cure fetal spirochetemia, pathologic changes may not be prevented completely.

Because the fetus becomes infected after the period of organogenesis (first trimester), organs develop normally. Congenital syphilis may stimulate preterm labor, but no evidence indicates that it causes IUGR. Organs affected later by congenital syphilis may include the liver, spleen, kidneys, adrenal glands, and bone covering and marrow. Disorders of the CNS, teeth, and cornea may not become evident until several months after birth.

The most severely affected infants are born to untreated mothers, and the newborn may be hydropic (edematous) and anemic, with enlarged liver and spleen. Hepatosplenomegaly probably results from extramedullary hematopoietic activity stimulated by the severe anemia. In some infants, signs of congenital syphilis do not appear until late in the neonatal period. In these newborns, early signs such as poor feeding, slight hyperthermia, and snuffles may be nonspecific. The term *snuffles* refers to the copious, clear, serosanguineous mucous discharge from the neonate's nose. A mucopurulent discharge indicates secondary infection, usually by streptococci or staphylococci.

By the end of the first week of life, a copper-colored maculopapular dermal rash appears in untreated newborns. The rash is characteristically first noticeable on the palms of the hands, soles of the feet (Fig. 27-4), and the diaper area and around the mouth and anus. The maculopapular lesions

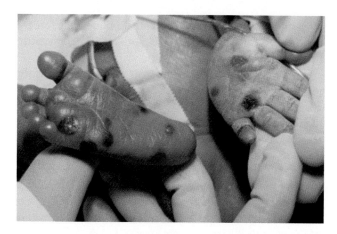

Fig. 27-4 Neonatal syphilis lesions on hands and feet. (Courtesy Mahesh Kotwal, MD, Phoenix, AZ.)

may become vesicular and confluent and extend over the trunk and extremities. Condylomata (i.e., elevated, wartlike lesions) may be seen around the anus. Rough, cracked, mucocutaneous lesions of the lips heal to form circumoral radiating scars known as *rhagades*.

If the mother was adequately treated before giving birth, and serologic testing of the infant does not show syphilis, generally the infant is not treated with antibiotics. The infant is checked for antibody titer (received from the mother through the placenta) every 2 weeks for 3 months, at which time the test result should be negative. Some physicians recommend antibiotic therapy for asymptomatic or inconclusive cases.

A 10-day course of aqueous penicillin G or procaine penicillin G (consult drug references for dosage and administration route for each) is the usual treatment for congenital syphilis (Boyer & Boyer, 2004). Erythromycin is the substitute antibiotic of choice for infants sensitive to penicillin.

NURSE ALERT *The infant born of a mother who has untreated syphilis at the time of labor and birth will be highly contagious until after the first bath. It is therefore imperative that caregivers use Standard Precautions with all newborns.*

In general, treatment of syphilis is more effective if it is begun early rather than later in the course of the disease. However, a recurrence rate of 5% can be expected. Even adequate treatment of congenital syphilis after birth does not always prevent late complication (e.g., 5 to 15 years after initial infection). Potential complications include neurosyphilis, deafness, Hutchinson's teeth (notched incisors), saber shins, joint involvement, saddle nose (depressed bridge), gummas (soft, gummy tumors) over the skin and other organs, and interstitial keratitis (inflammation of the cornea).

Varicella-zoster

The varicella-zoster virus, responsible for chickenpox and shingles, is a member of the herpes family. About 90% of women in their childbearing years are immune; therefore the risk of infection in pregnancy is low—5 per 10,000 births (Cowles & Gonik, 2002).

Varicella transmission to the fetus may occur across the placenta when the disease is contracted in the first half of pregnancy, but this is relatively infrequent. When transmission to the fetus does occur in the early part of pregnancy, especially between weeks 13 and 20, the effects on the fetus include limb atrophy, neurologic abnormalities, eye abnormalities, and IUGR.

When maternal infection occurs in the last few days of pregnancy, 20% of infants born to these mothers will develop clinical varicella (Boyer & Boyer, 2004). The severity of the infant's illness increases greatly if maternal infection occurred within 5 days before or 2 days after birth. The mortality in severe illness is 30% (Gibbs, Sweet, & Duff, 2004).

Infants born to mothers who develop chickenpox between 5 days before birth and 48 hours after birth should be given varicella-zoster immune globulin (VZIG) at birth because of the risk of severe disease. Acyclovir can be used to treat infants with generalized involvement and pneumonia (Myers, Stanberry, & Seward, 2004).

Term infants exposed to chickenpox after birth will have either a mild infection or no infection if they are born to immune mothers. Those born to nonimmune mothers may develop chickenpox, but the course is not usually severe. Experts are divided as to whether this group of infants should receive VZIG. Infants younger than 28 weeks of age are at risk regardless of their mother's status and probably benefit from VZIG if exposed to chickenpox.

Hepatitis B virus

HBV infection during pregnancy is not associated with an increase in malformations, stillbirths, or IUGR; however, about a 32% increase in risk exists for preterm birth. The transmission rate of HBV to the newborn is as high as 90% when the mother is seropositive for both hepatitis B surface antigen (HBsAg) and hepatitis B e antigen (HBeAg) (Duff, 1998). Transmission occurs transplacentally; serum to serum; and by contact with contaminated blood, urine, feces, saliva, semen, or vaginal secretions during birth. Infants are most commonly infected during birth or in the first few days of life. The rate of transmission is highest when the mother contracts the virus immediately before birth. These mothers will be positive for HBsAg. Transmission may occur through breast milk, but antigens also develop in formula-fed infants at the same or a higher rate. Diagnosis is made by viral culture of amniotic fluid as well as the presence of HBsAg and IgM in the cord blood or newborn's serum.

Neonatal and fetal effects are serious. Preterm birth exposes the neonate to the problems of prematurity. Infants may be symptom free at birth or may show evidence of acute hepatitis with changes in liver function. The mortality for full-blown hepatitis is 75%. Infants who become carriers are at high risk for chronic hepatitis, cirrhosis of the liver, or liver cancer even years later (Cowles & Gonik, 2002).

Infants whose mothers have antibodies for HBsAg or who have developed hepatitis during pregnancy or the postpartum period should be treated with hepatitis B immunoglobulin (HBIG), 0.5 milliliter IM, as soon as possible after birth or within the first 12 hours of life. The hepatitis B vaccine should also be given concurrently, but at a different site (AAP Committee on Infectious Diseases, 2003). The second dose of vaccine is given at 1 month, and the third dose at 6 months. The vaccine should protect the child for up to 9 years. After the infant has been cleansed thoroughly and has received the vaccine, breastfeeding may be initiated. Vaccination for infants not exposed to maternal HBV is recommended before discharge from the birth hospital; breastfeeding for these infants may begin before the vaccine is given.

Human immunodeficiency virus (HIV)

There were 700,000 children newly affected with HIV in 2003, mostly through mother-to-child transmission of HIV. Most (90%) of these infections occurred in sub-Saharan Africa. Fewer than 1000 children were estimated to become infected in North America and Western Europe during the same time. Globally, about 2.5 million children are living with the virus (World Health Organization, 2004). Universal counseling and screening of pregnant women is recommended in the United States and Canada.

Transmission of HIV from the mother to the infant may occur transplacentally at various gestational ages. The risk of infection in an infant born to an HIV-positive mother (not treated) is approximately 13% to 39% (AAP Committee on Infectious Diseases, 2003). Globally the rate of maternal transmission of the virus is estimated to be 25%. With antepartum, intrapartum, and neonatal zidovudine (ZDV) treatment the incidence of neonatal HIV infection is decreased to 5% to 8%, and compliance with highly active antiretroviral therapy (HAART) is said to further reduce newborn infection rates to 1% to 2% (Cooper et al., 2002; Kriebs, 2002). A critical factor in perinatal transmission is the maternal viral load; a high viral load creates a greater chance for perinatal transmission of the virus. Postpartum transmission may also occur, with an additional risk of 14% attributed to breast milk contact (Weinberg, 2000).

Diagnosis of HIV infection in the neonate is complicated by the presence of maternal IgG antibodies, which cross the placenta after 32 weeks of gestation. The most accurate test for newborns and infants younger than 18 months is the HIV DNA PCR (deoxyribonucleic acid polymerase chain reaction) assay, which is performed on neonatal blood, not cord blood; results may be obtained by 24 hours (AAP Committee on Infectious Diseases, 2003). Follow-up testing for infants born to HIV-positive mothers is recommended at several intervals within the first year of life.

Typically the HIV-infected neonate is asymptomatic at birth. Early-onset illness (i.e., virus detected within 48 hours of birth) is attributed to prenatal infection and occurs in 10%

to 15% of infected infants. These infants develop opportunistic infections (*Candida* and *Pneumocystis carinii* pneumonia [PCP]) and rapid progression of immunodeficiency, which progresses to death in the first 1 to 2 years of life.

The remainder of infants seroconvert over a period of months to years. By 1 year of life, 80% to 90% of perinatally infected infants show signs of infection. Some children infected at birth show no signs of disease 8 to 10 years later. The age of onset of symptoms predicts the length of survival.

The presenting signs and symptoms of HIV infection vary from severe immunodeficiency to nonspecific findings such as failure to thrive, parotitis, and recurrent or persistent upper respiratory infections. In the first year of life, lymphadenopathy and hepatosplenomegaly are common. The infant may have fever, chronic diarrhea, chronic dermatitis, interstitial pneumonitis, persistent thrush, and AIDS-defining secondary infections. Common secondary infections include PCP, candidiasis, CMV infection, cryptosporidiosis, herpes simplex or herpes zoster, and disseminated varicella.

Although it is rare for an infant to be born with symptoms of HIV infection, all infants born to seropositive mothers should be presumed to be HIV positive until proven otherwise. Management begins by implementing Standard Precautions. Measures should also be undertaken to protect the infant from further exposure to maternal blood and body fluids. Regimens for the prevention of HIV transmission include antepartum, intrapartum, and neonatal treatment with HAART. Neonates may be treated with a combination of ZVD, didanosine, and nevirapine. In some cases lamivudine or stavudine may be used instead of didanosine for neonatal treatment (Bell, 2004). If the infant is diagnosed with HIV infection, the family should be counseled about conventional and investigational treatment options.

Counseling regarding the care of the mothers themselves, the family's care of the infant, and future pregnancies should be provided. Social services are required in these cases. If the parent chooses to keep the infant, home health care may be arranged. The risk for transmission among members of the same household is minimal. For more information and updated information, parents are offered the following resource: the National AIDS hotline, 1-800-342-AIDS.

In the United States, breastfeeding in the HIV-positive mother is contraindicated; however, in developing countries, the issue of risks versus benefits in relation to number of infant deaths attributed to poor sanitary conditions and availability of an appropriate food supply for infants and the theoretic risk of HIV transmission via breast milk is less clear (Kriebs, 2002). HIV infected women should avoid breastfeeding when replacement feeding is available, affordable, and safe. Otherwise, the recommendation is for exclusive breastfeeding during the first months of life (WHO, 2005).

The family must be counseled about vaccinations. Children with symptomatic or asymptomatic HIV infection should receive all routine vaccines. Although data regarding children with HIV and varicella vaccine are limited, the AAP Committee on Infectious Diseases (2003) recommends that children with no or mild symptoms be immunized for varicella.

Rubella infection

Since rubella vaccination was begun in 1969, cases of congenital rubella have been reduced dramatically; however, it is still seen occasionally in the newborn. Vaccination failures, lack of compliance, and the immigration of nonimmunized persons result in periodic outbreaks of rubella, also known as *German measles* or *3-day measles.*

The risk for congenital anomalies varies with the gestational age of the fetus at the time maternal infection occurs. Abnormalities are most severe if the mother contracts the virus during the first trimester.

More than two-thirds of infected infants have no symptoms apparent at birth, but sequelae may develop years later. Hearing loss, the most common result, appears to be progressive after birth. Initially the newborn may present with hepatosplenomegaly, lymphedema, IUGR, jaundice, hepatitis, thrombocytopenic purpura with petechiae, and the characteristic blueberry muffin lesions. Congenital rubella syndrome often includes chronic problems such as cataracts or glaucoma, sensorineural hearing impairment, hypogammaglobulinemia, peripheral pulmonary stenosis, and diabetes mellitus type 1 (Boyer & Boyer, 2004). The rubella virus has been cultured in infants for up to 18 months after their birth. These infants are a serious source of infection to susceptible individuals, particularly women in the childbearing years. Extended pediatric isolation is mandatory until the noncontagious stage of rubella has been reached (i.e., the infant should be isolated until pharyngeal mucus and the urine are free of virus).

Cytomegalovirus infection

Cytomegalovirus (CMV) infection during pregnancy may result in miscarriage, stillbirth, or congenital illness. It is the most common cause of congenital viral infections in the United States (Boyer & Boyer, 2004). Most (90% to 95%) of the affected infants are asymptomatic at birth; however, sensorineural hearing impairment and learning disabilities have been reported in previously asymptomatic infants.

The neonate with classic, full-blown CMV displays IUGR and has microcephaly. The neonate may also have a rash, jaundice, and hepatosplenomegaly (Fig. 27-5). Anemia, thrombocytopenia, and hyperbilirubinemia are common in the early stages of the illness. Intracranial, periventricular calcification often is noted on radiography. Inclusion bodies ("owl's eye" figures) in cells sedimented from freshly voided urine or in liver biopsy specimens are typical.

The virus may be isolated from urine or saliva of the newborn using the PCR assay. Differential diagnosis includes other causes of jaundice, syphilis (positive Venereal Disease Research Laboratories [VDRL] findings), toxoplasmosis (positive Sabin-Feldman dye test result), hemolytic disease of the newborn (positive Coombs' test reaction), or coxsackievirus infection (positive culture).

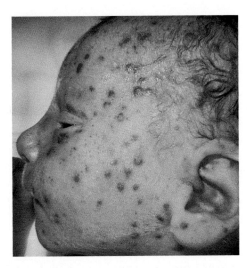

Fig. 27-5 Neonatal cytomegalovirus (CMV) infection. Typical rash seen in a severely affected infant. (Courtesy David A. Clarke, Philadelphia, PA.)

Despite the extensive, endemic nature of the disease in women and men and its potential for havoc in perinatal life, only occasionally are critically affected newborns seen. Milder forms of the disease often result when the fetus is affected late in pregnancy. CMV can be transmitted through breast milk while the mother is experiencing acute CMV syndrome. CMV infections acquired after birth are often asymptomatic and have no sequelae. Exceptions to this occur in preterm infants, in whom postnatal acquisition of CMV can result in pneumonia, hepatitis, thrombocytopenia, and long-term neurologic sequelae.

Antenatally infected infants who are asymptomatic at birth are at risk for late sequelae. Hearing loss may not be apparent until after the first year of life. Chorioretinitis, microcephaly, mental retardation, and neuromuscular deficits may occur by 2 years of age. Some children are at risk for a defect in tooth enamel, resulting in severe caries.

Treatment of the infected newborn with ganciclovir demonstrates a decrease in viral replication and severity of neurologic damage. Such treatment demands careful monitoring of the infant because the drug is toxic to bone marrow (Modlin, Grant, Makar, Roberts, & Krishnamoorthy, 2003).

Herpes simplex virus

Herpes simplex virus (HSV) infections among newborns are being diagnosed more frequently and are estimated to occur in as many as 1 in 3000 to 1 in 20,000 births (AAP Committee on Infectious Diseases, 2003).

The neonate may acquire the virus by any of four modes of transmission:

- Transplacental infection
- Ascending infection by way of the birth canal
- Direct contamination during passage through an infected birth canal
- Direct transmission from infected personnel or family

Congenital infection is rare and is characterized by in utero destruction of normally formed organs. Affected infants are growth restricted. They have severe psychomotor restriction, with intracranial calcifications, microcephaly, hypertonicity, and seizures. They suffer eye involvement, including microphthalmus, cataracts, chorioretinitis, blindness, and retinal dysplasia. Some infants have patent ductus arteriosus, limb anomalies, and recurrent skin vesicles, with a short life expectancy.

Most infants are infected directly during passage through the birth canal. The risk of infection during vaginal birth in the presence of genital herpes has not been clearly delineated. It may be as high as 33% to 50%, with active primary infection at term. Primary maternal infections after 32 weeks of gestation carry a higher risk for the fetus and newborn than do recurrent infections (Baley & Toltzis, 2002). The transmission rate of chronic vaginal herpes from the pregnant woman to her newborn is low. Passive intrauterine immunity to herpes may be responsible.

Postnatal acquisition of the virus and spread within a nursery have been documented by DNA analysis. Both mother and father, as well as maternal breast lesions, have been implicated in neonatal infections. There also is concern regarding symptomatic and asymptomatic shedding among hospital personnel. Nursery personnel with cold sores should practice strict handwashing and wear a mask, but no evidence indicates they should be removed from the nursery unless they have a herpetic whitlow (primary HSV infection of the terminal segment of a finger).

Clinically, neonatal HSV infections are classified as disseminated infection; localized CNS disease; or localized infection of the skin, eye, or mouth. Disseminated infections may involve virtually every organ system, but those primarily involved are the liver, adrenal glands, and lungs. Affected infants exhibit initial symptoms usually in the first week of life but sometimes in the second week, with signs of bacterial sepsis or shock. Clinical manifestations include skin vesicles in about 33% of infants (Fig. 27-6). Death results from progression of CNS involvement, respiratory distress and pneumonitis, shock, DIC, and bleeding. The risk of serious sequelae or death in disseminated infections is approximately 50% (Gibbs, Sweet, & Duff, 2004).

Standard Precautions should be observed when caregivers have contact with these infants. The neonate's eyes, oral cavity, and skin are inspected carefully for the presence of any lesions (Fig. 27-7). Cultures are obtained from the mouth, eyes, and lesions. Circumcision, if performed, is delayed until the infant is ready to be discharged. The infant may be discharged with the mother if the infant's cultures are negative for the virus. As long as no suspicious lesions are on the mother's breasts, breastfeeding is allowed. For the infant at risk, a prophylactic topical eye ointment (vidarabine or trifluridine) is administered for 5 days to prevent keratoconjunctivitis. Acyclovir should also be given to infants with ocular manifestation. No current recommendations exist for prophylactic systemic therapy; each case should be consid-

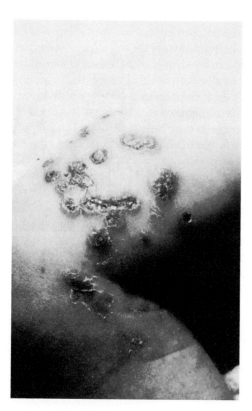

Fig. 27-6 Neonatal herpes simplex virus (HSV) skin infection. (From Behrmann, R. [1973]. *Neonatology: Diseases of the fetus and infant.* St. Louis: Mosby.)

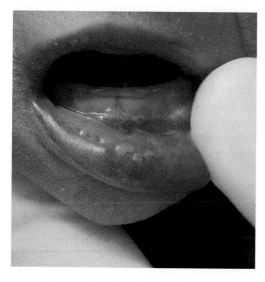

Fig. 27-7 Herpes simplex virus (HSV) oral lesions. (Courtesy David A. Clarke, Philadelphia, PA.)

ered individually. Blood, urine, and CSF specimens should be cultured when indicated clinically. If herpetic lesions first occur after 6 weeks of life, the risk of dissemination and severe illness is very low (Baley & Toltzis, 2002).

Therapy includes general supportive measures, as well as treatment with IV acyclovir. Acyclovir is the most commonly used and recommended drug for treatment of HSV. It is con-

sidered safe because only viral replication is inhibited, although long-term sequelae are not yet known. Although acyclovir is easier to administer than vidarabine, there is no difference between the two drugs regarding treatment of HSV. Continuing therapy may be required in recurrences. Ophthalmic ointment should be administered simultaneously.

Parvovirus B19

Parvovirus B19 is well-known in older children as *fifth disease* or "slapped-cheek illness" because of the characteristic facial appearance of the affected child. During pregnancy infection may result in fetal miscarriage or the development of nonimmune fetal hydrops. The estimated risk of transplacental transmission is approximately 30%, and fetal death may occur in about 9% of those affected (Boyer & Boyer, 2004). Protocols for intrauterine management have not been well developed, but intrauterine transfusion has offered limited success. Serial ultrasounds to detect fetal hydrops are possible. The virus may be isolated from amniotic fluid, fetal blood, or tissues using DNA PCR assay (Boyer & Boyer, 2004). Pericardial, pleural, and peritoneal effusions are common and fatal if not treated immediately, with cardiac failure from anemia being the most common cause of death.

Bacterial Infections
Group B streptococcus

Until recently GBS has been the most common cause of neonatal sepsis and meningitis in the United States; however, antepartum maternal screening and administration of penicillin has significantly decreased the incidence of GBS. Early-onset GBS infection in the neonate occurs in the first 7 days of life but most commonly manifests in the first 24 hours following birth. Risk factors for the development of early-onset GBS infection include low birth weight, preterm birth, rupture of membranes of more than 18 hours, maternal fever, previous GBS-infected infant, maternal GBS bacteriuria, and multiple gestation. Usually resulting from vertical transmission from the birth canal, early-onset disease results in a respiratory illness that mimics the symptoms of severe respiratory distress syndrome. The infant may rapidly develop septic shock, which has a significant mortality rate.

Late-onset GBS infection manifests between 1 week and 3 months of age, with an average age of onset of 24 days. Of infants with late-onset GBS, 85% have meningitis; this population has a mortality rate of 0% to 23%. Fifty percent of the survivors develop neurologic damage.

Escherichia coli

E. coli is the second most common cause of neonatal sepsis and meningitis in the United States, although some preliminary reports suggest that this organism has increased in some NICUs (Stoll et al., 2002). *E. coli* is found in the GI tract soon after birth and makes up the bulk of human fecal flora. In addition to meningitis, *E. coli* can also cause infections in other body systems, including the urinary tract. There is concern that increasing the use of ampicillin in labor as prophylaxis against GBS infection will result in more virulent *E. coli* infection because of ampicillin-resistant organisms.

Tuberculosis

The incidence of tuberculosis (TB), which is caused by *Mycobacterium tuberculosis*, is increasing in Canada and the United States. Congenitally acquired TB, although rare, can cause otitis media, pneumonia, hepatosplenomegaly, enlarged lymph glands, or disseminated disease. After birth, exposed infants contract TB through droplets expelled by infected individuals, which results in pneumonia and necrosis of lung tissue. Untreated neonatal TB is almost always fatal.

Chlamydia infection

Chlamydia trachomatis is an intracellular bacterium that causes neonatal conjunctivitis and pneumonia. The conjunctivitis, with minimal watery discharge, develops 5 days to 2 weeks after birth. Inclusion conjunctivitis is usually self-limiting, but if untreated, chronic follicular conjunctivitis (trachoma) with conjunctival scarring and corneal microgranulations has been reported. The organism may spread to the lungs from nasal secretions if left untreated, causing chlamydial pneumonia in about 33% of infected infants with symptoms of a repetitive staccato cough, tachypnea, rales, hyperinflation, and bilateral diffuse infiltrates on radiographic examination (Popovich & McAlhany, 2004).

Ophthalmic silver nitrate, 0.5 % erythromycin, and 1% tetracycline are not effective against *C. trachomatis;* therefore it is recommended that infants born to mothers who are positive for *Chlamydia* be followed closely for the development of symptoms. The neonate with positive cultures should be treated with oral erythromycin (AAP Committee on Infectious Diseases, 2003) or oral sulfonamide for 2 to 3 weeks. Erythromycin administration in infants younger than 6 weeks has been associated with an increased risk of infantile hypertrophic pyloric stenosis (IHPS); therefore, parents should be educated regarding the symptoms of the condition (feeding intolerance, projectile vomiting, and abdominal distention).

Fungal Infections
Candidiasis

Candida infections, formerly known as *moniliasis*, may occur in the newborn. *Candida albicans*, the organism usually responsible, may cause disease in any organ system. It is a yeastlike fungus (producing yeast cells and spores) that can be acquired from a maternal vaginal infection during birth; by person-to-person transmission; or from contaminated hands, bottles, nipples, or other articles. It usually is a benign disorder in the neonate, often confined to the oral and diaper regions. Diaper dermatitis caused by *Candida* presents as a moist, erythematous eruption with small white or yellow pebbly pustules. Small areas of skin erosion may also be seen.

Candidal diaper dermatitis appears on the perianal area, inguinal folds, and lower portion of the abdomen. The affected area is intensely erythematous, with a sharply demarcated, scalloped edge, often with numerous satellite lesions that extend beyond the larger lesion. The source of the infection can be through the GI tract or caretakers' hands.

Oral candidiasis (thrush or mycotic stomatitis) is characterized by the appearance of white plaques on the oral mucosa, gums, and tongue. The white patches are easily differentiated from milk curds; the patches cannot be removed and tend to bleed when touched. In most cases the infant does not seem to be in discomfort from the infection; however, some will pull away from the breast or bottle and cry. The child may be brought to the health care provider with a complaint of poor oral intake.

Infants who are sick, debilitated, or receiving prolonged antibiotic therapy are more susceptible to thrush. Those with conditions such as cleft lip or palate, neoplasms, and hyperparathyroidism seem to be more vulnerable to mycotic infection.

The objectives of management are to eradicate the causative organism and to control exposure to *C. albicans*. Interventions include maintenance of scrupulous cleanliness (by nursing personnel, parents, and others) to prevent reinfection. Good handwashing technique is imperative. Clean surfaces should be provided for neonates. Proper cleanliness of the equipment and environment is critical. Diaper dermatitis is treated with a topical fungicide at each diaper change. When possible, exposing the perineal area to dry air is recommended because yeast prefers a moist environment.

Topical application of 1 ml of nystatin (Mycostatin) over the surfaces of the oral cavity four times a day, or every 6 hours, is usually sufficient to prevent spread of the disease or prolongation of its course. Several other drugs may be used, including amphotericin B (Fungizone), clotrimazole (Lotrimin, Mycelex), fluconazole (Diflucan), or miconazole (Monistat, Micatin) given intravenously, orally, or topically. To prevent relapse, therapy should be continued for at least 2 days after the lesions disappear (Zenk, 2000). Gentian violet solution may be used in addition to one of the antifungal drugs in chronic cases of oral thrush; however, the former does not treat GI *Candida* and may be irritating to the oral mucosa.

NURSE ALERT *Nystatin is best absorbed when given either 1 hour before feeding or after a feeding. Using a needleless syringe or medicine dropper, apply the medication to each side of the infant's mouth for optimal absorption.*

Infants who are breastfed may acquire thrush from the mother; in the event that the mother is colonized, treatment for mother and infant is recommended. There is no need to stop breastfeeding even if the mother is receiving systemic antifungal medications (Lawrence & Lawrence, 2005).

SUBSTANCE ABUSE

Certain maternal behaviors result in perinatal risk. Maternal habits hazardous to the fetus and neonate include recreational drug abuse, smoking, and alcohol abuse. Physiologic signs of withdrawal have been reported in neonates of mothers who use to excess such drugs as barbiturates, alcohol, or amphetamines. Prescription opioids such as oxycodone (Percodan) have been identified as increasingly popular drugs of abuse that may cause withdrawal symptoms in neonates (Rao & Desai, 2002). Serious withdrawal reactions are seen in neonates whose mothers abuse psychoactive drugs. Mothers receiving methadone in substance abuse treatment may give birth to an infant who exhibits withdrawal symptoms requiring treatment. Almost 50% of pregnancies of women addicted to opioids result in low-birth-weight (LBW) infants who are not necessarily preterm. Alcohol is a teratogen that produces CNS effects that may not be evident for years.

It is important to note that the term *addiction* is often associated with behaviors whereby the person seeks the drug(s) to experience a high or euphoria, to escape from reality, or to satisfy a personal need. Newborns who have been exposed to drugs in utero are not addicted in a behavioral sense, yet they may experience mild to strong physiologic signs as a result of the exposure. Therefore, to say that an infant born to a mother who uses substances is addicted is incorrect; *drug-exposed newborn*, which implies intrauterine drug exposure, is a better term.

The adverse effects of exposure of the fetus to drugs are varied. They include transient behavioral changes such as fetal breathing movements and irreversible effects such as fetal death, IUGR, structural malformations, cognitive and motor delay, and behavioral problems. Critical determinants of the effect of the drug on the fetus include the specific drug, the dosage, the route of administration, the genotype of the mother or fetus, and the timing of the drug exposure.

Fig. 27-8 shows critical periods in human embryogenesis and the teratogenic effects of drugs. Table 27-5 summarizes the effects of commonly abused substances on the fetus and neonate.

Alcohol

Maternal ethanol abuse during gestation can lead to readily identifiable alcohol-related birth defects (ARBD) (formerly fetal alcohol syndrome [FAS]) or a constellation of neurobehavioral and cognitive problems which may only be identified by maternal history and behavioral characteristics.

The incidence of ARBD in the United States is about 0.2 to 1.5 per 1000 live births (CDC, 2004). ARBD is based on minimum criteria of signs in each of three categories: prenatal and postnatal growth restriction; CNS malfunctions, including mental retardation; and craniofacial features such as microcephaly, small eyes or short palpebral fissures, thin upper lip, flat midface, and an indistinct philtrum (Fig. 27-9) (Dunbar, 2005). Neurologic problems in ARBD children include some degree of intelligence quotient (IQ) deficit, attention deficit disorder, diminished fine motor skills, and poor speech (Jones & Bass, 2003). Infants exposed prenatally to alcohol who are affected but do not meet the criteria for ARBD may be said to have alcohol-related neurodevelopmental disorder (ARND), previously referred to as fetal alcohol effects (FAE) (CDC, 2004). These effects range from learning disabilities and behavioral problems to speech or language problems and hyperactivity. Often these problems are not detected until the child goes to school and learning problems become evident. Predictable abnormal patterns of fetal and neonatal morphogenesis are often attributed to severe, chronic alcoholism in women who continue to drink heavily

CD: Critical Thinking Exercise—Fetal Alcohol Syndrome

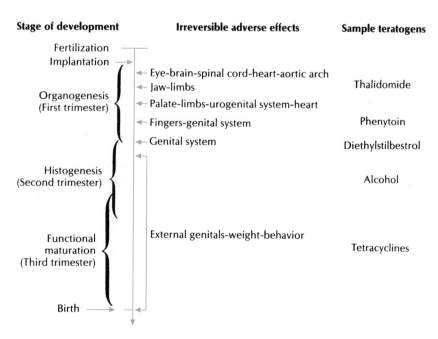

Fig. 27-8 Critical periods in human embryogenesis. (From Aranda, J., Edwards, D., Hales, B., & Rieder, M. [2002]. Developmental pharmacology. In A. Fanaroff & R. Martin [Eds.], *Neonatal-perinatal medicine: Diseases of the fetus and infant,* (7th ed.). St. Louis: Mosby.)

TABLE 27-5

Summary of Neonatal Effects of Commonly Abused Substances

SUBSTANCE	NEONATAL EFFECTS
Alcohol	*Alcohol-related birth defects (ARBD) (formerly fetal alcohol syndrome [FAS]):* craniofacial features vary, may include short eyelid opening, flat midface, flat upper lip groove, thin upper lip; microcephaly; hyperactivity; developmental delays; attention deficits *Alcohol-related neurodevelopmental disorder (ARND):* varying forms of ARBD, cognitive, behavioral and psychosocial problems without typical physical features
Cocaine	Prematurity, small size for gestational age, microcephaly, poor feeding, irregular sleep patterns, diarrhea, visual attention problems, hyperactivity, difficulty in consoling, hypersensitivity to noise and external stimuli, irritability, developmental delays, congenital anomalies such as prune belly syndrome (i.e., distended, flabby, wrinkled abdomen caused by lack of abdominal muscles)
Heroin	Low birth weight, small size for gestational age, irritability, tachypnea, feeding difficulties, vomiting, high-pitched cry, seizures
Methamphetamine	Small size for gestational age, prematurity, poor weight gain, lethargy, behavioral problems later in childhood
Tobacco	Prematurity; low birth weight; increased risk for sudden infant death syndrome; increased risk for bronchitis, pneumonia, developmental delays
Marijuana	Possible neonatal tremors, low birth weight, growth restriction

during pregnancy; however, the amount of alcohol consumption does not always correlate with identifiable features. Rather, it is the amount of alcohol consumed in excess of the maternal liver's ability to detoxify alcohol that defines what manifestations or effects will be evidenced from one child to another. The pattern of growth restriction begun in prenatal life persists after birth, especially in the linear growth rate, rate of weight gain, and growth of head circumference.

Ocular structural anomalies are common findings. Limb anomalies and various cardiocirculatory anomalies, especially ventricular septal defects, pose problems for the child. Table 27-6 outlines physical findings in ARBD. Mental retardation (e.g., IQ of 79 or below at 7 years of age), hyperactivity, and fine motor dysfunction (e.g., poor hand-to-mouth coordination, weak grasp) add to the handicapping problems that maternal alcoholism can impose. Genital abnormalities are seen in daughters of alcohol-addicted mothers. Two thirds of newborns with ARBD are girls; the cause of this altered fetal sex ratio is unknown. Severe and chronic alcoholism (ethanol toxicity), not maternal malnutrition, is responsible for the severity and consistency of postnatal performance problems. High alcohol levels are lethal to the developing embryo. Lower levels cause brain and other malformations. Long-term prognosis is discouraging even in an optimum psychosocial environment, when one considers the combination of growth failure and mental retardation.

Alcohol effects depend not only on the amount of alcohol consumed but also on the interaction of quantity, frequency, type of alcohol, and other drug abuse (polydrug use). Other drugs, such as cigarettes (nicotine), caffeine, opiates, and marijuana, may potentiate the fetal effects of alcohol consumption during gestation.

The infant of a mother who abuses alcohol is faced with many clinical problems. Identification of the problems leads to the medical diagnosis of ARBD. The infant may suffer respiratory distress related to preterm birth, neurologic damage, and a "floppy" epiglottis and small trachea. Tracheoepiglottal anomalies may cause cardiopulmonary arrest. Other disorders include recurrent otitis media and hearing loss. Craniofacial features may be important in diagnosing craniofacial and oral anomalies, dental development abnormalities, and long-term body growth patterns. Feeding difficulties are related to preterm birth, poor sucking ability, and possible

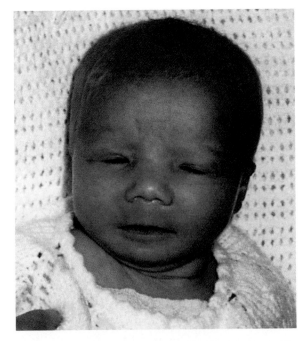

Fig. 27-9 Infant with alcohol-related birth defects. (From Markiewicz, M., & Abrahamson, E. [1999]. *Diagnosis in color: Neonatology.* St. Louis: Mosby.)

TABLE 27-6

Features of Alcohol-Related Birth Defects

AFFECTED PART	CHARACTERISTICS
Eyes	Epicanthal folds, strabismus, ptosis, hypoplastic retinal vessels
Mouth	Poor suck, cleft lip, cleft palate, small teeth
Ears	Sensorineural hearing deficits
Skeleton	Radioulnar synostosis, fusion of cervical vertebrae, restricted bone growth
Heart	Atrial and ventricular septal defects, tetralogy of Fallot, patent ductus arteriosus
Kidney	Renal hypoplasia, hydronephrosis, urogenital sinus
Liver	Extrahepatic biliary atresia, hepatic fibrosis
Immune system	Increased infections: otitis media, upper respiratory infections, immune deficiencies
Tumors	Nonspecific neoplasms
Skin	Abnormal palmar creases, irregular hair, whorls

From Weiner, L., & Morse, B. (1991). FAS: Clinical perspectives and prevention. In Chasnoff, I. (Ed.), *Drugs, alcohol, pregnancy and parenting.* Boston: Kluwer.

cleft palate. The infant may exhibit CNS dysfunction, microcephaly, and irritability.

Long-term effects into childhood may include impaired visual-motor perception and performance, lowered IQ scores, and delayed receptive and expressive language, as well as reduced capacity to process and store factual data (Dunbar, 2005). ARBD is now recognized as one of the leading, yet entirely preventable, causes of mental retardation in the United States. Although the distinctive facial features of the infant tend to become less evident, the mental capacities never become normal.

Nursing care involves many of the same strategies used for the care of preterm infants or drug-exposed infants, depending on the clinical manifestations. Special efforts are made to involve the parents in their child's care and to encourage opportunities for parent-infant attachment.

Placing infants in a warm, caring environment with understanding caregivers who can deal with the infant's hyperirritability can lead to improved emotional development and social functioning. These caregivers provide extensive cuddling and human contact and can deal with the eating problems that typically lead to a diagnosis of failure to thrive. However, these infants may not go home to an optimal environment because many affected families are dysfunctional.

Tobacco

Cigarette smoking in pregnancy is associated with birth weight deficits of up to 250 g for a full-term neonate (Aranda,

Edwards, Hales, & Rieder, 2002). Maternal cigarette smoking is implicated in 21% to 39% of LBW infants. Passive exposure to secondhand smoke by a pregnant woman may also result in the birth of an LBW infant. The rate of miscarriage and preterm birth is increased in the smoking population. Nicotine and cotinine, the two pharmacologically active substances in tobacco, are found in higher concentrations in infants whose mothers smoke. These substances can be secreted in breast milk for up to 2 hours after the mother has smoked. Cigarette smoke contains more than 2000 compounds, including carbon monoxide, dioxin, cyanide, and cadmium. Deficits in growth and intellectual and emotional development, poor auditory responsiveness, increased fine motor tremors, hypertonicity, and decreased verbal comprehension have been observed in infants exposed to smoke. There is also a positive dose-response relationship between the amount of tobacco exposure and newborn neurobehavior; increased tobacco exposure in utero is related to increasing negative neurobehavioral effects (Law et al., 2003). In addition, it is now recognized that neonates may experience withdrawal symptoms after exposure to nicotine. Pregnant women must be informed about the harmful effects of smoking on their unborn baby's health. These include IUGR, miscarriage, PROM, placenta previa, perinatal death, LBW, deficits in learning and behavior, and sudden infant death syndrome (SIDS) (Law et al., 2003). The positive association between maternal smoking and SIDS reflects in utero exposure and passive exposure postnatally. Mothers and all others should refrain from smoking near the infant. Smoking cessation during pregnancy greatly decreases the chance of fetal complications; therefore women should be counseled regarding smoking cessation programs.

Marijuana

Marijuana has replaced cocaine as the most common illicit drug used by women ages 18 to 44 years (nonpregnant and pregnant) in the United States (Ebrahim & Gfroerer, 2003). Marijuana crosses the placenta. Its use during pregnancy may result in a shortened gestation and a higher incidence of IUGR. A strong association has been reported between the use of marijuana and a decrease in fetal growth and infant birth weight and length (Hurd et al., 2005). Other investigators have found a higher incidence of meconium staining (Rosen & Bateman, 2002). Compounding the issue of the effects of marijuana, especially among women ages 18 to 30 years (Ebrahim & Gfroerer, 2003), is polydrug use, which combines the harmful effects of marijuana, tobacco, alcohol, opiates, and cocaine. Long-term follow-up studies on exposed infants are needed.

Cocaine

Cocaine, a common illicit drug used in the United States, has multiple modes of use. However, use of the relatively inexpensive and easily administered "crack" form is increasingly common, especially among women of childbearing age. Because crack vaporizes at relatively low temperatures, it is smoked and absorbed in large quantities through pulmonary vasculature. The drug readily crosses the placenta, placing the fetus at risk.

Cocaine is a CNS stimulant and peripheral sympathomimetic. Legally it is classified as a narcotic, but it is not an opioid. The effects on the fetus are secondary to maternal effects—increased BP, decreased uterine blood flow, and increased vascular resistance. Consequently, the fetus suffers decreased blood flow and oxygenation because of placental and fetal vasoconstriction. The difficulties encountered by cocaine-exposed infants are compounded when the mother is taking the drug in conjunction with other illicit drugs (Askin & Diehl-Jones, 2001). Researchers have concluded that variables such as the mother's lack of prenatal care; poor nutrition; and use of tobacco, alcohol, and other drugs during pregnancy compound the effects of cocaine exposure in the infant (Miller-Loncar et al., 2005).

Infants may appear normal, or they may show neurologic problems at birth that may continue during the neonatal period. Fortunately, these findings are transient, and there has been little evidence of permanent sequelae (Messinger et al., 2004). However, cocaine exposure is an additional risk for the development of disadvantaged children (Arendt et al., 2004; Lewis, Misra, Johnson, & Rosen, 2004; Singer et al., 2004). Either of two types of behavior may emerge as a result of cocaine effects on fetal development: neurobehavioral depression or excitability. The behaviors of the depressed infant include lethargy, poor suck, hypotonia, weak cry, and difficulty in arousal. The behaviors of the excitable neonate may include a high-pitched cry, hypertonicity, rigidity, irritability, inability to be consoled, and intolerance to a change in routine (Gewolb, Fishman, Qureshi, & Vice, 2004). Other behaviors may include frequent startling, poor awake state, sleeping difficulties, and persistent primitive reflexes. Some infants develop late onset of symptoms (2 to 8 weeks). They may become irritable and hypertonic, experience sleep-awake disruptions, and demonstrate an inability to tolerate change; they may also be slightly febrile. However, these findings have been refuted in other studies (e.g., Messinger et al., 2004).

Sequelae of prenatal cocaine exposure include a smaller head circumference, decreased birth length, and decreased weight. Head growth may be one of the best predictors of long-term development (Bateman & Chiriboga, 2000). Other neonatal effects of cocaine exposure include increased incidence of gastroschisis, genitourinary anomalies, and periventricular and intraventricular hemorrhage. Long-term sequelae for newborns exposed to cocaine include lower language, motor, and cognitive scores in some studies (Singer et al., 2002); however, in one study there were no significant differences in the expressive, receptive, and total language scores (Singer et al., 2004). In a large controlled study of children exposed to cocaine and opiates in utero, only subtle deficiencies in mental and psychomotor functioning were noted at 3 years of age (Messinger et al., 2004). No significant differences were noted in mental, psychomotor, or

behavioral functioning. The environmental factors to which these children were exposed were perceived as an important factor in their development. Further long-term studies of exposed infants were recommended (Messinger et al., 2004).

Nursing care of cocaine-exposed infants is the same as that for other drug-exposed infants. Because they have increased flexor tone, these infants respond to swaddling in a semiflexed position (Askin & Diehl-Jones, 2001). Positioning, infant massage, and limited tactile stimulation have been shown to be effective interventions. Cocaine enters the breast milk; mothers should be cautioned about this hazard to their infants.

Referral to early intervention programs that offer comprehensive care, including child health care, parental drug treatment, individualized developmental care, and parenting education, is essential in promoting the optimum outcome for these children. Because affected children often live in an impoverished environment, they are at high risk for cognitive delays, lack of child health care, and inadequate nutrition.

Phencyclidine ("Angel Dust")

Phencyclidine (PCP) increases the risk of injury to the pregnant woman and therefore also to her fetus. The user may be unaware that she is ingesting PCP because it often is misrepresented as another drug of abuse or is mixed with other drugs.

PCP crosses the placenta and is found in breast milk. Literature about the effects on infants is limited. Infants exposed to PCP may exhibit abnormal motor behavior such as irritability, jitteriness, and hypertonicity.

Heroin

Heroin crosses the placenta and often results in IUGR. Heroin may have a direct growth-inhibiting effect on the fetus, but the exact mechanisms of growth inhibition are not clear. There is an increased rate of stillbirths but not of congenital anomalies.

Many of the medical complications attributed to heroin ingestion result from prematurity. Other risks include physical dependence in the fetus and the risk of exposure to infections, including hepatitis B and C virus and HIV.

Drug withdrawal in the mother is accompanied by fetal withdrawal, which can lead to fetal death. Maternal detoxification in the first trimester carries an increased risk of miscarriage. Detoxification is not recommended after the thirty-second week because of possible withdrawal-induced fetal distress.

Heroin withdrawal occurs in 50% to 75% of infants born to addicted mothers, usually within the first 24 to 48 hours of life (Rosen & Bateman, 2002). The signs depend on the length of maternal addiction, the amount of drug taken, and the time of injection before birth. The infant whose mother is taking methadone may not demonstrate signs of withdrawal until a week or so after birth. The symptoms of

EVIDENCE-BASED PRACTICE
Kangaroo Care for Low-Birth-Weight Infants

BACKGROUND

- Low-birth-weight (LBW) babies (<2500 g, regardless of gestational age) are at greater risk for diseases; mortality; and possibly diseases as adults. Most infant deaths occur in this group worldwide. Medical care is costly and scarce in developing countries. A low-technologic, low-cost intervention to improve the outcomes for LBW infants would be an important advance. Kangaroo mother care (KMC) combines skin-to-skin contact between mother and infant, frequent breastfeeding, and early discharge from the hospital. Skin-to-skin contact has been shown to significantly increase and stabilize infant temperature, decrease respirations, increase blood glucose, and improve breastfeeding duration and lasting maternal-infant bonding. (See "Early Maternal Skin-to-Skin Contact with Healthy Infants," the Evidence-Based Practice box in Chapter 18.) Babies in KMC are secured between their mother's breasts in an upright position, day and night. Infants are not eligible for this intervention until they have demonstrated respiratory, temperature, and feeding stabilization (exclusive breastfeeding or a combination of gavage and breastfeeding).

OBJECTIVES

- The review committee sought evidence that would assess the beneficial and adverse effects of KMC on infants born weighing less than 2500 g, regardless of gestational age. Specific research questions included the effect of KMC on mortality, illness, infant growth, infection, admission to neonatal intensive care units (NICUs), breastfeeding, length of stay, costs, and satisfaction of parents and staff.

METHODS
Search Strategy

- The reviewers searched the Cochrane Library, MEDLINE, EMBASE, LILACS, POPLINE, and CINAHL databases. Keywords were *kangaroo mother care, skin-to-skin, infants,* and *low-birth-weight infants.* The reviewers found three randomized, controlled trials, involving 1362 infants from Ecuador, Colombia, Ethiopia, Indonesia, and Mexico, published from 1994 to 1998. All three studies used skin-to-skin contact and exclusive or nearly exclusive breastfeeding. Early hospital discharge was considered in only one study. Controls received standard neonatal care, including incubator use.

Statistical Analyses

- Statistical analyses allowed comparison of data at 41 weeks corrected gestational age, discharge, 6 months corrected age, and 12 months corrected age. Discharge may have occurred before 41 weeks corrected gestational age. "Corrected age" is counted not from the preterm birth, but from 41 weeks corrected gestational age, which would have been the term due date. Reviewers calculated relative risks for dichotomous (categoric) data, and weighted mean differences for continuous data. The authors accepted differences outside the 95% confidence intervals as significant.

FINDINGS

- No difference was found in infant mortality between the KMC and the control groups. Most mortality occurred during the stabilization process before eligibility for the study.
- Reviewers found a significant decrease in nosocomial (hospital acquired) infection at 41 weeks corrected gestational age. There was significantly less severe illness and lower respiratory tract disease in the KMC group at 6 months. There was no difference in other severe infections at 41 weeks corrected gestational age, or 12 months. Breastfeeding was significantly better established as exclusive, or nearly exclusive, at discharge from hospital, but no difference was noted at term or 1, 6, or 12 months corrected age. No difference in readmissions between groups was noted. Weight and head circumference at discharge were significantly higher in the KMC group, but the difference was lost by term and 12 months. There was no difference between psychomotor skills at 12 months. Mothers felt competent and significantly more satisfied with their caregiving in the KMC group, but felt less social support regarding the NICU, although both groups were similar in perception of social support from the hospital, worry, stress, sensitivity, and infant responsiveness from mother. Infant temperatures were more stable in the KMC group. Hospital length of stay was variable, with one study reporting the KMC group had a shorter stay, and another study reporting longer stays than controls. Cost was lower for KMC, but there was not enough information to determine if this was significant. Most of the cost came during the stabilization period before enrollment in the study.

LIMITATIONS

- Patients, staff, and evaluators were fully aware of the group into which they were randomized, which could introduce bias or some other confounding influence. The definition of stabilization was not clarified. This could affect the outcomes because a more immature infant is more fragile. Missing and incomplete information regarding costs limited the ability to analyze this important outcome. All three studies were carried out in developing countries.

CONCLUSIONS

- The authors conclude that KMC appears to both reduce severe infant morbidity and to have no adverse outcomes, but the available research has methodologic problems that limit its usefulness.

IMPLICATIONS FOR PRACTICE

- The reviewers conclude that evidence to recommend the routine use of KMC in LBW infants is insufficient.

IMPLICATIONS FOR FURTHER RESEARCH

- Well-designed, randomized controlled trials that account for lack of concealment and dropouts can provide higher quality evidence to recommend this promising intervention. While developing countries stand to benefit from evidence that this low-technologic, low-cost method can benefit LBW infants, it would be informative to have data from developed countries for comparison.

Reference: Conde-Aqudelo, A., Diaz-Rosello, J., & Belizan, J. (2003). Kangaroo mother care to reduce morbidity and mortality in low birth weight infants (Cochrane Review). In *The Cochrane Library*, Issue 2, 2004. Chichester, UK: John Wiley & Sons.

infants whose mothers used heroin or methadone are similar. Initially the infant may be depressed. The withdrawal syndrome may manifest as a combination of any of the following signs:

- Infant may be jittery and hyperactive.
- Cry is shrill and persistent.
- Infant may yawn or sneeze frequently.
- Tendon reflexes are increased, but the Moro reflex is decreased.
- Neonate may exhibit poor feeding and sucking, tachypnea, vomiting, diarrhea, hypothermia or hyperthermia, and sweating.
- Infant may exhibit abnormal sleep cycle, with absence of quiet sleep and disturbance of active sleep.

The risk of SIDS is 5 to 10 times higher for infants with significant withdrawal problems than for infants in the general population.

If withdrawal is not treated, vomiting, diarrhea, dehydration, apnea, and convulsions may develop. Death may follow. Therapy is individualized. Dehydration and electrolyte imbalance are prevented or treated. Usually the following drugs are given, singly or in combination: phenobarbital, diluted tincture of opium (paregoric), methadone, or morphine.

Buprenorphine, a partial morphine agonist, reduces opiate use. It is being used in Europe and will soon be used in the United States. Infants born to mothers on buprenorphine have a lower incidence of small size for gestational age and a milder and shorter course of abstinence syndrome (Rosen & Bateman, 2002).

> **NURSE ALERT** *The use of naloxone (Narcan) is contraindicated in infants born to narcotic addicts because it may exacerbate narcotic abstinence syndrome and cause seizures.*

Methadone

Methadone, a synthetic opiate, has been the therapy of choice for heroin addiction since 1965. Methadone crosses the placenta. An increasing number of infants have been born to methadone-maintained mothers, who seem to have better prenatal care and a somewhat better lifestyle than those taking heroin.

Some question exists concerning the benefits of methadone therapy during pregnancy because of its effect on the fetus. Methadone withdrawal resembles heroin withdrawal but tends to be more severe and prolonged. Signs of methadone withdrawal include tremors, irritability, state lability, hypertonicity, hypersensitivity, vomiting, mottling, and nasal stuffiness (Jansson, Velez, & Harrow, 2004). These infants exhibit a disturbed sleep pattern similar to that seen in heroin withdrawal. They have a higher birth weight than those infants in heroin withdrawal, usually appropriate for gestational age. No increased incidence of congenital anomalies is seen. The AAP Committee on Drugs (2001) has revised its statement regarding breastfeeding for mothers who are in a

methadone treatment program, suggesting that such mothers be allowed to breastfeed regardless of the methadone treatment dosage. Follow-up counseling and monitoring of the mother and infant are recommended.

Late-onset withdrawal occurs at age 2 to 4 weeks and may continue for weeks or months. A higher incidence of SIDS also has been reported in these infants (Rosen & Bateman, 2002). This factor is important for perinatal nurses who coordinate follow-up care for the infant and education for the mother or other caregiver. Community health nurses must know about the potential for withdrawal symptoms to occur.

Therapy for methadone withdrawal is similar to that for heroin withdrawal. The few available follow-up studies of these infants reveal a high incidence of hyperactivity, learning and behavior disorders, and poor social adjustment.

Miscellaneous Substances
Methamphetamines

The fetal and neonatal effects of maternal use of methamphetamines in pregnancy are not well known but appear to be dose related (Smith et al., 2003). LBW, preterm birth, and perinatal mortality may be consequences of higher doses used throughout pregnancy. In addition, a higher incidence of cleft lip and palate and cardiac defects has been reported in infants exposed to methamphetamines in utero (Plessinger, 1998).

Methamphetamine use has increased significantly in the past 10 years in certain regions of the United States. In Smith and colleagues' (2003) study, 63% of pregnant women reported using methamphetamine throughout the pregnancy. A higher incidence of preterm delivery and placental abruption was associated with methamphetamine use. In addition, fetal growth restriction (small size for gestational age) was slightly higher in methamphetamine-exposed offspring; however, 80% of these neonates' mothers also had significant intake of alcohol and tobacco use (Smith et al., 2003).

Study reports vary in the time of clinical manifestations of withdrawal from this drug; one study did not identify any signs of withdrawal in the first 3 days after birth, but long-term data were not collected (Smith et al., 2003). After birth, infants may experience bradycardia or tachycardia that resolves as the drug is cleared from the infant's system. Lethargy may continue for several months, along with frequent infections and poor weight gain. Emotional disturbances and delays in gross and fine motor coordination may be seen during early childhood.

Phenobarbital

Phenobarbital crosses the placenta readily and is subsequently found in high levels in the fetal liver and brain. Because of its slow metabolic rate, withdrawal onset is generally 2 to 14 days after birth and duration is about 2 to 4 months. Irritability, crying, hiccups, and sleepiness mark the initial response. During the second stage, the infant is extremely hungry, regurgitates and gags frequently, and demonstrates episodic irritability, sweating, and a disturbed sleep pattern.

Caffeine

Caffeine has not been implicated as a teratogen in humans. After a thorough review of the literature in print, Christian and Brent (2001) concluded that caffeine is a potential teratogen only when used with alcohol or tobacco or in very large amounts. Most published studies indicate an increased risk of fetal growth delay in women who consume more than 300 mg/day (three to four cups of coffee) (Andres, 2004).

Polydrug use

D'Apolito and Hepworth (2001) studied a small group (14) of infants exposed to multiple drugs (polydrug) in utero; these included opioids, stimulants, depressants, and sedatives. The most common symptoms observed were increased tone, increased respiratory rate, disturbed sleep, fever, frantic and increased sucking, and loose or watery stools. These findings are significant for nurses working in neonatal and obstetric areas; the presence of such findings may alert the nurse so documentation of events (using the Neonatal Abstinence Scoring [NAS] tool or other objective measure) may take place and therapy may be promptly implemented. Initial nursing interventions such as providing a quiet environment and offering a pacifier for frantic and excessive sucking may be implemented independently. It is important not to overfeed infants who demand frequent sucking as part of the withdrawal process.

CARE MANAGEMENT

Assessment and Nursing Diagnoses

Assessment of the newborn requires a review of the mother's prenatal record. A medical and social history of drug abuse and detoxification is noted. The infant may have IUGR or be preterm with LBW.

The woman who is abusing chemical substances may have infections that compound the risk to the infant, including hepatitis B; septicemia; and STIs, including HIV-positive status.

The nurse often is the first to observe the signs of drug withdrawal in the infant. In many cases the newborn may be discharged before the appearance of any manifestations of withdrawal. The infant is assessed by means of the guidelines discussed in Chapter 19. The infant's gestational age and maturity are noted. In utero exposure to some drugs results in observable malformations or dysmorphism (abnormality of shape). Neonatal behavior may arouse suspicion. Neonatal abstinence syndrome is the term used to describe the set of behaviors exhibited by the infant exposed to chemical substances in utero (Table 27-7). Fig. 27-10 provides an example of a Neonatal Abstinence Scoring system for assessing withdrawal symptoms. Because many women are polydrug users, the newborn initially may exhibit a variety of withdrawal manifestations.

Another scoring tool has been recently developed specifically aimed at measuring neurologic behavior and resultant

TABLE 27-7	
Signs of Neonatal Abstinence Syndrome	
SYSTEM	**SIGNS**
Gastrointestinal	Poor feeding, vomiting, regurgitation, diarrhea, excessive sucking
Central nervous	Irritability, tremors, shrill cry, incessant crying, hyperactivity, little sleep, excoriations on face, convulsions
Metabolic, vasomotor, respiratory	Nasal congestion, tachypnea, sweating, frequent yawning, increased respiratory rate >60/min, fever >37.2° C

effects on the neonate when substances are used during pregnancy. The NICU Network Neurobehavioral Scale (NNNS) was developed by the National Institutes of Health (NIH) and provides an assessment of neurologic, behavioral, and stress-abstinence function in the neonate. The test combines items from other tests such as the Neonatal Behavioral Assessment Scale (NBAS), stress-abstinence items developed by Finnegan (see Fig. 27-10), and a complete neurologic examination, which includes evaluation of primitive reflexes and active and passive tone (Law et al., 2003).

Newborn urine, hair, or meconium sampling may be required to identify drug exposure and implement appropriate early interventional therapies aimed at minimizing the consequences of intrauterine drug exposure. Meconium sampling for fetal drug exposure is reported to provide more screening accuracy than urine, because drug metabolites accumulate in meconium (Ostrea, 2001). Urine toxicology screening has less accuracy because it reflects only recent substance intake by the mother (Huestis & Choo, 2002). Meconium and hair testing for drug metabolites have the advantages of ease of collection, noninvasiveness, and greater accuracy.

Nursing diagnoses, which depend on the assessment findings, are tailored to the individual needs of the neonate and the family. Following are examples of nursing diagnoses.

Neonate

- *Risk for infection related to*
  - —Maternal risk behaviors that include sexual activity
  - —Prolonged rupture of membranes
  - —IUGR, preterm birth
- *Risk for disorganized infant behavior related to*
  - —Chemical effects of maternal substance abuse
  - —Caregiver cue misreading
  - —Caregiver cue deficient knowledge
  - —Sensory overstimulation
- *Disturbed sleep pattern related to*
  - —Drug, chemical withdrawal

NEONATAL ABSTINENCE SCORING SYSTEM

SYSTEM	SIGNS AND SYMPTOMS	SCORE	AM					PM				COMMENTS
CENTRAL NERVOUS SYSTEM DISTURBANCES	Excessive High Pitched (Or Other) Cry Continuous High Pitched (Or Other) Cry	2 3										Daily Weight:
	Sleeps <1 Hour After Feeding Sleeps <2 Hours After Feeding Sleeps <3 Hours After Feeding	3 2 1										
	Hyperactive Moro Reflex Markedly Hyperactive Moro Reflex	2 3										
	Mild Tremors Disturbed Moderate-Severe Tremors Disturbed	1 2										
	Mild Tremors Undisturbed Moderate-Severe Tremors Undisturbed	3 4										
	Increased Muscle Tone	2										
	Excoriation (Specific Area)	1										
	Myoclonic Jerks	3										
	Generalized Convulsions	5										
METABOLIC/VASOMOTOR/RESPIRATORY DISTURBANCES	Sweating	1										
	Fever <101° (99-100.8° F./37.2-38.2° C.) Fever >101° (38.4° C. and Higher)	1 2										
	Frequent Yawning (>3 or 4 Times/Interval)	1										
	Mottling	1										
	Nasal Stuffiness	1										
	Sneezing (>3 or 4 Times/Interval)	1										
	Nasal Flaring	2										
	Respiratory Rate >60/min Respiratory Rate >60/min with Retractions	1 2										
GASTROINTESTINAL DISTURBANCES	Excessive Sucking	1										
	Poor Feeding	2										
	Regurgitation Projectile Vomiting	2 3										
	Loose Stools Watery Stools	2 3										
	TOTAL SCORE											
	INITIALS OF SCORER											

Fig. 27-10 Neonatal Abstinence Scoring (NAS) system, developed by L. Finnegan. (From Nelson, N. [1990]. *Current therapy in neonatal-perinatal medicine* [2nd ed.]. St. Louis: Mosby.)

Parent(s)

- *Anxiety related to deficient knowledge regarding*
  —Care needs of an affected infant
- *Risk for impaired parenting related to*
  —Continuation of substance abuse or detoxification program
  —Guilt about infant's condition
  —Inability to cope with care needs of a special infant
- *Violence: self-directed or other-directed (toward infant) related to*
  —Drug-dependent lifestyle

Expected Outcomes of Care
Neonate

- The neonate will remain free of infection.
- Early manifestations of infection (viral or bacterial) will be recognized, and appropriate therapy to minimize effects of disease will be implemented.
- Newborn manifestation of withdrawal (NAS) will be recognized and appropriate therapy implemented to provide infant state regulation.
- Infant will receive appropriate physical and emotional care to minimize effects of maternal chemical substance use.
- Neonate will have steady patterns of uninterrupted sleep throughout the day.
- Neonate will demonstrate appropriate growth and development.

Parent(s)

- Parent(s) will demonstrate ability to consistently meet basic caregiving needs of neonate.
- Parent(s) will continue to participate in substance abuse program to enhance ability to cope with life and effectively parent the newborn.
- Parent(s) will receive counseling and information from health care staff regarding infant behavior, cues requiring comfort and feeding, signs of withdrawal, and general baby care.
- Parent(s) will recognize pattern of self destructive behavior (substance abuse) and seek intervention.

Plan of Care and Interventions

Planning for care of the infant born to a substance-abusing mother presents a challenge to the health care team. Parents are included in the planning for the newborn's care and are also encouraged to plan for their own care. A multidisciplinary approach is needed that includes home health or community resource personnel (e.g., regulatory agencies such as child protective services). Education and social support to prevent the abuse of drugs provide the ideal approach. However, given the scope of the drug abuse problem, total prevention is unrealistic.

Nursing care of the drug-exposed neonate involves supportive therapy for fluid and electrolyte balance, nutrition, infection control, and respiratory care. Swaddling, holding, reducing environmental stimuli, and feeding as necessary may be helpful in easing withdrawal (Plan of Care). Specific suggestions for providing care to infants experiencing withdrawal are listed in the Teaching Guidelines box.

Pharmacologic treatment is usually based on the severity of withdrawal symptoms, as determined by an assessment tool (see Fig. 27-10). Drug therapies to decrease withdrawal side effects include administration of phenobarbital, morphine, diluted tincture of opium, or methadone (Coyle, Ferguson, Lagasse, Oh, & Lester, 2002; Johnson, Gerada, & Greenough, 2003). A combination of these drugs may be necessary to treat infants exposed to multiple drugs in utero, and careful attention should be given to possible adverse effects of the treatment drugs (Johnson, Gerada, & Greenough, 2003).

After the presence of neonatal abstinence syndrome is identified in an infant, nursing care is directed toward treatment of the presenting signs, decreasing stimuli that may precipitate hyperactivity and irritability (e.g., dimming the lights, decreasing noise levels), providing adequate nutrition and hydration, and promoting maternal-infant relationships. Appropriate individualized developmental care is implemented to facilitate self-consoling and self-regulating behaviors. Irritable and hyperactive infants have been found to respond to physical comforting, movement, and close contact. Wrapping infants snugly and rocking and holding them tightly limits their ability to self-stimulate. The infant's arms should remain flexed with hands in close proximity of the mouth for sucking as is appropriate; sucking on fingers or hands is a form of self-control and comfort. Arranging nursing activities to reduce the amount of disturbance helps decrease exogenous stimulation.

Loose stools, poor intake, and regurgitation after feeding predispose infants with neonatal abstinence syndrome to malnutrition, dehydration, and electrolyte imbalance. Frequent weighing to detect fluid losses or caloric intake, careful monitoring of intake and output, electrolytes, and additional caloric supplementation may be necessary. In addition, these infants burn up energy with continual activity and increase oxygen consumption at the cellular level. It takes considerable time and patience to ensure that they receive a sufficient caloric and fluid intake.

Hyperactive infants must be protected from skin abrasions on the knees, toes, and cheeks that are caused by rubbing on bed linens while in a prone position while awake. The incidence of SIDS in children who have experienced neonatal abstinence syndrome is high, and parents should be reminded that the supine position for sleep is preferred. Monitoring and recording the activity level and its relationship to other activities, such as feeding and preventing complications, are important nursing functions.

Breastfeeding is encouraged in mothers who are not using illicit substances, are negative for HIV infection, and are compliant with a methadone program. Breastfeeding promotes maternal-infant bonding, and the small amount of methadone

PLAN OF CARE *The Drug-Exposed Newborn*

NURSING DIAGNOSIS Risk for injury related to hyperactivity, irritability, and disorganized state
Expected Outcome *Infant exhibits age-appropriate state modulation regulation and stability (i.e., quiet alert state, deep sleep state, drowsy) with minimal irritability and inability to modulate state.*

Nursing Interventions/*Rationales*

- Use an objective measure or tool such as the Neonatal Abstinence Scoring system *to verify and document behaviors associated with withdrawal.*
- Perform a comprehensive neurobehavioral assessment of the infant *to gather individual assessment data to assist in planning individualized care appropriate for the infant experiencing withdrawal as a result of intrauterine drug exposure.* NOTE: These first two interventions take precedence over all others because manifestations of withdrawal may vary from one infant to another.
- Administer medications *to decrease CNS irritability.*
- Decrease environmental stimuli *that may trigger irritability and hyperactive behaviors.*
- Plan care activities carefully *to allow for appropriate interaction as per infant's behavioral clues.*
- Wrap infant snugly and hold infant tightly *to reduce self-stimulation behaviors.*
- Position to avoid eye contact, swaddle infant, use vertical rocking techniques, and use a pacifier *to counter poor organizational response to stimuli and depressed interactive behaviors.*
- Monitor activity level, note the relationship between activity level and external stimulation, and stop external stimulation *if it causes activity increase.*
- Provide scheduled periods of rest, decreased overhead lighting, and no physical care *to allow time for recovery of quiet state after periods of care.*
- Help mother understand that infant behavioral cues are not a sign of rejection of her caretaking abilities *to facilitate long-lasting maternal-infant interaction, decrease maternal guilt, and enhance environment conducive to infant growth (promote infant's sense of trust).*

NURSING DIAGNOSIS Imbalanced nutrition: less than body requirements related to central nervous system (CNS) irritability, disorganized sucking pattern, vomiting, and loose or watery stools
Expected Outcome *Infant exhibits appropriate weight gain.*

Nursing Interventions/*Rationales*

- Observe for feeding cues indicating readiness for interaction (quiet alertness, rooting) and feed frequent small amounts and burp well *to diminish vomiting and aspiration.*
- Monitor weight daily and maintain strict intake and output *to evaluate success of feeding.*
- If intake is insufficient, feed by oral gavage per physician order *to ensure ingestion of needed nutrients.*
- Modify environment of feeding area as necessary *to decrease stimuli that detract from feeding process and interaction with caregiver.*

NURSING DIAGNOSIS Risk for impaired skin integrity related to hyperactivity, rubbing knees, elbows and face against linen, and loose, watery stools
Expected Outcome *Infant exhibits evidence of intact skin.*

Nursing Interventions/*Rationales*

- Position infant supine with knees and arms flexed and place a blanket roll *to promote containment and comfort and minimize frantic irritable activity.*
- Monitor hydration and nutritional status (i.e., skin turgor, weight, mucous membranes, fontanels, urine specific gravity, electrolytes) *to evaluate for evidence of poor skin integrity.*
- Administer medications intended to decrease hyperactivity, irritability and frantic posturing *to decrease exposure of skin to surfaces that may cause skin breakdown.*
- Wrap infant snugly in blanket and place hands in midline next to face *to promote self-comforting and decrease frantic activity.*

NURSING DIAGNOSIS Ineffective maternal coping, anxiety, powerlessness, related to drug use, and infant distress during withdrawal
Expected Outcome *Mother will accept newborn's condition and participate in care activities, showing evidence of maternal-infant bonding process.*

Nursing Interventions/*Rationales*

- Explain effects of maternal drug use on newborn and the withdrawal process *to facilitate understanding of the effects of drug use.*
- Encourage open communication (e.g., inform mother of ongoing condition, procedures, and treatment; answer questions; correct misperceptions; actively listen to her concerns) *to provide a sense of respect, provide support, and encourage a sense of control.*
- Encourage mother to interact with infant and to become involved in care routines *to foster emotional connection.*
- Explain how to perform care procedures, how to avoid overstimulation, and how to hold and comfort infant *to enhance mother's care abilities and her sense of confidence and control.*
- If the infant demonstrates signs of withdrawal, explain to mother the infant's inability to interact, gaze aversion, arching back, and lack of response to cuddling *to enhance understanding of infant behaviors.*
- Make appropriate referrals to social agencies for treatment of maternal substance abuse, infant development programs, and other needed support services *to ensure adequate resources for care of self and infant.*
- Encourage maternal participation in a substance abuse counseling (and methadone maintenance, as appropriate) program *to enhance maternal coping skills for effective caretaking of affected newborn.*
- Involve family in care of infant *to provide support for the mother.*

---

passed through breast milk has not proved to be harmful to the neonate (Hale, 2002; Berghella et al., 2003; Philipp, Merewood, & O' Brien, 2003). Because many new drugs are being manufactured, it is recommended that the reader consult with updated references regarding the safety of medications for breastfeeding infants (see Table 20-4 on p. 631) (Lawrence & Lawrence, 2005; see also AAP [2001] for a complete list of drugs that should be avoided with breastfeeding).

TEACHING GUIDELINES
Care of the Infant Experiencing Withdrawal

- Place the infant in a side-lying position with the spine and legs flexed.
- Position the infant's hands in midline with the arms at the side.
- Carry the infant in a flexed position.
- When interacting with the infant, introduce one stimulus at a time when the infant is in a quiet, alert state. Watch for time-out or distress signals (e.g., gaze aversion, yawning, sneezing, hiccups, arching, mottled color).
- When the infant is distressed, swaddle in a flexed position and rock in a slow, rhythmic fashion.
- Put the infant in a sitting position with chin tucked down for feeding.

Evaluation

Evaluation of the care of the drug-exposed newborn is based on the previously stated outcomes of care.

HEMOLYTIC DISORDERS

Hyperbilirubinemia and physiologic jaundice are discussed in Chapters 18 and 19.

Hemolytic Disease of the Newborn

Hemolytic disease occurs when the blood groups of the mother and newborn are different; the most common of these are RhD factor and ABO incompatibilities. Hemolytic disorders occur when maternal antibodies are present naturally or form in response to an antigen from the fetal blood crossing the placenta and entering the maternal circulation. The maternal antibodies of the IgG class cross the placenta, causing hemolysis of the fetal RBCs, resulting in fetal anemia and often neonatal jaundice and hyperbilirubinemia.

Rh incompatibility

Rh incompatibility, or isoimmunization, occurs when an RhD-negative mother has an RhD-positive fetus who inherits the dominant Rh-positive gene from the father. The Rh blood group consists of several antigens (because D is the most prevalent Rh antigen, the following discussion focuses on RhD isoimmunization). If the mother is Rh negative, and the father is Rh positive and homozygous for the Rh factor, all the offspring will be Rh positive. If the father is heterozygous for the factor, there is a 50% chance that each infant born of the union will be Rh positive and a 50% chance that each will be Rh negative. An Rh-negative fetus is in no danger because it has the same Rh factor as the mother. An Rh-negative fetus with an Rh-positive mother is also in no danger. Only the Rh-positive offspring of an Rh-negative mother is at risk. From 10% to 15% of all Caucasian couples and about 5% of African-American couples have Rh

incompatibility. Incompatibility is rare in Asian couples. The incidence of Rh sensitization and resulting hemolytic disease of the newborn have decreased dramatically since the development of $Rh_o(D)$ immune globulin in 1968.

The pathogenesis of Rh incompatibility is as follows: hematopoiesis in the fetus, or the formation of blood cells, begins as early as the eighth week of gestation; in up to 40% of pregnancies, these cells pass through the placenta into the maternal circulation. When the fetus is Rh positive and the mother Rh negative, the mother forms antibodies against the fetal blood cells: first IgM antibodies, which are too large to pass through the placenta, and then IgG antibodies, which can cross the placenta. The process of antibody formation is called *maternal sensitization.* Sensitization may occur during pregnancy, birth, miscarriage or abortion, amniocentesis, CVS, and PUBS. Usually women become sensitized in their first pregnancy with an Rh-positive fetus but do not produce enough antibodies to cause lysis (destruction) of the fetal blood cells. In subsequent pregnancies, antibodies form in response to repeated contact with the antigen from the fetal blood, and lysis results. In approximately 10% to 15% of sensitized mothers, there is no hemolytic reaction in the newborn. In addition, some Rh-negative women, even though exposed to Rh-positive fetal blood, are immunologically unable to produce antibodies to the foreign antigen (Neal, 2001).

Severe Rh incompatibility results in marked fetal hemolytic anemia because the fetal erythrocytes are destroyed by maternal Rh-positive antibodies. Although the placenta usually clears the bilirubin generated by the RBC breakdown, in extreme cases fetal bilirubin levels increase. The fetus compensates for the anemia by producing large numbers of immature erythrocytes to replace those hemolyzed—hence the name for this condition: erythroblastosis fetalis. In hydrops fetalis, the most severe form of this disease, the fetus has marked anemia, as well as cardiac decompensation, cardiomegaly, and hepatosplenomegaly. Hypoxia results from the severe anemia. In addition, because of the decreased intravascular oncotic pressure involved, fluid leaks out of the intravascular space, resulting in generalized edema as well as effusions into the peritoneal (ascites), pericardial, and pleural (hydrothorax) spaces. The placenta is often edematous, which, along with the edematous fetus, can cause the uterus to rupture.

Intrauterine or early neonatal death may occur as a result of hydrops fetalis, although intrauterine transfusions and early birth of the fetus may avert this. Intrauterine transfusion involves the infusion of Rh-negative, type O blood into the umbilical vein. The frequency of intrauterine transfusions may vary according to institution and fetal hydropic status, but it may be as often as every 2 weeks until the fetus reaches pulmonary maturity at approximately 37 to 38 weeks of gestation (Moise, 2002).

ABO incompatibility

ABO incompatibility is more common than Rh incompatibility but causes less severe problems in the affected infant. It occurs if the fetal blood type is A, B, or AB and the maternal type is O. It occurs rarely in infants with type B blood born to mothers with type A blood. The incompatibility arises because naturally occurring anti-A and anti-B antibodies are transferred across the placenta to the fetus. Unlike the situation that pertains to Rh incompatibility, first-born infants may be affected because mothers with type O blood already have anti-A and anti-B antibodies in their blood. Such a newborn may have a weakly positive direct Coombs' test (also referred to as a *direct antiglobulin test* [DAT]). The cord bilirubin level usually is less than 4 mg/dl, and any resulting hyperbilirubinemia usually can be treated with phototherapy. Exchange transfusion is required only occasionally. Although ABO incompatibility is a common cause of hyperbilirubinemia, it rarely precipitates significant anemia resulting from the hemolysis of RBCs.

Other

It is not within the scope of this text to discuss the many potential causes of hemolytic jaundice in childhood. However, in some populations there is a high incidence of glucose-6-phosphate dehydrogenase deficiency (G6PD), which may cause an exaggerated jaundice in a newborn within 24 to 48 hours of birth. G6PD red cells hemolyze at a greater rate than healthy red cells, thus overwhelming the immature neonatal liver's ability to conjugate the indirect bilirubin. Some of the triggers that potentiate hemolysis include vitamin K, acetaminophen, aspirin, sepsis, and exposure to certain chemicals (Reiser, 2004). Treatment is the same as for any newborn with rapidly rising serum bilirubin levels. Other metabolic and inherited conditions that increase hemolysis and may cause jaundice in the infant include galactosemia, Criglar-Najjar syndrome and hypothyroidism.

COLLABORATIVE CARE ■

At the first prenatal visit of an Rh-negative woman with a fetus who may be Rh positive, an indirect Coombs' test should be done to determine whether she has antibodies to the Rh antigen. In this test the maternal blood serum is mixed with Rh-positive RBCs. If the Rh-positive RBCs agglutinate or clump, this indicates that maternal antibodies are present or that the mother has been sensitized. The dilution of the specimen of blood at which clumping occurs determines the titer, or level, of maternal antibodies. This titer indicates the degree of maternal sensitization. A level of 1:8 rarely results in fetal jeopardy. If the titer reaches 1:16, amniocentesis is performed to determine the delta optical density (ΔOD) of the amniotic fluid to estimate fetal hemolytic process. Rising bilirubin levels may indicate the need for an intrauterine transfusion. Genetic testing allows early identification of paternal zygosity at the RhD gene locus, thereby allowing earlier detection of the potential for isoimmunization and precluding further maternal or fetal testing (Moise, 2002).

The indirect Coombs' test is repeated at 28 weeks. If the result remains negative, indicating that sensitization has not occurred, the woman is given an IM injection of $Rh_o(D)$ immune globulin. If the test result is positive, showing that sensitization has occurred, the test is repeated at 4- to 6-week intervals to monitor the maternal antibody titer as just described.

At birth the neonate's cord blood is sent to the laboratory to determine the infant's blood type and Rh status. A direct Coombs' test is performed on this cord blood to determine whether there are maternal antibodies in the fetal blood. If antibodies are present, the titer, which indicates the degree of maternal sensitization, is measured. If the titer is 1:64, an exchange transfusion is indicated. In addition, the prevention of or prompt therapy for perinatal asphyxia, acidosis, cold stress, sepsis, and hypoglycemia will decrease the newborn's risk for severe hemolytic disease and his or her susceptibility to kernicterus. Early feeding is also initiated to stimulate stooling and thus facilitate the removal of bilirubin.

If jaundice is present, the cause is determined and therapeutic management is begun. Phototherapy is used to reduce rapidly increasing serum bilirubin levels. See Chapter 19 for a discussion of phototherapy.

Exchange Transfusion

Exchange transfusions are needed infrequently because of the decrease in the incidence of severe hemolytic disease in newborns resulting from isoimmunization. Other factors must always be considered as well, particularly the clinical condition of the infant, because it is a procedure with potential complications. Guidelines for the initiation of exchange transfusion in relation to serum bilirubin levels in infants of ≥35 weeks of gestation may be found in the 2004 AAP Clinical Practice Guideline.

Exchange transfusion is accomplished by alternately removing a small amount of the infant's blood and replacing it with an equal amount of donor blood. If the infant has Rh incompatibility, type O Rh-negative blood is used for transfusion, so the maternal antibodies still present in the infant do not hemolyze the transfused blood. Depending on the infant's size, maturity, and condition, amounts of 5 to 20 ml of the infant's blood are removed at one time and replaced with warmed donor blood. The total amount of blood exchanged approximates 170 ml/kg of body weight, or 75% to 85% of the infant's total blood volume. Preservatives in donor blood lower the infant's serum calcium level; therefore, calcium gluconate is often given during the exchange transfusion. The neonate is monitored closely for signs of a blood transfusion reaction as well as hypotension, temperature instability, and cardiorespiratory compromise.

CONGENITAL ANOMALIES ■

Congenital anomalies (structural defects) occur in approximately 2% of all live births (Hudgins & Cassidy, 2002), but this number increases to about 6% by 5 years, when more anomalies are diagnosed. In addition, the incidence of congenital malformations in fetuses that are miscarried is higher than that in infants who are born alive, thus also adding to the overall incidence. Major congenital defects are the leading cause of death in infants younger than 1 year of age in the United States and account for 20% of neonatal deaths. Although the incidences of other causes of neonatal mortality have decreased, the death rate associated with most congenital anomalies has essentially remained stable since 1932.

The most common major congenital anomalies that cause serious problems in the neonate are congenital heart disease, choanal atresia, neural tube defects, cleft lip or palate, clubfoot, and developmental dysplasia of the hip (DDH). These are thought to result from the interaction of multiple genetic and environmental factors. Some of the most common malformations include lack of a helical fold of the pinna, complete or incomplete simian creases, and a capillary hemangioma other than on the face or posterior aspect of the neck.

Ways of detecting and preventing some of these anomalies are being improved continuously, as are some surgical techniques for the care of the fetus with certain anomalies. Promoting the availability of these services to populations at risk challenges community health care systems. An interdisciplinary team approach is vital for providing holistic care: the surgical treatment, rehabilitation, and education of the child, as well as psychosocial and financial assistance for the parents. Parental disappointment and disillusion add to the complexity of the nursing care needed for these infants.

Central Nervous System Anomalies

Most congenital anomalies of the CNS result from defects in the closure of the neural tube during fetal development. Although the cause of NTDs is unknown, they are thought to stem from the interaction of many genes that may be influenced by factors in the fetal environment. Environmental influences such as treatment with valproic acid (an anticonvulsant) or methotrexate (a chemotherapeutic agent) and alcohol and tobacco consumption have been implicated. Maternal folic acid deficit has a direct bearing on failure of the neural tube to close; therefore, folic acid supplementation is recommended for women of childbearing age. In the United States, rates of NTDs have declined from 1.3 per 1000 births (1970) to 0.3 per 1000 births after the introduction of mandatory food fortification with folic acid in 1998 (Honein, 2001). Increased use of prenatal diagnostic techniques and termination of pregnancies have also affected the overall incidence of NTDs. Although a neural tube defect is usually an isolated defect, it can occur with some chromosomal abnormalities and syndromes and also with other defects such as cleft palate, ventricular septal defect, tracheoesophageal fistula, congenital diaphragmatic hernia, imperforate anus, and renal anomalies.

Encephalocele and anencephaly

Encephalocele and anencephaly are abnormalities resulting from failure of the anterior end of the neural tube to close. An encephalocele is a herniation of the brain and meninges through a skull defect. Treatment consists of sur-

gical repair and shunting to relieve hydrocephalus, unless a major brain malformation is present. Some of these infants will have some degree of cognitive deficit. **Anencephaly** is the absence of both cerebral hemispheres and of the overlying skull. It is a condition that is incompatible with life; many of the infants are stillborn or die within a few days of birth. Comfort measures are provided until the infant eventually dies of temperature instability and respiratory failure.

Spina bifida

Spina bifida, the most common defect of the CNS, results from failure of the neural tube to close at some point. There are two categories of spina bifida: spina bifida occulta and spina bifida cystica. Spina bifida occulta is a malformation in which the posterior portion of the laminas fails to close but the spinal cord or meninges do not herniate or protrude through the defect (Fig. 27-11, *B*). It is usually asymptomatic and may not be diagnosed unless there are associated problems. Spina bifida cystica includes meningocele and

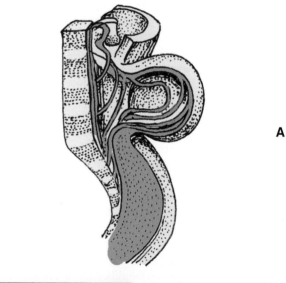

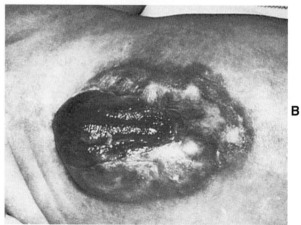

Fig. 27-11 **A,** Myelomeningocele. Note absence of vertebral arches. **B,** Myelomeningocele (ruptured sac exposing defect). (From Zitelli, B., & Davis, H. [2002]. *Atlas of pediatric physical diagnosis* [4th ed.]. St. Louis: Mosby.)

myelomeningocele. A meningocele is an external sac that contains meninges and CSF and that protrudes through a defect in the vertebral column. A myelomeningocele is similar, except that it also contains nerves; therefore the infant has motor and sensory deficits below the lesion. A myelomeningocele is visible at birth, most often in the lumbosacral area. It is usually covered with a very fragile, thin membrane (Fig. 27-11, *A*). The sac can tear easily, allowing cerebrospinal fluid to leak out and providing an entry for infectious agents into the CNS. Myelomeningocele usually is associated with an Arnold-Chiari malformation, which results from the improper development and downward displacement of part of the brain into the cervical spinal canal. This in turn results in hydrocephalus, which affects about 90% of children with myelomeningocele, although it is usually not present at birth. The long-term prognosis in an affected infant can be determined to a large extent at birth, with the degree of neurologic dysfunction related to the level of the lesion, which determines the nerves involved. Many physicians recommend that treatment be instituted regardless of the level of the lesion unless there is a severe CNS anomaly, advanced hydrocephalus at birth, severe anoxic brain damage, active CNS infection, or a malformation or syndrome incompatible with long-term survival. Prenatal diagnosis makes possible a scheduled cesarean birth, allowing for more careful delivery of the infant's back to try to prevent rupture of the meningeal sac.

A major preoperative nursing intervention for a neonate with a myelomeningocele is to protect the protruding sac from injury, rupture, and resultant risk of CNS infection. Such infants should be positioned in a side-lying or prone position to prevent pressure on the sac until surgical repair is done. If the infant is able to be held, the nurse or parent must be careful to keep the defect from being injured. The sac should be covered with a sterile, moist, nonadherent dressing and cared for using sterile technique. The skin around the defect must be cleansed and dried carefully to prevent breakdown, which would establish a portal of entry for infectious agents. A major nursing intervention is providing support and needed information to parents as they begin to learn to cope with an infant who has immediate needs for intensive care and who probably will have long-term needs as well. Surgical repair is performed in the neonatal period, often within the first 24 to 48 hours. Very early closure can prevent CNS infection and trauma to the exposed nerves. It can also prevent stretching of other nerve roots, which can occur as the sac continues to enlarge after birth. Surgical shunt procedures to prevent increasing hydrocephalus may be needed. Other problems, such as infection, are treated as they occur.

Hydrocephalus

Hydrocephalus is a condition in which the ventricles of the brain are enlarged as a result of an imbalance between the production and absorption of the CSF. Congenital hydrocephalus usually arises as a result of a malformation in the brain or an intrauterine infection. About one third of all cases of congenital hydrocephalus result from stenosis of the aqueduct of Sylvius in the brain. Hydrocephalus often occurs in conjunction with a myelomeningocele, which blocks the flow of CSF.

An infant with congenital hydrocephalus initially has a bulging anterior fontanel and a head circumference that increases at an abnormal rate, resulting from the increase in CSF pressure. Enlargement of the forehead with depressed eyes that are rotated downward, causing a "setting sun" sign, occurs as the condition worsens. If the surgical shunting of excess CSF from the brain is not done soon after birth, the resulting increasing ICP will lead to irreversible neurologic damage, as evidenced by palpably widening sutures and fontanels, distended scalp veins, lethargy, poor feeding, vomiting, irritability, opisthotonic positioning, and a high-pitched, shrill cry.

Nursing actions appropriate to the needs of a newborn with hydrocephalus include care similar to that for any high risk newborn. Measurement of the head circumference and neurologic assessments are done frequently. If the infant's head is large, the placement of sheepskin or a special pressure-sensitive air mattress under the infant and frequent position changes are necessary to prevent skin breakdown.

Microcephaly

Microcephaly refers to a head circumference that measures more than three standard deviations below the mean for age and sex. Brain growth is usually restricted, and there-

---

? Critical Thinking Exercise

Birth of a Child with a Congenital Anomaly

Marjorie, a 43-year-old mother, has just given birth to a daughter, Monica, who has a small ventricular septal defect (VSD). The infant has a loud murmur and circumoral cyanosis when crying vigorously but is pink at all other times. Marjorie knows that Monica has a heart defect but has not yet seen her. You are taking Marjorie to the nursery to see the baby for the first time. How will you introduce Monica to Marjorie? How will you describe Monica's defect and its treatment?

1 Evidence—Is there sufficient evidence to draw conclusions about what you should tell Marjorie?
2 Assumption—What assumptions can be made about the following factors:
   a. The parents' feelings about the infant and her physical defect
   b. Marjorie's initial reaction to the sight of her daughter
   c. Treatment for the defect
   d. Long-term outcome for Monica
3 What implications and priorities for nursing care can be drawn at this time?
4 Does the evidence objectively support your conclusion?
5 Are there alternative perspectives to your conclusion?

fore mental retardation is common. Microcephaly can be the result of an autosomal dominant disorder; a chromosomal abnormality; fetal exposure to teratogens such as radiation; and congenital infections such as rubella, toxoplasmosis, or CMV. Infants with microcephaly require supportive nursing care and medical observation to determine the extent of the psychomotor retardation that almost always accompanies this abnormality. There is no treatment. Parents need support to learn to care for a child with cognitive impairment.

Cardiovascular System Anomalies

Congenital heart defects (CHDs) are anatomic abnormalities of the heart that are present at birth, although they may not be diagnosed immediately. Some type of congenital cardiovascular problem is present in approximately 3.7 to 8 of every 1000 live births (Carey, 2002) and approximately two or three newborns will be symptomatic with heart disease in the first year of life (Bernstein, 2004). Ventricular septal defects, constituting more than 20% to 25% of all CHDs, are the most common type of acyanotic lesion. Tetralogy of Fallot, constituting 5% to 7% of all CHDs, is the most common type resulting in cyanosis (Fig. 27-12). After prematurity, CHDs, often in association with other congenital anomalies, are the next major cause of death in the first year of life.

The cause of the CHD is unknown in more than 90% of the cases. Maternal factors associated with a higher incidence of CHD include maternal rubella, alcohol intake, diabetes mellitus, systemic lupus erythematosus, phenylketonuria, poor nutrition, and antiepileptic medication use.

Genetic factors are implicated in the pathogenesis of CHD. As a general rule, these defects are thought to be multifactorial in origin, involving both genetic and environmental influences; however, a familial occurrence of virtually all forms of CHD has been noted.

Chromosomal abnormalities may also be associated with CHDs. For example, 50% of children with trisomy 21, or Down syndrome, have a cardiac defect. Most children who have trisomy 18, the second most common chromosomal abnormality, have a cardiac anomaly.

Some CHDs are often evident immediately after birth, especially those defects that cause central cyanosis (e.g., transposition of the great vessels) despite 100% oxygen administration. Infants with these anomalies are transferred directly to a neonatal intensive care nursery or pediatric intensive care unit.

Affected newborns may be cyanotic which is unrelieved by oxygen treatment, with the cyanosis increasing whenever the child cries. Pulse oximetry readings that remain low (below 89%) despite oxygen administration are not unusual, and respiratory distress may or may not be present. In many cases the infant's color is unrelated to the severity of the defect. Other infants may be acyanotic and pale, with or without mottling on exertion, such as crying, feeding, or stooling.

The affected newborn's activity level varies from restlessness to lethargy and possible unresponsiveness, except to pain. Persistent bradycardia (i.e., resting heart rate of <80 to 100 beats/min) or tachycardia (i.e., rate exceeding 160 to 180 beats/min) may be noted. The infant born to a mother with systemic lupus may exhibit bradycardia with normal sinus rhythm and good perfusion; eventually cardioversion may be required if the rhythm persists. The cardiac rhythm may be abnormal, and a murmur may or may not be heard. In many cases, however, ductal (ductus arteriosus) dependent defects or large shunts will not present with a murmur. Signs of congestive heart failure (CHF), diminished cardiac output, and poor tissue perfusion may be evident.

Because the cardiac and respiratory systems function together, cardiac disease may also be manifested by respiratory signs and symptoms. The respiratory rate should be determined when the newborn is in a resting state. Abnormal findings may include tachypnea, which is a rate of 60 breaths/min or more; retractions with nasal flaring; grunting occurring with or without exertion; and dyspnea, which may worsen with crying and activity.

A major role of the nurse is to assess infants for abnormal findings such as central cyanosis and poor perfusion. Newborns exhibiting these symptoms require prompt attention and appropriate therapy in a neonatal or pediatric intensive care unit. Interventions planned when a nursing diagnosis of decreased cardiac output is made include administering oxygen as ordered, although oxygen content is usually decreased once the defect is identified; administering cardiotonic medications to increase cardiac output, and medications designed to prevent closure of the ductus arteriosus (prostaglandin), and diuretics agents as needed for CHF; decreasing the work load of the heart by maintaining a thermoneutral environment; and feeding using the gavage method if necessary. Various diagnostic tests such as echocardiography and cardiac catheterization are performed to obtain specific information about the defect and the need for surgical intervention.

Respiratory System Anomalies

Screening for congenital anomalies of the respiratory system is necessary even in infants who are apparently normal at birth. Respiratory distress at birth or shortly thereafter may be the result of lung immaturity or anomalous development. Congenital laryngeal web and bilateral choanal atresia are readily apparent at birth. Respiratory distress caused by congenital diaphragmatic hernia and TEF may appear immediately or be delayed, depending on the severity of the defect.

Laryngeal web and choanal atresia

A laryngeal web, which is uncommon, results from the incomplete separation of the two sides of the larynx and is most often between the vocal cords. Choanal atresia (Fig. 27-13) is the most common congenital anomaly of the nose; it is a bony or membranous septum located between the nose and the pharynx. Inability to pass a suction catheter through the nose into the pharynx or cyanosis without

Atrial septal defect (ASD)

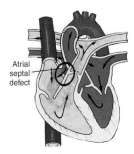

An ASD is an abnormal opening between the right and left atria. Basically, three types of abnormalities result from incorrect development of the atrial septum. An incompetent foramen ovale is the most common defect. The high ostium secundum defect results from abnormal development of the septum secundum. Improper development of the septum primum produces a basal opening known as an *ostium primum defect,* frequently involving the atrioventricular valves. In general, left-to-right shunting of the blood occurs in all atrial septal defects.

Ventricular septal defect (VSD)

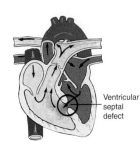

A VSD is an abnormal opening between the right and left ventricles. VSDs vary in size and may occur in either the membranous or muscular portion of the ventricular septum. Because of higher pressure in the left ventricle, a shunting of blood from the left to the right ventricle occurs during systole. If pulmonary vascular resistance produces pulmonary hypertension, the shunt of blood is then reversed from the right to the left ventricle, with cyanosis resulting.

Atrioventricular canal (AVC) defect

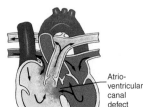

An AVC is an incomplete fusion of the endocardial cushions. It consists of a low atrial septal defect that is continuous, with a high ventricular septal defect and clefts of the mitral and tricuspid valves, creating a large central atrioventricular valve that allows blood to flow between all four chambers of the heart. Flow is generally from left to right. It is the most common cardiac defect in children with Down syndrome.

Patent ductus arteriosus (PDA)

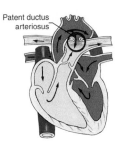

PDA is a vascular connection that, during fetal life, bypasses the pulmonary vascular bed and directs blood from the pulmonary artery to the aorta. Functional closure of the ductus normally occurs soon after birth. If the ductus remains patent after birth, the direction of blood flow in the ductus is reversed by the higher pressure in the aorta.

Coarctation of the aorta (COA)

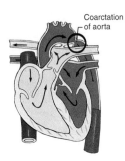

COA is characterized by localized narrowing of the aorta near the insertion of the ductus arteriosus, resulting in increased pressure proximal to the defect (head and upper extremities) and decreased pressure distal to the defect (body and lower extremities).

Aortic stenosis (AS)

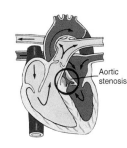

AS is a narrowing or stricture of the aortic valve, causing resistance to blood flow in the left ventricle, decreased cardiac output, left ventricular hypertrophy, and pulmonary vascular congestion. AS can be valvular, subvalvular, or supravalvular (rare). The most serious sequelae relate to the left ventricular hypertrophy (increased end-diastolic pressure, pulmonary hypertension, decreased coronary artery perfusion).

Pulmonic stenosis (PS)

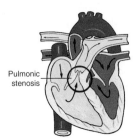

PS is a narrowing at the entrance to the pulmonary artery. Resistance to blood flow causes right ventricular hypertrophy and decreased pulmonary blood flow. Pulmonary atresia is the extreme form of PS; no blood flows to the lungs.

Tetralogy of Fallot (TOF)

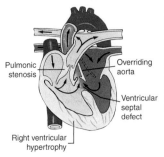

TOF is characterized by the combination of four defects: (1) pulmonary stenosis, (2) ventricular septal defect, (3) overriding aorta, and (4) hypertrophy of the right ventricle. It is the most common defect, causing cyanosis in children surviving beyond 2 years of age. The severity of symptoms depends on the degree of pulmonary stenosis, the size of the ventricular septal defect, and the degree to which the aorta overrides the septal defect.

Fig. 27-12 Congenital heart abnormalities. (Modified from Hockenberry, M. [2003]. *Wong's nursing care of infants and children* [7th ed.]. St. Louis: Mosby.)

Tricuspid atresia

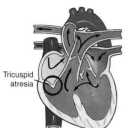

Tricuspid valvular atresia is characterized by a small right ventricle, a large left ventricle, and usually a diminished pulmonary circulation. Blood from the right atrium passes through an atrial septal defect into the left atrium, mixes with oxygenated blood returning from the lungs, flows into the left ventricle, and is propelled into the systemic circulation. The lungs may receive blood through one of three routes: (1) a small ventricular septal defect, (2) a patent ductus arteriosus, or (3) bronchial vessels.

Tricuspid atresia

Transposition of the great vessels (TGV)

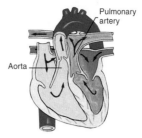

Pulmonary artery

Aorta

TGV is an embryologic defect caused by a straight division of the bulbar trunk without normal spiraling. As a result, the aorta originates from the right ventricle and the pulmonary artery from the left ventricle. An abnormal communication between the two circulations must be present to sustain life.

Total anomalous pulmonary venous connection (TAPVC)

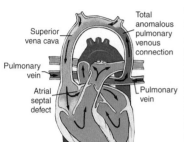

Total anomalous pulmonary venous connection

Superior vena cava

Pulmonary vein

Atrial septal defect

Pulmonary vein

TAPVC is a rare defect characterized by a failure of the pulmonary veins to join the left atrium. Instead, the pulmonary veins are abnormally connected to the systemic venous circuit via the right atrium or various veins draining toward the right atrium (e.g., superior vena cava). The abnormal attachment results in mixed blood being returned to the right atrium and shunted from the right to the left through an atrial septal defect.

Truncus arteriosus (TA)

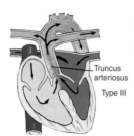

Truncus arteriosus

Type III

TA is a retention of the embryologic bulbar trunk. It results from the failure of normal septation and division of this trunk into an aorta and pulmonary artery. This single arterial trunk overrides the ventricles and receives blood from them through a ventricular septal defect. The entire pulmonary and systemic circulation is supplied from this common arterial trunk.

Hypoplastic left heart syndrome (HLHS)

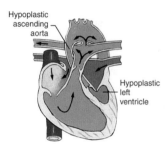

Hypoplastic ascending aorta

Hypoplastic left ventricle

HLHS is characterized by underdevelopment of the left side of the heart, resulting in a hypoplastic left ventricle and aortic atresia. Most blood from the left atrium flows across the patent foramen ovale to the right atrium, to the right ventricle, and out the pulmonary artery. The descending aorta receives blood from the patent ductus arteriosus supplying systemic blood flow.

Fig. 27-12   cont'd

obvious respiratory distress usually leads to its detection. Nearly half of the infants with choanal atresia have other anomalies. Infants with either a laryngeal web or choanal atresia require emergency surgery.

Congenital diaphragmatic hernia

Congenital diaphragmatic hernia (CDH) results from a defect in the formation of the diaphragm, allowing the abdominal organs to be displaced into the thoracic cavity. It occurs in approximately 1 in 5000 live births. However, if stillbirths resulting from this defect are included, the incidence increases to 1 in 2000 (Hartman, 2004). Herniation of the abdominal viscera into the thoracic cavity may cause severe respiratory distress and constitutes a neonatal emergency (Fig. 27-14). The defect and herniation may be minimal and easily repaired, or the defect may be so extensive that the viscera present in the thoracic cavity during embryonic life have prevented the normal development of pulmonary tissue. The defect is usually on the left because that is the side of the diaphragm that fuses last.

Most CDHs are discovered prenatally on ultrasound. Hernias may be repaired by fetal surgery in some research institutions. Intrauterine surgical correction of CDH has met with poor neonatal outcomes in many cases, primarily as a result of tocolysis failure and preterm birth. At birth, most affected infants have severe respiratory distress, and respiratory assessment reveals worsening distress as the bowel fills with air. Typically the breath sounds are diminished and bowel sounds are heard in the chest. Heart sounds may be heard on the right side of the chest because the heart has been displaced there by the abdominal contents. Physical examination reveals a flat or scaphoid abdomen and a prominent ipsilateral chest. Diagnosis can be made on the basis of the x-ray finding of loops of intestine in the thoracic cavity and the absence of intestine in the abdominal cavity.

Preoperative nursing interventions include participating in the stabilization of the infant's condition until surgical repair can be done. Inhaled nitric oxide (NO) has been used in many centers with moderate success to treat the accompanying persistent pulmonary hypertension (Bradshaw,

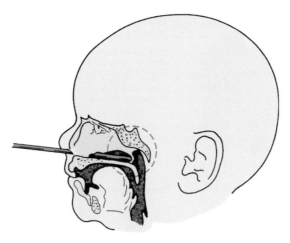

Fig. 27-13 Choanal atresia. Posterior nares are obstructed by membrane or bone, either bilaterally or unilaterally. Infant becomes cyanotic at rest. With crying, newborn's color improves. Nasal discharge is present. Snorting respirations often are observed with increased respiratory effort. Newborn may be unable to breathe and eat at the same time. Diagnosis is made by noting inability to pass small feeding tube through one or both nares. (Used with permission of Ross Products Division, Abbott Laboratories, Inc., Columbus, OH 43216. From Clinical Education Aid no. 6, Copyright © 1963, Ross Products Division, Abbott Laboratories, Inc.)

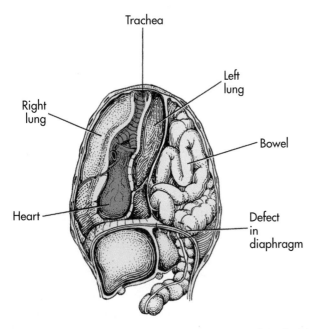

Fig. 27-14 Congenital diaphragmatic hernia. (Used with permission of Ross Products Division, Abbott Laboratories, Inc., Columbus, OH 43216. From Clinical Education Aid no. 6, Copyright © 1963, Ross Products Division, Abbott Laboratories, Inc.)

2004). Gastric contents are aspirated and suction applied to decompress the GI tract and prevent further cardiothoracic compromise. Oxygen therapy, mechanical ventilation, and the correction of acidosis are necessary in infants with early

clinical respiratory distress from CDH. Extracorporeal membrane oxygenation (ECMO) may be used in infants with severe circulatory and respiratory complications.

The prognosis depends largely on the degree of fetal pulmonary development, but the prognosis in severe cases is often poor. The overall survival rate for infants who are symptomatic within the first few hours of life is about 50%, although it has improved recently with the advent of inhaled NO, improved management of high-frequency ventilation, and ECMO.

Gastrointestinal System Anomalies

Anomalies in the GI system can occur anywhere along the GI tract, from the mouth to the anus. Some anomalies, such as cleft lip, omphalocele, and gastroschisis, are apparent at birth. Others, including cleft palate, esophageal atresia, intestinal obstruction, and imperforate anus become apparent as the infant is further assessed or becomes symptomatic.

Cleft lip and palate

Cleft lip or cleft palate is a commonly occurring congenital midline fissure, or opening, in the lip or palate resulting from failure of the primary palate to fuse (Fig. 27-15). One or both deformities may occur. Multiple genetic and, to a lesser extent, environmental factors (e.g., maternal infection, radiation exposure, alcohol ingestion, and treatment with medications such as corticosteroids, some tranquilizers, and antiepileptics) appear to be involved in their development.

Cleft lip with or without cleft palate occurs approximately 1 in 800 live births. The incidence of cleft palate alone is 1 in 2000 live births. Cleft lip with or without cleft palate is more common in males, and cleft palate alone is more common in females. The defect appears more often in Asians and certain tribes of Native Americans than in Caucasians, and less often in African-Americans.

Treatment of the infant with cleft lip is surgical; repair usually occurs between 6 and 12 weeks of age. Cleft palate repair is generally postponed until 12 to 18 months of age to take advantage of palatal changes that take place with normal growth.

Feeding is difficult because the cleft lip renders the newborn unable to maintain a seal around a nipple; the cleft palate renders the infant unable to form a vacuum to maintain suction when feeding. In addition, the inability to suck and swallow normally allows milk to pool in the nasopharynx, which increases the likelihood of aspiration. Furthermore, as the infant attempts to suck, milk often comes out through the cleft and out of the nares. Although the degree of difficulty depends on the size of the cleft, feeding problems are greater in infants with a cleft palate than in those with a cleft lip alone (Fig. 27-15, *D*). Breastfeeding can be successful in some infants. There are special nipples, bottles, and appliances available to aid in feeding (Fig. 27-16). In

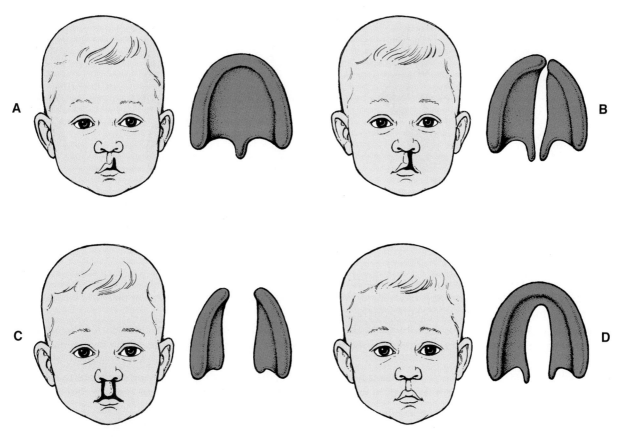

Fig. 27-15 Variations in clefts of lip and palate at birth. **A,** Notch in vermilion border. **B,** Unilateral cleft lip and cleft palate. **C,** Bilateral cleft lip and cleft palate. **D,** Cleft palate.

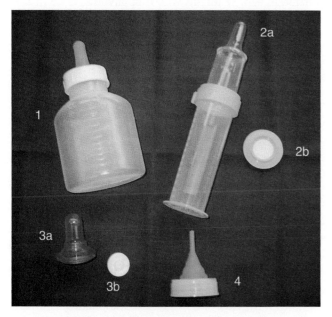

Fig. 27-16 *1,* Mead Johnson bottle and nipple for cleft palate. Cleft palate nipple system *(2a)* with valve *(2b)* to regulate flow. Haberman feeder *(3a)* with disc *(3b)* to control flow of milk. *4,* Ross cleft palate assembly. Nipple can be trimmed to accommodate palate size. (Courtesy Shannon Perry, Phoenix, AZ.)

general, parents of infants with these defects need a great deal of education and support as they learn to feed their baby, to prevent what should be a normal part of infant care from becoming a very frustrating experience.

Parents of infants with a cleft lip or palate need much support, particularly in the case of a cleft lip because this is both a cosmetic and functional defect. Recognizing that this may interfere with normal parent-infant bonding in the neonatal period, the nurse must assess for this and intervene appropriately.

Esophageal atresia and tracheoesophageal fistula

Esophageal atresia (EA) and tracheoesophageal fistula (TEF) often occur together, although they can also occur singly. EA is a congenital anomaly in which the esophagus ends in a blind pouch or narrows into a thin cord, thus failing to form a continuous passageway to the stomach (Fig. 27-17). TEF is an abnormal connection between the esophagus and trachea.

Maternal hydramnios is a common finding, particularly if the fetus has an EA without TEF. The infant with EA or TEF may also show some fetal growth restriction and will therefore be SGA; in addition, the presence of a midline defect such as EA or TEF is often accompanied by another significant embryonic defect such as a cardiac anomaly, cleft

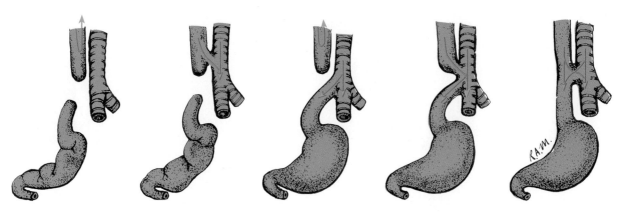

Fig. 27-17 Five most common types of esophageal atresia (EA) and tracheoesophageal fistula (TEF).

lip and/or palate, or vertebral, genitourinary, or abdominal wall defect (Bensard, Calkins, Partrick, & Price, 2002). Variations of the anomalies are possible, depending on the presence or absence of a TEF, the site of the fistula, and the location and degree of the esophageal obstruction (see Fig. 27-17).

Infants with EA and TEF may show significant respiratory difficulty immediately after birth. EA with or without TEF results in excessive oral secretions, drooling, and feeding intolerance. When fed, the infant may swallow, but then cough and gag and return the fluid through the nose and mouth. Respiratory distress can result from aspiration or from the acute gastric distention produced by the TEF. Choking, coughing, and cyanosis occur after even a small amount of fluid is taken by mouth.

Nursing interventions are supportive until surgery is performed. Any infant with excessive oral secretions and respiratory distress should not be fed orally until further evaluation is carried out. The infant is placed in the position least likely to cause aspiration of either mouth or stomach secretions. A double-lumen catheter is placed in the proximal esophageal pouch and attached to continuous suction to remove secretions and decrease the possibility of aspiration. Other supportive measures include maintaining thermoregulation, fluid and electrolyte balance intravenously, and acid-base balance and prevention of any further complications as a result of an associated defect. Surgical correction, done in one stage if possible, consists of ligating the fistula and anastomosing the two segments of the esophagus. The chances for survival in infants in a good risk category exceed 95%, depending on the presence of associated defects and the infant's birth weight. Many EA and TEF infants will have postoperative issues related to feeding difficulties such as gastroesophageal reflux (GER) and esophageal strictures requiring periodic dilation.

Omphalocele and gastroschisis

Omphalocele and gastroschisis are two of the more common congenital defects that occur in the abdominal wall. They are rare, however, with omphalocele occurring in approximately 1 in 3000 to 10,000 live births, whereas the incidence of gastroschisis is 1 in 6000 live births (Blackburn, 2003).

An **omphalocele** is a covered defect of the umbilical ring into which varying amounts of the abdominal organs may herniate (Fig. 27-18). Although it is covered with a peritoneal sac, the sac may rupture during or after birth. Many infants born with an omphalocele are preterm, and more than half have other serious syndromes or defects involving the GI, cardiac, genitourinary, musculoskeletal, and nervous systems.

Gastroschisis is the herniation of the bowel through a defect in the abdominal wall to the right of the umbilical cord. No membrane covers the contents, as occurs with an omphalocele. Unlike infants with omphalocele, these infants have less than a 10% to 15% likelihood of associated anomalies, most of which are cardiac.

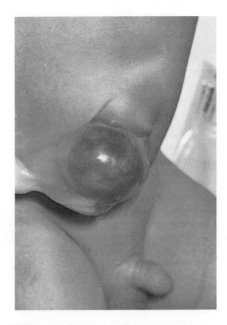

Fig. 27-18 Omphalocele. (From O'Doherty, N. [1986]. *Neonatology: Micro atlas of the newborn.* Nutley, NJ: Hoffmann-La Roche.)

The preoperative nursing care is similar for infants with either defect. Exposure of the viscera causes problems with thermoregulation and fluid and electrolyte balance. Until closure is performed, the exposed viscera are covered with a moistened saline gauze and plastic wrap. In some cases the infant may be placed in an impermeable, clear plastic bowel bag to decrease insensible water losses, maintain thermoregulation, and prevent contamination of the exposed viscera (Bensard et al., 2002). Antibiotics, fluid and electrolyte replacement, gastric decompression, and thermoregulation are needed for physiologic support. If complete closure is impossible because of the small size of the abdominal cavity and the large amount of viscera to be replaced, a Silastic silo pouch (Dow Corning, Midland, MI) is created and sewn to the fascia of the abdominal defect. The defect is closed surgically after the reduction of contents is complete, which usually takes 7 to 10 days. Gastric decompression is necessary preoperatively to prevent aspiration pneumonia and to allow as much bowel as possible to be placed into the abdomen during surgery. Surgery is usually performed soon after birth. With surgical treatment, nutritional support, and medical management, the prognosis has improved for infants born with an abdominal wall defect. It is estimated that more than 80% of infants born with omphalocele survive, as do more than 90% of those born with gastroschisis, although residual feeding difficulties such as GER are not uncommon.

Gastrointestinal obstruction

Congenital intestinal obstruction can occur anywhere in the GI tract and takes one of the following forms: atresia, which is a complete obliteration of the passage; partial obstruction, in which the symptoms may vary in severity and sometimes not be detected in the neonatal period; or malrotation of the intestine, which leads to twisting of the intestine (volvulus) and obstruction. Esophageal atresia, discussed previously, is a type of GI obstruction. Meconium ileus is an obstruction caused by impacted meconium and is the earliest symptom of cystic fibrosis, a life-threatening chronic illness. Infants with this type of obstruction should be tested for cystic fibrosis because 95% of infants with meconium ileus have cystic fibrosis.

In addition to polyhydramnios in the pregnant woman, the infant shows the following cardinal signs and symptoms: bilious vomiting, abdominal distention, and failure to pass normal amounts of meconium in the first 24 hours.

Nursing care is aimed at supporting the infant until surgical intervention can be carried out to eliminate the obstruction. Oral feedings are withheld, a nasogastric tube is placed for suction, and IV therapy is initiated to provide needed fluid and electrolytes. In infants with an intestinal obstruction, surgery consists of resecting the obstructed area of bowel and anastomosing the nonaffected bowel. In recent years the survival rate for these infants has risen to 90% to 95% as a result of better treatments, improved neonatal intensive care, and an increased understanding of the total problem.

Imperforate anus

Imperforate anus is a term used to describe a wide range of congenital disorders involving the anus and rectum and, in many cases, the genitourinary system (Fig. 27-19). These anomalies have an incidence of approximately 1 in 5000 live births (Bensard et al., 2002). Occurring more in male than in female infants, they result from the failure of anorectal development in weeks 7 and 8 of gestational life. Such infants have no anal opening, and commonly there is also a fistula from the rectum to the perineum or genitourinary system. Types of anorectal malformations include the typical cloaca in females, which involves the vagina, colon, and urethra forming a single common passage in the perineum. Others include the low rectovaginal fistula (female) and rectourethral bulbar fistula (male). Extensive surgical repair is often required in stages for the more complex types of anorectal malformations. In some cases the anomaly may involve stenotic areas, or there may be a thin translucent membrane covering the anal opening. Treatment for such a membrane is excision followed by daily dilation, which parents are taught to do.

Musculoskeletal System Anomalies
Developmental dysplasia of the hip

The broad term developmental dysplasia of the hip (DDH) describes a spectrum of disorders related to abnormal development of the hip that may develop at any time during fetal life, infancy, or childhood. A change in terminology from *congenital hip dysplasia* and *congenital dislocation of the hip* to developmental dysplasia of the hip more properly reflects a variety of hip abnormalities in which there is a shallow acetabulum, subluxation, or dislocation.

The incidence of hip instability of some kind is approximately 10 per 1000 live births. The incidence of frank dislocation or a dislocatable hip is 1 per 1000 live births (Wall,

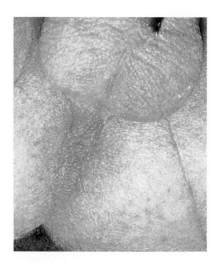

Fig. 27-19 Imperforate anus. (From Chessell, G. et al. [1984]. *Diagnostic picture tests in clinical medicine* [Vol. 2]. St. Louis: Mosby.)

2000), and approximately 30% to 50% of infants with DDH are born in breech presentation (Thompson, 2004).

The cause of DDH is unknown, but certain factors such as sex, birth order, family history, intrauterine position, birth type, joint laxity, and postnatal positioning are believed to affect the risk of DDH. Predisposing factors associated with DDH may be divided into three broad categories: (1) physiologic factors, which include maternal hormone secretion and intrauterine positioning; (2) mechanical factors, which involve breech presentation, multiple fetus, oligohydramnios, and large infant size; other mechanical factors may include continued maintenance of the hips in adduction and extension that will in time cause a dislocation; and (3) genetic factors, which entail a higher incidence (6%) of DDH in siblings of affected infants and an even greater incidence (36%) of recurrence if a sibling and one parent were affected.

Three degrees of DDH are illustrated in Fig. 27-20 and are described as follows:

Acetabular dysplasia (or preluxation)—mildest form of DDH, in which there is neither subluxation nor dislocation. There is a delay in acetabular development evidenced by osseous hypoplasia of the acetabular roof that is oblique and shallow, although the cartilaginous roof is comparatively intact. The femoral head remains in the acetabulum.

Subluxation—The largest percentage of DDH, subluxation; implies incomplete dislocation of the hip and is sometimes regarded as an intermediate stage in the development from primary dysplasia to complete dislocation. The femoral head remains in contact with the acetabulum, but a stretched capsule and ligamentum teres cause the head of the femur to be partially displaced. Pressure on the cartilaginous roof inhibits ossification and produces a flattening of the socket.

Dislocation—The femoral head loses contact with the acetabulum and is displaced posteriorly and superiorly over the fibrocartilaginous rim. The ligamentum teres is elongated and taut.

DDH is often not detected at the initial examination after birth; therefore all infants should be carefully monitored for hip dysplasia at follow-up visits throughout the first year of life. In the newborn period dysplasia usually appears as hip joint laxity rather than as outright dislocation. Subluxation and the tendency to dislocate can be demonstrated by the Ortolani or Barlow tests. The Ortolani and Barlow tests are most reliable from birth to 2 or 3 months of age. Other signs of DDH are shortening of the limb on the affected side (Galeazzi sign, Allis sign), asymmetric thigh and gluteal folds, and broadening of the perineum (in bilateral dislocation) (see also Fig. 18-12).

NURSE ALERT *The Ortolani and Barlow tests must be performed by an experienced clinician to prevent fracture or other damage to the hip. If these tests are performed too vigorously in the first 2 days of life, when the hip subluxates freely, persistent dislocation may occur.*

Treatment is begun as soon as the condition is recognized, because early intervention is more favorable to the restoration of normal bony architecture and function. The longer treatment is delayed, the more severe the deformity, the more difficult the treatment, and the less favorable the prognosis. The treatment varies with the age of the child and the extent of the dysplasia. The goal of treatment is to obtain and maintain a safe, congruent position of the hip joint to promote normal hip joint development and ambulation.

The hip joint is maintained by dynamic splinting in a safe position with the proximal femur centered in the acetabulum in an attitude of flexion. Of the numerous devices available, the Pavlik harness is the most widely used, and with time, motion, and gravity, the hip works into a more abducted, reduced position (Fig. 27-21). The harness is worn continuously until the hip is proved stable on clinical and radiographic examination, usually in about 3 to 5 months.

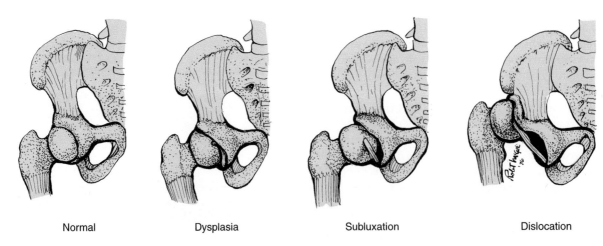

| Normal | Dysplasia | Subluxation | Dislocation |

Fig. 27-20 Configuration and relationship of structures in developmental dysplasia of the hip.

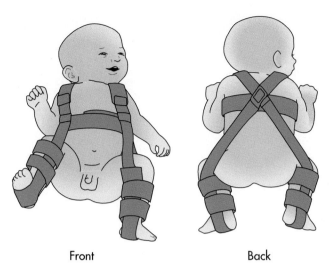

Fig. 27-21 Treatment for developmental hip dysplasia with Pavlik harness. (From Ball, J. [1998]. *Mosby's pediatric patient teaching guides.* St. Louis: Mosby.)

Front   Back

NURSE ALERT *The former practice of double- or triple-diapering for DDH is not recommended because it promotes hip extension, thus preventing proper hip development.*

Clubfoot

Congenital clubfoot is a complex deformity of the ankle and foot that includes forefoot adduction, midfoot supination, hindfoot varus, and ankle equinus. Deformities of the foot and ankle are described according to the position of the ankle and foot. The more common positions involve the following variations:

Talipes varus—An inversion or a bending inward

Talipes valgus—An eversion or bending outward

Talipes equines—Plantar flexion in which the toes are lower than the heel

Talipes calcaneus—Dorsiflexion, in which the toes are higher than the heel

Most cases of clubfoot are a combination of these positions, and the most frequently occurring type of clubfoot (approximately 95%) is the composite deformity talipes equinovarus, in which the foot is pointed downward and inward in varying degrees of severity. Unilateral clubfoot is somewhat more common than bilateral clubfoot and may occur as an isolated defect or in association with other disorders or syndromes, such as chromosomal aberrations, arthrogryposis (a generalized immobility of the joints), cerebral palsy, or spina bifida.

The goal of treatment for clubfoot is to achieve a painless, plantigrade (able to walk on the sole of the foot with the heel on the ground), and stable foot. Treatment of clubfoot involves three stages: (1) correction of the deformity, (2) maintenance of the correction until normal muscle balance is regained, and (3) follow-up observation to avert possible recurrence of the deformity. Some feet respond to

treatment readily; some respond only to prolonged, vigorous, and sustained efforts; and the improvement in others remains disappointing even with maximum effort on the part of all concerned.

Serial casting is begun shortly after birth, before discharge from the nursery. Successive casts allow for gradual stretching of skin and tight structures on the medial side of the foot. Manipulation and casting are repeated frequently (every week) to accommodate the rapid growth of early infancy. In some cases daily manipulation and stretching of tissues is accomplished with taping and splinting of the affected extremity; a continuous passive motion machine may be used several hours daily to stretch and strengthen muscle groups involved (Faulks & Luther, 2005). The extremity or extremities are often casted or splinted until maximum correction is achieved, usually within 8 to 12 weeks. A Denis Browne splint may be used to manage feet that correct with casting and manipulation.

Polydactyly

Occasionally hands or feet have extra digits. In some instances, polydactyly is hereditary. If there is little or no bone involvement, the extra digit is tied with silk suture soon after birth. The finger falls off within a few days, leaving a small scar. When there is bone involvement, surgical repair is indicated.

Genitourinary System Anomalies
Hypospadias and epispadias

Hypospadias constitutes a range of penile anomalies associated with an abnormally located urinary meatus. The meatus can open below the glans penis or anywhere along the ventral surface of the penis, the scrotum, or the perineum (Fig. 27-22). It is the most common anomaly of the penis, affecting approximately 1 in 125 live births (Stokowski, 2004). It is classified according to the location of the meatus and the presence or absence of chordee, which is a ventral curvature of the penis.

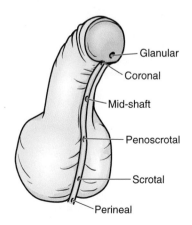

Glanular
Coronal
Mid-shaft
Penoscrotal
Scrotal
Perineal

Fig. 27-22 Classification of hypospadias by position of the urethral meatus.

Mild cases of hypospadias (Fig. 27-23) are often repaired for cosmetic reasons and involve a single surgical procedure. In more severe cases, several operations are required to reconstruct the urethral opening and correct the chordee, thereby straightening the penis. The goals are to improve the appearance of the genitalia and make it possible for the child to be able to urinate in a standing position and have a sexually adequate organ. These infants are not circumcised because the foreskin may be needed during surgical repair. Repair is done early, between 4 and 8 months of life (Stokowski, 2004).

Epispadias, a rare anomaly, results from failure of urethral canalization. About 55% of the affected infants are males who have a widened pubic symphysis and a broad spadelike penis with the urethra opened on its dorsal surface. In females there is a wide urethra and a bifid (split in two) clitoris. Severity ranges from mild anomaly to a severe one that is associated with exstrophy of the bladder. Surgical correction is necessary, and affected male infants should not be circumcised.

Exstrophy of the bladder

The most common bladder anomaly is exstrophy (Fig. 27-24), which often occurs in conjunction with epispadias. It is rare, occurring in only about 1 in 35,000 to 40,000 live births (Elder, 2004). It results from the abnormal development of the bladder, the abdominal wall, and the symphysis pubis that causes the bladder, urethra, and ureteral orifices to all be exposed. The bladder is visible in the suprapubic area as a red mass with numerous folds, with urine draining from it onto the infant's skin.

Immediately after birth the exposed bladder is covered with a sterile, nonadherent dressing to protect it until closure can be performed. It is recommended that reconstructive surgery be started in the neonatal period, preferably with the bladder being closed during the first or second day of life.

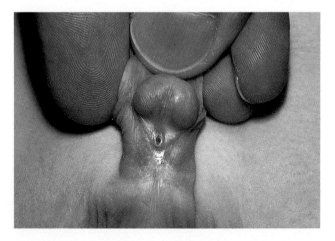

Fig. 27-23 Hypospadias. (Courtesy H. Gil Rushton, MD, Children's National Medical Center, Washington, DC.)

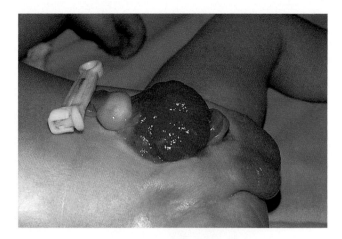

Fig. 27-24 Exstrophy of bladder. (Courtesy H. Gil Rushton, MD, Children's National Medical Center, Washington, DC.)

Ambiguous genitalia

Ambiguous genitalia in the newborn (Fig. 27-25) often is discovered by the nurse during a physical assessment. Erroneous or abnormal sexual differentiation may be a genetic defect, such as congenital adrenal hypoplasia, which can be life-threatening because it involves deficiency of all adrenocortical hormones. Other possible causes of sexual ambiguity include chromosomal abnormalities, defective sex hormone synthesis in males, and the placental transfer of masculinizing agents to female fetuses. Gender assignment should be based on data gathered from the following sources: maternal and family history, including the ingestion of steroids during pregnancy and relatives with ambiguous genitalia or who died during the neonatal period; physical examination; chromosomal analysis (results are available in 2 to 3 days); endoscopy, ultrasonography, and radiographic contrast studies; biochemical tests, such as analysis of urinary steroid excretion, which helps detect several of the adrenal cortical syndromes; and, in some instances, laparotomy or gonad biopsy.

Therapeutic intervention, including any counseling and surgery, should be started as soon as possible. Any child born with ambiguous genitalia should not receive sex assignment until the appropriate sex of rearing may be properly assessed and assigned. An appropriate sex assignment should be based on the following: age at presentation, potential for mature sexual function, potential fertility, and the long-term psychologic and intellectual impact on the child and family. Parents need much support as they learn to deal with this very challenging situation.

Teratoma

A teratoma is an embryonal tumor that may be solid, cystic, or mixed. It is composed of at least two and usually three types of embryonal tissue: ectoderm, mesoderm, and endoderm. A teratoma in the newborn may occur in the skull, mediastinum, abdomen, or sacral area; more than half are

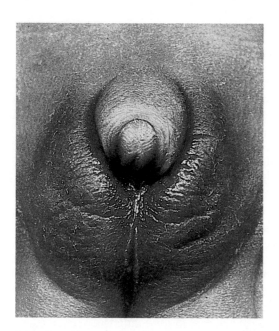

Fig. 27-25 Ambiguous external genitalia (i.e., structure may be enlarged clitoral hood and clitoris or micropenis and bifid scrotum). (Courtesy Edward S. Tank, MD, Division of Urology, Oregon Health Sciences University, Portland, OR.)

located in the sacrococcygeal area. The treatment of choice for such neonates is complete surgical resection. Approximately 80% of all teratomas are benign, and no additional therapy is needed after complete resection done in the neonatal period. If the tumor is not surgically resected before the infant is 1 to 2 months old, the likelihood of the teratoma becoming malignant increases rapidly.

COLLABORATIVE CARE

Any deviations from normal are reported to the primary health provider immediately. A thorough assessment of all body systems follows, with identification of both visible anomalies and those that might not be visible.

Some infants have multiple congenital anomalies. A recognized pattern of malformations is referred to as a *syndrome.* The most common is Down syndrome, with the diagnosis confirmed early in the neonatal period.

Genetic Diagnosis

Diagnostic procedures for the detection of genetic disorders are performed after birth at any time from the postnatal period through adulthood. Many tests are available for various disorders; only the most commonly used ones are discussed here.

Newborn Screening

The most widespread use of postnatal testing for genetic disease is the routine screening of newborns for inborn errors of metabolism (IEMs) such as phenylketonuria (PKU),

galactosemia, hemoglobinopathy (sickle cell disease and thalassemias) and hypothyroidism; these are the minimum mandatory newborn screening tests in most states in the United States. An *inborn error of metabolism* is the term applied to a large group of disorders caused by a metabolic defect that results from the absence of or change in a protein, usually an enzyme, and mediated by the action of a certain gene. These defects can involve any substrate produced from protein, carbohydrate, or fat metabolism. IEMs are recessive disorders, and a person must receive a defective gene from each parent for them to occur. The parents usually are unaffected because their normal dominant gene directs the synthesis of sufficient protein to meet their metabolic needs under normal circumstances. With the advent of new biochemical techniques, it is now possible to detect the abnormal gene responsible for causing an increasing number of these disorders early in the neonatal period so appropriate therapies to prevent further morbidity may be implemented.

A new screening test, tandem mass spectrometry, has the potential for identifying more than 20 IEMs, in addition to the standard ones. With tandem mass spectrometry, earlier identification of IEMs may prevent further developmental delays and morbidities in affected children.

PKU results from a deficiency of the enzyme phenylalanine dehydrogenase. The test for PKU is not reliable until the newborn has ingested an ample amount of the amino acid phenylalanine, a constituent of both human and cow's milk. The nurse must document the initial ingestion of milk and perform the test at least 24 hours after that time. Early infant discharge from the hospital has the potential to cause neonates with a disorder such as PKU not to be screened as often as in the past. In response to this, the AAP (1996) made the following recommendations:

- Collect the initial specimen as close as possible to discharge and no later than 7 days after birth.
- Designate a primary care provider for all newborns before discharge for adequate newborn screening follow-up.
- Obtain a subsequent sample before 2 weeks of age if the initial specimen is collected before the newborn is 24 hours old.

If the infant is found to have PKU, a diet low in phenylalanine is begun soon after birth. Breastfeeding or partial breastfeeding may be possible for some infants if the phenylalanine levels are monitored carefully and remain within acceptable limits. Many affected children have some intellectual impairment. Successful management and outcome is largely dependent on early identification of the condition, modifying the diet, and compliance with the treatment regimen throughout the entire life cycle.

Galactosemia, caused by a deficiency of the enzyme galactose-1-phosphate uridyltransferase, results in the inability to convert galactose to glucose. Galactosemia can be detected by measuring the blood levels of galactose in the urine of newborns suspected of having the disease who have ingested formula containing galactose. Early symptoms are vomiting, weight loss, and CNS symptoms, including poor feeding, drowsiness, and seizures. If the disorder goes untreated, the galactose levels will continue to increase and the affected infant will show failure to thrive, mental retardation, cataracts, jaundice, hepatomegaly, and cirrhosis of the liver, with death possibly occurring in the first month of life. Therapy consists of eliminating galactose from the diet; this condition precludes breastfeeding because lactose is present in breast milk.

Congenital hypothyroidism results from a deficiency of thyroid hormones; it affects approximately 1 of every 3500 to 4000 newborns (Rose, 2002). All states in the United States routinely screen for hypothyroidism. This involves measuring thyroxine (T_4) in a drop of blood obtained from a heel stick at 2 to 5 days of age. At this time the normally expected increase in T_4 would be lacking in newborns with hypothyroidism. It is more often included as part of the newborn screen done in the first 24 to 48 hours or before discharge. Neonatal screening consists of an initial filter paper blood spot T_4 measurement followed by measurement of thyroid-stimulating hormone (TSH) in specimens with low T_4 values. Early screening may have false-positive results. Treatment is thyroid replacement. In the newborn, thyroid function test results are elevated in comparison with values in older children; therefore it is important to document the timing of the tests. In preterm and sick full-term infants thyroid function test results are usually lower than in the healthy full-term infant; T_4 and TSH levels may be evaluated again after 30 weeks (corrected age) in newborns born before that time and after resolution of the acute illness in the sick full-term infant.

Cytogenetic Studies

Abnormalities can occur in either the autosomes or the sex chromosomes. Chromosomal disorders may sometimes be diagnosed on the basis of the clinical manifestations alone. However, an infant may have a clinical appearance that is only suggestive of a problem. Cytogenetic studies then need to be done to confirm or rule out a suspected diagnosis. Newer techniques in molecular cytogenetic analysis make possible a more precise identification of risk for having a fetus affected with a genetic defect such as PKU.

Disorders in the number or structure of chromosomes can be diagnosed by a karyotype (see Fig. 8-1, *B*), which is a photographic enlargement of the chromosomes arranged by their numbered pairs.

Dermatoglyphics

Dermatoglyphics is the study of the patterns formed by the ridges in the skin on the digits, palms, and soles. These patterns, formed early in development, are strongly correlated with the effects of chromosomes. Many disorders that affect multiple body systems also affect these dermal ridges. The addition or deletion of genetic material produces alterations in the loops, swirls, and arches of the finger and toe prints,

in the palm lines, and in the flexion creases on the palms of the hands and soles of the feet. Characteristic dermatoglyphic patterns have been noted for almost all the chromosomal abnormalities, such as Down syndrome.

An infant with Down syndrome may have a single, palmar crease; a single flexion crease of the fifth digit; and an increased distance between the first and second toes (Matthews & Robin, 2002). The characteristic dermatoglyphic feature in a child with Turner syndrome is the large size of the dermal patterns on the fingers and toes. Certain fingerprint patterns may also be found in those people who have cardiac valvular problems later in life. Asymmetry of palmar ridges has been reported in congenital anomalies such as cleft lip and palate and congenital vertebral anomaly.

Interventions

A collaborative health team approach that includes specialists and community service representatives is needed in the care of infants with some disorders. Surgical intervention in the neonatal period may be necessary for the infant requiring either immediate correction or a palliative procedure to relieve the symptoms of the anomaly until definitive correction can be done. There is a higher morbidity and mortality in neonates than in older children or adults undergoing similar procedures. However, despite these problems unique to neonates, advances in surgical techniques, anesthesia, and the nursing care given in intensive care nurseries have together been responsible for decreasing the risk of surgery in neonates.

The health care team must be highly skilled to meet the needs of these infants. These needs are similar to those of other high risk infants. In addition to stabilization of the infant's condition (oxygenation and perfusion of tissues), other preoperative interventions, such as nasogastric tube placement for abdominal decompression, pain management, and the maintenance of fluid and electrolyte balance, are implemented to manage specific problems.

Postoperative care of the newborn

Postoperatively, the infant is returned to the intensive care nursery, where close monitoring is maintained. The infant's respiratory efforts are supported; this often requires mechanical ventilation. Constant surveillance is necessary to detect any respiratory complications resulting from the anesthesia. A pulse oximeter is attached to measure the oxygen saturation in hemoglobin, which closely correlates with arterial oxygen saturation. Oxygen is provided as needed. An indwelling gastric catheter attached to intermittent suction is placed to remove gastric secretions, thereby preventing aspiration and distention of the abdomen. The infant's fluid, electrolyte, and acid-base balances are monitored and adjusted as needed. Urinary output is monitored and should equal 1 to 2 ml/kg/hr. Other nursing interventions are focused on caring for the surgical site, maintaining thermoregulation, managing pain, and promoting comfort.

Needs of parents and family

While the infant is receiving optimal care, the parents also have needs that must be met as they deal with the crisis of having an infant with an abnormal condition. Their reactions are carefully assessed and are likely to be those typical of a grief response. Facilitating their understanding of the information given them about their infant's condition is a vital nursing intervention. A newly diagnosed disorder often implies the need for the implementation of a therapeutic regimen. For example, the disorder may be an inborn error of metabolism, such as PKU, which requires consistent and rigid adherence to a diet. The family may need help with securing the required formula and in receiving counseling from a clinical dietitian. The importance of maintaining the diet, keeping an adequate supply of special preparations, and avoiding the use of unauthorized substitutions must be impressed on the family.

Referral to appropriate agencies is another essential component of the follow-up management, and the nurse should make the parents aware of all possible sources of aid, including pertinent literature, parent groups, and national organizations. Many organizations and foundations, such as the March of Dimes, provide services and counseling for families of affected children. There are also numerous parent groups the family can join. There they can share experiences and derive mutual support in coping with problems similar to those of other group members. Nurses must be familiar with the services available in their communities that provide assistance and education to families with these special problems.

A major nursing function is providing emotional support to the family during all aspects of the care of the child born with a defect or disorder. The feelings stemming from the real or imagined threat posed by a congenital anomaly are as varied as the people being counseled. Responses may include apathy, denial, anger, hostility, fear, embarrassment, grief, and loss of self-esteem.

Parents benefit from seeing before-and-after pictures of other babies born with the same defect. Coupled with other verbal and nonverbal supportive care, this visual reassurance may be effective in allaying their concerns.

Families need much information, guidance, and support as they make decisions regarding the care of their infant. Once they have been given the facts and possible consequences and all the assistance they need in problem solving, the final decision regarding a course of action must be their own. It is then incumbent on health care providers to support the decision of the family.

Nurses frequently encounter children with genetic diseases and families in which there is a risk that a disorder may be transmitted to or occur in an offspring. It is a responsibility of nurses to be alert to situations in which persons could benefit from a genetic evaluation and counseling to be aware of the local genetic resources, to aid the family in finding services, and to offer support and care for children and families affected by genetic conditions. Local genetic clinics can be located through several sites, such as Gene Tests (www.genetests.org), a publicly funded medical genetics information resource developed for physicians and other health care providers, which is available at no cost to all interested persons. Another resource is the National Society of Genetic Counselors (www.nsgc.org), which lists genetic counselors by states in the United States. See also Chapter 7.

COMMUNITY ACTIVITY

Using the local telephone directory, identify sources of referral in your community for infants with congenital anomalies or who have been exposed to drugs such as cocaine or heroin. How many sources were you able to find? How difficult was it for you to locate these sources? Select one of the agencies and call to inquire (after identifying yourself as a nursing student) about (a) their source of funding, (b) whether those without insurance can access their services, (c) who can make referrals, (d) the number of children seen each year, and (e) the major problems seen. What have you learned from this exercise? Are there enough services available in your community to assist parents who need these services?

Key Points

- The identification of maternal and fetal risk factors in the antepartum and intrapartum periods is vital for planning adequate care of high risk infants.

- A small percentage of significant birth injuries may occur despite skilled and competent obstetric care.

- Infection in the newborn may be acquired in utero, at birth, in breast milk, and from within the nursery.

- The most common maternal infections during early pregnancy that are associated with various congenital malformations are represented by the acronym TORCH.

- HIV transmission from mother to infant occurs transplacentally at various gestational ages, perinatally through maternal blood and secretions, and through breast milk.

- Preterm infants are at risk for problems related to the immaturity of organ systems.

- Hyperbilirubinemia has a variety of etiologic factors, including maternal-fetal Rh and ABO incompatibility.

- The injection of $Rh_o(D)$ immune globulin in Rh-negative and Coombs' test–negative women minimizes the possibility of isoimmunization.

Key Points—cont'd

- The nurse often first observes signs of newborn drug withdrawal (neonatal abstinence syndrome) and acquires information from the maternal history.
- Major congenital defects are now the leading cause of death in infants under one year of age.
- The curative and rehabilitative problems of a child with a congenital disorder are often complex, requiring a multidisciplinary approach to care.

- Parents often need special instruction (e.g., cardiopulmonary resuscitation, oxygen therapy, or meeting nutrition requirements) before they take a high risk infant home.
- The supportive care given to the parents of infants with an abnormal condition must begin at birth or at the time of diagnosis and continue for years.

Answer Guidelines to Critical Thinking Exercise

Birth of a Child with a Congenital Anomaly

1 Yes, evidence is sufficient to draw conclusions about what you should tell Marjorie about the treatment and prognosis for Monica. The defect is not visible; symptoms are minimal. Breastfeeding is possible if Marjorie desires.

2 a. While a VSD is not visible, it can be serious. At times, parents may think a defect is not serious if they cannot see it. In Monica's case the pediatrician thinks that the small defect will close spontaneously.

b. When the infant is quiet and has good color, Marjorie may find it hard to believe that anything is wrong; she may use denial to cope with the situation. The nurse can assist Marjorie to accept the reality of the defect.

c. Many small defects close spontaneously during the first year of life. Most children with small defects remain asymptomatic and require no treatment.

d. Infective endocarditis is a long term risk. Some adults with small VSDs have an increased incidence of subaortic stenosis, arrhythmias, and exercise intolerance.

3 The priority for nursing care at this time is to explain the VSD and possible sequelae. Marjorie will need assurance that follow-up will occur. She should be educated about the symptoms of adverse events including congestive heart failure and endocarditis. It is important to include the father of the baby and her family in the teaching. Reassurance and support is essential. Referral to a social worker may be useful if Marjorie does not have the resources to pay for the follow-up care.

4 Treatment of the child with a small VSD is symptomatic and supportive.

5 Although unlikely, parents may reject children with defects or be overprotective and not permit them to participate in activities of children without similar defects even when there is no reason to limit such activities.

Resources

Advances in Neonatal Care
Elsevier
360 Park Ave., South
New York, NY 10010

AIDS Network Hotline
800-342-2437

American Academy of Pediatrics (AAP)
141 Northwest Point Blvd.
Elk Grove, IL 60007-1098
847-228-5005
www.aap.org

American Cleft Palate Association
1218 Grandview Ave.
Pittsburgh, PA 15211
412-681-1376
800-242-5338 (800-24-CLEFT)
www.cleftline.org

American Society of Plastic Surgeons
Plastic Surgery Educational Foundation
Plastic Surgery Information Service: FAQs
www.plasticsurgery.org/faq/cleft.htm

Centers for Disease Control and Prevention (CDC)
1600 Clifton Rd., NE
Atlanta, GA 30333
404-329-1819
404-329-3286
www.cdc.gov

Gene Tests (funded by the NIH)
9725 Third Ave., NE
Suite 602
Seattle, WA 98115
206-616-4033
206-221-4679 (fax)
genetests@genetests.org
www.genetests.org

HEST (Helga's European Specialty Toys) (Down syndrome dolls used to teach children about disabilities and for children with Down syndrome)
www.downsyndromedolls.com

Journal of Genetic Counseling
Kluwer Academic Publishers
P.O. Box 322
3300 AH Dordrecht
The Netherlands
+31 (0) 78 657 60 50
+31 (0) 78 657 64 74 (fax)
frontoffice@wkap.nl
www.wkap.nl

Journal of Perinatal and Neonatal Nursing
Lippincott Williams & Wilkins
530 Walnut St.
Philadelphia, PA 19106-3621
215-521-8300
215-521-8902 (fax)
www.lww.com

March of Dimes Birth Defects Foundation
National Foundation/March of Dimes
1275 Mamaroneck Ave.
White Plains, NY 10605
914-663-4637 (800-MODIMES)
www.modimes.org

National AIDS Information Clearinghouse
P.O. Box 6003
Rockville, MD 20849-6003
800-458-5231 (English and Spanish)

National Association of Neonatal Nurses
4700 W. Lake Ave.
Glenview, IL 60025-145
800-451-3795
888-477-6266 (fax)
www.nann.org
info@nann.org

National Clearinghouse for Alcohol and Drug Abuse Information
P.O. Box 426
Dept. DQ
Kensington, MD 20795
800-729-6686
www.health.org

National Down Syndrome Congress
1800 Dempster St.
Park Ridge, IL 60069-1146
708-823-7550
800-232-6372
www.ndsccenter.org

National Down Syndrome Society Hotline
666 Broadway
New York, NY 10012
800-221-4602
www.ndss.org

National Society of Genetic Counselors
233 Canterbury Dr.
Wallingford, PA 19086-6617
610-872-7608
FYI@nsgc.org
www.nsgc.org

Neonatal Network
2270 Northpoint Pkwy.
Santa Rosa, CA 95407-7398
707-569-1415
707-569-0786 (fax)
www.neonatalnetwork.com

Spina Bifida Association of America
4590 McArthur Blvd., NW, Suite 250
Washington, DC 20007-4226
800-621-3141
www.sbaa.org

References

American Academy of Pediatrics (AAP) Committee on Drugs. (2001). The transfer of drugs and other chemicals into human milk. *Pediatrics, 108*(3), 776-789.

American Academy of Pediatrics (AAP) Committee on Genetics. (1996). Newborn screening fact sheets. *Pediatrics, 98*(3), 473-481.

American Academy of Pediatrics (AAP) Committee on Infectious Diseases. (2003). *Red book: 2003 report of the committee on infectious diseases* (26th ed.). Elk Grove Village, IL: AAP.

American Academy of Pediatrics (AAP) Subcommittee on hyperbilirubinemia. (2004). Clinical Practice Guideline: Management of hyperbilirubinemia in the newborn infant 35 or more weeks of gestation. *Pediatrics, 114*(1), 297-316.

American Academy of Pediatrics (AAP) & American College of Obstetricians and Gynecologists (ACOG). (2002). *Guidelines for perinatal care* (5th ed.). Elk Grove Village, IL: AAP.

Andres, R. (2004). Effects of therapeutic, diagnostic, and environmental agents and exposure to social and illicit drugs. In R. Creasy, R. Resnik, & J. Iams (Eds.), *Maternal-fetal medicine: Principles and practice* (5th ed.). Philadelphia: Saunders.

Aranda, J., Edwards, D., Hales, B., & Rieder, M. (2002). Developmental pharmacology. In A. Fanaroff & R. Martin (Eds.), *Neonatal-perinatal medicine: Diseases of the fetus and infant* (7th ed.). St. Louis: Mosby.

Arendt, R. et al. (2004). Children prenatally exposed to cocaine: Developmental outcomes and environmental risks at seven years of age. *Journal of Developmental and Behavioral Pediatrics, 25*(2), 83-90.

Askin, D. (1995). Bacterial and fungal sepsis in the neonate. *Journal of Obstetric, Gynecologic, and Neonatal Nursing, 24*(7), 635-643.

Askin, D., & Diehl-Jones, W. (2001). Cocaine: Effects of in utero exposure on the fetus and newborn. *Journal of Perinatal and Neonatal Nursing, 14*(4), 83-102.

Association of Women's Health, Obstetric and Neonatal Nursing (AWHONN). (2001). *Evidence-based clinical practice guideline: Neonatal skin care*. Washington, DC: AWHONN.

Baley, J., & Toltzis, P. (2002). Viral infections. In A. Fanaroff & R. Martin (Eds.), *Neonatal-perinatal medicine: Diseases of the fetus and infant* (7th ed.). St. Louis: Mosby.

Ball, J. (1998). *Mosby's pediatric patient teaching guides*. St. Louis: Mosby.

Bateman, D., & Chiriboga, C. (2000). Dose-response effect of cocaine on newborn head circumference. *Pediatrics, 106*(3), e33.

Behrmann, R. (1973). *Neonatology: Diseases of the fetus and infant*. St. Louis: Mosby.

Bell, S. (2004). Pointers in practical pharmacology: Highly active antiretroviral therapy in neonates and young infants. *Neonatal Network, 23*(2), 55-64.

Bensard, D., Calkins, C., Partrick. D., & Price, F. (2002). Neonatal surgery. In G. Merenstein & S. Gardner (Eds.), *Handbook of neonatal intensive care* (5th ed.). St. Louis Mosby.

Berghella, V., Lim, P., Hill, M., Cherpes, J., Chennat, J., & Kaltenback, K. (2003). Maternal methadone dose and neonatal withdrawal. *American Journal of Obstetrics and Gynecology, 189*(2), 312-317.

Bernstein, D. (2004). Congenital heart disease. In R. Behrman, R. Kliegman, & H. Jenson (Eds.), *Nelson textbook of pediatrics* (17th ed.). Philadelphia: Saunders.

Blackburn, S. (2003). *Maternal, fetal, and neonatal physiology: A clinical perspective* (2nd ed.). St. Louis: Saunders.

Boyer, S., & Boyer, K. (2004). Update on TORCH infections in the newborn infant. *Newborn and Infant Nursing Reviews, 4*(1), 70-80.

Bradshaw, W. (2004). The use of nitric oxide in neonatal care. *Critical Care Nursing Clinics of North America, 16*(2), 249-255.

Buus-Frank, M. (2004). Hands that heal—hands that harm. *Advances in Neonatal Care, 4*(5), 251-255.

Carey, B. (2002). Incidence and epidemiology of congenital cardiovascular malformation in the newborn infant. *Newborn and Infant Nursing Reviews, 2*(2), 54-59.

Centers for Disease Control and Prevention (CDC). (2002). Prevention of perinatal group B streptococcal disease. *Morbidity and Mortality Weekly Report, 51*(RR-11), 1-231.

Centers for Disease Control and Prevention (CDC). (2004). *Fetal alcohol syndrome, fetal alcohol information.* Internet document available at www.cdc.gov/ncbd/fas/fasak.htm (accessed June 15, 2004).

Chessell, G. et al. (1984). *Diagnostic picture tests in clinical medicine* (Vol. 2). St. Louis: Mosby.

Christian, M., & Brent, R. (2001). Teratogen update: Evaluation of the reproductive and developmental risks of caffeine. *Teratology, 64*(1), 51-78.

Conde-Aqudelo, A., Diaz-Rosello, J., & Belizan, J. (2003). Kangaroo mother care to reduce morbidity and mortality in low birth weight infants (Cochrane Review). In *The Cochrane Library*, Issue 2, 2004. Chichester, UK: John Wiley & Sons.

Cooper, E. et al. (2002). Combination antiretroviral strategies for the treatment of pregnant of HIV-1 infected women and prevention of perinatal HIV-1 transmission. *Journal of Acquired Immune Deficiency Syndrome, 29*(5), 484-494.

Cowles, T., & Gonik, B. (2002). Perinatal infections. In A. Fanaroff & R. Martin (Eds.), *Neonatal-perinatal medicine: Diseases of the fetus and infant* (7th ed.). St. Louis: Mosby.

Coyle, M., Ferguson, A., Lagasse, L., Oh, W., & Lester, B. (2002). Diluted tincture of opium (DTO) and phenobarbital versus DTO alone for neonatal opiate withdrawal in term infants. *Journal of Pediatrics, 140*(5), 561-564.

D'Apolito, K., & Hepworth, J. (2001). Prominence of withdrawal symptoms in polydrug-exposed infants. *Journal of Perinatal and Neonatal Nursing, 14*(4), 46-60.

Duff, P. (1998). Hepatitis in pregnancy. *Seminars in perinatology, 22*(4), 277-283.

Dunbar, C. (2005). One drink can last a lifetime. *NurseWeek,* May 9, 30-32.

Dunham, E. (2003). Obstetrical brachial plexus palsy. *Orthopedic Nursing, 22*(2), 106-116.

Ebrahim, S., & Gfroerer, J. (2003). Pregnancy-related substance use in the United States during 1996-1998. *Obstetrics and Gynecology, 101*(2), 374-379.

Edwards, R., Jamie, W., Sterner, D., Gentry, S., Counts, K., & Duff, P. (2003). Intrapartum antibiotic prophylaxis and early-onset neonatal sepsis patterns. *Infectious Diseases in Obstetrics and Gynecology, 11*(4), 221-224.

Elder, J. (2004). Urologic disorders in infants and children: Anomalies of the bladder. In R. Behrman, R. Kliegman, & H. Jenson (Eds.), *Nelson textbook of pediatrics* (17th ed.). Philadelphia: Saunders.

Faulks, S., & Luther, B. (2005). Changing paradigm for the treatment of clubfeet. *Orthopedic Nursing, 24*(1), 25-30.

Frenkel, L. (2005). Challenges in the diagnosis and management of neonatal herpes simplex virus encephalitis. *Pediatrics, 115*(3), 795-797.

Gewolb, I., Fishman, D., Qureshi, M., & Vice, F. (2004). Coordination of suck-swallow-respiration in infants born to mothers with drug-abuse problems. *Developmental Medicine and Child Neurology, 46*(10), 700-705.

Gibbs, R., Sweet, R., & Duff, W. (2004). Maternal and fetal infectious disorders. In R. Creasy, R. Resnik, & J. Iams (Eds.), *Maternal-fetal medicine: Principles and practice* (5th ed.). Philadelphia: Saunders.

Hale, T. (2002). *Medications and mothers' milk.* Amarillo, TX: Pharmasoft Medical Publishing.

Hartman, G. (2004). Diaphragmatic hernia. In R. Behrman, R. Kliegman, & H. Jenson (Eds.), *Nelson textbook of pediatrics* (17th ed.). Philadelphia: Saunders.

Hockenberry, M. (2003). *Wong's nursing care of infants and children* (7th ed.). St. Louis: Mosby.

Honein, M. (2001). Impact of folic acid fortification of the U.S. food supply and occurrence of neural tube defects. *Journal of the American Medical Association, 285*(23), 2981-2986.

Hudgins, L., & Cassidy, S. (2002). Congenital anomalies. In A. Fanaroff & R. Martin (Eds.), *Neonatal-perinatal medicine: Diseases of the fetus and infant* (7th ed.). St. Louis: Mosby.

Huestis, M., & Choo, R. (2002). Drug abuse's smallest victims: In utero drug exposure. *Forensic Science International, 128*(1-2), 20-30.

Hurd, Y., Wang, X., Anderson, V., Beck, O., Minkoff, H., & Dow-Edwards, D. (2005). Marijuana impairs growth in mid-gestation fetuses. *Neurotoxicology and Teratology, 27*(2), 221-229.

Jansson, L., Velez, M., & Harrow, C. (2004). Methadone maintenance and lactation: A review of the literature and current management guidelines. *Journal of Human Lactation, 20*(1), 62-71.

Johnson, K., Gerada, C., & Greenough, A. (2003). Treatment of neonatal abstinence syndrome. *Archives of Disease in Childhood. Fetal and Neonatal Edition, 88*(1), F2-F5.

Jones, M., & Bass, W. (2003). Fetal alcohol syndrome. *Neonatal Network, 22*(3), 63-70.

Kriebs, J. (2002). The global reach of HIV: Preventing mother-to-child transmission. *Journal of Perinatal and Neonatal Nursing, 16*(3), 1-10.

Law, K., Stroud, L., LaGasse, L., Niaura, R., Liu, J., & Lester, B. (2003). Smoking during pregnancy and newborn neurobehavior. *Pediatrics, 111*(6), 1318-1323.

Lawrence, R., & Lawrence, R. (2005). *Breastfeeding: A guide for the medical profession* (6th ed). St. Louis: Mosby.

Lewis, M., Misra, S., Johnson, H., & Rosen, T. (2004). Neurological and developmental outcomes of prenatally cocaine-exposed offspring from 12 to 36 months. *American Journal of Drug and Alcohol Abuse, 30*(2), 299-320.

Mangurten, H. (2002). Birth injuries. In A. Fanaroff & R. Martin (Eds.), *Neonatal-perinatal medicine: Diseases of the fetus and infant* (7th ed.). St. Louis: Mosby.

Markiewicz, M., & Abrahamson, E. (1999). *Diagnosis in color: Neonatology.* St. Louis: Mosby.

Matthews, A., & Robin, N. (2002). Genetic disorders, malformations, and inborn errors of metabolism. In G. Merenstein & S. Gardner (Eds.), *Handbook of neonatal intensive care* (5th ed.). St. Louis: Mosby.

Merenstein, G., Adams, K., & Weisman, L. (2002). Infection in the neonate. In G. Merenstein & S. Gardner (Eds.), *Handbook of neonatal intensive care* (5th ed.). St. Louis: Mosby.

Messinger, D. et al. (2004). The maternal lifestyle study: Cognitive, motor, and behavioral outcomes of cocaine-exposed and opiate-exposed infants through three years of age. *Pediatrics, 113*(6), 1677-1685.

Miller-Loncar, C. et al. (2005). Predictors of motor development in children prenatally exposed to cocaine. *Neurotoxicology and Teratology, 27*(2), 213-220.

Modlin, J., Grant, P., Makar, R., Roberts, D., & Krishnamoorthy, K. (2003). Case records of the Massachusetts General Hospital. Weekly clinicopathological exercises. Case 25-2003. A newborn boy with petechiae and thrombocytopenia. *New England Journal of Medicine, 349*(16), 1575-1576.

Moise, K. (2002). Management of rhesus alloimmunization in pregnancy. *Obstetrics and Gynecology, 100*(3), 600-611.

Moolenaar, R. et al. (2000). A prolonged outbreak of *Pseudomonas aeruginosa* in a neonatal intensive care unit: Did staff fingernails play a role in disease transmission? *Infection Control and Hospital Epidemiology, 21*(2), 80-85.

Myers, M., Stanberry, L., & Seward, J. (2004). Varicella-zoster virus. In R. Behrman, R. Kliegman, & H. Jenson (Eds.), *Nelson textbook of pediatrics* (17th ed.). Philadelphia: Saunders.

Neal, J. (2001). RhD isoimmunization and current management modalities. *Journal of Obstetric, Gynecologic, and Neonatal Nursing, 30*(6), 589-607.

Nelson, N. (1990). *Current therapy in neonatal-perinatal medicine* (2nd ed.). St. Louis: Mosby.)

O'Doherty, N. (1986). *Neonatology: Micro atlas of the newborn.* Nutley, NJ: Hoffmann-La Roche.

Ostrea, E. (2001). Understanding drug testing in the neonate and the role of meconium analysis, *Journal of Perinatal and Neonatal Nursing, 14*(4), 61-82.

Paige, P., & Carney, P. (2002). Neurologic disorders. In G. Merenstein & S. Gardner (Eds.), *Handbook of neonatal intensive care* (5th ed.). St. Louis: Mosby.

Philipp, B., Merewood, A., & O'Brien, S. (2003). Commentary: Methadone and breastfeeding: New horizons. *Pediatrics, 111*(6 Pt 1), 1429-1430.

Plessinger, M. (1998). Prenatal exposure to amphetamines. *Obstetrics and Gynecology Clinics of North America, 25*(1), 119-138.

Polak, J., Ringler, N., & Daugherty, B. (2004). Unit based procedures: Impact on the incidence of nosocomial infections in the newborn intensive care unit. *Newborn and Infant Nursing Reviews, 4*(1), 38-45.

Popovich, D., & McAlhany, A. (2004). Practitioner care and screening guidelines for infants born to *Chlamydia*-positive mothers. *Newborn and Infant Nursing Reviews, 4*(1), 51-55.

Rao, R., & Desai, N. (2002). OxyContin and neonatal abstinence syndrome. *Journal of Perinatology, 22*(4), 324-325.

Reiser, D. (2004). Neonatal jaundice: Physiologic variation or pathologic process. *Critical Care Nursing Clinics of North America, 16*(2), 257-269.

Rollnik, J. et al. (2000). Botulinum toxin treatment of cocontractions after birth-related brachial plexus lesions. *Neurology, 55*(1), 112-114.

Rose, S. (2002). Thyroid disorders. In A. Fanaroff & R. Martin (Eds.), *Neonatal-perinatal medicine: Diseases of the fetus and infant* (7th ed.). St. Louis: Mosby.

Rosen, T., & Bateman, D. (2002). Infants of addicted mothers. In A. Fanaroff & R. Martin (Eds.), *Neonatal-perinatal medicine: Diseases of the fetus and infant* (7th ed.). St. Louis: Mosby.

Singer, L. et al. (2002). Cognitive and motor outcomes of cocaine-exposed infants. *Journal of the American Medical Association, 287*(15), 1952-1960.

Singer, L. et al. (2004). Cognitive outcomes of preschool children with prenatal cocaine exposure. *Journal of the American Medical Association, 291*(20), 2448-2456.

Smith, L. et al. (2003). Effects of prenatal methamphetamine exposure on fetal growth and drug withdrawal symptoms in infants born at term. *Journal of Developmental and Behavioral Pediatrics, 24*(1), 17-23.

Stoll, B. et al. (2002). Changes in pathogens causing early-onset sepsis in very-low-birth-weight infants. *New England Journal of Medicine, 347*(4), 240-247.

Stokowski, L. (2004). Hypospadias in the neonate. *Advances in Neonatal Care, 4*(4), 206-215.

Strodtbeck, F. (2003). The role of early enteral nutrition in protecting premature infants from sepsis. *Critical Care Nursing Clinics of North America, 15*(1), 79-87.

Tappero, E. (2003). Musculoskeletal system assessment. In E. Tappero & M. Honeyfield (Eds.), *Physical assessment of the newborn* (3rd ed.). Santa Rosa, CA: NICU Ink.

Thompson, G. (2004). The hip. In R. Behrman, R. Kliegman, & H. Jenson (Eds.), *Nelson textbook of pediatrics* (17th ed.). Philadelphia: Saunders.

Volpe, J. (2001). *Neurology of the newborn* (4th ed.). Philadelphia: Saunders.

Wall, E. (2000). Practical primary pediatric orthopaedics. *Nursing Clinics of North America, 35*(1), 95-113.

Weinberg, G. (2000). The dilemma of postnatal mother-to-child transmission of HIV: To breastfeed or not? *Birth, 27*(3), 199-205.

Weiner, L., & Morse, B. (1991). FAS: Clinical perspectives and prevention. In I. Chasnoff (Ed.), *Drugs, alcohol, pregnancy and parenting.* Boston: Kluwer.

World Health Organization. (2005). *Antiretroviral drugs and the prevention of mother-to-child transmission of HIV infection in resource-limited settings. Recommendations for a public health approach (2005 revision).* Internet document available at www.who.int/3by5/PMTCTreport_June2005.pdf (accessed September 18, 2005).

World Health Organization (2004). *Antiretroviral drugs for treating pregnant women and preventing HIV infection in infants. Guidelines on care, treatment and support for women living with HIV/AIDS and their children in resource-constrained settings.* Internet document available at www.who.int/hiv/pub/mtct/en/arvdrugsguidelines.pdf (accessed September 18, 2005).

Zenk, K. (2000). *Neonatal medications and nutrition.* Petaluma, CA: NICU Ink.

Zitelli, B., & Davis, H. (2002). *Atlas of pediatric physical diagnosis* (4th ed.). St. Louis: Mosby.

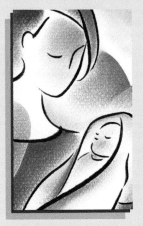

CHAPTER 28

Perinatal Loss and Grief

SHANNON E. PERRY

LEARNING OBJECTIVES

- Describe emotional, behavioral, cognitive, and physical responses commonly experienced during the grieving process associated with perinatal loss.
- Understand the personal and societal issues that may complicate responses to perinatal loss.
- Formulate appropriate nursing diagnoses for parents and their families experiencing perinatal loss.

- Identify specific nursing interventions to meet the special needs of parents and their families related to perinatal loss and grief.
- Differentiate among helpful and nonhelpful responses in caring for parents experiencing loss and grief.

KEY TERMS AND DEFINITIONS

bereavement The feelings of loss, pain, desolation, and sadness that occur after the death of a loved one

bittersweet grief The resurgence of feelings and emotions that occur on remembering a loved one after the bereavement process has lessened

complicated bereavement The persistent feelings of anger, guilt, loss, pain, and sadness over time

that lead to feelings of hopelessness, helplessness, and diminishing self-worth

grief Physical, emotional, social, and cognitive response to death of a loved one

perinatal loss Death of a fetus or infant through the twenty-eighth day after birth

ELECTRONIC RESOURCES

Additional information related to the content in Chapter 28 can be found on

the companion website at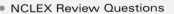
http://evolve.elsevier.com/Lowdermilk/Maternity/
- NCLEX Review Questions
- WebLinks

or on the interactive companion CD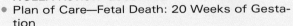
- NCLEX Review Questions
- Plan of Care—Fetal Death: 20 Weeks of Gestation

Becoming a parent is an important developmental milestone that is anticipated by most men and women in our society. However, loss can be associated with pregnancy and birth. During pregnancy, parents plan for the birth, imagine what the birth will be like, and develop an image of the appearance of the baby. The reality of childbirth may not be what the parents have dreamed of or hoped for. In particular, the experience of premature labor and preterm birth or cesarean birth all involve a loss of the expected pregnancy and birth plans. Parents may grieve over the sex or ap-

pearance of their child. For some parents, loss is associated with the birth of an infant who has a birth defect or chronic illness.

Although having children can be a strong desire for women and men, not everyone is successful in achieving parenthood. For some couples, infertility may thwart their plans and desires for parenthood and cause intense feelings of grief. When couples undergo infertility treatments, feelings of loss may intensify, especially when treatments fail and/or a pregnancy ends in a miscarriage. Women, in particular, experience high distress during this time.

Many women and their partners, whether infertile or not, experience miscarriage in the early months of pregnancy. Miscarriage affects the personal identity of the woman and causes guilt, depression, and anxiety. Others may have an ectopic pregnancy or experience a fetal death. Women and their partners also may suddenly be confronted with stillbirth, the birth of an infant who shows no signs of life. All of these experiences may be called perinatal loss. Others may experience intense grief after infant death. These others include women who give birth prematurely to an infant who survives only a few hours or who dies after days, weeks, or months in an intensive care unit. A woman may give birth to an infant with severe congenital anomalies or other serious health problems; these infants also may die after a few hours, days, weeks, or months in an intensive care unit.

The statistics on perinatal loss and death of an infant are grim. Approximately 2% of pregnancies are ectopic pregnancies, taking place outside the uterus, usually in a uterine tube. Ectopic pregnancies account for 9% of maternal deaths (Luciano, Jain, Roy, Solima, & Luciano, 2004). A miscarriage—a pregnancy that ends before 20 weeks of gestation—is reported to account for 10% to 15% of all pregnancies (Simpson, 2002). In addition, each year approximately 5 of every 1000 births end in stillbirth or fetal death (those occurring after 20 weeks of gestation). Newborn death, death of a baby born showing signs of life such as respiratory effort, heart rate, pulsating cord at birth, and/or muscle irritability, regardless of gestational age, accounts for approximately 28,000 deaths per year in the United States (Martin, Kochanek, Strobino, Guyer, & MacDorman, 2005). Of those, 20% die of congenital malformations and chromosomal abnormalities, 17% of short gestation and low birth weight (LBW), and 8% of sudden infant death syndrome (SIDS) (Martin et al., 2005). African-American women experience pregnancy and infant losses at rates more than twice those of Caucasian women and women of other ethnic minority groups (Martin et al., 2005).

Parents can experience grief before or during the childbearing experience. Grief involves the painful emotions and related behavioral and physical responses to a major loss. Grief can be particularly difficult with perinatal losses for a number of reasons: the societal belief that there are no barriers to getting pregnant, and the expectation that once a woman is pregnant, the result will be a healthy live infant. As a result, our society tends to minimize perinatal loss and to lack understanding of the associated pain. Women and men who undergo perinatal losses struggle with these issues themselves, and because of these societal attitudes, they may not receive the support they need. In addition, many perinatal losses are hidden or private, in that others may not know about the infertility or the early pregnancy that ended in miscarriage.

Perinatal losses may be intensified for couples who delay pregnancy until the woman's career and the family's financial status are at the right point for the responsibilities of a child to be undertaken. Feelings of helplessness and loss of control can be very difficult when the couple experiences infertility or miscarriage. In many instances of perinatal loss, the lack of an identified cause for the loss can complicate grief. This is particularly difficult for women, who often feel personally responsible for infertility, miscarriage, and infant death. Some couples endure repeated losses; 4% of married women in the United States have had two fetal losses, and 3% have had three or more (Simpson, 2002). Such losses can be devastating. Furthermore, society allows far too little time for mothers grieving a perinatal loss and even less time for men. All of these issues can reduce the support to bereaved parents. Parents in a Canadian study reported that social support from families and friends fell short of expectations, and they interpreted this inattention as an indication that the death of their baby was not an important life event. Some also reported a lack of understanding and support from health care professionals (Malacrida, 1999).

Nurses have a powerful influence on how parents experience and cope with perinatal loss (Corbet-Owen & Kruger, 2001; Saflund, Sjogren, & Wredling, 2004). Nurses encounter these parents in a variety of settings, including the antepartum, labor and birth, neonatal, postpartum, and gynecologic units of hospitals, and obstetric, gynecologic, and infertility outpatient clinics and offices, as well as emergency rooms. In these settings, nurses have opportunities to provide sensitive and caring interventions to parents. Parents have reported that their nurses were an important resource in helping them cope with their grief.

Nurses in many inpatient settings have developed protocols that provide clear direction to all staff with regard to how to help parents through this difficult process. In some units, experienced nurses, social workers, or hospital chaplains who are particularly comfortable in helping bereaved parents are designated as perinatal grief consultants. They are available to help parents but also to help prepare the staff for their role with parents. In addition, many institutions now have follow-up programs involving telephone calls, home visits, and support groups that are effective in helping parents after discharge. It is important, then, that dealing with perinatal loss be included in nursing curricula and in-service training for staff nurses.

The focus of this chapter is to prepare the beginning nurse to provide sensitive, supportive, and therapeutic interventions to parents experiencing perinatal loss in a variety of settings. An overview of the grief process is presented as a guide for assessing and understanding the responses of bereaved women, men, and their families. Guidelines for intervention are given, and specific intervention approaches are discussed.

GRIEF RESPONSES

Grief or bereavement has been described as a cluster of painful responses experienced by individuals coping with the death of someone with whom they had a close relationship, generally a relative or close friend (Lindemann, 1944; Osterweis, Solomon, & Green, 1984; Parkes, 1972; Parkes &

Weiss, 1983). Many authors believe there are overlapping phases in the grief process, but most do not believe that grief is experienced in "stages." There is an early period of acute distress and shock followed by a period of intense grief that includes emotional, cognitive, behavioral, and physical responses. The phase of reorganization is reached when the individuals return to their usual level of functioning in society, although the pain associated with the death remains. The duration of grief varies with the individual, but there is general agreement that grief is a long-term process that can extend for months and years. With a very close relationship such as with one's baby, some aspects of grief never truly end. Another way of conceptualizing the grief process is through the achievement of certain tasks of mourning. Worden (1991) identified four tasks: (1) accepting the loss, (2) working through the pain, (3) adjusting to the environment, and (4) moving on. He proposed that these four "tasks of mourning" must be completed to resolve grief.

Miles (1984) and Miles and Demi (1986, 1997) proposed a conceptual model of parental grief, based on the work of Lindemann (1944), Parkes (1972), Parkes and Weiss (1983), and Worden (1991). The model proposes that the grief responses of a parent are closely linked to self-image as a mother or father. Parental grief responses occur in three overlapping phases of grief—acute distress, intense grief, and reorganization (Box 28-1).

BOX 28-1

Conceptual Model of Parental Grief

PHASE OF ACUTE DISTRESS
- Shock
- Numbness
- Intense crying
- Depression

PHASE OF INTENSE GRIEF
- Loneliness, emptiness, and yearning
- Guilt
- Anger, resentment, bitterness, irritability
- Fear and anxiety (especially about getting pregnant again)
- Disorganization
- Difficulties with cognitive processing
- Sadness and depression
- Physical symptoms

REORGANIZATION
- Search for meaning
- Reduction of distress
- Reentering normal life activities with more enthusiasm
- Ability to make future plans, including decision about another pregnancy

Adapted from Miles, M. (1980). *The grief of parents . . . when a child dies.* Oak Brook, IL: Compassionate Friends, Inc.; Miles, M. (1984). Helping adults mourn the death of a child. In H. Wass & C. Corr (Eds.), *Childhood and death.* New York: Hemisphere.

Acute Distress

The loss of a pregnancy or death of an infant is an acute and distressing experience for mothers and fathers who planned for and expected a normal healthy infant as the outcome. The loss encompasses a loss of their identity as a mother or father and the loss of their many dreams related to parenthood. The immediate reaction to news of a perinatal loss or infant death encompasses a period of acute distress. Parents generally are in a state of shock and numbness. They may feel a sense of unreality and confusion, as though they were in a bad dream or in a fog or trancelike state. Disbelief and denial can occur. However, parents also feel very sad and depressed. Intense outbursts of emotion and crying are common. However, lack of affect, euphoria, and calmness may occur and may reflect numbness, denial, or a personal way of coping with stress.

Much of the literature and research on grief after perinatal loss and infant death has focused on the mother. Likewise, much of the attention during the time of a loss is on the mother; the father is expected to be her main support but is often not acknowledged as grieving too. The response of fathers may be more variable than that of mothers and depends on the level of identification with the pregnancy. With early miscarriage or ectopic pregnancy, some fathers may not have a strong investment in the wished-for child. However, many fathers do grieve deeply for a miscarriage. Fathers are profoundly affected by a stillbirth or death of an infant. They have feelings of self-blame, a loss of identity and a need to hide feelings of grief and anger, and to appear strong (McCreight, 2004). Fathers also are distressed by the grief of the mother and often feel helpless with regard to how to help her with the intense pain. It is important to realize that fathers may be experiencing deep pain beneath their calm and quiet appearance and need help in acknowledging these feelings. Because fathers do not easily share feelings or ask for help, special efforts are needed to help them realize that they too have a right to support from others in their pain.

During this time of acute distress, parents face the first task of grief, accepting the reality of the loss. The pregnancy has ended or the baby has died, and their life has changed. Although parents are often required to make many decisions, such as having an autopsy, naming the infant, and funeral arrangements, normal functioning is impeded, and decisions are difficult to make. These decisions are especially painful and difficult for young couples who have limited or no previous experience with death. Grandparents are often called on to help make difficult decisions regarding funeral arrangements and/or disposition of the body because they have more life experience with taking care of these painful, yet required arrangements. However, some well-meaning grandparents and other family members may try to take over with all the decisions that must be made. It is critical that the nurse remember that a very important role is always to be a patient advocate and that the parents themselves should approve the final decisions.

Intense Grief

The phase of intense grief encompasses many difficult emotions, including loneliness, emptiness, yearning; guilt, anger, and fear; disorganization and depression; and physical symptoms. During this time, parents are working on two additional tasks of mourning: working through the pain and adjusting to life without the wished-for child. Being able to adjust to the environment after the loss means learning how to accommodate the changes that the loss has brought.

In the early months after the loss, parents often experience feelings of loneliness, emptiness, and yearning. The mother may report that her arms ache to hold or nurse her baby and that she wakes to the sound of a baby crying. When her milk comes in, it is particularly poignant when there is no baby to take to breast. Both mothers and fathers may be preoccupied with thoughts about the wished-for child. Some women cope with these feelings by avoiding memories and by not talking about the baby, whereas others want to reminisce and discuss their loss over and over. Deciding what to do about the nursery and baby clothes is particularly difficult during this period. Some women want the room taken down before they go home, whereas others want the room left intact until they have had time to grieve their loss. It is not unusual for a grandparent or other family member to want to rush home to take down the nursery with the thought that they would be sparing additional painful grief. In fact, their actions might only complicate the grief if parents were not involved in the decision. The bereaved parents, in their own time frame, must go through these types of experiences so that healing can take place.

During this phase of intense grief, guilt may emerge from the deep feelings of helplessness in not somehow preventing the pregnancy loss or the death of the infant. Mothers are particularly vulnerable to feel guilt because of their sense of responsibility for the well-being of the fetus and baby. With many perinatal losses, there is no clear cause of the event, leaving the woman to speculate about what she might have done or not done to cause the loss. Guilt also may be intense if a mother thinks she is being punished for some unrelated event such as having had a prior induced abortion. Such self-blame is torture for mothers, and they need repeated emotional reassurance that they were not at fault. Guilt can occur when one is enjoying life again and experiencing happiness despite the loss of the infant.

Another common response during this phase of grief is anger, resentment, bitterness, or irritability. Anger is particularly poignant if the loss is perceived as senseless, and there is a felt need to blame others. Anger may be focused on the health care team who failed to save the pregnancy or infant. For some parents, anger is vented toward a God who allowed the loss to occur. This can lead to a spiritual crisis. Anger also occurs toward family, friends, and peers when they do not provide the support bereaved parents need and want. Some parents focus their resentment on parents who do not appreciate their children or who neglect and abuse them. A

sense of bitterness or generalized irritability, rather than frank anger, may be another response.

Fear and anxiety can occur during the grief process as a profound worry that something else bad might happen to another. Fear and anxiety are particularly poignant when the couple thinks about another pregnancy. Whereas some parents, especially mothers, are almost obsessed with the desire to become pregnant again, others struggle with whether they can cope with another potential loss. A prior loss increases parents' stress in a subsequent pregnancy; parents experience a mixture of hope and fear (Armstrong, 2004).

Deep sadness and depression occur when the parent is faced with the full awareness of the reality of the loss. This often occurs several months after a perinatal loss and can continue for some time. Sadness and depression are often accompanied by disorganization and problems with cognitive processing. This leads to behavioral changes such as difficulty in getting things done, an inability to concentrate, restlessness, confused thought processes, difficulty in solving problems, and poor decision making. Disorganization and depression often cause difficulties in keeping up with work and family expectations. Additionally, parents returning to work face issues such as handling well-meaning but painful comments or the silence of co-workers.

Physical symptoms of grief include fatigue, headaches, dizziness, or backaches. Parents are at risk for developing health problems, such as colds or hypertension. The grieving process makes it difficult for bereaved parents to sleep. Their appetites may be depressed or voracious. Lack of sleep and inadequate nutrition and fluids can complicate other grief responses.

Grief responses are very personal, ongoing, and difficult to cope with. Some parents may suppress or deny their feelings because of societal indifference toward pregnancy loss and infant death. Suppression of feelings may, on the surface, be more socially acceptable. However, denying the pain of grief may lead to eventual physical and emotional distress or illness. Many parents, especially mothers, want to tell their story over and over. This helps them actualize the loss and face their feelings. Sometimes parents begin to think they are the only individuals who have ever had such a rough time and that they may be going crazy. Although bereaved parents have many ups and downs for many months and even years after a child's death, few parents actually become mentally ill or commit suicide. Knowing that these feelings are normal and that others have felt the same is helpful. The grief process during this phase is often difficult for fathers. Some may continue to have difficulty sharing their feelings. A rift can occur if one parent, usually the mother, wants to talk about the loss and pain, and the other parent, often but not always the father, withdraws. Other signs of problems of the father include reliance on alcohol and drugs, extramarital affairs, prolonged hours at work, and overinvolvement in diversional and other activities outside the home as an escape. The Perinatal Grief Scale is an instrument that can be used to quantify the grief parents experience (Fig. 28-1).

EVIDENCE-BASED PRACTICE
Measuring the Unmeasurable: Perinatal Grief Scale

BACKGROUND

- With the decrease in infant mortality during the last century and increased parental expectations, response to perinatal loss became a topic for investigation. Cultural changes in the 1970s created increased patient expectations of control during childbirth, self-help movements, and increased awareness of the stages of dying and grieving. With increasing interest in understanding the grief of perinatal loss, social scientists faced the challenge of measuring this powerful and profound emotion. Since the introduction of the Perinatal Grief Scale (PGS) in 1988, it has been used in many studies to quantify and predict the impact of perinatal loss. The PGS is a 33-item test, using Likert-type responses ("strongly agree" to "strongly disagree") to various statements of grief (see Fig. 28-1).

OBJECTIVES

- The original authors' goals were to compare the internal consistency of the tool, establish normative ranges so as to be able to identify the parent who may be experiencing extreme duress, and compare groups across cultures and times.

METHODS
Search Strategy

- The reviewers searched PsycLit, SciSearch, and Social SciSearch. Keywords included *pregnancy loss* and *grief*. Every article that referenced the original publications about PGS was evaluated. The reviewers also searched WorldCat for relevant dissertations and followed up on all studies that had requested the use of the PGS tool.
- The authors identified 22 empirical studies, presented from 1988 to 1999, representing 1803 women and 654 men (total 2457) from the United States, the United Kingdom, the Netherlands, and Germany. The types of losses included miscarriage, stillbirth, newborn loss, ectopic pregnancy, adoption, and elective abortion.

Statistical Analysis

- Metaanalysis indicated strong internal consistency (all items seem to measure the same phenomenon similarly) and external validity (generalizability) of the PGS tool. The number of subjects enabled the establishment of a normal range of grief by determining that 97.5% of newly bereaved parents' scores fell below 91. Therefore a score above 91 was accepted as reflecting severe distress. No normal low range was established. It was speculated that grief scores would decline across time. Group scores were compared, as were stages of pregnancy and birth at time of loss.
- High benchmarks were also set for the three subscale groups that showed progressive psychologic decline: active grief, difficulty coping (more severe), and despair (most severe).

FINDINGS

- Between-group comparisons revealed that women's scores exceeded men's scores, but not to the level of significance. Grief does decrease across 2 years. There were significantly higher grief scores in groups recruited from grief groups or advertisements than from parents referred by health care workers. This may account for the significantly higher scores in the U.S. samples, who were mostly recruited through advertisements and groups, as compared to the European cohorts, who were mostly referrals from hospitals. Strong marriages and the perception of social support were consistently related to lower grief scores. Preloss poor mental health, such as neuroticism, led to significantly higher grief. Grief scores showed a pattern of increasing with increasing gestation, but not to the level of significance. In the United States, low socioeconomic status was significantly associated with higher grief scores; this disparity was less marked in Europe.

LIMITATIONS

- Diversity was lacking in the U.S. samples, which were largely composed of Caucasian and middle class subjects. Groups and advertisements may attract people seeking relief from more severe grief; this sample bias may confound the comparison of scores in the United States and Europe. Cultural bias and wording may also influence results.

CONCLUSIONS

- The PGS is a valuable tool for clinical and research purposes, across time and countries.

IMPLICATIONS FOR PRACTICE

- Nurses can identify those at risk for poor adaptation and can counsel bereaved parents that healing will take years, and requires much marital and social support. Patients with high PGS scores that do not improve across time or who seem to be slipping into measurable despair on the subscale can be referred to grief specialists.

IMPLICATIONS FOR FUTURE RESEARCH

- Deeper understanding would be derived from more diverse cohorts and from exploring the grief patterns of men and other family or support members. Researchers can explore the lower end of the grief scale to distinguish functional results from denial, which may prove to be a bigger problem later. Research can determine whether those seeking groups have higher baseline scores or whether self-help groups are not as effective for alleviating grief as some hospital interventions. In-depth research is still needed on ectopic pregnancy, second trimester abortions for genetic abnormalities, and elective abortion.

Reference: Toedter, L., Lasker, J., & Janssen, H. (2001). International comparison of studies using the Perinatal Grief Scale: A decade of research on pregnancy loss. *Death Studies, 25*(3), 205-228.

Presents Thoughts and Feelings About Your Loss

Each of the items is a statement of thoughts and feelings that some people have concerning a loss such as yours. There are no right or wrong responses to these statements. For each item, circle the number that best indicated the extent to which you agree or disagree with it at the present time. If you are not certain, use the "neither" category. Please try to use this category only when you truly have no opinion.

	Strongly Agree	Agree	Neither Agree nor Disagree	Disagree	Strongly Disagree
1. I feel depressed.	1	2	3	4	5
2. I find it hard to get along with certain people.	1	2	3	4	5
3. I feel empty inside.	1	2	3	4	5
4. I can't keep up with my normal activities.	1	2	3	4	5
5. I feel a need to talk about the baby.	1	2	3	4	5
6. I am grieving for the baby.	1	2	3	4	5
7. I am frightened.	1	2	3	4	5
8. I have considered suicide since the loss.	1	2	3	4	5
9. I take medicine for my nerves.	1	2	3	4	5
10. I very much miss the baby.	1	2	3	4	5
11. I feel I have adjusted well to the loss.	1	2	3	4	5
12. It is painful to recall memories of the loss.	1	2	3	4	5
13. I get upset when I think about the baby.	1	2	3	4	5
14. I cry when I think about him/her.	1	2	3	4	5
15. I feel guilty when I think about the baby.	1	2	3	4	5
16. I feel physically ill when I think about the baby.	1	2	3	4	5
17. I feel unprotected in a dangerous world since he/she died.	1	2	3	4	5
18. I try to laugh, but nothing seems funny anymore.	1	2	3	4	5
19. Time passes so slowly since the baby died.	1	2	3	4	5
20. The best part of me died with the baby.	1	2	3	4	5
21. I have let people down since the baby died.	1	2	3	4	5
22. I feel worthless since he/she died.	1	2	3	4	5
23. I blame myself for the baby's death.	1	2	3	4	5
24. I get cross at my friends and relatives more than I should.	1	2	3	4	5
25. Sometimes I feel like I need a professional counselor to help me get my life back together again.	1	2	3	4	5
26. I feel as though I'm just existing and not really living since he/she died.	1	2	3	4	5
27. I feel so lonely since he/she died.	1	2	3	4	5
28. I feel somewhat apart and remote, even among friends.	1	2	3	4	5
29. It's safer not to love.	1	2	3	4	5
30. I find it difficult to make decisions since the baby died.	1	2	3	4	5
31. I worry about what my future will be like.	1	2	3	4	5
32. Being a bereaved parent means being a "Second-Class Citizen."	1	2	3	4	5
33. It feels great to be alive.	1	2	3	4	5

Scoring Instructions

The total PGS score is arrived at by first reversing all of the items except 11 and 33. By reversing the items, higher scores now reflect more intense grief. Then add the scores together. The result is a total scale consisting of 33 items with a possible range of 33-165.

The three subscales consist of the sum of the scores of 11 items each, with a possible range of 11-55.

Subscale 1 *Active Grief*	Subscale 2 *Difficulty Coping*	Subscale 3 *Despair*
1	2	9
3	4	15
5	8	16
6	*11	17
7	21	18
10	24	20
12	25	22
13	26	23
14	28	29
19	30	31
27	*33	32

*Do not reverse.

Fig. 28-1 The Perinatal Grief Scale (33-Item Short Version). From Toedter, L., Lasker, J., & Janssen, H. (2001). International comparison of studies using the Perinatal Grief Scale: A decade of research on pregnancy loss. *Death Studies, 25*(3), 205-228.

Reorganization

From the time of the pregnancy loss or infant death, parents attempt to understand "why?" This leads to a long and intense "search for meaning." At first the "why" is focused on the cause of death. Finding few good answers, parents focus next on "why me, why mine?" These questions lead some parents into an existential search about the meaning of life and death. "What does my loss mean to my life?" "What is life all about?" "What do I do with the rest of my life?" This search continues into the phase of reorganization and may lead to profound changes in the parents' views about the fragility of life. Internal (hardiness) and external (marital support and social support) factors are predictors of health in bereaved parents (Lang, Goulet, & Amsel, 2004).

Time helps to ease slowly the painful feelings of grief. Over time the pain becomes less frequent. Reorganization occurs when the parent is better able to function at home and work, experiences a return of self-esteem and confidence, can cope with new challenges, and has placed the loss in perspective. Reorganization begins to peak sometime after the first year as parents begin to achieve the task of moving on with their lives. Enjoying the simple pleasures of life without feeling guilty, nurturing self and others, developing new interests, and reestablishing relationships are all signs of moving on. For some women and families, another pregnancy and the birth of a subsequent child is an important step in moving on with their lives; however, the term "recovery" is used because the grief related to perinatal loss can continue in varying degrees for life. Parents have shared that they will never forget the baby who has died, and they are not the same persons as before the loss. The term "bittersweet grief," invented by Kowalski (1984), refers to the grief response that occurs with reminders of the loss. This typically happens at special anniversary dates related to the loss (Box 28-2). Grief feelings also can be triggered after a subsequent live birth.

Resuming the sexual relationship is an extremely important aspect of recovery but can be very complicated. Many parents are comforted with the belief that their babies were conceived in love, lived in love, and died in love. The result of love and intimacy created this child, and parents may believe that they may never experience joy and closeness again. Once the doctor has given permission for resumption of sexual activities, parents may find it emotionally very difficult. Some couples may have an increased need for sexual activity in an attempt for closeness and healing, whereas others have a decreased desire for sexual intimacy. It is important that parents be aware of some possible deep need from inside themselves to stop the emotional pain. Difficulties arise when the needs of the couple differ.

Sexuality also brings with it decisions about a future pregnancy. Some couples are eager to have another child, although one child cannot replace the one who died, and the grief will continue despite pregnancy. Other parents have a deep fear of experiencing the pain of loss again, which can make the resumption of sexual activity difficult. These ambivalent feelings are normal, and couples will find themselves moving back and forth between the emotions of exhilaration and fear. The subsequent pregnancy after a loss is often filled with guarded emotions and great anxiety. The excitement that many others experience with a pregnancy is very different for previously bereaved parents. Fathers also reported anxiety about the outcome of the next pregnancy and increased their vigilance (Armstrong, 2001). Couples often mark the progress of the pregnancy in terms of fetal development, waiting anxiously until the number of weeks before the previous loss have passed. In some cases the fear of repeated loss, especially after a stillbirth, is so great that induction of labor is considered if lung maturity studies can confirm that the baby is mature. Parents may have anxiety in caring for the surviving infant. Burkhammer, Anderson, and Chiu (2004) reported assisting a young, anxious mother whose first child was stillborn and the second born alive, but small-for-dates, to use skin-to-skin breastfeedings to overcome her grief, guilt, and anxiety when feeding difficulties emerged.

BOX 28-2

Bittersweet Grief

To Jessica Mayo—on her eleventh birthday
  Sunday, November 18, 1990
"The child who is born on the Sabbath day,
is bonny and blithe and good and gay."
    Sundays are special days.
    . . . a day of rest, a day to play.
    A day to reflect on days past.
. . . a day to thank God for all that we bless.
    I bless your memory.
    I wish you were here.
On your eleventh birthday I still want to share.
    . . . Your dreams of the future.
    . . . Our memories past.
    My baby's first cry.
    My daughter's first laugh.
I was told you were an angel in heaven above.
    Eleven years later, I'm an expert . . .
    At long-distance love.
    On your third birthday I wrote my first poem
to you.
    Eight years later, it's still true
" . . . no birthday cake,
    no presents unwrapped . . .
no pictures of you in your party hat.
    But the candles are lit,
    Never to go out
For they burn forever in my heart.
    Love, Mom"
Kathie Rataj Mayo
1990

Used with permission of Bereavement Services. Copyright Lutheran Hospital-La Crosse, Inc., a Gundersen Lutheran Affiliate, La Crosse, WI.

Family Aspects of Grief: Grandparents and Siblings

It is extremely important for the nurse taking care of these parents to keep in mind that they have an entire family to minister to, including especially grandparents and siblings. Grandparents have hopes and dreams for a grandchild; these have been shattered. The grief of grandparents is often complicated by the fact that they are experiencing intense emotional pain by witnessing and feeling the immense grief of their own child. It is extremely difficult to watch their son or daughter experience unimaginable emotional trauma with very few ways to comfort and end their pain. As a result, the grief response may be complicated or delayed for grandparents. On occasions, some grandparents experience immense "survival guilt" because they feel the death is out of order. They are angry that they are alive and their grandchild is not.

The siblings of the expected infant also experience a profound loss. Most children have been prepared for having another child in the family once the pregnancy is confirmed. These children come in all ages and stages of development, and this must be considered in understanding how they view the event and their loss experience. A young child will respond more to the response of their parents, picking up on the fact that they are behaving differently and are extremely sad. This can cause clinging, altered eating and sleeping patterns, or acting-out behaviors, yet it is a time when parents have limited patience for responding to and meeting the needs of the child. Older children have a more complete understanding of the loss. School-aged children may be frightened by the entire event, whereas teens may understand fully but feel awkward in responding. Older siblings need to be included in grieving rituals to the extent the parents and the child feel comfortable. They may need to see the baby to actualize the loss. Nurses need to have a basic understanding about how children view death and grieve to reach out to siblings in an appropriate and sensitive manner. Nurses also need to help parents understand and be sensitive to the needs of their other children despite their own deep pain.

CARE MANAGEMENT

Nursing care of mothers and fathers experiencing a perinatal loss begins the first time the parents are faced with the potential loss of their pregnancy or death of their infant. Supportive interventions are important both at the time of the loss and after the parents have returned home.

Assessment and Nursing Diagnoses

An important step in the nursing process involves assessment. Several key areas to address include the following:

- The nature of the parental attachment with the pregnancy or infant, the meaning of the pregnancy and infant to the parents, and the related losses they are experiencing. Each pregnancy and birth has a special meaning to parents. Whether a woman has experienced a miscarriage or ectopic pregnancy, stillbirth, or death of an infant, it is important to gain some understanding of parents' perceptions of their unique loss. The meaning of the loss is determined by familial and cultural systems of the parents. In one study, feelings about perinatal loss ranged from devastation to relief (Corbet-Owen & Kruger, 2001). Listening to parents tell their stories and being sensitive to the language used to describe their experience can help one gain an understanding of the meaning of the loss. Open-ended questions are helpful: "Tell me about your labor and birth with Mia." Or "When did you know you were miscarrying?" Mothers who have had a previous pregnancy loss may feel less attached, which can increase their feelings of guilt when a loss occurs.

- The circumstances surrounding the loss, including the level of preparation for the loss and the parents' level of understanding about the cause of the loss or death, and any related unresolved issues are important. While listening to the parents' stories, it is important to uncover any special experiences that may make their losses even more poignant. A history of infertility, repeated pregnancy losses, a previous stillbirth, or infant death can make this loss even more painful. In addition, other life circumstances such as illness of another family member, loss of a job, or other family stresses can increase the distress of parents. It also is helpful to know whether the mother and father perceived the loss to be totally unexpected or whether they had some forewarning or preparation.

- The immediate response of the mother and father to the loss, whether their responses are complementary or problematic, and how their responses match with their past experiences, personalities, and behavioral and cultural backgrounds. An understanding of the usual responses to grief described earlier can be helpful in attempting to understand the unique grief responses of the mother and father and other family members. As nurses work with families, they may uncover information about how the individual or family responded to a previous loss, or a personality or behavioral trait that may interact in their responses to this grief. In particular, it is important to know about any history of infertility, previous pregnancy losses, or infant deaths and evaluate how that might affect parental responses. It also is important to be sensitive to different expectations during grief for men and women from different cultural groups (see section on cultural and spiritual needs of parents later in this chapter).

- The social support network of the parent (e.g., extended family, friends, co-workers, church) and the extent to which it has been activated. Support during a perinatal loss is important to most couples. However, it is important to assess the amount of support and the type of support from others that a couple wants. Some prefer to handle the tragedy alone for a time. Others want assistance in calling other family members, friends, and clergy to be with them and to help them with decisions.

Nursing diagnoses may include physiologic and psychosocial problems experienced by the mother or father or problems occurring within the couple or family because of the loss and subsequent grief. Examples of nursing diagnoses include the following:

- *Anxiety related to*
  - lack of experience regarding how to manage the loss
  - worry about the partner
  - intense concern over not achieving a pregnancy
  - becoming pregnant again with risk of another loss
- *Ineffective family or individual coping related to*
  - inability to make decisions as a family
  - difficulties in communication within the family
  - conflicting coping patterns between mother and father
- *Powerlessness related to*
  - high risk pregnancy and birth
  - unexpected cesarean birth
  - inability to prevent the infant's death
- *Interrupted family processes related to*
  - maternal depression leading to changes in role function
  - inadequate communication of feelings between the grieving mother and father
  - lack of expected support from family
  - behavioral and emotional reactions of siblings
  - grief within the family system including grandparents and other relatives
- *Ineffective sexuality patterns between the mother and father related to*
  - guilt and fear associated with sexuality
  - loss of pleasure in sexual intercourse
  - differences in desires of each partner
  - fear of getting pregnant again
- *Fatigue and disturbed sleep pattern related to*
  - inability to fall asleep because of grief
  - waking in the night and thinking about the loss
  - loss of sleep
- *Dysfunctional grieving related to*
  - prolonged denial or avoidance of the loss
  - intense guilt related to the loss
  - continued anger about the loss
  - serious depressive symptoms and despair
  - loss of self-esteem
  - intense grieving patterns that continue for more than a year

  - social isolation resulting from grief
- *Situational low self-esteem related to*
  - prolonged feelings of poor self-worth because of the loss
  - feeling unworthy of having a child
- *Spiritual distress related to*
  - anger with God
  - confusion about why prayers were not answered
- *Disturbed thought processes related to*
  - difficulty making decisions
  - inability to get organized
  - poor work performance
  - confused thinking

Expected Outcomes of Care

Expected outcomes are set and priorities assigned in patient-centered terms according to the mutual goals chosen by the patient and the nurse. Nursing actions are then selected to meet the expected outcomes, which may include that the woman or family will do the following:

- Actualize the loss
- Share experiences and verbalize feelings of grief as much as is culturally and personally appropriate
- Understand the normal grief responses they and others in the family may experience at the time of and after the loss
- Demonstrate increasing independence in participating in and making decisions that meet their needs and reflect their religious and cultural beliefs
- Identify family, spiritual, health care, and community resources for support
- Discuss problems or issues involving relationships with each other and family
- Verbalize satisfaction with the care and support provided by their health care professionals

Plan of Care and Interventions

Interventions and support for parents from the nursing and medical staff before and after a perinatal loss or infant death are extremely important in their healing. Although parents often cannot recall details of their experiences at the time of death, they may recall vividly minor events that were perceived as particularly painful or particularly helpful. When parents know before birth that the baby will not survive, they can make arrangements to spend time with the baby, even if for just a short time (Cole, 2004). However, care must be individualized to each parent and family. Parents appreciate the opportunity to make choices about their needs. Providers should not try to influence parents or make presumptions that would limit their choices or force them to make choices they do not want. Furthermore, the cultural and spiritual beliefs and practices of individual parents and families must be considered. The interventions discussed later are general ideas about what may be helpful to parents.

Help the mother, father, and other family members actualize the loss

When a loss or death occurs, the nurse should be sure that parents have been honestly told about the situation by their physician or others on the health care team. It is important for their nurse to be with them during this time. With infant death, caregivers must use the words "dead" and "died," rather than "lost" or "gone," to assist the bereaved in accepting this reality. Parents need opportunities to tell their story about the events, experiences, and feelings surrounding the loss. This can help them come to terms with the reality of their loss. Listening to their pain and allowing time for them to absorb the information are important.

One way of actualizing the loss is to tell the parents the sex of the baby (if not already known) and give them the option of naming the fetus or to help them to name an infant who has died. Choosing a name helps make the baby a member of their family so that the baby can be remembered in a special way. Once the baby is named, the nurse should use the name when referring to the baby. Although naming can be helpful, it is important not to create the sense that the parents have to name the "baby," especially in the case of a miscarriage when the sex is not known.

NURSE ALERT *A caution about naming is important. Cultural taboos and rules in some religious faiths prohibit the naming of an infant who has died. It is very important to be sensitive to this possibility and not impose naming on such parents.*

It may be helpful for mothers and fathers to see the fetus or baby. Many professionals, based on vast clinical experiences with parents, believe that seeing the fetus or baby helps parents face the reality of the loss, reduces painful fantasies, and offers an opportunity for closure. This has been questioned as the result of a longitudinal study of a small group of mothers in England (Hughes, Turton, Hopper, & Evans, 2002). These authors suggest that the wishes of the parents should be respected. Parents should never be made to feel they "should" see or hold their baby when this is something that they do not really want. Encouraging reluctant parents to hold or see their dead child by telling them that not seeing the child could make mourning more difficult is inappropriate. Obviously, this subject must be approached very carefully. A question such as, "Some parents have found it helpful to see their baby. Would you like time to consider this?" Because the need or willingness to see also may vary between the mother and father, it is extremely important to determine what each parent really wants. This should not be a joint decision made by one person or a decision made for the parents by grandparents or others. It is a good policy for the nurse to first tell them about this option and then give them time to think about it. Later the nurse can return and ask each parent individually what they decided. In preparation for the visit with the baby, parents appreciate explanations about what to expect. Descriptions

of how their baby looks is important. For example, babies may have red, peeling skin like a bad sunburn, dark discoloration similar to bruises, molding of the head that makes the head look soft and swollen, or birth defects. The nurse should make the baby look as normal as possible, and remember that parents and health care professionals view the baby differently. Bathing the baby, applying lotion to the baby's skin, combing hair, placing identification bracelets on the arm and leg, dressing the baby in a diaper and special outfit, sprinkling powder in the baby's blanket, and wrapping the baby in a pretty blanket convey to the parents that their baby has been cared for in a special way. The use of powder and lotion stimulates the parent's senses and provides pleasant memories of their baby.

It is more complicated if the fetus died several days or weeks before birth or if decapitation or dismemberment occurred. Consultation with a local funeral director can help the nurse prepare the baby to be seen by his or her parents. If the baby has been in the morgue, he or she can be placed underneath a warmer for 20 to 30 minutes and wrapped in a warm blanket before being brought to the parents. Cold cream rubbed over stiffened joints can help in positioning the baby.

When bringing the baby to the parents, it is important to treat the baby as one would a live baby. Holding the baby close, touching a hand or cheek, using the baby's name, and talking with the parents about the special features of their child convey that it is all right for them to do likewise. If a baby has a congenital anomaly, the nurse can desensitize the family by pointing out aspects of the baby that are normal. Nurses can help parents explore the baby's body as they desire. Parents often seek to identify family resemblance. A good question might be: "Who in your family does Michael resemble?"

Some families may like to have the opportunity to bathe and dress their baby. Although the skin may be fragile, parents can still apply lotion with cotton balls, sprinkle powder, tie ribbons, fasten the diaper, and place amulets, medallions, rosaries, or special toys or mementos in their baby's hands or alongside their baby. They may want to perform other parenting activities, such as combing hair, dressing the baby in a special outfit, wrapping the baby in a blanket, or placing the baby in a crib.

Parents need to be offered time alone with their baby if they wish. They also need to know when the nurse will return and how to call if they need anything. If at all possible the family should be placed in a private room, and when possible the room should have a rocking chair for the parents to sit in when holding their baby. This offers the mother and father special time together with their baby and with other family members (Fig. 28-2). Marking the door to the room with a special card can be helpful for reminding the staff that this family has experienced a loss (Fig. 28-3).

It is difficult to predict how long and how often parents will need to spend time with their baby. These moments are

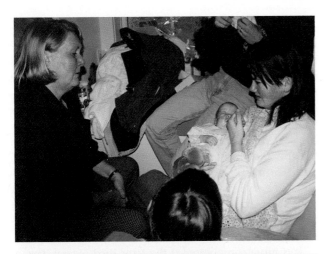

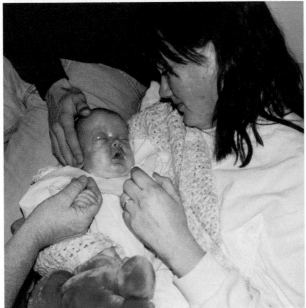

Fig. 28-2 Laura's family members say a special good-bye. (Courtesy Amy and Ken Turner, Cary, NC.)

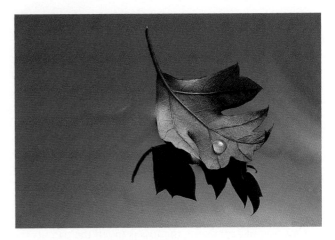

Fig. 28-3 Door card for room of mother who has had a perinatal loss. (Used with permission of Bereavement Services. Copyright Lutheran Hospital-La Crosse, Inc., A Gundersen Lutheran Affiliate, La Crosse, WI.)

the only ones they will have to parent their child while their child's physical presence is still with them. Some parents need only a few minutes; others need hours. It is extremely painful for some parents to say good-bye to their baby. They will tell the nurse when they are ready verbally and nonverbally. The nurse should watch for cues that the parents have had enough time with their baby, such as when parents are no longer holding their child close to them or have placed the baby back in the crib. Asking parents whether they have had enough time may make parents feel that the nurse thinks they have had enough time, which may not be the case. When a baby is taken too soon from parents, it leaves them feeling as though the baby was "ripped from their arms too soon." Heiman, Yankowitz, and Wilkins (1997) found that 85% of parents in their study would have appreciated additional opportunities to see their baby, and 44% felt they did not have adequate time with the baby. Therefore sensi-

tivity to parental needs in actualizing the loss and coping with the reality of the death is essential for their healing. Grandparents should be offered the same opportunities to hold, rock, swaddle, and love their grandchildren so that their grief is started in a healthy way.

Help the parents with decision making

At the time of a perinatal loss, and especially if the loss was of an infant, parents have many decisions to make when they are experiencing great distress. Mothers, fathers, and extended families look to the medical and nursing staff for guidance in knowing what decisions they must and can make and in understanding the options related to those decisions. Therefore it is a primary responsibility of the nurse to help them and to advocate for them because decisions made during the time of their loss will provide their memories for a lifetime.

One decision might be related to conducting an autopsy (Box 28-3). An autopsy can be very important in answering the question "why" if there is a chance that the cause of death can be determined. This information can be helpful in processing grief and perhaps preventing another loss. However, the cost of an autopsy must be considered. Autopsies may not be covered by insurance and are expensive. However, if the autopsy is done under the jurisdiction of the medical examiner's office, there is no charge. Some parents may feel that their baby has been through enough and prefer not to have further information about the cause of death. Some religions prohibit autopsy or limit the choice to times when it may help prevent another loss. Options for the type of autopsy, such as excluding the head, are available to parents. Parents may need time to make this decision. There is no need to rush them, unless there was evidence of contagious disease or maternal infection at the time of death.

Organ donation can be an aid to grieving and an opportunity for the family to see something positive associated

Autopsies

Autopsies are the best method to investigate perinatal deaths. However, the improvement in diagnostic techniques may make the autopsy seem unnecessary to the clinician (Steigman, 2002).

Autopsies are expensive, and third-party payers do not pay hospitals or pathologists directly for them; payment is bundled into general hospital payments. Current charge for an autopsy is $3200 (Vidal Herrera, personal communication, May 25, 2005).

The rate of neonatal autopsies remains higher than that for adults, with the rate ranging from 59% to 81% (Brodlie, Laing, Keeling, & McKenzie, 2002). Parents agree to an autopsy to answer questions about "Why?" and to help others. Parents may refuse autopsy because they do not want the child mutilated and feel that the baby has already been through enough and when they have no questions that were not answered (Lyon, 2004). Rankin, Wright, and Lind

(2002) investigated the experience and views of autopsy by parents. They found that 7% of parents who agreed to the examination and 14% who refused the examination regretted their decision.

When parents refuse autopsy, magnetic resonance imaging is a noninvasive alternative with the major disadvantage of a lack of tissue sampling (Huisman, 2004). In cases of the death of a neonate with congenital anomalies, the probability of identifying the etiologic diagnosis is increased when clinical geneticists and fetal pathologists work together (Cernach, Patricio, Galera, Moron, & Brunoni, 2004).

Nurses may be involved in seeking consent for autopsy or in answering parents' questions about the examination. They can provide support for the decision the parents make. They should be aware of agency policies where they are employed and pertinent regulations dictated by the community.

with their experience. The federal "Gift of Life Act" and HCFA-3005-F, enacted in 1998, shifted the responsibility for determining organ donation potential from the hospital staff to the state's organ procurement organization (OPO). States and hospitals have clear procedures for how and when to call OPO. Generally, if a death certificate is issued, a call must be made to the OPO. Once contacted, the organization will decide whether to talk to the family, and either an OPO representative or a designated requester will contact them. This allows requests to be made by trained personnel in a consistent and compassionate manner. The most common donation is of cornea; donation of cornea from a baby can occur if the baby was born alive at 36 weeks of gestation or later.

Another important decision relates to spiritual rituals that may be helpful and important to parents. Support from clergy is an option that should be offered to all parents. Parents may wish to have their own pastor, priest, rabbi, or spiritual leader contacted, or they may wish to see the hospital's chaplain. They may choose to do neither. Members of the clergy may offer the parents the opportunity for baptism when appropriate. Other rituals that may be important include a blessing, a naming ceremony, anointing, ritual of the sick, memorial service, or prayer.

One of the major decisions parents must make has to do with disposition of the body. Parents should be given information about the choices for the final disposition of their baby, regardless of gestational age. The nurses must be aware, however, of cultural and spiritual beliefs that may dictate the choices of parents. A baby younger than 20 weeks of gestation is considered a product of conception, whereas embryos, uterine tubes removed with an ectopic pregnancy, and tissue from a pregnancy obtained during a dilation and curettage are all considered tissue. Many hospitals will make

arrangements for the cremation of these babies. The nurse should know the hospital's policies and procedures and answer the parents' questions honestly. In most states, if a baby is at least 20 weeks and 1 day of gestational age or is born alive, it is the parents' responsibility to make the final arrangements for their baby, although some hospitals will offer free cremation. In this case, the family would not get the ashes.

LEGAL TIP   Defining Live Birth

Laws in all states govern what constitutes a live birth. In most states a live birth is considered to be any products of conception expelled from a woman that show any signs of life. Signs of life are considered to be any muscle irritability, respiratory effort, or heart rate, regardless of gestational age. All nurses should be knowledgeable about their state laws regarding what constitutes a live birth and what forms must be completed and filed in the case of fetal death, stillbirth, or newborn death.

Provide postmortem care

Preparation of the baby's body and transport to the morgue depends on the procedures and protocols developed by individual hospitals. The Joint Committee on Accreditation of Healthcare Organizations requires that we offer appropriate care to the body after death. A sensitive and respectful approach for taking the fetus or infant to the morgue is the use of a "burial cradle" (Fig. 28-4). These miniature coffins have a quilted lining and replace wrapping the baby in a Chux pad (see Resources at end of chapter). Postmortem care can be an emotional and sometimes difficult task for the nurse. However, nurses may find that providing postmortem care helps them find closure in their own grief related to a perinatal loss. This is particularly true for neonatal

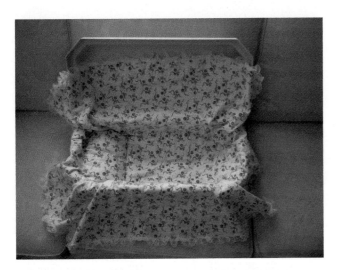

Fig. 28-4 Burial cradle for newborn infant. (Courtesy Shannon Perry, Phoenix, AZ.)

intensive care nurses who have cared for an infant for several hours, days, or weeks.

Final disposition of all identifiable babies, regardless of gestational age, includes burial or cremation. Depending on the cemetery's policies, babies in caskets or the ashes from cremated babies can be buried in a special place designated for babies, at the foot of a deceased relative, in a separate plot, or in a mausoleum. Ashes also may be scattered in a designated area; many states have regulations regarding where ashes can be scattered. A local funeral director or a state's Vital Statistics Bureau should have information about the state's rules, codes, and regulations regarding live births, burial requirements, transportation of the deceased by parents, and cremation.

In making final arrangements for their baby, parents may want a special service. They may choose to have a service in the hospital chapel, visitation at a funeral home or their own home, a funeral service, or a graveside service. Parents can make any of these services as special, personal, and memorable as they like. They can choose special music, poetry, or prose written by themselves or others.

If the family has decided on a funeral and burial, they still have decisions about what funeral home to call and where to bury the baby. Many couples may be living in an area distant from their family homes, and they may want to bury their child in their hometown or family cemetery. If the family desires cremation, they may want to have the option of obtaining the ashes. It is important to determine whether this will be done by the facility conducting the cremation.

Parents' hopes, dreams, self-esteem, and role expectations have been shattered with a perinatal loss; thus they may have many needs. Unmet needs can form the basis of "if only" that may plague a mother or family for a lifetime and can be the foundation for the development of complicated bereavement. However, it is difficult for parents to know ex-

actly what they can expect or what they need; thus the nurse as an advocate should lead by offering various options that might meet specific needs. When a mother or family is able to verbalize needs, it is extremely important for the nurse to respond positively and do everything to see that the request is met.

Families become unaware of time frames and do not care about the change of shifts or any needs the hospital system might have in "moving things along." When families are pushed or rushed into making decisions, in most cases, they make a decision in response to the health care system's needs, not their own. The timing for actions such as naming the baby, seeing and holding the baby, disposition of the body, and funeral arrangements should never be rushed. In some cases the mother may be discharged home before these decisions are made. Then the family can think about them in the comfort of their home and contact the hospital in the following days to give their answers.

Help the bereaved to acknowledge and express their feelings

One of the most important goals of the nurse is to validate the experience and feelings of the parents by encouraging them to tell their stories and to listen with care (Corbet-Owen & Kruger, 2001). At the very least, the nurse should acknowledge the loss with a simple but sincere comment such as "I'm sorry about the baby," or "I'm sorry about your loss." Helping the parents to talk about their loss and the meaning it has for their lives and to share their emotional pain is the next step. "Tell me about what happened." Because nurses tend to be very focused on the physical and emotional needs of the mother, it is especially important to ask the father directly about his views of what happened and his feelings of loss.

The nurse should listen patiently during the story of loss or grief, but listening is hard work and can be painful for the helper. The feelings and emotions of expressed grief can overwhelm health care professionals. Being with someone who is terribly sad and crying or sobbing can be extremely difficult. The initial impulse to reduce one's sense of helplessness is to say or do something that you think will reduce their pain. Although such a response may seem supportive at the time, it can stifle the further expression of emotion. Bereaved parents have identified many unhelpful responses made to them by well-meaning health care professionals, family, and friends. The nurse should resist the temptation to give advice or to use clichés in offering support to the bereaved (Box 28-4). Nurses need to be comfortable with their own feelings of grief and loss to support and care for bereaved persons effectively. The nurse should have a presence of self, the willingness to be alongside, quietly supporting the bereaved in whatever expressions of feelings or emotions are appropriate for them. This presence leaves parents feeling that they were cared for. Leaning forward, nodding the head, and saying "Uh-huh" or "Tell me more" is often en-

What to Say and What Not to Say to Bereaved Parents

WHAT TO SAY

"I'm sad for you."

"How are you doing with all of this?"

"This must be hard for you."

"What can I do for you?"

"I'm sorry."

"I'm here, and I want to listen."

WHAT NOT TO SAY

"God had a purpose for her."

"Be thankful you have another child."

"The living must go on."

"I know how you feel."

"It's God's will."

"You have to keep on going for her sake."

"You're young; you can have others."

"We'll see you back here next year, and you'll be happier."

"Now you have an angel in heaven."

"This happened for the best."

"Better for this to happen now, before you knew the baby."

"There was something wrong with the baby anyway."

Used with permission of Bereavement Services. Copyright Lutheran Hospital–La Crosse, Inc., a Gundersen Lutheran Affiliate, La Crosse, WI.

couragement enough for the bereaved person to tell his or her story. Sitting through the silence can be therapeutic; silence gives the bereaved person an opportunity to collect thoughts and to process what he or she is sharing. Furthermore, careful assessment is important before using touch as a therapeutic technique. For some, touch is a meaningful expression of concern, but for others it is an invasion of privacy.

Bereaved parents have many questions surrounding the event of their loss that can leave them feeling guilty. This is particularly true for mothers. Such questions include "What did I do?" "What caused this to happen?" "What do you think I should have, could have done?" Part of the grief process for bereaved parents is figuring out what happened, their role in the loss, why it happened to them, and why it happened to their baby. The nurse should recognize that the answers to these questions must be answered by the bereaved themselves; it is part of their healing. For example, a bereaved mother might ask, "Do you think that this was caused by painting the baby's room?" An appropriate response might be, "I understand you need to find an answer for why your baby died, but we really don't know why she died. What are some of the other things you have been thinking about?" Trying to give bereaved parents answers when there are no clear answers or trying to squelch their guilt feelings by telling them they should not feel guilty does not help them process their grief. In reality, many times there are no definite an-

swers to the question of why this terrible thing has happened to them. However, factual information, such as data about the frequency of miscarriages in pregnant women or the fact that there usually is no clear cause for a stillbirth, can be helpful.

Stillbirth can create intense feelings of incompleteness and failure. There may be culturally bound taboos against talking about death, taking part in events related to death, or expressing grief in public that can influence the grieving process (Hsu, Tseng, Banks, & Kuo, 2004).

Feelings of anger, guilt, and sadness can occur immediately but often become more problematic in the early days and months after a loss. When a bereaved person expresses feelings of anger, it can be helpful to identify the feeling by simply saying, "You sound angry," or "You look angry." The nurse's willingness to sit down and listen to these feelings of anger can help the bereaved move past those surface feelings into the underlying feelings of powerlessness and helplessness in not being able to control the many aspects of the situation.

Normalize the grief process and facilitate positive coping

While helping parents share their feelings of pain, it is critical to help them understand their grief responses and feel they are not alone in these painful responses. Most parents are not prepared for the raw feelings that they experience or the fact that these painful, complex feelings and related behavioral reactions continue for many weeks or months. Reassuring them of the normality of their responses and preparing them for the length of their grief is important. The nurse can help the parent be prepared for the emptiness, loneliness, and yearning; for the feelings of helplessness that can lead to anger, guilt, and fear; and for the cognitive processing problems, disorganization, difficulty making decisions; and sadness and depression that are part of the grief process. Books and pamphlets about grief, if short and sensitive, can be given to parents to take home. Many parents have reported feelings of fear that they were going crazy because of the many emotions and behavioral responses that leave them feeling totally out of control in the months after the loss. It is essential for the nurse to reassure and educate bereaved parents about the grief process, including the physical, social, and emotional responses of individuals and families. Offering health teaching on the bereavement process alone is not enough, however. In the initial days after a loss, other strategies might include follow-up phone calls, referrals to a perinatal grief support group, or provision of a list of publications or websites intended to help parents who have experienced a perinatal loss (see Community Activity). As with any referral, however, the nurse should first read the materials or check out the websites (see Resources at the end of the chapter).

To reduce relationship problems that can occur in couples who are grieving, it is particularly important to help them understand that they may respond and grieve in very different ways. Differences in grieving can lead to serious marital problems and be a risk factor for complicated bereavement. Remind the couple of the importance of being understanding and patient with each other. Nurses can reinforce positive coping efforts and attempt to prevent negative coping. They can remind the parents of the importance of being patient and being good to themselves during the grief process. In particular, nurses should discourage dependence on drugs and alcohol.

Meet the physical needs of the postpartum bereaved mother

Coping with loss and grief after childbirth can be an overwhelming experience for the woman and her family. One particularly difficult aspect of the loss is the sound of crying babies and the happiness of other families on the unit who have given birth to healthy infants. The mother should be given the opportunity to decide if she wants to remain on the maternity unit or be moved to another hospital unit. She also should be helped to understand the advantages and disadvantages of each choice. Postpartum care as well as grief support may not be as good on another hospital unit where the staff are not experienced in postpartum and bereavement care. The physical needs of a bereaved mother are the same as those of any woman who has given birth. The cruel reality for many bereaved mothers is that their milk may come in with no baby to nurse, their afterpains remind them of their emptiness, and gas pains feel as though a baby is still moving inside. The nurse should ensure that the mother receives appropriate medications to reduce these physical signs and symptoms. Adequate rest, diet, and fluids must be offered to replenish her physical strength. Mothers need postpartum care instructions on discharge. They also need ideas about how to cope with problems with sleep such as decreasing food or fluids that contain caffeine, limiting alcohol and nicotine consumption, exercising regularly, using strategies for rest, taking a warm bath or drinking warm milk before bedtime, doing relaxation exercises, listening to restful music, or getting a massage. Furthermore, the couple needs to be encouraged and supported in maintaining their relationship and keeping open channels of communication. They also need to be prepared for some of the issues related to resuming sexual intimacy after perinatal loss.

Assist the bereaved in communicating with, supporting, and getting support from family

Providing sensitive care to bereaved parents means including their families in the grief process. Grandparents and siblings are particularly important when a perinatal loss has occurred. However, it is up to the parents to decide to what extent they want family involved in their grief process. If it is the parents' desire, children, grandparents, extended family members, and friends should be allowed to be involved in the rituals surrounding the death, such as seeing and hold-

ing the baby. Such visits afford others the opportunity to become acquainted with the baby, to understand the parents' loss, to offer their support, and to say good-bye (see Fig. 28-2). This experience helps parents explain to their surviving children who their brother or sister was and what death means, offers the children answers to their questions in a concrete manner, and helps the children in expressing their grief. Involving extended family and friends enables the parents to mobilize their social support system of people who will support the family not only at the time of loss but also in the future.

Parents also need information about how grief affects a family. They may need help in understanding and coping with the potential differing responses of various family members. Frustrations may arise because of the insensitive or inadequate responses of other family members. Parents may need help in determining ways to let family members know how they feel and what they need.

Create memories for parents to take home

Parents may want tangible mementos of their baby to allow them to actualize the loss. Some may want to bring in a previously purchased baby book. Special memory books, cards, and information about grief and mourning are available for purchase by parents or hospitals or clinics through national perinatal bereavement organizations (Fig. 28-5).

The nurse can provide information about the baby's weight, length, and head circumference to the family. Footprints and handprints can be taken and placed with the other information on a special card or in a memory or baby book. Sometimes it is difficult to obtain good handprints or footprints. Application of alcohol or acetone on the palms or soles can help the ink adhere to make the prints clearer, es-

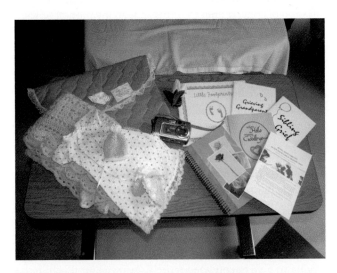

Fig. 28-5 A memory kit assembled at John C. Lincoln Hospital, Phoenix, AZ. Memory kits may include pictures of the infant, clothing, death certificate, footprints, identification bands, fetal monitor printout, and ultrasound picture. (Courtesy Julie Perry Nelson, Gilbert, AZ.)

pecially for small babies. When making prints, have a hard surface underneath the paper to be printed. The baby's heel or palm is placed down first, the foot or hand is rolled forward, keeping the toes or fingers extended. It may be helpful to have assistance with the procedure. If the print does not turn out, tracing around the baby's hands and feet can be done, although this distorts the actual size. A form of plaster of paris can also be used to make an imprint of the baby's hand or foot.

Parents often appreciate articles that were in contact with or used in caring for the baby. This might include the tape measure used to measure the baby, baby lotions, combs, clothing, hats, blankets, crib cards, and identification bands. The identification band helps the parents remember the size of the baby and personalizes the mementos. The nurse should ask parents if they wish to have these articles before giving them to the parents. A lock of hair may be another important keepsake. Parents must be asked for permission before cutting a lock of hair, which can be removed from the nape of the neck where it is not noticeable.

For some, pictures are the most important memento. Photographs should be taken whenever there is an identifiable baby and when it is culturally acceptable to the family. It does not matter how tiny the baby is, what the baby looks like, or how long the baby has been dead. Pictures should include close-ups of the baby's face, hands, and feet. Pictures should be taken of the baby clothed and wrapped in a blanket as well as unclothed. If there are any congenital anomalies, close-ups of the anomalies also should be taken. Flowers, blocks, stuffed animals, or toys can be placed in the background to make the picture more special. Parents may want their pictures taken holding the baby. Keeping a camera nearby and taking pictures when parents are spending special time with their baby can provide special memories. Some parents may have their own camera or video camera and would like the nurse to record them as they bathe, dress, hold, or diaper their baby.

Communicate using a caring framework

Mothers, fathers, and extended families look to the nursing staff for support and understanding during the time of loss. Nurses have an important role in providing sensitive care to parents at the time of a perinatal loss. The nurse needs to take the time to understand the meaning of the loss to the woman and her family. The nurse provides physical care, comfort, and safety for the woman and her family. Offers of information, anticipatory guidance, choices for decision making, and support during hospitalization and after discharge help the family feel more in control of a situation in which they feel very much out of control. The woman and her family are encouraged to believe in their own ability to begin the process of healing. The nurse spends time with the family, learns their inner strengths and coping abilities, and points out these inner resources to the family by saying, "I know this is a difficult time for you, but I have seen some of your inner strength and know that you will be able to make it through all of this."

Be concerned about cultural and spiritual needs of parents

Parents who experience perinatal loss can be from widely diverse cultural and ethnic groups. In addition, parents belong to many different religious groups. Many of the responses that are described and the interventions suggested in this chapter are based on European-American views of perinatal grief and loss. Although it is thought that there are no particular differences in the individual, intrapersonal experiences of grief based on culture, ethnicity, or religion, many differences are found in mourning rituals, traditions, and behavioral expressions of grief that are often ignored or misunderstood. Therefore the practices suggested earlier may not be appropriate for parents from other cultural, ethnic, and religious groups, and the nurse must consider the potential unique responses and needs of parents from different groups. This involves understanding the cultural orientation and beliefs of the individual parent, the partner, the extended family, and the larger community to which they belong.

Cultural and religious differences can affect the way parents respond to a perinatal loss. This includes their way of

---

 ### *Critical Thinking Exercise*

The Bereaved Couple

Marsha gave birth to a stillborn 17-week fetus. This is her second miscarriage. She has been diagnosed with premature dilation of the cervix. She and her husband, Andrew, are in the LDRP room 1 hour after the birth. Both are crying softly. Andrew has his arm around Marsha and is trying to comfort her. You have just come on duty and are assigned to care for the couple. When you enter the room, Marsha says, "Why did this happen? I want a baby so badly. I did everything right; I did exactly what the doctor told me to do. My sister has five children and she didn't even want the last one. What is the matter with me? Why is God doing this to us?" How should you respond to Marsha's questions? What can you do to comfort the couple? Should they see the baby?

1 Evidence—Is there sufficient evidence to draw conclusions about factors interfering with healthy bereavement? About appropriate support related to accepting the death of the baby? Is the fact that this is Marsha's second miscarriage a factor in her grief?
2 Assumptions—What assumptions can be made about the following factors?
  a. A diagnosis of premature dilation of the cervix
  b. A second miscarriage
  c. The importance of the father's support
  d. Andrew's need for an outlet for his grief
3 What implications and priorities for nursing care can be drawn at this time?
4 Does the evidence objectively support your conclusion?
5 Are there alternative perspectives to your conclusion?

communicating with health care professionals, as well as their emotional and behavioral responses and family interaction patterns. Some groups, such as Orthodox Jews, may not support the notion of grieving for perinatal loss because the fetus or stillborn infant is not considered a person. Some African-American women were found to use self-healing strategies that reflect inner processes, resources, and remedies (Van, 2001). Mothers from some cultural groups may have intense somatic symptoms. In some cultures, such as the Muslim culture, decisions are communal (Arshad, Horsfall, & Yasin, 2004). Expressions of grief may range from quiet and stoic to dramatic and hysterical for different Native American groups. Native Americans from many tribes would not respond well to an "interviewing" or "questioning" approach (Lawson, 1990). Mexican mothers may be very demonstrative in their grief, while also struggling with the view that hardship is "God's will" (Lawson, 1990).

With perinatal loss, culture and religious beliefs can affect issues such as seeing the child, naming the child, and taking pictures. Some cultural and religious groups do not believe in naming an infant who dies before 30 days of age. Picture taking can conflict with beliefs of some cultures, such as some Native American, Eskimo, Amish, Hindu, and Muslim cultures. Families from these cultures should be sensitively offered this opportunity but not pushed into having a picture taken.

Many different taboos and expectations are related to death for different religious groups. Autopsies are not allowed by some religions except under unusual circumstances. Cremation is forbidden by the Jewish religion, Baha'is, and the Greek Orthodox Church (Harakas, 1999). It is discouraged or allowed only under unusual circumstances in the Church of Jesus Christ of Latter-Day Saints. Embalming is not allowed for Jews, Baha'is, and Muslims.

Culture and religious beliefs also influence the customs surrounding death. Many religious groups have rituals, such as prayers, ritualistic washing and shrouding, or anointing with oil, that are performed at the time of death. Baptism is extremely important for Roman Catholics and some Protestant groups. Baptism can be performed by a lay person, such as a nurse, in an emergency situation when a priest cannot be there in a timely fashion (Box 28-5).

Many Protestant groups believe that baptism is conducted at the age of reason, and parents from these religions would not want their baby baptized. When bereaved parents need a referral for grief counseling, cultural considerations are paramount. Native Americans, for example, are best referred to native healers and counselors rather than to Western biomedical therapists (Lawson, 1990).

Provide sensitive care at and after discharge

When leaving the hospital, mothers are often taken out in a wheelchair. This can be a devastating experience for the mother who has experienced a pregnancy loss. Leaving the hospital without a baby in her arms is a very empty and

---

BOX 28-5

Infant Baptism

In an emergency, Christian baptism may be performed by anyone by pouring water over the forehead (or products of conception) and saying "I baptize you in the name of the Father and of the Son and of the Holy Spirit." The person performing the baptism needs only to have the intention of baptizing and does not necessarily have to believe in infant baptism for the baptism to be valid. If the infant has no signs of life, the person performing the baptism can add "If you are alive, I baptize you . . . " In the Greek Orthodox tradition, baptism is only for the living; thus a miscarried or stillborn infant would not be baptized. If the infant is born alive and in serious danger of death, the infant can be lifted up while saying "The servant of God is baptized in the name of the Father and the Son and the Holy Spirit" (Harakas, 1999).

---

painful experience. It is especially difficult if others are seen leaving with babies; therefore the discharge of mothers and fathers who have experienced a perinatal loss should be done with great sensitivity to their feelings. They should not be discharged at a time when other mothers with live babies are leaving. Giving the mother a special flower to carry in her arms can be a thoughtful gesture.

The grief of the mother and her family does not end with discharge; rather it really begins once they return home, attend the funeral, and start to live their lives without their baby. Follow-up phone calls after a loss may be helpful to some parents. However, it must be determined when parents do not want a follow-up call, which often is the case after early loss. Follow-up calls let the parents know they are still thought of and cared about. The calls are made at predictably difficult times such as the first week at home, 1 month to 6 weeks later, 4 to 6 months after the loss, and at the anniversary of the death. Families who experienced a miscarriage, ectopic pregnancy, or death of a premature baby may appreciate a phone call on the estimated date of birth. The calls provide an opportunity for parents to ask questions, share their feelings, seek advice, and receive information to help them in processing their grief.

A grief conference can be planned when parents return for an appointment with their doctor, nurses, and other health care providers. At the conference, the loss or death of the infant is discussed in detail, parents are given information about the baby's autopsy report and genetic studies, and they have opportunities to ask the questions that have arisen since their baby's death. Parents appreciate the opportunity to review the events of hospitalization, go over the baby's and/or mother's chart with their primary health care provider, and talk with those who cared for them and their baby during hospitalization. This is an important time to help parents understand the cause of the loss, or to accept the fact that the cause will forever be unknown. This gives health care professionals the opportunity to assess how the family is coping with their loss and provide additional information and education on grief.

Some parents are very interested in finding a perinatal or parental grief support group. They appreciate the opportunity to talk with others who have been through similar experiences. A grief support group also can be helpful for sharing feelings and gaining an understanding of the normality of the grief process. An online perinatal loss listserv is a way to connect women who are geographically distant but share similar stories and pain (Capitulo, 2004). A group for women experiencing pregnancy after loss is also useful (Cote-Arsenault & Freije, 2004).

Over time, a support group may be the only place where bereaved parents can talk about the wished-for child and their grief. However, not all parents find such groups helpful. When referring to a group, it is important to know something about the group and how it operates. For example, if a group has a religious basis for their interventions, a non-religious parent would not be likely to find the group helpful. If parents experiencing a perinatal loss are referred to a parental grief group, they might feel overwhelmed with the grief of parents whose older children have died of cancer, suicide, or homicide. In addition, their grief might be minimized by participants; therefore the needs of the parents must be matched with the focus of the group.

Evaluation

The evaluation of nursing care is made more difficult by the shock and numbness of the bereavement process and the varied grief responses of the parents and other family members during hospitalization. The achievement of expected outcomes is assured when the positive integration of the perinatal loss is expressed by the family (Plan of Care).

One approach to evaluation is the use of checklists. Many hospitals have checklists used in providing care, mobilizing members of the multidisciplinary health care team, communicating options the family has chosen, and keeping track of all the details in meeting the needs of bereaved parents (Fig. 28-6). Such checklists may be a permanent part of the chart. Documentation in the nursing notes of primary concerns, grief responses, health teaching, health care advice, and any referrals of the mother or other family members is essential to ensure continuity and consistency of care.

✍ PLAN OF CARE   *Fetal Death: 20 Weeks of Gestation*

NURSING DIAGNOSIS Dysfunctional grieving related to fetal death, as evidenced by intense expressions of grief for prolonged period of time
Expected Outcome *Parents will identify appropriate ways to deal with grief.*

Nursing Interventions/*Rationales*

- Prepare family for viewing fetus by cleaning body and wrapping in clean blanket *to initiate and support the grieving process in a supportive setting.*
- Allow family quiet time to hold and view fetus. Take pictures for family to keep *to provide sense of reality regarding the death and support the grieving process.*
- Provide a certificate for the family with vital statistics, along with identification bands, lock of hair, and footprints *to emphasize reality of situation and support the grieving process.*
- Provide spiritual support as needed to assist with religious services such as baptism and memorial services *to provide spiritual support and assist with religious practices.*
- Refer to appropriate community support groups *to facilitate grieving with group input and to share experiences.*

NURSING DIAGNOSIS Situational low self-esteem related to fetal death as evidenced by mother's or family's intense feelings of guilt
Expected Outcomes *Mother and family will exhibit positive self-image and adapt to death of fetus in a timely manner.*

Nursing Interventions/*Rationales*

- Provide private time for expressions of feelings through therapeutic communication and active listening *to validate feelings.*
- Identify mother's and family's perception and feelings about fetal death *to correct any misconceptions and alleviate guilt.*

- Assist mother and family to identify positive coping mechanisms and support systems *to promote feelings of self-worth.*
- Refer to appropriate health professionals for further evaluation and counseling, such as social service, *to provide ongoing assistance as needed.*

NURSING DIAGNOSIS Spiritual distress related to perinatal loss
Expected Outcome *Parents will verbalize a decrease in spiritual distress.*

Nursing Interventions/*Rationales*

- Assess parent's spiritual preference *to reinforce parent's own beliefs.*
- Assist with spiritual rituals for parents and infant *to promote comfort for parents.*
- Provide opportunity for parents to express feelings about perinatal loss *to facilitate the grief process.*
- Assist parents in contacting the facility's chaplain or personal spiritual advisor *to provide spiritual support.*

NURSING DIAGNOSIS Ineffective family coping
Expected Outcome *Family will use coping strategies to accept death of fetus.*

Nursing Interventions/*Rationales*

- Encourage parents to seek emotional support from each other *to improve coping ability.*
- Assist grandparents to participate in grieving with their son/daughter *to demonstrate understanding and support.*
- Refer parents to grief support group *to provide ongoing assistance and support.*
- Listen to parents' expressions of grief *to enhance understanding of factors creating distress and give direction to support.*

CD: Plan of Care—Fetal Death: 20 Weeks of Gestation

RTS Bereavement Services
CHECKLIST FOR ASSISTING PARENT(S) EXPERIENCING STILLBIRTH OR NEWBORN DEATH

SAMPLE

Mother's discharge date: _____
Mother's name: _____
Address: _____
Phone number: ( ) _____
Father's name: _____
Address: _____
Phone number: ( ) _____
Optimal call time: _____
RTS Counselor: _____
Unit: _____ Ext _____
Regular OB MD/Midwife: _____
Religion: _____

Age _____ Gr ___ Para ___ L.C. ___ Due date _____
Previous loss: _____
Date/Time delivered: _____
Date/Time death: _____
Baby's name: _____ Sex: _____
Children's name(s): _____ Age: _____
_____ Age: _____
_____ Age: _____
Support people
Attending MD &/or Pediatrician _____
Notify Peds Nurse Practitioner _____

Date	Time		Comments	Initials
		Notify/Assign RTS counselor ☐ Yes ☐ No		
		Pastoral Care notified ☐ Yes ☐ No		
		Funeral Home notified: ☐ Yes ☐ No Family Burial: ☐ Yes ☐ No		
		Saw baby when born and/or after delivery: ☐ Mother ☐ Father		
		Touched and/or held baby: ☐ Mother ☐ Father		
		☐ Siblings ☐ Grandparents ☐ Friends		
		Offered private time with their baby: ☐ Yes ☐ No		
		Baptism offered: (use seashell as vessel, give to parents) ☐ Yes ☐ No		
		Remembrance of Blessing offered: ☐ Yes ☐ No		
		(can offer for any perinatal loss) ☐ Given to parents		
		Given option to transfer off Maternity Unit: ☐ Yes ☐ No		
		Patient's room flagged with door card ☐ Yes ☐ No		
		Autopsy: ☐ Yes ☐ No Genetic studies: ☐ Yes ☐ No		
		Genetic Associate notified: ☐ Yes ☐ No		
		Regular Physician/Midwife notified of death: ☐ Yes ☐ No		
		Memo sent to Physician/Midwife: ☐ Yes ☐ No		
		Section of Fetal monitor strip: ☐ Given to parents ☐ On file		
		ID Bands/Crib cards/Tape measure: ☐ Given to parents ☐ On file		
		Footprints/Handprints/Weight/Length recorded on "In Memory Of" sheet: ☐ Given to parents ☐ On file		
		Lock of hair offered: (ask permission) ☐ Yes ☐ No		
		☐ Given to parents ☐ On file		
		Mementos (clothing, hat, blanket, pacifier, crib cards, basin, baby ring, bear, thermometer, silk flower) ☐ Given to parents ☐ On file		
		Complimentary birth keepsake ☐ Given to parents ☐ On file		
		RTS Photos taken: (clothed, unclothed, w. props, family photo)		
		1) Polaroid - 3 or more ☐ Given to parents ☐ On file		
		2) 35 mm (6-12 pictures) ☐ Given to parents ☐ On file		
		3) Medical photos: ☐ Yes ☐ No		

Fig. 28-6 Sample checklist for assisting parents experiencing stillbirth or newborn death. (Used with permission of Bereavement Services. Copyright Lutheran Hospital–La Crosse, Inc., A Gundersen Lutheran Affiliate, La Crosse, WI.)

Date	Time		Comments	Initials
		Informed about postponing funeral until mother is able to attend: ☐ Yes ☐ No		
		Services/Funeral arrangements, options discussed: ☐ Self-transport ☐ Gravesite service ☐ Visitation ☐ Hospital chapel ☐ Cremation ☐ Funeral home ☐ Burial at foot or head of relative's grave ☐ Specific area for babies in cemetery ☐ Plan own service		

		Funeral arrangements made by: ☐ Mother ☐ Father
		Discussed: ☐ Seeing baby at funeral home
		  ☐ Taking pictures there
		  ☐ Providing outfit/toy for baby
		  ☐ Dressing baby at funeral home		

		Grief information packet given to: ☐ Mother ☐ Father		
		Discussed grief process/incongruent grief with: ☐ Mother ☐ Father		
		Discussed grief conference: ☐ Yes ☐ No		
		RTS Parents Support Group brochure given to: ☐ Mother ☐ Father		
		RTS business card given to: ☐ Mother ☐ Father		
		Pregnancy & Infant Loss Card sent to RTS secretary: ☐ Yes ☐ No		
		Follow-up calls: 1 week: . . . . 3 weeks:. . . . . Due date:. . . . . 6-10 months: . . . . Anniversary date:		
		Grief conference planned with parents: Date _____ Time _____ Place _____ Letter of confirmation sent: ☐ Yes ☐ No		
		Parent Support Group, first meeting attended: Date: _____ Follow-up meetings attended: Dates _____		
		Would like another parent to call: ☐ Yes ☐ No ☐ Ask later Parent contact: _____		

Forms Needed: Report of fetal death (Photocopy and save for mother.)
  Autopsy if ordered
  Record of death
  Genetics protocol (folder) if ordered
  Notice of removal of a human corpse from an institution
  Final disposition form
  If funeral home involved - Final disposition will be completed by them.
  Original certificate of death (for NB death only)

Note: <u>Family Burial</u> - Check with your funeral home.

** You may wish to list your hospital and state forms that are necessary, as required by your state laws and your institution.

Fig. 28-6 cont'd

SPECIAL LOSSES ■

Prenatal Diagnoses with Negative Outcome

Early prenatal diagnostic tests such as ultrasonography, chorionic villus sampling, and amniocentesis can determine the well-being of the embryo or fetus. Reasons for prenatal testing include history of chromosomal abnormality in the family; three or more miscarriages; maternal age over 35 years; lack of fetal growth, movement, or heart beat; and diabetes mellitus or other chronic illnesses. If the health care provider is certain that the baby has a serious genetic defect that would lead to death in utero or after birth (congenital anomalies incompatible with life or genetic disorders with severe mental retardation), the choice of interruption of a pregnancy may be offered. Abortion is controversial, and this may prevent parents from sharing this decision with other family members or friends. This limits their support systems after their loss.

The decision to terminate a pregnancy paves the way for feelings such as guilt, despair, sadness, depression, and anger. The nurse's role is to be a good listener. It is important to assess how these families feel about the experience and to offer options for their memories as appropriate. Healing can take place when words can be given to feelings and needs can be met.

The parent who decides to continue the pregnancy also requires emotional support. The time of labor and birth can be particularly difficult. The nurse should remember that parents may be grieving not only the loss of the perfect child but the loss of expectations for their child's future.

Loss of One in a Multiple Birth

The death of a twin or baby in a multifetal gestation during pregnancy, labor, or birth or after birth requires parents to parent and grieve at the same time. Such a death results in a confusing and ambivalent induction into parenthood. Parents feel that they cannot do anything right. They cannot parent their surviving child with all the joy and enthusiasm of new parents because their surviving child reminds them of what they have lost. They cannot give over completely and grieve in the manner they need to because their surviving child demands their attention. These parents are at risk for altered parenting and complicated bereavement.

It is important to help the parents acknowledge the birth of all their babies. Parents should be treated as bereaved families, and all the options previously discussed should be offered. Pictures should be taken of the babies, and parents should be offered the opportunity to hold their babies in their arms and have time to say good-bye to the baby who has died.

Bereaved parents should be warned that well-meaning family members or friends may say, "Well, at least you have the other baby," implying that there should be no grief because they are lucky to have one at all. Parents need to be able to anticipate insensitivity to their loss and be empowered to say to those people, "That is not how I feel." By simply setting a boundary on what their feelings are, they are able to acknowledge the baby who died and then have an opportunity to share more about their feelings if they so choose.

Bereaved parents of multiples have special problems in coping with life without their anticipated "extra special" family, telling their surviving child about his or her twin, dealing with the possibility of that child's feelings of survivor guilt, and deciding on how to celebrate birthdays, death days, or special holidays.

Adolescent Grief

Adolescent pregnancy accounts for many births in the United States. Each year, many adolescents experience perinatal loss, including as elective abortion or miscarriage. Although adolescent participants have been included in the samples of research done in all areas of perinatal bereavement, their unique responses to perinatal loss have not been identified. Adolescents grieve the loss of their babies and need the emotional support from the nurses who care for them. However, nurses and other health care professionals, as well as family members, often believe that the adolescent's loss of her baby was for the best, so that the adolescent can

move on with her life. Adolescent girls, then, may not receive the support they need from staff and family. In addition, adolescent girls usually do not have the support from the father of the baby as compared with older women who have a perinatal loss; therefore there is a great need to provide sensitive care to all adolescents who experience any type of perinatal loss.

The first step for the nurse in caring for a bereaved adolescent is to acknowledge the significance of giving birth, no matter what the mother's age. Second, the nurse should make additional efforts to develop a trusting relationship with the adolescent. Third, the nurse should offer options for saying goodbye, anticipatory guidance, support, and information to meet the adolescent at the point of her need. It may take longer for adolescents to process their grief because of their level of cognitive and emotional maturation. Being patient, saving mementos, and giving the adolescent information on how to contact the nurse are interventions that can help the adolescent accept the reality of the loss and process her grief.

COMPLICATED BEREAVEMENT ■

Although most parents cope adequately with the pain of their grief and return to some level of normal functioning, some parents have extremely intense grief reactions that last for a very long time; this response is complicated bereavement. Other parents have grief from one loss that is exaggerated or intensified by other past losses. A long preloss pregnancy (e.g., the fetus died in late gestation), a more neurotic personality, more preexisting psychiatric symptoms, and a lack of other living children are important risk factors for stronger grief reactions for either parent (Janssen, Cuisinier, de Graauw, Hoogduin, 1997).

Evidence of complicated grief includes continued obsession with yearning and loneliness, intense and continued guilt or anger, relentless depression or anxiety that interferes with role functioning, abuse of drugs (including prescription medications) or alcohol, severe relationship difficulties, continued feelings of inadequacy and low self-esteem, and suicidal thoughts or threats. Feelings of inadequacy, in particular, were strongly and positively related to distress after 4 years (Hunfeld, Wladimiroff, & Passchier, 1997). Parents showing signs of complicated grief should be referred for counseling. It is the responsibility of a qualified mental health professional to determine whether the parents are experiencing a normal, albeit intense grief response or whether they are also having a serious mental health problem such as depression. However, it is important to refer to a therapist or counselor who is experienced in grief counseling and knows how to help the bereaved, because some therapists and counselors do not have an understanding of the special needs related to grief.

Therapy is a big step. The highest number of cancellations and "no shows" in a therapist's practice are intakes, or first visits; therefore, anything the nurse can do for a family or individual to help with that major hurdle would be useful. However, it also is important to remember that people may have symptoms but may not, for whatever reason, be ready to deal directly with these symptoms or may not have the energy to make the call. Enlisting a family member to encourage parents to seek such assistance may be helpful.

COMMUNITY ACTIVITY

1. Identify community resources and support groups for parents who have experienced the following:
   a. Infertility
   b. Birth of a less-than-perfect child
   c. Death of a baby through miscarriage, stillbirth, or newborn death
   What services do each of these resources or groups provide?
2. Interview a mother, father, or couple who have experienced a perinatal loss.
   a. Ask them to tell you their story and then listen intently for their story lines.
   b. Ask them who or what helped them the most.
   c. Ask who or what made their experience more difficult.
   d. Ask what they would want nursing students caring for such parents to know so they may help parents.

Key Points

- Parental and infant attachment can begin before pregnancy with many hopes and dreams for the future.
- The gestational age of the baby influences neither the severity of the grief response nor the bereavement process.
- When a baby dies, all members of a family are affected, but no two family members grieve in the same way.
- When birth represents death, the role of the nurse is critical in caring for the woman and her family, regardless of the age of the woman or stage of gestation.
- An understanding of the grief process is fundamental in the implementation of the nursing process.

- Assessment of each family member's perception and experience of the loss is important.
- Therapeutic communication and counseling techniques can help families identify their feelings, feel comfortable in expressing their grief, and understand their bereavement process.
- Follow-up after discharge can be an important component in providing care to families who have experienced a loss.
- Nurses need to be aware of their own feelings of grief and loss to provide a nonjudgmental environment of care and support for bereaved families.

Answer Guidelines to Critical Thinking Exercise

The Bereaved Couple

1. Yes, there is sufficient evidence to draw conclusions about factors interfering with healthy bereavement. Marsha may feel guilty about the death of her baby in spite of the fact that many stillbirths are unexplainable. She also may feel shame or incomplete as a woman because of the inability of her cervix to stay closed to permit pregnancy to continue. Women who have previously experienced a stillbirth have higher stress and anxiety than other pregnant women. There are excellent sources on appropriate support related to accepting the death of the baby and suggestions for what to say and what not to say (see Resources).
2. a. Some women with premature dilation of the cervix experience pregnancies that attain a longer gestation each time until finally a viable infant is born. She may be a candidate for a cerclage.
   b. Women who have experienced miscarriage often are anxious until the current pregnancy exceeds the gestation at which the previous miscarriage occurred.
   c. Support of the father is very important, as is that of the family.

d. Andrew will also need support and understanding. He needs to be able to be vulnerable and express his feelings about the loss. Parents may express grief differently; they require good communication and understanding to resolve their differences.
3. The priority for nursing care at this time is to allow the couple to express their feelings: grief, anger, and sadness. They should be offered the opportunity to view, hold, and care for the baby. A memory kit should be assembled. The couple should be given the choice of moving off the maternity floor to another one. They may need assistance with contacting clergy, arranging for burial, etc. (A 17-week fetus does not have to be buried, but the parents may choose to do so.)
4. There is considerable information derived from research on death and dying, including appropriate support for bereaved parents.
5. Various cultures and religions may view a 17-week baby as a fetus and may not choose to name the baby, have it baptized, or buried. Some parents may choose cremation.

Resources

American Association of Pastoral Counselors (AAPC)
www.aapc.org

Bay Memorials
321 S. 15th Street
Escanaba, MI 49829
www.baymemorialsbabycaskets.com
906-786-2609

The Compassionate Friends (self-help organization for bereaved parents and siblings)
www.compassionatefriends.org

Griefnet (collection of resources of value to those who are experiencing loss and grief)
www.griefnet.org

Growth House, Inc. (grief related to pregnancy, including miscarriage, stillbirth, termination of pregnancy, and neonatal death)
www.growthhouse.org

Hannah's Prayer (Christian support for fertility challenges)
www.hannah.org

Houston's Aid in Neonatal Death (HAND): Supporting grieving parents in the greater Houston area with the rest of the world via the Internet
www.hern.org/~hand

Hygeia (online journal for pregnancy and neonatal loss: Dr. Michael Berman)
www.connix.com/~hygeia/

Miscarriage Support and Information Resources (comprehensive resource list)
www.pinelandpress.com/support/miscarriage.html

NAME, the National Association of Medical Examiners
430 Pryor St., SW
Atlanta, GA 30312
404-730-4781
404-730-4420 (fax)
www.thename.org

OBGYN.net (list of resources for loss and bereavement)
www.obgyn.net/woman/loss/loss.htm

Pen-Parents, Inc. (international nonprofit support network for bereaved parents)
www.penparents.org

A Place to Remember (uplifting resources for those who have been touched by a crisis in pregnancy or the birth of a baby)
www.aplacetoremember.com

SHARE
Pregnancy and Infant Loss Support, Inc.
www.nationalshareoffice.com

SIDS NETWORK
Sudden infant death syndrome (SIDS) information website
www.sids-network.org
1-800Autopsy.com
1-800-autopsy (1-800-288-6779)
info@1800autopsy.com

References

Armstrong, D. (2001). Exploring fathers' experiences of pregnancy after a prior perinatal loss. *MCN American Journal of Maternal Child Nursing, 26*(3), 147-153.

Armstrong, D. (2004). Impact of prior perinatal loss on subsequent pregnancies. *Journal of Obstetric, Gynecologic, and Neonatal Nursing, 33*(6), 765-773.

Arshad, M., Horsfall, A., & Yasin, R. (2004). Pregnancy loss—the Islamic perspective. *British Journal of Midwifery, 12*(8), 481-484.

Brodlie, M., Laing, I., Keeling, J., & McKenzie, K. (2002). Ten years of neonatal autopsies in tertiary referral centre: Retrospective study. *British Medical Journal, 324*(7340), 761-763.

Burkhammer, M., Anderson, G., & Chiu, S. (2004). Grief, anxiety, stillbirth, and perinatal problems: Healing with kangaroo care. *Journal of Obstetric, Gynecologic, and Neonatal Nursing, 33*(6), 774-782.

Capitulo, K. (2004). Perinatal grief online. *MCN American Journal of Maternal Child Nursing, 29*(5), 305-311.

Cernach, M., Patricio, F., Galera, M., Moron, A., & Brunoni, D. (2004). Evaluation of a protocol for postmortem examination of stillbirths and neonatal deaths with congenital anomalies. *Pediatric Developmental Pathology, 7*(4), 335-341.

Cole, M. (September 20, 2004). Born breathless—The tragedy of stillborn births. *Nursing Spectrum, New York/New Jersey Metro Edition, 19*, 16A.

Corbet-Owen, C., & Kruger, L. (2001). The health system and emotional care: Validating the many meanings of spontaneous pregnancy loss. *Family Systems of Health, 19*, 411-417.

Cote-Arsenault, D., & Freije, M. (2004). Support groups helping women through pregnancies after loss. *Western Journal of Nursing Research, 26*(6), 650-670.

Harakas, S. (1999). Personal communication by E-mail to M. Miles.

Heiman, J., Yankowitz, J., & Wilkins, J. (1997). Grief support programs: Patients' use of services following the loss of a desired pregnancy and degree of implementation in academic centers. *American Journal of Perinatology, 14*(10), 587-591.

Hsu, M., Tseng, Y., Banks, J., & Kuo, L. (2004). Interpretations of stillbirth. *Journal of Advanced Nursing, 47*(4), 408-416.

Hughes, P., Turton, P., Hopper, E., Evans, C. (2002). Assessment of guidelines for good practice in psychosocial care of mothers after stillbirth: A cohort study. *Lancet, 360*(9327), 114-118.

Huisman, T. (2004). Magnetic resonance imaging: An alternative to autopsy in neonatal death? *Seminars in Perinatology, 9*(4), 347-353.

Hunfeld, J., Wladimiroff, J., & Passchier, J. (1997). Prediction and course of grief four years after perinatal loss due to congenital anomalies: A follow-up study. *British Journal of Medical Psychology, 70*(Pt 1), 85-91.

Janssen, H., Cuisinier, M., de Graauw, K., Hoogduin, K. (1997). A prospective study of risk factors predicting grief intensity following pregnancy loss. *Archives of General Psychiatry, 54*(1), 56-61.

Kowalski, K. (1984). *Perinatal death: An ethnomethodological study of factors influencing parental bereavement.* Doctoral dissertation, University of Colorado.

Lang, A., Goulet, C., & Amsel, R. (2004). Explanatory model of health in bereaved parents post–fetal/infant death. *International Journal of Nursing Studies, 41*(8), 869-880.

Lawson, L. (1990). Culturally sensitive support for grieving parents. *MCN American Journal of Maternal Child Nursing, 15*(2), 76-79.

Lindemann, E. (1944). Symptomatology and management of acute grief. *American Journal of Psychiatry, 101*, 141-148.

Luciano, D., Jain, A., Roy, G., Solima, E., & Luciano, A. (2004). Ectopic pregnancy—From surgical emergency to medical management. *Journal of the American Association of Gynecologic Laparoscopists, 11*(1), 109-122.

Lyon, A. (2004). Perinatal autopsy remains the "gold standard." *Archives of Disease in Childhood. Fetal and Neonatal Edition, 89*(4), F284.

Malacrida, C. (1999). Complicating mourning: The social economy of perinatal death. *Qualitative Health Research, 9*, 504-519.

Martin, J., Kochanek, K., Strobino, D., Guyer, B., & MacDorman, M. (2005). Annual summary of vital statistics—2003. *Pediatrics, 115*(3), 619-634.

McCreight, B. (2004). A grief ignored: Narratives of pregnancy loss from a male perspective. *Sociology of Health and Illness, 26*(3), 326-350.

Miles, M. (1980). *The grief of parents . . . when a child dies.* Oak Brook, IL: Compassionate Friends, Inc.

Miles, M. (1984). Helping adults mourn the death of a child. In H. Wass & C. Corr (Eds.), *Childhood and death.* New York: Hemisphere Publishing.

Miles, M., & Demi, A. (1986). Guilt in bereaved parents. In T. Rando (Ed.), *Parental loss of a child: Clinical and research considerations.* Champaign, IL: Research Press.

Miles, M., & Demi, A. (1997). Historical and contemporary theories of grief. In I. Corless, B. Germino, & M. Pittman-Lindeman (Eds.), *Dying, death and bereavement.* Boston, MA: Jones and Bartlett.

Osterweis, M., Solomon, F., & Green, M. (Eds.). (1984). *Bereavement: Reactions, consequences, and care.* Washington, DC: National Academy Press.

Parkes, C. (1972). *Bereavement: Studies of grief in adult life.* New York: International Universities Press.

Parkes, C., & Weiss, R. (1983). *Recovery from bereavement.* New York: Basic Books.

Rankin, J., Wright, C., & Lind, T. (2002). Cross sectional survey of parents' experience and views of the postmortem examination. *British Medical Journal, 324*(7341), 816-818.

Saflund, K., Sjogren, B., & Wredling, R. (2004). The role of caregivers after a stillbirth: Views and experiences of parents. *Birth, 31*(2), 132-137.

Simpson, J. (2002). Fetal wastage. In S. Gabbe, J. Niebyl, & J. Simpson (Eds.), *Obstetrics: Normal and problem pregnancies* (4th ed.). New York: Churchill Livingstone.

Toedter, L., Lasker, J., & Janssen, H. (2001). International comparison of studies using the Perinatal Grief Scale: A decade of research on pregnancy loss. *Death Studies, 25*(3), 205-228.

Van, P. (2001). Breaking the silence of African American women: Healing after pregnancy loss. *Health Care for Women International, 22*(3), 229-243.

Worden, W. (1991). *Grief counseling and grief therapy: A handbook for the mental health practitioner.* New York: Springer.

Glossary

ABO incompatibility Hemolytic disease that occurs when the mother's blood type is O and the newborn's is A, B, or AB

abruptio placentae Partial or complete premature separation of a normally implanted placenta

acceleration Increase in fetal heart rate; usually interpreted as a reassuring sign

acculturation Changes that occur within one group or among several groups when people from different cultures come in contact with one another

acoustic stimulation test Antepartum test to elicit fetal heart rate response to sound; performed by applying sound source (laryngeal stimulator) to maternal abdomen over the fetal head

acquaintance Process used by parents to get to know or become familiar with their new infant; an important step in attachment

acrocyanosis Peripheral cyanosis; blue color of hands and feet in most infants at birth that may persist for 7 to 10 days

active phase Phase in the first stage of labor when the cervix dilates from 4 to 7 cm

adequate intakes (AIs) Recommended nutrient intakes estimated to meet the needs of almost all healthy people in the population; provided for nutrients or age-group categories where the available information is not sufficient to warrant establishing recommended dietary allowances

afterbirth pains (afterpains) Painful uterine cramps that occur intermittently for approximately 2 or 3 days after birth and that result from contractile efforts of the uterus to return to its normal involuted condition

alcohol-related birth defects (ARBD) Congenital abnormality or anomaly resulting from excessive maternal alcohol intake during pregnancy. Newer terminology for fetal alcohol syndrome (FAS)

alcohol-related neurodevelopmental disorder (ARND) Infants affected by prenatal exposure to alcohol but do not meet the criteria for ARBD; previously referred to as fetal alcohol effects (FAE)

alpha-fetoprotein (AFP) Fetal antigen; elevated levels in amniotic fluid and maternal blood are associated with neural tube defects

amenorrhea Absence or cessation of menstruation

amniocentesis Procedure in which a needle is inserted through the abdominal and uterine walls to obtain amniotic fluid; used for assessment of fetal health and maturity

amnioinfusion Infusion of normal saline warmed to body temperature through an intrauterine catheter into the uterine cavity in an attempt to increase the fluid around the umbilical cord and prevent compression during uterine contractions

amniotic fluid embolism (AFE) Embolism resulting from amniotic fluid entering the maternal bloodstream during labor and birth after rupture of membranes; often fatal to the woman if it is a pulmonary embolism

amniotic fluid index (AFI) Estimation of amount of amniotic fluid by means of ultrasound to determine excess or decrease

amniotomy Artificial rupture of the fetal membranes (AROM), using a plastic Amnihook or surgical clamp

analgesia Absence of pain without loss of consciousness

anencephaly Congenital deformity characterized by the absence of cerebrum, cerebellum, and flat bones of the skull

anesthesia Partial or complete absence of sensation with or without loss of consciousness

antenatal glucocorticoids Medications administered to the mother for the purpose of accelerating fetal lung maturity when there is increased risk for preterm birth between 24 and 34 weeks of gestation

anthropometric measurements Body measurements, such as height and weight

Apgar score Numeric expression of the condition of a newborn obtained by rapid assessment at 1 and 5 minutes of age; developed by Dr. Virginia Apgar

assimilation Occurs when a cultural group loses its identity and becomes part of the dominant culture

assisted reproductive therapies (ARTs) Treatments for infertility, including in vitro fertilization procedures, embryo adoption, embryo hosting, and therapeutic insemination

asynclitism Oblique presentation of the fetal head at the superior strait of the pelvis; the pelvic planes and those of the fetal head are not parallel

attachment A specific and enduring affective tie to another person

attitude Relation of fetal parts to each other in the uterus (e.g., all parts flexed, or all parts flexed except neck is extended)

augmentation of labor Stimulation of ineffective uterine contractions after labor has started spontaneously but is not progressing satisfactorily

autoimmune disorders Group of diseases that disrupt the function of the immune system, causing the body to produce antibodies against itself, resulting in tissue damage

autolysis The self-destruction of excess hypertrophied tissue

ballottement Diagnostic technique using palpation: a floating fetus, when tapped or pushed, moves away and then returns to touch the examiner's hand

barotrauma Physical injury due to changing air pressure; often associated with ventilatory assistance in preterm infants

basal body temperature (BBT) Lowest body temperature of a healthy person taken immediately after awakening and before getting out of bed

baseline fetal heart rate Average fetal heart rate during a 10-minute period that excludes periodic and episodic changes and periods of marked variability

becoming a mother Transformation and growth of the mother identity

bereavement The feelings of loss, pain, desolation, and sadness that occur after the death of a loved one

best practice A program or service that has been recognized for excellence

binuclear family Family after divorce, in which the child is a member of both the maternal and paternal nuclear households

biophysical profile (BPP) Noninvasive assessment of the fetus and its environment using ultrasonography and fetal monitoring; includes fetal breathing movements, gross body movements, fetal tone, reactive fetal heart rate, and qualitative amniotic fluid volume

biorhythmicity Cyclic changes that occur with established regularity, such as sleeping and eating patterns

biparietal diameter Largest transverse diameter of the fetal head; measured between the parietal bones

birth plan A tool by which parents can explore their childbirth options and choose those that are most important to them

Bishop score Rating system to evaluate inducibility (ripeness) of the cervix; a higher score increases the likelihood of a successful induction of labor

bittersweet grief The resurgence of feelings and emotions that occur on remembering a loved one after the bereavement process has lessened

blastocyst Stage in development of a mammalian embryo, occurring after the morula stage, that consists of an outer layer, or trophoblast, and a hollow sphere of cells enclosing a cavity

bloody show Vaginal discharge that originates in the cervix and consists of blood and mucus; increases as cervix dilates during labor

body mass index (BMI) Method of calculating appropriateness of weight for height (BMI = Weight [kilograms]/Height^2 [meters])

bonding A process by which parents, over time, form an emotional relationship with their infant

Bradley method Husband-coached childbirth preparation method using labor breathing techniques and environmental modification

bradycardia Baseline fetal heart rate below 110 beats per minute (beats/min)

Braxton Hicks sign Mild, intermittent, painless uterine contractions that occur during pregnancy; occur more frequently as pregnancy advances but do not represent true labor; however, they should be distinguished from preterm labor

breast self-examination (BSE) Systematic examination of the breasts by the woman

brown fat Source of heat unique to neonates that is capable of greater thermogenic activity than ordinary fat; deposits are found around the adrenals, kidneys, and neck, between the scapulae, and behind the sternum for several weeks after birth

caput succedaneum Swelling of the tissue over the presenting part of the fetal head caused by pressure during labor

cardiac decompensation Condition of heart failure in which the heart is unable to maintain a sufficient cardiac output

carpal tunnel syndrome Pressure on the median nerve at the point at which it goes through the carpal tunnel of the wrist; causes soreness, tenderness, and weakness of the muscles of the thumb

cephalhematoma Extravasation of blood from ruptured vessels between a skull bone and its external covering, the periosteum; swelling is limited by the margins of the cranial bone affected (usually parietals)

cephalopelvic disproportion (CPD) Condition in which the infant's head is of such a shape, size, or position that it cannot pass through the mother's pelvis or the maternal pelvis is too small, abnormally shaped, or deformed to allow the passage of a fetus of average size

cerclage Use of nonabsorbable suture to keep a premature dilating cervix closed; removed when pregnancy is at term

cervical funneling Effacement of the internal cervical os

cesarean birth Birth of a fetus by an incision through the abdominal wall and uterus

Chadwick sign Violet color of vaginal mucous membrane that is visible from approximately the fourth week of pregnancy; caused by increased vascularity

chloasma Increased pigmentation over bridge of nose and cheeks of pregnant women and some women taking oral contraceptives; also known as "mask of pregnancy"

chorioamnionitis Inflammatory reaction in fetal membranes to bacteria or viruses in the amniotic fluid, which then become infiltrated with polymorphonuclear leukocytes

chorionic villi Tiny vascular protrusions on the chorionic surface that project into the maternal blood sinuses of the uterus and that help form the placenta and secrete human chorionic gonadotropin

chorionic villus sampling (CVS) Removal of fetal tissue from placenta for genetic diagnostic studies

chromosomes Elements within the cell nucleus carrying genes and composed of DNA and proteins

chronic hypertension Systolic pressure of 140 mm Hg or higher or diastolic pressure of 90 mm Hg or higher that is present preconceptually or presents before 20 weeks of gestation

chronic lung disease (bronchopulmonary dysplasia [BPD]) Pulmonary condition affecting preterm infants who have experienced respiratory failure and have been oxygen dependent for more than 28 days

circumcision Excision of the prepuce (foreskin) of the penis, exposing the glans

claiming process Process by which the parents identify their new baby in terms of likeness to other family members, differences, and uniqueness

cleft lip Incomplete closure of the lip; lay term is *harelip*

cleft palate Incomplete closure of the palate or roof of the mouth; a congenital fissure

climacteric The period of a woman's life when she is passing from a reproductive to a nonreproductive state, with regression of ovarian function; the cycle of endocrine, physical, and psychosocial changes that occurs during the termination of the reproductive years; also called *climacterium* or *perimenopause*

clinical benchmarking Standards based on results achieved by others

clonus Spasmodic alternation of muscular contraction and relaxation; counted in beats

Cochrane Pregnancy and Childbirth Database Database of up-to-date systematic reviews and dissemination of reviews of randomized controlled trials of health care

cold stress Excessive loss of heat that results in increased respirations and nonshivering thermogenesis to maintain core body temperature

colostrum The fluid in the breast from pregnancy into the early postpartal period; rich in antibodies, which provide protection from many diseases; high in protein, which binds bilirubin; and laxative acting, which speeds the elimination of meconium and helps loosen mucus

complicated bereavement The persistent feelings of anger, guilt, loss, pain, and sadness over time that lead to feelings of hopelessness, helplessness, and diminishing self-worth

conception Union of the sperm and ovum resulting in fertilization; formation of the one-celled zygote

continuous positive airway pressure (CPAP) Infuses oxygen or air under a preset pressure by means of nasal prongs, a face mask, or an endotracheal tube

continuum of care Range of clinical services provided for an individual or group that reflects care given during a single hospitalization or care for multiple conditions over a lifetime

contraction stress test (CST) Test to stimulate uterine contractions for the purpose of assessing fetal response; a healthy fetus does not react to contractions, whereas a compromised fetus demonstrates late decelerations in the fetal heart rate that are indicative of uteroplacental insufficiency

Coombs' test Indirect: determination of Rh-positive antibodies in maternal blood; direct: determination of maternal Rh-positive antibodies in fetal cord blood; positive test result indicates the presence of antibodies or titer

corrected age Taking into account the gestational age and the postnatal age of a preterm infant when determining expectations for development

counterpressure Pressure applied to the sacral area of the back during uterine contractions

couplet care One nurse, educated in both mother and infant care, functions as the primary nurse for both mother and infant (also known as *mother-baby care* or *single-room maternity care*)

couvade syndrome The phenomenon of expectant fathers' experiencing pregnancy-like symptoms

Couvelaire uterus Interstitial myometrial hemorrhage after premature separation (abruption) of placenta; purplish-bluish discoloration of the uterus and boardlike rigidity of the uterus are noted

crowning Phase in the descent of the fetus when the top of the head can be seen at the vaginal orifice as the widest part of the head (biparietal diameter) distends the vulva just before birth

cultural competence Awareness, acceptance, and knowledge of cultural differences and adaptation of services to acknowledge and support the culture of the patient

cultural context Setting in which one considers the individual's and the family's beliefs and practices (culture)

cultural knowledge Includes beliefs and values about each facet of life and is passed from one generation to the next

cultural prescriptions Practices that are expected or acceptable

cultural proscriptions Forbidden; taboo practices

cultural relativism Refers to learning about and applying the standards of another person's culture to activities within that culture

cycle of violence Violence against a woman (usually) occurring in a pattern consisting of three phases: period of increasing tension, the abusive episode, and a period of contrition and kindness

daily fetal movement count (DFMC) Maternal assessment of fetal activity; the number of fetal movements within a specified time are counted; also called "kick count"

deceleration Slowing of fetal heart rate attributed to a parasympathetic response and described in relation to uterine contractions

    early deceleration A visually apparent gradual decrease of fetal heart rate before the peak of a contraction and return to baseline as the contraction ends; caused by fetal head compression

    late deceleration A visually apparent gradual decrease of fetal heart rate with the lowest point of the deceleration occurring after the peak of the contraction and returning to baseline after the contraction ends; caused by uteroplacental insufficiency

    variable deceleration A visually apparent abrupt decrease in fetal heart rate below the baseline occurring any time during the uterine contracting phase and caused by compression of the umbilical cord

decidua basalis Maternal aspect of the placenta made up of uterine blood vessels, endometrial stroma, and glands; shed in lochial discharge after birth

demand feeding Feeding a newborn when feeding cues are exhibited by the baby, indicating that hunger is present

developmental dysplasia of the hip Abnormal development of the hip joint, resulting in instability of the hip causing one or both of the femoral heads to be displaced from the acetabulum (hip socket)

developmentally appropriate care Care that takes into consideration the gestational age and condition of the infant and promotes the development of the infant

diastasis recti abdominis Separation of the two rectus muscles along the median line of the abdominal wall; often seen in women with repeated childbirths or with a multiple gestation (e.g., triplets)

Dick-Read method A prepared childbirth approach based on the premise that fear of pain produces muscular tension, producing pain, and greater fear; includes teaching physiologic processes of labor, exercise to improve muscle tone, and techniques to assist in relaxation and prevent the fear-tension-pain mechanism

dietary reference intakes (DRIs) Nutritional recommendations for the United States, consisting of the recommended dietary allowances, adequate intakes, and tolerable upper intake levels; the upper limit of intake associated with low risk in almost all members of a population

dilation Stretching of the external cervical os from an opening a few millimeters in size to an opening large enough to allow the passage of the fetus

disseminated intravascular coagulation (DIC) Pathologic form of coagulation in which clotting factors are consumed to such an extent that generalized bleeding can occur; associated with abruptio placentae, eclampsia, intrauterine fetal demise, amniotic fluid embolism, and hemorrhage

Doppler blood flow analysis Use of ultrasound for noninvasive measurement of blood flow in the fetus and placenta

doula Trained assistant hired to give the woman support during pregnancy, labor and birth, and/or postpartum

dysfunctional labor Abnormal uterine contractions that prevent normal progress of cervical dilation, effacement, or descent

dysfunctional uterine bleeding (DUB) Excessive uterine bleeding with no demonstrable organic cause

dysmenorrhea Painful menstruation beginning 2 to 6 months after menarche, related to ovulation or to organic disease such as endometriosis, pelvic inflammatory disease, or uterine neoplasm

dystocia Prolonged, painful, or otherwise difficult labor caused by various conditions associated with the five factors affecting labor (powers, passage, passenger, maternal position, and maternal emotions)

eclampsia Severe complication of pregnancy of unknown cause and occurring more often in the primigravida; characterized by new onset grand mal seizures in a woman with preeclampsia occurring during pregnancy or shortly after birth

ectopic pregnancy Implantation of the fertilized ovum outside of the uterine cavity; locations include the uterine tubes, ovaries, and abdomen

effacement Thinning and shortening or obliteration of the cervix that occurs during late pregnancy or labor or both

effleurage Gentle stroking used in massage, usually on the abdomen

electronic fetal monitoring (EFM) Electronic surveillance of fetal heart rate by external and internal methods

embryo Conceptus from day 15 of development until approximately the eighth week after conception

endometriosis Tissue closely resembling endometrial tissue but located outside the uterus in the pelvic cavity

endometritis Postpartum uterine infection, often beginning at the site of the placental implantation

en face Face-to-face position in which the parent's and infant's faces are approximately 20 cm apart and on the same plane

engagement In obstetrics, the entrance of the fetal presenting part into the superior pelvic strait and the beginning of the descent through the pelvic canal

engorgement Swelling of the breast tissue brought about by an increase in blood and lymph supplied to the breast, occurring as early milk (colostrum) transitions to mature milk at about 72 to 96 hours after birth

engrossment A parent's absorption, preoccupation, and interest in his or her infant; term typically used to describe the father's intense involvement with his newborn

entrainment Phenomenon observed in the microanalysis of sound films in which the speaker moves several parts of the body and the listener responds to the sounds by moving in ways that are coordinated with the rhythm of the sounds (infants have been observed to move in time to the rhythms of adult speech but not to random noises or disconnected words or vowels); believed to be an essential factor in the process of maternal-infant bonding

epidural block Type of regional anesthesia produced by injection of a local anesthetic alone or in combination with a narcotic analgesic into the epidural (peridural) space

epidural blood patch A patch formed by a few milliliters of the mother's blood occluding a tear in the dura mater around the spinal cord that occurs during induction of spinal block; its purpose is to relieve headache associated with leakage of spinal fluid

episodic changes Changes from baseline patterns in the fetal heart rate that are not associated with uterine contractions

episiotomy Surgical incision of the perineum at the end of the second stage of labor to facilitate birth and to avoid laceration of the perineum

epulis Tumorlike benign lesion of the gingiva seen in pregnant women

erythema toxicum Innocuous pink papular neonatal rash of unknown cause, with superimposed vesicles appearing within 24 to 48 hours after birth and resolving spontaneously within a few days

erythroblastosis fetalis Hemolytic disease of the newborn usually caused by isoimmunization resulting from Rh incompatibility or ABO incompatibility

ethnocentrism Belief in the rightness of one's culture's way of doing things

euglycemia Pertaining to a normal blood glucose level; also called *normoglycemia*

evidence-based practice Practice based on knowledge that has been gained through research and clinical trials

exchange transfusion Replacement of 75% to 85% of circulating blood by withdrawal of the recipient's blood and injection of a donor's blood in equal amounts, the purposes of which are to prevent an accumulation of bilirubin in the blood above a dangerous level, to prevent the accumulation of other by-products of hemolysis in hemolytic disease, and to correct anemia and acidosis

extended family Includes nuclear family and other people related by blood

external cephalic version (ECV) Turning of the fetus to a vertex presentation by external exertion of pressure on the fetus through the maternal abdomen

extracorporeal membrane oxygenation (ECMO) Oxygenation of blood external to body using cardiopulmonary bypass and a membrane oxygenator; used primarily for newborns with refractory respiratory failure or meconium aspiration syndrome

failure to rescue Concept that the quality and quantity of nursing care can be measured by comparing the number of surgical patients who develop common complications who survive versus those who do not survive

family dynamics Interaction and communication among family members

family functions Affective, socialization, reproductive, economic, and health care functions that contribute to the well-being of the family

feeding-readiness cues Infant responses (mouthing motions, sucking fist, awakening, and crying) that indicate optimal times to begin a feeding

Ferguson reflex Reflex contractions (urge to push) of the uterus after stimulation of the cervix

fern test The appearance of a fernlike pattern found on microscopic examination of certain fluids such as amniotic fluid

fertility awareness methods (FAMs) Methods of family planning that identify the beginning and end of the fertile period of the menstrual cycle

fertilization Union of an ovum and a sperm

fetal alcohol effects (FAE) See alcohol-related neurodevelopmental disorder

fetal alcohol syndrome (FAS) See alcohol-related birth defects

fetal membranes Amnion and chorion surrounding the fetus

fetus Child in utero from approximately the ninth week after conception until birth

fibroadenoma Firm, freely movable solitary, solid, benign breast tumor

fibrocystic changes Benign changes in breast tissue

first stage of labor Stage of labor from the onset of regular uterine contractions to full effacement and dilation of the cervix

fontanels Broad areas, or soft spots, consisting of a strong band of connective tissue contiguous with cranial bones and located at the junctions of the bones

forceps-assisted birth Vaginal birth in which forceps (i.e., curved-bladed instruments) are used to assist in the birth of the fetal head

fourth stage of labor The first 1 or 2 hours after birth

funic souffle Soft, muffled, blowing sound produced by blood rushing through the umbilical vessels and synchronous with the fetal heart sounds

gamete Mature male or female germ cell; the mature sperm or ovum

gastroschisis Abdominal wall defect at the base of the umbilical stalk

gate-control theory of pain Pain theory used to explain the neurophysiologic mechanism underlying the perception of pain: the capacity of nerve pathways to transmit pain is reduced or completely blocked by using distraction techniques

genetics Study of single gene or gene sequences and their effects on living organism

genogram Pictorial representation of family relationships and health history

genome Complete copy of genetic material in an organism

genomics Study of the entire DNA structure of all of an organism's genes including functions and interactions of genes

gestational diabetes mellitus (GDM) Glucose intolerance first recognized during pregnancy

gestational hypertension Onset of hypertension without proteinuria after week 20 of pregnancy

glycosylated hemoglobin A_{1c} Glycohemoglobin, a minor hemoglobin with glucose attached; the glycosylated hemoglobin concentration represents the average blood glucose level over the previous several weeks and is a measurement of glycemic control in diabetic therapy

Goodell sign Softening of the cervix, a probable sign of pregnancy, occurring during the second month

grief Physical, emotional, social, and cognitive response to death of a loved one

growth spurts Times of increased neonatal growth that usually occur at approximately 6 to 10 days, 6 weeks, 3 months, and 4 to 5 months; increased caloric needs necessitate more frequent feedings to increase the amount of milk produced

habituation Psychologic and physiologic phenomenon whereby the response to a constant or repetitive stimulus is decreased

Hegar sign Softening of the lower uterine segment that is classified as a probable sign of pregnancy, may be present during the second and third months of pregnancy, and is palpated during bimanual examination

HELLP syndrome Condition characterized by hemolysis, elevated liver enzymes, and low platelet count; a complication of severe preeclampsia

hemorrhagic (hypovolemic) shock Clinical condition in which the peripheral blood flow is inadequate to return sufficient blood to the heart for normal function, particularly oxygen transport to the organs or tissue

Homans' sign Early sign of phlebothrombosis of the deep veins of the calf in which there are complaints of pain when the leg is in extension and the foot is dorsiflexed

home birth Planned birth of the child at home, usually done under the supervision of a midwife

home health care Providing care within the home

homosexual (lesbian or gay) family Consists of same-sex adults and children from previous heterosexual unions, conceived through therapeutic insemination, or adopted

human chorionic gonadotropin (hCG) Hormone that is produced by chorionic villi; the biologic marker in pregnancy tests

hydatidiform mole (molar pregnancy) Gestational trophoblastic neoplasm usually resulting from fertilization of egg that has no nucleus or an inactivated nucleus

hydramnios (polyhydramnios) Amniotic fluid in excess of 2000 ml

hydrocephalus Accumulation of fluid in the subdural or subarachnoid spaces

hydrops fetalis Most severe expression of fetal hemolytic disorder, a possible sequela to maternal Rh isoimmunization; infants exhibit gross edema (anasarca), cardiac decompensation, and profound pallor from anemia, and seldom survive

hyperbilirubinemia Elevation of unconjugated serum bilirubin concentrations

hyperemesis gravidarum Abnormal condition of pregnancy characterized by protracted vomiting, weight loss, and fluid and electrolyte imbalance

hyperglycemia Excess glucose in the blood, usually caused by inadequate secretion of insulin by the islet cells of the pancreas or inadequate control of diabetes mellitus

hypertonic uterine dysfunction Uncoordinated, painful, frequent uterine contractions that do not cause cervical dilation and effacement; primary dysfunctional labor

hyperthyroidism Excessive functional activity of the thyroid gland

hypoglycemia Less than normal amount of glucose in the blood; usually caused by administration of too much insulin, excessive secretion of insulin by the islet cells of the pancreas, or dietary deficiency

hypothermia Temperature that falls below normal range, that is, below 35° C, usually caused by exposure to cold

hypothyroidism Deficiency of thyroid gland activity with underproduction of thyroxine

hypotonic uterine dysfunction Weak, ineffective uterine contractions usually occurring in the active phase of labor; often related to cephalopelvic disproportion or malposition of the fetus; secondary uterine inertia

hypoxemia Reduction in arterial Po_2 resulting in metabolic acidosis by forcing anaerobic glycolysis, pulmonary vasoconstriction, and direct cellular damage

hypoxia Insufficient availability of oxygen to meet the metabolic needs of body tissue

implantation Embedding of the fertilized ovum in the uterine mucosa; nidation

induced abortion Intentionally produced termination of pregnancy

infertility Decreased capacity to conceive

insensible water loss Evaporative water loss that occurs mainly through the skin and respiratory tract

integrative health care Complementary and alternative therapies in combination with conventional Western modalities of treatment

intermittent auscultation Listening to fetal heart sounds at periodic intervals using nonelectronic or ultrasound devices placed on the maternal abdomen

intrauterine growth restriction (IUGR) Fetal undergrowth from any cause

inversion of the uterus Condition in which the uterus is turned inside out so that the fundus intrudes into the cervix or vagina

inverted nipples Nipples invert rather than evert when stimulated; interferes with latch-on

in vitro fertilization Fertilization in a culture dish or test tube

involution Reduction in size of the uterus after birth and its return to its nonpregnant condition

kangaroo care Skin-to-skin infant care, especially for preterm infants, that provides warmth to infant; infant is placed naked or diapered against mother's or father's bare chest and is covered with parent's shirt or a warm blanket

karyotype Schematic arrangements of the chromosomes within a cell to demonstrate their numbers and morphology

kcal Kilocalorie; unit of heat content or energy equal to 1000 small calories

Kegel exercises Pelvic muscle exercises to strengthen the pubococcygeal muscles

ketoacidosis The accumulation of ketone bodies in the blood as a consequence of hyperglycemia; leads to metabolic acidosis

key informants Individuals in positions of leadership who can provide information about a situation

lactation consultant Health care professional who has specialized training in breastfeeding

lactogenesis Beginning of milk production

lactose intolerance Inherited absence of the enzyme lactase

Lamaze (psychoprophylaxis) method Childbirth preparation method developed in the 1950s by a French obstetrician, Fernand Lamaze, that gained popularity in the United States in the 1960s; requires practice at home and coaching during labor and birth; goals are to minimize fear and the perception of pain and to promote positive family relationships by using both mental and physical preparation, including breathing and relaxation techniques, effleurage, and focusing

latch-on Attachment of the infant to the breast for feeding

latent phase Phase in the first stage of labor when the cervix dilates from 0 to 3 cm

leiomyoma Benign smooth muscle tumor; e.g., fibroid tumor of the uterine muscle

Leopold maneuvers Four maneuvers for diagnosing the fetal position by external palpation of the mother's abdomen

let-down reflex Release of milk caused by the contraction of the myoepithelial cells within the milk glands in response to oxytocin; also called *milk ejection reflex (MER)*

letting-go phase Interdependent phase after birth in which the mother and family move forward as a system with interacting members

leukorrhea White or yellowish mucus discharge from the cervical canal or the vagina that may be normal physiologically or caused by pathologic states of the vagina and endocervix

levels of prevention Consists of three levels; primary prevention is promoting general health and well-being; secondary prevention involves early detection of health problems so that treatment can begin before significant disability occurs; tertiary prevention is the treatment and rehabilitation of persons who have developed disease

lie Relationship existing between the long axis of the fetus and the long axis of the mother; in a longitudinal lie, the fetus is lying lengthwise or vertically, whereas in a transverse lie, the fetus is lying crosswise or horizontally in the uterus

lightening Sensation of decreased abdominal distention produced by uterine descent into the pelvic cavity as the fetal presenting part settles into the pelvis; usually occurs 2 weeks before the onset of labor in nulliparas

linea nigra Line of darker pigmentation seen in some women during the latter part of pregnancy that appears on the middle of the abdomen and extends from the symphysis pubis toward the umbilicus

lithotomy position Position in which the woman lies on her back with her knees flexed and with abducted thighs drawn up toward her chest; stirrups attached to an examination table can be used to facilitate assuming and maintaining this position

local perinaeal infiltration anesthesia Process by which a substance such as a local anesthetic medication is deposited within the tissue to anesthetize a limited region of the body

lochia Vaginal discharge during the puerperium consisting of blood, tissue, and mucus

    lochia alba Thin, yellowish to white, vaginal discharge that follows lochia serosa on approximately the tenth day after birth and that may last from 2 to 6 weeks postpartum

    lochia rubra Red, distinctly blood-tinged vaginal flow that follows birth and lasts 2 to 4 days

    lochia serosa Serous, pinkish brown, watery vaginal discharge that follows lochia rubra until approximately the tenth day after birth

low-birth-weight (LBW) infants Babies born weighing less than 2500 g

lumpectomy Removal of a wide margin of normal breast tissue surrounding a breast cancer

macrosomia Large body size as seen in infants of diabetic or prediabetic mothers

magnetic resonance imaging (MRI) Noninvasive nuclear procedure for imaging tissues with high fat and water content; in obstetrics, uses include evaluation of fetal structures, placenta, and amniotic fluid volume

mastitis Infection in a breast, usually confined to a milk duct, characterized by influenza-like symptoms and redness and tenderness in the affected breast

mechanical ventilation Technique used to provide predetermined amount of oxygen; requires intubation

meconium Greenish black viscous first stool formed during fetal life from the amniotic fluid and its constituents;

intestinal secretions (including bilirubin) and cells (shed from the mucosa)

meconium aspiration syndrome (MAS) Function of fetal hypoxia; with hypoxia, the anal sphincter relaxes and meconium is released; reflex gasping movements draw meconium and other particulate matter in the amniotic fluid into the infant's bronchial tree, obstructing the airflow after birth

meiosis Process by which germ cells divide and decrease their chromosomal numbers by one half

menarche Onset, or beginning, of menstrual function

menopause From the Greek words *mensis* (month) and *pausis* (cessation), the actual permanent cessation of menstrual cycles; so diagnosed after 1 year without menses

menorrhagia Abnormally profuse or excessive menstrual flow

menstrual cycle A complex interplay of events that occur simultaneously in the endometrium, the hypothalamus and pituitary glands, and the ovaries that results in ovarian and uterine preparation for pregnancy

menstruation Periodic vaginal discharge of bloody fluid from the nonpregnant uterus that occurs from the age of puberty to menopause

metrorrhagia Abnormal bleeding from the uterus, particularly when it occurs at any time other than the menstrual period

microcephaly Abnormal smallness of the head in relation to the rest of the body and underdevelopment of the brain, resulting in some degree of mental retardation

milia Small, white sebaceous glands, appearing as tiny, white, pinpoint papules on the forehead, nose, cheeks, and chin of the neonate

milk ejection reflex (MER) Release of milk caused by the contraction of the myoepithelial cells within the milk glands in response to oxytocin; also called *let-down reflex*

miscarriage Loss of pregnancy that occurs naturally without interference or known cause; also called *spontaneous abortion*

mitosis Process of somatic cell division in which a single cell divides, but both of the new cells have the same number of chromosomes as the first

modified radical mastectomy Surgery that includes removal of the breast and fascia over the pectoralis major muscle

molding Overlapping of cranial bones or shaping of the fetal head to accommodate and conform to the bony and soft parts of the mother's birth canal during labor

mongolian spots Bluish gray or dark nonelevated pigmented areas usually found over the lower back and buttocks present at birth in some infants, primarily non-white; usually fade by school age

monosomy Chromosomal aberration characterized by the absence of one chromosome from the normal diploid complement

Montgomery tubercles Small, nodular prominences (sebaceous glands) on the areolas around the nipples of the breasts that enlarge during pregnancy and lactation

mood disorders Disorders that have a disturbance in the prevailing emotional state as the dominant feature; cause is unknown

morning sickness Nausea and vomiting that affect some women during the first few months of their pregnancy; may occur at any time of day

morula Developmental stage of the fertilized ovum in which there is a solid mass of cells resembling a mulberry

mosaicism Condition in which some somatic cells are normal, whereas others show chromosomal aberrations

multifetal pregnancy Pregnancy in which there is more than one fetus in the uterus at the same time; multiple pregnancy

mutuality Parent-infant interaction in which the infant's behaviors and characteristics call forth a corresponding set of maternal behaviors and characteristics

myelomeningocele External sac containing meninges, spinal fluid, and nerves that protrudes through defect in vertebral column

Nägele's rule One method for calculating the estimated date of birth, or "due date"

necrotizing enterocolitis (NEC) Acute inflammatory bowel disorder that occurs primarily in preterm or low-birth-weight neonates; characterized by ischemic necrosis (death) of the gastrointestinal mucosa, which may lead to perforation and peritonitis; formula-fed infants are at higher risk for this disease

neonatal abstinence syndrome Signs and symptoms associated with drug withdrawal in the neonate

neonatal narcosis Central nervous system depression in the newborn caused by an opioid (narcotic); may be exhibited by respiratory depression, hypotonia, lethargy, and delay in temperature regulation

neutral thermal environment (NTE) Environment that enables the neonate to maintain a normal body temperature with minimum use of oxygen and energy

nipple confusion Difficulty experienced by some infants in mastering breastfeeding after having been given a pacifier or bottle

nitrazine test Evaluation of body fluids using a test strip to determine the fluid's pH; urine will exhibit an acidic result and amniotic fluid will exhibit an alkaline result

nonnutritive sucking Use of a pacifier by infants

nonreassuring FHR patterns Fetal heart rate pattern that indicates the fetus is not well oxygenated and requires intervention

nonstress test (NST) Evaluation of fetal response (fetal heart rate) to natural contractile uterine activity or to an increase in fetal activity

nuchal cord Encircling of fetal neck by one or more loops of umbilical cord

nuclear family Consists of parents and their dependent children

oligomenorrhea Abnormally light or infrequent menstruation

omphalocele Congenital defect resulting from failure of closure of the abdominal wall or muscles and leading to herniation of abdominal contents through the navel

operculum Plug of mucus that fills the cervical canal during pregnancy

ophthalmia neonatorum Infection in the neonate's eyes usually resulting from gonorrheal, chlamydial, or other infection contracted when the fetus passes through the birth canal (vagina)

opioid (narcotic) agonist analgesics Medications that relieve pain by activating opioid receptors

opioid (narcotic) agonist-antagonist analgesics Medications that combine agonist activity (activates or stimulates a receptor to perform a function) and antagonist activity (blocks a receptor or medication designed to activate a receptor) to relieve pain without causing significant maternal or fetal/newborn respiratory depression

opioid (narcotic) antagonists Medications used to reverse the CNS depressant effects of an opioid; especially respiratory depression

outcomes-oriented care Measures effectiveness of care against benchmarks or standards

ovulation Periodic ripening and discharge of the ovum from the ovary, usually 14 days before the onset of menstrual flow

oxytocin Hormone produced by the posterior pituitary gland that stimulates uterine contractions and the release of milk in the mammary glands (let-down reflex); synthetic oxytocin is a medication that mimics the uterine stimulating action of oxytocin

palmar erythema Rash on the surface of the palms sometimes seen in pregnancy

Papanicolaou (Pap) test or smear Microscopic examination using scrapings from the cervix, endocervix, or other mucous membranes that will reveal, with a high degree of accuracy, the presence of premalignant or malignant cells

patent ductus arteriosus (PDA) Failure of the fetal ductus arteriosus to close after birth

pelvic inflammatory disease (PID) Infection of internal reproductive structures and adjacent tissues usually secondary to sexually transmitted infections

pelvic relaxation Lengthening and weakening of the fascial supports of pelvic structures

pelvic tilt (rock) Exercise used to help relieve low back discomfort during menstruation and pregnancy

percutaneous umbilical blood sampling (PUBS) Procedure during which a fetal umbilical vessel is accessed for blood sampling or for transfusions

perimenopause Period of transition of changing ovarian activity before menopause and through the first few years of amenorrhea

perinatal loss Death of a fetus or infant through the twenty-eighth day after birth

periodic abstinence Contraceptive method in which a woman abstains from sexual intercourse during the fertile period of her menstrual cycle; also referred to as natural family planning (NFP) because no other form of birth control is used during this period

periodic changes Changes from baseline of the fetal heart rate that occur with uterine contractions

peripartum cardiomyopathy Inability of the heart to maintain an adequate cardiac output; congestive heart failure occurring during the peripartum

periventricular-intraventricular hemorrhage (PV-IVH) Hemorrhage into the ventricles of the brain; a common type of brain injury in preterm infants; prognosis depends on the severity of hemorrhage

phototherapy Use of lights to reduce serum bilirubin levels by oxidation of bilirubin into water-soluble compounds that are processed in the liver and excreted in bile and urine

physiologic anemia Relative excess of plasma leading to a decrease in hemoglobin concentration and hematocrit; normal adaptation during pregnancy

physiologic jaundice Yellow tinge to skin and mucous membranes in response to increased serum levels of unconjugated bilirubin; not usually apparent until after

24 hours; also called *neonatal jaundice, physiologic hyperbilirubinemia*

pica Unusual oral craving during pregnancy (e.g., for laundry starch, dirt, red clay)

pinch test Determines whether nipples are everted or inverted by placing thumb and forefinger on areola and pressing inward; the nipple will stand erect or will invert

placenta previa Placenta that is abnormally implanted in the thin, lower uterine segment and that is typed according to proximity to cervical os: total-completely occludes os; partial-does not occlude os completely; marginal-placenta encroaches on margin of internal cervical os

plugged milk ducts Milk ducts blocked by small curds of dried milk

position In pregnancy, relationship of a reference point on the presenting part of the fetus, such as the occiput, sacrum, chin, or scapula, to its location in the front, back, or sides of the maternal pelvis

postpartum blues A let-down feeling, accompanied by irritability and anxiety, which usually begins 2 to 3 days after giving birth and disappears within a week or two; sometimes called "baby blues"

postpartum depression (PPD) Depression occurring within 4 weeks of childbirth, lasting longer than postpartum blues and characterized by a variety of symptoms that interfere with activities of daily living and care of the baby

postpartum hemorrhage (PPH) Excessive bleeding after childbirth; traditionally defined as a loss of 500 ml or more after a vaginal birth and 1000 ml after a cesarean birth

postterm pregnancy Pregnancy prolonged past 42 weeks of gestation

precipitous labor Rapid or sudden labor lasting less than 3 hours from the onset of uterine contractions to complete birth of the fetus

preconception care Care designed for health maintenance and health promotion for the general and reproductive health of all women of childbearing potential

preeclampsia Disease encountered after 20 weeks of gestation or early in the puerperium; a vasospastic disease process characterized by increasing hypertension, and proteinuria (0.3 g protein or higher in a 24-hour urine)

  superimposed preeclampsia New onset proteinuria in a woman with hypertension before 20 weeks of gestation, sudden increase in proteinuria if already present in early gestation, sudden increase in hypertension, or the development of HELLP syndrome

pregestational diabetes mellitus Diabetes mellitus type 1 or type 2 that exists before pregnancy

premature dilation of the cervix Cervix that is unable to remain closed until a pregnancy reaches term because of a mechanical defect in the cervix; also called *incompetent cervix*

premature rupture of membranes (PROM) Rupture of the amniotic sac and leakage of amniotic fluid beginning at least 1 hour before the onset of labor at any gestational age

premenstrual syndrome (PMS) Syndrome of nervous tension, irritability, weight gain, edema, headache, mastalgia, dysphoria, and lack of coordination occurring during the last few days of the menstrual cycle preceding the onset of menstruation

presentation That part of the fetus that first enters the pelvis and lies over the inlet; may be head, face, breech, or shoulder

presenting part That part of the fetus that lies closest to the internal os of the cervix

preterm birth Birth occurring before the completion of 37 weeks of gestation

preterm infants Infants born before 38 weeks of gestation

preterm labor Cervical changes and uterine contractions occurring between 20 weeks and 37 weeks of pregnancy

preterm premature rupture of membranes (PPROM) PROM that occurs before 37 weeks of gestation

prolapse of the umbilical cord Protrusion of the umbilical cord in advance of the presenting part

prostaglandins (PGs) Substances present in many body tissues; have roles in many reproductive tract functions; used to induce abortions and for cervical ripening for labor induction

ptyalism Excessive salivation

pudendal block Injection of a local anesthetic at the pudendal nerve root to produce numbness of the genital and perianal region

puerperal infection Infection of the pelvic organs during the postbirth period; also called *postpartum infection*

puerperium Period after the third stage of labor and lasting until involution of the uterus takes place, usually approximately 3 to 6 weeks; fourth trimester of pregnancy

pyrosis Burning sensation in the epigastric and sternal region from stomach acid (heartburn)

quickening Maternal perception of fetal movement; usually occurs between weeks 16 and 20 of gestation

radical mastectomy Surgery that includes total removal of the breast, as well as underlying pectoralis major and pectoralis minor muscles

reciprocity Type of body movement or behavior that provides the observer with cues, such as the behavioral cues infants provide to parents and parents' responses to cues

recommended dietary allowances (RDAs) Recommended nutrient intakes estimated to meet the needs of almost all (97% to 98%) of the healthy people in the population

reconstituted family Also called *blended, combined,* or *remarried* family; includes stepparents and stepchildren

reflex bradycardia Slowing of the heart in response to a particular stimulus

respiratory distress syndrome (RDS) Condition resulting from decreased pulmonary gas exchange, leading to retention of carbon dioxide (increase in arterial PCO_2); most common neonatal causes are prematurity, perinatal asphyxia, and maternal diabetes mellitus; also called *hyaline membrane disease*

retinopathy of prematurity (ROP) Complex, multicausal disorder that affects the developing retinal vessels of premature infants resulting in capillary hemorrhages, fibrotic resolution, and possible retinal detachment; visual impairment may be mild or severe

Ritgen maneuver Technique used to control the birth of the head; upward pressure from the coccygeal region to extend the head during the actual birth

rooting reflex Normal response of the newborn to move toward whatever touches the area around the mouth and to attempt to suck; usually disappears by 3 to 4 months of age

rupture of membranes (ROM) Integrity of the amniotic membranes is broken either spontaneously or artificially (amniotomy)

second stage of labor Stage of labor from full dilation of the cervix to the birth of the baby

semen analysis Examination of semen specimen to determine liquefaction, volume, pH, sperm density, and normal morphology

sex chromosomes Chromosomes associated with determination of sex: the X (female) and Y (male) chromosomes; the normal female has two X chromosomes, the normal male has one X and one Y chromosome

sexual response cycle The phases of physical changes that occur in response to sexual stimulation and sexual tension release

shoulder dystocia Condition in which the head is born but the anterior shoulder cannot pass under the pubic arch

sibling rivalry A sibling's jealousy of and resentment toward a new child in the family

simple mastectomy Surgery that includes removal of the breast without underlying muscle or fascial tissue

single-parent family Child living with one parent resulting from divorce, separation, or desertion; birth to a single parent; or adoption

sleep-wake states Variation in states of newborn consciousness

spinal block Regional anesthesia induced by injection of a local anesthetic agent into the subarachnoid space at the level of the third, fourth, or fifth lumbar interspace

spontaneous rupture of membranes (SROM, SRM) Rupture of membranes by natural means, most often during labor

squamocolumnar junction Site in the endocervical canal where columnar epithelium and squamous epithelium meet; also called *transformation zone*

standard of care Level of practice that a reasonable, prudent nurse would provide

station Relationship of the presenting fetal part to an imaginary line drawn between the ischial spines of the pelvis

sterilization Procedure meant to be a permanent form of birth control, e.g., vasectomy, bilateral tubal ligation

striae gravidarum "Stretch marks"; shining reddish lines caused by stretching of the skin, often found on the abdomen, thighs, and breasts during pregnancy; these streaks turn to a fine pinkish white or silver tone in time in fair-skinned women and brownish in darker-skinned women

subculture Group existing within a larger cultural system that retains its own characteristics

subinvolution Failure of the uterus to reduce to its normal size and condition after pregnancy

suboccipitobregmatic diameter Smallest diameter of the fetal head; follows a line drawn from the middle of the anterior fontanel to the undersurface of the occipital bone

supine hypotension Shock; fall in blood pressure caused by impaired venous return when gravid uterus presses on ascending vena cava, when woman is lying flat on her back; vena cava syndrome

supply-meets-demand system Physiologic basis for determining milk production; the volume of milk produced equals the amount removed from the breast

surfactant Phosphoprotein necessary for normal respiratory function that prevents alveolar collapse (atelectasis)

synchrony Fit between the infant's cues and the parent's response

systemic analgesia Pain relief induced when an analgesic is administered parenterally (e.g., subcutaneous, intramuscular, or intravenous route) and crosses the blood-brain barrier to provide central analgesic effects

tachycardia Baseline fetal heart rate above 160 beats/min

taking-hold phase Period after birth characterized by a woman becoming more independent and more interested in learning infant care skills; learning to be a competent mother is an important task

taking-in phase Period after birth characterized by the woman's dependency; maternal needs are dominant, and talking about the birth is an important task

telemedicine Use of communication technologies and electronic information to provide or support health care when participants are separated by distance

telephonic nursing Services such as warm lines, nurse advice lines, and telephonic nursing assessments

teratogens Environmental substances or exposures that result in functional or structural disability

therapeutic donor insemination (TDI) Introduction of donor semen by instrument injection into the vagina or uterus for impregnation

therapeutic rest Administration of analgesics and implementation of comfort/relaxation measures to decrease pain and induce rest for management of hypertonic uterine dysfunction

thermogenesis Creation or production of heat, especially in the body

thermoregulation Control of temperature

third stage of labor Stage of labor from the birth of the baby to the separation and expulsion of the placenta

thrombophlebitis Inflammation of a vein with secondary clot formation

thrombus Blood clot obstructing a blood vessel that remains at the place it was formed

thrush Fungal infection of the mouth or throat characterized by the formation of white patches on a red, moist, inflamed mucous membrane; caused by *Candida albicans*

tocolysis Inhibition of uterine contractions through administration of medications; used to suppress preterm labor, for version, or as an adjunct to other interventions in the management of fetal compromise related to increased uterine activity

tocolytics Medications used to suppress uterine activity and relax the uterus in cases of hyperstimulation or preterm labor

TORCH infections Infections caused by organisms that damage the embryo or fetus; acronym for *t*oxoplasmosis, *o*ther (e.g., syphilis), *r*ubella, *c*ytomegalovirus, and *h*erpes simplex

transition period Period from birth to 4 to 6 hours later; infant passes through period of reactivity, sleep, and second period of reactivity

transition phase Phase in the first stage of labor when the cervix dilates from 8 to 10 cm

transition to parenthood Period of time from the preconception parenthood decision through the first months after birth of the baby during which parents define their parental roles and adjust to parenthood

trial of labor (TOL) Period of observation to determine whether a laboring woman is likely to be successful in progressing to a vaginal birth

trimesters One of three periods of approximately 3 months each into which pregnancy is divided

trophic feedings Very small feedings given to stimulate maturation of the gut

urinary incontinence (UI) Uncontrollable leakage of urine

uterine atony Relaxation of uterine muscle; leads to postpartum hemorrhage

uterine contractions Primary powers of labor that act involuntarily to dilate and efface the cervix, expel the fetus, facilitate separation of the placenta, and prevent hemorrhage

uterine souffle Soft, blowing sound made by the blood in the arteries of the pregnant uterus and synchronous with the maternal pulse

uteroplacental insufficiency Decline in placental function (exchange of gases, nutrients, and wastes) leading to fetal hypoxia and acidosis; evidenced by late fetal heart rate decelerations in response to uterine contractions

vacuum-assisted birth Birth involving attachment of a vacuum cap to the fetal head (occiput) and application of negative pressure to assist in birth of the fetus

vaginal birth after cesarean (VBAC) Giving birth vaginally after having had a previous cesarean birth

Valsalva maneuver Any forced expiratory effort against a closed airway such as holding one's breath and tightening the abdominal muscles (e.g., pushing during the second stage of labor)

variability Normal irregularity of fetal cardiac rhythm or fluctuations from the baseline fetal heart rate of two cycles or more

vernix caseosa Protective gray-white fatty substance of cheesy consistency covering the fetal skin

vertex Crown, or top, of the head

vulnerable populations Groups who are at higher risk of developing physical, mental, or social health problems or who are more likely to have worse outcomes from these health problems than the population as a whole

vulvar self-examination (VSE) Systematic examination of the vulva by the woman

walking survey Using one's senses while traveling through a community to obtain information about sociocultural characteristics and the environment, housing, transportation, and local community agencies

warm line A help line, or consultation service, for families to access; most often for support of newborn care and postpartum care after hospital discharge

zygote Cell formed by the union of two reproductive cells or gametes; the fertilized ovum resulting from the union of a sperm and an ovum

Index

Page numbers followed by f indicate figures; t, tables; b, boxes.

Hemorrhoids
  interventions for, 478b
  postpartal, 457, 462, 477
  during pregnancy, 218, 218f
Hemostasis, postpartal, 455
Hepatic system
  fetal, 197
  neonatal
    adaptations of, 541-543, 541f
    potential problems in, 543
Hepatitis A infection, 118-119
  during pregnancy, effects, prevention,
    management, 758t
Hepatitis B immune globulin, guidelines for,
  597
Hepatitis B infection, 118-119
  maternal transmission of, 560
  neonatal, 896
  during pregnancy
    effects, prevention, management, 758t
    treatment of, 757t
Hepatitis B vaccination, recommendations
  for, 596
Hepatitis C infection, 119
Herbal remedies
  for dysmenorrhea, 104, 106t
  for infertility, 166
  during pregnancy, 263
Herbal tea during breastfeeding, 636
Hernia, congenital diaphragmatic, 917-918,
  918f
Heroin abuse
  health risks associated with, 77
  maternal
    methadone treatment for, 708
    neonatal effects of, 902t, 904, 906
Heroin withdrawal, neonatal, 904, 906
Herpes gestationis, 223b
Herpes simplex infection
  genital, 117-118, 117f
  neonatal, 894, 898-899, 899f
  during pregnancy
    effects, prevention, management, 759t
    effects and care, 756t
    treatment of, 757t
  preventing spread of, 476
High-frequency jet ventilation, description
  and mechanism, 860t
High-frequency oscillation, description and
  mechanism, 860t
High-frequency ventilation for preterm infant, 861
Highly active antiretroviral therapy. See
  HAART
Hip dysplasia
  congenital, 921-922, 922f
    nurse alert for, 922
    treatment of, 922-923, 923f
  developmental, defined, 886
Hispanic cultures
  beliefs about childbearing and parenting,
    35t
  beliefs about pain, 339
  birth control and, 488
  food patterns in, 311t
  parent-child bonding in, 499
  parenting behaviors in, 511
HIV infection, 119-120
  in adolescent girls, 43
  antepartum care, 706
  condom use and, 142
  as contraindication to breastfeeding, 256
  intrapartum care, 706
  legal aspects of, 120

management, 120
maternal, as breastfeeding contraindication, 619
maternal transmission of, 560
neonatal, 6, 896-897
nonoxynol-9 spermicides and, 143
opportunistic infections associated with,
  119
perinatal transmission of, factors increasing risk, 705b
postpartum/newborn care, 706
preconception counseling for, 705
pregnancy risks due to, 705-706
in pregnant women, 6
  screening for, 247, 249b
protection against, 113
spermicide use and, 142
standard precautions for, 124b
testing and counseling, 119-120
transmission of, 119
treatment of, 705
Hmong culture
  birth control and, 488
  and father's presence during labor, 403
Homans sign
  defined, 466
  as indicator of thromboembolism, 482
Home birth, 282-283
  critical thinking exercise, 283, 284
  defined, 231
Home care. See also Community/home care
  AWHONN definition of, 52
  defined, 41
  high-technology, 53
Home care agencies, government/profes-
  sional regulation of, 52-53
Home environment
  physical assessment of, 55-56
  unsafe situations in, 58
Home Oriented Maternity Experience, 283
Home uterine activity monitoring, use and
  effectiveness of, 776
Home visits, 490
  initial, 55
  preparing for, 53, 54b
Homeless women, nursing implications,
  45-46
Homelessness, 44
Homosexual family
  characteristics of, 24
  defined, 21
Hon, Edward, 3b
Hormonal antagonists for endometriosis, 108
Hormonal contraception methods, 147-152.
  See also Oral contraceptives
  male, 156
  types, administration, duration, 148t
Hormonal therapy, breast cancer and, 126
Hormones
  changes during pregnancy, 227-228
  "mothering," 624
  ovarian, 69-71
  pituitary, postpartal levels of, 458
  pituitary/placental, changes during preg-
    nancy, 227-228
  placental, 194
    postpartal changes in, 457
  reproductive, during pregnancy, 675
Hospital
  as data source, 46
  infant abduction from, 476
  neonatal security in, 5
HUAM. See Home uterine activity
  monitoring

Human chorionic gonadotropin
  defined, 208
  placental production of, 194
  pregnancy testing of, 210
  for treating infertility, 166t
β-Human chorionic gonadotropin, postpartal
  levels of, 457
Human chorionic somatomammotropin
  functions during pregnancy, 228
  placental production of, 194
Human Developmental Ecology, family theory in, 27t
Human Genome Project
  ethical, legal, social implications, 179
  findings of, 179
  gene therapy and, 179
  genetic testing and, 179
  pharmacogenomics and, 179
Human immunodeficiency virus. See HIV;
  HIV infection
Human milk. See Breast milk; Breastfeeding
Human Milk Banking Association of North
  America, 635
Human papillomavirus, gynecologic cancers
  associated with, 79
Human papillomavirus infection, 116-117,
  116f
  during pregnancy
    effects and care, 756t
    treatment of, 757t
Human placental lactogen, 194
Huntington disease, 183
  genetic testing for, 179
Husband-coached childbirth, 341
Hutchinson's teeth, 895
Hydatidiform mole, 747-748, 747f
  chromosomal origin of, 747f
  defined, 715
  uterine rupture from, 747f
Hydralazine (Apresoline) for hypertension in
  pregnancy, 733t
Hydramnios
  defined, 192, 673
  fetal, assessing for, 250
  maternal, congenital esophageal
    atresia/tracheoesophageal fistula and,
    919
Hydration. See also Fluids
  of preterm infant, 863
Hydrocephalus
  cause and treatment of, 914
  defined, 886
Hydrops fetalis
  characteristics of, 911
  defined, 886
Hydrotherapy. See also Water therapy
  critical thinking exercise, 365-366
Hydroxyzine (Vistaril), effects of, 349
Hygiene
  during first stage of labor, 419, 420t
  during pregnancy, 255
Hymenal tags, 547
Hyperbilirubinemia. See also Jaundice
  in cephalhematoma, 545
  defined, 531
  in infants of diabetic mothers, 880
  in neonate, 542-543
  therapy for, 597
Hypercapnia, permissive, for chronic lung
  disease, 861
Hyperemesis gravidarum, 735-737. See also
  Vomiting
  collaborative care, 736-737
  defined, 715

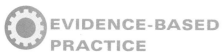

EVIDENCE-BASED PRACTICE

 ## Critical Thinking Exercise

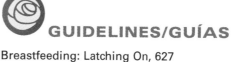 # GUIDELINES/GUÍAS

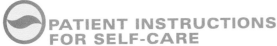
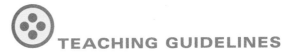